CHILD PSYCHOPATHOLOGY

CHILD PSYCHOPATHOLOGY

SECOND EDITION

Edited by
Eric J. Mash
and
Russell A. Barkley

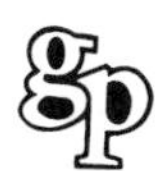

THE GUILFORD PRESS
New York London

A Division of Guilford Publications, Inc.
72 Spring Street, New York, NY 10012
www.guilford.com

Printed in the United States of America

This book is printed on acid-free paper.

Last digit is print number: 9 8 7 6 5 4 3 2 1

Library of Congress Cataloging-in-Publication Data

Child psychopathology / edited by Eric J. Mash and Russell A. Barkley. — 2nd ed.
p. cm.
Includes bibliographical references and index.
ISBN 1-57230-609-2
1. Child psychopathology. I. Mash, Eric J. II. Barkley, Russell A., 1949– .
RJ499 .C4863 2002
618.92'89—dc21 2002009086

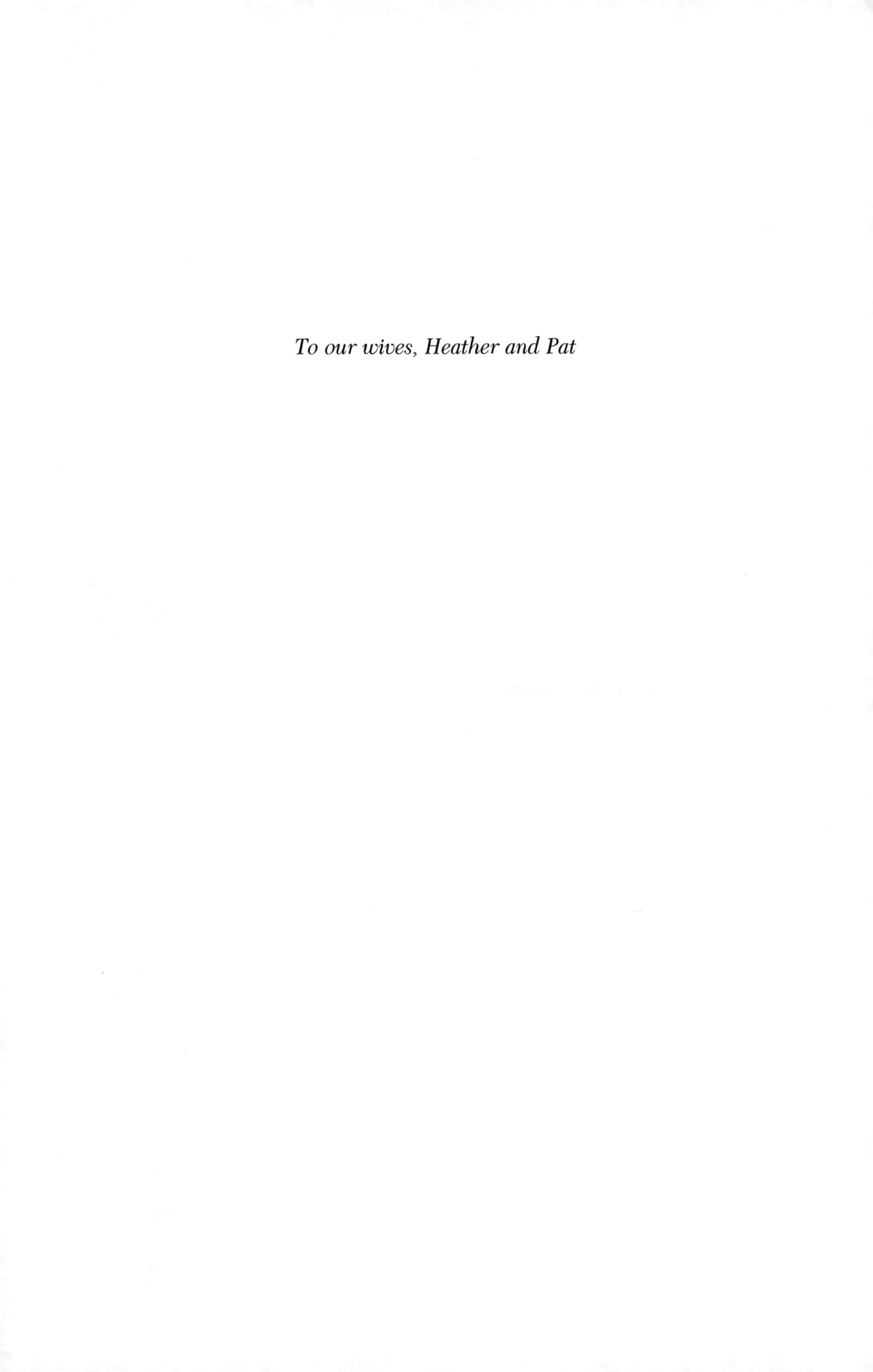

To our wives, Heather and Pat

About the Editors

Eric J. Mash, PhD, is Professor in the Department of Psychology at the University of Calgary. He completed his undergraduate studies at City University of New York, his doctorate in clinical psychology at Florida State University, and his postdoctoral work at the Oregon Health Sciences University. Dr. Mash is a fellow of the American and Canadian Psychological Associations and has served as an editorial board member and consultant for numerous scientific and professional journals. His research interests are in child and adolescent psychopathology, assessment, and therapy, and he has published many books and journal articles on these topics. His research has focused on interaction patterns in families of children with different problems including attention-deficit and oppositional disorders and children who have been maltreated.

Russell A. Barkley, PhD, is Professor in the College of Health Professions at the Medical University of South Carolina, Charleston, South Carolina. He is a Diplomate in both Clinical Psychology and Clinical Neuropsychology, has written more than 200 scientific articles and book chapters dealing with ADHD and related topics, and is author, editor, or coeditor of 15 books. Dr. Barkley is the founding Editor of *The ADHD Report*, a newsletter for clinicians, and creator of seven professional videos, two of which have won national awards. He has served as President of the International Society for Research in Child and Adolescent Psychopathology and the Section of Clinical Child Psychology of the American Psychological Association (now Division 53).

Contributors

Anne Marie Albano, PhD, Institute for the Study of Child and Adolescent Anxiety Disorders, New York University Child Study Center, New York, New York

Joan Rosenbaum Asarnow, PhD, Department of Psychiatry, Neuropsychiatric Institute, University of California, Los Angeles, School of Medicine, Los Angeles, California

Robert F. Asarnow, PhD, Department of Psychiatry, Neuropsychiatric Institute, University of California, Los Angeles, School of Medicine, Los Angeles, California

Russell A. Barkley, PhD, College of Health Professions, Medical University of South Carolina, Charleston, South Carolina

David H. Barlow, PhD, Center for Anxiety and Related Disorders, Department of Psychology, Boston University, Boston, Massachusetts

Marcia C. Barnes, PhD, Department of Pediatrics, University of Toronto and The Hospital for Sick Children, Toronto, Ontario, Canada

Carolyn Black Becker, PhD, Graduate School of Professional and Applied Psychology, Rutgers University, Piscataway, New Jersey

Diane Benoit, MD, FRCPC, Department of Psychiatry, University of Toronto and The Hospital for Sick Children, Toronto, Ontario, Canada

Kim B. Burgess, PhD, Department of Human Development, University of Maryland, College Park, Maryland

Laurie Chassin, PhD, Department of Psychology, Arizona State University, Tempe, Arizona

Bruce F. Chorpita, PhD, Department of Psychology, University of Hawaii, Honolulu, Hawaii

Geraldine Dawson, PhD, Department of Psychology, University of Washington, Seattle, Washington

David J. A. Dozois, PhD, Department of Psychology, University of Western Ontario, London, Ontario, Canada

Elisabeth M. Dykens, PhD, Neuropsychiatric Institute, Department of Child Psychiatry, University of California, Los Angeles, Los Angeles, California

Jack M. Fletcher, PhD, Department of Pediatrics/Center for Academic and Reading Skills, University of Texas–Houston Health Science Center, Houston, Texas

Kenneth E. Fletcher, PhD, University of Massachusetts Medical School, Worcester, Massachusetts

Shelly Grabe, MA, Department of Psychological Sciences, University of Missouri–Columbia, Columbia, Missouri

Constance Hammen, PhD, Department of Psychology, University of California, Los Angeles, Los Angeles, California

Karen Heffernan, PhD, private practice, New York, New York

Stephen P. Hinshaw, PhD, Department of Psychology, University of California, Berkeley, Berkeley, California

Robert M. Hodapp, PhD, Department of Education, University of California, Los Angeles, Los Angeles, California

Amy E. Kennedy, BA, Department of Human Development, University of Maryland, College Park, Maryland

Kevin M. King, MA, Department of Psychology, Arizona State University, Tempe, Arizona

Laura Grofer Klinger, PhD, Department of Psychology, University of Alabama, Tuscaloosa, Alabama

Steve S. Lee, MA, Department of Psychology, University of California, Berkeley, Berkeley, California

G. Reid Lyon, Child Development and Behavior Branch, National Institute of Child Health and Human Development, Bethesda, Maryland

Karlen Lyons-Ruth, PhD, Department of Psychiatry, Harvard Medical School, Cambridge, Massachusetts

Eric J. Mash, PhD, Department of Psychology, University of Calgary, Calgary, Alberta, Canada

Lizette Peterson, PhD, (deceased), Department of Psychological Sciences, University of Missouri–Columbia, Columbia, Missouri

Kelle Reach, BA, Department of Psychological Sciences, University of Missouri–Columbia, Columbia, Missouri

Peggy Renner, PhD, Department of Psychology, University of Alabama, Tuscaloosa, Alabama

Jennifer Ritter, MA, Department of Psychology, Arizona State University, Tempe, Arizona

Kenneth H. Rubin, PhD, Department of Human Development, University of Maryland, College Park, Maryland

Karen D. Rudolph, PhD, Department of Psychology, University of Illinois, Champaign, Illinois

Shannon L. Stewart, PhD, Child and Parent Resource Institute, Ministry of Community, Family, and Children's Services, London, Ontario, Canada

Ryan S. Trim, MA, Department of Psychology, Arizona State University, Tempe, Arizona

Christine Wekerle, PhD, Department of Psychiatry, University of Toronto and Child Psychiatry Program, Centre for Addiction and Mental Health, Toronto, Ontario, Canada

G. Terence Wilson, PhD, Graduate School of Applied and Professional Psychology, Rutgers University, Piscataway, New Jersey

David A. Wolfe, PhD, Department of Psychology, The University of Western Ontario, London, Ontario, Canada

Charles H. Zeanah, MD, Department of Psychiatry and Pediatrics, Tulane University School of Medicine, New Orleans, Louisiana

Preface

Research in child, adolescent, and developmental psychopathology continues to flourish, even more so than when the first edition of this text was published. Previously recognized disorders are even better delineated than they were only a few years ago, and a few new ones seem to have been discovered along the way. The publication rate in this field is extraordinary, with many journals now focusing exclusively on childhood mental illness and health, and numerous articles on children appearing each month in journals that were once the exclusive domains of adult psychopathology. To those of us who take a developmental view of psychopathology, this is a most gratifying state of affairs as we come to recognize the roots of many adult disorders in childhood and adolescence. The down side, of course, is that even the expert researchers in the various disorders that constitute this field find it harder than ever to keep abreast of research findings appearing at such a rapid clip. And woe to the clinical professionals who must deal with these childhood disorders: They may find themselves quickly and hopelessly behind in the advancements occurring in the understanding of these clinical conditions. Hence the need for a volume such as this, and especially for its second edition, to assist the clinical professional, student, and even expert in remaining current on child and adolescent psychopathological disorders.

Now more than ever, the field of child psychopathology epitomizes the dynamic, accumulative, and self-correcting nature of the scientific enterprise, as new findings expand upon and are assimilated with the established facts in any given disorder. Often these new findings challenge older theoretical or conceptual assumptions or more explicit models of these disorders, at times even leading to small-scale paradigm shifts in perspective. In short, the literature on child and adolescent psychopathology is alive, well, prosperous, and rapidly advancing. Old questions undoubtedly get answered, but along the way those answers raise new questions for researchers to pursue in ever more complex programs of research on each of the childhood disorders covered here. Although the pace and excitement levels vary considerably across different areas of child psychopathology, within each area the eager anticipation of new knowledge remains palpable as new lines of research and methodologies—such as neuroimaging, behavioral and molecular genetics, structural equation modeling, and longitudinal designs—come to overlap old ones and so provide greater opportunities to better understand these disorders.

The challenge remains for this second edition as it was for the first: How are we to capture the current status of this rapidly evolving field? Our answer was again to identify those experts who have dedicated their professional careers to these disorders, and let them—unfettered by fashion or the editors' pet perspectives—tell us what they have learned. In other words, we tried to find the most knowledgeable professionals on particular disorders and asked them to provide up-to-date and comprehensive summaries of the nature of the disorders in which they have specialized. We asked only that their discussions be grounded in their respective bodies of scientific literature, eschewing clinical lore, dogmatic wisdom, the sayings of the guru *du jour*, or political agendas. We also asked that they set aside the concerns of assessment and treatment of their respective disorders, so as to have ample room for the burgeoning findings on the disorders themselves. These other topics are the focus of related books (Mash & Barkley, 1998; Mash & Terdal, 1997).

In essence, each author or group of authors was once more challenged to answer these basic questions: "What do we know about this disorder?", "What are the implications for future research into further understanding the disorder?", and, just as important, "Where are the current limitations or gaps in our knowledge that deserve future attention?" If sound, scientifically grounded theoretical or conceptual models of the disorder exist, then these were also to be reviewed. In addressing these questions, the experts assembled here were directed to cover (1) the nature of the behavior, symptoms, and/or cognitive and emotional deficits that typify the core of each disorder; (2) a brief historical perspective; (3) any criteria that exist to establish its presence (diagnosis) and a candid appraisal of those criteria; (4) epidemiological knowledge pertaining to the prevalence, gender distribution, and ethnic and cultural factors associated with the disorder; (5) the developmental course and varied pathways shown to be associated with the disorder; (6) the psychiatric, psychological, and social disorders or difficulties that most often coexist with the disorder (comorbidity); and (7) a survey of those things believed to give rise to the disorder (etiology). Once more, we believe that the many authors assembled here have done a marvelous job accomplishing their charge. We trust the reader will concur.

As before, we are indebted to the professionals who agreed to write for this second edition on their respective disorders. We genuinely appreciate the substantial time commitment they have made to writing their chapters, many of which are major updates of their previous work. Many others deserve our gratitude as well, including Jeannie Tang, Judith Grauman, Marie Sprayberry, Carolyn Graham, Kim Miller, and Alison Wiigs, for shepherding the manuscript through the production process. Special thanks are also owed to our long-time friends and founders of The Guilford Press, Seymour Weingarten (Editor-in-Chief) and Bob Matloff (President), for more than 20 years of support for our various books, including this one. Last, but hardly least, we thank our families—Heather Mash, and Pat, Ken, and Steve Barkley—for relinquishing the family time such a project requires, and for their support, patience, and encouragement of our careers in this field.

Eric J. Mash, PhD
Department of Psychology
University of Calgary

Russell A. Barkley, PhD
College of Health Professions
Medical University of South Carolina

REFERENCES

Mash, E. J., & Barkley, R. A. (Eds.). (1998). *Treatment of childhood disorders* (2nd ed.). New York: Guilford Press.

Mash, E. J., & Terdal, L. G. (Eds.). (1997). *Assessment of childhood disorders* (3rd ed.). New York: Guilford Press.

Contents

I

INTRODUCTION

CHAPTER ONE

Child Psychopathology

A Developmental–Systems Perspective

Eric J. Mash
David J. A. Dozois

This volume provides a comprehensive account of the characteristics, definitions, developmental course, correlates, causes, contexts, and outcomes of psychopathology in children.[1] Our knowledge base of child and developmental psychopathology has grown exponentially over the past decade (Cicchetti & Cohen, 1995a, 1995b; Cicchetti & Sroufe, 2000; Mash & Wolfe, 2002; Ollendick & Hersen, 1998). New conceptual frameworks, research methods, and findings continue to advance our understanding of childhood disorders (Cicchetti & Rogosch, 1999; Rutter & Sroufe, 2000; Sameroff, Lewis, & Miller, 2000), as well as our ability to assess and treat children with problems (Mash & Barkley, 1998; Mash & Terdal, 1997a; Orvaschel, Faust, & Hersen, 2001; Shaffer, Lucas, & Richters, 1999). However, this knowledge base is compromised by the frequently atheoretical, unsystematic, and fragmented fashion in which research findings in child psychopathology have accrued, and by the conceptual and research complexities inherent in the study of such a rapidly changing and socially embedded organism as the child (Hinshaw, 2001; Jensen et al., 1993; Kazdin & Kagan, 1994). In this introductory chapter, we address several central themes and issues related to conceptualizing childhood dysfunction and its many determinants. In doing so, we provide a developmental–systems framework for understanding child psychopathology—one that emphasizes the role of developmental processes, the importance of context, and the influence of multiple and interacting events and processes in shaping adaptive and maladaptive development.

FACTORS COMPLICATING THE STUDY OF CHILD PSYCHOPATHOLOGY

Almost since modern views of mental illness began to emerge in the late 18th and early 19th centuries, far less attention has been given to the study of psychopathology in children than in adults (Silk, Nath, Siegel, & Kendall, 2000). For example, in 1812 Benjamin Rush, the first American psychiatrist, suggested that children were less likely to suffer from mental illness than adults, because the immaturity of their developing brains would prevent them from retaining the mental events that caused insanity (Silk et al., 2000). More recently, interest in the study of child psychopathology has increased dramatically. This is due to a growing realization that (1) many childhood problems have lifelong consequences and costs both for children and for society; (2) most adult disorders are rooted in early childhood conditions and/or experiences; and (3) a better understanding of childhood disorders offers promise for developing effective intervention and prevention programs (National Advisory Mental Health Council [NAMHC] Workgroup, 2001).

Issues concerning the conceptualization and definition of psychopathology in children continue to be vigorously debated. Such debates are fueled by the relative absence of well-controlled research studies with children as compared with adults. Until recently, much of the field's accumulated knowledge about child psychopathology, its causes, and its outcomes was extrapolated from theory and research on adult disorders. For example, only in the last 5–10 years have child-focused models and research into such disorders as depression and anxiety emerged (Zahn-Waxler, Klimes-Dougan, & Slattery, 2000).

Even in studies conducted with children, much of our knowledge is based on findings obtained at a single point in a child's development and in a single context. Although useful, such findings provide still photographs of moving targets and fail to capture the dynamic changes over time that characterize most forms of child psychopathology (Achenbach & Dumenci, 2001; Lewis & Granic, 2000; Patterson, 1993). In addition, prior studies have not given sufficient attention to the social and cultural milieu in which atypical child development occurs (Cicchetti & Aber, 1998; García Coll & Garrido, 2000). Contextual models (e.g., Bronfenbrenner, 1977) and longitudinal approaches (e.g., Robins, 1966) have been available in the field of child study for some time. However, only in the past decade has the research enterprise taken seriously the need for developmentally sensitive systems-oriented models to account for the emergence of psychopathology in children (del Carmen & Huffman, 1996; Sameroff, 2000a), or the need to study developmental trajectories utilizing longitudinal methods (e.g., Emery, Waldron, Kitzmann, & Aaron, 1999; Hauser-Cram, Warfield, Shonkoff, & Krauss, 2001; Kotler, Cohen, Davies, Pine, & Walsh, 2001; Maughan & Rutter, 2001; Verhulst & Koot, 1991).

The study of child psychopathology is further complicated by the facts that childhood problems do not come in neat packages, and that most forms of psychopathology in children are known to overlap and/or to coexist with other disorders (Angold, Costello, & Erkanli, 1999). For example, there is much overlap among such problems as violence, emotional and behavioral disorders, child maltreatment, substance abuse, delinquency, and learning difficulties (e.g., Greenbaum, Prange, Friedman, & Silver, 1991); between childhood anxiety and depression (e.g., Compas & Oppedisano, 2000; Seligman & Ollendick, 1998); and between reading disabilities and anxiety and depression (Willcutt & Pennington, 2000b). Many behavioral and emotional disturbances in children are also associated with specific physical symptoms and/or medical conditions (Egger, Costello, Erkanli, & Angold, 1999; Meltzer, Gatward, Goodman, & Ford, 2000).

It is also the case that distinct boundaries between many commonly occurring childhood difficulties (e.g., noncompliance, defiance) and those problems that come to be labeled as "disorders" (e.g., oppositional defiant disorder) are not easily drawn (e.g., Loeber, Burke, Lahey, Winters, & Zera, 2000). Judgments of deviancy often depend as much on other child characteristics (e.g., age, sex, intelligence), the situational appropriateness of a child's behavior, the social and cultural context in which judgments are made, and the characteristics and decision rules of adults who make these judgments as they do on any specific behaviors displayed by the child (Achenbach, 2000; Mash & Terdal, 1997b).

There is a growing recognition that all current diagnostic categories of child psychopathology are heterogeneous with respect to etiology and outcome, and will need to be broken down into subtypes (Kagan, 1997). Although these diagnostic systems make some allowances for subtypes, designations are rudimentary at best, given the many different subgroups and types that have been identified for children with such disorders as attention-deficit/ hyperactivity disorder (ADHD), conduct disorder, oppositional defiant disorder, anxiety disorders, and mood disorders (e.g., Milich, Balentine, & Lynam, 2001).

It has become increasingly evident that most forms of child psychopathology cannot be attributed to a single unitary cause. Although certain rare disorders (e.g., phenylketonuria, fragile-X mental retardation, or Rett's disorder) may be caused by single genes, current models in behavioral and molecular genetics recognize that more common and complex disorders are the result of the operation of multigene systems containing varying effect sizes (Goldsmith, Gottesman, & Lemery, 1997; McGuffin, Riley, & Plomin, 2001; O'Conner & Plomin, 2000). Most forms of child psychopathology are polygenic, involving a number of susceptibility genes that interact with one another and with environmental influences to result in observed levels of impairment (Rutter, 2000a; State, Lombroso, Pauls, & Leckman, 2000). Child and family disturbances are likely to result from multiple, frequently co-occurring, reciprocal, and interacting risk factors, causal events, and processes (e.g., Eaves et al., 1997; Ge, Conger, Lorenz, Shanahan, & Elder, 1995; Rende, 1999; Rutter et al., 1997). Contextual events exert considerable influence in producing child and adolescent disorders—an influence that is almost always equivalent to or greater than those factors usually thought of as residing "within" the child (Caspi, Taylor, Moffitt, & Plomin, 2000; Reiss & Neiderhiser, 2000; Rutter, 2000b).

Numerous determinants of child psychopathology have been identified, including genetic influences (e.g., State et al., 2000); hypo- or hyperreactive early infant dispositions (e.g., Hirshfeld, Biederman, Brody, & Faraone, 1997); insecure child–parent attachments (e.g., Bretherton, 1995; Sroufe, Carlson, Levy, & Egeland, 1999); difficult child behavior (e.g., Costello & Angold, 2001); social-cognitive deficits (e.g., Crick & Dodge, 1994; Schwartz & Proctor, 2000); deficits in social learning (e.g., Patterson, 1982; Patterson, Reid, & Dishion, 1992), emotion regulation (e.g., Keenan, 2000), and/or impulse control and response inhibition (Barkley, 1997; Nigg, 2000, 2001); neuropsychological and/or neurobiological dysfunction (e.g., Cicchetti & Cannon, 1999); maladaptive patterns of parenting (e.g., Lovejoy, Graczyk, O'Hare, & Neuman, 2000); parental psychopathology, such as maternal depressed mood (e.g., Goodman & Gotlib, 1999); parental or couple discord (e.g., Grych & Fincham, 2001); limited family resources and other poverty-related life stressors (e.g., Rutter, 1999); institutional deprivation (e.g., Kreppner et al., 2001); and a host of other potential factors. These factors cannot be understood in isolation, and for most disorders, research does not support granting central etiological status to any single risk or causal factor (e.g., Seifer, Sameroff, Baldwin, & Baldwin, 1992).

Since the many causes and outcomes of child psychopathology operate in dynamic and interactive ways over time, they are not easy to disentangle. The designation of a specific factor as a cause or an outcome of child psychopathology usually reflects (1) the point in an ongoing developmental process at which the child is observed, and (2) the perspective of the observer. For example, a language deficit may be viewed as a disorder in its own right (e.g., mixed receptive–expressive language disorder), the cause of other difficulties (e.g., impulsivity), or the outcome of some other condition or disorder (e.g., autistic disorder). In addition, biological and environmental determinants interact at all periods of development. Dawson, Hessl, and Frey (1994), for example, noted that the characteristic styles parents use in responding to their infants' emotional expressions may influence how patterns of cortical mappings and connections within the limbic system are established in the infants. Similarly, J. Hart, Gunnar, and Cicchetti (1995) reported that maltreated preschoolers showed reduced cortisol activity in response to stress relative to controls—a finding that suggests altered activity of the stress-regulating hypothalamic–pituitary–adrenocortical (HPA) system among children who have been maltreated. These and other findings suggest that early experiences may shape neural structure and function, which may then create dispositions that direct and shape a child's later experiences and behavior (Cicchetti & Walker, 2001; Dawson et al., 1999; Glaser, 2000; Kaufman & Charney, 2001; Post & Weiss, 1997).

As will be discussed throughout this volume, current models of child psychopathology seek to incorporate the role of evolved mechanisms, neurobiological factors, early parent–child relationships, attachment processes, a long-term memory store that develops with age and experience, micro- and macrosocial influences, cultural factors, age and gender, and reactions from the social environment as variables and processes that interact and transform one another over time. In short, then, current approaches view the roots of developmental and psychological disturbances in children as the result of complex interactions over the course of development between the biology of brain maturation and the multidimensional nature of experience (Cicchetti & Toth, 1997; Cicchetti & Tucker, 1994; Reiss & Neiderhiser, 2000; Rutter et al., 1997).

The experience and the expression of psychopathology in children are known to have cognitive, affective, physiological, and behavioral components; in light of this, many differing descriptions and definitions of dysfunctionality in children have been proposed. As we discuss in a later section, a common theme in defining child psychopathology has been that of "adaptational failure" in one or more of these components or in the ways in which these components are organized and integrated (Sameroff, 2000a; Sroufe,

1997; Sroufe & Rutter, 1984). Adaptational failure may involve deviation from age-appropriate norms (Achenbach, 2001), exaggeration or diminishment of normal developmental expressions, interference in normal developmental progress, failure to master developmental tasks, failure to develop a specific function or regulatory mechanism, and/or the use of non-normative skills (e.g., rituals, dissociation) as a way of adapting to regulatory problems or traumatic experiences (Fischer et al., 1997; Sroufe, 1997).

A multitude of etiological models and treatment approaches have been proposed to explain and remediate psychopathology in children. Unfortunately, most of these have yet to be substantiated—or, for that matter, even tested (Kazdin, 2000, 2001). These models and approaches have differed in their relative emphasis on certain causal mechanisms and constructs, often using very different terminology and concepts to describe seemingly similar child characteristics and behaviors. Although useful, many of these models have been based on what seem to be faulty premises concerning singular pathways of causal influence that do not capture the complexities of child psychopathology (Kazdin & Kagan, 1994).

In this regard, evolutionary models have emphasized the role of selection pressures operating on the human species over millions of years; biological paradigms have emphasized genetic mutations, neuroanatomy, and neurobiological mechanisms as factors contributing to psychopathology; psychodynamic models have focused on intrapsychic mechanisms, conflicts, and defenses; attachment models have emphasized the importance of early relationships and the ways in which internal representations of these relationships provide the foundation for constructing working models of self, others, and relationships more generally; behavioral/reinforcement models have emphasized excessive, inadequate, or maladaptive reinforcement and/or learning histories; social learning models have emphasized the importance of observational learning, vicarious experience, and reciprocal social interactions; cognitive models generally focus on the child's distorted or deficient cognitive structures and processes; affective models have emphasized dysfunctional emotion-regulating mechanisms; and family systems models have conceptualized child psychopathology within a framework of intra- and intergenerational family systems and subsystems and have emphasized the structural and/or functional elements that surround family relational difficulties.

The distinctiveness of each model mentioned above is in the relative importance it attaches to certain events and processes. However, it should be emphasized that despite these variations in the relative emphasis given to certain causes versus others, most models recognize the role of multiple interacting influences. For example, although differing in emphasis, social learning and affective models both place importance on the role of symbolic representational processes in explaining childhood dysfunction.

There is a growing recognition of the need to integrate currently available models through intra- and interdisciplinary research efforts. Such integration generally requires looking beyond the emphasis of each single-cause theory to see what can be learned from other approaches, as well as a general openness to relating concepts and findings from diverse theories (cf. Arkowitz, 1992). Recent studies suggest that theoretical integration is becoming more common in psychopathology research (e.g., Beauchaine, 2001). Attachment theory has, for instance, been increasingly integrated with cognitive models (e.g., Ingram & Ritter, 2000). Theoretical integration is also apparent in studies combining proximal cognitive and interpersonal factors with distal variables, such as the early home environment and patterns of attachment (e.g., Lara, Klein, & Kasch, 2000). The link between cognitive and neuropsychological functioning is likewise being tested more frequently (e.g., Nigg, Blaskey, Huang-Pollack, & Rappley, 2002; Pine & Grun, 1999). Thus it appears as though researchers are beginning to recognize the importance of combining theoretical approaches, and are accepting the monumental task of incorporating increased complexity into their research designs.

Interdisciplinary perspectives on child psychopathology mirror the considerable investment in children on the part of many different disciplines and professions. The study of the etiology and maintenance of psychopathology in children has been and continues to be the subject matter of psychology, medicine, psychiatry, education, and numerous other disciplines. Clearly, no one discipline has proprietary rights to the study of childhood disturbances. Each discipline has formulated child psychopathology in terms of its own unique perspective. Particularly relevant, in the context of this chapter, is that child psychopathology and normality in medicine and psychiatry have typically been conceptualized and defined categorically in terms of the presence or absence of a particular disorder or syndrome that is believed to exist "within the child." In contrast, psychology has more often conceptualized psychopathology–normality as representing extremes on a continuum or dimension of characteristics, and has also focused on the role of environmental influences that operate "outside the child." However, the boundaries between categories and dimensions, or between inner and outer conditions and causes, are arbitrarily drawn, and there is a continuing need to find workable ways of integrating the two different world views of psychiatry/medicine and psychology (Richters & Cicchetti, 1993; Scotti & Morris, 2000; Shaffer et al., 1999).

As the subsequent chapters in this volume attest, research into child psychopathology is accelerating at a remarkable rate. This in turn has resulted in a rapidly expanding and changing knowledge base. Each chapter in this volume provides a comprehensive review of current research and theory for a specific form of child psychopathology, and a discussion of new developments and directions related to this disorder. In the remainder of this introductory chapter, we provide a brief overview and discussion of the following: historical developments in the study of child psychopathology; epidemiological considerations; basic issues; approaches to the definition and classification of childhood disorders; common types of psychopathology in children; important philosophical and epistemological assumptions that have guided theory and research; predominant theories regarding etiology; and prevalent and recurrent conceptual and methodological issues that cut across the wide spectrum of disorders represented in this volume. Particular emphasis is given to concepts, methods, and strategies capturing the complexities, reciprocal influences, and divergent pathways that current models and research have identified as crucial for understanding child psychopathology.

HISTORICAL CONTEXT FOR CHILD PSYCHOPATHOLOGY

Brief Historical Overview

Historical developments surrounding the emergence of child psychopathology as a field of study have been documented in a number of excellent sources and are considered only briefly here (see Achenbach, 1982; Cicchetti, 1990; Donohue, Hersen, & Ammerman, 2000; Kanner, 1962; Rie, 1971; Rubinstein, 1948; Silk et al., 2000). In general, the emergence of concepts of child psychopathology was inextricably related to the broader philosophical and societal changes in the ways children have been viewed and treated by adults over the course of history (Aries, 1962; Borstelmann, 1983; French, 1977; Postman, 1994). Several overlapping perspectives for conceptualizing and dealing with deviant child behavior emerged, including the religious, the legal, the medical, the social, and the educational (Costello & Angold, 2001).

In ancient Greek and Roman societies, child behavior disorders were believed to result from organic imbalances, and children with physical or mental handicaps, disabilities, or deformities were viewed as sources of economic burden and/or social embarrassment. As such, they were usually scorned, abandoned, or put to death (French, 1977). This mistreatment, by today's standards, was common throughout the Middle Ages (A.D. 500–1300). In colonial America, as many as two-thirds of all children died prior to the age of 5 years, and those who survived continued to be subjected to harsh treatment by adults. For example, the Massachusetts Stubborn Child Act of 1654 permitted a father to petition a magistrate to put a "stubborn" or "rebellious" child to death (fortunately, no sentences were carried out); in Massachusetts and elsewhere, mentally ill children were kept in cages and cellars into the mid-1800s (Silk et al., 2000).

The historical record indicates that prior to the 18th century, when references to disordered child behavior were made at all, they were usually presented in terms of the problem child's behavior as inherently evil (Kanner, 1962). Bizarre behaviors in children were attributed to Satanic possession and evil spirits during the Spanish Inquisition, and both John Calvin and Martin Luther viewed mentally retarded children as filled with Satan. And, as noted by Rie (1971), "No distinct concept of disordered behavior in children could emerge so long as possession by the devil excluded other notions of causality" (p. 8).

Although nearly all varieties of aberrant behavior in children have existed for millennia, the formal study of such behavior is relatively recent. Following a comprehensive review of historical developments in child psychopathology, Rie

(1971) concluded: "There is a consensus, then, about the absence of any substantial body of knowledge—prior to the twentieth century—concerning disordered behavior in childhood; about the inconsistencies and discontinuities of efforts on behalf of disturbed children; and about the relative absence of those professional specialties which now concern themselves with such problems" (p. 6). Rubinstein (1948) noted that (1) there was not a single article dealing with insanity in childhood in any of the first 45 volumes of the *Journal of Insanity*; (2) there was no discovery or theory of importance to child psychiatry in the American literature prior to 1900, and no research today stems from any of these writings; and (3) the only significant work with children prior to the 20th century focused on the care, treatment, and training of "mental defectives."

Increased concern for the plight and welfare of children with mental and behavioral disturbances was the result of two important influences. First, advances in general medicine, physiology, and neurology led to the reemergence of the organic disease model and a concomitant emphasis on more humane forms of treatment. Second, the growing influence of the philosophies of John Locke, Johann Pestalozzi, and Jean-Jacques Rousseau led to the view that children needed moral guidance and support. With these changing views came an increased concern for moral education, compulsory education, and improved health practices. These early influences also provided the foundation for evolving views of child psychopathology as dependent on both organic and environmental causes.

Masturbatory Insanity: An Example

Societal and clinical views regarding masturbation in children can be used to illustrate the ways in which conceptualizations of child psychopathology have changed over time, as well as several general issues related to its definition, study, and treatment. In addition to the historical significance of masturbation as the first disorder described as unique to children and adolescents (Rie, 1971), early conceptualizations of masturbatory insanity illustrate a view of mental illness as residing within the child (Cattell, 1938; Hare, 1962; Rees, 1939; Rie, 1971; Szasz, 1970).

Society's objections to masturbation originated from Orthodox Jewish codes and from Judeo-Christian dogmata (Patton, 1985; Szasz, 1970). It was not until the 18th century—with a decline in the domination of religious thought, coupled with the augmented influence of science—that masturbation came to be viewed as particularly harmful (Rie, 1971; Szasz, 1970). An anonymous clergyman who later became a physician wrote a dissertation entitled *Onania, or the Heinous Sin of Self-Pollution* (circa 1710, cited in Szasz, 1970). It was this manuscript that initially transformed the moral convictions regarding the wrongfulness of masturbation into a physiological explanation with severe medical ramifications. Following this exposition, numerous books appeared claiming that masturbation was a predominant etiological cause of both physical disease and mental illness. Thus the notion that sexual overindulgence was deleterious to one's health was accepted, "virtually unaltered, first by the Church and then by Medicine" (Szasz, 1970, p. 182). Although the medical view of masturbation first emphasized the adverse impact upon physical health, the dominant thinking shifted by the middle of the 19th century to a focus on the presumed negative effects on mental health and nervous system functioning. By the latter part of the 19th century, masturbation was the most frequently mentioned "cause" of psychopathology in children. In fact, Spitzka (1890; cited in Rie, 1971) attributed at least 25% of all psychiatric cases to this etiological factor.

Views of masturbatory insanity emerged and were maintained in the absence of any thought to the contrary, and without any consideration of the base rate of masturbation in the general population. Although interest in masturbatory insanity began to wane in the latter half of the 19th century, the argument endured (albeit in milder forms) during the early 20th century, when psychoanalytic theory gained rapid acceptance. Freud suggested that masturbation was one of the precipitants of neurasthenia, hypochondriasis, and anxiety neurosis (Rees, 1939). Apart from his own theories regarding the pathogenesis of neuroses, however, Freud did not present any real evidence for this view (Szasz, 1970). Eventually the notion of masturbatory insanity gave way to the concept of neurosis, but it was still not until much later in the 20th century that the misguided and illusory belief in a relationship between masturbation and mental illness was dispelled.

As conceptualizations of childhood psychopathology evolved, and several variants of psychotherapy and residential treatments were developed (see Grellong, 1987, and Roberts & Kurtz,

1987), the search for determinants of psychiatric disorders in children became increasingly sophisticated, thorough, and systematic (Rie, 1971). With this increased refinement of theory and research, there remained only fragments of the etiological hypothesis of masturbation. For example, in some psychoanalytic circles, enuresis was thought to symbolize suppressed masturbation (Rees, 1939; Walker, Kenning, & Faust-Campanile, 1989). Eventually masturbation came to be viewed as entirely harmless (Szasz, 1970) and even as usefully adaptive (Baker, 1996).

This brief historical review illustrates a number of points. First, it shows how the political and social climates influence our definitions of child psychopathology. The impact of religious thought was clearly reflected in the transformation from the moral judgment against the sins of the flesh, to the medical opinion that masturbation was harmful to one's physical health, to the psychiatric assertion that sexual overindulgence caused insanity.

Second, the review points out the need to be cognizant of the ways in which moral convictions, idiosyncratic definitions of normality or pathology, and personal expectations influence what investigators look for and ultimately find in the name of science. In the case of masturbation, misleading findings resulted because hypotheses were "tested" with a mentality of confirmation rather than falsification (see Maxwell & Delaney, 1990). Szasz (1970), in writing about the powerful authority of America's historical psychiatric figures such as Benjamin Rush, noted that there is a tendency among scientists to "attend only to those of their observations that confirm the accepted theories of their age, and reject those that refute them" (p. 187).

Third, masturbatory insanity illustrates the potential dangers that ensue when treatment decisions are made on the basis of deficient theoretical exposition and in the absence of empirical data. For example, early treatments consisted of clitoridectomies for women and spike-toothed rings placed on the penises of men (Szasz, 1970). Finally, the example of masturbatory insanity portrays the long-standing view of psychopathology as residing within the child and the essential neglect of the role of his or her surroundings, context, relationships, and the interactions among these variables.

Current theory, research, and practice reflect a shift toward acknowledging developmental factors and including the family, peer group, school, and other sources of influence in conceptualizing and understanding child psychopathology (Luthar, Burack, Cicchetti, & Weisz, 1997; Mash & Wolfe, 2002). Additional developments have included an increased research emphasis on examining the interactions of multiple proximal and distal vulnerability factors (Ingram, Miranda, & Segal, 1998; Price & Lento, 2001), understanding psychopathology across the life span (Ingram & Price, 2001), identifying empirically supported treatments for various childhood problems (Kazdin & Weisz, 1998; Lonigan, Elbert, & Johnson, 1998), and a focus on prevention (Greenberg, Domitrovich, & Bumbarger, 2001; National Institute of Mental Health, 2001).

SIGNIFICANCE OF CHILD PSYCHOPATHOLOGY

There has been and continues to be a great deal of misinformation and folklore concerning disorders of childhood. Many unsubstantiated theories have existed in both the popular and scientific literatures. These have ranged from mid-19th-century views that overstimulation in the classroom causes insanity (see Makari, 1993), to mid-20th-century views that inadequate parenting causes autism (Bettelheim, 1967) or that chemical food additives cause hyperactivity (Feingold, 1975). In addition, many of the constructs used to describe the characteristics and conditions of psychopathology in children have been globally and/or poorly defined (e.g., "adjustment problem," "emotional disturbance"). Despite the limitations, uncertainties, and definitional ambiguities that exist in the field, it is also evident that psychopathology during childhood represents a frequently occurring and significant societal concern that is gradually coming to the forefront of the political agenda.

In the United States, the approach of the new millennium witnessed the first Surgeon General's report on mental health (U.S. Public Health Service, 1999), which was followed by White House meetings on mental health in young people and on the use of psychotropic medications with children. A Surgeon General's conference on children's mental health resulted in an extensive report and recommendations (U.S. Public Health Service, 2001a), a similar report on youth violence (U.S. Public Health Service, 2001b), and a "blueprint" for research on child and adolescent mental health (NAMHC Workgroup, 2001).[2]

Increasingly, researchers in the fields of developmental psychopathology, child psychiatry, and clinical child psychology are considering the social policy implications of their work and striving to effect improvements in the identification of and services for youths with mental health needs (Cicchetti & Toth, 2000; Weisz, 2000). Greater recognition is also being given to factors that contribute to children's successful mental functioning, personal well-being, productive activities, fulfilling relationships, and ability to adapt to change and cope with adversity (Cicchetti, Rappaport, Sandler, & Weissberg, 2000; Thompson & Ontai, 2000; U.S. Department of Health and Human Services, 2000b; U.S. Public Health Service, 2001a).

The growing attention to children's mental health problems and competencies arises from a number of sources. First, many young people experience significant mental health problems that interfere with normal development and functioning. As many as 1 in 5 children in the United States experience some type of difficulty (Costello & Angold, 2000; Roberts, Attkisson, & Rosenblatt, 1998), and 1 in 10 have a diagnosable disorder that causes some level of impairment (Burns et al., 1995; Shaffer et al., 1996). These numbers probably underestimate the magnitude of the problem, since they do not include a substantial number of children who manifest subclinical or undiagnosed disturbances that may place them at high risk for the later development of more severe clinical problems. For example, McDermott and Weiss (1995) reported that of the children in their national sample who were classified as adjusted, 34.4% were classified as being only "marginally" adjusted. In addition, although not meeting formal diagnostic criteria, many subclinical conditions (e.g., depressed mood, eating problems) are also associated with significant impairment in functioning (e.g., Angold, Costello, Farmer, Burns, & Erkanli, 1999; Lewinsohn, Striegel-Moore, & Seeley, 2000). Evidence gathered by the World Health Organization (WHO) suggests that by the year 2020, childhood neuropsychiatric disorders will rise by over 50% internationally, to become one of the five most common causes of morbidity, mortality, and disability among children (U.S. Public Health Service, 2001a).

Second, a significant proportion of children do not grow out of their childhood difficulties, although the ways in which these difficulties are expressed change in both form and severity over time (Offord et al., 1992). Even when diagnosable psychopathology is not evident at later ages, a child's failure to adjust during earlier developmental periods may still have a lasting negative impact on later family, occupational, and social adjustment. And some forms of child psychopathology—for example, an early onset of antisocial patterns of behavior in boys—can be highly predictive of various negative psychosocial, educational, and health outcomes in adolescence and adulthood (see Hinshaw & Lee, Chapter 3, this volume).

Third, recent social changes and conditions may place children at increasing risk for the development of disorders, and also for the development of more severe problems at younger ages (Duncan, Brooks-Gunn, & Klebanov, 1994; Kovacs, 1997). These social changes and conditions include multigenerational adversity in inner cities; chronic poverty in women and children; pressures of family breakup, single parenting, and homelessness; problems of the rural poor; direct and indirect exposure to traumatic events (e.g., terrorist attacks or school shootings); adjustment problems of children in immigrant families; difficulties of Native American children; and conditions associated with the impact of prematurity, HIV, cocaine, and alcohol on children's growth and development (McCall & Groark, 2000; National Commission on Children, 1991; Shonkoff & Phillips, 2000). In addition to sociocultural changes, medical advances associated with higher rates of fetal survival may also contribute to a greater number of children showing serious behavior problems and learning disorders at a younger age.

Fourth, for a majority of children who experience mental health problems, these problems go unidentified: Only about 20% receive help, a statistic that has not changed for some time (Burns et al., 1995). Even when children are identified and receive help for their problems, this help may be less than optimal. For example, only about half of children with identified ADHD seen in real-world practice settings receive care that conforms to recommended treatment guidelines (Hoagwood, Kelleher, Feil, & Comer, 2000). The fact that so few children with mental health problems receive appropriate help is probably related to such factors as a lack of screening, inaccessibility, cost, a lack of perceived need on the part of parents, parental dissatisfaction with services, and the stigmatization and exclusion often experienced by these children and their families (Hinshaw & Cicchetti, 2000; Kroes et al., 2001). Empirically supported prevention and treatment programs for many childhood disorders are only now becoming available (Kazdin & Weisz, 1998; Lonigan et al., 1998), and there is a pressing need for the development and evaluation of prevention and intervention programs that are grounded in theory and research on child development in general, and developmental psychopathology in particular (Greenberg et al., 2001; Kazdin, 2001; Kurtines & Silverman, 1999; NAMHC Workgroup, 2001; Rapport, 2001).[3]

Fifth, a majority of children with mental health problems who go unidentified and unassisted often end up in the criminal justice or mental health systems as young adults (Loeber & Farrington, 2000). They are at much greater risk for dropping out of school and of not being fully functional members of society in adulthood; this adds further to the costs of childhood disorders in terms of human suffering and financial burdens. For example, average costs of medical care for youngsters with ADHD are estimated to be double those for youngsters without ADHD (Leibson, Katusic, Barberesi, Ransom, & O'Brien, 2001). Moreover, allowing just *one* youth to leave high school for a life of crime and drug abuse is estimated to cost society from $1.7 to $2.3 million (Cohen, 1998).

Finally, a significant number of children in North America are being subjected to maltreatment, and chronic maltreatment during childhood is associated with psychopathology in children and later in adults (Emery & Laumann-Billings, 1998; MacMillan et al., 2001). Based on a review of the evidence, De Bellis (2001) has proposed that the psychobiological outcomes of abuse be viewed as "an environmentally induced complex developmental disorder" (p. 539). Although precise estimates of the rates of occurrence of maltreatment are difficult to obtain, due to the covert nature of the problem and other sampling and reporting biases (see Cicchetti & Manly, 2001; Mash & Wolfe, 1991), the numbers appear to be large. Nearly 3 million suspected cases of child abuse and neglect are investigated each year by child protective service agencies, and about 1 million children in the United States were confirmed as victims of child maltreatment in 1998 (U.S. Department of Health and Human Services, 2000a). It has been estimated that each year as many as 2,000 infants and young children die from abuse or neglect at the hands of their parents or caregivers (U.S. Advisory Board on Child Abuse and Neglect, 1995). Moreover, many reports of "accidental" injuries in children may be the result of unreported mistreatment by parents or siblings (Peterson & Brown, 1994). It would appear, then, that the total number of children who show adverse psychological and physical effects of maltreatment in North American society is staggering.

EPIDEMIOLOGICAL CONSIDERATIONS

Prevalence

Epidemiological studies seek to determine the prevalence and distribution of disorders and their correlates in particular populations of children who vary in age, sex, socioeconomic status (SES), ethnicity, or other characteristics (Costello & Angold, 2000). The overall lifetime prevalence rates for childhood problems are estimated to be high and on the order of 14–22% of all children (Rutter, 1989). Rutter, Tizard, and Whitmore (1970), in the classic Isle of Wight Study, found the overall rate of child psychiatric disorders to be 6–8% in 9- to 11-year-old children. Richman, Stevenson, and Graham (1975), in the London Epidemiological Study, found moderate to severe behavior problems for 7% of the population, with an additional 15% of children having mild problems. Boyle et al. (1987) and Offord et al. (1987), in the Ontario Child Health Study, reported that 19% of boys and 17% of girls had one or more disorders. Many other epidemiological studies have reported similar rates of prevalence (e.g., Brandenburg, Friedman, & Silver, 1990; Costello, Farmer, Angold, Burns, & Erkanli, 1997; Earls, 1980; Hewitt et al., 1997; Lapouse & Monk, 1958; MacFarlane, Allen, & Honzik, 1954; Shaffer et al., 1996; Verhulst & Koot, 1992; Werner, Bierman, & French, 1971). Perhaps the most consistent general conclusions to be drawn from these studies are that prevalence rates for childhood problems are generally high, but that rates vary with the nature of the disorder; the age, sex, SES, and ethnicity of the child; the criteria used to define the problem; the method used to gather information (e.g., interview, questionnaire); the informant (e.g., child, parent, teacher);

sampling considerations; and a host of other factors.

Age Differences

Bird, Gould, Yager, Staghezza, and Camino (1989) reported no significant age differences for children aged 4 to 16 years in the total number of *Diagnostic and Statistical Manual of Mental Disorders*, third edition (DSM-III) disorders diagnosed at each age. Some studies of nonclinical samples of children have found a general decline in overall problems with age (e.g., Achenbach & Edelbrock, 1981), whereas similar studies of clinical samples have found an opposite trend (e.g., Achenbach, Howell, Quay, & Conners, 1991). Some studies have reported interactions among number of problems, age, sex of child, problem type, clinical status, and source of information (e.g., Simonoff et al., 1997). For example, Achenbach et al. (1991) found that externalizing problems showed a decline with age relative to internalizing problems, but only for those children who had been referred for treatment; Offord, Boyle, and Racine (1989) found complex interactions between age and sex of the child, with the results also depending on whether the informant was a child, parent, or teacher.

These and other findings raise numerous questions concerning age differences in children's problem behaviors. Answers to even a seemingly simple question such as "Do problem behaviors decrease (or increase) with age?" are complicated by (1) a lack of uniform measures of behavior that can be used across a wide range of ages; (2) qualitative changes in the expression of behavior with development; (3) the interactions between age and sex of the child; (4) the use of different informants; (5) the specific problem behavior(s) of interest; (6) the clinical status of the children being assessed; and (7) the use of different diagnostic criteria for children of different ages.

Notwithstanding these difficulties, both longitudinal (MacFarlane et al., 1954) and cross-sectional (Achenbach & Edelbrock, 1981; Achenbach et al., 1991) general population surveys are informative in depicting changes in the proportions of specific parent-, teacher-, or child-reported problem behaviors with age (e.g., "hyperactive," "argues," "cries"), as well as the manner in which the age changes vary as a function of problem type, sex, and clinical status of the child. However, it should be emphasized that general age trends are based on group statistics, which may obscure the nonlinear and nonnormative changes that often occur for individual children. In addition, general surveys do not provide information concerning the processes underlying age changes. Studies of change in individual children over time and of the context in which this change occurs are needed if such processes are to be understood (e.g., Bergman & Magnusson, 1997; Francis, Fletcher, Stuebing, Davidson, & Thompson, 1991).

Socioeconomic Status

Although most children with mental health problems are from the middle class, mental health problems are overrepresented among the very poor. It is estimated that 20% or more of children in North America are poor, and that as many as 20% of children growing up in inner-city poverty are impaired to some degree in their social, behavioral, and academic functioning (Duncan et al., 1994; Institute of Medicine, 1989; Schteingart, Molnar, Klein, Lowe, & Hartmann, 1995).

Lower-SES children have been reported to display more psychopathology and other problems than upper-SES children (e.g., Keenan, Shaw, Walsh, Delliquadri, & Giovannelli, 1997; Samaan, 2000). However, although the reported relationships between SES and child psychopathology are statistically significant, the effects are small and should be interpreted cautiously (Achenbach et al., 1991). More importantly, global estimates of SES often tell us little about the associated processes through which SES exerts its influence on a child. Knowledge of such processes is needed to inform our understanding of disorders. For example, the effects of SES on aggression can be explained mostly by stressful life events and by beliefs that are accepting of aggression (Guerra, Tolan, Huesmann, Van Acker, & Eron, 1995).

The impact of socioeconomic disadvantage on children derives from the fact that SES is a composite variable that includes many potential sources of negative influence (Bradley, Corwyn, McAdoo, & García Coll, 2001). In addition to low income, low SES is often characterized by low maternal education, a low level of employment, single-parent status, parental psychopathology, limited resources, and negative life events (e.g., poor nutrition, exposure to violence). Since overall indices of SES may include one or more of these variables in any given study, the relationship that is reported between SES and child psychopathology may vary as a function of the particular index used, as well as ethnic factors (McLeod & Nonnemaker, 2000). In short, SES may serve as a proxy or indicator of other more active factors that influence risk for child psychopathology.

Some research findings in child psychopathology are confounded by a failure to control for SES. For example, although physically abused children show higher levels of externalizing problems than nonabused children (Mash, Johnston, & Kovitz, 1983), it is not clear that physical abuse and externalizing problems are associated when the effects of SES are controlled for (Cummings, Hennessy, Rabideau, & Cicchetti, 1994; Wolfe & Mosk, 1983). The relationships among SES, maltreatment, and behavior disorders are further complicated by other findings that the effects of physical abuse on internalizing disorders may be independent of SES, whereas the effects of abuse on externalizing disorders may be dependent on SES-related conditions (Okun, Parker, & Levendosky, 1994).

Sex Differences

Although sex differences in the expression of psychopathology have been formally recognized since the time that Freud presented his views at the beginning of the 20th century, psychopathology in girls has received far less research attention than psychopathology in boys (Bell-Dolan, Foster, & Mash, in press; Eme, 1979). In the past, many studies have either excluded girls from their samples entirely or have examined all children together without considering findings for girls separately. For example, until recently there were relatively few studies on disruptive behavior disorders in girls (e.g., Moffitt, Caspi, Rutter, & Silva, 2001; Silverthorn & Frick, 1999; Zoccolillo, 1993). This omission was related to the perception that such disorders are much more common in boys than in girls; to sampling biases in which boys, who are more severely disruptive, are also more likely to be referred and studied; and to the use of inclusionary diagnostic criteria that were derived and validated largely from studies with boys (Spitzer, Davies, & Barkley, 1990).

Research has confirmed that there are important differences in the prevalence, expression, accompanying disorders, underlying processes, outcomes, and developmental course of psychopathology in boys versus girls (Eme, 1979, 1992; Hops, 1995; Keenan & Shaw, 1997; Willcutt & Pennington, 2000a; Zahn-Waxler, 1993). ADHD, autism, childhood disruptive behavior disorders, and learning and communication disorders are all more common in boys than girls, whereas the opposite is true for most anxiety disorders, adolescent depression, and eating disorders (Hartung & Widiger, 1998). Although these sex differences are well established, their meaning is not well understood. For example, it is difficult to determine whether observed sex differences are a function of referral or reporting biases, the way in which disorders are currently defined, differences in the expression of the disorder (e.g., direct vs. indirect aggressive behavior), sex differences in the genetic penetrance of disorders, or sex differences in biological characteristics and environmental susceptibilities. All are possible, and there is a need for research into the processes underlying observed differences. Clearly the mechanisms and causes of sex differences may vary for different disorders (e.g., ADHD vs. depression), or for the same disorder at different ages (e.g., child vs. adolescent obsessive–compulsive disorder or early- vs. late-onset conduct disorder).

Early research into sex differences focused mainly on descriptive comparisons of the frequencies of different problems for boys versus girls at different ages. In general, differences in problem behaviors between the sexes are small in children of preschool age or younger (e.g., Briggs-Gowan, Carter, Skuban, & Horwitz, 2001; Gadow, Sprafkin, & Nolan, 2001), but become increasingly common with age. For example, Weisz and Suwanlert (1989) studied children in the United States and Thailand, and found that boys were rated higher than girls on every problem for which there was a significant sex difference—including total problems, undercontrolled problems, overcontrolled problems, and culture-specific problems. Across cultures, boys have been found to display more fighting, impulsivity, and other uncontrolled behaviors than girls (Olweus, 1979).

It has been found that boys show greater difficulties than girls during early or middle childhood, particularly with respect to ADHD and disruptive behavior disorders (MacFarlane et al., 1954). Girls' problems may increase during adolescence, with higher prevalence rates for depression and dysphoric mood from midadolescence through adulthood. For example, conduct disorder and hyperactivity have been found to be more frequent in 12- to 16-year-old boys than girls, whereas emotional problems have been found to be more frequent for girls than boys in this age group (Boyle et al., 1987; Offord et al., 1987). In addition, early signs of aggression have been found to predict later antisocial behavior for boys but not for girls (Tremblay et al., 1992).

However, not all studies have reported significant sex differences in overall rates of problem behavior (e.g., Achenbach & Edelbrock, 1981; Velez, Johnson, & Cohen, 1989), and even when significant overall sex differences have been found, they tend to be small and to account for only a small proportion of the variance. It has also been found that although there is a much larger predominance of externalizing problems in boys and of internalizing problems in adolescent girls in samples of children who are referred for treatment, sex differences in externalizing versus internalizing problems are minimal in nonreferred samples of children (Achenbach et al., 1991).

Comparisons of the behavioral and emotional problems in boys versus girls over time can provide useful information about sex-related characteristics. However, taken in isolation, such global comparisons do not address possible qualitative differences in (1) expressions of psychopathology in boys versus girls; (2) the processes underlying these expressions; (3) the long-term consequences of certain behaviors for boys versus girls; and/or (4) the impact of certain environmental events on boys versus girls (Zahn-Waxler, 1993). As noted by Hops (1995), it seems likely that "the pathways from childhood to adolescence and adult pathology are age and gender specific and that these differences may be the result of different social contexts that nurture the development of health or pathology for female and male individuals" (p. 428). In addition to differential socialization practices, there are likely to be differences in the expression and outcome of psychopathology in boys versus girls as a function of biologically based differences. For example, in a study of the psychophysiology of disruptive behavior in boys versus girls, Zahn-Waxler, Cole, Welsh, and Fox (1995) found that disruptive girls showed high electrodermal responding relative to disruptive boys and were also highly activated by a sadness mood induction. These investigators suggested that girls' disruptive behavior may be more closely connected than boys' disruptive behavior to experiences of anxiety. Other research has found that increases in depression in females during adolescence are related mostly to accompanying changes in levels of estrogen and androgen (Angold, Costello, Erkanli, & Worthman, 1999). It is also possible that for some disorders (e.g., ADHD), girls may require a higher genetic loading for the disorders than boys before the disorders are likely to express themselves (Rhee, Waldman, Hay, & Levy, 1999).

There may also be differences in the processes underlying the expression of psychopathology and distress in boys versus girls. For example, findings suggest that the an adolescent's emergent sexuality may create special difficulties with the parent of the opposite sex, and that distress in adolescent males may be particularly disruptive for mothers and daughters (Ge et al., 1995). Others studies have found that daughters of depressed mothers may be at greater risk than sons for the development of internalizing disorders (Gelfand & Teti, 1990) and that sons of fathers showing avoidant patterns of adjustment to marital distress may be particularly susceptible to internalizing disorders (Katz & Gottman, 1993). Finally, depression in adolescent females has been found to be strongly associated with maternal depression, whereas a lack of supportive early care appears to be more strongly associated with depression in adolescent males (Duggal, Carlson, Sroufe, & Egeland, 2001).

It has also been found that the types of childrearing environments predicting resilience to adversity may differ for boys and girls. Resilience in boys is associated with households in which there is a male model (e.g., father, grandfather, older sibling), structure, rules, and some encouragement of emotional expressiveness. In contrast, resilient girls come from households that combine risk taking and independence with support from a female caregiver (e.g., mother, grandmother, older sister) (Werner, 1995).

Zahn-Waxler et al. (1995) refer to the "gender paradox of comorbidities," which is that although the prevalence of disruptive behavior is lower in females than in males, the risk of comorbid conditions such as anxiety is higher in female samples. In explaining this paradox, Zahn-Waxler et al. (1995) suggest that girls' heightened level of interpersonal sensitivity, caring, and empathy may be a protective factor in insulating them from developing antisocial behavior. At the same time, girls' overreceptivity to the plight of others, and their reluctance to assert their own needs in situations involving conflict and distress, may elevate their risk for the development of internalizing problems. However, the relations between gender and comorbidity are likely to vary with the disorders under consideration, the age of the child, the source of referral, and other factors. For example, in contrast to Zahn-Waxler et al. (1995), Biederman et al. (2002) found that girls with ADHD had a significantly *lower* rate of comorbid major depression than did boys with ADHD.

Although findings relating to sex differences and child psychopathology are complex, inconsistent, and frequently difficult to interpret, the cumulative findings from research strongly indicate that the effects of gender are critical to understanding the expression and course of most forms of childhood disorder (Bell-Dolan et al., in press; Kavanagh & Hops, 1994). It is particularly important to understand the processes and mechanisms underlying these gender effects, and to recognize that biological influences and differential socialization practices are likely to interact throughout development in accounting for any differences between the sexes that are found.

Rural versus Urban Differences

Although there is a general belief that rates of child behavior disorder are higher in urban than in rural areas, research findings in support of this view are weak and/or inconsistent. Findings from the Isle of Wight, Inner London Borough, and Ontario Child Health Studies reveal prevalence rates of problem behavior that were higher for urban than rural children (Offord et al., 1987; Rutter, 1981). On the other hand, in a cross-cultural investigation, Weisz and Suwanlert (1991) found few differences in parent or teacher ratings of child problems as a function of rural versus urban status in either of the cultures that were studied (United States and Thailand). In a detailed analysis that controlled for the effects of SES and ethnicity and also looked at gradations of urbanization, Achenbach et al. (1991) found few differences in children's behavior problems or competencies as a function of rural versus urban status, although there was a significant but very small effect indicating higher delinquency scores for children in urban environments. These investigators concluded that earlier findings of higher rates of problem behavior in urban than in rural areas "may have reflected the tendency to combine areas of intermediate urbanization with large urban areas for comparison with rural areas as well as a possible lack of control for demographic differences" (p. 86). Even in studies in which rural versus urban differences have been found, for the most part these differences were associated with economic and cultural differences between sites, and not with urbanization per se (Zahner, Jacobs, Freeman, & Trainor, 1993).

Ethnicity and Culture

Ethnicity

Numerous terms have been used to describe ethnic influences. These include "ethnicity," "race," "ethnic identity," "ethnic orientation," "acculturation," "bicultural orientation," and "culture." As pointed out by Foster and Martinez (1995), there is a need to recognize the diversity of terminology that has been used in describing ethnicity, and the fact that these terms refer to related but different things. Despite the growing ethnic diversity of the North American population, ethnic representation in research studies and the study of ethnicity-related issues more generally have received relatively little attention in studies of child psychopathology (García Coll, Akerman, & Cicchetti, 2000; U.S. Public Health Service, 2001c). In lamenting this state of affairs, Foster and Martinez (1995) state: "The underrepresentation of children from diverse backgrounds is accompanied by a dearth of empirical literature on the origins, correlates, and treatment of child psychopathology in different ethnic groups within the United States. Instead, investigators have based theories of child behavior, both normal and deviant, on data drawn largely from European-American culture" (p. 214).

Research into child psychopathology has generally been insensitive to possible differences in prevalence, age of onset, developmental course, and risk factors related to ethnicity (Kazdin & Kagan, 1994), and to the considerable heterogeneity that exists within specific ethnic groups (Murry, Bynum, Brody, Willert, & Stephens, 2001; Murry, Smith, & Hill, 2001). In addition, few studies have compared ethnic groups while controlling for other important variables, such as SES, sex, age, and geographic region. In recent comparisons that have controlled for these variables, African American and Hispanic American children are identified and referred at the same rates as other children, but they are much less likely to actually receive specialty mental health services or psychotropic medications (García Coll & Garrido, 2000). European American and Native American children have been found to display similar mental health problems with the exception of substance abuse, where rates are higher for Native American youngsters (Costello, Farmer, & Angold, 1999).

Some studies that have included a small number of African American children in their samples have reported somewhat higher rates of externalizing problems for this group (Costello, 1989; Velez et al., 1989). However, other studies with much larger national samples that included European American, African American, and Hispanic American children have reported either no or very small differences related to race or ethnicity when SES, sex, age, and referral status were controlled for (Achenbach & Edelbrock, 1981; Achenbach et al., 1991; Lahey et al., 1995). So, although externalizing problems have been reported to be more common among African American children, this finding is probably an artifact related to SES. Externalizing disorder is associated with both ethnicity and SES, and since there is an overrepresentation of minority status children in low-SES groups in North America, caution must be exercised in interpreting the relationships among SES, ethnicity, and aggression (Guerra et al., 1995; Lahey et al., 1995).

Ethnicity has not been found to be strongly associated with risk for eating disorders (Leon, Fulkerson, Perry, & Early-Zald, 1995), although differences between European Americans and other groups have been reported for such subclinical eating disturbances as dietary restraint, ideal body shape, and body dissatisfaction (Wildes & Emery, 2001). Differing patterns of substance abuse as a function of ethnicity have also been reported (Catalano et al., 1993). More research is needed, but these and other findings suggest that the effects of ethnicity are likely to vary with the problem under consideration and its severity.

As is the case for SES and sex differences, global comparisons of the prevalence of different types of problems for different ethnic groups are not likely to be very revealing. On the other hand, studies into the processes affecting the form, associated factors, and outcomes of different disorders for various ethnic groups hold promise for increasing our understanding of the relationship between ethnicity and child psychopathology (e.g., Bird et al., 2001; Bradley, Corwyn, Burchinal, McAdoo, & García Coll, 2001).

Culture

The values, beliefs, and practices that characterize a particular ethnocultural group contribute to the development and expression of childhood distress and dysfunction, which in turn are organized into categories through cultural processes that further influence their development and expression (Harkness & Super, 2000; Wong & Ollendick, 2001). Through shared views about causality and intervention, culture also structures the way in which people and institutions react to a child's problems. Since the meaning of children's social behavior is influenced by cultural beliefs and values, it is not surprising that the form, frequency, and predictive significance of different forms of child psychopathology vary across cultures, or that cultural attitudes influence diagnostic and referral practices (Lambert & Weisz, 1992). For example, shyness and oversensitivity in children have been found to be associated with peer rejection and social maladjustment in Western cultures, but with leadership, school competence, and academic achievement in Chinese children in Shanghai (Chen, Rubin, & Li, 1995). Similarly, Lambert and Weisz (1989) found that overcontrolled problems were reported significantly more often for Jamaican than for American youngsters—a finding consistent with Afro-British Jamaican cultural attitudes and practices that discourage child aggression and other undercontrolled behavior, and that foster inhibition and other overcontrolled behavior.

Weisz and Sigman (1993), using parent reports of behavioral and emotional problems in 11- to 15-year-old children from Kenya, Thailand, and the United States, found that Kenyan children were rated particularly high on overcontrolled problems (e.g., fears, feelings of guilt, somatic concerns), due primarily to numerous reports of somatic problems. In this mixed-race sample, whites were rated particularly high on undercontrolled problems (e.g., "arguing," "disobedient at home," "cruel to others"). Weisz and Suwanlert (1987) compared 6- to 11-year-old children in the Buddhist-oriented, emotionally controlled culture of Thailand with American 6- to 11-year-olds. Parent reports revealed Thai–U.S. differences in 54 problem behaviors, most of which were modest in magnitude. Thai children were rated higher than American children on problems involving overcontrolled behaviors such as anxiety and depression, whereas American children were rated higher than Thai children on undercontrolled behaviors such as disobedience and fighting.

Weisz and Suwanlert (1991) compared ratings of behavior and emotional problems of 2- to

9-year-old children in Thailand and the United States. Parents and teachers in Thailand rated both overcontrolled and undercontrolled problems as less serious, less worrisome, less likely to reflect personality traits, and more likely to improve with time. These findings suggest that there may be cultural differences in the meanings ascribed to problem behaviors across cultures.

Findings from these and other studies suggest that the expression of, and tolerance for, many child behavioral and emotional disturbances are related to social and cultural values. The processes that mediate this relationship are in need of further investigation. In this regard, it is important that research on child psychopathology not be generalized from one culture to another, unless there is support for doing so. There is some support for the notion that some processes—for example, those involved in emotion regulation and its relation to social competence—may be similar across diverse cultures (Eisenberg, Pidada, & Liew, 2001). The rates of expression of some disorders, particularly those with a strong neurobiological basis (e.g., ADHD, autistic disorder), may be less susceptible to cultural influences than others. However, even so, social and cultural beliefs and values are likely to influence the meaning given to these behaviors, the ways in which they are responded to, their forms of expression, and their outcomes.

An important distinction to be made with respect to cross-cultural comparisons is whether or not there are real differences in the rates of the disorder, or differences in the criteria used to make judgments about these problems. For example, Weisz and Suwanlert (1989) compared the teacher-reported behavioral/emotional problems of Thai and U.S. children (ages 6–11 years). It was found that Thai teachers were confronted with students who were more prone to behavioral and emotional problems at school than were teachers in the United States, but that they applied different judgments to the behaviors they observed.

Cultural factors are known to influence not only informal labeling processes but formal diagnostic practices as well. For example, reported prevalence rates of ADHD in Britain are much lower than in the United States, because of differences in the way in which diagnostic criteria for ADHD are applied in the two countries. Such differences in diagnostic practices may lead to spurious differences in reported prevalence rates for different forms of child psychopathology across cultures.

Cross-cultural research on child psychopathology would suggest that the expression and experience of mental disorders in children are not universal (Fisman & Fisman, 1999). Patterns of onset and duration of illness and the nature and relationship among specific symptoms vary from culture to culture, and across ethnic groups within cultures (Hoagwood & Jensen, 1997). However, few studies have compared the attitudes, behaviors, and biological and psychological processes of children with mental disorders across different cultures. Such information is needed to understand how varying social experiences and contexts influence the expression, course, and outcome of different disorders across cultures. For example, greater social connectedness and support in more traditional cultures, and greater access to resources and opportunities in industrialized societies, are examples of mechanisms that may alter outcomes across cultures. Sensitivity to the role of cultural influences in child psychopathology has increased (Evans & Lee, 1998; Lopez & Guarnaccia, 2000), and is likely to continue to do so as globalization and rapid cultural change become increasingly more common (García Coll et al., 2000).

BASIC ISSUES IN CHILD PSYCHOPATHOLOGY

Several recurrent and overlapping issues have characterized the study of psychopathology in children (Rutter & Garmezy, 1983; Rutter & Sroufe, 2000). A number of these are highlighted in this section, including (1) difficulties in conceptualizing psychopathology and normality; (2) the need to consider healthy functioning and adjustment; (3) questions concerning developmental continuities and discontinuities; (4) the concept of developmental pathways; (5) the notions of risk and resilience; (6) the identification of protective and vulnerability factors; and (7) the role of contextual influences.

Psychopathology versus Normality

Conceptualizing child psychopathology and attempting to establish boundaries between what constitutes abnormal and normal functioning are arbitrary processes at best (Achenbach, 1997). Traditional approaches to mental disorders in children have emphasized concepts such as symptoms, diagnosis, illness, and treatment; by doing so, they have strongly influenced the way we think about child psychopathology and related questions (Richters & Cicchetti, 1993). Childhood disorders have most commonly been conceptualized in terms of deviancies involving breakdowns in adaptive functioning, statistical deviation, unexpected distress or disability, and/or biological impairment.

Wakefield (1992, 1997, 1999a) has proposed an overarching concept of mental disorder as "harmful dysfunction." This concept encompasses a child's physical and mental functioning, and includes both value- and science-based criteria. In the context of child psychopathology, a child's condition is viewed as a disorder only if (1) it causes harm or deprivation of benefit to the child, as judged by social norms; and (2) it results from the failure of some internal mechanism to perform its natural function (e.g., "an effect that is part of the evolutionary explanation of the existence and structure of the mechanism"; Wakefield, 1992, p. 384). This view of mental disorder focuses attention on internally evolved mechanisms—for example, executive functions in the context of self-regulation (Barkley, 2001). Nevertheless, as pointed out by Richters and Cicchetti (1993), this view only identifies the decisions that need to be made in defining mental disorders; it does not specify *how* such decisions are to be made.

As is the case for most definitions of mental disorder that have been proposed, questions related to defining the boundaries between normal and abnormal, understanding the differences between normal variability and dysfunction, defining what constitute "harmful conditions," linking dysfunctions causally with these conditions, and circumscribing the domain of "natural" or of other proposed mechanisms are matters of considerable controversy (Lilienfeld & Marino, 1995; Richters & Cicchetti, 1993).[4] Categories of mental disorder stem from human-made linguistic distinctions and abstractions, and boundaries between what constitutes normal and abnormal conditions, or between different abnormal conditions, are not easily drawn. Although it may sometimes appear that efforts to categorize mental disorders are carving "nature at its joints," whether or not such "joints" actually exist is open to debate (e.g., Cantor, Smith, French, & Mezzich, 1980; Lilienfeld & Marino, 1995). However, clear joints do not necessarily need to exist for categorical distinctions to have utility. For instance, there is no joint at which one can carve day from night; yet distinguishing the two has proven incredibly useful to humans in going about their social discourse and engagements. Likewise, although the threshold for determining disorder from merely high levels of symptoms may be fuzzy, it could be stipulated as being at that point along a dimension where impairment in a major, culturally universal life activity befalls the majority of people at or exceeding that point. Thus, despite the lack of clear boundaries between what is normal and abnormal, categorical distinctions are still useful.

Healthy Functioning

The study of psychopathology in children requires concomitant attention to adaptive developmental processes for several reasons. First, judgments of deviancy require knowledge of normative developmental functioning, both with respect to a child's performance relative to same-age peers and with respect to the child's own baseline of development. Second, maladaptation and adaptation often represent two sides of the same coin, in that dysfunction in a particular domain of development (e.g., the occurrence of inappropriate behaviors) is usually accompanied by a failure to meet developmental tasks and expectations in the same domain (e.g., the nonoccurrence of appropriate behaviors). It is important to point out, however, that adaptation should not be equated with the mere absence of psychopathology. Kendall and his colleagues (Kendall, Marrs-Garcia, Nath, & Sheldrick, 1999; Kendall & Sheldrick, 2000), for instance, contend that it is important to use normative comparisons to evaluate treatment outcome; they suggest that improvement involves falling within a certain range of healthy functioning, in addition to the amelioration of one's symptom presentation. Moreover, adaptation involves the presence and development of psychological, physical, interpersonal, and intellectual resources (see Fredrickson, 2001). Third, in addition to the specific problems that lead to referral and diagnosis, disturbed children are likely to show impairments in other areas of adaptive functioning. For example, in addition to their core symptoms of impulsivity and inattention, children with ADHD also show lower-than-average levels of functioning in their socialization, communication, and activities of daily living (e.g., Stein, Szumowski, Blondis, & Roizen, 1995). Fourth, most children with specific disorders are known to cope effectively in some areas of their lives. Understanding a child's strengths informs our knowledge of the child's disorder and provides a basis for the development of effective treatment strategies. Fifth, children move between pathological and nonpathological forms of functioning over the course of their development. Individual children may have their "ups and downs" in problem type and frequency over time. Sixth, many child behaviors that are not classifiable as deviant at a particular point in time may nevertheless represent less extreme expressions or compensations of an already existing disorder or early expressions of a later progression to deviant extremes as development continues (Adelman, 1995). Finally, no theory of a childhood disorder is complete if it cannot be linked with a theory of how the underlying normal abilities develop and what factors go awry to produce the disordered state. Therefore, understanding child psychopathology requires that we also attend to these less extreme forms of difficulty and develop more complete models of the normal developmental processes underlying the psychopathology.

For these and other reasons to be discussed, the study of child psychopathology requires an understanding of both abnormal and healthy functioning. As noted by Cicchetti and Richters (1993), "it is only through the joint consideration of adaptive and maladaptive processes within the individual that it becomes possible to speak in meaningful terms about the existence, nature, and boundaries of the underlying psychopathology" (p. 335). To date, far greater attention has been devoted to the description and classification of psychopathology in children than to healthy child functioning; to nonpathological psychosocial problems related to emotional upset, misbehavior, and learning; or to factors that promote the successful resolution of developmental tasks (Adelman, 1995; Sonuga-Barke, 1998). In light of this imbalance, there is a need for studies of normal developmental processes (Lewis, 2000), for investigations of normative and representative community samples of children (Ialongo, Kellam, & Poduska, 2000; Kazdin, 1989), and for studies of "resilient" children who show normal development in the face of adversity (Masten, 2001).

Developmental Continuities and Discontinuities

A central issue for theory and research in child psychopathology concerns the continuity of disorders identified from one time to another and the relationship between child, adolescent, and adult disorders (Caspi, 2000; Garber, 1984; Kazdin & Johnson, 1994; Rutter & Rutter, 1993; Sroufe & Jacobvitz, 1989). Over the past two decades, research into early attachment has stimulated general interest in the roles of relational processes and internalized representational systems as the bases for understanding continuities and discontinuities in psychopathology over time and across generations (Cassidy & Shaver, 1999; Lyons-Ruth, 1995; Sroufe, Duggal, Weinfeld, & Carlson, 2000).

Some childhood disorders, such as mental retardation and autistic disorder, are chronic conditions that will persist throughout childhood and into adulthood. Other disorders, such as functional enuresis and encopresis, occur during childhood and only rarely manifest themselves in adults (Walker et al., 1989). And other disorders (e.g., mood disorders, schizophrenia, generalized anxiety disorder) are expressed, albeit in modified forms, in both childhood and adulthood and exhibit varying degrees of continuity over time.

Evidence in support of the continuity between child and adult disorders is equivocal and depends on a number of methodological factors related to research design, assessment instruments, the nature of the study sample, and the type and severity of the disorder (Garber, 1984). In general, the literature suggests that child psychopathology is continuous with adult disorders for some, but not all, problems. As we discuss below, there is evidence that appears to favor the stability of externalizing problems over internalizing problems. However, previous findings may reflect the severity and pervasiveness of the disorders assessed, referral biases, and the fact that longitudinal investigations of children with internalizing and other disorders are just beginning to emerge. For example, one study found that first-grade anxious symptoms predicted levels of anxious symptoms and adaptive functioning in fifth grade (Ialongo, Edelsohn, Werthamer-Larsson, Crockett, & Kellam, 1995). In another report, early-onset bulimia nervosa was associated with a 9-fold increase in risk for late-adolescent bulimia nervosa and a 20-fold increase in risk for adult bulimia nervosa (Kotler et al., 2001).

The possible mechanisms underlying the relationships between early maladaptation and later disordered behavior are numerous and can operate in both direct and indirect ways (Garber, 1984; Rutter, 1994a; Sroufe & Rutter, 1984). Some examples of *direct* relationships between early and later difficulties include (1) the development of a disorder during infancy or childhood, which then persists over time; (2) experiences that alter the infant's or child's physical status (e.g., neural plasticity), which in turn influences later functioning (Courchesne, Chisum, & Townsend, 1994; Johnson, 1999; Nelson, 2000); and (3) the acquisition of early patterns of responding (e.g., compulsive compliance, dissociation) that may be adaptive in light of the child's current developmental level and circumstances, but may result in later psychopathology when circumstances change and new developmental challenges arise.

Some examples of *indirect* associations between child and adult psychopathology may involve early predispositions that eventually interact with environmental experiences (e.g., stressors), the combination of which leads to dysfunction. For example, Egeland and Heister (1995) found that the impact of day care on disadvantaged high-risk children at 42 months of age was related to the children's attachment quality at 12 months of age, with securely attached children more likely to be negatively affected by early out-of-home care. Other examples of indirect links between child and adult disturbance include (1) experiences (e.g., peer rejection) that contribute to an altered sense of self-esteem (DuBois & Tevendale, 1999), or that create a negative cognitive set, which then leads to later difficulties; and (2) experiences providing various opportunities or obstacles that then lead to the selection of particular environmental conditions, and by doing so guide a child's course of development (Rutter, 1987; Sroufe & Rutter, 1984).

Research efforts have focused not only on the continuities and discontinuities in childhood disorders, but also on the identification of factors that predict them. One factor that has been studied in the context of conduct disorder is age of onset, with early onset usually viewed as the occurrence of conduct disorder symptoms prior to age 12 years (Loeber & Dishion, 1983; O'Donnell, Hawkins, & Abbott, 1995). It has been found that early onset of symptoms is associated with higher rates and more serious antisocial acts over a longer period of time for both boys and girls (Lavigne et al., 2001). However, psychosocial variables that are present prior to and following onset may influence the seriousness and chronicity more than age of onset per se does (Tolan & Thomas, 1995). A question that needs to be addressed is this: Does early age of onset operate in a causal fashion for later problems, and if so, how? Another issue is whether the causal processes that are associated with an early onset of a disorder (e.g., depression) are different from those that serve to maintain the disorder. Even then, the specification of an age of onset need not be made so precisely that it creates a false distinction that only valid cases meet that precise threshold, as may have happened with ADHD (see Barkley, chapter 2, this volume). Such efforts to impose precision where none exists may have backfired in hampering studies of teens and adults having the same disorder who cannot adequately recall such a precise onset, and in presuming that cases having qualitatively identical symptoms and impairments but later onsets are invalid instances of a disorder.

Although research supports the notion of continuity of disorders, it does not support the continuity of identical symptoms over time (i.e., "homotypic correspondence"). Continuity over time for patterns of behavior rather than for specific symptoms is the norm. For example, although externalizing disorders in boys are stable over time, the ways in which these behavioral patterns are expressed are likely to change dramatically over the course of development (Olweus, 1979). Even with wide fluctuations in the expression of behavior over time, "children may show consistency in their general adaptive or maladaptive pattern of organizing their experiences and interacting with the environment" (Garber, 1984, p. 34). Several research findings can be used to illustrate this notion of consistent "patterns of organization." For example, early heightened levels of behavioral inhibition may affect later adjustment by influencing the way in which a child adapts to new and unfamiliar situations and the ensuing person–environment interactions over time (Kagan, 1994a). Another example of a consistent pattern of organization involves early attachment quality and the development of internal working models that children carry with them into their later relationships (Bowlby, 1988; Goldberg, 1991). Internal working models of self and relationships may remain relatively stable over time, at the same time that the behavioral expressions of these internal models change with development. From a neuroscientific perspective, Pennington and Ozonoff (1991) argue that certain genes and neural systems also play a significant predisposing role in influencing the continuity of psychopathology, and that the "discontinuities at one level of analyses—that of observable behavior—may mask continuities at deeper levels of analysis; those concerned with the mechanisms underlying observable behavior" (p. 117).

Given that developmental continuity is reflected in general patterns of organization over time rather than in isolated behaviors or symptoms, the relationships between early adaptation and later psychopathology are not likely to be direct or uncomplicated. The connections between psychopathology in children and adults are marked by *both* continuities and discontinuities. The degree of continuity–discontinuity will vary as a function of changing environmental circumstances and transactions between a child and the environment that affect the child's developmental trajectory.

Developmental Pathways

The concept of "developmental pathways" is crucial for understanding continuities and discontinuities in psychopathology. Such pathways are not directly observable, but function as metaphors that are inferred from repeated assessments of individual children over time (Loeber, 1991). A pathway, according to Loeber (1991), "defines the sequence and timing of behavioral continuities and transformations and, ideally, summarizes the probabilistic relationships between successive behaviors" (p. 98). In attempting to identify developmental pathways as either "deviant" or "normal," it is important to recognize that (1) different pathways may lead to similar expressions of psychopathology (i.e., "equifinality"); and (2) similar initial pathways may result in different forms of dysfunction (i.e., "multifinality"), depending on the organization of the larger system in which they occur (Cicchetti & Rogosch, 1996; Lewis, 2000; Loeber, 1991).

Research findings related to child maltreatment provide an example of a possible developmental pathway. It has been found that physically abused children are more likely to develop insecure attachments, view interpersonal relationships as being coercive and threatening, become vigilant and selectively attend to hostile cues, instantly classify others as threatening or nonthreatening, and acquire aggressive behavioral strategies for solving interpersonal problems (see Cicchetti & Manly, 2001). These children bring representational models to peer relationships that are negative, conflictual, and unpredictable. They process social information in a biased and deviant manner, and develop problems with peer relationships that involve social withdrawal, unpopularity, and overt social rejection by peers (Dodge, Pettit, & Bates, 1994). In another example of a developmental pathway, the diagnosis of conduct disorder typically precedes the initiation of use of various substances, and this use in turn precedes the diagnosis of alcohol dependence in adolescents (Kuperman et al., 2001).

The systematic delineation of developmental pathways not only offers several advantages for the study of the etiology and outcomes of childhood disorders, but may also suggest strategies for intervention. Loeber (1991, p. 99) describes these advantages as "attempts to capture the changing manifestations and variable phenotype of a given disorder" over time. In this way, the study of developmental pathways includes etiological considerations, the assessment of comorbidities as they accrue over time, and a sensitivity to diverse outcomes (e.g., White, Bates, & Buyske, 2001).

Risk and Resilience

Previous studies of child psychopathology focused on elucidating the developmental pathways for deviancy and maladjustment to the relative exclusion of those for competency and adjustment (but see Luthar, 1993; Rutter, 1985, 1987, 1994b; and Rutter & Rutter, 1993, for exceptions). However, a significant number of children who are at risk do *not* develop later problems. There is a growing recognition of the need to examine not only risk factors, but also those conditions that protect vulnerable children from dysfunction and lead to successful adaptations despite adversity (Cicchetti & Garmezy, 1993).

"Resilience," which refers to successful adaptations in children who experience significant adversity, has now received a good deal of attention (Luthar, Cicchetti, & Becker, 2000). Early patterns of adaptation influence later adjustment in complex and reciprocal ways. Adverse conditions, early struggles to adapt, and failure to meet developmental tasks do not inevitably lead to a fixed and unchanging abnormal path. Rather, many different factors, including chance events and encounters, can provide turning points whereby success in a particular developmental task (e.g., educational advances, peer relationships) shifts a child's course onto a more adaptive trajectory. Conversely, there are numerous events and circumstances and underlying dynamic biological systems that may deflect the child's developmental trajectory toward maladaptation (e.g., a dysfunctional home environment, peer rejection, difficulties in school, parental psychopathology, intergenerational conflict, and even late-onset genetic effects).

Although the term "resilience" has not been clearly operationalized, it is generally used to describe children who (1) manage to avoid negative outcomes and/or to achieve positive outcomes despite being at significant risk for the development of psychopathology; (2) display sustained competence under stress; or (3) show recovery from trauma (Werner, 1995). Risk is usually defined in terms of child characteristics that are known to be associated with negative outcomes—for example, difficult temperament (Ingram & Price, 2001; Rothbart, Ahadi, & Evans, 2000)—and/or in terms of a child's exposure to extreme or disadvantaged environmental conditions (e.g., poverty or abuse). Individual children who are predisposed to develop psychopathology and who show a susceptibility to negative developmental outcomes under high-risk conditions are referred to as "vulnerable." Genetic makeup and temperament are two factors that are presumed to contribute to susceptibility for children who are exposed to high-risk environments (Rutter, 1985; Seifer, 2000).

Research on resilience has lacked a consistent vocabulary, conceptual framework, and methodological approach (Luthar et al., 2000; Rutter, 2000c; Zimmerman & Arunkumar, 1994). It is particularly important to ensure that resilience is not defined as a universal, categorical, or fixed attribute of a child, but rather as a number of different types of dynamic processes that operate over time. Individual children may be resilient in relation to some specific stressors but not others, and resilience may vary over time and across contexts (Freitas & Downey, 1998). As noted by Zimmerman and Arunkumar (1994, p. 4), "research on resiliency can only identify those particular risk circumstances when environmental conditions, individual factors, and developmental tasks interact to help children and adolescents avoid negative consequences." Fortunately, models of resilience have increasingly begun to address the complex and dynamic relationships between the child and his or her environment, to incorporate the theoretical and empirical contributions of developmental psychology, and to acknowledge the multiple factors related to normal and deviant behavior (Glantz & Johnson, 1999; Walden & Smith, 1997; Tebes, Kaufman, Adnopoz, & Racusin, 2001).

One problem in research on resilience has been an absence of agreed-upon criteria for defining positive developmental outcomes (see Kaufman, Cook, Arny, Jones, & Pittinsky, 1994, for a review of the ways in which positive outcomes in studies of resilience have been operationalized). For example, there is currently debate as to whether the criteria for defining resilience and adaptation should be based on evidence from external criteria (e.g., academic performance), internal criteria (e.g., subjective well-being), or some combination of these (see Masten, 2001). Variations across studies in the source of information (e.g., parent or teacher); the type of assessment method (e.g., interview, questionnaire, observation); the adaptational criteria used; and the number and timing of assessments can easily influence the proportion of children who are designated as resilient or not in any particular investigation (Kaufman et al., 1994; Masten, 2001). And there is also some confusion about and circularity in how the term "resilience" has been used, in that it has been used to refer to both an outcome and to the cause of an outcome. Several different models of resilience have also been proposed, the most common ones being a compensatory model, a challenge model (e.g., stress inoculation), and a protective-factors model (Garmezy, Masten, & Tellegen, 1984).

Years of research suggest that resilience is not indicative of any rare or special qualities of the child per se (as implied by the term "the invulnerable child"), but rather is the result of the interplay of normal developmental processes such as brain development, cognition, caregiver–child relationships, regulation of emotion and behavior, and the motivation for learning (Masten, 2001). Some researchers have argued that resilience may be more ubiquitous than previously thought, and that this phenomenon is part of the "ordinary magic" and makeup of basic human adaptation (Masten, 2001; Sheldon & King, 2001). It is when these adaptational systems are impaired, usually through prolonged or repeated adversity, that the risk for childhood psychopathology increases.

Protective and Vulnerability Factors

Various protective and vulnerability factors have been found to influence children's reactions to potential risk factors or stressors. These include factors within the child, the family, and the community (Osofsky & Thompson, 2000; Werner &

Smith, 1992). Common risk factors that have been found to have adverse effects on a child encompass both acute stressful situations and chronic adversity; they include such events as chronic poverty, serious caregiving deficits, parental psychopathology, death of a parent, community disasters, homelessness, reduced social support, decreased financial resources, family breakup, parental marital/couple conflict, and perinatal stress (Deater-Deckard & Dunn, 1999; Rutter, 1999; Tebes et al., 2001; Walden & Smith, 1997).

Protective factors within a child that have been identified include an "easy" temperament (i.e., a child who is energetic, affectionate, cuddly, good-natured, and/or easy to deal with), which makes the child engaging to other people; early coping strategies that combine autonomy with help seeking when needed; high intelligence and scholastic competence; effective communication and problem-solving skills; positive self-esteem and emotions; high self-efficacy; and the will to be or do something (Fredrickson, 2001; Gilgun, 1999; Werner, 1995). An example of a possible protective factor within the child is seen in findings that high vagal tone and vagal suppression—taken as indices of a child's ability to regulate emotion via self-soothing, focused attention, and organized and goal-directed behavior—can buffer children from the increases in externalizing behaviors, internalizing behaviors, and social problems often associated with exposure to parental marital/couple hostility and discord (Katz & Gottman, 1995) or parental problem drinking (El-Sheikh, 2001).

At a family level, protective factors that have been identified include the opportunity to establish a close relationship with at least one person who is attuned to the child's needs, positive parenting, availability of resources (e.g., child care), a talent or hobby that is valued by adults or peers, and family religious beliefs that provide stability and meaning during times of hardship or adversity (Werner & Smith, 1992). Protective factors in the community include extrafamilial relationships with caring neighbors, community elders, or peers; an effective school environment, with teachers who serve as positive role models and sources of support; and opening of opportunities at major life transitions (e.g., adult education, voluntary military service, church or community participation, a supportive friend or marital/relationship partner).

In summary, early patterns of adaptation influence later adjustment in complex and reciprocal ways. Adverse conditions, early adaptational struggles, and failure to meet developmental tasks do not inevitably lead to a fixed and unmalleable dysfunctional path. Rather, as noted earlier, many different factors can act to alter a child's developmental course for the better. Conversely, numerous events and circumstances may serve to alter this course for the worse.

The interrelated issues of developmental continuities–discontinuities, developmental pathways, risk and resilience, and vulnerability and protective factors are far from being resolved or clearly understood. The multitude of interdependent and reciprocal influences, mechanisms, and processes involved in the etiology and course of child psychopathology clearly suggest a need for more complex theories (e.g., chaos theory, nonlinear dynamic models) (Barton, 1994; Glantz & Johnson, 1999; Gottman, Guralnick, Wilson, Swanson, & Murray, 1997; Haynes & Blaine, 1995), research designs, and data-analytic strategies (Kazdin & Kagan, 1994; Mash & Krahn, 2000; Richters, 1997).

Contextual Influences

Messick (1983) cogently argues that any consideration of child psychopathology must consider and account for three sets of contextual variables: (1) the child *as* context—the idea that unique child characteristics, predispositions, and traits influence the course of development; (2) the child *of* context—the notion that the child comes from a background of interrelated family, peer, classroom, teacher, school, community, and cultural influences; and (3) the child *in* context—the understanding that the child is a dynamic and rapidly changing entity, and that descriptions taken at different points in time or in different situations may yield very different information.

Research has increasingly come to recognize the reciprocal transactions between the developing child and the multiple social and environmental contexts in which development occurs (Cicchetti & Aber, 1998; Deater-Deckard, 2001). Understanding context requires a consideration of events that impinge directly on the child in a particular situation at a particular point in time; extrasituational events that affect the child indirectly (e.g., a parent's work-related stress); and temporally remote events that continue to affect the child through their representation in the child's current cognitive–affective data base.

Defining context has been, and continues to be, a matter of some complexity. The context of maltreatment provides an illustration of difficulties in definition. Maltreatment can be defined in terms of its type, timing, frequency, severity, and chronicity in the family (e.g., Manly, Kim, Rogosch, & Cicchetti, 2001). Each of these parameters and their interaction may contribute to child outcomes, but in different ways. For example, Manly, Cicchetti, and Barnett (1994) studied different types of maltreatment and found that outcomes generally did not differ for children who were categorized as neglected versus abused. However, a regression analysis indicated that neglect accounted for more of the variance in child problems than other types of abuse did. In this study, sexually abused children were also found to be more socially competent than children exposed to other forms of maltreatment. This may reflect a lack of chronicity associated with sexual abuse, or it may suggest that problems related to sexual abuse may not reveal themselves until later periods in a child's development, when issues concerning sexuality become more salient. Other studies have found that psychological maltreatment and emotional abuse account for most of the distortions in development attributed to maltreatment in general, and have the most negative consequences for a child (Crittenden, Claussen, & Sugarman, 1994).

The example of maltreatment illustrates how contexts for development encompass heterogeneous sets of circumstances, and how child outcomes may vary as a function of (1) the configuration of these circumstances over time, (2) when and where outcomes are assessed, and (3) the specific aspects of development that are affected. More precise definitions are needed if the impact of maltreatment, or for that matter any contextual event (e.g., parent disciplinary styles, family support, intellectual stimulation), is to be understood.

Even for those forms of child psychopathology for which there are strong neurobiological influences, the expression of the disorder is likely to interact with contextual demands. For example, Iaboni, Douglas, and Baker (1995) found that although the overall pattern of responding shown by children with ADHD was indicative of a generalized inhibitory deficit, the self-regulatory problems of these children became more evident with continuing task demands for inhibition and/or deployment of effort. Likewise, tasks having high interest value or high external incentives may moderate these children's typically deficient performance on less interesting or low incentive tasks (Carlson & Tamm, 2000; Slusarek, Velling, Bunk, & Eggers, 2001).

Child psychopathology research has increasingly focused on the role of the family system, the complex relationships within families, and the reciprocal influences among various family subsystems (Fiese, Wilder, & Bickham, 2000). There is a need to consider not only the processes occurring within disturbed families, but the common and unique ways in which these processes affect both individual family members and subsystems. Within the family, the roles of the mother–child and marital/couple subsystems have received the most research attention to date, with less attention given to the roles of siblings (Hetherington, Reiss, & Plomin, 1994) and fathers (Lamb & Billings, 1997; Phares & Compas, 1992). For the most part, research into family processes and child psychopathology has not kept pace with family theory and practice, and there is a need for the development of sophisticated methodologies and valid measures that will capture the complex relationships hypothesized to be operative in disturbed and normal family systems (Bray, 1995; Bray, Maxwell, & Cole, 1995). This task is complicated by a lack of consensus concerning how dysfunctional or healthy family functioning should be defined, what specific family processes are important to assess (Bray, 1994; Mash & Johnston, 1995), or the extent to which such measures of family environment reflect true environmental effect or shared genetic influences between parent and child (Plomin, 1995).

DEFINING CHILD PSYCHOPATHOLOGY

There has been, and continues to be, a lack of consensus concerning how psychopathology in children should be defined (Silk et al., 2000; Sonuga-Barke, 1998). Although the situation is improving, comparisons of findings across studies are extremely difficult to make, because of the idiosyncratic ways in which samples of children have been constituted. For example, children described as "hyperactive" in previous studies have varied widely with respect to their symptoms and conditions, problem severities, comorbidities, and levels of cognitive functioning.

More recently, researchers and clinicians have come to define child psychopathology using standardized diagnostic systems such as DSM-IV (American Psychiatric Association [APA], 1994, 2000) and the *International Classification of Diseases*, 10th revision (ICD-10; WHO, 1992). The diagnostic criteria utilized in DSM-IV are the ones most commonly used in North America, and these are presented for the individual disorders described in each of the chapters of this volume. However, the increased use and acceptance of DSM-IV should not be taken as an indication of widespread agreement regarding the fundamental nature of what constitutes psychopathology in children or the specific criteria used to define it (cf. Achenbach, 1997; Cantwell, 1996; Follette & Houts, 1996; Scotti, Morris, McNeil, & Hawkins, 1996). In many ways, the increased use of DSM-IV seems to reflect a degree of resignation on the part of researchers and clinicians concerning the prospects for developing a widely agreed-upon alternative approach, combined with a growing consensus regarding the need to achieve a greater level of standardization (albeit an imperfect one) in defining childhood disorders.

Several fundamental questions have characterized most discussions concerning how child psychopathology should be defined:

1. Should child psychopathology be viewed as a disorder that occurs within the individual child, as a relational disturbance, as a reaction to environmental circumstances, or as some combination of all of these?
2. Does child psychopathology constitute a condition qualitatively different from normality (aberration), an extreme point on a continuous trait or dimension, a delay in the rate at which a normal trait would typically emerge, or some combination of the three? How are "subthreshold" problems to be handled?
3. Can homogeneous disorders be identified, or is child psychopathology best defined as a configuration of co-occurring disorders or as a profile of traits and characteristics?
4. Can child psychopathology be defined as a static entity at a particular point in time, or do the realities of development necessitate that it be defined as a dynamic and ongoing process that expresses itself in different ways over time and across contexts?
5. Is child psychopathology best defined in terms of its current expression, or do definitions also need to incorporate nonpathological conditions that may constitute risk factors for later problems?

There are currently no definitive answers to these questions. More often, the way in which they are answered reflects theoretical or disciplinary preferences and specific purposes and goals (e.g., defining samples for research studies, or determining program or insurance eligibility).

Psychopathology as Adaptational Difficulty

As we have noted earlier, a common theme in defining child psychopathology has been that of adaptational difficulty or failure (Garber, 1984; Mash, 1998). Sroufe and Rutter (1984) note that regardless of whether "particular patterns of early adaptation are to a greater or lesser extent influenced by inherent dispositions or by early experience, they are nonetheless patterns of adaptation" (p. 23). Developmental competence is reflected in a child's ability to use internal and external resources to achieve a successful adaptation (Masten & Curtis, 2000; Waters & Sroufe, 1983), and problems occur when the child fails to adapt successfully. Even with wide variations in terminology and proposed explanatory mechanisms across theories, there is general agreement that maladaptation represents a pause, a regression, or a deviation in development (Garber, 1984; Simeonsson & Rosenthal, 1992).

In conceptualizing and defining psychopathology as adaptational difficulty, it is also essential to conceptualize and identify the specific developmental tasks that are important for children at various ages and periods of development, and the many contextual variables that derive from and surround the child (Garber, 1984; Luthar et al., 1997; Mash, 1998). In this regard, the study of psychopathology in children and the study of development and context are for all intents and purposes inseparable (Cicchetti & Aber, 1998).

In determining whether a given behavior should be considered to be deviant in relation to stage-salient developmental issues, Garber (1984) stresses the need to understand several important parameters. The first, "intensity," refers to the magnitude of behavior as excessive or deficient. The second, "frequency," refers to the severity of the problem behavior, or how often it does or does not occur. Third, the "duration" of behavior must be considered. Some difficulties are transient and spontaneously remit, whereas others persist over time. To these parameters, we would add a qualitative parameter reflecting how grossly atypical the behavior may be (e.g., some of the complex compulsions seen in Tourette's disorders), such that even low-intensity, low-frequency, and short-duration behavior may be so bizarre as to constitute "psychopathology." It is crucial that the intensity, frequency, duration, and atypicality of the child's behavior be appraised with respect to what is considered normative for a given age. The final parameter of deviance concerns the "number of different symptoms" and their "configuration." Each of these parameters is central to research and theory, and to one's specific definition of adaptational failure, regression, stagnation, or deviation.

Social Judgment

The diagnosis of psychopathology in children is almost always a reflection of both the characteristics and behavior of the child *and* of significant adults and professionals (Lewis, 2000). Research findings utilizing behavior problem checklists and interviews indicate that there can be considerable disagreement across informants (e.g., parents, teachers, professionals) concerning problem behaviors in children (Achenbach, McConaughy, & Howell, 1987; Feiring & Lewis, 1996). Mothers typically report more problems than do fathers (e.g., Achenbach et al., 1991), and across a range of domains, teachers identify more problems than other informants do in assessing the same domains. For example, in a study with maltreated children, only 21% of children were classified as resilient by teachers, whereas 64% of children were so classified based on reports from other sources (Kaufman et al., 1994).

Issues regarding disagreement–agreement among informants are complicated by the fact that the amount of agreement will vary with the age and sex of the child (Offord et al., 1989), the nature of the problem being reported on (e.g., internalizing vs. externalizing), the method used to gather information (e.g., interview vs. questionnaire), and the informants being compared. For example, Tarullo, Richardson, Radke-Yarrow, and Martinez (1995) found that both mother–child and father–child agreement was higher for preadolescent than for adolescent children and, in a meta-analysis, Duhig, Renk, Epstein, and Phares (2000) reported higher mother–father agreement for externalizing than for internalizing problems. Disagreements among informants create methodological difficulties in interpreting epidemiological data when such data are obtained from different sources, and also in how specific diagnoses are arrived at in research and practice.

Also of importance is how disagreements among informants are interpreted. For example, disagreements may be viewed as (1) reflections of bias or error on the part of one informant; (2) evidence for the variability of children's behavior across the situations in which they are observed by others; (3) lack of access to certain types of behavior (i.e., private events) on the part of one informant; (4) denial of the problem; or (5) active distortion of information in the service of some other goal (e.g., defensive exclusion, treatment eligibility).

Parental psychopathology may "color" descriptions of child problems—as may occur when abusive or depressed mothers provide negative or exaggerated descriptions of their children (Gotlib & Hammen, 1992; Mash et al., 1983; Richters, 1992), or when dismissive/avoidant adult informants deny the presence of emotional problems at the same time that professionals observe a high level of symptoms (Dozier & Lee, 1995). These latter types of problems in reporting may be especially likely, given the frequent lack of correspondence between the expression and the experience of distress for many child and adult disturbances. Hypothesized relationships between parental psychopathology and reports of exaggerated child symptoms have received mixed support. For example, some studies have failed to find evidence for distorted reports by depressed mothers (Tarullo et al., 1995).

TYPES OF CHILD PSYCHOPATHOLOGY

The types of problems for which children are referred for treatment are reflected in the different approaches that have been used to conceptualize and classify these problems. Among the more common of these approaches are the following:

1. General and specific behavior problem checklists, which enumerate individual child symptoms—for example, the Child Behavior Checklist (Achenbach, 1991) and the Children's Depression Inventory (Kovacs & Beck, 1977).
2. Dimensional approaches, which focus on symptom clusters or syndromes derived from behavior problem checklists—for example, the Child Behavior Checklist and Profile (Achenbach, 1993).

3. Categorical approaches, which use predetermined diagnostic criteria to define the presence or absence of particular disorders—for example, the DSM-IV (APA, 1994) and ICD-10 (WHO, 1992).
4. A multiple-pathway, developmental approach, which emphasizes developmental antecedents and competencies both within the child and the environment that contribute to (mal)adjustment and (mal)adaptation (Sroufe, 1997).

Issues related to the use of these different classification approaches are discussed in a later section of this chapter. What follows is a brief overview of the types of problem behaviors, dimensions, and disorders that occur during childhood and that are the topics of this volume's other chapters.

Individual Symptoms

The individual behavioral and emotional problems (i.e., symptoms) that characterize most forms of child psychopathology have been found to occur in almost all children at one time or another during their development (e.g., Achenbach & Edelbrock, 1981; Achenbach et al., 1991; MacFarlane et al., 1954). When taken in isolation, specific symptoms have generally shown little correspondence to a child's overall current adjustment or to later outcomes. This is the case even for many symptoms previously hypothesized to be significant indicators of psychopathology in children—for example, thumbsucking after 4 years of age (Friman, Larzelere, & Finney, 1994). Usually the age-appropriateness, clustering, and patterning of symptoms are what serve to define child psychopathology, rather than the presence of individual symptoms.

Many of the individual behavior problems displayed by children referred for treatment are similar to those that occur in less extreme forms in the general population or in children of younger ages. For example, Achenbach et al. (1991) found that although referred children scored higher than nonreferred children on 209 of 216 parent-rated problems, only 9 of the 209 items showed effects related to clinical status that were considered to be large (accounting for more than 13.8% of the variance), according to criteria specified by Cohen (1988). To illustrate the kinds of individual symptoms that are more common in referred than in nonreferred children, individual parent-reported symptoms that accounted for 10% or more of the variance in clinical status in the Achenbach et al. (1991) study are shown in Table 1.1. It can be seen that even the problems that best discriminated between referred and nonreferred children are relatively common behaviors that occur to some extent in all children—they are not particularly strange or unusual behaviors. In addition, most *individual* problem behaviors (approximately 90% of those on behavior problem checklists) do not, by themselves, discriminate between groups of clinic-referred and nonreferred children. Nondiscriminating items include some problems for children in both groups that are relatively common (e.g., "brags," "screams") and others that occur less frequently (e.g., "sets fires," "bowel movements outside the toilet").

Dimensions of Child Psychopathology

A second approach to describing child psychopathology identifies symptom clusters or "syndromes" derived through the use of multivariate statistical procedures, such as factor analysis or cluster analysis (e.g., Achenbach, 1993, 1997; McDermott, 1993; McDermott & Weiss, 1995). Research has identified two broad dimensions of child psychopathology—one reflecting "externalizing" or "undercontrolled" problems, and the other reflecting "internalizing" or "overcontrolled" problems (Reynolds, 1992). The externalizing dimension encompasses behaviors often thought of as directed at others, whereas the internalizing dimension describes feelings or states that are commonly viewed as "inner-directed."

Within the two broad dimensions of externalizing and internalizing disorders are specific subdimensions or syndromes. Some subdimensions of child psychopathology that have commonly been identified in research are presented in Table 1.2. They include "withdrawn," "somatic complaints," "anxious/depressed," "social problems," "thought problems," "attention problems," "delinquent behavior," and "aggressive behavior" (Achenbach, 1993). Examples of the specific problem behaviors constituting each of these subdimensions are also included in Table 1.2. The particular subdimensions that are identified may vary from study to study as a function of the item pool from which they are derived, the age and sex of children in the sample, the methods of assessment, and the informants.

TABLE 1.1. Individual Parent-Rated Problems Accounting for More than 10% of the Variance in Clinical Status of Children Aged 4–16

Poor school work (19%)[a,b]
Can't concentrate, can't pay attention for long (18%)[b]
Lacks self-confidence (17%)[b]
Punishment doesn't change his/her behavior (17%)[b]
Disobedient at home (15%)[b]
Has trouble following directions (15%)[b]
Sad or depressed (15%)[b]
Uncooperative (14%)[b]
Nervous, high-strung, or tense (14%)[b]
Feels he/she can't succeed (13%)
Feels worthless or inferior (13%)
Disobedient at school (13%)
Easily distracted (13%)
Lies (13%)
Looks unhappy without good reason (13%)
Fails to finish things he/she starts (12%)
Defiant (12%)
Doesn't get along with other kids (12%)
Has a hard time making friends (12%)
Doesn't seem to feel guilty after misbehavior (12%)
Needs constant supervision (12%)
Sudden changes in mood or feelings (12%)
Angry moods (11%)
Impulsive or acts without thinking (11%)
Irritable (11%)
Temper tantrums or hot temper (10%)
Does things slowly and incorrectly (10%)
Loses train of thought (10%)
Loss of ability to have fun (10%)
Passive or lacks initiative (10%)

Note. Data from Achenbach, Howell, Quay, and Conners (1991, pp. 107–115).
[a]Number in parentheses indicates the percentage of variance accounted for by this problem behavior.
[b]Items accounting for 14% or more of the variance are designated as having a large effect size, according to criteria presented by Cohen (1988).

Taxometric efforts have also described groups of children in terms of consistently identified profiles of scores on the various syndromes (Achenbach, 1993). Such profiles have been reliably identified and appear to have promise in addressing problems related to comorbidity (see the section on comorbidity, below). At present, however, our nomenclature for describing these profiles is limited, and they have yet to be widely validated or used in clinical research and practice.

Categories of Child Psychopathology

The DSM-IV diagnostic system (APA, 1994, 2000) provides comprehensive coverage of the general types of symptom clusters displayed by children characterized as having mental disorders. To illustrate, DSM-IV categories that apply to children are listed in Tables 1.3 to 1.6. These tables are not intended to be exhaustive of all DSM-IV diagnoses that may apply to children. Rather, they are intended to provide an overview of the range and variety of disorders that typically occur during childhood. Specific DSM-IV disorders and their subtypes are discussed in detail in the subsequent chapters of this volume.

Table 1.3 lists the DSM-IV categories for developmental and learning disorders, including mental retardation, pervasive developmental disorders (e.g., autistic disorder), specific problems related to reading and mathematics, and communication difficulties. Many of these disorders constitute chronic conditions that often reflect deficits in capacity rather than performance difficulties per se.

Table 1.4 lists DSM-IV categories for other disorders that are usually first diagnosed in infancy, childhood, or adolescence. These disorders have traditionally been thought of as first occurring in childhood or as exclusive to childhood and as requiring operational criteria different from those used to define disorders in adults.

Table 1.5 lists disorders that can be diagnosed in children or adolescents (e.g., mood disorders, anxiety disorders), but that are not listed in DSM-IV as distinct disorders first occurring during childhood, or requiring operational criteria that are different from those used for adults. In many ways, the DSM-IV distinction between child and adult categories is an arbitrary one; it is more a reflection of our current lack of knowledge concerning the continuities between child and adult disorders than of the existence of qualitatively distinct conditions. Recent efforts to diagnose ADHD in adults illustrate this problem. Although the criteria for ADHD were derived from work with children, and the disorder is included in the "infancy, childhood, or adolescence" section of DSM-IV, these criteria are being used to diagnose adults even though they do not fit the expression of the disorder in adults very well.

The more general issue here is whether there is a need for separate diagnostic criteria for children versus adults, or whether one can use the same criteria by adjusting them to take into account differences in developmental level. For instance, the childhood category of overanxious disorder in DSM-III-R (APA, 1987) was subsumed under the category of generalized anxiety disorder in DSM-IV (APA, 1994). With this

TABLE 1.2. Commonly Identified Dimensions of Child Psychopathology and Examples of Items Reflecting Each of the Dimensions

Withdrawn

Would rather be alone
Refuses to talk
Secretive
Shy, timid
Stares blankly
Sulks
Underactive
Unhappy, sad, depressed
Withdrawn

Somatic complaints

Feels dizzy
Overtired
Aches, pains
Headaches
Nausea
Eye problems
Rashes, skin problems
Stomachaches
Vomiting

Anxious/depressed

Lonely
Cries a lot
Fears impulses
Needs to be perfect
Feels unloved
Feels persecuted
Feels worthless
Nervous, tense
Fearful, anxious
Feels too guilty
Self-conscious
Suspicious
Unhappy, sad, depressed
Worries
Harms self
Thinks about suicide
Overconforms
Hurt when criticized
Anxious to please
Afraid of mistakes

Social problems

Acts too young
Too dependent
Doesn't get along with peers
Gets teased
Not liked by peers
Clumsy
Prefers younger children
Overweight
Withdrawn
Lonely
Cries
Feels unloved
Feels persecuted
Feels worthless
Accident-prone

Thought problems

Can't get mind off thoughts
Hears things
Repeats acts
Sees things
Strange behavior
Strange ideas
Stares blankly
Harms self
Fears
Stores up things

Attention problems

Acts too young
Can't concentrate
Can't sit still
Confused
Daydreams
Impulsive
Nervous, tense
Poor school work
Clumsy
Stares blankly
Twitches
Hums, odd noises
Fails to finish
Fidgets
Difficulty with directions
Difficulty learning
Apathetic
Messy work
Inattentive
Underachieving
Fails to carry out tasks

Delinquent behavior

Lacks guilt
Bad companions
Lies
Prefers older kids
Runs away from home
Sets fires
Steals at home
Swearing, obscenity
Truancy
Alcohol, drugs
Thinks about sex too much
Vandalism
Tardy

Aggressive behavior

Argues
Brags
Mean to others
Demands attention
Destroys own things
Destroys others' things
Disobedient at school
Jealous
Fights
Attacks people
Screams
Shows off
Stubborn, irritable
Sudden mood changes
Talks too much
Teases
Temper tantrums
Threatens
Loud
Disobedient at home
Defiant
Disturbs others
Talks out of turn
Disrupts class
Explosive
Easily frustrated

Note. Dimensions are based on analyses across informants (e.g., parents, teachers, and children) and assessment methods (Child Behavior Checklist, Youth Self-Report Form, and Teacher Report Form). Adapted from Achenbach (1993, pp. 41–43). Copyright 1993 by T. M. Achenbach. Adapted by permission.

TABLE 1.3. DSM-IV Categories for Developmental and Learning Disorders Usually First Diagnosed in Infancy, Childhood, or Adolescence

Mental retardation
Mild, moderate, severe, profound, severity unspecified

Learning disorders
Reading disorder
Mathematics disorder
Disorder of written expression
Learning disorder not otherwise specified

Motor skills disorder
Developmental coordination disorder

Communication disorders
Expressive language disorder
Mixed receptive–expressive language disorder
Phonological disorder
Stuttering
Communication disorder not otherwise specified

Pervasive developmental disorders
Autistic disorder
Rett's disorder
Childhood disintegrative disorder
Asperger's disorder
Pervasive developmental disorder not otherwise specified

change, the number of criteria required for children to meet this diagnosis was also altered.

Finally, Table 1.6 lists DSM-IV categories for other conditions that are not defined as mental disorders, but that may be a focus of clinical attention during childhood or adolescence. The categories that are included are the ones that seem especially relevant to children, in that they emphasize relational problems, maltreatment, and academic and adjustment difficulties.

APPROACHES TO THE CLASSIFICATION AND DIAGNOSIS OF CHILD PSYCHOPATHOLOGY

The formal and informal classification systems that have been used by psychiatrists, psychologists, and educators to categorize the different forms of child psychopathology have played a central role in defining the field. For example, in referring to these systems, Adelman (1995) states: "They determine the ways individuals are described, studied, and served; they shape prevailing practices related to intervention, professional training, and certification; and they influence decisions about funding. It is not surprising, therefore, that debates about classification schemes, specific diagnostic procedures, and the very act of labeling are so heated" (p. 29).

Although early conceptualizations of psychopathology included underdeveloped and global descriptions of childhood disorders (e.g., "adjustment problem"), this state of affairs has been steadily improving. Nevertheless, problems and issues in describing and classifying childhood disorders continue to plague the field (e.g., Quay, Routh, & Shapiro, 1987). As noted by Rutter and Garmezy (1983), "All too frequently findings have been inconclusive because the measures employed have been weak, nondiscriminating, or open to systematic bias. Similarly, comparisons

TABLE 1.4. DSM-IV Categories for Other Disorders Usually First Diagnosed in Infancy, Childhood, or Adolescence

Attention-deficit and disruptive behavior disorders
Attention-deficit/hyperactivity disorder
  Predominantly inattentive type
  Predominantly hyperactive–impulsive type
  Combined type
  Attention-deficit/hyperactivity disorder not otherwise specified
Disruptive behavior disorders
  Conduct disorder
  Oppositional defiant disorder
  Disruptive behavior disorder not otherwise specified

Feeding and eating disorders of infancy or early childhood
Pica
Rumination disorder
Feeding disorder of infancy or early childhood

Tic disorders
Tourette's disorder
Chronic motor or vocal tic disorder
Tic disorder not otherwise specified

Elimination disorders
Encopresis
Enuresis

Other disorders of infancy, childhood, or adolescence
Separation anxiety disorder
Selective mutism
Reactive attachment disorder of infancy or early childhood
Stereotypic movement disorder
Disorder of infancy, childhood, or adolescence not otherwise specified

TABLE 1.5. Selected Categories for Disorders of Childhood or Adolescence That Are Not Listed Separately in DSM-IV as Those Usually First Diagnosed in Infancy, Childhood, or Adolescence

Mood disorders
Depressive disorders
  Major depressive disorder
  Dysthymic disorder
Bipolar disorders

Anxiety disorders
Specific phobia, social phobia, obsessive–compulsive disorder, posttraumatic stress disorder, acute stress disorder, generalized anxiety disorder, anxiety disorder due to . . . (specific medical condition)

Somatoform disorders
Factitious disorders
Dissociative disorders
Sexual and gender identity disorders
Eating disorders
Sleep disorders
Schizophrenia and other psychotic disorders
Substance-related disorders
Impulse-control disorders not elsewhere classified
Adjustment disorders
Personality disorders

between studies have often been vitiated because cases have been defined differently, because the settings have been noncomparable, or because the measures focused on different aspects of behavior" (p. 865).

There is general agreement in medicine, psychiatry, and psychology regarding the need for a system of classifying for childhood disorders. However, major areas of contention have arisen around such issues as which disorders should be included in the system, what the optimal strategies are for organizing and grouping disorders, and what specific criteria should be used to define a particular disorder (Achenbach, 1985; Achenbach & Edelbrock, 1989; Mash & Terdal, 1997a; Sonuga-Barke, 1998).

The two most common approaches to the diagnosis and classification of child psychopathology involve the use of (1) "categorical" classification systems that are based primarily on informed clinical consensus, an approach that has dominated and continues to dominate the field (APA, 1994, 2000); and (2) empirically based "dimensional" classification schemes derived through the use of multivariate statistical techniques (Achenbach, 1993, 1997). In addition, alternative and/or derivative approaches to classification have been proposed to address perceived deficiencies associated with the use of categorical and dimensional approaches. These have included developmentally based measures (Garber, 1984; Mohr & Regan-Kubinski, 1999; Sroufe, 1997); laboratory and performance-based measures (Frick, 2000); prototype classification (Cantor et al., 1980); and behavioral classification based on behavioral excesses, deficits, and faulty stimulus control (Adams, Doster, & Calhoun, 1977; Kanfer & Saslow, 1969; Mash & Hunsley, 1990). Although each of these alternative approaches has something to offer to the classification of childhood disorders, they are generally underdeveloped and unstandardized, and have not been widely accepted or used in either research or practice.

To date, no single classification scheme for childhood disorders has established adequate reliability and validity (Cantwell, 1996; Mash & Terdal, 1997a). Many researchers and clinicians continue to express concerns that current diagnostic and classification systems (1) underrepresent disorders of infancy and childhood; (2) are inadequate in representing the interrelationships and overlap that exist among many childhood disorders; (3) are not sufficiently sensitive to the developmental, contextual, and relational parameters that are known to characterize most forms of psychopathology in children; and (4) are heterogeneous with respect to etiology (Jensen & Hoagwood, 1997; Kagan, 1997).

TABLE 1.6. Selected DSM-IV Categories for Other Conditions That May Be a Focus of Clinical Attention during Childhood or Adolescence, but Are Not Defined as Mental Disorders

Relational problems
Relational problem related to a general mental disorder or general medical condition
Parent–child relational problem
Partner relational problem
Sibling relational problem
Relational problem not otherwise specified

Problems related to abuse or neglect
Physical abuse of child
Sexual abuse of child
Neglect of child

Bereavement
Borderline intellectual functioning
Academic problem
Child or adolescent antisocial behavior
Identity problem

Categorical Approaches

Categorical approaches to the classification of childhood disorders have included systems developed by the Group for the Advancement of Psychiatry (1974), the WHO (1992), the APA (1994), and the Zero to Three/National Center for Clinical Infant Programs (1994). Although a detailed review of all these systems is beyond the scope of this chapter, a brief history of the APA's development of the DSM approach is presented to illustrate the issues associated with categorical approaches, the growing concern for more reliable classification schemes for childhood disorders, and the evolving conceptualizations of childhood disorders over the past 50 years. Also, the *Diagnostic Classification of Mental Health and Developmental Disorders of Infancy and Early Childhood,* or *Diagnostic Classification: 0–3* (DC:0–3; Zero to Three/National Center for Clinical Infant Programs, 1994), is described to illustrate a categorical approach that attempts to integrate developmental and contextual information into the diagnosis of infants' and young children's problems.

Development of the DSM Approach

One of the first efforts to collect data on mental illness was in the U.S. census of 1840, which recorded the frequency of a single category of "idiocy/insanity." Forty years later, seven categories of mental illness were identified: dementia, dipsomania, epilepsy, mania, melancholia, monomania, and paresis (APA, 1994). Much later (in the 1940s), the WHO classification system emerged with the manuals of the ICD, whose 6th revision included, for the first time, a section for mental disorders (APA, 1994; Cantwell, 1996).

In response to perceived inadequacies of the ICD system for classifying mental disorders, the APA's Committee on Nomenclature and Statistics developed the DSM-I in 1952 (APA, 1952). There were three major categories of dysfunction in the DSM-I—"organic brain syndromes," "functional disorder," and "mental deficiency" (Kessler, 1971)—under which were subsumed 106 categories (by contrast, DSM-IV consists of 407 separate categories; Cantwell, 1996). The term "reaction" was used throughout the text, which reflected Adolf Meyer's psychobiological view that mental illness involves reactions of the personality to psychological, social, and biological factors (APA, 1987). Children were virtually neglected in the early versions of DSM, with most childhood disorders relegated to the adult categories (Cass & Thomas, 1979; Silk et al., 2000). In fact, DSM-I included only one child category of "adjustment reactions of childhood and of adolescence," which was included under the heading of "transient situational disorders."

As reflected in the use of the term "reaction," psychoanalytic theory had a substantial influence on the classification of both child and adult psychopathology (Clementz & Iacono, 1993). In part, this was due to the fact that the first classification system to focus on childhood psychopathology was developed by Anna Freud in 1965 (see Cantwell, 1996). Although the term "reaction" was eliminated from DSM-II (APA, 1968), a separate section was reserved for classifying neuroses, and diagnoses could be based on either an assessment of the client's presenting symptomatology or inferences about his or her unconscious processes (Clementz & Iacono, 1993). Once again, apart from conditions subsumed under the adult categories, DSM-II gave little recognition to childhood difficulties except for mental retardation and schizophrenia—childhood type (Cass & Thomas, 1979).

As a formal taxonomy, DSM-III (APA, 1980) represented a significant advance over the earlier editions of the DSM. The first and second editions contained only narrative descriptions of symptoms, and clinicians had to draw on their own definitions for making a diagnosis (APA, 1980). In DSM-III, these descriptions were replaced by explicit criteria, which in turn enhanced diagnostic reliability (Achenbach, 1985; APA, 1980). Moreover, unsubstantiated inferences that were heavily embedded in psychoanalytic theory were dropped; more child categories were included; a multiaxial system was adopted; and a greater emphasis was placed on empirical data (Achenbach, 1985). These changes reflected the beginnings of a conceptual shift in both diagnostic systems and etiological models away from an isolated focus of psychopathology as existing within the child alone, and toward an increased emphasis on his or her surrounding context. DSM-III was revised in 1987 (DSM-III-R) to help clarify the numerous inconsistencies and ambiguities that were noted in its use. For example, empirical data at that time did not support the category of attention deficit disorder *without* hyperactivity as a unique symptom cluster (Routh, 1990), and this category was removed from DSM-III-R. DSM-III-R was also developed to be polythetic, in that a child could be diagnosed with a certain subset of symptoms without having to meet all criteria. This was an important change, especially in light of the heterogeneity and rapidly changing nature of most childhood disorders (Mash & Terdal, 1997a). Relative to its predecessors, far greater emphasis was also placed on empirical findings in the development of the DSM-IV, particularly for the child categories.

In order to bridge the planned 12-year span between the DSM-IV and DSM-V, a revision (DSM-IV-TR) of the DSM was published in 2000 (APA, 2000). The DSM-IV-TR was limited to text revisions (e.g., associated features and disorders, prevalence) and was designed mainly to correct any factual errors in DSM-IV, make sure that information is still current, and incorporate new information since the time the original DSM-IV literature reviews were completed in 1992. Substantive changes in diagnostic criteria were not considered or made; nor were there any changes in relation to new disorders or subtypes. Thus DSM-IV and DSM-IV-TR are equivalent with respect to specific diagnostic criteria.

DSM-IV is a multiaxial system that includes five different axes. Axis I is used to report clinical disorders and other conditions that may be a focus of clinical attention. The various Axis I diagnostic categories that apply to infants, children, and adolescents have been listed in Tables 1.3 to 1.6 of this chapter. Axis II includes personality disorders and mental retardation. The remaining axes pertain to general medical conditions (Axis III), psychosocial and environmental problems (Axis IV), and global assessment of functioning (Axis V).

Although DSM-III-R (APA, 1987) and DSM-IV (APA, 1994) include numerous improvements over the previous DSMs—with their greater emphasis on empirical research, and more explicit diagnostic criteria sets and algorithms—criticisms have also been raised (e.g., Mohr & Regan-Kubinski, 1999; Nathan & Lagenbucher, 1999; Sonuga-Barke, 1998; Sroufe, 1997). One major criticism is the static nature of DSM categories, especially when one considers the dynamic nature of development in children (Mash & Terdal, 1997a; Routh, 1990). Another source of dissatisfaction is that the DSM-IV categorical scheme may contribute minimally to meeting children's needs. For example, it may be necessary for a child to meet specific diagnostic criteria for a learning disability in order to qualify for a special education class. However, if the child's problems are subclinical, or the child's problems relate to more than one DSM category, then he or she may be denied services (Achenbach, 2000). However, even if one were to adopt a more dimensional approach to classification, there would nonetheless continue to be a categorical interpretation of the data (e.g., distinguishing between individuals who require help and those who do not) (Sonuga-Barke, 1998).

Another problem with DSM-IV relates to the wording and the lack of empirical adequacy for certain criterion sets. For example, the words "often" in the criteria for ADHD and conduct disorder, and "persistent" and "recurrent" in the criteria for separation anxiety disorder, are not clearly defined. This ambiguity poses a particular problem when one considers that the primary sources of assessment information are often a child's parents, whose perception and understanding of these terms may be idiosyncratic or inaccurate. This ambiguity and other factors may contribute to the unreliability or unsuitability of the DSM for diagnosing certain childhood disorders (e.g., Nicholls, Chater, & Lask, 2000). A further difficulty with DSM-IV diagnostic criteria is the lack of emphasis on the situational or contextual factors surrounding and contributing to various disorders. This is a reflection of the fact that DSM-IV continues to view mental disorder as individual psychopathology or risk for psychopathology, rather than in terms of problems in psychosocial adjustment. One problem with respect to the atheoretical nature of DSM is that it has perhaps mistakenly fostered the assumption that a description of symptoms is sufficient for diagnosis, without taking into account natural history, psychosocial correlates, biological factors, or response to treatment (Cantwell, 1996). However, the consideration in DSM-IV of such factors as culture, age, and gender associated with the expression of each disorder is laudable, as is the increased recognition of the importance of family problems and extrafamilial relational difficulties.

The changes in the DSMs from 1952 to 2000 reflect increasing diagnostic accuracy and sophistication. The transition from "reactive" diagnoses (DSM-I) and the virtual neglect of childhood criteria (DSM-I, DSM-II) to an increased number of child categories, more explicit criteria, and multiaxial evaluation (DSM-III, DSM-III-R), and then to an even greater emphasis on empirical research to guide nomenclature as well as the increased awareness (and inclusion) of contextual and developmental considerations (DSM-IV, DSM-IV-TR), exemplify important shifts in how psychopathology in children has come to be conceptualized. However, along with increased complexity has come a new set of problems. For example, the extent to which comorbidity is an artifact of the DSM's polythetic criteria or truly differentiated nosological entities is unclear (Angold, Costello, & Erkanli, 1999; Nottelmann & Jensen, 1995), or whether the pendulum has swung too far from not recognizing psychopathology in children to identifying and diagnosing too much (Silk et al., 2000).

It is also the case that ongoing changes in diagnostic criteria based on new findings and other considerations (e.g., eligibility for services) are likely to influence prevalence estimates for many childhood disorders. For example, current estimates of autistic disorder are about three times higher than previous ones (Fombonne, 1999; Tanguay, 2000); this increase is primarily due to a broadening of the criteria used to diagnose autism, as well as increased recognition of milder forms of the disorder (Bryson & Smith, 1998; Gillberg & Wing, 1999). There is also ongoing debate about whether Asperger's disorder is a variant of autism or simply describes higher-functioning individuals with autism (Schopler, Mesibov, & Kunce, 1998; Volkmar & Klin, 2000). The resolution of this debate and prevalence estimates for both autism and Asperger's disorder will depend on how the diagnosis of Asperger's disorder is used, since no "official" definition for this disorder existed until it was introduced in DSM-IV (Volkmar & Klin, 1998).

Development of the DC:0–3 System

In addition to the limitations noted above, DSM-IV does not provide in-depth coverage of the mental health and developmental problems of infants and young children, for whom family relationships are especially salient. To address this perceived deficiency, the DC:0–3 was developed by the Diagnostic Classification Task Force of the Zero to Three/National Center for Clinical Infant Programs (Zero to Three/National Center for Clinical Infant Programs, 1994). DC:0–3 is intended to provide a comprehensive system for classifying problems during the first 3–4 years of life (Greenspan & Wieder, 1994; Lieberman, Wieder, & Fenichel, 1997). Unlike DSM-IV, DC:0–3 is based on the explicit premise that diagnosis must be guided by the principle that all infants and young children are active participants in relationships within their families. Hence descriptions of infant–caregiver interaction patterns, and of the links between these interaction patterns and adaptive and maladaptive patterns of infant and child development, constitute an essential part of the diagnostic process.

In explicitly recognizing the significance of relational problems, DC:0–3 includes a relationship disorder classification as a separate axis (Axis II) in its multiaxial approach (Axis I, primary diagnosis; Axis III, medical and developmental disorders and conditions; Axis IV, psychosocial stressors; Axis V, functional emotional developmental level). The diagnosis of relationship disturbances or disorders is based on observations of parent–child interaction and the parent's verbal report regarding his or her subjective experience of the child. Relational difficulties are rated with respect to their intensity, frequency, and duration, and classified as perturbations, disturbances, or disorders. In making the DC:0–3 Axis II relationship disorder diagnosis, three aspects of the relationship are considered: (1) behavioral quality of the interaction (e.g., sensitivity or insensitivity in responding to cues); (2) affective tone (e.g., anxious/tense, angry); and (3) psychological involvement (e.g., parents' perceptions of the child and of what can be expected in a relationship).

Axis V of DC:0–3, functional emotional development level, includes the ways in which infants or young children organize their affective, interactive, and communicative experiences. Axis V assessment is based in large part on direct observations of parent–child interaction. The various levels include social processes such as mutual attention, mutual engagement or joint emotional involvement, reciprocal interaction, and affective/symbolic communication. Problems may reflect constrictions in range of affect within levels or under stress, or failure to reach expected levels of emotional development.

DC:0–3 is of note in recognizing (1) the significance of early relational difficulties; (2) the need to integrate diagnostic and relational approaches in classifying child psychopathology (Lyons-Ruth, 1995); and (3) the need to apply both quantitative and qualitative criteria in describing relational problems. In addition, the dimensions and specific processes that are used for classification (e.g., negative affect, unresponsivity, uninvolvement, lack of mutual engagement, lack of reciprocity in interaction) include those that have been identified as important in many developmental and clinical research studies on early relationships, and the system is decidedly more sensitive to developmental and contextual parameters than DSM-IV. However, although promising, DC:0–3 is relatively untested, was generated on the basis of uncontrolled clinical observations, is of unknown reliability and validity, and suffers from many of the same criticisms that have been noted for DSM-IV (Eppright, Bradley, & Sanfacon, 1998). Nevertheless, the scheme provides a rich descriptive base for exploring the ways in which psychopathology is expressed during the first few years of life, and it calls attention to the need to examine potential continuities between early problems and later individual and/or family disorders (Keren, Feldman, & Tyano, 2001; Thomas & Clark, 1998; Thomas & Guskin, 2001).

Dimensional Approaches

Dimensional approaches to classification assume that a number of relatively independent dimensions or traits of behavior exist, and that all children possess these to varying degrees. These traits or dimensions are typically derived through the use of multivariate statistical methods, such as factor analysis or cluster analysis (Achenbach, 1993). Empirically derived schemes are more objective, are potentially more reliable, and allow for a greater description of multiple symptom patterns than clinically derived classification systems. However, there are also a number of problems associated with their use, including the dependency of the derived dimensions on sampling, method, and informant characteristics, and on the age and sex of the child (Mash & Terdal, 1997a). As a result, there can be difficulties in integrating information obtained from different methods, from different informants, over time, or across situations. Dimensional approaches have also shown a lack of sensitivity to contextual influences, although there have been efforts to develop dimensional classification schemes based on item pools that include situational content (e.g., McDermott, 1993).

The growth in the use of multivariate classification approaches in child and family assessment has been fueled by the extensive work of Thomas Achenbach and his colleagues (see the Achenbach System of Empirically Based Assessment [ASEBA]: http://www.ASEBA.org) with the various parent, teacher, youth, observer, and interview versions of the Child Behavior Checklist and Profile (Achenbach, 1993), and by the development of similar assessment batteries (e.g., the Behavior Assessment System for Children [BASC]: Kamphaus et al., 1999; Reynolds & Kamphaus, 1992). For a comprehensive discussion of these approaches and the use of empirically derived classification schemes more generally, the reader is referred to Achenbach (1985, 1993), Hart and Lahey (1999), and Mash and Terdal (1997a),

It should also be noted that there has been a trend toward greater convergence of the categorical and dimensional approaches to classification. Many of the items that were retained in DSM-IV child categories were derived from findings from multivariate studies, and the process that led to the development of DSM-IV treated most childhood disorders as dimensions, albeit the use of cutoff scores on item lists arbitrarily created categories out of these dimensions (Spitzer et al., 1990).

Performance-Based Diagnostic Information

Performance-based information and/or observational measures provide additional sources of diagnostic information that may be sensitive to differences among children exhibiting similar self- or other-reported symptoms (Frick, 2000; Kazdin & Kagan, 1994). These measures assess children's performance on standardized tasks, usually ones that reflect basic biological, cognitive, affective, or social functioning. For example, tasks involving behavioral observations of fear and avoidance, recall memory under stressful conditions, delayed response times to threatening stimuli, and the potentiation of the blink reflex following exposure to a threatening stimulus have all been suggested as potentially useful in diagnosing groups and/or subgroups of children with anxiety disorders (Kazdin & Kagan, 1994; Vasey & Lonigan, 2000). Similarly, tests of behavioral inhibition (e.g., the stop-signal paradigm) and tasks involving sustained attention (e.g., the continuous-performance test) have proven useful with children with ADHD (Rapport, Chung, Shore, Denney, & Isaacs, 2000). Measures of low resting heart rate as an early biological marker for later aggressive behavior (Raine, Venables, & Mednick, 1997); facial emotion recognition tasks and gambling tasks in identifying children with psychopathic tendencies (Blair, Colledge, & Mitchell, 2001; Blair, Colledge, Murray, & Mitchell, 2001); and a variety of cognitive tasks for children with autism (Klinger & Renner, 2000) have also been found to have diagnostic value.

A study by Rubin, Coplan, Fox, and Calkins (1995) illustrates the utility of performance-based diagnostic information. These researchers differentiated groups of preschool children based on the two dimensions of "emotionality" (i.e., threshold and intensity of emotional response) and "soothability" (i.e., recovery from emotional reaction based on soothing by self and others), and on their amount of social interactions with peers. Children's dispositional characteristics and behavioral styles were used to predict outcomes. Asocial children with poor emotion regulation had more internalizing problems. In contrast, social children with poor emotion regulation were rated as having more externalizing difficulties. When behavioral and emotional dimensions were incorporated into classification, it was possible to make finer predictions—for example, that only a certain type of asocial children (i.e., reticent children with poor emotion regulation) would display later problems.

The use of performance-based measures in diagnosis is predicated on the availability of reliable and valid performance indicators for groups of children with known characteristics. Although such data are available in varying amounts for a wide range of disorders, there is a need to validate such findings for the purposes of diagnosis and against other sources of information. It is also the case that performance criteria for these measures are based on information obtained from children who were themselves previously identified using other diagnostic procedures. This raises the question of nonindependence and representativeness of data sources. There is also little normative information available regarding the base rates of children in the general population who exhibit certain patterns of responding on these tasks.

ISSUES IN CLASSIFICATION

Categories, Dimensions, or Both?

Psychological studies of child psychopathology have tended to conceptualize behavior, affect, and cognition on quantitative/continuous dimensions, whereas child psychiatry has tended to conceptualize child psychopathology in categorical terms. Both approaches are relevant to classifying childhood disorders, in that some disorders may be best conceptualized as qualitatively distinct conditions and others as extreme points on one or more continuous dimensions. Kazdin and Kagan (1994) argue for greater research attention to qualitatively distinct categories of disorder, based on illustrative findings from studies suggesting that the emotional arousal generated by unfamiliarity, threat, and attack is not a continuous dimension, and that it is possible to identify different subgroups of aggressive children based on varying levels of adrenaline in their urine.

There is currently little agreement as to which childhood disorders are best conceptualized as categories and which as dimensions. It has been suggested that many childhood disorders, such as anxiety, depression, ADHD, and the disruptive behavior disorders, appear to reflect dimensions of personality rather than categorical problems (e.g., Werry, 2001). For example, childhood ADHD symptom clusters of inattention–disorganization and hyperactivity–impulsivity have been found to be related to adult personality dimensions of low conscientiousness and low agreeableness, respectively (Nigg et al., 2001). Even a disorder such as autism, which has traditionally been viewed as "categorical" in nature, can be conceptualized as an extreme on a continuum of social behavior (Baron-Cohen, 2000). For dimensional disorders, children who score just below the cutoff for a diagnosis may one day meet criteria, and often show impairment comparable to that of children who score above the cutoff. Similarly, those above the cutoff may one day move below it. Since any classification scheme represents a construction rather than a reality, it seems unlikely that most disorders will fall neatly into one designation or the other (Lilienfeld & Marino, 1995). Whether or not particular conditions are construed as qualitatively distinct categories, as continuous dimensions, or as both will probably depend on the utility, validity, and predictive value of particular groupings and subgroupings for certain purposes related to understanding and remediating child psychopathology. Research into such subgroupings is just beginning to emerge (e.g., Kendall, Brady, & Verduin, 2001).

Regardless of the particular approach one adopts for the classification of childhood psychopathology, diagnostic decisions need to be based on a comprehensive assessment of the individual child—one that incorporates sensitivity to and understanding of the complexity of multiple antecedents, developmental considerations, comorbidity, continuity–discontinuity, and the constantly changing nature of the child (Orvaschel, Ambrosini, & Rabinovich, 1993).

Comorbidity

An issue that has important ramifications for theory and research in defining and classifying child psychopathology is comorbidity (Achenbach, 1995; Angold, Costello, & Erkanli, 1999; Carey & DiLalla, 1994; Caron & Rutter, 1991; Sonuga-Barke, 1998). "Comorbidity" generally refers to the manifestation of two or more disorders that co-occur more often than would be expected by chance alone. For example, although the base rates for ADHD and conduct disorder in the general population are less than 10% for each disorder, epidemiological studies have found that among children diagnosed with ADHD, approximately 50% are also diagnosed with conduct disorder (Kazdin & Johnson, 1994; Loeber & Keenan, 1994). Comorbidity has been reported to be as high as 50% in community samples and even higher in clinic samples (Anderson, Williams, McGee, & Silva, 1987; Bird et al., 1988; Caron & Rutter, 1991). Some of the more commonly co-occurring child and adolescent disorders include conduct disorder and ADHD, autistic disorder and mental retardation, and childhood depression and anxiety.

There is continuing debate regarding the definition and nature of "comorbidity" (Angold, Costello, & Erkanli, 1999; Blashfield, McElroy, Pfohl, & Blum, 1994; Caron & Rutter, 1991; Lilienfeld, Waldman, & Israel, 1994; Meehl, 2001; Robins, 1994; Rutter, 1994b; Sameroff, 2000a; Spitzer, 1994; Widiger & Ford-Black, 1994). Some researchers contend that the term is wholly inadequate, because it does not distinguish accurately between manifest conditions seen in organic medicine (e.g., diseases) and latent conditions described in mental health (e.g., syndromes and disorders (Lilienfeld et al., 1994). Others argue that the dispute over whether one should use the term "comorbidity," "co-occurrence," or "covariation" is largely a semantic one (Rutter, 1994b; Spitzer, 1994; Widiger & Ford-Black, 1994).

Several possible reasons why comorbidity may be exaggerated or artificially produced have been identified in the literature (Angold, Costello, & Erkanli, 1999; Caron & Rutter, 1991; Lilienfeld et al., 1994; Rutter, 1994b; Verhulst & van der Ende, 1993). There may be a sampling bias that occurs whenever there are fewer numbers of individuals who are referred to clinics than who exhibit a given disorder. In such cases, the clinic samples will contain a disproportionately large number of subjects who display comorbid conditions. This phenomenon occurs because the probability of being referred to mental health services is higher for a child with a comorbid condition than for a child with only one disorder. Related to this sampling bias are various other referral factors that may inflate the degree of co-occurring disorders among clinic samples. Clinics that and clinicians who specialize in treating more complicated cases, for example, may be more likely to receive referrals in which comorbid conditions are present. In addition, children with internalizing difficulties such as depression are more likely to be referred by their parents or the school system if they also show externalizing symptoms, largely because externalizing problems are viewed as more disruptive by referral sources.

Comorbidity may also reflect various sources of nosological confusion arising from the manner in which different childhood disorders have been conceptualized and organized. For instance, Widiger and Ford-Black (1994) claim that excessive rates of co-occurrence seemed to appear concomitantly with the changes that occurred in DSM-III (e.g., increased coverage, divisions of diagnostic categories, the provision of separate and multiple axes). Another example is that DSM-IV makes it possible to have multiple diagnoses in the absence of multiple syndromes (Cantwell, 1996; Robins, 1994). One source of confusion stems from the overlapping criterion sets within contemporary classification schemes. In DSM-IV, diagnoses are based on a set of polythetic criteria that includes specific symptom constellations. In many cases, the presence of concomitant symptoms of a different kind are ignored, resulting in an increased likelihood that the accompanying symptoms will be represented in a different diagnostic category (Caron & Rutter, 1991). Sonuga-Barke (1998) argues, however, that although earlier diagnostic systems steered clear of comorbidity by using a hierarchical set of exclusionary criteria, "these approaches were abandoned because they clearly led to a misrepresentation of the structure of disorder" (p. 119). For example, they led to low base rates of disorders and poor interrater agreement.

Apart from the various artifactual contributors to comorbidity, there are also indicators in support of "true" comorbidity (Rutter, 1994b). It is possible that general propensities toward and/or struggles with adaptation are at the core of every disorder, but how the phenotype is expressed is contingent upon a myriad of environmental conditions and person–environment interactions (Caron & Rutter, 1991). Consistent with this notion, Lilienfeld et al. (1994) maintain that comorbidity in childhood disorders may be partly a function of developmental level—that is, of underlying processes that have not yet achieved full differentiation. Differing rates of comorbidity with age may also reflect the fact that the appearance of one disorder or problem may precede the appearance of the other, as is the case for anxiety preceding depression (Brady & Kendall, 1992) or for impulsivity preceding attentional problems (E. L. Hart et al., 1995). Still another possibility is that comorbidity reflects "a more amorphous early expression of psychopathology in young children that does not crystallize into more definitive psychopathology until later in life" (Cantwell, 1996, p. 4). Comorbidity can also arise as a result of a causal association in which the severity of one disorder may lead to or greatly increase the later risk for another disorder (e.g., ADHD and oppositional defiant disorder) or a shared underlying cause, such as common genetic effects (e.g., conduct disorder and depression) or shared environmental effects (oppositional defiant disorder and conduct disorder).

In summary, it would appear that some cases of comorbidity are the result either of ambiguity in the definition of dysfunctionality that is used, or of artifactual/methodological issues. However, as Kazdin and Kagan (1994) note, "the broader point is still relevant and not controverted with specific diagnostic conundrums—namely, multiple symptoms often go together in packages" (p. 40). This is not to suggest that *all* disorders cluster together into packages; rather, the fact that many frequently do has important implications for how child psychopathology is conceptualized and treated. The complexity of comorbidity behooves researchers to move beyond singular models and to examine multiple expressions, etiologies, and pathways of childhood dysfunction (Burt, Krueger, McGue, & Iacono, 2001; Kazdin & Johnson, 1994).

THEORY AND CHILD PSYCHOPATHOLOGY

The Role of Theory in Child Psychopathology

Every step in the research process is influenced by the investigator's preconceptions and ideologies (Kuhn, 1962; Maxwell & Delaney, 1990). As the history of child psychopathology has shown, an overemphasis on a grand theory or explanatory model in the absence of data can perpetuate false ideas and seriously impede our understanding of childhood disorders. On the other hand, "data gathering in the absence of hypotheses can become an inconsequential exercise in gathering inconsequential facts" (Rutter & Garmezy, 1983, p. 870). The value of theory lies not just in providing answers but also in raising new questions, which arise not only from addressing new problems but also from looking at familiar problems in different ways. One cannot consider theory, research, and practice in childhood psychopathology without also having some understanding of the underlying philosophical and epistemological assumptions that have guided work in this area. In this context, Overton and Horowitz (1991) discuss four levels of science: (1) epistemology; (2) guidelines, rules, and definitions of scientific knowing; (3) metatheoretical principles; and (4) theory.

The first level, "epistemology," defined as a theory about the nature of knowledge itself, has to do with the general rules of science, the metatheoretical assumptions about the nature of humankind, and the specific theoretical models and research designs that arise out of such assumptions. One epistemological stance (i.e., "realism") asserts that knowledge exists independently of one's own perceptual and cognitive processes (Maxwell & Delaney, 1990; Overton & Horowitz, 1991). "Logical positivism," a view that has guided most of our past and present research efforts in child psychopathology, reflects this stance. A second philosophical position is that of "rationalism." Rationalists contend that the knower of scientific knowledge actively constructs what is known (Maxwell & Delaney, 1990). Instead of there being a fixed and absolute knowledge base to unveil, rationalists assume that knowledge derives from the exercise of relating and interpreting observables to latent constructs (Overton & Horowitz, 1991). Within this metatheoretical position, there lies a continuum between the belief at one end that our knowledge base will always be uncertain, and the conviction at the other end that some universal truth must lie beyond our interpretive schemes.

At the second level of scientific knowledge—that of "guidelines, rules, and definitions"—it becomes evident that epistemology exerts a strong influence. Logical positivism, for instance, distinguishes scientific knowledge from knowledge that accumulates from other modes of knowing by requiring that all theoretical constructs be reducible to stable, objective, and observable knowledge (Maxwell & Delaney, 1990; Overton & Horowitz, 1991). This view maintains that theoretical constructs are to be mathematically related (via correspondence rules) to directly observable behavior and events. Theory, under this argument, advances by means of the empirical method. A hypothesis is tested and when enough hypotheses have been independently and empirically supported, generalizations can be made (via the inductive process) to form a theoretical model.

At the third level of scientific knowledge identified by Overton and Horowitz (1991), "metatheoretical principles" guide the development of more specific theories. Two metaphors have been dominant in guiding scientific metatheory: the "machine" and the "organic" metaphors (Overton & Horowitz, 1991; Simeonsson & Rosenthal, 1992). The machine metaphor adopts a metatheoretical principle that views the child as reactive and influences as linear. The organic metaphor, on the other hand, underlies theories that view the child as an active construer of and contributor to his or her circumstances. These basic assumptions regarding human nature, in turn, guide the conceptualizations and research strategies of child psychopathology (Sonuga-Barke, 1998). One example of the way in which metatheory guides research may be highlighted from the mechanistic view. Mechanistic models attempt to resolve or eliminate apparent paradoxes within the data by controlling for superfluous variance (i.e., "error") through experimental (e.g., random selection and random assignment) or statistical means (e.g., analysis of covariance), or by transforming them into linear conjunctives or disjunctives (Kazdin & Kagan, 1994; Overton & Horowitz, 1991).

In a manner that parallels the mechanistic–organismic distinction, theoretical models have also varied according to whether the role of the child and/or the environment is viewed as passive or active (Lewis, 2000; Sameroff, 1993, 2000b). The "passive child, passive environment" view stems from the ideas of John Locke and David Hume. According to this view, the environment does not actively seek to influence the child's behavior, and the child passively receives information from his or her world. Such models currently receive little attention.

A second view emphasizes an active environment and the child as a passive recipient of external influences. Radical behaviorists would assert, for instance, that behavior is strictly a function of the contingencies of reinforcement (Lewis, 2000). The Watsonian belief that, given enough time, one can turn a child into anything (e.g., a thief or a doctor) is indicative of this position. A third view is of the child as active and the environment as passive. Constructivist theories, which regard the child's reality as socially and cognitively constructed, are representative of this view. A fourth and final view regards both the child and the environment as active contributors to adaptive and maladaptive behavior (Lewis, 2000). Examples of this approach include interactive and transactional models (Sameroff, 1993), the goodness-of-fit model (Lewis, 2000; Thomas & Chess, 1977), and models of risk and resilience (Rutter, 1985, 1987, 1994a, 1994b; Rutter & Rutter, 1993).

There is currently a shift in child psychopathology toward the integration of divergent metatheoretical foundations under the "active child, active environment" position. This trend is reflected in the emergence of integrative theoretical paradigms such as developmental psychopathology, the increased use of research designs incorporating a larger number of reciprocally related variables, and the emergence of statistical techniques that permit the analysis of such complex processes (e.g., structural equation modeling, latent growth curve analyses).

Finally, the aforementioned levels of scientific knowledge (epistemology, scientific guidelines, and metatheory) contribute to the development of "theories," or the specific systems of explanatory concepts in child psychopathology. Some of these theories are highlighted in the following discussion. There is no single integrative theory that fully captures the diversity of perspectives and findings represented by current research in child psychopathology. Although the overarching theories (e.g., psychodynamic, cognitive-structural, behavioral) that have guided the study of child development and psychopathology during its formative stage have contributed to our knowledge base, at present these theories seem insufficient to account for the dynamic and interacting contextual, developmental, and system influences that have been identified as important in recent research. Many of the existing theories do not take into account the broader developmental, social, cognitive, affective, biological, family, community, and cultural context in which psychopathology develops.

As noted earlier, logical positivism dominated the early scientific scene, and concomitant scientific goals set out to simplify and isolate variables, provide operational definitions to test the reliability and validity of constructs, and experimentally or statistically control for unwanted variance (e.g., the theory of "true" and "error" score; Ghiselli, Campbell, & Zedeck, 1981; Kazdin & Kagan, 1994; Overton & Horowitz, 1991). This has perpetuated an oversimplified view of the etiology of child psychopathology in terms of singular pathways and outcomes. Beck's notion of a "cognitive triad" consisting of a negative view of oneself, the world, and the future as the causal source of major depression is one of many such examples (Beck, Rush, Shaw, & Emery, 1979). Rather than identifying and allowing for several possible pathways leading to depression (e.g., genetic factors, early loss, reinforcement history, peer relational difficulties), the cognitive model assumes that maladaptive thought processes are the principal antecedent factors of depression for virtually all individuals. It is becoming increasingly evident, however, that similar outcomes may be associated with heterogeneous influences and that similar risk factors may be related to disparate outcomes (e.g., Alloy et al., 2001; Hammen & Rudolph, Chapter 5, this volume).

Related to the notion of singular causal pathways has been the emphasis in models of child psychopathology on main effects and linear relations. "Main effects and linear relations" models assume that the impact of a single variable will be the same across varying conditions (e.g., outcomes associated with parental marital/couple discord will be the same for children of all ages and both sexes) and across a wide range of values (e.g., more severe stressors will lead to poorer outcomes in a continuous and graded fashion), respectively. Although such models may apply to some aspects of child psychopathology, when they become the primary focus of theory and research (amidst much evidence for interactive effects and nonlinearity) they may obscure important trends in the data, oversimplify or mask salient relations, and become detrimental to research progress (Kazdin & Kagan, 1994).

As noted by Rutter and Garmezy (1983), "the limitations inherent in the current data base render premature any effort to construct a global overarching theory of the psychopathology of development" (p. 870). Furthermore, any single overarching theory is unlikely to be appropriate to explain all forms of child psychopathology or to account for the full range of contributory child and family influences. Nevertheless, the developmental psychopathology perspective described below provides a useful working framework for conceptualizing and understanding child psychopathology. This perspective integrates and coordinates a wide range of theories (e.g., psychodynamic, behavioral, cognitive, biological, family systems, and sociological), each of which focuses on different sets of variables, methods, and explanations (Achenbach, 2000).

Developmental Psychopathology Perspective

A developmental psychopathology perspective provides a broad template and general principles for understanding the range of processes and mechanisms underlying how and why psychopathology in children emerges, how it changes over time, and how it is influenced by a child's developmental capacities and by the contexts in which development occurs (Cicchetti & Richters, 1993). Viewed as a macroparadigm that subsumes several theoretical approaches (Cicchetti, 1984; Cicchetti & Cohen, 1995a; Lewis, 2000; Luthar et al., 1997; Sameroff, 2000a; Rutter & Sroufe, 2000), "developmental psychopathology" has been defined as "*the study of the origins and course of individual patterns of behavioral maladaptation,* whatever the age of onset, whatever the causes, whatever the transformations in behavioral manifestation, and however complex the course of the developmental pattern may be" (Sroufe & Rutter, 1984, p. 18; emphasis in original). Put simply, developmental psychopathology provides a general framework from which to understand both normal development and its maladaptive deviations. Its main focus is an elucidation of developmental processes and their functioning through an examination of extremes in developmental outcome and of variations between normative outcomes and negative and positive extremes. Developmental psychopathology does not focus exclusively on the study of childhood disorders, but serves to inform the understanding and treatment of disorders through the study of a full range of developmental processes and outcomes.

A developmental psychopathology perspective is consistent with both transactional and ecological views, and assumes that within ongoing change and transformation there exist coherence and predictability for adaptive and maladaptive development (Cicchetti & Toth, 1997; Campbell, 1989). This perspective also emphasizes the importance of family, social, and cultural factors in predicting and understanding developmental changes (Achenbach, 2000; Lewis, 2000). In this way, developmental psychopathology attempts to address the complex influences surrounding the development of the child across the life span. In attempting to do so, it draws on knowledge from multiple fields of inquiry (including psychology, psychiatry, sociology, education, criminology, epidemiology, and neuroscience) and attempts to integrate this knowledge within a developmental framework (Rutter & Sroufe, 2000).

The focus of developmental psychopathology is on normal developmental patterns, continuities and discontinuities in functioning, and transformational interactions over different developmental periods that produce adaptive or maladaptive outcomes. The processes underlying both healthy and pathological development are seen as stemming from idiosyncratic transactions between a child and his or her unique context (Achenbach, 2000; Sroufe & Rutter, 1984). Thus a central tenet of this approach is that to understand maladaptive behavior adequately, one needs to view it in relation to what may be considered normative for a given period of development (Edelbrock, 1984). Significant challenges for research, then, are to differentiate those developmental deviations that are within normative ranges from those that are not, and to ascertain which among the plethora of interacting variables account for developmental deviation.

A developmental psychopathology perspective is also guided by a number of the assumptions that characterize organizational theories of development more generally (Cicchetti & Tucker, 1994). These include the following:

1. The individual child plays an active role in his or her own developmental organization (consciously or not).
2. Self-regulation and self-organization occurs at multiple levels, and the quality of integration within and among the child's biological, cognitive, emotional, and social systems needs to be considered.
3. There is a dialectic between canalization of developmental process and ongoing changes through the life process.
4. Developmental outcomes are best predicted through consideration of prior experience and recent adaptations examined in concert.
5. Individual choice and self-organization play an important role in determining the course of development.
6. Transitional turning points or sensitive periods in development represent times when developmental processes are most susceptible to positive and/or negative self-organizational efforts.

Until recently, the developmental psychopathology perspective has been more of a conceptual enterprise than a well-validated approach (Lewis, 2000). However, in a very short period of time, it has proven to be an enormously useful framework for understanding and guiding research in child psychopathology, and it represents an important shift in thinking away from single causal hypotheses toward a view based on complex and multiple pathways of influence: "After each effort to support an explanatory model by collecting a set of data, the results have required modifications in the model, forcing the field to evolve from a concern with causes and effects to an increasing appreciation of the probabilistic interchanges between dynamic individuals and dynamic contexts that comprise human behavior" (Sameroff, 2000a, p. 297).

Disorder-Specific Models

In addition to a need for an integrative framework such as developmental psychopathology, there is a parallel need for more focused disorder- and problem-specific theories and hypotheses to account for the different forms of psychopathology in children, the different pathways through which similar forms of psychopathology emerge, and the reasons why seemingly similar developmental pathways may lead to different outcomes. Kazdin and Kagan (1994) rightfully argue that the best explanatory models are likely to be different, depending on the specific disorder and/or on differences related to gender, ethnicity, SES, and a host of other conditions. A key issue is to identify the range of conditions under which particular models are or are not applicable.

Numerous disorder- and problem-focused theories have been proposed. These models are empirically based and are sensitive to the specific characteristics and processes that research has identified as important for understanding a particular disorder or problem. A few examples of representative models include Barkley's (1997) theory of "inhibitory dysfunction," which proposes that behavioral inhibition is the primary and central deficit underlying the attentional, cognitive, affective, and social difficulties of children with ADHD; Cummings and Davies's (1995; Davies & Cummings, 1994) "emotional security hypothesis," which proposes that emotional insecurity resulting from a number of sources (e.g., maternal depression, marital conflict) may lead to child difficulties in self-regulation, efforts to overregulate others, and maladaptive relational representations; Feldman and Downey's (1994) proposal that the impact of family violence on adult attachment behavior is mediated by an increased sensitivity to rejection, which is a motive to avoid rejection that is evidenced in social encoding biases, expectancies, values, and regulatory plans; Crick and Dodge's (1994) model of social information-processing deficits in aggressive children, which views aggression as a outcome of a child's use of biased or distorted interpretational processes in social situations Bugental's (1993) model of abusive parent–child relationships, which focuses on "low personal control over failure," perceived power disadvantage, and a maladaptive defensive coping style to child behaviors that are perceived by the parent as potentially threatening; and Mundy's (1995) proposed "social-emotional approach disturbance" in children with autism, a disturbance hypothesized to be related to the compromised integrity of the neurological system that mediates social stimulus approach behaviors. This dysfunction is hypothesized to lead to an attenuation of the tendency to initiate affectively positive social behaviors, which in turn restricts the interactions that are needed to develop the social-cognitive capacities regulating adaptive social interchange.

Many other theories that have been proposed to account for these and other problems and disorders are presented in the subsequent chapters of this volume. The growth in the number of such theories reflects an increasing trend toward models that focus on the processes underlying specific forms of child psychopathology rather than on child psychopathology in general, and a concomitant recognition of the importance of disorder-specific theories to guide research and practice. Recent research findings indicate that there are likely to be both common factors (e.g., insecure models of attachment, executive function deficits) that apply across many different types of disorder, and specific factors that play a particularly crucial role in understanding individual disorders (e.g., impulsivity and ADHD). Identifying both common and specific factors and their relationship to one another is an important task for future research.

INFLUENCES ON CHILD PSYCHOPATHOLOGY

All forms of child psychopathology are influenced by the complex interactions among person variables (e.g., genetics) and the environmental context for development and behavior. Adelman and Taylor (1993, p. 64) have presented a useful conceptual framework that describes a representative range of factors related to emotional, behavioral, and learning problems in children. This framework is shown in Table 1.7. In elaborating on this framework, Adelman (1995) has described children's emotional, behavioral, and learning problems based on paradigmatic causes that include those that are primarily within a child, primarily within the environment, or in mismatches between the child and the environment. Many theories of child psychopathology have differed in the emphasis given to the influences and interactions described in Table 1.7.

GENERAL THEORIES OF CHILD PSYCHOPATHOLOGY

Several major theories have been proposed to account for the emergence of psychopathology in children. These are listed in Table 1.8 and include psychodynamic (Dare, 1985; Fonagy & Target, 2000; Shapiro & Esman, 1992), attachment (Bowlby, 1973, 1988; Sroufe, Carlson, Levy, & Egeland, 1999), behavioral/reinforcement (Bijou & Baer, 1961; Skinner, 1953), social learning (Bandura, 1977, 1986), interpersonal (Joiner & Coyne, 1999; Gotlib & Hammen, 1992); cognitive (Beck, 1964; Beck et al., 1979; Clark, Beck, & Alford, 1999; Ingram et al., 1998), constitutional/neurobiological (e.g., Pennington & Ozonoff, 1991; Raine, 1997; Torgersen, 1993), affective (Cicchetti & Izard, 1995; Fox, 1994b;

TABLE 1.7. Factors Instigating Emotional, Behavioral, and Learning Problems

Environment (E)

1. Insufficient stimuli (e.g., prolonged periods in impoverished environments; deprivation of learning opportunities at home or school, such as lack of play and practice situations and poor instruction; inadequate diet)
2. Excessive stimuli (e.g., overly demanding home, school, or work experiences, such as overwhelming pressure to achieve and contradictory expectations; overcrowding)
3. Intrusive and hostile stimuli (e.g., medical practices, especially at birth, leading to physiological impairment; contaminated environments; conflict in home, school, workplace; faulty child-rearing practices, such as long-standing abuse and rejection; dysfunctional family; migratory family; language used is a second language; social prejudices related to race, sex, age, physical characteristics and behavior)

Person (P)

1. Physiological insult (e.g., cerebral trauma, such as accident or stroke, endocrine dysfunctions and chemical imbalances; illness affecting brain or sensory functioning)
2. Genetic anomaly (e.g., genes that limit, slow down, or lead to any atypical development)
3. Cognitive activity and affective states experienced by self as deviant (e.g., lack of knowledge or skills such as basic cognitive strategies; lack of ability to cope effectively with emotions, such as low self-esteem)
4. Physical characteristics shaping contact with environment and/or experienced by self as deviant (e.g., visual, auditory, or motoric deficits; excessive or reduced sensitivity to stimuli; easily fatigued; factors such as race, sex, age or unusual appearance that produce stereotypical responses)
5. Deviant actions of the individual (e.g., performance problems, such as excessive errors in performing; high or low levels of activity)

Interactions and transactions between E and P[a]

1. Severe to moderate personal vulnerabilities and environmental defects and differences (e.g., a person with extremely slow development in a highly demanding environment), all of which simultaneously and equally instigate the problem
2. Minor personal vulnerabilities not accommodated by the situation (e.g., person with minimal CNS disorders resulting in auditory perceptual disability trying to do auditory-loaded tasks; very active person forced into situations at home, school, or work that do not tolerate this level of activity)
3. Minor environmental defects and differences not accommodated by the individual (e.g., person is in the minority racially or culturally and is not participating in many social activities because he or she thinks others may be unreceptive)

Note. From *Learning Problems and Learning Disabilities: Moving Forward*, 1st edition, by H. S. Adelman and L. Taylor © 1993. Reprinted with permission of Wadsworth, an imprint of the Wadsworth Group, a division of Thomson Learning, Fax 800 730-2215.
[a]May involve only one P and one E variable, or may involve multiple combinations.

Rubin, Cheah, & Fox, 2001), and family systems (Fiese et al., 2000; Grych & Fincham, 2001; Jacob, 1987) models. A detailed discussion of the basic tenets of each of these general theories is beyond the scope of this chapter. For comprehensive discussions of these theories, the reader is directed to original sources and to specific references cited throughout this volume. What follows is a discussion of several general points related to some of these theories.

Each general theoretical approach reflects a diversity of viewpoints. For example, psychodynamic theory encompasses traditional Freudian and Kleinian psychoanalytic constructs and their many derivatives as reflected in ego-analytic and object relations theory (Fonagy & Target, 2000; Lesser, 1972). Behavioral/reinforcement perspectives include traditional operant/classical conditioning constructs, mediational models, and contemporary theories of learning (Klein & Mower, 1989; Krasner, 1991; Viken & McFall, 1994). Cognitive theories include cognitive-structural models, models of cognitive distortion, and models of faulty information processing (Clark et al., 1999; Ingram et al., 1998; Kendall & Dobson, 1993). Family systems theories include systemic, structural, and social learning models (Jacob, 1987). Therefore, when one is discussing any theory, it is critical to distinguish among the different perspectives encompassed by the approach.

Many theories of child psychopathology are derivatives of earlier approaches. For example, psychodynamic theories dominated thinking about child psychopathology for the first half of the 20th century. These theories contributed to our understanding of child psychopathology

TABLE 1.8. General Models Used to Conceptualize Child Psychopathology

Psychodynamic models
Inborn drives, intrapsychic mechanisms, conflicts, defenses, psychosexual stages, fixation, and regression.
Attachment models
Early attachment relationships, internal working models of self, others, and relationships in general.
Behavioral/reinforcement models
Excessive, inadequate, or maladaptive reinforcement and/or learning histories.
Social learning models
Vicarious and observational experience, reciprocal parent–child interactions.
Interpersonal models
Interactional styles, social skills deficits, social difficulties, stressful interpersonal environments.
Cognitive models
Distorted or deficient cognitive structures and processes.
Constitutional/neurobiological models
Temperament, genetic mutations, neuroanatomy, neurobiological mechanisms.
Affective models
Dysfunctional emotion-regulating mechanisms.
Family systems models
Intra- and intergenerational family systems, and the structural and/or functional elements within families.

Note. Models are highlighted in terms of their relative emphasis.

through their emphasis on the importance of relationships, early life experiences, mental mechanisms, and unconscious processes, and they spawned a number of other models—for example, attachment theory (Rutter, 1995). The emergence of attachment theory reflected a shifting of attention from the more traditional psychoanalytic role of intrapersonal defenses to that of interpersonal relationships (Bretherton, 1995). Similarly, the emergence of social learning theory reflected disenchantment with nonmediational models of learning and a growing interest in the role of symbolic processes.

A number of general points can be made regarding theories of child psychopathology:

1. Each theory offers an explanation regarding the etiology of child psychopathology. The strength of each theory rests on its specificity in predicting various forms of psychopathology and its degree of empirical support.
2. The varying degrees of support for each conceptualization suggest that no single model can fully explain the complexities involved in understanding child psychopathology. In light of this, increased understanding may accrue if greater integrative and collaborative efforts are undertaken.
3. Many explanations of childhood disorders implicitly or explicitly assume a simple association between a limited number of antecedents and a given disorder. However, as we have discussed, the concept of multiple pathways that lead to different outcomes depending on the circumstances represents a more viable framework in light of current research findings.
4. Although the testing of specific models is consistent with the spirit of parsimony, far greater attention needs to be given to the unique contexts and conditions under which a particular model does or does not apply.
5. Research on dysfunction frequently examines static conditions and influences such as the expression of a disorder at a given age or the influence of a specific stressor. However, evidence indicates that the expression and etiology of psychopathology in children are continuously changing over time, and theories need to account for these types of changes.

Current models are becoming increasingly sensitive to the many different components of childhood dysfunction. Indeed, constitutional, behavioral, cognitive, emotional, and social factors cross a number of theoretical domains; this is reflected in the emergence of hybrid models (e.g., cognitive-behavioral, social information processing, cognitive-neuropsychological), as well as the inclusion of family and ecological constructs across many different theories. Behavioral models, which have frequently been characterized as having a narrow emphasis on conditioning principles, are also becoming increasingly sensitive to systems influences (Viken & McFall, 1994).

Four interrelated theoretical approaches have received increased attention in current research on child psychopathology: (1) attachment theory, (2) cognitive theories, (3) emotion theories, and (4) constitutional/neurobiological theories. Each of these approaches is highlighted in the sections that follow.

Attachment Theory

Bowlby's (1973, 1988) theory of attachment is based on both an ethological and a psychoanalytic perspective (Cassidy & Shaver, 1999; Cicchetti, Toth, & Lynch, 1995). Nevertheless, Bowlby rejected the psychoanalytic ideas that individuals pass through a series of stages where fixation at or regression to an earlier state can occur, and that emotional bonds are derived from drives based on food or sex. Drawing on ethology and control theory, Bowlby and his successors replaced Freudian concepts of motivation based on psychic energy with cybernetically controlled motivational–behavioral systems organized as plan hierarchies (Bowlby, 1973; Bretherton, 1995). Within attachment theory, instinctive behaviors are not rigidly predetermined, but rather become organized into flexible goal-oriented systems through learning and goal-corrected feedback. Motivational–behavioral systems (e.g., attachment, exploration) regulate time-limited consummatory behaviors and time-extended instinctive behaviors that maintain an organism in relation to its environment. Attachment belongs to a group of stress-reducing behavioral systems that operate in conjunction with physiological arousal-regulating systems. The child is motivated to maintain a balance between familiarity-preserving, stress-reducing behaviors, and exploratory and information-seeking behaviors. Self-reliance develops optimally when an attachment figure provides a secure base for exploration (Bretherton, 1995).

It is via the attachment relationship that the infant develops an "internal working model" of the self and others. Bowlby (1988) argued that the development of psychopathology is directly related to the inability of the caregiver to respond appropriately to the child's needs. This assertion is, however, a point of contention among researchers. Sroufe (1985), for example, has questioned the direct role of parental influence, arguing that infant temperament and the reciprocal interaction of a "difficult temperament" with parental response may better account for the variance in the attachment relationship and its ensuing insecure attachment difficulties. On the basis of a review of several studies examining infant temperament and attachment, Sroufe (1985) suggests that although some studies have supported the notion that differences between secure and insecure attachments may be due to temperament, the bulk of evidence suggests that infants change their attachment patterns with different caregivers.

In postulating an association between early attachment and later psychopathology, one must exercise caution, in that there does not appear to be one specific subtype of attachment that leads to one particular childhood disorder. Rather, the trajectory for developmental pathways and manifestations of psychopathology emerges as the result of environmental experience, biological predispositions, and learning. When one is identifying possible developmental paths as factors related to subsequent psychopathology, the concept of the child's internal working model is useful; however, it is important to bear in mind that the internal working model represents a set of active constructions that are subject to change, and that the association with later psychopathology is probabilistic rather than absolute.

Rutter (1995) has highlighted a number of key issues surrounding attachment, including (1) the need to identify mechanisms involved in proximity-seeking behavior; (2) broadening the basis for measuring attachment to include dimensions as well as categories; (3) studying relationship qualities that may not be captured by "insecurity"; (4) understanding the relationship between temperament and attachment; (5) dealing with how discrepant relationships are translated into individual characteristics; (6) operationalizing internal working models; (7) defining attachment quality across the life span, and determining whether or not meanings are equivalent at different ages; (8) determining how one relationship affects others; and (9) identifying the boundaries of attachment vis-à-vis other aspects of relationships. Understanding the association between attachment and later functioning, the linkage between parenting and attachment quality, the adaptive value of secure attachment (e.g., insecure attachment does not equal psychopathology), disorders of attachment associated with abuse and neglect, and the diffuse attachments associated with institutionalization are all issues in need of further investigation.

Bowlby's attachment theory has played an important role in focusing attention on the quality of parent–child relationships, the interaction between security in relationships and the growth of independence, the importance of placing emergent human relationships within a biological/evolutionary context (e.g., Kraemer, 1992), the concept of internal working models, and insecure early attachments (e.g., Barnett & Vondra, 1999) as the basis for the development of psychopathology (Rutter, 1995).

Cognitive Theories

Considerable research has focused on the role of cognitions in both adult and child psychopathology (Clark et al., 1999; Ingram et al., 1998; Ingram & Price, 2001). Several theoretical perspectives have been concerned with childhood cognitions. These have included cognitive-structural models (Ingram et al., 1998; Selman, Beardslee, Schultz, Krupa, & Poderefsky, 1986), information-processing approaches (Crick & Dodge, 1994; Ingram & Ritter, 2000; Taylor & Ingram, 1999), and cognitive-behavioral approaches (Braswell & Kendall, 2001; Dobson & Dozois, 2001; Meichenbaum, 1977). Representative examples of the information-processing and cognitive-behavioral approaches are described below. Recently cognitive theories have focused on the importance of positive cognitions, the role of cognitive specificity, the role of context on cognitions, the impact of comorbidity, the use of information-processing risk paradigms, a movement away from simple cognitive diathesis–stress models to looking at information-processing mediators, and the need for theoretical integration.

Information Processing

Faulty information processing has been implicated in a number of childhood disorders. For example, socially aggressive children have been found to display negative attributional biases (Dodge & Crick, 1990; Schwartz & Proctor, 2000); children with anxiety disorders show attentional biases to threatening stimuli (Vasey, Daleiden, Williams, & Brown, 1995; Waters, Lipp, & Cobham, 2000); and depressed children exhibit greater encoding biases for negative material, and less endorsement and recall of positive information (Gencoez, Voelz, Gencoez, Pettit, & Joiner, 2001). Research into faulty information processing and child psychopathology has emanated from three streams: one focusing on deficits in basic information processing related to attention, memory, and other cognitive functions (e.g., Carter & Swanson, 1995); another related to social information processing (Crick & Dodge, 1994); and a third focusing on maladaptive cognition (e.g., Ingram et al., 1998; Ingram & Ritter, 2000; Taylor & Ingram, 1999).

Dodge's model as applied to socially aggressive boys illustrates the social information-processing approach (Dodge & Newman, 1981; Dodge & Somberg, 1987). In this model, a series of thought processes and behaviors (i.e., encoding, interpretation, response search, response decision, and enactment) is postulated to occur during the course of appropriate social interactions and to be absent or distorted during inappropriate social interactions. Crick and Dodge (1994) have expanded this conceptual framework to reflect more accurately theoretical and empirical advances in the domains of developmental psychopathology, clinical psychology, and cognitive psychology. The reformulated model continues to posit the same basic information-processing steps, but at each stage there is ongoing reciprocal interaction between the information-processing skills required during social transactions in context and the individual's "data base" (a collection of social schemas, memories, social knowledge, and cultural values or rules) (Crick & Dodge, 1994). Instead of a linear processing model, there are postulated to be cyclical feedback loops connecting all stages of processing. Increased recognition of the influence of peer appraisal and response, emotional processes, and the development and acquisition of cognitive skill as important contributors to social adjustment are meaningful additions to the reformulated model. In addition to the enhanced sensitivity to developmental trajectories, the reformulated model emphasizes the role of early dispositions (e.g., temperament) and other factors (e.g., age, gender, social context) that serve to moderate the relationship between information processing and social adjustment. Specifically, the model asserts that parent–child interactions and the quality of early attachments may be important contributors to the ongoing formulation of the child's data base. A number of recent studies have provided empirical support for the expanded model (Contreras, Kerns, Weimer, Getzler, & Tomich, 2000; Gomez & Gomez, 2000; Gomez, Gomez, DeMello, & Tallent, 2001). The reformulated model is a good illustration of the current trend toward models of child psychopathology that attempt to integrate the structural aspects of cognition with ongoing cognitive processes, and with emotions, as they interact with one another across time and contexts.

Cognitive-Behavioral Theories

Cognitive-behavioral theories stem from a rational epistemological viewpoint: "a purposeful attempt to preserve the positive features of the behavioral approaches, while also working to incorporate into a model the cognitive activity and information-processing factors of the individual" (Kendall & MacDonald, 1993, p. 387; see also Braswell & Kendall, 2001). Importantly, cognitive-behavioral models also consider the role of affect and recognize the importance of contextual variables (e.g., family, peers) in both the etiology and maintenance of psychopathology (Dobson & Kendall, 1993; Kendall, 1991, 1993; Kendall & Dobson, 1993; Kendall & Morris, 1991; Short, Barrett, Dadds, & Fox, 2001).

Cognitive-behavioral theories assert that maladaptive cognitive processes predispose an individual to psychopathology and maintain the dysfunctional patterns and developmental anomalies (Beck et al., 1979). Four elements of cognition are distinguished for the purpose of understanding the pathogenesis of psychiatric disturbances: cognitive structures, content, operations, and products (Beck et al., 1979; Dozois & Dobson, 2001; Ingram et al., 1998; Kendall & Dobson, 1993). "Cognitive structures" represent the way in which information is organized and stored in memory, and serve the function of filtering or screening ongoing experiences. "Cognitive content" (or propositions) refers to the information that is stored in memory (i.e., the substance of the cognitive structures). Together, cognitive structures and content make up what is termed a "schema." A schema stems from a child's processing of life experiences and acts as a guideline or core philosophy influencing expectations and filtering information in a fashion consistent with the child's core philosophy. As such, cognitive schemas have also been referred to as "filters" or "templates" (see Kendall & MacDonald, 1993). A schema is postulated to effect the relative observed consistency in the child's cognition, behavior, and affect (Stark, Rouse, & Livingston, 1991). According to Beck's model, maladaptive schemas develop in early childhood and remain dormant until some untoward event triggers the latent schemas, and the individual begins to encode, process, and interpret information in a schema-congruent way. Individuals with a depression schema, for instance, process and interpret information about themselves, the world, and the future in a negatively biased fashion, whereas persons with an anxiety schema interpret environmental stimuli with a cognitive focus on future threat. In addition, what appears to be specific to depression is a lack of positive cognition (Dozois & Dobson, 2001; Gencoez et al., 2001).

"Cognitive processes" or "cognitive operations" pertain to the manner by which the cognitive system functions. Thus cognitive processes, which are guided by schemas, suggest the mode by which an individual perceives and interprets both internal and external stimuli. Finally, "cognitive products" are the ensuing thoughts that stem from the simultaneous and reciprocal interactions among the various components of the cognitive system.

According to the cognitive model, each (or all) of these components may become dysfunctional and precipitate the expression of psychopathology (Kendall, 1991, 1993; Stark et al., 1991). Consistent with this model, a number of studies have found that children who either experience psychopathology themselves (e.g., Epkins, 2000; Lewinsohn, Joiner, & Rohde, 2001; Waters et al., 2000) or have a parent with a psychiatric disorder (e.g., Moradi, Neshat-Doost, Taghavi, Yule, & Dalgleish, 1999; Taylor & Ingram, 1999) demonstrate disorder-congruent information-processing biases. For instance, Taylor and Ingram (1999) found that nondepressed children of depressed mothers showed negative cognitive patterns similar to those of their mothers. This resultant early vulnerability, which may be due to impaired attachment patterns and/or the modeling of negative cognition, may lead to the development of core negative self-schemas or internal working models that contribute to subsequent depression (Garber & Flynn, 2001; Ingram et al., 1998; Ingram & Ritter, 2000).

An important distinction can be made between "cognitive deficits" and "cognitive distortions." Kendall (1993) argues that this distinction is useful in describing, classifying, and understanding a variety of juvenile disorders. "Deficits" refer to an absence of thinking where it would be beneficial. Aggressive youths, for example, frequently lack the ability to encode interpersonal information (Coy, Speltz, DeKlyen, & Jones, 2001; Pakaslahti, 2000; Schwartz & Proctor, 2000) or to solve social problems adequately (Crick & Dodge, 1994; Lochman & Dodge, 1994), and impulsive children often fail to think before they respond (Moore & Hughes, 1988). Conversely, children who display "distortions" typically do not lack the ability to organize or process information; rather, their thinking is described as biased, dysfunctional, or misguided (Kendall, 1993; Kendall & MacDonald, 1993). A depressed individual's negative view of him- or herself, the world, and the future is an example of distorted thinking. Kendall (1985, 1993) notes that the distinction between deficient and distorted thinking is relevant to the distinction that has been made between externalizing and internalizing disorders (cf. Achenbach, 2000). Generally, internalizing disorders are related to distortions in thinking, whereas externalizing disorders are more commonly associated with cognitive deficits. However, empirical evidence suggests that aggressive behaviors usually include both distortions and deficits (e.g., Lochman, White, & Wayland, 1991).

Various strengths and limitations of cognitive models may be delineated. A particularly important strength of cognitive-behavioral theory is that it examines the areas of cognition, affect, behavior, and social functioning as indicators of the etiology and maintenance of childhood disorders, and thus possesses strong theory-to-assessment-to-treatment links (Stark et al., 1991). Based on the theoretical model that a latent schema develops in childhood and remains dormant until an event triggers its structure, assessment functions to determine the severity and content of the maladaptive cognitive processes and products, and therapy serves to build new cognitive structures that serve as templates for coping (Braswell & Kendall, 2001; Kendall, 1993).

One important limitation of cognitive-behavioral approaches pertains to tests of their etiological assumptions. Although there is research support for faulty cognition as a concomitant of various adult (Dobson & Shaw, 1987; Lewinsohn, Steinmetz, Larson, & Franklin, 1981; Silverman, Silverman, & Eardley, 1984) and child disorders (Tems, Stuart, Skinner, Hughes, & Emslie, 1993), evidence for the causal hypothesis is equivocal. For example, Tems et al. (1993) examined the cognitive patterns of depressed children and adolescents. Although depressed children displayed more cognitive distortions than controls, no significant differences between groups remained upon remission. This finding is unique neither to the childhood literature (for similar findings with adult depression, see Lewinsohn et al., 1981; Dobson & Shaw, 1987; or Silverman et al., 1984) nor to internalizing disorders. On the other hand, some researchers have evidence to support the notion that stable patterns of cognition exist. Dozois and Dobson (2001a), for example, found that depressed adults continued to demonstrate well-interconnected negative schematic structures into remission. A series of studies have also shown that individuals with remitted depression do show biased information processing, but only when their core schemas have become activated via cognitive challenges or mood-priming paradigms (e.g., Miranda & Persons, 1988; Miranda, Persons, & Byers, 1990; Persons & Miranda, 1992; Solomon, Haaga, Brody, Kirk, & Friedman, 1998).

Emotion Theories

Emotion and its regulatory functions are constructs that cross several conceptual models—including psychodynamic theory, with its concept of defense mechanisms; cognitive-behavioral theory, which stresses the role of thought patterns and behavior as determinants of emotion; attachment theory, with its premise that an internal working model is formed on the basis of early relations and continues to regulate emotion in subsequent relationships (Cassidy, 1994); and biological theories, which emphasize the structural and neurochemical correlates of emotion regulation (Pennington & Ozonoff, 1991; Posner & Rothbart, 2000). Emotion and its regulation–dysregulation played a central role in the conceptual paradigms of early models of child psychopathology. For example, psychoanalytic theory emphasized the regulation of emotions through the use of defense mechanisms, with an absence of such regulation leading to anxiety and psychopathology (see Cole, Michel, & Teti, 1994). By affording individuals the opportunity to avoid, minimize, or convert emotions, defense mechanisms were hypothesized to serve the function of regulating emotional experiences that are too difficult to deal with at the conscious level.

Although the advent and growth of cognitive and behavioral models shifted attention away from an interest in affective processes, the study of emotional processes in child psychopathology has experienced a resurgence of interest (Arsenio & Lemerise, 2001; Belsky, Friedman, & Hsieh, 2001; Cicchetti & Izard, 1995; Cummings & Davies, 1996; Fox, 1994b; Kagan, 1994b; Keenan, 2000; Rubin et al., 2001). In part, this renewed interest reflects the growing recognition that children's emotional experience, expression, and regulation are likely to affect the quality of their thinking, social interactions, and relationships (e.g., Flavell, Flavell, & Green, 2001; Garber & Dodge, 1991; Gottman et al., 1997; Schultz, Izard, Ackerman, & Youngstrom, 2001; Rubin et al., 2001). From a functionalist perspective, emotions are viewed as playing a causal role in organizing and directing the way in which children react to environmental events. This perspective is illustrated by findings showing that induced negative child emotions increase children's distress, negative expectations, and appraisals of adult conflict, whereas induced positive emotions have the opposite effect (Davies & Cummings, 1995). Several discussions have focused on the development of emotion regulation and its ability to influence both adaptive and maladaptive functioning (Cassidy, 1994; Cole et al., 1994; Fredrickson, 2001; Kagan, 1994b; Mayer & Salovey, 1995; Thompson, 1994). In general, there is growing support for the the view that emotionality and regulation are related to children's concurrent and long-term social competence and adjustment (Eisenberg, Fabes, Guthrie, & Reiser, 2000).

Emotion systems have as their primary functions the motivation/organization of behavior and communication with self and with others. Emotions represent patterns that include at least several of the following components: (1) activating neural, sensory–motor, cognitive, and/or affective stimulus events; (2) dedicated neural processes; (3) changes in physiological responses; (4) changes in motoric/expressive behavior; (5) related cognitive appraisals; and (6) concomitant alterations in subjective experiences or feeling states (Cicchetti, Ackerman, & Izard, 1995; Izard, 1993; Kagan, 1994b).

Different theories have viewed child psychopathology as emanating from the following: (1) unrestrained emotions (i.e., emotions that are unconnected to cognitive or affective–cognitive control processes); (2) deficits or distortions in cognitions and behaviors that interfere with emotion modulation (i.e., emotions connected to cognitive processes and behavior that are situationally inappropriate); (3) emotional interference with planful cognitive processes (i.e., emotional flooding); (4) dysfunctional patterns of emotion processing and communication, involving problems with recognition, interpretation, and expression; and (5) difficulties in coordinating emotional and cognitive processes in the regulation of emotion (Cicchetti, Ackerman, & Izard, 1995).

Emotion dysfunction may emanate from several sources, including variations in biological vulnerability and stress. In studying child psychopathology, it is important not to focus on negative emotions without also recognizing the beneficial and buffering effects of positive emotions (Fredrickson, 2001; Masten, 2001), the adaptive value and facilitating effects of negative emotions of moderate or at times even extreme intensity, and the ongoing importance of emotion content and meaning for a child's behavior. Also, since negative emotions are neither topographically nor functionally unidimensional, it is important to identify the *discrete* emotions and emotional patterns underlying different forms of child psychopathology (Cicchetti, Ackerman, & Izard, 1995). For example, the negative affect that is associated with depression may involve sadness, anger, or guilt, in the same way that negative behaviors in depressed children may be both aggressive/confrontational and depressive/distressed (Hops, 1995).

It is useful to distinguish between the two dimensions of "emotion reactivity" and "emotion regulation." "Reactivity" refers to individual differences in the threshold and intensity of emotional experience, whereas "regulation" describes processes that operate to control or modulate reactivity (e.g., attention, inhibition, approach–avoidance, coping styles) (Rubin et al., 1995). According to Rubin et al. (1995), this distinction is important because it highlights the need to focus on the dynamic interaction between general temperament and specific regulatory mechanisms, and in turn the need to recognize that emotional arousal (reactivity) can serve to inhibit, facilitate, or disrupt behavior. The distinction can also be made between problems in regulation and problems in dysregulation, with regulation problems involving weak or absent control structures or structures overwhelmed by disabling input, and dysregulation involving existing control structures that operate in a maladaptive manner and direct emotion toward inappropriate goals (Cicchetti, Ackerman, & Izard, 1995). Functions of emotion involve the emotion knowledge of self and others in identifying feelings and behavior, including monitoring of self and environment. Absent or weak monitoring may result in dissociated emotional and cognitive processes and emotional leakage, whereas excessive monitoring may lead to a narrow sampling of emotional signals and excessive use of specific emotions in communication (Cicchetti Ackerman, & Izard, 1995).

Of interest to the present chapter is the manner in which emotion regulation has been defined and conceptualized with respect to psychopathology (Keenan, 2000). The processes of emotion regulation include the attenuation or deactivation of an ongoing emotion, the amplification of an ongoing emotion, the activation of a desired emotion, and the masking of emotional states (Cicchetti, Ackerman, & Izard, 1995). Thompson (1994) defines emotion regulation as consisting of "the extrinsic and intrinsic processes responsible for monitoring, evaluating, and modifying emotional reactions, especially their intensive and temporal features, to accomplish one's goals" (p. 27). This definition highlights several important characteristics of emotion regulation. First, it involves enhancing, maintaining, or inhibiting emotional arousal for the purpose of meeting one's goals. Second, there are both internal and external factors that influence the development and use of emotion-regulating strategies. Finally, there is a temporal dimension: Sometimes there are sudden and transitory changes in emotional arousal that must be dealt with (e.g., acute or state anxiety), whereas at other times there are longer-lasting ramifications of emotional arousal created by years of experience (e.g., chronic or trait anxiety; Kagan, 1994b; Terr, 1991).

The development of emotion regulation or dysregulation is thought to derive both from innate predispositions and from socialization. At the level of constitutional factors are various neural circuits and temperamental characteristics. For example, inhibited children appear to bring a high state of reactivity into their environment, particularly in novel or unfamiliar situations. This biological propensity is thought to be the result of a number of neurological factors that include interrelating messages sent to and from neuroanatomical structures (vis-à-vis neuroelectricity and neuropharmacology) to the central and peripheral nervous system (Fox, 1994a; Kagan, 1994b; Posner & Rothbart, 2000).

Cognitive and language development also contributes to emotion regulation. Growth in cognitive development allows the child increasingly to differentiate and cope with a diverse set of emotion-arousing stimuli. The development of emotion language also affords an opportunity for the communication of emotion meaning to others and its management through self-regulatory mechanisms (Cole et al., 1994; Thompson, 1994).

Finally, emotion regulation is also embedded within the unique context of the child. Socialization influences within the family, peer group, and culture are important in the development and expression of emotion, and may support or hinder emotion regulation in a variety of ways. One important influence is the way in which parents respond to the child's initial expressions of emotion, and how emotions are communicated in the context of the ongoing interactions between the parents and child (Cassidy, 1994; Volling, 2001). The development of emotion regulation may also come about through the modeling of appropriate or inappropriate emotional expression (e.g., Shipman & Zeman, 2001). Finally, the rules or boundaries of emotional expression, which are established by both the family and the community at large, also impact upon the development of emotion regulation (Cole et al., 1994).

Emotion dysregulation begins with contextually bound regulatory events, which may then develop into more stable patterns of responding and thereby contribute to the development of psychopathology. The determination of emotion regulation as adaptive or maladaptive varies with the circumstances, but it generally involves the degree of flexibility of the response, the perceived conformity of the response to cultural and familial rules and boundaries, and the outcome of the response relative to the child's and parents' short- and long-term goals (Thompson, 1994).

Some forms of emotion dysregulation may be adaptive in one environment or at one time, but maladaptive in other situations or at other points in development (Fischer et al., 1997; Thompson & Calkins, 1996). For example, in discussing children who have been emotionally and sexually abused, Terr (1991) describes the process of "numbing" (a symptom of a posttraumatic stress reaction), which serves to protect the child from overwhelming pain and trauma. However, when numbing becomes a characteristic way of coping with stressors later in life, it may interfere with adaptive functioning and with long-term goals. Another example stems from studies on attachment quality. In response to attachment figures that are rejecting or inconsistent, infants may develop an insecure/avoidant attachment in which emotional expression is minimized. Such an infant's reduced emotional expression, while serving the strategic function within the attachment relationship of minimizing loss by reducing investment in the relationship, may establish a pattern of emotional responding that is maladaptive for the development of subsequent relationships (Cassidy, 1994).

In summary, emotion theorists conceptualize the development of emotion regulation as involving a variety of increasingly complex developmental tasks. The degree of interference with these tasks depends on the characteristics of the child and his or her environment, as well as on their interaction. Emotion dysregulation is believed to be the consequence of interference in the associated developmental processes. Dysregulation is associated with a wide range of emotions; depending on the overall context, it may or may not become a stylistic pattern, and it may or may not lead to later psychopathology.

Constitutional/Neurobiological Theories

In attempting to understand child psychopathology, constitutional/neurobiological theories recognize the physical makeup and tendencies of humans in general, as well as variations and individual differences in neurobiologically based characteristics and processes. These theories have emphasized evolutionary mechanisms, genetic influences, constitutional factors, neuroanatomy, neurochemical mechanisms, and rates of maturation (e.g., onset of puberty). From a neurobiological perspective, all mental disorders are represented in the brain as a biological entity. Somehow, numerous biochemicals and neurohormones interact to influence several brain regions, causing the individual to experience emotional and/or behavioral dysfunction (Kaplan & Sadock, 1991). The goals of research in this field are to ascertain what specific genetic mutations are associated with structural and biochemical impairments and psychopathology.

In considering general human characteristics for behavior, emotion, and cognition, Richters and Cicchetti (1993) specify a number of important functions of the human nervous system. These include the capacity for emotion recognition and expression, cooperation, formation of attachments, self-awareness, learning from experience, withholding or delaying a response, anticipating the future, recognizing and avoiding danger, generating strategies for action and choosing among them, and social communication. Since there are an unlimited number of ways to conceptualize the adaptive functions of the nervous system and its dysfunctions, it becomes necessary to circumscribe which of these and other functions of the nervous system are the most causally relevant to a particular childhood disorder (e.g., recognizing and avoiding danger in the case of anxiety disorders, or delaying a response in the case of ADHD).

Genetic, neurobiological, neurophysiological, and neuroanatomical evidence suggests a neurobiological basis for many childhood disorders, including ADHD, autistic disorder, adolescent depression, social withdrawal, and some anxiety disorders (e.g., obsessive–compulsive disorder), to name a few. Research on brain structure and function using neuroimaging procedures has implicated specific brain regions for ADHD (e.g., Semrud-Clikeman et al., 2000), anxiety disorders (Pine & Grun, 1999), autism, and many other disorders. Neuroimaging studies tell us that one region or another may be involved, but they do not tell us why, and the findings for particular disorders are not always consistent from study to study, for children of different ages, or boys versus girls. Research into specific neurotransmitters has also provided promising leads, although findings have also been inconsistent. One of the difficulties in research in this area is that many forms of child psychopathology involve the same brain structures and neurotransmitters, making it difficult to assess the specificity of their contributions to particular disorders. Such findings may reflect the limitations of existing categorical diagnostic systems, as we have discussed earlier. Another limitation, until recently, has been the inability to link structural changes with functional changes. The further developmental and refinement of functional neuroimaging techniques, such as functional magnetic resonance imaging, has helped to improve this state of affairs.

Recent findings and technological advances in genetics have established the central role of these influences in understanding child psychopathology (e.g., Lombroso, Pauls, & Leckman, 1994; Rutter, Silberg, O'Connor, & Simonoff, 1999a, 1999b; Skuse, 2000; State et al., 2000). Clearly, both constitutional and environmental factors contribute to children's behavioral and emotional disorders (Rutter et al., 1997). As Torgersen (1993) states, "No behavior is independent of inborn endowments, and any behavior requires an environment in order to take place" (p. 42). Thus asking whether a specific form of child psychopathology is due to genetics or to environmental influences is both naive and futile. Rather, the more appropriate question is this: To what extent are given behaviors due to variations in genetic endowment, variations within the environment, or the interaction between these two factors?

Over the past decade, research in behavioral and molecular genetics has greatly increased our understanding of the mechanisms involved in a plethora of medical, neurological, and psychiatric disorders (Lombroso et al., 1994; State et al., 2000). Genetic influences have been implicated in most forms of child psychopathology (e.g., autistic disorder, ADHD, conduct disorder, Tourette's disorder, mood disorders, and schizophrenia; see State et al., 2000, for a review). There is also evidence to support the role of genetic influences in important developmental processes, such as temperament (Kagan & Snidman, 1991), emotion regulation (Baum, Grunberg, & Singer, 1992; Fox, 1994a), and executive functioning (Coolidge, Thede, & Young, 2000). However, despite increasing research support and enthusiasm for the role of genetic influences in childhood dysfunction (see, e.g., Faraone, Doyle, Mick, & Biederman, 2001), no specific mutations have yet been conclusively isolated or identified in their pathogenesis (State et al., 2000).

Familial aggregation is frequently an initial step in understanding the function of genetic mechanisms. Once familial clustering is demonstrated, more in-depth and costly twin studies, adoption studies, segregation analyses, and linkage studies can be conducted (cf. Szatmari, Boyle, & Offord, 1993). "Familial aggregation" refers to the nonrandom clustering of disorders or characteristics within a given family, relative to the random distribution of these disorders or characteristics in the general population (Szatmari et al., 1993). This paradigm rests on the premise that if there is a genetic component to a given disorder, the frequency of the phenotype (or manifest pathology) will be higher among biological relatives of the proband than in the general population (Lombroso et al., 1994).

Twin studies are beneficial in helping to ascertain the contribution of genetic factors in the etiology of child psychopathology. The twin study approach emerged from the long-standing "nature versus nurture" or "genes versus environment" debate (Lombroso et al., 1994). Although twin studies provide a powerful research strategy for examining the role of genetic influences in both psychiatric and nonpsychiatric disorders, numerous methodological issues necessitate that caution be exercised in interpreting findings. For example, although Willerman (1973) found a concordance rate for hyperactivity of approximately 70%, this does not necessarily mean that 70% of the variance in hyperactivity is accounted for by genetic variation. Research suggests, for instance, that monozygotic twins spend more time together, frequently engage in similar activities, and have many of the same friends in common (Torgersen, 1993). Thus the common or shared environment presents a potential confound in any twin study, and unless twins are reared apart, or dizygotic twins are employed as the comparison group, it becomes difficult to separate the effects of genetic and environmental influences. Representativeness and generalizability to the general population are other problems with twin studies (Lombroso et al., 1994; Torgersen, 1993). Growing up with a sibling of an identical age, for example, introduces its own special challenges (e.g., competition between siblings, greater dependency on each other) that make the twin environment unique.

Adoption studies have been used to circumvent some of the problems with twin and familial aggregation studies. They explicitly attempt to control for environmental variation in the heritability equation. The assumption behind this strategy is that when a disorder has a genetic etiology, the frequency of its expression should be greater among biological relatives than among adoptive relatives. Conversely, when environmental factors assume a larger role in the etiology of psychopathology, the frequency of the disorder would be expected to be greater among the parents of adoptive relatives than among biological parents (Lombroso et al., 1994; Torgersen, 1993). Lombroso and his collaborators reviewed the extant adoptive studies of childhood psychopathology as of 1984 and concluded that there was a paucity of research in this important area.

Several reasons may be advanced to account for the sparse number of investigations using the adoptive strategy. One obstacle has been the difficulty of attaining reliable information regarding the biological parents of adoptees. The timing of adoption placements also represents a potential confound. Since children are typically adopted at different ages, it is difficult to determine what environmental influences the biological parents may have had during the earliest years of life (Lombroso et al., 1994). Similarly, many children are placed in residential settings prior to adoption; these conditions, which may affect a child's development, would be unaccounted for by an adoptive strategy. A confound analogous to the problem of timing is the high probability of being placed in an adoptive home that is similar to the home environment of the biological family. For instance, adoption agencies are quite strict in their criteria for adequate placements, and the adoptive home must, at a minimum, meet current middle-class standards (Torgersen, 1993).

Recent research using molecular genetics has identified specific genes for autism (International Molecular Genetic Study of Autism Consortium, 1998), ADHD (Kuntsi & Stevenson, 2000), and Rett's disorder (Amir et al., 1999). The identification of specific genes has the potential to greatly enhance our understanding of a disorder, as well as its specific components (Stodgell, Ingram, & Hyman, 2000). However, the initial steps in identifying a specific gene for any disorder address only a small part of the genetic risk. Similar searches will be needed to identify other genes, and multiple interacting genes are a far more likely cause than is a single gene (Rutter, 2000a). Moveover, genetic influences are probabilistic rather than deterministic, and environmental and genetic factors are generally of about equal importance (Plomin & Rutter, 1998). Most forms of child psychopathology are polygenic, involving a number of susceptibility genes that interact with one another and with environmental influences to result in observed levels of impairment (State et al., 2000).

Many genetic research strategies are still in their technological infancy, and the goal of translating information from behavioral genetics to the implementation of treatment strategies (e.g., psychopharmacology) is far from being realized. Nevertheless, as discussed in subsequent chapters of this volume, genetic factors have been clearly implicated in many disorders, including autism, personality disorders, substance abuse and dependence, anxiety disorders, mood disorders, schizophrenia, ADHD, and reading disorders (State et al., 2000). There is also a broadened interest in including environmental considerations in genetic models of child psychopathology (Rutter et al., 1997, 1999a, 1999b).

SUMMARY AND CONCLUSIONS

In this introductory chapter, we have described a developmental–systems framework for child psychopathology that emphasizes three central themes: (1) the need to study child psychopathology in relation to ongoing normal and pathological developmental processes; (2) the importance of context in determining the expression and outcome of childhood disorders; and (3) the role of multiple and interacting events and processes in shaping both adaptive and maladaptive development. The research findings presented in the subsequent chapters of this volume illustrate the importance of these themes for understanding children and adolescents displaying a wide range of problems and/or conditions.

A developmental–systems framework eschews simple linear models of causality and advocates for a greater emphasis on systemic and developmental factors and their interactions in understanding child psychopathology. Multiple etiologies and their interplay represent the norm for most forms of child psychopathology. For example, in the study of conduct disorder, genetic influences, constitutional factors, insecure attachment relationships, impulsivity, biased cognitive processing, parental rejection, a lack of parental supervision, interpersonal difficulties, and many other influences have been implicated. However, many of these influences have also been implicated in other disorders, and not all children who experience them display conduct disorder. There is a need for research that will help to disentangle the role of these multiple sources of influence and their interactions in relation to different childhood disorders.

We have argued that all forms of child psychopathology are best conceptualized in terms of developmental trajectories, rather than as static entities, and that the expression and outcome for any problem will depend on the configuration and timing of a host of surrounding circumstances that include events both within and outside a child. For any dynamically changing developmental trajectory there also exists some degree of continuity and stability of structure, process, and function across time. Understanding such continuity and stability in the context of change represents a challenge for future research; it necessitates that psychopathology in children be studied over time, from a number of different vantage points, utilizing multiple methods, and drawing on knowledge from a variety of different disciplines.

Given the complexities associated with a developmental–systems framework for understanding child psychopathology, there is a clear need for theories to guide our research efforts. We have argued that a developmental psychopathology perspective provides a broad macroparadigm for conceptualizing and understanding childhood disorders in general, and that complementary disorder- and problem-specific theories are also needed to account for the specific configurations of variables commonly associated with particular disorders. Such problem-specific theories are presented in the subsequent chapters of this volume. The conceptualization of child psychopathology in terms of developmental trajectories, multiple influences, probabilistic relationships, and diverse outcomes suggests that some influences are likely to be common to many different disorders and that others are probably specific to particular problems. Our theories need to account for both types of influence.

The problems of childhood are universal; as a result, much folklore and many unsubstantiated theories exist about the causes of childhood difficulties and their remedies. As we have seen, childhood disorders constitute a significant societal problem, and in the absence of an empirically grounded knowledge base, unsubstantiated theories have frequently been used as the basis for developing solutions to these problems. There is a pressing need for longitudinal research to inform our intervention and prevention efforts. Such research is likely to require new ways of conceptualizing childhood disorders; far greater collaboration among disciplines than has previously been the case; and the use of more sophisticated design strategies and statistical tools, which will be sensitive to the multiple interacting influences and changes over time outlined in this chapter. Considerable advances have been made in all of these areas since the first edition of this book. The chapters in this volume provide a state-of-the-art review and critique of current definitions, theories, and research for a wide range of childhood disorders. They also identify current needs and forecast likely future directions for research into child psychopathology.

ACKNOWLEDGMENTS

During the preparation of this chapter, Eric J. Mash was supported by a University of Calgary Killam Resident Fellowship and by a sabbatical fellowship from the University of Calgary. David J. A. Dozois was supported by a fellowship from the Ontario Mental Health Foundation. This support is gratefully acknowledged.

NOTES

1. As a matter of convenience, we use the terms "children" and "child" in this chapter and volume to refer to children of all ages, from infancy through adolescence. The diversity within this wide age range will necessitate the use of more specific designations of age and developmental level as appropriate to each discussion. We have also opted to use the term "child psychopathology" rather than "developmental psychopathology." Either term would have been appropriate, since we view all disorders of childhood and adolescence as embedded in developmental processes and sequences. However, we use "child psychopathology" as the more general and theoretically neutral term to describe the full range of problems occurring during childhood and adolescence. For the most part, the two terms are used interchangeably in this volume. Other terms that have been used to describe problems during childhood are "abnormal child psychology," "childhood disorders," "atypical child development," "childhood behavior disorders," and "exceptional child development." These differences in terminology reflect the many disciplines and theoretical perspectives that are concerned with understanding and helping disturbed children.

2. These important and comprehensive reports are available at the following Web sites:

U.S. Public Health Service (1999): http://www.surgeongeneral.gov/library/mentalhealth/home.html
U.S. Public Health Service (2001a): http://www.surgeongeneral.gov/cmh/childreport.htm
U.S. Public Health Service (2001b): http://www.surgeongeneral.gov/library/youthviolence/
NAMHC Workgroup (2001): http://www.nimh.nih.gov/child/blueprint.cfm

3. We recognize that theory and research in child psychopathology need to be put to the test in the applied arena. However, in this volume we do not consider in any detail the range of assessment, treatment, or prevention strategies available for the problems under discussion. Our decision not to address assessment, treatment, and prevention in this volume was based on two factors. First, we perceived a need for a substantive review of what we currently know about childhood disorders. Many current treatments for childhood disorders are untested (Kazdin, 2000; Mash & Barkley, 1998), and it was felt that future efforts to test treatment approaches would benefit from a detailed discussion of our current knowledge base for child psychopathology. Second, we wished not to dilute the discussion of theory and research in child psychopathology by attempting to provide cursory coverage of assessment and intervention. Instead, we refer the reader to companion volumes to this one, which have as their primary focus child assessment (Mash & Terdal, 1997a) and child treatment (Mash & Barkley, 1998), respectively.

4. A complete discussion of the scope and complexity of issues surrounding the concept of harmful dysfunction is beyond the scope of this chapter. The reader is referred to papers in the *Journal of Abnormal Psychology* (see Clark, 1999, for an overview) and in *Behaviour Research and Therapy* (Houts, 2001; McNally, 2001; Wakefield, 1999a, 1999b, 2001) for excellent discussions of these and related issues.

REFERENCES

Achenbach, T. M. (1982). *Developmental psychopathology* (2nd ed.). New York: Wiley.

Achenbach, T. M. (1985). *Assessment and taxonomy of child and adolescent psychopathology*. Beverly Hills, CA: Sage.

Achenbach, T. M. (1991). *Manual for the Child Behavior Checklist/4–18 and 1991 Profile.* Burlington: University of Vermont, Department of Psychiatry.

Achenbach, T. M. (1993). *Empirically based taxonomy: How to use syndromes and profile types derived from the CBCL/4–18, TRF, and YSR.* Burlington: University of Vermont, Department of Psychiatry.

Achenbach, T. M. (1995). Diagnosis, assessment, and comorbidity in psychosocial treatment research. *Journal of Abnormal Psychology, 23,* 45–65.

Achenbach, T. M. (1997). What is normal? What is abnormal?: Developmental perspectives on behavioral and emotional problems. In S. S. Luthar, J. A. Burack, D. Cicchetti, & J. R. Weisz (Eds.), *Developmental psychopathology: Perspectives on adjustment, risk, and disorder* (pp. 93–114). Cambridge, England: Cambridge University Press.

Achenbach, T. M. (2000). Assessment of psychopathology. In A. J. Sameroff, M. Lewis, & S. M. Miller (Eds.), *Handbook of developmental psychopathology* (2nd ed., pp. 41–56). New York: Kluwer Academic/Plenum.

Achenbach, T. M. (2001). What are norms and why do we need valid ones? *Clinical Psychology: Science and Practice, 8,* 446–450.

Achenbach, T. M., & Dumenci, L. (2001). Advances in empirically based assessment: Revised cross-informant syndromes and new DSM-oriented scales for the CBCL, YSR, and TRF. Comment on Lengua, Sadowski, Friedrich, and Fisher (2001). *Journal of Consulting and Clinical Psychology, 69,* 699–702.

Achenbach, T. M., & Edelbrock, C. (1981). Behavioral problems and competencies reported by parents of normal and disturbed children aged four through sixteen. *Monographs of the Society for Research in Child Development, 46*(1, Serial No. 188).

Achenbach, T. M., & Edelbrock, C. (1989). Diagnostic, taxonomic, and assessment issues. In T. H. Ollendick & M. Hersen (Eds.), *Handbook of child psychopathology* (2nd ed., pp. 53–73). New York: Plenum Press.

Achenbach, T. M., Howell, C. T., Quay, H. C., & Conners, C. K. (1991). National survey of problems and competencies among four- to sixteen-year-olds. *Monographs of the Society for Research in Child Development, 56*(3, Serial No. 225).

Achenbach, T. M., McConaughy, S. H., & Howell, C. T. (1987). Child/adolescent behavioral and emotional problems: Implications of cross-informant correlations for situational specificity. *Psychological Bulletin, 101,* 213–232.

Adams, H. E., Doster, J. A., & Calhoun, K. S. (1977). A psychologically-based system of response classification. In A. R. Ciminero, K. S. Calhoun, & H. E. Adams (Eds.), *Handbook of behavioral assessment* (pp. 47–78). New York: Wiley.

Adelman, H. S. (1995). Clinical psychology: Beyond psychopathology and clinical interventions. *Clinical Psychology: Science and Practice, 2,* 28–44.

Adelman, H. S., & Taylor, L. (1993). *Learning problems and learning disabilities: Moving forward.* Pacific Grove, CA: Brooks/Cole.

Alloy, L. B., Abramson, L. T., Tashman, N. A., Berrebbi, D. S., Hogan, M. E., Whitehouse, W. G., Crossfield, A. G., & Moroco, A. (2001). Developmental origins of cognitive vulnerability to depression: Parenting, cognitive, and inferential feedback styles of the parents of individuals at high and low cognitive risk for depression. *Cognitive Therapy and Research, 25,* 397–423.

American Psychiatric Association (APA). (1952). *Diagnostic and statistical manual of mental disorders.* Washington, DC: Author.

American Psychiatric Association (APA). (1968). *Diagnostic and statistical manual of mental disorders* (2nd ed.). Washington, DC: Author.

American Psychiatric Association (APA). (1980). *Diagnostic and statistical manual of mental disorders* (3rd ed.). Washington, DC: Author.

American Psychiatric Association (APA). (1987). *Diagnostic and statistical manual of mental disorders* (3rd ed., rev.). Washington, DC: Author.

American Psychiatric Association (APA). (1994). *Diagnostic and statistical manual of mental disorders* (4th ed.). Washington, DC: Author.

American Psychiatric Association (APA). (2000). *Diagnostic and statistical manual of mental disorders* (4th ed. *text rev.*). Washington, DC: Author.

Amir, R. E., Van den Veyver, I. B., Wan, M., Tran, C. Q., Francke, U., & Zoghbi, H, Y. (1999). Rett syndrome is caused by mutations in *X-linked MECP2, encoding methyl-CpG-binding protein 2. Nature Genetics, 23,* 185–188.

Anderson, J. C., Williams, S., McGee, R., & Silva, P. A. (1987). DSM-III disorders in preadolescent children: Prevalence in a large sample from the general population. *Archives of General Psychiatry, 44,* 69–76.

Angold, A., Costello, E. J., & Erkanli, A. (1999). Comorbidity. *Journal of Child Psychology and Psychiatry, 40,* 57–87.

Angold, A., Costello, E. J., Erkanli, A., & Worthman, C. M. (1999). Pubertal changes in hormone levels and depression in girls. *Psychological Medicine, 29,* 1043–1053.

Angold, A., Costello, E. J., Farmer, E. M. Z., Burns, B. J., & Erkanli, A. (1999). Impaired but undiagnosed. *Journal of the American Academy of Child and Adolescent Psychiatry, 38,* 129–137.

Aries, P. (1962). *Centuries of childhood.* New York: Vintage Books.

Arkowitz, H. (1992). Integrative theories of therapy. In D. K. Freedheim (Ed.), *History of psychotherapy: A century of change* (pp. 261–303). Washington, DC: American Psychological Association.

Arsenio, W. F. & Lemerise, E. A. (2001). Varieties of childhood bullying: Values, emotion processes, and social competence. *Social Development, 10,* 59–73.

Baker, R. (1996). *Sperm wars: The science of success.* New York: Basic Books.

Bandura, A. (1977). *Social learning theory.* Englewood Cliffs, NJ: Prentice Hall.

Bandura, A. (1986). *Social foundations of thought and action: A social cognitive theory.* Englewood Cliffs, NJ: Prentice-Hall.

Barkley, R. A. (1997). *ADHD and the nature of self-control.* New York: Guilford Press.

Barkley, R. A. (2001). The executive functions and self-regulation: An evolutionary neuropsychological perspective. *Neuropsychology Review, 11,* 1–29.

Barnett, D., & Vondra, J. I. (Eds.). (1999). Atypical attachment in infancy and early childhood among children at developmental risk. *Monographs of the Society for Research in Child Development, 64*(3, Serial No. 258), 1–24.

Baron-Cohen, S. (2000). Is Asperger syndrome/high functioning autism necessarily a disability? *Development and Psychopathology, 12,* 489–500.

Barton, S. (1994). Chaos, self-organization, and psychology. *American Psychologist, 49,* 5–14.

Baum, A., Grunberg, N. E., & Singer, J. E. (1992). Biochemical measurements in the study of emotion. *Psychological Science, 3,* 56–59.

Beauchaine, T. P. (2001). Vagal tone, development, and Gray's motivational theory: Toward an integrated model of autonomic nervous system functioning in psychopathology. *Development and Psychopathology, 13,* 183–214.

Beck, A. T. (1964). Thinking and depression: Theory and therapy. *Archives of General Psychiatry, 10,* 561–571.

Beck, A. T., Rush, A. J., Shaw, B. F., & Emery, G. (1979). *Cognitive therapy of depression.* New York: Guilford Press.

Bell-Dolan, D., J., Foster, S. L., & Mash, E. J. (in press). *Handbook of behavioral and emotional problems in girls.* New York: Kluwer Academic/Plenum.

Belsky, J., Friedman, S. L., & Hsieh, K. H. (2001). Testing a core emotion-regulation prediction: Does early attentional persistence moderate the effect of infant negative emotionality on later development? *Child Development, 72,* 123–133.

Bergman, L. R., & Magnusson, D. (1997). A person-oriented approach in research on developmental psychopathology. *Development and Psychopathology, 9,* 291–319.

Bettelheim, B. (1967). *The empty fortress.* New York: Free Press.

Biederman, J., Mick, E., Faraone, S. V., Doyle, A., Spencer, T., Wilens, T. E., Frazier, E., & Johnson, M. A. (2002). Influence of gender on attention deficit hyperactivity disorder in children referred to a psychiatric clinic. *American Journal of Psychiatry, 159,* 36–42.

Bijou, S. W., & Baer, D. M. (1961). *Child development: Systematic and empirical theory.* New York: Appleton-Century-Crofts.

Bird, H. R., Canino, G. J., Davies, M., Zhang, H., Ramirez, R., & Lahey, B. B. (2001). Prevalence and correlates of antisocial behavior among three ethnic groups. *Journal of Abnormal Child Psychology, 29,* 465–478.

Bird, H. R., Canino, G., J. Rubio-Stipec, M., Gould, M. S., Ribera, J., Sesman, M., Woodbury, M., Huertas-Goldman, S., Pagan, A., Sanchez-Lacay, A., & Moscoso, M. (1988). Estimates of the prevalence of childhood maladjustment in a community survey of Puerto Rico: The use of combined measures. *Archives of General Psychiatry, 45,* 1120–1126.

Bird, H. R., Gould, M. S., Yager, T., Staghezza, B., & Camino, G. (1989). Risk factors for maladjustment in Puerto Rican children. *Journal of the American Academy of Child and Adolescent Psychiatry, 28,* 847–850.

Blair, R. J. R., Colledge, E., & Mitchell, D. V. G. (2001). Somatic markers and response reversal: Is there orbitofrontal cortex dysfunction in boys with psychopathic tendencies. *Journal of Abnormal Child Psychology, 29,* 499–511.

Blair, R. J. R., Colledge, E., Murray, L., & Mitchell, D. V. G. (2001). A selective impairment in the processing of sad and fearful expressions in children with psychopathic tendencies. *Journal of Abnormal Child Psychology, 29,* 491–498.

Blashfield, R. K., McElroy, R. A., Jr., Pfohl, B., & Blum, N. (1994). Comorbidity and the prototype model. *Clinical Psychology: Science and Practice, 1,* 96–99.

Borstelmann, L. J. (1983). Children before psychology: Ideas about children from antiquity to the late 1800s. In P. H. Mussen (Series Ed.) & W. Kessen (Vol. Ed.), *Handbook of child psychology: Vol. 1. History, theory, and methods* (4th ed., pp. 1–40). New York: Wiley.

Bowlby, J. (1973). *Attachment and loss: Vol. 2. Separation: Anxiety and anger.* New York: Basic Books.

Bowlby, J. (1988). *A secure base: Parent–child attachment and healthy human development.* New York: Basic Books.

Boyle, M. H., Offord, D. R., Hoffman, H. G., Catlin, G. P., Byles, J. A., Cadman, D. T., Crawford, J. W., Links, P. S., Rae-Grant, N. I., & Szatmari, P. (1987). Ontario Child Health Study: I. Methodology. *Archives of General Psychiatry, 44,* 826–831.

Bradley, R. H., Corwyn, R. F., Burchinal, M., McAdoo, H. P., & Garcia Coll, C. (2001). The home environments of children in the United States: II. Relations with behavioral development through age thirteen. *Child Development, 72,* 1868–1886.

Bradley, R. H., Corwyn, R. F., McAdoo, H. P., & García Coll, C. (2001). The home environments of children in the United States: I. Variations by age, ethnicity, and poverty status. *Child Development, 72,* 1844–1867.

Brady, E. U., & Kendall, P. C. (1992). Comorbidity of anxiety and depression in children and adolescents. *Psychological Bulletin, 111,* 244–255.

Brandenburg, N. A., Friedman, R. M., & Silver, S. E. (1990). The epidemiology of childhood psychiatric disorders: Prevalence findings from recent studies. *Journal of the American Academy of Child and Adolescent Psychiatry, 29,* 76–83.

Braswell, L., & Kendall, P. C. (2001). Cognitive-behavioral therapy with youth. In K. S. Dobson (Ed.), *Handbook of cognitive-behavioral therapies* (2nd ed., pp. 246–294). New York: Guilford Press.

Bray, J. H. (1994). *Family assessment: Current issues in evaluating families.* Unpublished manuscript, Department of Family Medicine, Baylor College of Medicine, Houston, TX.

Bray, J. H. (1995). Methodological advances in family psychology research: Introduction to the special section. *Journal of Family Psychology, 9,* 107–109.

Bray, J. H., Maxwell, S. E., & Cole, D. (1995). Multivariate statistics for family psychology research. *Journal of Family Psychology, 9,* 144–160.

Bretherton, I. (1995). Attachment theory and developmental psychopathology. In D. Cicchetti & S. L. Toth (Eds.), *Emotion, cognition, and representation* (Vol. 6, pp. 231–260). Rochester, NY: University of Rochester Press.

Briggs-Gowan, M. J., Carter, A. S., Skuban, E., & Horwitz, S. (2001). Prevalence of social-emotional and behavioral problems in a community sample of 1- and 2-year-old children. *Journal of the American Academy of Child and Adolescent Psychiatry, 40*, 811–819.

Bronfenbrenner, U. (1977). Toward an experimental ecology of human development. *American Psychologist, 32*, 513–531.

Bryson, S. E., & Smith, I. M. (1998). Epidemiology of autism: Prevalence, associated characteristics, and implications for research and service delivery. *Mental Retardation and Developmental Disabilities Research Reviews, 4*, 97–103.

Bugental, D. B. (1993). Communication in abusive relationships: Cognitive constructions of interpersonal power. *American Behavioral Scientist, 36*, 288–308.

Burns, B. J., Costello, E. J., Angold, A., Tweed, D., Stangl, D., Farmer, E. M. Z., & Erkanli, A. (1995). Data watch: Children's mental health service use across service sectors. *Health Affairs, 14*, 147–159.

Burt, S. A., Krueger, R. F., McGue, M., & Iacono, W. G. (2001). Sources of covariation among attention-deficit/hyperactivity disorder, oppositional defiant disorder, and conduct disorder: The importance of shared environment. *Journal of Abnormal Psychology, 110*, 516–525.

Campbell, S. B. (1989). Developmental perspectives. In T. H. Ollendick & M. Hersen (Eds.), *Handbook of child psychopathology* (2nd ed., pp. 5–28). New York: Plenum Press.

Cantor, N., Smith, E. E., French, R. S., & Mezzich, J. (1980). Psychiatric diagnosis as prototype categorization. *Journal of Abnormal Psychology, 89*, 181–193.

Cantwell, D. P. (1996). Classification of child and adolescent psychopathology. *Journal of Child Psychology and Psychiatry, 37*, 3–12.

Carey, G., & DiLalla, D. L. (1994). Personality and psychopathology: Genetic perspectives. *Journal of Abnormal Psychology, 103*, 32–43.

Carlson, C. L., & Tamm, L. (2000). Responsiveness of children with attention deficit-hyperactivity disorder to reward and response cost: Differential impact on performance and motivation. *Journal of Consulting and Clinical Psychology, 68*, 73–83.

Caron, C., & Rutter, M. (1991). Comorbidity in child psychopathology: Concepts, issues, and research strategies. *Journal of Child Psychology and Psychiatry, 32*, 1063–1080.

Carter, J. D., & Swanson, H. L. (1995). The relationship between intelligence and vigilance in children at risk. *Journal of Abnormal Child Psychology, 23*, 201–220.

Caspi, A. (2000). The child is father of the man: Personality continuities from childhood to adulthood. *Journal of Personality and Social Psychology, 78*, 158–172.

Caspi, A., Taylor, A., Moffitt, T. E., & Plomin, R. (2000). Neighborhood deprivation affects children's mental health: Environmental risks idenitified in a genetic design. *Psychological Science, 11*, 338–342.

Cass, L. K., & Thomas, C. B. (1979). *Childhood pathology and later adjustment.* New York: Wiley.

Cassidy, J. (1994). Emotion regulation: Influences of attachment relationships. In N. A. Fox (Ed.), The development of emotion regulation: Biological and behavioral considerations. *Monographs of the Society for Research in Child Development, 59*(2–3, Serial No. 240), 228–249.

Cassidy, J., & Shaver, P. R. (Eds.). (1999). *Handbook of attachment: Theory, research, and clinical applications.* New York: Guilford Press.

Catalano, R. F., Hawkins, J. D., Krenz, C., Gilmore, M., Morrison, D., Wells, E., & Abbott, R. (1993). Using research to guide culturally appropriate drug abuse prevention. *Journal of Consulting and Clinical Psychology, 61*, 804–811.

Cattell, R. B. (1938). *Crooked personalities in childhood and after.* New York: Appleton-Century.

Chen, X., Rubin, K. H., & Li, Z. Y. (1995). Social functioning and adjustment in Chinese children: A longitudinal study. *Developmental Psychology, 31*, 531–539.

Cicchetti, D. (1984). The emergence of developmental psychopathology. *Child Development, 55*, 1–7.

Cicchetti, D. (1990). An historical perspective on the discipline of developmental psychopathology. In J. Rolf, A. Masten, D. Cicchetti, K. Nuechterlein, & S. Weintraub (Eds.), *Risk and protective factors in the development of psychopathology* (pp. 2–28). New York: Cambridge University Press.

Cicchetti, D., & Aber, J. L. (Eds.). (1998). Contextualism and developmental psychopathology [Special issue]. *Development and Psychopathology, 10*(2).

Cicchetti, D., Ackerman, B. P., & Izard, C. E. (1995). Emotions and emotion regulation in developmental psychopathology. *Development and Psychopathology, 7*, 1–10.

Cicchetti, D., & Cannon, T. D. (1999). Neurodevelopmental processes in the ontogenesis and epigenesis of pychopathology. *Development and Psychopathology, 11*, 375–393.

Cicchetti, D., & Cohen, D. J. (1995a). *Developmental psychopathology: Risk, disorder, and adaptation* (Vol. 2). New York: Wiley.

Cicchetti, D., & Cohen, D. J. (1995b). *Developmental psychopathology: Theory and methods* (Vol. 1). New York: Wiley.

Cicchetti, D., & Garmezy, N. (1993). Prospects and promises in the study of resilience. *Development and Psychopathology, 4*, 497–502.

Cicchetti, D., & Izard, C. E. (Eds.). (1995). Emotions in developmental psychopathology [Special issue]. *Developmental Psychopathology, 7*(1).

Cicchetti, D., & Manly, J. T. (Eds.). (2001). Operationalizing child maltreatment: Developmental processes and outcomes [Special issue]. *Development and Psychopathology, 13*(4).

Cicchetti, D., Rappaport, J., Sandler, I., & Weissberg, R. P. (Eds.). (2000). *The promotion of wellness in children and adolescents.* Washington, DC: Child Welfare League of America.

Cicchetti, D., & Richters, J. E. (1993). Developmental considerations in the investigation of conduct disorder. *Development and Psychopathology, 5*, 331–344.

Cicchetti, D., & Rogosch, F. A. (1996). Equifinality and multifinality in developmental psychopathology. *Development and Psychopathology, 8*, 597–600.

Cicchetti, D., & Rogosch, F. A. (1999). Conceptual and methodological issues in developmental psychopathology research. In P. C. Kendall & J. N. Butcher (Eds.), *Handbook of research methods in clinical psychology* (2nd ed., pp. 433–465). New York: Wiley.

Cicchetti, D., & Sroufe, L. A. (2000). The past as prologue to the future: The times, they've been a-changin'. *Development and Psychopathology, 12*, 255–264.

Cicchetti, D., & Toth, S. L. (1997). Transactional ecological systems in developmental psychopathology. In S. S. Luthar, J. A. Burack, D. Cicchetti, & J. R. Weisz (Eds.), *Developmental psychopathology: Perspectives on adjustment, risk, and disorder* (pp. 317–349). Cambridge, England: Cambridge University Press.

Cicchetti, D., & Toth, S. L. (2000). Social policy implications of research in developmental psychopathology, *Developmental Psychopathology, 12*, 551–554.

Cicchetti, D., Toth, S. L., & Lynch, M. (1995). Bowlby's dream comes full circle: The application of attachment theory to risk and psychopathology. *Advances in Clinical Child Psychology, 17*, 1–75.

Cicchetti, D., & Tucker, D. (1994). Development and self-regulatory structures of the mind. *Development and Psychopathology, 6,* 533–549.

Cicchetti, D., & Walker, E. F. (2001). Stress and development: Biological and psychological consequences [Editorial]. *Development and Psychopathology, 13*, 413–418.

Clementz, B. A., & Iacono, W. G. (1993). Nosology and diagnosis. In A. S. Bellack & M. Hersen (Eds.), *Psychopathology in adulthood* (pp. 3–20). Boston: Allyn & Bacon.

Clark, D. A., Beck, A. T., & Alford, B. A. (1999). *Scientific foundations of cognitive theory and therapy of depression.* New York: Wiley.

Clark, L. A. (1999). Introduction to the special section on the concept of disorder. *Journal of Abnormal Psychology, 108*, 371–373.

Cohen, J. (1988). *Statistical power analysis for the behavioral sciences* (2nd ed.). New York: Academic Press.

Cohen, M. (1998). The monetary value of saving a high risk youth. *Journal of Quantitative Criminology, 14*, 5–34.

Cole, P. M., Michel, M. K., & Teti, L. O. (1994). The development of emotion regulation and dysregulation: A clinical perspective. In N. A. Fox (Ed.), The development of emotion regulation: Biological and behavioral considerations. *Monographs of the Society for Research in Child Development, 59*(2–3, Serial No. 240), 53–72.

Compas, B. E., & Oppedisano, G. (2000). Mixed anxiety/depression in childhood and adolescence. In A. J. Sameroff, M. Lewis, & S. M. Miller (Eds.), *Handbook of developmental psychopathology* (2nd ed., pp. 531–548). New York: Kluwer Academic/Plenum.

Coolidge, F. L., Thede, L. L., & Young, S. E. (2000). Heritability and the comorbidity of attention deficit hyperactivity disorder with behavioral disorders and executive function deficits: A preliminary investigation. *Developmental Neuropsychology, 17*, 273–287.

Contreras, J. M., Kerns, K. A., Weimer, B. L., Gentzler, A., & Tomich, P. L. (2000). Emotion regulation as a mediator of associations between mother–child attachment and peer relationships in middle childhood. *Journal of Family Psychology, 14,* 111–124.

Costello, E. J. (1989). Developments in child psychiatric epidemiology. *Journal of the American Academy of Child and Adolescent Psychiatry, 28,* 836–841.

Costello, E. J., & Angold, A. (2000). Developmental epidemiology: A framework for developmental psychopathology. In A. J. Sameroff, M. Lewis, & S. M. Miller (Eds.), *Handbook of developmental psychopathology* (2nd ed., pp. 57–73). New York: Kluwer Academic/Plenum.

Costello, E. J., & Angold, A. (2001). Bad behaviour: An historical perspective on disorders of conduct. In J. Hill & B. Maughan (Eds.), *Conduct disorders in childhood and adolescence* (pp. 1–31). New York: Cambridge University Press.

Costello, E. J., Farmer, E. M. Z. & Angold, A. (1999). Same place, different children: White and American Indian children in the Appalachian Mountains. In P. Cohen & C. Slomkowski (Eds.), *Historical and geographical influences on psychopathology* (pp. 279–298). Mahwah, NJ: Erlbaum.

Costello, E. J., Farmer, E. M. Z., Angold, A., Burns, B. J., & Erkanli, A. (1997). Psychiatric disorders among American Indian and white youth in Appalachia: The Great Smoky Mountains Study. *American Journal of Public Health, 87*, 827–832.

Courchesne, E., Chisum, H., & Townsend, J. (1994). Neural-activity-dependent brain changes in development: Implications for psychopathology. *Development and Psychopathology, 6,* 697–722.

Coy, K., Speltz, M. L., DeKlyen, M., & Jones, K. (2001). Social-cognitive processes in preschool boys with and without oppositional defiant disorder. *Journal of Abnormal Child Psychology, 29,* 107–119.

Crick, N. R., & Dodge, K. A. (1994). A review and reformulation of social information-processing mechanisms in children's social adjustment. *Psychological Bulletin, 115,* 73–101.

Crittenden, P. M., Claussen, A. H., & Sugarman, D. B. (1994). Physical and psychological maltreatment in middle childhood and adolescence. *Development and Psychopathology, 6,* 145–164.

Cummings, E. M., & Davies, P. T. (1995). The impact of parents on their children: An emotional security perspective. *Annals of Child Development, 10,* 167–208.

Cummings, E. M., & Davies, P. T. (1996). Emotional security as a regulatory process in normal development and the development of psychopathology. *Development and Psychopathology, 8,* 123–139.

Cummings, E. M., Hennessy, K. D., Rabideau, G. J., & Cicchetti, D. (1994). Responses of physically abused boys to interadult anger involving their mothers. *Development and Psychopathology, 6,* 31–41.

Dare, C. (1985). Psychoanalytic theories of development. In M. Rutter & L. Hersov (Eds.), *Child and adolescent psychiatry: Modern approaches* (2nd ed., pp. 205–215). Oxford: Blackwell Scientific.

Davies, P. T., & Cummings, E. M. (1994). Marital conflict and child adjustment: An emotional security hypothesis. *Psychological Bulletin, 116,* 387–411.

Davies, P. T., & Cummings, E. M. (1995). Children's emotions as organizers of their reactions to interadult anger: A functionalist perspective. *Developmental Psychology, 31,* 677–684.

Dawson, G., Frey, K., Self, J., Panagiotides, H., Hessl, D., Yamada, E., & Rinaldi, J. (1999). Frontal brain electrical activity in infants of depressed and nondepressed mothers: Relations to variations in infant behavior. *Development and Psychopathology, 11*, 589–605.

Dawson, G., Hessl, D., & Frey, K. (1994). Social influences on early developing biological and behavioral systems related to risk for affective disorder. *Development and Psychopathology, 6,* 759–779.

Deater-Deckard, K. (2001). Annotation: Recent research examining the role of peer relationships in the development of psychopathology. *Journal of Child Psychology and Psychiatry, 42*, 565–579.

Deater-Deckard, K., & Dunn, J. (1999). Multiple risks and adjustment in young children growing up in different family settings: A British community study of stepparent, single mother, and nondivorced families. In E. M. Hetherington (Ed.), *Coping with divorce, single parenting, and remarriage: A risk and resiliency perspective* (pp. 47–64). Mahwah, NJ: Erlbaum.

De Bellis, M. D. (2001). Developmental traumatology: The psychobiological development of maltreated children and its implications for research, treatment, and policy. *Development and Psychopathology, 13*, 539–564.

del Carmen, R., & Huffman, L. (1996). Epilogue: Bridging the gap between research on attachment and psychopathology. *Journal of Consulting and Clinical Psychology, 64*, 291–294.

Dobson, K. S., & Dozois, D. J. A. (2001). Historical and philosophical bases of the cognitive-behavioral therapies. In K. S. Dobson (Ed.), *Handbook of cognitive-behavioral therapies* (2nd ed., pp. 3–39). New York: Guilford Press.

Dobson, K. S., & Kendall, P. C. (1993). Future trends for research and theory in cognition and psychopathology. In K. S. Dobson & P. C. Kendall (Eds.), *Psychopathology and cognition* (pp. 475–486). San Diego, CA: Academic Press.

Dobson, K. S., & Shaw, B. F. (1987). Specificity and stability of self-referent encoding in clinical depression. *Journal of Abnormal Psychology, 96*, 34–40.

Dodge, K. A., & Crick, N. R. (1990). Social information-processing bases of aggressive behavior in children. *Personality and Social Psychology Bulletin, 16*, 8–22.

Dodge, K. A., & Newman, J. P. (1981) Biased decision-making processes in aggressive boys. *Journal of Abnormal Psychology, 90*, 375–379.

Dodge, K. A., Pettit, G. S., & Bates, J. E. (1994). Effects of physical maltreatment on the development of peer relations. *Development and Psychopathology, 6*, 43–55.

Dodge, K. A., & Somberg, D. R. (1987). Hostile attributional biases among aggressive boys are exacerbated under conditions of threats to the self. *Child Development, 58*, 213–224.

Donohue, B., Hersen, M., & Ammerman, R. T. (2000). Historical overview. In M. Hersen & R. T. Ammerman (Eds.), *Advanced abnormal child psychology* (2nd ed., pp. 3–14). Mahwah, NJ: Erlbaum.

Dozier, M., & Lee, S. (1995). Discrepancies between self- and other-report of psychiatric symptomatology: Effects of dismissing attachment strategies. *Development and Psychopathology, 7*, 217–226.

Dozois, D. J. A., & Dobson, K. S. (2001b). Information processing and cognitive organization in unipolar depression: Specificity and comorbidity issues. *Journal of Abnormal Psychology, 110*, 236–246.

Dozois, D. J. A., & Dobson, K. S. (2001a). A longitudinal investigation of information processing and cognitive organization in clinical depression: Stability of schematic interconnectedness. *Journal of Consulting and Clinical Psychology, 69*, 914–925.

DuBois, D. L., & Tevendale, H. D. (1999). Self-esteem in childhood and adolescence: Vaccine or epiphenomenon? *Applied and Preventive Psychology, 8*, 103–117.

Duggal, S., Carlson, E. A., Sroufe, A., & Egeland, B. (2001). Depressive symptomatology in childhood and adolescence. *Development and Psychopathology, 13*, 143–164.

Duhig, A. M., Renk, K., Epstein, M. K., & Phares, V. (2000). Interparental agreement on internalizing, externalizing, and total behavior problems: A meta-analysis. *Clinical Psychology: Science and Practice, 7*, 435–453.

Duncan, G. J., Brooks-Gunn, J., & Klebanov, P. K. (1994). Economic deprivation and early-childhood development. *Child Development, 65*, 296–318.

Earls, F. J. (1980). Prevalence of behavior problems in 3-year-old children. *Archives of General Psychiatry, 37*, 1153–1157.

Eaves, L. J., Silberg, J. L., Maes, H. H., Simonoff, E., Pickles, A., Rutter, M., Neale, M. C., Reynolds, C. A., Erikson, M. T., Heath, A. C., Loeber, R., Truett, K. R., & Hewitt, J. K. (1997). Genetics and developmental psychopathology: 2. The main effects of genes and environment on behavioral problems in the Virginia Twin Study of Adolescent Behavioral Development. *Journal of Child Psychology and Psychiatry, 38*, 965–980.

Edelbrock, C. (1984). Developmental considerations. In T. H. Ollendick & M. Hersen (Eds.), *Child behavioral assessment: Principles and procedures* (pp. 20–37). New York: Pergamon Press.

Egeland, B., & Heister, M. (1995). The long-term consequences of infant day-care and mother–infant attachment. *Child Development, 66*, 474–485.

Egger, H. L., Costello, E. J., Erkanli, A., & Angold, A. (1999). Somatic complaints and psychopathology in children and adolescents: Stomach aches, musculoskeletal pains, and headaches. *Journal of the American Academy of Child and Adolescent Psychiatry, 38*, 852–860.

Eisenberg, N., Fabes, R. A., Guthrie, I. K., & Reiser, M. (2000). Dispositional emotionality and regulation: Their role in predicting quality of social functioning. *Journal of Personality and Social Psychology, 78*, 136–157.

Eisenberg, N., Pidada, S., & Liew, J. (2001). The relations of regulation and negative emotionality to Indonesian children's social functioning. *Child Development, 72*, 1747–1763.

El-Sheikh, M. (2001). Parental drinking problems and children's adjustment: Vagal regulation and emotional reactivity as pathways and moderators of risk. *Journal of Abnormal Psychology, 110*, 499–515.

Eme, R. F. (1979). Sex differences in childhood psychopathology: A review. *Psychological Bulletin, 86*, 574–595.

Eme, R. F. (1992). Selective female affliction in development of disorders of childhood: A literature review. *Journal of Clinical Child Psychology, 21*, 354–364.

Emery, R. E., & Laumann-Billings, L. (1998). An overview of the nature, causes, and consequences of abusive family relationships: Toward differentiating maltreatment from violence. *American Psychologist, 53*, 121–135.

Emery, R. E., Waldron, M., Kitzmann, K. M., & Aaron, J. (1999). Delinquent behavior, future divorce or nonmarital childbearing, and externalizing behavior among offspring: A 14-year prospective study. *Journal of Family Psychology, 13*, 568–579.

Epkins, C. C. (2000). Cognitive specificity in internalizing and externalizing problems in community and clinic-referred children. *Journal of Clinical Child Psychology, 29*, 199–208.

Eppright, T. D., Bradley, S., & Sanfacon, J. A. (1998). The diagnosis of infant psychopathology: Current challenges and recent contributions. *Child Psychiatry and Human Development, 28*, 213–222.

Evans, B., & Lee, B. K. (1998). Culture and child psychopathology. In S. S. Kazarian & D. R. Evans (Eds.), *Cultural clinical psychology: Theory, research, and practice* (pp. 289–315). New York: Oxford University Press.

Faraone, S. V., Doyle, A. E., Mick, E., & Biederman, J. (2001). Meta-analysis of the association between the 7-Repeat allele of the dopamine D4 receptor gene and attention deficit hyperactivity disorder. *American Journal of Psychiatry, 158*, 1052–1057.

Feingold, B. (1975). *Why your child is hyperactive*. New York: Random House.

Feldman, S., & Downey, G. (1994). Rejection sensitivity as a mediator of the impact of childhood exposure to family violence on adult attachment behavior. *Development and Psychopathology, 6,* 231–247.

Feiring, C., & Lewis, M. (1996). Finality in the eye of the beholder: Multiple sources, multiple time points, multiple paths. *Development and Psychopathology, 8,* 721–733.

Fiese, B. H., Wilder, J., & Bickham, N. L. (2000). Family context in developmental psychopathology. In A. J. Sameroff, M. Lewis, & S. M. Miller (Eds.), *Handbook of developmental psychopathology* (2nd ed., pp. 115–134). New York: Kluwer Academic/Plenum.

Fischer, K. W., Ayoub, C., Singh, I., Noam, G., Maraganore, A., & Rayna, P. (1997). Psychopathology as adaptive development along distinctive pathways. *Development and Psychopathology, 9,* 749–779.

Fisman, S., & Fisman, R. (1999). Cultural influences on symptom presentation in childhood. *Journal of the American Academy of Child and Adolescent Psychiatry, 38,* 782–783.

Flavell, J. H., Flavell, E. R., & Green, F. L. (2001). Development of children's understanding of connections between thinking and feeling. *Psychological Science, 12,* 430–432.

Follette, W. C., & Houts, A. C. (1996). Models of scientific progress and the role of theory in taxonomy development: A case study of the DSM. *Journal of Consulting and Clinical Psychology, 64,* 1120–1132.

Fombonne, E. (1999). The epidemiology of autism: A review. *Psychological Medicine, 29,* 769–786.

Fonagy, P., & Target, M. (2000). The place of psychodynamic theory in developmental psychopathology. *Development and Psychopathology, 12,* 407–425.

Foster, S. L., & Martinez, C. R., Jr. (1995). Ethnicity: Conceptual and methodological issues in child clinical research. *Journal of Clinical Child Psychology, 24,* 214–226.

Fox, N. A. (1994a). Dynamic cerebral processes underlying emotion regulation. In N. A. Fox (Ed.), The development of emotion regulation: Biological and behavioral considerations. *Monographs of the Society for Research in Child Development, 59*(2–3, Serial No. 240), 152–166.

Fox, N. A. (Ed.). (1994b). The development of emotion regulation: Biological and behavioral considerations. *Monographs of the Society for Research in Child Development, 59*(2–3, Serial No. 240).

Francis, D. J., Fletcher, J. M., Stuebing, K. K., Davidson, K. C., & Thompson, N. M. (1991). Analysis of change: Modeling individual growth. *Journal of Consulting and Clinical Psychology, 59,* 27–37.

Fredrickson, B. L. (2001). The role of positive emotions in positive psychology: The broaden-and-build theory of positive emotions. *American Psychologist, 56,* 218–226.

Freitas, A. L., & Downey, G. (1998). Resilience: A dynamic perspective. *International Journal of Behavioral Development, 22,* 263–285.

French, V. (1977). History of the child's influence: Ancient Mediterranean civilizations. In R. Q. Bell & L. V. Harper (Eds.), *Child effects on adults* (pp. 3–29). Hillsdale, NJ: Erlbaum.

Frick, P. J. (2000). Laboratory and performance-based measures of childhood disorders. *Journal of Clinical Child Psychology, 29,* 475–478.

Friman, P. C., Larzelere, R., & Finney, J. W. (1994). Exploring the relationship between thumbsucking and psychopathology. *Journal of Pediatric Psychology, 19,* 431–441.

Gadow, K. D., Sprafkin, J., & Nolan, E. E. (2001). DSM-IV symptoms in community and clinic preschool children. *Journal of the American Academy of Child and Adolescent Psychiatry, 40,* 1383–1392.

Garber, J. (1984). Classification of childhood psychopathology: A developmental perspective. *Child Development, 55,* 30–48.

Garber, J., & Dodge, K. A. (Eds.). (1991). *The development of emotion regulation and dysregulation.* New York: Cambridge University Press.

Garber, J., & Flynn, C. (2001). Vulnerability to depression in childhood and adolescence. In R. E. Ingram & J. M. Price (Eds.), *Vulnerability to psychopathology: Risk across the lifespan* (pp. 175–225). New York: Guilford Press.

García Coll, C., Akerman, A., & Cicchetti, D. (2000). Cultural influence on developmental processes and outcomes: Implications for the study of development and psychopathology. *Development and Psychopathology, 12,* 333–356.

García Coll, C., & Garrido, M. (2000). Minorities in the United States: Sociocultural context for mental health and developmental psychopathology. In A. J. Sameroff, M. Lewis, & S. M. Miller (Eds.), *Handbook of developmental psychopathology* (2nd ed., pp. 177–195). New York: Kluwer Academic/Plenum.

Garmezy, N., Masten, N. S., & Tellegen, A. (1984). The study of stress and competence in children: A building block of developmental psychopathology. *Child Development, 55,* 97–111.

Ge, X., Conger, R. D., Lorenz, F. O., Shanahan, M., & Elder, G. H., Jr. (1995). Mutual influences in parent and adolescent distress. *Developmental Psychology, 31,* 406–419.

Gelfand, D. M., & Teti, D. M. (1990). The effects of maternal depression on children. *Clinical Psychology Review, 10,* 329–353.

Gencoez, T., Voelz, Z. R., Gencoez, F., Pettit, J. W., & Joiner, T. E. (2001). Specificity of information processing styles to depressive symptoms in youth psychiatric inpatients. *Journal of Abnormal Child Psychology, 29,* 255–262.

Ghiselli, E. E., Campbell, J. P., & Zedeck, S. (1981). *Measurement theory for the behavioral sciences.* New York: Freeman.

Gillberg, C., & Wing, L. (1999). Autism: Not an extremely rare disorder. *Acta Psychiatrica Scandinavica, 99,* 399–406.

Gilgun, J. F. (1999). Mapping resilience as process among adults with childhood adversities. In H. I. McCubbin, E. A. Thompson, A. I. Thompson, & J. A. Futrell (Eds.), *Resiliency in families: Vol. 4. The dynamics of resilient families* (pp. 41–70). Thousand Oaks, CA: Sage.

Glantz, M. D., & Johnson, J. L. (Eds.). (1999). *Resilience and development: Positive life adaptations.* New York: Kluwer Academic/Plenum.

Glaser, D. (2000). Child abuse and neglect and the brain: A review. *Journal of Child Psychology and Psychiatry, 41,* 97–116.

Goldberg, S. (1991). Recent developments in attachment theory and research. *Canadian Journal of Psychiatry, 36,* 393–400.

Goldsmith, H. H., Gottesman, I. I., & Lemery, K. S. (1997). Epigenetic approaches to developmental psychopathology. *Development and Psychopathology, 9,* 365–397.

Gomez, R., & Gomez, A. (2000). Perceived maternal control and support as predictors of hostile–biased attribution of intent and response selection in aggressive boys. *Aggressive Behavior, 26,* 155–168.

Gomez, R., Gomez, A., DeMello, L., & Tallent, R. (2001). Perceived maternal control and support: Effects on hostile biased social information processing and aggression among clinic-referred children with high aggression. *Journal of Child Psychology and Psychiatry, 42,* 513–522.

Goodman, S. H., & Gotlib, I. H. (1999). Risk for psychopathology in the children of depressed mothers: A developmental model for understanding mechanisms of transmission. *Psychological Review, 106,* 458–490.

Gotlib, I. H., & Hammen, C. L. (1992). *Psychological aspects of depression: Toward a cognitive–interpersonal integration.* Chichester, England: Wiley.

Gottman, J. M., Guralnick, M. J., Wilson, B., Swanson, C., & Murray, J. D. (1997). What should be the focus of emotion regulation in children?: A nonlinear dynamic mathematical model of children's peer interaction in groups. *Development and Psychopathology, 9,* 421–452.

Greenbaum, P. E., Prange, M. E., Friedman, R. M., & Silver, S. E. (1991). Substance abuse prevalence and comorbidity with other psychiatric disorders among adolescents with severe emotional disturbances. *Journal of the American Academy of Child and Adolescent Psychiatry, 30,* 575–583.

Greenberg, M. T., Domitrovich, C., & Bumbarger, B. (2001). The prevention of mental disorders in school-aged children: Current state of the field. *Prevention and Treatment* [Online], *4,* Article 0001a. Available: http://www.journals.apa.org/prevention/volume4/pre0040001a.html [2001, April 30].

Greenspan, S. I., & Wieder, S. (1994). Diagnostic classification of mental health and developmental disorders of infancy and early childhood. *Zero to Three, 14*(6), 34–41.

Grellong, B. A. (1987). Residential care in context: Evolution of a treatment process in response to social change. *Residential Treatment for Children and Youth, 4,* 59–70.

Group for the Advancement of Psychiatry. (1974). *Psychopathological disorders in childhood: Theoretical considerations and a proposed classification.* New York: Jason Aronson.

Grych, J. H., & Fincham, F. D. (Eds.). (2001). *Interparental conflict and child development: Theory, research, and applications.* Cambridge, England: Cambridge University Press.

Guerra, N. G., Tolan, P. H., Huesmann, L. R., Van Acker, R., & Eron, L. D. (1995). Stressful events and individual beliefs as correlates of economic disadvantage and aggression among urban children. *Journal of Consulting and Clinical Psychology, 63,* 518–528.

Hare, E. H. (1962). Masturbatory insanity: The history of an idea. *Journal of Mental Science,* 1–25.

Harkness, S., & Super, C. M. (2000). Culture and psychopathology. In A. J. Sameroff, M. Lewis, & S. M. Miller (Eds.), *Handbook of developmental psychopathology* (2nd ed., pp. 197–214). New York: Kluwer Academic/Plenum.

Hart, E. L., & Lahey, B. B. (1999). General child behavior rating scales. In D. Shaffer, C. P. Lucas, & J. Richters (Eds.), *Diagnostic assessment in child and adolescent psychopathology* (pp. 65–87). New York: Guilford Press.

Hart, E. L., Lahey, B. B., Loeber, R., Applegate, B., Green, S. M., & Frick, P. J. (1995). Developmental change in attention-deficit hyperactivity disorder in boys: A four-year longitudinal study. *Journal of Abnormal Child Psychology, 23,* 729–749.

Hart, J., Gunnar, M., & Cicchetti, D. (1995). Salivary cortisol in maltreated children: Evidence of relations between neuroendocrine activity and social competence. *Development and Psychopathology, 7,* 11–26.

Hartung, C. M., & Widiger, T. A. (1998). Gender differences in the diagnosis of mental disorders: Conclusions and controversies of DSMIV. *Psychological Bulletin, 123,* 260–278.

Hauser-Cram, P., Warfield, M. E., Shonkoff, J. P., & Krauss, M. W. (2001). Children with disabilities: A longitudinal study of child development and parent well-being. *Monographs of the Society for Research in Child Development, 66*(Whole No. 3), 1–131.

Haynes, S. N., & Blaine, D. (1995). Dynamical models for psychological assessment: Phase space functions. *Psychological Assessment, 7,* 17–24.

Hetherington, E. M., Reiss, D., & Plomin, R. (Eds.). (1994). *Separate social worlds of siblings: The impact of nonshared environment on development.* Hillsdale, NJ: Erlbaum.

Hewitt, J. K., Silberg, J. L., Rutter, M., Simonoff, E., Meyer, J. M., Maes, H., Pickles, A., Neale, M. C., Loeber, R., Erickson, M. T., Kendler, K. S., Heath, A. C., Truett, K. R., Reynolds, C. A., & Eaves, L. J. (1997). Genetics and developmental psychopathology: 1. Phenotypic assessment in the Virginia Twin Study of Adolescent Behavioral Development. *Journal of Child Psychology and Psychiatry, 38,* 943–963.

Hinshaw, S. P. (2001, June). *Process, mechanism, and explanation related to externalizing behavior.* Presidential address to the International Society for Research in Child and Adolescent Psychopathology, Vancouver, Canada.

Hinshaw, S. P., & Cicchetti, D. (2000). Stigma and mental disorder: Conceptions of illness, public attitudes, personal disclosure, and social policy. *Development and Psychopathology, 12,* 555–598.

Hirshfeld, D. R., Biederman, J., Brody, L., & Faraone, S. V. (1997). Associations between expressed emotion and child behavioral inihibition and psychopathology: A pilot study. *Journal of the American Academy of Child and Adolescent Psychiatry, 36,* 205–213.

Hoagwood, K., & Jensen, P. (1997). Developmental psychopathology and the notion of culture. *Applied Developmental Science, 1,* 108–112.

Hoagwood, K., Kelleher, K. J., Feil, M., & Comer, D. M. (2000). Treatment services for children with ADHD: A national perspective. *Journal of the American Academy of Child and Adolescent Psychiatry, 39,* 198–206.

Hops, H. (1995). Age- and gender-specific effects of parental depression: A commentary. *Developmental Psychology, 31,* 428–431.

Houts, A. C. (2001). The diagnostic and statistical manual's new white coat and circularity of plausible dysfunctions: Response to Wakefield, Part 1. *Behaviour Research and Therapy, 39,* 315–345.

Iaboni, F., Douglas, V. I., & Baker, A. G. (1995). Effects of reward and response costs on inhibition in ADHD children. *Journal of Abnormal Psychology, 104,* 232–240.

Ialongo, N., Edelsohn, G., Werthamer-Larsson, L., Crockett, L., & Kellam, S. (1995). The significance of self-reported anxious symptoms in first grade children: Prediction to anxious symptoms and adaptive functioning in fifth grade. *Journal of Child Psychology and Psychiatry, 36,* 427–437.

Ialongo, N. S., Kellam, S. G., & Poduska, J. (2000). A developmental epidemiological framework for clinical child and pediatric psychology research. In D. Drotar (Ed.), *Handbook of research in pediatric and clinical child psy-*

chology: Practical strategies and methods (pp. 3–19). New York: Kluwer Academic/Plenum.

Ingram, R. E., Miranda, J., & Segal, Z. V. (1998). *Cognitive vulnerability to depression*. New York: Guilford Press.

Ingram, R. E., & Price, J. M. (Eds.). (2001). *Vulnerability to psychopathology: Risk across the lifespan*. New York: Guilford Press.

Ingram, R. E., & Ritter, J. (2000). Vulnerability to depression: Cognitive reactivity and parental bonding in high-risk individuals. *Journal of Abnormal Psychology, 109,* 588–596.

Institute of Medicine. (1989). *Research on children and adolescents with mental, behavioral and developmental disorders*. Washington, DC: National Academy Press.

International Molecular Genetic Study of Autism Consortium. (1998). A full genome screen for autism with evidence for linkage to a region on chromosome 7q. *Human Molecular Genetics, 7,* 571–578.

Izard, C. E. (1993). Four systems for emotion activation: Cognitive and noncognitive processes. *Psychological Review, 100,* 68–90.

Jacob, T. (Ed.). (1987). *Family interaction and psychopathology: Theories, methods, and findings*. New York: Plenum Press.

Jensen, P. S., & Hoagwood, K. (1997). The book of names: DSM-IV in context. *Development and Psychopathology, 9,* 231–249.

Jensen, P. S., Koretz, D., Locke, B. Z., Schneider, S., Radke-Yarrow, M., Richters, J. E., & Rumsey, J. M. (1993). Child and adolescent psychopathology research: Problems and prospects for the 1990s. *Journal of Abnormal Child Psychology, 21,* 551–580.

Johnson, M. H. (1999). Coritcal plasticity in normal and abnormal cognitive development: Evidence and working hypotheses. *Development and Psychopathology, 11,* 419–437.

Joiner, T., & Coyne, J. C. (Eds.). (1999). *The interactional nature of depression*. Washington, DC: American Psychological Association.

Kagan, J. (1994a). *Galen's prophecy: Temperament in human nature*. New York: Basic Books.

Kagan, J. (1994b). On the nature of emotion. In N. A. Fox (Ed.), The development of emotion regulation: Biological and behavioral considerations. *Monographs of the Society for Research in Child Development, 59*(2–3, Serial No. 240), 7–24.

Kagan, J. (1997). Conceptualizing psychopathology: The importance of developmental profiles. *Development and Psychopathology, 9,* 321–334.

Kagan, J., & Snidman, N. (1991). Temperamental factors in human development. *American Psychologist, 46,* 856–862.

Kamphaus, R. W., Petoskey, M. D., Cody, A. H., Rowe, E. W., Huberty, C. J., & Reynolds, C. R. (1999). A typology of parent rated child behavior for a national U.S. sample. *Journal of Child Psychology and Psychiatry, 40,* 607–616.

Kanfer, F. H., & Saslow, G. (1969). Behavioral diagnosis. In C. M. Franks (Ed.), *Behavior therapy: Appraisal and status* (pp. 417–444). New York: McGraw-Hill.

Kanner, L. (1962). Emotionally disturbed children: A historical review. *Child Development, 33,* 97–102.

Kaplan, H. I., & Sadock, B. J. (1991). *Synopsis of psychiatry* (6th ed.). Baltimore: Williams & Wilkins.

Katz, L. F., & Gottman, J. M. (1993). Patterns of marital conflict predict children's internalizing and externalizing behaviors. *Developmental Psychology, 29,* 940–950.

Katz, L. F., & Gottman, J. M. (1995). Vagal tone protects children from marital conflict. *Development and Psychopathology, 7,* 83–92.

Kaufman, J., & Charney, D. (2001). Effects of early stress on brain structure and function: Implications for understanding the relationship between child maltreatment and depression. *Development and Psychopathology, 13,* 451–471.

Kaufman, J., Cook, A., Arny, L., Jones, B., & Pittinsky, T. (1994). Problems defining resiliency: Illustrations from the study of maltreated children. *Development and Psychopathology, 6,* 215–229.

Kavanagh, K., & Hops, H. (1994). Good girls? Bad boys?: Gender and development as contexts for diagnosis and treatment. In T. H. Ollendick & R. J. Prinz (Eds.), *Advances in clinical child psychology* (Vol. 16, pp. 45–79). New York: Plenum Press.

Kazdin, A. E. (1989). Developmental psychopathology: Current research, issues and directions. *American Psychologist, 44,* 180–187.

Kazdin, A. E. (2000). *Psychotherapy for children and adolescents: Directions for research and practice*. New York: Oxford University Press.

Kazdin, A. E. (2001). Bridging the enormous gaps of theory with therapy research and practice. *Journal of Clinical Child Psychology, 30,* 59–66.

Kazdin, A. E., & Johnson, B. (1994). Advances in psychotherapy for children and adolescents: Interrelations of adjustment, development, and intervention. *Journal of School Psychology, 32,* 217–246.

Kazdin, A. E., & Kagan, J. (1994). Models of dysfunction in developmental psychopathology. *Clinical Psychology: Science and Practice, 1,* 35–52.

Kazdin, A. E., & Weisz, J. R. (1998). Identifying and developing empirically supported child and adolescent treatments. *Journal of Consulting and Clinical Psychology, 66,* 19–36.

Keenan, K. (2000). Emotion dysregulation as a risk factor for child psychopathology. *Clinical Psychology: Science and Practice, 7,* 418–434.

Keenan, K., & Shaw, D. (1997). Developmental and social influences on young girls' early problem behavior. *Psychological Bulletin, 121,* 95–113.

Keenan, K., Shaw, D. S., Walsh, B., Delliquadri, E., & Giovannelli, J. (1997). DSM-III-R disorders in preschool children from low-income families. *Journal of the American Academy of Child and Adolescent Psychiatry, 36,* 620–627.

Kendall, P. C. (1985). Toward a cognitive-behavioral model of child psychopathology and a critique of related interventions. *Journal of Abnormal Child Psychology, 13,* 357–372.

Kendall, P. C. (1991). Guiding theory for therapy with children and adolescents. In P. C. Kendall (Ed.), *Child and adolescent therapy: Cognitive-behavioral procedures* (pp. 3–22). New York: Guilford Press.

Kendall, P. C. (1993). Cognitive-behavioral therapies with youth: Guiding theory, current status, and emerging developments. *Journal of Consulting and Clinical Psychology, 61,* 235–247.

Kendall, P. C., Brady, E. U., & Verduin, T. L. (2001). Comorbidity in childhood anxiety disorders and treatment outcome. *Journal of the American Academy of Child and Adolescent Psychiatry, 40,* 787–794.

Kendall, P. C., & Dobson, K. S. (1993). On the nature of cognition and its role in psychopathology. In K. S. Dobson & P. C. Kendall (Eds.), *Psychopathology and cognition* (pp. 3–17). San Diego, CA: Academic Press.

Kendall, P. C., & MacDonald, J. P. (1993). Cognition in the psychopathology of youth and implications for treatment. In K. S. Dobson & P. C. Kendall (Eds.), *Psychopathology and cognition* (pp. 387–427). San Diego, CA: Academic Press.

Kendall, P. C., Marrs-Garcia, A., Nath, S. R., & Sheldrick, R. C. (1999). Normative comparisons for the evaluation of clinical significance. *Journal of Consulting and Clinical Psychology, 67,* 285–299.

Kendall, P. C., & Morris, R. J. (1991). Child therapy: Issues and recommendations. *Journal of Consulting and Clinical Psychology, 59,* 777–784.

Kendall, P. C., & Sheldrick, R. C. (2000). Normative data for normative comparisons. *Journal of Consulting and Clinical Psychology, 68,* 767–773.

Keren, M., Feldman, R., & Tyano, S. (2001). Diagnoses and interactive patterns of infants referred to a community-based infant mental health clinic. *Journal of the American Academy of Child and Adolescent Psychiatry, 40,* 27–35.

Kessler, J. W. (1971). Nosology in child psychopathology. In H. E. Rie (Ed.), *Perspectives in child psychopathology* (pp. 85–129). Chicago: Aldine-Atherton.

Klein, S. B., & Mower, R. R. (Eds.). (1989). *Contemporary learning theories: Instrumental conditioning theory and the impact of biological constraints on learning*. Hillsdale, NJ: Erlbaum.

Klinger, L. G., & Renner, P. (2000). Performance-based measures in autism: Implications for diagnosis, early detection, and identification of cognitive profiles. *Journal of Clinical Child Pychology, 29,* 479–492.

Kotler, L. A., Cohen, P., Davies, M., Pine, D. S., & Walsh, B. T. (2001). Longitudinal relationships between childhood, adolescent, and adult eating disorders. *Journal of the American Academy of Child and Adolescent Psychiatry, 40,* 1434–1440.

Kovacs, M. (1997). Depressive disorders in childhood: An impressionistic landscape. *Journal of Child Psychology and Psychiatry, 38,* 287–298.

Kovacs, M., & Beck, A. T. (1977). An empirical clinical approach towards a definition of childhood depression. In J. G. Schulterbrandt & A. Raskin (Eds.), *Depression in children: Diagnosis, treatment, and conceptual models* (pp. 1–25). New York: Raven Press.

Kraemer, G. W. (1992). A psychobiological theory of attachment. *Behavioral and Brain Sciences, 15,* 493–541.

Krasner, L. (1991). History of behavior modification. In A. S. Bellack & M. Hersen (Eds.), *International handbook of behavior modification and therapy* (2nd ed., pp. 3–25). New York: Plenum Press.

Kreppner, J. M., O'Connor, T. G., Rutter, M., & the English and Romanian Adoptees Study Team. (2001). Can inattention/overactivity be an institutional deprivation syndrome? *Journal of Abnormal Child Psychology, 29,* 513–528.

Kroes, M., Kalff, A. C., Kessels, A. G. C., Steyaert, J., Feron, F. J. M., van Someren, A. J. W. G. M., Hurks, P. P. M., Hendriksen, J. G. M., van Zeben, T. M. C. B., Rozendal, N., Crolla, I. F. A. M., Troost, J., Jolles, J., & Vles, J. S. H. (2001). Child psychiatric diagnosis in a population of Dutch schoolchildren aged 6 to 8 years. *Journal of the American Academy of Child and Adolescent Psychiatry, 40,* 1401–1409.

Kuhn, T. S. (1962). *The structure of scientific revolutions.* Chicago: University of Chicago Press.

Kuntsi, J., & Stevenson, J. (2000). Hyperactivity in children: A focus on genetic research and psychological theories. *Clinical Child Family Psychology Review, 3,* 1–23.

Kuperman, S., Schlosser, S. S., Kramer, J. R., Bucholz, K., Hesselbrock, V., & Reich, T. (2001). Developmental sequence from disruptive behavior diagnosis to adolescent alcohol dependence. *American Journal of Psychiatry, 158,* 2022–2026.

Kurtines, W. M., & Silverman, W. K. (1999). Emerging views of the role of theory. *Journal of Clinical Child Psychology, 28,* 558–562.

Lahey, B. B., Loeber, R., Hart, E. L., Frick, P. J., Applegate, B., Zhang, Q., Green, S. M., & Russo, M. F. (1995). Four-year longitudinal study of conduct disorder in boys: Patterns and predictors of persistence. *Journal of Abnormal Psychology, 104,* 83–93.

Lamb, M. E., & Billings, L. A. (1997). Fathers of children with special needs. In M. E. Lamb (Ed.), *The role of the father in child development* (3rd ed., pp. 179–190). New York: Wiley.

Lambert, M. C., & Weisz, J. R. (1989). Over- and under-controlled clinic referral problems in Jamaican clinic-referred children: Teacher reports for ages 6–17. *Journal of Abnormal Child Psychology, 17,* 553–562.

Lambert, M. C., & Weisz, J. R. (1992). Jamaican and American adult perspectives on child psychopathology: Further exploration of the threshold model. *Journal of Consulting and Clinical Psychology, 60,* 146–149.

Lapouse, R., & Monk, M. A. (1958). An epidemiologic study of behavior characteristics in children. *American Journal of Public Health, 48,* 1134–1144.

Lara, M. E., Klein, D. N., & Kasch, K. L. (2000). Psychosocial predictors of the short-term course and outcome of major depression: A longitudinal study of a nonclinical sample with recent-onset episodes. *Journal of Abnormal Psychology, 109,* 644–650.

Lavigne, J. V., Cicchetti, C., Gibbons, R. D., Binns, H. J., Larsen, L., & DeVito, C. (2001). Oppositional defiant disorder with onset in preschool years: Longitudinal stability and pathways to other disorders. *Journal of the American Academy of Child and Adolescent Psychiatry, 40,* 1393–1400.

Leibson, C. L., Katusic, S. K., Barberesi, W. J., Ransom, J., & O'Brien, P. (2001). Use and costs of medical care for children and adolescents with and without attention-deficit/hyperactivity disorder (ADHD). *Journal of the American Medical Association, 285,* 60–66.

Leon, G. R., Fulkerson, J. A., Perry, C. L., & Early-Zald, M. B. (1995). Prospective analysis of personality and behavioral vulnerabilities and gender influences in later development of disordered eating. *Journal of Abnormal Psychology, 104,* 140–149.

Lesser, S. T. (1972). Psychoanalysis of children. In B. B. Wolman (Ed.), *Manual of child psychopathology* (pp. 847–864). New York: McGraw-Hill.

Lewinsohn, P. M., Joiner, T. E., & Rohde, P. (2001). Evaluation of cognitive diathesis–stress models in predicting major depressive disorder in adolescents. *Journal of Abnormal Psychology, 110,* 203–215.

Lewinsohn, P. M., Steinmetz, J. L., Larson, D. W., & Franklin, J. (1981). Depression-related cognitions: Antecedent or consequence? *Journal of Abnormal Psychology, 90,* 213–219.

Lewinsohn, P. M., Striegel-Moore, R., & Seeley, J. (2000). Epidemiology and natural course of eating disorders in young women from adolescence to young adulthood.

Journal of the American Academy of Child and Adolescent Psychiatry, 39, 1284–1292.

Lewis, M. (2000). Toward a development of psychopathology: Models, definitions, and prediction. In A. J. Sameroff, M. Lewis, & S. M. Miller (Eds.), *Handbook of developmental psychopathology* (2nd ed., pp. 3–22). New York: Kluwer Academic/Plenum.

Lewis, M. D., & Granic, I. (Eds.). (2000). *Emotion, development, and self-organization: Dynamic systems approaches to emotional development*. New York: Cambridge University Press.

Lieberman, A. F., Wieder, S., & Fenichel, E. (Eds.). (1997). *The DC:0–3 casebook: A guide to the use of 0 to 3's Diagnostic Classification of Mental Health and Developmental Disorders of Infancy and Early Childhood in assessment and treatment planning*. Washington, DC: Zero to Three/National Center for Infants, Toddlers and Families.

Lilienfeld, S. O., & Marino, L. (1995). Mental disorder as a Roschian concept: A critique of Wakefield's "harmful dysfunction" analysis. *Journal of Abnormal Psychology, 104*, 411–420.

Lilienfeld, S. O., Waldman, I. D., & Israel, A. C. (1994). A critical examination of the use of the term and concept of comorbidity in psychopathology research. *Clinical Psychology: Science and Practice, 1*, 71–83.

Lochman, J. E., & Dodge, K. A. (1994). Social-cognitive processes of severely violent, moderately aggressive, and nonaggressive boys. *Journal of Consulting and Clinical Psychology, 62*, 366–374.

Lochman, J. E., White, K. J., & Wayland, K. K. (1991). Cognitive-behavioral assessment with aggressive children. In P. C. Kendall (Ed.), *Child and adolescent therapy: Cognitive-behavioral procedures* (pp. 25–65). New York: Guilford Press.

Loeber, R. (1991). Questions and advances in the study of developmental pathways. In D. Cicchetti & S. L. Toth (Eds.), *Rochester Symposium on Developmental Psychopathology: Vol. 3. Models and integrations* (pp. 97–116). New York: University of Rochester Press.

Loeber, R., Burke, J. D., Lahey, B. B., Winters, A., & Zera, M. (2000). Oppositional defiant and conduct disorder: A review of the past 10 years, Part I. *Journal of the American Academy of Child and Adolescent Psychiatry, 39*, 1468–1484.

Loeber, R., & Dishion, T. (1983). Early predictors of male delinquency: A review. *Psychological Bulletin, 93*, 68–99.

Loeber, R., & Farrington, D. P. (2000). Young children who commit crime: Epidemiology, developmental origins, risk factors, early interventions, and policy implications. *Development and Psychopathology, 12*, 737–762.

Loeber, R., & Keenan, K. (1994). Interaction between conduct disorder and its comorbid conditions: Effects of age and gender. *Clinical Psychology Review, 14*, 497–523.

Lombroso, P. J., Pauls, D. L., & Leckman, J. F. (1994). Genetic mechanisms in childhood psychiatric disorders. *Journal of the American Academy of Child and Adolescent Psychiatry, 33*, 921–938.

Lonigan, C. J., Elbert, J. C., & Johnson, S. B. (1998). Empirically supported psychosocial interventions for children: An overview. *Journal of Clinical Child Psychology, 27*, 138–145.

Lopez, S. R., & Guarnaccia, P. J. (2000). Cultural psychopathology: Uncovering the social world of mental illness. *Annual Review of Psychology, 51*, 571–598.

Lovejoy, M. C., Graczyk, P. A., O' Hare, E., & Neuman, G. (2000). Maternal depression and parenting behavior: A meta-analytic review. *Clinical Psychology Review, 20*, 561–592.

Luthar, S. S. (1993). Annotation: Methodological and conceptual issues in research on childhood resilience. *Journal of Child Psychology and Psychiatry, 34*, 441–453.

Luthar, S. S., Burack, J. A., Cicchetti, D., & Weisz, J. R. (Eds.). (1997). *Developmental psychopathology: Perspectives on adjustment, risk, and disorder*. Cambridge, England: Cambridge University Press.

Luthar, S. S., Cicchetti, D., & Becker, B. (2000). The construct of resilience: A critical evaluation and guidelines for future work. *Child Development, 71*, 543–562.

Lyons-Ruth, K. (1995). Broadening our conceptual frameworks: Can we reintroduce relational strategies and implicit representational systems to the study of psychopathology? *Developmental Psychology, 31*, 432–436.

MacFarlane, J. W., Allen, L., & Honzik, M. P. (1954). *A developmental study of the behavior problems of normal children between twenty-one months and fourteen years.* Berkeley: University of California Press.

MacMillan, H. L., Fleming, J. E., Streiner, D. L., Lin, E., Boyle, M. H., Jamieson, E., Duku, E. K., Walsh, C. A., Wong, M. Y. Y., & Beardslee, W. R. (2001). Childhood abuse and lifetime psychopathology in a community sample. *American Journal of Psychiatry, 158*, 1878–1883.

Makari, G. J. (1993). Educated insane: A nineteenth-century psychiatric paradigm. *Journal of the History of the Behavioral Sciences, 29*, 8–21.

Manly, J. T., Cicchetti, D., & Barnett, D. (1994). The impact of subtype, frequency, chronicity, and severity of child maltreatment on social competence and behavior problems. *Development and Psychopathology, 6*, 121–143.

Manly, J. T., Kim, J. E., Rogosch, F. A., & Cicchetti, D. (2001). Dimensions of child maltreatment and children's adjustment: Contributions of developmental timing and subtype. *Development and Psychopathology, 13*, 759–782.

Mash, E. J. (1998). Treatment of child and family disturbance: A behavioral–systems perspective. In E. J. Mash & R. A. Barkley (Eds.), *Treatment of childhood disorders* (2nd ed., pp. 3–38). New York: Guilford Press.

Mash, E. J., & Barkley, R. A. (Eds.). (1998). *Treatment of childhood disorders* (2nd ed.). New York: Guilford Press.

Mash, E. J., & Hunsley, J. (1990). Behavioral assessment: A contemporary approach. In A. S. Bellack & M. Hersen (Eds.), *International handbook of behavior modification and behavior therapy* (2nd ed., pp. 87–106). New York: Plenum Press.

Mash, E. J., & Johnston, C. (1995). Family relational problems. In V. E. Caballo, G. Buela-Casal, & J. A. Carrobles (Eds.), *Handbook of psychopathology and psychiatric disorders.* (Vol. 2). Madrid: Siglo XXI.

Mash, E. J., Johnston, C., & Kovitz, K. (1983). A comparison of the mother-child interactions of physically abused and non-abused children during play and task situations. *Journal of Clinical Child Psychology, 12*, 337–346.

Mash, E. J., & Krahn, G. L. (2000). Research strategies in child psychopathology. In M. Hersen & R. T. Ammerman (Eds.), *Advanced abnormal child psychology* (2nd ed., pp. 101–130). Mahwah, NJ: Erlbaum.

Mash, E. J., & Terdal, L. G. (Eds.). (1997a). *Assessment of childhood disorders* (3rd ed.). New York: Guilford Press.

Mash, E. J., & Terdal, L. G. (1997b). Assessment of child and family disturbance: A behavioral–systems approach. In E. J. Mash & L. G. Terdal (Eds.), *Assessment of child-*

hood disorders (3rd ed., pp. 3–68). New York: Guilford Press.

Mash, E. J., & Wolfe, D. A. (1991). Methodological issues in research on physical child abuse. *Criminal Justice and Behavior, 18,* 8–30.

Mash, E. J., & Wolfe, D. A. (2002). *Abnormal child psychology* (2nd ed.). Belmont, CA: Wadsworth.

Masten, A. S. (2001). Ordinary magic: Resilience processes in development. *American Psychologist, 56,* 227–238.

Masten, A. S., & Curtis, W. J. (2000). Integrating competence and psychopathology: Pathways toward a comprehensive science of adaption in development. *Development and Psychopathology, 12,* 529–550.

Maxwell, S. E., & Delaney, H. D. (1990). *Designing experiments and analyzing data: A model comparison perspective.* Belmont, CA: Wadsworth.

Maughan, B., & Rutter, M. (2001). Antisocial children grown up. In J. Hill & B. Maughan (Eds.), *Conduct disorders in childhood and adolescence* (pp. 507–552). New York: Cambridge University Press.

Mayer, J. D., & Salovey, P. (1995). Emotional intelligence and the construction and regulation of feelings. *Applied and Preventive Psychology, 4,* 197–208.

McCall, R. B., & Groark, C. J. (2000). The future of applied child development research and public policy. *Child Development, 71,* 197–204.

McDermott, P. A. (1993). National standardization of uniform multisituational measures of child and adolescent behavior pathology. *Psychological Assessment, 5,* 413–424.

McDermott, P. A., & Weiss, R. V. (1995). A normative typology of healthy, subclinical, and clinical behavior styles among American children and adolescents. *Psychological Assessment, 7,* 162–170.

McGuffin, P., Riley, B., & Plomin, R. (2001). Toward behavioral genomics. *Science, 291,* 1232–1249.

McLeod, J. D., & Nonnemaker, J. M. (2000). Poverty and child emotional and behavioral problems: Racial/ethnic differences in processes and effects. *Journal of Health and Social Behavior, 41,* 137–161.

McNally, R J. (2001). On Wakefield's harmful dysfunction analysis of mental disorder. *Behaviour Research and Therapy, 39,* 309–314.

Meehl, P. E. (2001). Comorbidity and taxometrics. *Clinical Psychology: Science and Practice, 8,* 507–519.

Meichenbaum, D. (1977). *Cognitive-behavior modification: An integrative approach.* New York: Plenum Press.

Meltzer, H., Gatward, H., Goodman, R., & Ford, T. (2000). *The mental health of children and adolescents in Great Britain: Summary report.* London: Office for National Statistics.

Messick, S. (1983). Assessment of children. In P. H. Mussen (Series Ed.) & W. Kessen (Vol. Ed.), *Handbook of child psychology: Vol. 1. History, theory, and methods* (4th ed., pp. 477–526). New York: Wiley.

Milich, R., Balentine, A. C., & Lynam, D. R. (2001). ADHD combined type and ADHD predominantly inattentive type are distinct and unrelated disorders. *Clinical Psychology: Science and Practice, 8,* 463–488.

Miranda, J., & Persons, J. B. (1988). Dysfunctional attitudes are mood-state dependent. *Journal of Abnormal Psychology, 97,* 76–79.

Miranda, J., Persons, J. B., & Byers, C. N. (1990). Endorsement of dysfunctional beliefs depends on current mood state. *Journal of Abnormal Psychology, 99,* 237–241.

Moffitt, T. E., Caspi, A., Rutter, M., & Silva, P. A. (2001). *Sex differences in antisocial behaviour: Conduct disorder, delinquency, and violence in the Dunedin longitudinal study.* Cambridge, England: Cambridge University Press.

Mohr, W. K., & Regan-Kubinski, M. J. (1999). The DSM and child psychiatric nursing: A cautionary reflection. *Scholarly Inquiry for Nursing Practice, 13,* 305–318.

Moore, L. A., & Hughes, J. N. (1988). Impulsive and hyperactive children. In J. N. Hughes (Ed.), *Cognitive behavior therapy with children in schools* (pp. 127–159). Toronto: Pergamon Press.

Moradi, A. R., Neshat-Doost, H. T., Taghavi, R., Yule, W., & Dalgleish, T. (1999). Performance of children of adults with PTSD on the Stroop color-naming task: A preliminary study. *Journal of Traumatic Stress, 12,* 663–671.

Mundy, P. (1995). Joint attention and social-emotional approach behavior in children with autism. *Development and Psychopathology, 7,* 137–162.

Murry, V. M., Bynum, M. S., Brody, G. H., Willert, A., & Stephens, D. (2001). African American single mothers and children in context: A review of studies on risk and resilience. *Clinical Child and Family Psychology Review, 4,* 133–155.

Murry, V. M., Smith, E. P., & Hill, N. E. (2001). Race, ethnicity, and culture in studies of families in context. *Journal of Marriage and the Family, 63,* 911–914.

Nathan, P. E., & Lagenbucher, J. W. (1999). Psychopathology: Description and classification. *Annual Review of Psychology, 50,* 79–107.

National Advisory Mental Health Council (NAMHC) Workgroup on Child and Adolescent Mental Health Intervention Development and Deployment. (2001). *Blueprint for change: Research on child and adolescent mental health.* Washington, DC: U.S. Government Printing Office.

National Commission on Children. (1991). *Beyond rhetoric: A new American agenda for children and families. The final report of the National Commission on Children.* Washington, DC: U.S. Government Printing Office.

National Institute of Mental Health. (2001). National Advisory Mental Health Council Workshop on Mental Disorders Prevention Research: Priorities for prevention research at NIMH. *Prevention and Treatment* [Online], *4,* NP. Available: http://www.journals.apa.org/prevention/volume 4/pre0040017a.html [2001, June 30].

Nelson, C. A. (2000). The neurobiological basis of early intervention. In J. P. Shonkoff & S. J. Meisels (Eds.), *Handbook of early childhood intervention* (2nd ed., pp. 204–227). New York: Cambridge University Press.

Nicholls, D., Chater, R., & Lask, B. (2000). Children into DSM don't go: A comparison of classification systems for eating disorders in childhood and early adolescence. *International Journal of Eating Disorders, 28,* 317–324.

Nigg, J. T. (2000). On inhibition/disinhibition in developmental psychopathology: Views from cognitive and personality psychology and a working inhibition taxonomy. *Psychological Bulletin, 126,* 220–246.

Nigg, J. T. (2001). Is ADHD a disinhibitory disorder? *Psychological Bulletin, 127,* 571–598.

Nigg, J. T., Blaskey, L. G., Huang-Pollack, C. L., & Rappley, M. D. (2002). Neuropsychological and executive functions in DSM-IV ADHD subtypes. *Journal of the American Academy of Child and Adolescent Psychiatry, 41,* 1–8.

Nigg, J. T., John, O. P., Blaskey, L., Huang-Pollack, C., Willcutt, E. G., Hinshaw, S. P., & Pennington, B. (2001). *Big five dimensions and ADHD symptoms: Links between personality traits and clinical symptoms.* Unpublished manuscript, Department of Psychology, Michigan State University.

Nottelmann, E. D., & Jensen, P. S. (1995). Comorbidity of disorders in children and adolescents: Developmental perspectives. In T. H. Ollendick & R. J. Prinz (Eds.), *Advances in clinical child psychology* (Vol. 17, pp. 109–155). New York: Plenum.

O'Conner, T. G., & Plomin, R. (2000). Developmental and behavioral genetics. In A. J. Sameroff, M. Lewis, & S. M. Miller (Eds.), *Handbook of developmental psychopathology* (2nd ed., pp. 197–214). New York: Kluwer Academic/Plenum.

O'Donnell, J., Hawkins, J. D., & Abbott, R. D. (1995). Predicting serious delinquency and substance abuse among aggressive boys. *Journal of Consulting and Clinical Psychology, 63,* 529–537.

Offord, D. R., Boyle, M. H., & Racine, Y. A. (1989). Ontario Child Health Study: Correlates of disorder. *Journal of the American Academy of Child and Adolescent Psychiatry, 28,* 856–860.

Offord, D. R., Boyle, M. H., Racine, Y. A., Fleming, J. E., Cadman, D. T., Blum, H. M., Byrne, C., Links, P. S., Lipman, E. L., MacMillan, H. L., Grant, N. I. R., Sanford, M. N., Szatmari, P., Thomas, H., & Woodward, C. A. (1992). Outcome, prognosis, and risk in a longitudinal follow-up study. *Journal of the American Academy of Child and Adolescent Psychiatry, 31,* 916–923.

Offord, D. R., Boyle, M. H., Szatmari, P., Rae-Grant, N. I., Links, P. S., Cadman, D. T., Byles, J. A., Crawford, J. W., Blum, H. M., Byrne, C., Thomas, H., & Woodward, C. A. (1987). Ontario Child Health Study: II. Six-month prevalence of disorder and rates of service utilization. *Archives of General Psychiatry, 44,* 832–836.

Okun, A., Parker, J. G., & Levendosky, A. A. (1994). Distinct and interactive contributions of physical abuse, socioeconomic disadvantage, and negative life events to children's social, cognitive, and affective adjustment. *Development and Psychopathology, 6,* 77–98.

Ollendick, T. H., & Hersen, M. (Eds.). (1998). *Handbook of child psychopathology* (3rd ed.). New York: Plenum Press.

Olweus, D. (1979). Stability of aggressive reaction patterns in males: A review. *Psychological Bulletin, 86,* 852–875.

Orvaschel, H., Ambrosini, P. J., & Rabinovich, H. (1993). Diagnostic issues in child assessment. In T. H. Ollendick & M. Hersen (Eds.), *Handbook of child and adolescent assessment* (pp. 26–40). Boston: Allyn & Bacon.

Orvaschel, H., Faust, J., & Hersen, M. (2001). *Handbook of conceptualization and treatment of child psychopathology*. New York: Pergamon Press.

Osofsky, J. D., & Thompson, M. D. (2000). Adaptive and maladaptive parenting: Perspectives on risk and protective factors. In J. P. Shonkoff & S. J. Meisels (Eds.), *Handbook of early childhood intervention* (2nd ed., pp. 54–75). New York: Cambridge University Press.

Overton, W. F., & Horowitz, H. A. (1991). Developmental psychopathology: Integrations and differentiations. In D. Cicchetti & S. L. Toth (Eds.), *Rochester Symposium on Developmental Psychopathology: Vol. 3. Models and integrations* (pp. 1–42). New York: University of Rochester Press.

Pakaslahti, L. (2000). Children's and adolescents' aggressive behavior in context: The development and application of aggressive problem-solving strategies. *Aggression and Violent Behavior, 5,* 467–490.

Patterson, G. R. (1982). *Coercive family process.* Eugene, OR: Castalia.

Patterson, G. R. (1993). Orderly change in a stable world: The antisocial trait as a chimera. *Journal of Consulting and Clinical Psychology, 61,* 911–919.

Patterson, G. R., Reid, J. B., & Dishion, T. J. (1992). *Antisocial boys.* Eugene, OR: Castalia.

Patton, M. S. (1985). Masturbation from Judaism to Victorianism. *Journal of Religion and Health, 24,* 133–146.

Pennington, B. F., & Ozonoff, S. (1991). A neuroscientific perspective on continuity and discontinuity in developmental psychopathology. In D. Cicchetti & S. L. Toth (Eds.), *Rochester Symposium on Developmental Psychopathology: Vol. 3. Models and integrations* (pp. 117–159). New York: University of Rochester Press.

Persons, J. B., & Miranda, J. (1992). Cognitive theories of vulnerability to depression: Reconciling negative evidence. *Cognitive Therapy and Research, 16,* 485–502.

Peterson, L., & Brown, D. (1994). Integrating child injury and abuse–neglect research: Common histories, etiologies, and solutions. *Psychological Bulletin, 116,* 293–315.

Phares, V., & Compas, B. (1992). The role of fathers in child and adolescent psychopathology: Make room for Daddy. *Psychological Bulletin, 111,* 387–412.

Pine, D. S., & Grun, J. (1999). Childhood anxiety: Integrating developmental psychopathology and affective neuroscience. *Journal of Child and Adolescent Psychopharmacology, 9,* 1–12.

Plomin, R. (1995). Genetics and children's experiences in the family. *Journal of Child Psychology and Psychiatry, 36,* 33–68.

Plomin, R., & Rutter, M. (1998). Child development, molecular genetics, and what to do with genes once they are found. *Child Development*, 69, 1223–1242.

Posner, M. I., & Rothbart, M. K. (2000). Developing mechanisms of self-regulation. *Development and Psychopathology, 12,* 427–441.

Post, R. M., & Weiss, S. R. B. (1997). Emergent properties of neural systems: How focal molecular neurobiological alterations can affect behavior. *Development and Psychopathology, 9,* 907–929.

Postman, N. (1994). *The disappearance of childhood.* New York: Vintage Books.

Price, J. M., & Lento, J. (2001). The nature of child and adolescent vulnerability: History and definitions. In R. E. Ingram & J. M. Price (Eds.), *Vulnerability to psychopathology: Risk across the lifespan* (pp. 20–38). New York: Guilford Press.

Quay, H. C., Routh, D. K., & Shapiro, S. K. (1987). Psychopathology of childhood: From description to validation. *Annual Review of Psychology, 38,* 491–532.

Raine, A. (1997). Antisocial behavior and psychophysiology: A biosocial perspective and a prefrontal dysfunction hypothesis. In D. M. Stoff, J. Breiling, & J. D. Maser (Eds.), *Handbook of antisocial behavior* (pp. 289–304). New York: Wiley.

Raine, A., Venables, P. H., & Mednick, S. A. (1997). Low resting heart rate at age 3 years predisposes to aggression at age 11 years: Evidence from the Mauritius Child Health Project. *Journal of the American Academy of Child and Adolescent Psychiatry, 36*, 1457–1464.

Rapport, M. D. (2001). Bridging theory and practice: Conceptual understanding of treatments for children with attention deficit hyperactivity disorder (ADHD), obsessive–compulsive disorder (OCD), autism, and depression. *Journal of Clinical Child Psychology, 30,* 3–7.

Rapport, M. D., Chung, K., Shore, G., Denney, C. B., & Isaacs, P. (2000). Upgrading the science and technology of assessment and diagnosis: Laboratory and clinic-based assessment of children with ADHD. *Journal of Clinical Child Psychology, 29*, 555–568.

Rees, J. R. (1939). Sexual difficulties in childhood. In R. G. Gordon (Ed.), *A survey of child psychiatry* (pp. 246–256). Oxford: Oxford University Press.

Reiss, D., & Neiderhiser, J. M. (2000). The interplay of genetic influences and social processes in developmental theory: Specific mechanisms are coming into view. *Development and Psychopathology, 12*, 357–374.

Rende, R. (1999). Adapative and maladaptive pathways in development: A quantitative genetic perspective. In M. C. LaBuda & E. L. Grigorenko (Eds.), *On the way to individuality: Current methodological issues in behavioral genetics* (pp. 1–21). New York: Nova Science.

Reynolds, W. M. (Ed.). (1992). *Internalizing disorders in children and adolescents*. New York: Wiley.

Reynolds, W. M., & Kamphaus, R. W. (1992). *Behavior Assessment System for Children (BASC)*. Circle Pines, MN: American Guidance Services.

Rhee, S. H., Waldman, I. D., Hay, D. A., & Levy, F. (1999). Sex differences in genetic and environmental influences on DSM-III-R attention-deficit/hyperactivity disorder. *Journal of Abnormal Psychology, 108*, 24–41.

Richman, N., Stevenson, J. E., & Graham, P. J. (1975). Prevalence of behaviour problems in 3-year-old children: An epidemiological study in a London borough. *Journal of Child Psychology and Psychiatry, 16*, 277–287.

Richters, J. E. (1992). Depressed mothers as informants about their children: A critical review of the evidence for distortion. *Psychological Bulletin,112*, 485–499.

Richters, J. E. (1997). The Hubble hypothesis and the developmentalist's dilemma. *Development and Psychopathology, 9*, 193–229.

Richters, J. E., & Cicchetti, D. (1993). Mark Twain meets DSM-III-R: Conduct disorder, development, and the concept of harmful dysfunction. *Development and Psychopathology, 5*, 5–29.

Rie, H. E. (1971). Historical perspective of concepts of child psychopathology. In H. E. Rie (Ed.), *Perspectives in child psychopathology* (pp. 3–50). Chicago: Aldine-Atherton.

Roberts, R. E., Attkisson, C. C., & Rosenblatt, A. (1998). Prevalence of psychopathology among children and adolescents. *American Journal of Psychiatry, 155*, 715–725.

Roberts, A. R., & Kurtz, L. F. (1987). Historical perspectives on the care and treatment of the mentally ill. *Journal of Sociology and Social Welfare, 14*, 75–94.

Robins, L. N. (1966). *Deviant children grown up*. Baltimore: Williams & Wilkins.

Robins, L. N. (1994). How recognizing "comorbidities" in psychopathology may lead to an improved research nosology. *Clinical Psychology: Science and Practice, 1*, 93–95.

Rothbart, M. K., Ahadi, S. A., & Evans, D. E. (2000). Temperament and personality. Origins and outcomes. *Journal of Personality and Social Psychology, 78*, 122–135.

Routh, D. K. (1990). Taxonomy in developmental psychopathology: Consider the source. In M. Lewis & S. M. Miller (Eds.), *Handbook of developmental psychopathology* (pp. 53–62). New York: Plenum Press.

Rubin, K. H., Cheah, C. S. L., & Fox, N. (2001). Emotion regulation, parenting and display of social reticence in preschoolers. *Early Education and Development, 12*, 97–115.

Rubin, K. H., Coplan, R. J., Fox, N. A., & Calkins, S. D. (1995). Emotionality, emotion regulation, and preschoolers' social adaptation. *Development and Psychopathology, 7*, 49–62.

Rubinstein, E. (1948). Childhood mental disease in America: A review of the literature before 1900. *American Journal of Orthopsychiatry, 18*, 314–321.

Rutter, M. (1981). The city and the child. *American Journal of Orthopsychiatry, 51*, 610–625.

Rutter, M. (1985). Resilience in the face of adversity: Protective factors and resistance to psychiatric disorder. *British Journal of Psychiatry, 147*, 598–611.

Rutter, M. (1987). Psychosocial resilience and protective mechanisms. *American Journal of Orthopsychiatry, 57*, 316–331.

Rutter, M. (1989). Isle of Wight revisited: Twenty-five years of child psychiatric epidemiology. *Journal of the American Academy of Child and Adolescent Psychiatry, 28*, 633–653.

Rutter, M. (1994a). Beyond longitudinal data: Causes, consequences, and continuity. *Journal of Consulting and Clinical Psychology, 62*, 928–940.

Rutter, M. (1994b). Comorbidity: Meanings and mechanisms. *Clinical Psychology: Science and Practice, 1*, 100–103.

Rutter, M. (1995). Clinical implications of attachment concepts: Retrospect and prospect. *Journal of Child Psychology and Psychiatry, 36*, 549–571.

Rutter, M. L. (1999). Psychosocial adversity and child psychopathology. *British Journal of Psychiatry, 174*, 480–493.

Rutter, M. L. (2000a). Genetic studies of autism: From the 1970s into the millennium. *Journal of Abnormal Child Psychology, 28*, 3–14.

Rutter, M. L. (2000b). Psychosocial influences: Critiques, findings, and research needs. *Development and Psychopathology, 12*, 375–405.

Rutter, M. (2000c). Resilience reconsidered: Conceptual considerations, empirical findings, and policy implications. In J. P. Shonkoff & S. J. Meisels (Eds.), *Handbook of early childhood intervention* (2nd ed., pp. 651–682). New York: Cambridge University Press.

Rutter, M., Dunn, J., Plomin, R., Simonoff, E., Pickles, A., Maughan, B., Ormel, J., Meyer, J., & Eaves, L. (1997). Integrating nature and nurture: Implications of person–environment correlations and interactions for developmental psychopathology. *Development and Psychopathology, 9*, 335–364.

Rutter, M., & Garmezy, N. (1983). Developmental psychopathology. In P. H. Mussen (Series Ed.) & E. M. Hetherington (Vol. Ed.), *Handbook of child psychology: Vol. 4. Socialization, personality, and social development* (4th ed., pp. 775–911). New York: Wiley.

Rutter, M., & Rutter, M. (1993). *Developing minds: Challenge and continuity across the life span*. New York: Basic Books.

Rutter, M., Silberg, J., O'Connor, T., & Simonoff, E. (1999a). Genetics and child psychiatry: I. Advances in quantitative and molecular genetics. *Journal of Child Psychology and Psychiatry, 40*, 3–18.

Rutter, M., Silberg, J., O'Connor, T., & Simonoff, E. (1999b). Genetics and child psychiatry: II. Empirical research findings. *Journal of Child Psychology and Psychiatry, 40*, 19–55.

Rutter, M., & Sroufe, L. A. (2000). Developmental psychopathology: Concepts and challenges. *Developmental and Psychopathology, 12*, 265–296.

Rutter, M., Tizard, J., & Whitmore, K. (Eds.). (1970). *Education, health, and behaviour*. London: Longman.

Samaan, R. A. (2000). The influences of race, ethnicity, and poverty on the mental health of children. *Journal of Health Care for the Poor and Underserved, 11*, 100–110.

Sameroff, A. J. (1993). Models of development and developmental risk. In C. H. Zeanah, Jr. (Ed.), *Handbook of infant mental health* (pp. 3–13). New York: Guilford Press.

Sameroff, A. J. (2000a). Developmental systems and psychopathology. *Development and Psychopathology, 12*, 297–312.

Sameroff, A. J. (2000b). Dialectical processes in developmental psychopathology. In A. J. Sameroff, M. Lewis, & S. M. Miller (Eds.), *Handbook of developmental psychopathology* (2nd ed., pp. 23–40). New York: Kluwer Academic/Plenum.

Sameroff, A. J., Lewis, M., & Miller, S. M. (Eds.). (2000). *Handbook of developmental psychopathology* (2nd ed.). New York: Kluwer Academic/Plenum.

Schopler, E., Mesibov, G. B., & Kunce, L. J. (Eds.). (1998). *Asperger syndrome or highfunctioning autism?* New York: Plenum.

Schteingart, J. S., Molnar, J., Klein, T. P., Lowe, C. B., & Hartmann, A. H. (1995). Homelessness and child functioning in the context of risk and protective factors moderating child outcomes. *Journal of Clinical Child Psychology, 24*, 320–331.

Schultz, D., Izard, C. E., Ackerman, B. P., & Youngstrom, E. A. (2001). Emotion knowledge in economically disadvantaged children: Self-regulatory antecedents and relations to social difficulties and withdrawal. *Development and Psychopathology, 13*, 53–67.

Schwartz, D., & Proctor, L. J. (2000). Community violence exposure and children's social adjustment in the school peer group: The mediating roles of emotion regulation and social cognition. *Journal of Consulting and Clinical Psychology, 68*, 670–683.

Scotti, J. R., & Morris, T. L. (2000). Diagnosis and classification. In M. Hersen & R. T. Ammerman (Eds.). *Advanced abnormal child psychology* (2nd ed., pp. 15–32). Mahwah, NJ: Erlbaum.

Scotti, J. R., Morris, T. L., McNeil, C. B., & Hawkins, R. P. (1996). DSM-IV and disorders of childhood and adolescence: Can structural criteria be functional? *Journal of Consulting and Clinical Psychology, 64*, 1177–1191.

Seifer, R. (2000). Temperament and goodness of fit: Implications for developmental psychopathology. In A. J. Sameroff, M. Lewis, & S. M. Miller (Eds.), *Handbook of developmental psychopathology* (2nd ed., pp. 257–276). New York: Kluwer Academic/Plenum.

Seifer, R., Sameroff, A. J., Baldwin, C. P., & Baldwin, A. (1992). Child and family factors that ameliorate risk between 4 and 13 years of age. *Journal of the American Academy of Child and Adolescent Psychiatry, 31*, 893–903.

Seligman, L. D., & Ollendick, T. H. (1998). Comorbidity of anxiety and depression in children and adolescents: An integrative review. *Clinical Child and Family Psychology Review, 1*, 125–144.

Selman, R. L., Beardslee, W., Schultz, L. H., Krupa, M., & Poderefsky, D. (1986). Assessing adolescent interpersonal negotiation strategies: Toward the integration of structural and functional models. *Developmental Psychology, 22*, 450–459.

Semrud-Clikeman, M., Steingard, R. J., Filipek, P., Biederman, J., Bekken, K., & Renshaw, P. F. (2000). Using MRI to examine brain-behavior relationships in males with attention deficit disorder with hyperactivity. *Journal of the American Academy of Child and Adolescent Psychiatry, 39*, 477–484.

Shaffer, D., Fisher, P., Dulcan, M. K., Davies, M., Piacentini, J., Schwab-Stone, M. E., Lahey, B. B., Bourdon, K., Jensen, P. S., Bird, H. R., Canino, G., & Regier, D. A. (1996). The NIMH Diagnostic Inverview Schedule for Children Version 2.3 (DISC-2.3): Description, acceptability, prevalence rates, and performance in the MECA study. *Journal of the American Academy of Child and Adolescent Psychiatry, 35*, 865–877.

Shaffer, D., Lucas, C. P., & Richters, J. E. (Eds.). (1999). *Diagnostic assessment in child and adolescent psychopathology*. New York: Guilford Press.

Shapiro, T., & Esman, A. (1992). Psychoanalysis and child and adolescent psychiatry. *Journal of the American Academy of Child and Adolescent Psychiatry, 31*, 6–13.

Sheldon, K. M., & King, L. (2001). Why positive psychology is necessary. *American Psychologist, 56*, 216–217.

Shipman, K. L. & Zeman, J. (2001). Socialization of children's emotion regulation in mother–child dyads: A developmental psychopathology perspective. *Development and Psychopathology, 13*, 317–336.

Shonkoff, J. P., & Phillips, D. A. (Eds.). (2000). *From neurons to neighborhoods: The science of early childhood development*. Washington, DC: National Academy Press.

Short, A. L., Barrett, P. M., Dadds, M. R., & Fox, T. L. (2001). The influence of family and experimental context on cognition in anxious children. *Journal of Abnormal Child Psychology, 29*, 585–596.

Silk, J. S., Nath, S. R., Siegel, L. R., & Kendall, P. C. (2000). Conceptualizing mental disorders in children: Where have we been and where are we going? *Development and Psychopathology, 12*, 713–735.

Silverman, J. S., Silverman, J. A., & Eardley, D. A. (1984). Do maladaptive attitudes cause depression? *Archives of General Psychiatry, 41*, 28–30.

Silverthorn, P., & Frick, P. J. (1999). Developmental pathways to antisocial behavior: The delayed-onset pathway in girls. *Development and Psychopathology, 11*, 101–126.

Simeonsson, R. J., & Rosenthal, S. L. (1992). Developmental models and clinical practice. In C. E. Walker & M. C. Roberts (Eds.), *Handbook of clinical child psychology* (2nd ed., pp. 19–31). New York: Wiley.

Simonoff, E., Pickles, A., Meyer, J. M., Silberg, J. L., Maes, H. H., Loeber, R., Rutter, M., Hewitt, J. K., & Eaves, L. J. (1997). The Virginia Twin Study of Adolescent Behavioral Development: Influence of age, sex, and impairment on rates of disorder. *Archives of General Psychiatry, 54*, 801–808.

Skinner, B. F. (1953). *Science and human behavior*. New York: Macmillan.

Skuse, D. H. (2000). Behavioural neuroscience and child psychopathology: Insights from model systems. *Journal of Child Psychology and Psychiatry, 41*, 3–31.

Slusarek, M., Velling, S., Bunk, D., & Eggers, C. (2001). Motivational effects on inhibitory control in children with ADHD. *Journal of the American Academy of Child and Adolescent Psychiatry, 40*, 355–363.

Solomon, A., Haaga, D. A. F., Brody, C., Kirk, L., & Friedman, D. G. (1998). Priming irrational beliefs in recovered-depressed people. *Journal of Abnormal Psychology, 107*, 440–449.

Sonuga-Barke, E. J. S. (1998). Categorical models of childhood disorder: A conceptual and empirical analysis. *Journal of Child Psychology and Psychiatry, 39*, 115–133.

Spitzer, R. L. (1994). Psychiatric "co-occurrence"? I'll stick with "comorbidity." *Clinical Psychology: Science and Practice, 1,* 88–92.

Spitzer, R. L., Davies, M., & Barkley, R. A. (1990). The DSM-III-R field trial of disruptive behavior disorders. *Journal of the American Academy of Child and Adolescent Psychiatry, 29,* 690–697.

Sroufe, L. A. (1985). Attachment classification from the perspective of infant–caregiver relationships and infant temperament. *Child Development, 56,* 1–14.

Sroufe, L. A. (1997). Psychopathology as an outcome of development. *Development and Psychopathology, 9,* 251–268.

Sroufe, L. A., Carlson, E. A., Levy, A. K., & Egeland, B. (1999). Implications of attachment theory for developmental psychopathology. *Development and Psychopathology, 11,* 1–13.

Sroufe, L. A., Duggal, S., Weinfeld, N., & Carlson, E. (2000). Relationships, development, and psychopathology. In A. J. Sameroff, M. Lewis, & S. M. Miller (Eds.), *Handbook of developmental psychopathology* (2nd ed., pp. 75–91). New York: Kluwer Academic/Plenum.

Sroufe, L. A., & Jacobvitz, D. (1989). Diverging pathways, developmental transformations, multiple etiologies and the problem of continuity in development. *Human Development, 32,* 196–203.

Sroufe, L. A., & Rutter, M. (1984). The domain of developmental psychopathology. *Child Development, 55,* 17–29.

Stark, K. D., Rouse, L. W., & Livingston, R. (1991). Treatment of depression during childhood and adolescence: Cognitive-behavioral procedures for the individual and family. In P. C. Kendall (Ed.), *Child and adolescent therapy: Cognitive-behavioral procedures* (pp. 165–206). New York: Guilford Press.

State, M. W., Lombroso, P. J., Pauls, D. L., & Leckman, J. F. (2000). The genetics of childhood psychiatric disorders: A decade of progress. *Journal of the American Academy of Child and Adolescent Psychiatry, 39,* 946–962.

Stein, M. A., Szumowski, E., Blondis, T. A., & Roizen, N. J. (1995). Adaptive skills dysfunction in ADD and ADHD children. *Journal of Child Psychology and Psychiatry, 36,* 663–670.

Stodgell, C. J., Ingram, J. L., & Hyman, S. L. (2000). The role of candidate genes in unraveling the genetics of autism. *International Review of Research in Mental Retardation, 23,* 57–82.

Szasz, T. S. (1970). *The manufacture of madness.* New York: Dell.

Szatmari, P., Boyle, M. H., & Offord, D. R. (1993). Familial aggregation of emotional and behavioral problems of childhood in the general population. *American Journal of Psychiatry, 150,* 1398–1403.

Tanguay, P. E. (2000). Pervasive developmental disorders: A 10-year review. *Journal of the American Academy of Child and Adolescent Psychiatry, 39,* 1079–1095.

Tarullo, L. B., Richardson, D. T., Radke-Yarrow, M., & Martinez, P. E. (1995). Multiple sources in child diagnosis: Parent–child concordance in affectively ill and well families. *Journal of Clinical Child Psychology, 24,* 173–183.

Taylor, L. & Ingram, R. E. (1999). Cognitive reactivity and depressotypic information processing in children of depressed mothers. *Journal of Abnormal Psychology, 108,* 202–210.

Tebes, J. K., Kaufman, J. S., Adnopoz, J., & Racusin, G. (2001). Resilience and family psychosocial processes among children of parents with serious mental disorders. *Journal of Child and Family Studies, 10,* 115–136.

Tems, C. L., Stewart, S. M., Skinner, J. R., Hughes, C. W., & Emslie, G. (1993). Cognitive distortions in depressed children and adolescents: Are they state dependent or traitlike? *Journal of Clinical Child Psychology, 22,* 316–326.

Terr, L. C. (1991). Childhood traumas: An outline and overview. *American Journal of Psychiatry, 148,* 10–20.

Thomas, A., & Chess, S. (1977). *Temperament and development.* New York: Brunner/Mazel.

Thomas, J. M., & Clark, R. (1998). Disruptive behavior in the very young child: Diagnostic Classification: 0–3 guides identification of risk factors and relational interventions. *Infant Mental Health Journal, 19,* 229–244.

Thomas, J. M., & Guskin, K. A. (2001). Disruptive behavior in young children: What does it mean? *Journal of the American Academy of Child and Adolescent Psychiatry, 40,* 44–51.

Thompson, R. A. (1994). Emotion regulation: A theme in search of definition. In N. A. Fox (Ed.), The development of emotion regulation: Biological and behavioral considerations. *Monographs of the Society for Research in Child Development, 59*(2–3, Serial No. 240), 25–52.

Thompson, R. A., & Calkins, S. D. (1996). The double-edged sword: Emotion regulation for children at risk. *Development and Psychopathology, 8,* 163–182.

Thompson, R. A., & Ontai, L. (2000). Striving to do well what come naturally: Social support, developmental psychopathology, and social policy. *Development and Psychopathology, 12,* 657–676.

Tolan, P., & Thomas, P. (1995). The implications of age of onset for delinquency risk: II. Longitudinal data. *Journal of Abnormal Child Psychology, 23,* 157–181.

Torgersen, S. (1993). Genetics. In A. S. Bellack & M. Hersen (Eds.), *Psychopathology in adulthood* (pp. 41–56). Boston: Allyn & Bacon.

Tremblay, R. E., Masse, B., Perron, D., LeBlanc, M., Schwartzman, A., & Ledingham, J. E. (1992). Early disruptive behavior, poor school achievement, delinquent behavior, and delinquent personality: Longitudinal analyses. *Journal of Consulting and Clinical Psychology, 60,* 64–72.

U.S. Advisory Board on Child Abuse and Neglect. (1995). *A nation's shame: Fatal child abuse and neglect in the United States.* Washington, DC: National Clearinghouse on Child Abuse and Neglect.

U.S. Department of Health and Human Services. (2000a). *Child maltreatment 1998: Reports from the states to the National Child Abuse and Neglect Data Systems.* Washington, DC: U.S. Government Printing Office.

U.S. Department of Health and Human Services. (2000b). *Healthy people 2010: Understanding and improving health* (2nd ed.). Washington, DC: U.S. Government Printing Office.

U.S. Public Health Service. (1999). *Mental health: A report of the Surgeon General.* Washington, DC: U.S. Department of Health and Human Services.

U.S. Public Health Service. (2001a). *Report of the Surgeon General's conference on children's mental health: A national action agenda.* Washington, DC: U.S. Department of Health and Human Services.

U.S. Public Health Service. (2001b). *Youth violence: Report from the Surgeon General.* Washington, DC: U.S. Department of Health and Human Services.

U.S. Public Heath Service. (2001c). *Culture, race, and ethnicity: A supplement to mental health: A report of the*

Surgeon General. Washington, DC: U.S. Department of Health and Human Services.

Vasey, M. W., Daleiden, E. L., Williams, L. L., & Brown, L. M. (1995). Biased attention in childhood anxiety disorders: A preliminary study. *Journal of Abnormal Child Psychology, 23,* 267–279.

Vasey, M. W., & Lonigan, C. J. (2000). Considering the clinical utility of performance-based measures of child anxiety. *Journal of Clinical Child Psychology, 29,* 493–508.

Velez, C. N., Johnson, J., & Cohen, P. (1989). A longitudinal analysis of selected risk factors for childhood psychopathology. *Journal of the American Academy of Child and Adolescent Psychiatry, 28,* 861–864.

Verhulst, F. C., & Koot, H. M. (1991). Longitudinal research in child and adolescent psychiatry. *Journal of the American Academy of Child and Adolescent Psychiatry, 30,* 361–368.

Verhulst, F. C., & Koot, H. M. (1992). *Child psychiatric epidemiology: Concepts, methods, and findings*. Newbury Park, CA: Sage.

Verhulst, F. C., & van der Ende, J. (1993). "Comorbidity" in an epidemiological sample: A longitudinal perspective. *Journal of Child Psychology and Psychiatry, 34,* 767–783.

Viken, R. J., & McFall, R. M. (1994). Paradox lost: Contemporary reinforcement theory for behavior therapy. *Current Directions in Psychological Science, 3,* 123–125.

Volkmar, F. R., & Klin, A. (1998). Asperger syndrome and nonverbal learning disabilities. In E. Schopler, G. B. Mesibov, & L. J. Kunce (Eds.), *Asperger syndrome or highfunctioning autism?* (pp. 107–121). New York: Plenum.

Volkmar, F. R., & Klin, A. (2000). Asperger's disorder and higher functioning autism: Same or different? *International Review of Research in Mental Retardation, 23,* 83–111.

Volling, B. L. (2001). Early attachment relationships as predictors of preschool children's emotion regulation with a distressed sibling. *Early Education and Development, 12,* 185–207.

Wakefield, J. C. (1992). The concept of mental disorder: On the boundary between biological facts and social values. *American Psychologist, 47,* 373–388.

Wakefield, J. C. (1997). When is development disordered?: Developmental psychopathology and the harmful dysfunction analysis of mental disorder. *Development and Psychopathology, 9,* 269–290.

Wakefield, J. C. (1999a). Evolutionary versus prototype analyses of the concept of disorder. *Journal of Abnormal Psychology, 108,* 374–399.

Wakefield, J. C. (1999b) The concept of disorder as a foundation for the DSM's theory-neutral nosology: Response to Follette and Houts, Part II. *Behaviour Research and Therapy, 37,* 1001–1027.

Wakefield, J. C. (2001). Evolutionary history versus current causal role in the definition of disorder: Reply to McNally. *Behaviour Research and Therapy, 39,* 347–366.

Walden, T. A., & Smith, M. C. (1997). Emotion regulation. *Motivation and Emotion, 21,* 7–25.

Walker, C. E., Kenning, M., & Faust-Campanile, J. (1989). Enuresis and encopresis. In E. J. Mash & R. A. Barkley (Eds.), *Treatment of childhood disorders* (pp. 423–448). New York: Guilford Press.

Waters, A. M., Lipp, O. V., & Cobham, V. E. (2000). Investigation of threat-related attentional bias in anxious children using the startle eyeblink modification paradigm. *Journal of Psychophysiology, 14,* 142–150.

Waters, E., & Sroufe, L. A. (1983). Social competence as a developmental construct. *Developmental Review, 3,* 79–97.

Weisz, J. R. (2000). Lab–clinic differences and what we can do about them: III. National policy matters. *Clinical Child Psychology Newsletter, 15*(3), 1–3, 6, 10.

Weisz, J. R., & Sigman, M. (1993). Parent reports of behavioral and emotional problems among children in Kenya, Thailand, and the United States. *Child Development, 64,* 98–109.

Weisz, J. R., & Suwanlert, S. (1987). Epidemiology of behavioral and emotional problems among Thai and American children: Parent reports for ages 6 to 11. *Journal of the American Academy of Child and Adolescent Psychiatry, 26,* 890–897.

Weisz, J. R., & Suwanlert, S. (1989). Over- and undercontrolled referral problems among children and adolescents from Thailand and the United States: The wat and wai of cultural differences. *Journal of Consulting and Clinical Psychology, 55,* 719–726.

Weisz, J. R., & Suwanlert, S. (1991). Adult attitudes toward over- and undercontrolled child problems: Urban and rural parents and teachers from Thailand and the United States. *Journal of Child Psychology and Psychiatry, 32,* 645–654.

Werner, E. E. (1995). Resilience in development. *Current Directions in Psychological Science, 4,* 81–85.

Werner, E. E., Bierman, J. M., & French, F. E. (1971). *The children of Kauai: A longitudinal study from the prenatal period to age ten.* Honolulu: University of Hawaii Press.

Werner, E. E., & Smith, R. S. (1992). *Overcoming the odds: High risk children from birth to adulthood.* Ithaca, NY: Cornell University Press.

Werry, J. S. (2001). Pharmacological treatments of autism, attention deficit hyperactivity disorder, oppositional defiant disorder, and depression in children and youth: Commentary. *Journal of Clinical Child Psychology, 30,* 110–113.

White, H. R., Bates, M. E., & Buyske, S. (2001). Adolescence-limited versus persistent delinquency: Extending Moffitt's hypothesis into adulthood. *Journal of Abnormal Psychology, 110,* 600–609.

Widiger, T. A., & Ford-Black, M. M. (1994). Diagnoses and disorders. *Clinical Psychology: Science and Practice, 1,* 84–87.

Wildes, J. E., & Emery, R. E. (2001). The roles of ethnicity and culture in the development of eating disturbance and body dissatisfaction: A meta-analytic review. *Clinical Psychology Review, 21,* 521–551.

Willcutt, E. G., & Pennington, B. F. (2000a). Comorbidity of reading disability and attention-deficit/hyperactivity disorder: Differences by gender and subtype. *Journal of Learning Disabilities,* 33, 179–191.

Willcutt, E. G., & Pennington, B. F. (2000b). Psychiatric comorbidity in children and adolescents with reading disability. *Journal of Child Psychology and Psychiatry, 41,* 1039–1048.

Willerman, L. (1973). Activity level and hyperactivity in twins. *Child Development, 44,* 1411–1415.

Wolfe, D. A., & Mosk, M. D. (1983). Behavioral comparisons of children from abusive and distressed families. *Journal of Consulting and Clinical Psychology, 51,* 702–708.

Wong, Y., & Ollendick, T. H. (2001). A cross-cultural and developmental analysis of self-esteem in Chinese and Western children. *Clinical Child and Family Psychology Review, 4,* 253–271.

World Health Organization (WHO). (1992). *The ICD-10 classification of mental and behavioural disorders: Clinical descriptions and diagnostic guidelines*. Geneva: Author.

Zahn-Waxler, C. (1993). Warriors and worriers: Gender and psychopathology. *Development and Psychopathology, 5*, 79–89.

Zahn-Waxler, C., Cole, C. M., Welsh, J. D., & Fox, N. A. (1995). Psychophysiological correlates of empathy and prosocial behaviors in preschool children with behavior problems. *Development and Psychopathology, 7*, 27–48.

Zahn-Waxler, C., Klimes-Dougan, B., & Slattery, M. J. (2000). Internalizing problems of childhood and adolescence. *Development and Psychopathology, 12*, 443–466.

Zahner, G. E., Jacobs, J. H., Freeman, D. H., & Trainor, K. F. (1993). Rural–urban child psychopathology in a northeastern U.S. state: 1986–1989. *Journal of the American Academy of Child and Adolescent Psychiatry, 32*, 378–387.

Zero to Three/National Center for Clinical Infant Programs. (1994). *Diagnostic classification of mental health and developmental disorders of infancy and early childhood (Diagnostic classification: 0–3)*. Washington, DC: Author.

Zimmerman, M. A., & Arunkumar, R. (1994). Resiliency research: Implications for schools and policy. *Social Policy Report, 8*(4), 1–17.

Zoccolillo, M. (1993). Gender and the development of conduct disorder. *Development and Psychopathology, 5*, 65–78.

II

BEHAVIOR DISORDERS

CHAPTER TWO

Attention-Deficit/ Hyperactivity Disorder

Russell A. Barkley

It is commonplace for children (especially preschoolers) to be active, energetic, and exuberant; to flit from one activity to another as they explore their environment and its novelties; and to act without much forethought, responding on impulse to events that occur around them, often with their emotional reactions readily apparent. But when children persistently display levels of activity that are far in excess of their age group; when they are unable to sustain attention, interest, or persistence as well as their peers do to their activities, longer-term goals, or the tasks assigned to them by others; or when their self-regulation lags far behind expectations for their developmental level, they are no longer simply expressing the *joie de vivre* that characterizes childhood. They are instead highly likely to be impaired in their social, cognitive, academic, familial, and eventually occupational domains of major life activities.

Highly active, inattentive, and impulsive youngsters will find themselves far less able than their peers to cope successfully with the universal developmental progressions toward self-regulation, cross-temporal organization, and preparation for their future so evident in our social species. And they will often experience the harsh judgments, punishments, moral denigration, and social ostracism reserved for those society views as lazy, unmotivated, selfish, thoughtless, immature, and willfully irresponsible. These heedless risk-taking children with the devil-may-care attitudes, and self-destructive ways have captured public and scientific interest for more than a century. Diagnostic labels for inattentive, impulsive children have changed numerous times over the last century; yet the actual nature of the disorder has changed little, if at all, from descriptions nearly a century ago (Still, 1902). This constellation of behavior problems may constitute one of the most well-studied childhood disorders of our time. Yet these children remain an enigma to most members of the public, who struggle to accept the notion that the disorder may be a biologically rooted developmental disability when nothing seems physically, outwardly wrong with them.

Children possessing the above-described attributes to a degree that is deviant for their developmental level sufficient to create impairments in major life activities are now diagnosed as having attention-deficit/hyperactivity disorder (ADHD; American Psychiatric Association, 1994). Their problematic behavior is thought to arise early in childhood, and to be persistent over development in most cases. This chapter provides an overview of the nature of this disorder; briefly considers its history; and describes its diagnostic criteria, its developmental course and outcomes, and its causes. Current critical issues related to these matters are raised along the way. Given the thousands of scientific papers on this topic, this chapter must of necessity concentrate on the most important topics in this literature. Readers interested in more detail can pursue other sources (Accardo, Blondis, Whitman, & Stein, 2001; Barkley, 1998; Weiss & Hechtman, 1993). My own theoretical model of ADHD is also presented, providing a more parsimonious accounting for the many cognitive and social deficits in the disorder; this model points to numerous promising directions for future research, while rendering a deeper appreciation for the developmental significance and seriousness of ADHD. As will become evident, continuing to refer to this disorder as one involving attention deficits understates a more central problem with inhibition, self-regulation, and the cross-temporal organization of social behavior.

HISTORICAL CONTEXT

Literary references to individuals having serious problems with inattention, hyperactivity, and poor impulse control date back to Shakespeare, who made reference to a malady of attention in *King Henry VIII*. A hyperactive child was the focus of a German poem, "Fidgety Phil," by physician Heinrich Hoffman (see Stewart, 1970). William James (1890/1950), in his *Principles of Psychology*, described a normal variant of character that he called the "explosive will," which resembles the difficulties experienced by those who today are described as having ADHD. But, more serious clinical interest in children with ADHD first occurred in three lectures of the English physician George Still (1902) before the Royal Academy of Physicians.

Still reported on a group of 20 children in his clinical practice whom he defined as having a deficit in "volitional inhibition" (p. 1008), which led to a "defect in moral control" (p. 1009) over their own behavior. Described as aggressive, passionate, lawless, inattentive, impulsive, and overactive, many of these children today would be diagnosed as having not only ADHD but also oppositional defiant disorder (ODD) (see Hinshaw & Lee, Chapter 3, this volume). Still's observations were quite astute, describing many of the associated features of ADHD that would come to be corroborated in research over the next century: (1) an overrepresentation of male subjects (ratio of 3:1 in Still's sample); (2) high comorbidity with antisocial conduct and depression; (3) an aggregation of alcoholism, criminal conduct, and depression among the biological relatives; (4) a familial predisposition to the disorder, likely of hereditary origin; and yet (5) the possibility of the disorder's also arising from acquired injury to the nervous system.

Interest in these children arose in North America after the great encephalitis epidemics of 1917–1918. Children surviving these brain infections had many behavioral problems similar to those seen in contemporary ADHD (Ebaugh, 1923; Hohman, 1922; Stryker, 1925). These cases and others known to have arisen from birth trauma, head injury, toxin exposure, and infections (see Barkley, 1998) gave rise to the concept of a "brain-injured child syndrome" (Strauss & Lehtinen, 1947), often associated with mental retardation, that would eventually be applied to children manifesting these same behavior features but without evidence of brain damage or retardation (Dolphin & Cruickshank, 1951; Strauss & Kephardt, 1955). This concept evolved into that of "minimal brain damage" and eventually "minimal brain dysfunction" (MBD), as challenges were raised to the label in view of the dearth of evidence of obvious brain injury in most cases (see Kessler, 1980, for a more detailed history of MBD).

By the late 1950s, focus shifted away from etiology and toward the more specific behavior of hyperactivity and poor impulse control characterizing these children, reflected in labels such as "hyperkinetic impulse disorder" or "hyperactive child syndrome" (Burks, 1960; Chess, 1960). The disorder was thought to arise from cortical overstimulation, due to poor thalamic filtering of stimuli entering the brain (Knobel, Wolman, & Mason, 1959; Laufer, Denhoff, & Solomons, 1957). Despite a continuing belief among clinicians and researchers of this era that the condition had some sort of neurological origin, the larger influence of psychoanalytic thought held sway. And so, when the second edition of the *Diagnostic and Statistical Manual of Mental Disorders* (DSM-II) appeared, all childhood disorders were described as "reactions," and the hyperactive child syndrome became "hyperkinetic reaction of childhood" (American Psychiatric Association, 1968).

The recognition that the disorder was not caused by brain damage seemed to follow a similar argument made somewhat earlier by the prominent child psychiatrist Stella Chess (1960). It set off a major rift between professionals in North America and those in Europe, which continues (to a lessening extent) to the present. Europe continued to view hyperkinesis for most of the latter half of the 20th century as a relatively rare condition of extreme overactivity, often associated with mental retardation or evidence of organic brain damage. This discrepancy in perspectives has been converging over the last decade, as evident in the similarity of the DSM-IV criteria (see below) with those of the *International Classification of Diseases*, 10th revision (ICD-10; World Health Organization, 1993). Nevertheless, the manner in which clinicians and educators view the disorder remains quite disparate; in North America, Canada, and Australia, such children are diagnosed with ADHD (a developmental disorder), whereas in Europe they are viewed as having a conduct problem or disorder (a behavioral disturbance believed to arise largely out of family dysfunction and social disadvantage).

By the 1970s, research emphasized the problems with sustained attention and impulse control in addition to hyperactivity (Douglas, 1972). Douglas (1980, 1983) theorized that the disorder involved major deficits in (1) the investment, organization, and maintenance of attention and effort; (2) the ability to inhibit impulsive behavior; and (3) the ability to modulate arousal levels to meet situational demands. Together with these deficits went an unusually strong inclination to seek immediate reinforcement. Douglas's emphasis on attention, along with the numerous studies of attention, impulsiveness, and other cognitive sequelae that followed (see Douglas, 1983; and Douglas & Peters, 1978, for reviews), eventually led to renaming the disorder "attention deficit disorder" (ADD) in 1980 (DSM-III; American Psychiatric Association, 1980). Historically significant was the distinction in DSM-III between two types of ADD: ADD with hyperactivity and without it. Little research existed at the time on the latter subtype that would have supported such a distinction being made in an official and increasingly prestigious diagnostic taxonomy. Yet, in hindsight, this bald assertion led to valuable research on the differences between these two supposed forms of ADD, which otherwise would never have taken place. That research may have been fortuitous, as it may be leading to the conclusion that a subset of those having ADD without hyperactivity may actually have a separate, distinct, and qualitatively unique disorder, rather than a subtype of ADHD (Milich, Balentine, & Lynam, 2001).

Even so, concern arose within a few years of the creation of the label ADD that the important features of hyperactivity and impulse control were being deemphasized,when in fact they were critically important to differentiating the disorder from other conditions and to predicting later developmental risks (Barkley, 1998; Weiss & Hechtman, 1993). In 1987, the disorder was renamed "attention-deficit hyperactivity disorder" in DSM-III-R (American Psychiatric Association, 1987), and a single list of items incorporating all three symptoms was specified. Also important here was the placement of the condition of ADD without hyperactivity, renamed "undifferentiated attention-deficit disorder," in a separate section of the manual from ADHD, with the specification that insufficient research existed to guide in the construction of diagnostic criteria for it at that time.

During the 1980s, reports focused instead on problems with motivation generally, and an insensitivity to response consequences specifically (Barkley, 1989a; Glow & Glow, 1979; Haenlein & Caul, 1987). Research was demonstrating that under conditions of continuous reward, the performances of children with ADHD were often indistinguishable from normal children on various lab tasks, but that when reinforcement patterns shifted to partial reward or to extinction (no-reward) conditions, the children with ADHD showed significant declines in their performance (Douglas & Parry, 1983, 1994; Parry & Douglas, 1983). It was also observed that deficits in the control of behavior by rules characterized these children (Barkley, 1989a).

Beginning in the late 1980s, researchers employed information-processing paradigms to study ADHD, and found that problems in perception and information processing were not so evident as were problems with motivation and response inhibition (Barkley, Grodzinsky, & DuPaul, 1992; Schachar & Logan, 1990; Sergeant, 1988; Sergeant & Scholten, 1985a, 1985b). The problems with hyperactivity and impulsivity also were found to form a single dimension of behavior (Achenbach & Edelbrock, 1983; Goyette, Conners, & Ulrich, 1978; Lahey et al., 1988), which others described as "disinhibition" (Barkley, 1990). All of this led to the creation of two separate lists of items and thresholds for ADHD when the DSM-IV was published later in the decade (American Psychiatric Association, 1994): one for inattention and another for hyperactive–impulsive behavior. Unlike its predecessor, DSM-III-R, DSM-IV thus once again permitted the diagnosis of a subtype of ADHD that consisted principally of problems with attention (ADHD predominantly inattentive type). It also permitted, for the first time, the distinction of a subtype of ADHD that consisted chiefly of hyperactive–impulsive behavior without significant inattention (ADHD, predominantly hyperactive–impulsive type). Children having significant problems from both item lists were described as having ADHD, combined type. The specific criteria from DSM-IV are discussed in more detail below (see "Diagnostic Criteria and Related Issues").

Healthy debate continues to the present over the core deficits in ADHD, with increasing weight being given to problems with behavioral inhibition, self-regulation, and the related domain of executive functioning (Barkley, 1997a, 1997b, 2001c; Douglas, 1999; Nigg, 2001; Quay, 1997). The symptoms of inattention may actually be evidence of impaired working memory and not of perceptual, filtering, or selection (input) problems (Barkley, 1997b). Likewise, controversy continues to swirl around the place of a subtype composed primarily of inattention within the larger condition of ADHD (see *Clinical Psychology: Science and Practice*, 2001, Vol. 8, No. 4, for a debate on this issue): Some argue for its being a distinct disorder from ADHD (Barkley, 2001a; Milich et al., 2001), and others argue that this distinction may be premature (Hinshaw, 2001; Lahey, 2001) or not especially important to treatment planning (Pelham, 2001). Relatively consistent across viewpoints, however, is the opinion that a subset of children with only high levels of inattention probably have a qualitatively different problem in attention (deficient selective attention and sluggish cognitive processing) than is seen in children with ADHD (poor persistence, inhibition, and resistance to distraction).

DESCRIPTION AND DIAGNOSIS

The Core Symptoms

Research employing factor analysis has repeatedly identified two distinct behavioral dimensions underlying the various behavioral problems (symptoms) thought to characterize ADHD (Burns, Boe, Walsh, Sommers-Flanagan, & Teegarden, 2001; DuPaul, Powers, Anastopoulos, & Reid, 1997; Lahey et al., 1994; Pillow, Pelham, Hoza, Molina, & Stultz, 1998). These two dimensions have been identified across various ethnic and cultural groups, including Native American children (Beiser, Dion, & Gotowiec, 2000).

Inattention

Attention represents a multidimensional construct (Bate, Mathias, & Crawford, 2001; Mirsky, 1996; Strauss, Thompson, Adams, Redline, & Burant, 2000), and thus several qualitatively distinct problems with attention may be evident in children (Barkley, 2001a). The dimension impaired in ADHD reflects an inability to sustain attention or persist at tasks or play activities, remember and follow through on rules and instructions, and resist distractions while doing so. I have elsewhere argued that this dimension is more likely to reflect problems with the executive function of working memory than poor attention per se (Barkley, 1997b), and evidence is becoming available to support this contention (Oosterlan, Scheres, & Sergeant, in press; Seguin, Boulerice, Harden, Tremblay, & Pihl, 1999; Wiers, Gunning, & Sergeant, 1998). Parents and teachers frequently complain that these children do not seem to listen as well as they should for their age, cannot concentrate, are easily distracted, fail to finish assignments, are forgetful, and change activities more often than others (DuPaul et al., 1998). Research employing objective measures corroborates these complaints through observations of exhibiting more "off-task" behavior and less work productivity, looking away more often from assigned tasks (including television), showing less persistence at tedious tasks (such as continuous-performance tasks), being slower and less likely to return to an activity once interrupted, being less attentive to changes in the rules governing a task, and being less capable of shifting attention across tasks flexibly (Borger & van der Meere, 2000; Hoza, Pelham, Waschbusch, Kipp, & Owens, 2001; Lorch et al., 2000; Luk, 1985; Newcorn et al., 2001; Seidman, Biederman, Faraone, Weber, & Ouellette, 1997; Shelton et al., , 1998). This inattentive behavior distinguishes these children from those with learning disabilities (Barkley, DuPaul, & McMurray, 1990) or other psychiatric disorders (Chang et al., 1999; Swaab-Barneveld et al, 2000), and does not appear to be a function of other disorders often comorbid with ADHD (anxiety, depression, or oppositional and conduct problems)

(Murphy, Barkley, & Bush, 2001; Klorman et al., 1999; Newcorn et al., 2001; Nigg, 1999; Seidman, Biederman, Faraone, et al., 1995).

Hyperactive–Impulsive Behavior (Disinhibition)

Like attention, inhibition is a multidimensional construct (Nigg, 2000; Olson, Schilling, & Bates, 1999), and thus various qualitatively distinct forms of inhibitory impairments may eventually be found in children. The problems with inhibition seen in ADHD are thought to involve voluntary or executive inhibition of prepotent responses, rather than impulsiveness that may be more motivationally controlled, as in a heightened sensitivity to available reward (reward seeking) or to excessive fear (Nigg, 2001). Some evidence suggests that an excess sensitivity to reward or to sensation seeking may be more associated with severity of conduct disorder (CD) or psychopathy than with severity of ADHD (Beauchaine, Katkin, Strassberg, & Snarr, 2001; Daugherty & Quay, 1991; Fischer, Barkley, Smallish, & Fletcher, in press-a; Matthys, van Goozen, de Vries, Cohen-Kettenis, & van Engeland, 1998). Evidence is less clear about deficits in automatic or involuntary inhibition, as in eye blinking or negative priming, being associated with ADHD (Nigg, 2001).

More specifically, children with ADHD manifest difficulties with excessive activity level and fidgetiness, less ability to stay seated when required, greater touching of objects, moving about, running, and climbing than other children, playing noisily, talking excessively, acting impulsively, interrupting others' activities, and being less able than others to wait in line or take turns in games (American Psychiatric Association, 1994). Parents and teachers describe them as acting as if driven by a motor, incessantly in motion, always on the go, and unable to wait for events to occur. Research objectively documents them to be more active than other children (Barkley & Cunningham, 1979a; Dane, Schachar, & Tannock, 2000; Luk, 1985; Porrino et al., 1983; Shelton et al., 1998); to have considerable difficulties with stopping an ongoing behavior (Schachar, Tannock, & Logan, 1993; Milich, Hartung, Matrin, & Haigler, 1994; Nigg, 1999, 2001; Oosterlaan, Logan, & Sergeant, 1998); to talk more than others (Barkley, Cunningham, & Karlsson, 1983); to interrupt others' conversations (Malone & Swanson, 1993); to be less able to resist immediate temptations and delay gratification (Anderson, Hinshaw, & Simmel, 1994; Barkley, Edwards, Laneiri, Fletcher, & Metevia, 2001; Olson et al., 1999; Rapport, Tucker, DuPaul, Merlo, & Stoner, 1986; Solanto et al., 2001); and to respond too quickly and too often when they are required to wait and watch for events to happen, as is often seen in impulsive errors on continuous-performance tests (Losier, McGrath, & Klein, 1996; Newcorn et al., 2001). Although less frequently examined, similar differences in activity and impulsiveness have been found between children with ADHD and those with learning disabilities (Barkley, DuPaul, & McMurray, 1990; Bayliss & Roodenrys, 2000; Klorman et al., 1999; Willcutt et al., 2001). Mounting evidence further shows that these inhibitory deficits are not a function of other psychiatric disorders that may overlap with ADHD (Barkley, Edwards, et al., 2001; Halperin, Matier Bedi, Sharpin, & Newcorn, 1992; Fischer et al., in press-a; Murphy et al., 2001; Nigg, 1999; Oosterlaan et al., 1998; Seidman Biederman, Faraone, et al., 1997).

Interestingly, recent research shows that the problems with inhibition arise first (at ages 3–4 years), ahead of those related to inattention (at ages 5–7 years), and that the sluggish cognitive tempo that characterizes the predominantly inattentive subtype of ADHD may arise even later (ages 8–10) (Hart, Lahey, Loeber, Applegate, & Frick, 1995; Loeber, Green, Lahey, Christ, & Frick, 1992; Milich et al., 2001). Whereas the symptoms of disinhibition in the DSM item lists seem to decline with age, perhaps owing to their heavier weighting with hyperactive than with impulsive behavior, those of inattention remain relatively stable during the elementary grades (Hart et al., 1995). They eventually decline by adolescence (Fischer, Barkley, Fletcher, & Smallish, 1993a), though not to normal levels. Why the inattention arises later than the disinhibitory symptoms and does not decline when the latter do over development remains an enigma. As noted above, it may simply reflect the different weightings of symptoms in the DSM. Those of hyperactivity may be more typical of preschool to early school-age children and are overrepresented in the DSM list, while those reflecting inattention may be more characteristic of school-age children. Another explanation comes from the theoretical model described below (Barkley, 1997b), in which inhibition and the two types of working memory (nonverbal and verbal) emerge at separate times in development.

Situational and Contextual Factors

The symptoms constituting ADHD are greatly affected in their level of severity by a variety of situational and task-related factors. Douglas (1972) commented on the greater variability of task performances by children with ADHD compared to control children. Many others since then have found that when a child with ADHD must perform multiple trials within a task assessing attention and impulse control, the range of scores around that child's own mean performance is frequently greater than in normal children (see Douglas, 1983). The finding is especially common in measures of reaction time (Chee, Logan, Schachar, Lindsay, & Wachsmuth, 1989; Fischer et al., in press-a; Kuntsi, Oosterlaan, & Stevenson, 2001; Murphy et al., 2001; Scheres, Oosterlaan, & Sergeant, 2001).

A number of other factors influence the ability of children with ADHD to sustain their attention to task performance, control their impulses to act, regulate their activity level, and/or produce work consistently. The performance of these children is worse (1) later in the day than earlier (Dane et al., 2000; Porrino et al., 1983; Zagar & Bowers, 1983); (2) in greater task complexity, such that organizational strategies are required (Douglas, 1983); (3) when restraint is demanded (Barkley & Ullman, 1975; Luk, 1985); (4) under low levels of stimulation (Antrop, Roeyers, Van Oost, & Buysse, 2000; Zentall, 1985); (5) under more variable schedules of immediate consequences in the task (Carlson & Tamm, 2000; Douglas & Parry, 1983, 1994; Slusarek, Velling, Bunk, & Eggers, 2001; Tripp & Alsop, 1999); (6) under longer delay periods prior to reinforcement availability (Solanto et al., 2001; Sonuga-Barke, Taylor, & Heptinstall, 1992; Tripp & Alsop, 2001); and (7) in the absence of adult supervision during task performance (Draeger, Prior, & Sanson, 1986; Gomez & Sanson, 1994).

Besides the aforementioned factors, which chiefly apply to task performance, variability has also been documented across more macroscopic settings. For instance, children with ADHD exhibit more problematic behavior when persistence in work-related tasks is required (chores, homework, etc.) or where behavioral restraint is necessary, especially in settings involving public scrutiny (in church, in restaurants, when a parent is on the phone, etc.), than in free-play situations (Altepeter & Breen, 1992; Barkley & Edelbrock, 1987; DuPaul & Barkley, 1992). Although they will be more disruptive when their fathers are at home than during free play, children with ADHD are still rated as much less problematic when their fathers are at home than in most other contexts. Fluctuations in the severity of ADHD symptoms have also been documented across a variety of school contexts (Barkley & Edelbrock, 1987; DuPaul & Barkley, 1992). In this case, contexts involving task-directed persistence and behavioral restraint (classroom) are the most problematic, with significantly fewer problems posed by contexts involving less work and behavioral restraint (at lunch, in hallways, at recess, etc.), and even fewer problems being posed during special events (field trips, assemblies, etc.) (Altepeter & Breen, 1992).

Associated Developmental Impairments

Children with ADHD often demonstrate deficiencies in many other cognitive and emotional abilities. Among these are difficulties with (1) physical fitness, gross and fine motor coordination, and motor sequencing (Breen, 1989; Denckla & Rudel, 1978; Harvey & Reid, 1997; Kadesjo & Gillberg, 1999; Mariani & Barkley, 1997); (2) speed of color naming (Tannock, Martinussen, & Frijters, 2000); (3) verbal and nonverbal working memory and mental computation (Barkley, 1997a; Mariani & Barkley, 1997; Murphy et al., 2001; Zentall & Smith, 1993); (4) story recall (Lorch et al., 2000; Sanchez, Lorch, Milich, & Welsh, 1999); (5) planning and anticipation (Grodzinsky & Diamond, 1992; Klorman et al., 1999); (6) verbal fluency and confrontational communication (Grodzinsky & Diamond, 1992; Zentall, 1988); (5) effort allocation (Douglas, 1983; Nigg, Hinshaw, Carte, & Treuting, 1998; Sergeant & van der Meere, 1994; Voelker, Carter, Sprague, Gdowski, & Lachar, 1989); (6) developing, applying, and self-monitoring organizational strategies (Clark, Prior, & Kinsella, 2000; Hamlett, Pellegrini, & Connors, 1987; Purvis & Tannock, 1997; Zentall, 1988); (7) internalization of self-directed speech (Berk & Potts, 1991; Copeland, 1979; Winsler, 1998; Winsler, Diaz, Atencio, McCarthy, & Chabay, 2000); (8) adhering to restrictive instructions (Danforth, Barkley, & Stokes, 1991; Roberts, 1990; Routh & Schroeder, 1976); and (9) self-regulation of emotion (Braaten & Rosen, 2000; Hinshaw, Buhrmeister, & Heller, 1989; Maedgen & Carlson, 2000). The last-mentioned difficulties, those with emotional control, may be especially salient in children having ADHD with comorbid

ODD (Melnick & Hinshaw, 2000). Several studies have also demonstrated that ADHD may be associated with less mature or diminished moral development (Hinshaw, Herbsman, Melnick, Nigg, & Simmel, 1993; Nucci & Herman, 1982; Simmel & Hinshaw, 1993). Many of these cognitive difficulties appear to be specific to ADHD and are not a function of its commonly comorbid disorders, such as learning disabilities, depression, anxiety, or ODD/CD (Barkley, Edwards, et al., 2001; Clark et al., 2000; Klorman et al., 1999; Murphy et al., 2001; Nigg, 1999; Nigg et al., 1998).

The commonality among most or all of these seemingly disparate abilities is that all have been considered to fall within the domain of "executive functions" in the field of neuropsychology (Barkley, 1997b; Denckla, 1994) or "metacognition" in developmental psychology (Flavell, 1970; Torgesen, 1994; Welsh & Pennington, 1988), or to be affected by these functions. All seem to be mediated by the frontal cortex, particularly the prefrontal lobes (Fuster, 1997; Stuss & Benson, 1986). "Executive functions" have been defined as those neuropsychological processes that permit or assist with human "self-regulation" (Barkley, 1997b, 2001a, 2001b), which itself has been defined as any behavior by a person that modifies the probability of a subsequent behavior by that person so as to alter the probability of a later consequence (Kanfer & Karoly, 1972). By classifying cognitive actions or thinking as private behavior, one can understand how these private, self-directed, cognitive (executive) actions fall within the definition of human self-regulation: They are private behaviors (cognitive acts) that modify other behaviors so as to alter the likelihood of later consequences for the individual. And when the role of the frontal lobes generally, and the prefrontal cortex particularly, in these executive abilities is appreciated, it is easy to see why researchers have repeatedly speculated that ADHD probably arises out of some disturbance or dysfunction of this brain region (Barkley, 1997b; Heilman, Voeller, & Nadeau, 1991; Levin, 1938; Mattes, 1980).

THEORETICAL FRAMEWORK

Many different theories of ADHD have been proposed over the past century to account for the diversity of findings so evident in this disorder (Barkley, 1999b). Some of these have been discussed above (see "Historical Context"), such as Still's (1902) notion of defective volitional inhibition and moral regulation of behavior; Douglas's (1972, 1983) theory of deficient attention, inhibition, arousal, and preference for immediate reward; and the attempts to view ADHD as a deficit in sensitivity to reinforcement (Haenlein & Caul, 1987) or rule-governed behavior (Barkley, 1981, 1989a). More recently, Quay (1997), relying on Gray's (1982) neuropsychological model of anxiety, has proposed that ADHD represents a deficit in the brain's behavioral inhibition system. Quay's hypothesis has resulted in increased research on inhibitory and activation (reinforcement) processes in both ADHD (Fischer et al., in press-a; Milich et al., 1994) and CD (see Hinshaw & Lee, Chapter 3, this volume). Relying on Logan's "race" model of inhibition, Schachar et al. (1993) have also argued for a central deficit in inhibitory processes in those with ADHD. In this model, an event or stimulus is hypothesized to trigger both an activating or primary response and an inhibitory response, creating a competition or race between the two as to which will be executed first. Disinhibited individuals, such as those with ADHD, are viewed as having slower initiation of inhibitory processes than normal children do.

There is little doubt that poor behavioral inhibition plays a central role in ADHD (see Barkley, 1997b, 1999a, and Nigg, 2001, for reviews). Although important in the progress of our understanding about ADHD, this conclusion still leaves at least two important questions on the nature of ADHD unresolved. First, how does this account for the numerous other associated symptoms found in ADHD (described above) and apparently subsumed under the concepts of motor control and executive functioning? Second, how does this account for the involvement of the separate problem with inattention (poor sustained attention) in the disorder? The theoretical model of ADHD I have developed over the past decade not only encompasses many of these earlier explanations, but may hold the answers to these questions as well some unexpected directions that future research on ADHD might wish to pursue (Barkley, 1994, 1997a, 1997b, 2001b).

Inhibition, Executive Functions, and Time

The model of ADHD set forth below and in Figure 2.1 places behavioral inhibition at a central point in its relation to four other executive func-

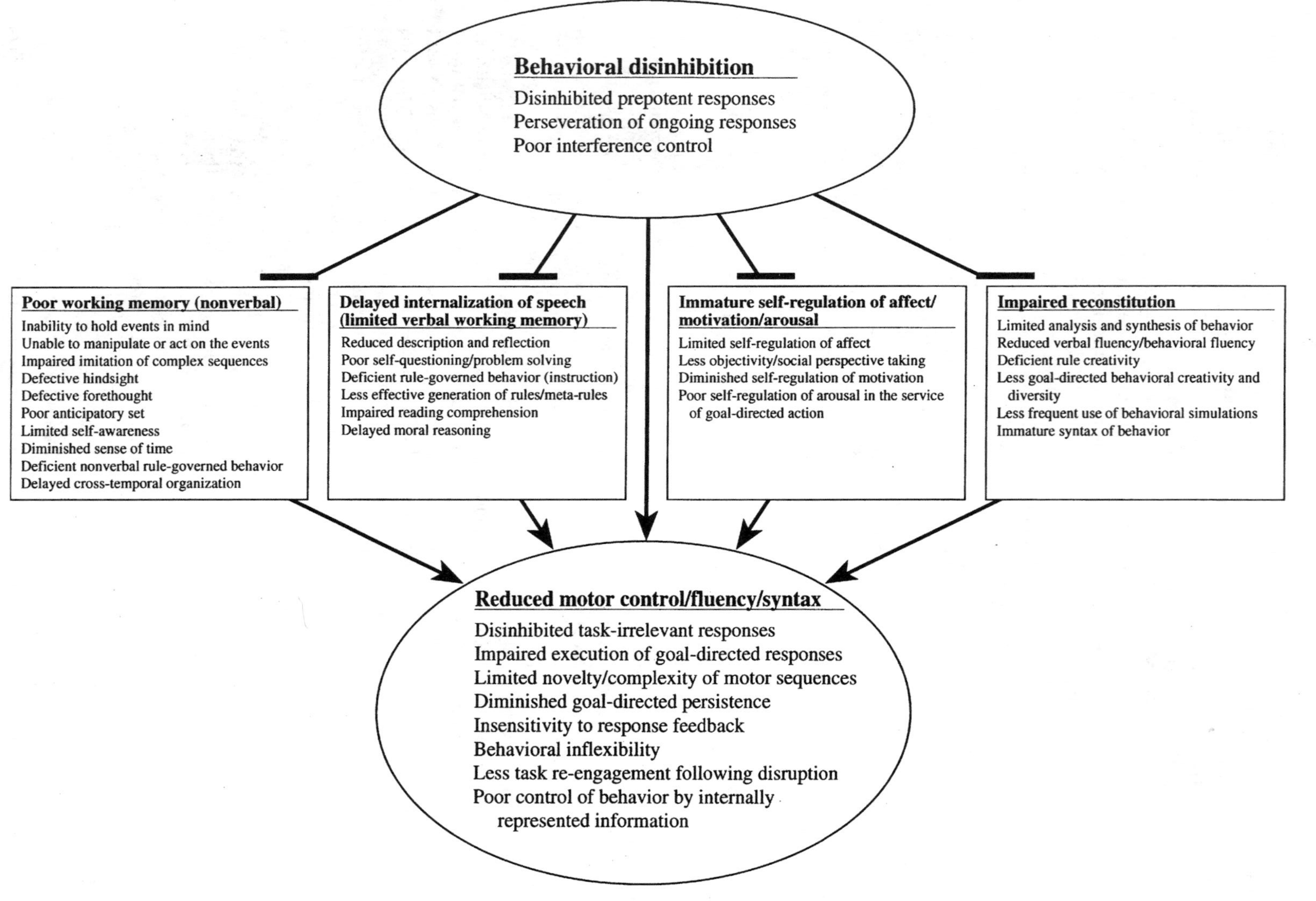

FIGURE 2.1. Diagram illustrating the complete hybrid model of executive functions (boxes) and the relationship of these four functions to the behavioral inhibition and motor control systems. From Barkley (1997b). Copyright 1997 by The Guilford Press. Reprinted by permission.

tions dependent upon it for their own effective execution. These four executive functions provide for self-regulation, bringing behavior progressively more under the control of time and the influence of future over immediate consequences. The interaction of these executive functions permits far more effective adaptive functioning toward the social future (social self-sufficiency).

Several assumptions are important in understanding the model as it is applied to ADHD: (1) The capacity for behavioral inhibition begins to emerge first in development, ahead of most or all these four executive functions but possibly in conjunction with the first, nonverbal working memory. (2) These executive functions emerge at different times in development, may have different developmental trajectories, and are interactive. (3) The impairment that ADHD creates in these executive functions is secondary to the primary deficit it creates in behavioral inhibition (improve the inhibition, and these executive functions should likewise improve). (4) The deficit in behavioral inhibition arises principally from genetic and neurodevelopmental origins rather than purely social ones, although its expression is certainly influenced by social factors over development. (5) The secondary deficits in self-regulation created by the primary deficiency in inhibition feed back to contribute further to poor behavioral inhibition, given that self-regulation contributes to the enhancement of self-restraint (inhibition). Finally, (6) the model does not apply to those having what is presently called the predominantly inattentive type of ADHD. The model has been derived from earlier theories on the evolution of human language (Bronowski, 1977), the internalization of speech (Vygotsky, 1966/1987), and the functions of the prefrontal cortex (Fuster, 1997). The evidence for the model as applied to ADHD is reviewed in detail elsewhere (Barkley, 1997b).

"Behavioral inhibition" is viewed as consisting of two related processes: (1) the capacity to inhibit prepotent responses, either prior to or once initiated, creating a delay in the response to an event (response inhibition); and (2) the protection of this delay, the self-directed actions occurring within it, and the goal-directed behaviors they create from interference by competing events and their prepotent responses (interference control). "Prepotent responses" are defined as those for which immediate reinforcement is available for their performance or for which there is a strong history of reinforcement in this context. Through the postponement of the prepotent response and the creation of this protected period of delay, the occasion is set for four other executive functions to act effectively in modifying the individual's eventual response(s) to the event. This is done to achieve a net maximization of temporally distant consequences rather than immediate consequences alone for the individual. The self-regulation is also protected from interference during its performance by a related form of inhibition (interference control).

The four executive functions are believed to develop via a common process. All represent private, covert forms of behavior that at one time in early child development (and in human evolution) were entirely publicly observable and were directed toward others and the external world at large. With maturation, this outer-directed behavior becomes turned on the self as a means to control one's own behavior. Such self-directed behaving then becomes increasingly less observable to others as the suppression of the public, peripheral, musculo-skeletal aspects of the behavior progresses. The child is increasingly able to act toward the self without publicly displaying the actual behavior being activated. This progressively greater capacity to suppress the publicly observable aspects of behavior is what is meant here by the terms "covert," "privatized," or "internalized." The child comes to be capable of behaving internally (in the brain) without showing that response through the peripheral muscles, at least not to the extent that it is visible to others. As I have discussed elsewhere (Barkley, 1997b, 2001c), this behavior-to-the-self can still be detected in very subtle, vestigial forms as slight shifts in muscle potential at those peripheral sites involving the muscles used in performing the public form of that behavior (e.g., when one engages in verbal thought, one still slightly moves the lips, tongue, larynx, etc.). In this sense, all of the executive functions follow the same general sequence as the internalization of speech (Diaz & Berk, 1992; Vygotsky, 1966/1987, 1978), which in this model forms the second executive function.

Each executive function is hypothesized to contribute to the following developmental shifts in the sources of control over human behavior:

- From external events to mental representations related to those events.
- From control by others to control by the self.
- From immediate reinforcement to delayed gratification.

- From the temporal now to the conjectured social future.

I have elsewhere asserted that the executive functions probably evolved in successive stages in our hominid ancestry from intraspecies competition for resources and reproduction in our group living speces. The sequence may resemble, to some extent, the same sequential development evident in children today. The first executive function (nonverbal working memory, which involves sensory–motor action to the self, especially visual imagery) begins its development so early in infancy that it must have been crucial to human survival. It may have evolved for the adaptive purposes of reciprocal altruism (social exchange) and generalized vicarious learning. These activities seem to be essential for the survival of our group-living species, contributing to cooperation, coalition formation (friendships), the construction of social hierarchies from these coalitions, and pedagogy (Barkley, 2001c). Vicarious learning can be considered a form of behavioral theft that, once having arisen in a species, would have set up strong selection pressure for the privatization of one's behavior—particularly during learning, rehearsal, and other forms of practice—so as not to have one's behavioral innovations readily appropriated by others (competitors). Other adaptive purposes that may have been served by this and the other three executive functions (which develop later) are verbal self-instruction, verbal self-defense against social manipulation by others, and self-innovation. Such evolutionary speculations permit this theory to hypothesize various social deficits that should be evident in ADHD, given the executive deficits associated with it, that can be tested in subsequent experiments. As is evident below, children with ADHD experience serious difficulties in their social relationships, some of which may arise from the deficits in executive functioning that interfere with reciprocal exchange, vicarious learning, social coalition formation, social self-defense, and self-innovation (improvement).

Nonverbal Working Memory (Sensory–Motor Action to the Self)

During the delay in responding created by inhibition, humans activate and retain a mental representation of events in mind (Bronowski, 1977), typically using visual imagery and private audition. The capacity for imagery may allow even infants to successfully perform delayed-response tasks to a limited degree (Diamond, 1990; Diamond, Cruttenden, & Niederman, 1994; Goldman-Rakic, 1987). As this capacity increases developmentally, it forms the basis for "nonverbal working memory," which has been defined as the ability to maintain mental information online so as to guide a later motor response. This activation of past images for the sake of preparing a current response is known as "hindsight" or the "retrospective function" of working memory (Bronowski, 1977; Fuster, 1997). It allows for the retention of events in a temporal sequence that contributes to the "subjective estimation of time" (Michon, 1985). Such temporal sequences can be analyzed for recurring patterns, and those patterns can then be used to conjecture hypothetical future events. Anticipating these hypothetical futures gives rise to a preparation to act, or "anticipatory set" (Fuster, 1997). This extension of hindsight forward into time also underlies "forethought" or the "prospective function" of working memory (Bronowski, 1977; Fuster, 1997). And from this sense of future probably emerges the progressively greater valuation of future consequences over immediate ones, which takes place throughout child development and early adult life (Green, Fry, & Meyerson, 1994).

Important in this model for understanding the linkage of inattention to disinhibition in ADHD is the critical role played by working memory in maintaining online (in mind) one's intentions to act ("plans"), so as to guide the construction and execution of complex goal-directed actions over time (Fuster, 1997). Such sustained chains of goal-directed actions create persistence of responding, giving rise to the capacity of humans to sustain attention (responding) for dramatically long periods of time in pursuit of future goals. As James (1890/1950) so eloquently described it: "The essential achievement of the will, in short, when it is most 'voluntary,' is to ATTEND to a difficult object and hold it fast before the mind" (p. 815); and "Everywhere then the function of the effort [voluntary or free will] is the same: to keep affirming and adopting a thought which, if left to itself, would slip away" (p. 818). Thus self-regulation relative to time arises as a consequence of inhibition acting in conjunction with nonverbal working memory. And since language is used in part to express cognitive content, references to time, sense of past, and sense of future can occur in verbal interactions with others; such references should become increasingly frequent in the developmental course of children as this sense of time develops.

As extrapolated to those with ADHD, the model predicts that deficits in behavioral inhibition lead to deficiencies in nonverbal working memory, and thus (1) particular forms of forgetfulness (forgetting to do things at certain critical points in time); (2) impaired ability to organize and execute actions relative to time (e.g., time management); and (3) reduced hindsight and forethought, leading to (4) a reduction in the creation of anticipatory action toward future events. Consequently, the capacity for the cross-temporal organization of behavior in those with ADHD is diminished, disrupting the ability to string together complex chains of actions directed, over time, to a future goal. The greater the degree to which time separates the components of the behavioral contingency (event, response, consequence), the more difficult the task will prove for those with ADHD, who cannot bind the contingency together across time so as to use it to govern their behavior as well as others.

Research is beginning to demonstrate some of these deficits in those with ADHD, such as nonverbal working memory, timing, and forethought (Barkley, 1997b; Barkley, Edwards, et al., 2001; Barkley, Murphy, & Bush, 2001; Murphy et al., 2001). Still unstudied is the prediction from this theory that children with ADHD will be delayed in making references to time, past, and future in their verbal interactions with others, relative to when normal children begin making such references in their development of sense of time.

Verbal Working Memory (Internalization of Speech)

One of the more fascinating developmental processes witnessed in children is the progressive internalization or privatization of speech (Diaz & Berk, 1992). During the early preschool years, speech, once developed, is initially employed for communication with others. By 3–5 years of age, language comes to be turned on the self. Such overt self-speech is readily observable in preschool and early school-age children. By 5–7 years of age, this speech becomes somewhat quieter and more telegraphic, and shifts from being more descriptive to being more instructive. Language is now a means of reflection (self-directed description), as well as a means for controlling one's own behavior. Self-directed speech progresses from being public to being subvocal to finally being private, all over the course of perhaps 6 to 10 years, thereby giving rise to verbal thought (Diaz & Berk, 1992; Kopp, 1982; Vygotsky, 1966/1987). I have conjectured (Barkley, 1997b) that this internalization of speech represents a larger process, in that various other forms of behavior may be internalized as well (sensory–motor action, emotion, and play).

For those with ADHD, the privatization of speech should be delayed, resulting in greater public speech (excessive talking), less verbal reflection before acting, less organized and rule-oriented self-speech, a diminished influence of self-directed speech in controlling one's own behavior, and difficulties following the rules and instructions given by others (Barkley, 1997b). Substantial evidence has accumulated to support this prediction of delayed internalization of speech (Berk & Potts, 1991; Landau, Berk, & Mangione, 1996; Winsler, 1998; Winsler et al., 2000). Given that such private self-speech is a major basis for verbal working memory, this domain of cognitive activity should be impaired in ADHD as well. Evidence suggests that this is so: Children with ADHD have difficulties with tasks such as backward digit span, mental arithmetic, paced auditory serial addition, paired-associate learning, and other tasks believed to reflect verbal working memory (Barkley, 1997b; Chang et al., 1999; Grodzinsky & Diamond, 1992; Kuntsi et al., 2001). Children with learning disabilities may also have difficulties with some of these tasks, making it unclear to what extent the deficits seen in working memory in ADHD are a function of the overlap of learning disabilities with this disorder (Cohen et al., 2000; Willcutt et al., 2001). ADHD may impair the actual internalization of speech, whereas reading disorders may reflect a normal internalization but of an impaired language ability.

Internalization and Self-Regulation of Affect

The inhibition of the initial prepotent response includes the inhibition of the initial emotional reaction that it may have elicited. It is not that the child does not experience emotion, but that the behavioral reaction to or expression of that emotion is delayed, along with any motor behavior associated with it. The delay in responding with this emotion allows the child time to engage in self-directed behavior that will modify both the eventual response to the event and the emotional reaction that may accompany it. This permits a moderating effect on the emotion being experienced subjectively by the child, as well as on the child's eventual public expression of emotional behavior (Keenan, 2000). But it is not just affect that is being managed by the development of self-regulation, but the underlying components of emotion as well, these being motivation (drive states) and arousal (Fuster, 1997; Lang, 1995). This internalization and self-regulation of motivation permit the child to induce drive states that may be required for the initiation and maintenance of goal-directed, future-oriented behavior, thereby permitting greater persistence toward tasks and activities that may offer little immediate reinforcement but for which there may be substantial delayed reinforcement.

Extending this model to ADHD leads to the following predictions. Those with ADHD should display (1) greater emotional expression in their reactions to events; (2) less objectivity in the selection of a response to an event; (3) diminished social perspective taking, as these children do not delay their initial emotional reaction long enough to take the view of others and their own needs into account; and (4) diminished ability to induce drive and motivational states in themselves in the service of goal-directed behavior. Those with ADHD remain more dependent upon the environmental contingencies within a situation or task to determine their motivation than do others (Barkley, 1997b). Preliminary work has begun to demonstrate that those with ADHD do have significant problems with emotion regulation (Braaten & Rosen, 2000; Maedgen & Carlson, 2000; Southam-Gerow & Kendall, 2002) and that this may be particularly so in that subset having comorbid oppositional defiant disorder (Melnick & Hinshaw, 2000).

Reconstitution (Internalization of Play)

The use of private visual imagery as well as private language to mentally represent objects, actions, and their properties provides a means by which the world can be taken apart and recombined cognitively rather than physically. The delay in responding allows time for an event to be held in mind and then disassembled, so as to extract more information about the event before preparing a response to it. Internal imagery and speech permit analysis, and out of this process comes its complement—synthesis. Just as the parts of speech can be recombined to form new sentences, the parts of the world represented in speech and imagery are likewise recombined to create entirely new ideas about the world and entirely new responses to that world (Bronowski, 1977). The world is seen as having parts rather than inviolate wholes—parts capable of multiple, novel recombinations. This permits humans a far greater capacity for creativity and problem solving than is evident in our closest primate relatives. I believe that this process results from the internalization of play. Just as speech goes from being overt to self-directed and then covert, so does manipulative and verbal play. This process of mental play, or reconstitution, is evident in everyday speech in its fluency and generativity (diversity); yet it is also evident in nonverbal expression as well, such as in motor and design fluency. The need for reconstitution becomes obvious when obstacles must be surmounted to accomplish a goal. In a sense, reconstitution provides for planning and problem solving to overcome obstacles and attain goals. This mental module produces rapid, efficient, and often novel combinations of speech or action into entirely new messages or behavioral sequences, and so gives rise to behavioral innovation.

As applied to ADHD, the model predicts a diminished use of analysis and synthesis in the formation of both verbal and nonverbal responses to events. The capacity to mentally visualize, manipulate, and then generate multiple plans of action (options) in the service of goal-directed behavior, and to select from among them those with the greatest likelihood of succeeding, should therefore be reduced. This impairment in reconstitution will be evident in everyday verbal fluency when a person with ADHD is required by a task or situation to assemble rapidly, accurately, and efficiently the parts of speech into messages (sentences), so as to accomplish the goal or requirements of the task. It will also be evident in tasks where visual information must be held in mind and manipulated to generate diverse scenarios to help solve problems (Barkley, 1997b). Evidence for a deficiency in verbal and nonverbal fluency, planning, problem solving, and strategy development more generally in children with ADHD is limited, but what exists is consistent with the theory (Barkley, 1997b; Clark et al., 2000; Klorman et al., 1999; Nigg et al., 1998; Oosterlaan et al., in press).

Motor Control/Fluency

If the deficit in behavioral inhibition proposed in the current model is housed within the brain's motor or output system, then its effects should also be evident in the planning and execution of motor actions. Complex fine and gross motor actions require inhibition to preclude the initiation of movements located in neural zones adjacent to those being activated. Inhibition provides an increasing "functional pruning" of the motor system such that only those actions required to accomplish the task are initiated by the individual. Lengthy, complex, and novel chains of goal-directed behavior can be constructed and protected from interference until they have been completed. The model stipulates that those with ADHD should display greater difficulties with the development of motor coordination, and especially in the planning and execution of complex, lengthy, and novel chains of goal-directed responses. There is substantial evidence already available for problems in motor development and motor execution in those with ADHD (see Barkley, 1997b; Harvey & Reid, 1997; Kadesjo & Gillberg, 2001). It remains to be determined whether those with ADHD have more difficulties in producing, executing, and sustaining lengthy and complex chains of novel responses toward goals.

Conclusion

I have recently theorized that this executive system may have evolved to support the social activities of reciprocal exchange and altruism, imitation and vicarious learning, self-sufficiency and innovation, and social self-defense (Barkley, 2001b). This theory implies that these larger, universally important domains of social development may be impaired by ADHD as well. If so, then deficits in adaptive functioning (self-sufficiency) more generally would be evident in ADHD, as seems to be the case (Barkley, Shelton, et al., 2002; Roizen, Blondis, Irwin, & Stein, 1994; Shelton et al., 1998; Stein, Szumowski, Blondis, & Roizen, 1995).

The present model of ADHD shows how the findings noted above under "Associated Developmental Impairments" can now be integrated into a more unifying theory of the disorder. Undoubtedly, this theory is imperfect. A great deal of research will be required to clarify the nature of each component in the model; to evaluate the strength of the relationship of each component to behavioral inhibition and to the other components; to elucidate the developmental progression of each component and their ordering; and to critically test some of the previously unexpected predictions of the model as applied to ADHD (e.g., diminished time management, reduced references to time in verbal interactions, the impact of ADHD on analysis/synthesis and self-innovation, etc.). All useful theories are imperfect and time-limited. What we ask of them is not perfection from birth, but the more pragmatic standard of greater utility than previously existing models or theories. Competing theories of ADHD have limited themselves to elucidating the nature of the inhibitory deficit (Quay, 1997; Sonuga-Barke, Lamparelli, Stevenson, Thompson, & Henry, 1994) while ignoring the associated cognitive, emotional, and social deficiencies associated with it and explaining why they exist. The present theory offers more utility, in that it addresses the origins of those associated problems, is more testable and hence falsifiable, provides a better link to normal child development, and yields a greater understanding of the basis for managing the disorder than do other extant models. Regardless of what theory may replace it in the future, that theory will likewise have to deal with the evidence that points to problems with inhibition and these four executive functions.

This appreciation of the linkage among the executive functions in the model, the self-regulation they permit, and the goal-directed persistence that derives from self-control explain several important findings about the link between disinhibition (hyperactive–impulsive behavior) and inattention. It is possible to see now why the problems with hyperactive–impulsive behavior arise first in the development of ADHD, to be followed within a few years by the problems with inattention. And it also explains the nature of that inattention as it arises. The inattention reflects a deficit in executive functioning, especially working memory, and so is really a form of intention deficit (attention to the future).

DIAGNOSTIC CRITERIA AND RELATED ISSUES

DSM-IV Criteria

The most recent diagnostic criteria for ADHD as defined in DSM-IV (American Psychiatric Association, 1994) are set forth in Table 2.1. These diagnostic criteria are some of the most rigorous and most empirically derived criteria ever available in the history of clinical diagnosis for this disorder. They were derived from a committee of some of the leading experts in the field, a literature review of ADHD, an informal survey of

TABLE 2.1. DSM-IV Criteria for Attention-Deficit/Hyperactivity Disorder (ADHD)

A. Either (1) or (2):

(1) six (or more) of the following symptoms of inattention have persisted for at least 6 months to a degree that is maladaptive and inconsistent with developmental level:

Inattention
(a) often fails to give close attention to details or makes careless mistakes in schoolwork, work, or other activities
(b) often has difficulty sustaining attention in tasks or play activities
(c) often does not seem to listen when spoken to directly
(d) often does not follow through on instructions and fails to finish schoolwork, chores, or duties in the workplace (not due to oppositional behavior or failure to understand instructions)
(e) often has difficulty organizing tasks and activities
(f) often avoids, dislikes, or is reluctant to engage in tasks that require sustained mental effort (such as schoolwork or homework)
(g) often loses things necessary for tasks or activities (e.g., toys, school assignments, pencils, books, or tools)
(h) is often easily distracted by extraneous stimuli
(i) is often forgetful in daily activities

(2) six (or more) of the following symptoms of hyperactivity–impulsivity have persisted for at least 6 months to a degree that is maladaptive and inconsistent with developmental level:

Hyperactivity
(a) often fidgets with hands or feet or squirms in seat
(b) often leaves seat in classroom or in other situations in which remaining seated is expected
(c) often runs about or climbs excessively in situations in which it is inappropriate (in adolescents or adults, may be limited to subjective feelings of restlessness)
(d) often has difficulty playing or engaging in leisure activities quietly
(e) is often "on the go" or often acts as if "driven by a motor"
(f) often talks excessively

Impulsivity
(g) often blurts out answers before the questions have been completed
(h) often has difficulty awaiting turn
(i) often interrupts or intrudes on others (e.g., butts into conversations or games)

B. Some hyperactive–impulsive or inattentive symptoms that caused impairment were present before age 7 years.

C. Some impairment from the symptoms is present in two or more settings (e.g., at school [or work] and at home).

D. There must be clear evidence of clinically significant impairment in social, academic, or occupational functioning.

E. The symptoms do not occur exclusively during the course of a Pervasive Developmental Disorder, Schizophrenia, or other Psychotic Disorder and are not better accounted for by another mental disorder (e.g., Mood Disorder, Anxiety Disorder, Dissociative Disorder, or a Personality Disorder).

Code based on type:
314.01 Attention-Deficit/Hyperactivity Disorder, Combined Type: if both Criteria A1 and A2 are met for the past 6 months
314.00 Attention-Deficit/Hyperactivity Disorder, Predominantly Inattentive Type: if Criterion A1 is met but Criterion A2 is not met for the past 6 months
314.01 Attention-Deficit/Hyperactivity Disorder, Predominantly Hyperactive–Impulsive Type: if Criterion A2 is met but Criterion A1 is not met for the past 6 months

Coding note: For individuals (especially adolescents and adults) who currently have symptoms that no longer meet full criteria, "In Partial Remission" should be specified.

Note. From American Psychiatric Association (1994, pp. 83–85).

empirically derived rating scales assessing the behavioral dimensions related to ADHD by the committee, and from statistical analyses of the results of a field trial of the items using 380 children from 10 different sites in North America (Lahey et al., 1994).

Despite its empirical basis, the DSM criteria have some problems. As noted earlier, evidence is mounting that the predominantly inattentive type of ADHD (hereafter abbreviated as ADHD-PI) may be a diagnosis applied to a rather heterogeneous mix of children, a subset of whom have a qualitatively different disorder of attention and cognitive processing (Milich et al., 2001). This subset is probably not a subtype of ADHD, but may represent a separate disorder (Barkley, 1998, 2001a; Milich et al., 2001)—one manifesting a sluggish cognitive style and selective attention deficit; having less comorbidity with ODD and CD; demonstrating a more passive style of social relationship; involving memory retrieval problems; and, owing to the lower level of impulsiveness, probably having a different, more benign developmental course. Other children consigned to this subtype may be children who formerly met the criteria for ADHD, combined type (hereafter abbreviated as ADHD-C), but with age have had a sufficient decline in their hyperactive symptoms that they no longer qualify for this subtype. For example, in our follow-up study of hyperactive children, all of whom probably had ADHD-C in childhood, we found that 16% of these cases (or 27% of persistent cases) now met criteria only for ADHD-PI as young adults (Barkley, Fischer, Fletcher, & Smallish, 2002). Such individuals might better be thought of as having residual ADHD-C than as having ADHD-PI. Likewise, some children diagnosed with ADHD-PI place just a single symptom or two short of ADHD-C status yet resemble children with ADHD-C, albeit in milder form, in all other respects. Mixing these children formerly diagnosed with ADHD-C and ones currently diagnosed with subthreshold ADHD-C together into the ADHD-PI group is likely to constrain research on the distinctive features of this subtype, its etiology, its response to treatments, and its developmental course. In agreement with Milich et al. (2001), I believe that the subset of children with hypoactivity, lethargy, and sluggish cognitive tempo should be set aside as having a separate disorder from ADHD (Barkley, 2001a).

It is also unclear whether ADHD, predominantly hyperactive–impulsive type (hereafter abbreviated as ADHD-PHI) is really a separate type from ADHD-C or simply an earlier developmental stage of it. The DSM-IV field trial found that those diagnosed with ADHD-PHI were primarily preschool-age children, whereas those with ADHD-C were primarily school-age children. As noted above, this is what one would expect to find, given that the hyperactive–impulsive symptoms appear first and are followed within a few years by those of inattention. If one is going to require that inattention symptoms be part of the diagnostic criteria, then the age of onset for such symptoms will necessitate that ADHD-C have a later age of onset than ADHD-PHI. It seems that these two types may actually be developmental stages of the same type of ADHD.

Are the two separate symptom lists in DSM-IV important, rather than the one combined list used in DSM-III-R? Apparently. In the field trial (Lahey et al., 1994), significant levels of inattention mainly predicted additional problems with completing homework that were not as well predicted by the hyperactive–impulsive behavior. Otherwise, the latter predicted most of the other areas of impairment studied in this field trial. Other studies find that childhood symptoms of hyperactivity are related to adverse adolescent outcomes, such as antisocial behavior, substance abuse, and school disciplinary actions, such as suspensions/expulsions (Babinski, Hartsough, & Lambert, 1999). Symptoms of inattention seem to be primarily predictive of impairment in academic achievement (particularly reading) and school performance (DuPaul, Power, et al., 1998; Fischer, Barkley, Fletcher, & Smallish, 1993b; Weiss & Hechtman, 1993; Rabiner, Coie, & the Conduct Problem Prevention Research Group, 2000). Severity of hyperactive–impulsive behavior is often found to be the dimension of ADHD that more strongly predicts later CD, and so risk for various forms of substance use and abuse (Molina, Smith, & Pelham, 1999). A recent study suggests that adolescent inattention, however, may contribute further to the risk for tobacco use beyond that risk contributed by severity of CD alone (Burke, Loeber, & Lahey, 2001).

Another critical issue deserving consideration is how well the diagnostic thresholds set for the two symptom lists apply to age groups outside of those used in the field trial (ages 4–16 years, chiefly). This concern arises out of the well-known findings that the behavioral items in these lists, particularly those for hyperactivity, decline significantly with age (DuPaul, Power, et al., 1998;

Hart et al., 1995). Applying the same threshold across such a declining developmental slope could produce a situation where a larger percentage of young preschool-age children (ages 2–3 years) would be inappropriately diagnosed as having ADHD (false positives), whereas a smaller than expected percentage of adults would meet the criteria (false negatives). Support of just such a problem with using these criteria for adults was found in a study (Murphy & Barkley, 1996b) collecting norms for DSM-IV item lists on a large sample of adults, ages 17–84 years. The threshold needed to place an individual at the 93rd percentile for that person's age group declined to four of nine inattention items and five of nine hyperactive–impulsive items for ages 17–29 years, then to four of nine on each list for the 30- to 49-year age group, then to three of nine on each list for those 50 years and older. Studies of the utility of the diagnostic thresholds to preschool children younger than 4 years remain to be done. Until then, it seems prudent to utilize the recommended symptom list thresholds only for children ages 4–16 years.

The issue of selecting symptom cutoff scores raises a related conceptual problem for ADHD as well. Is ADHD a static psychopathology, the symptoms of which remain essentially the same regardless of age? Or is it a developmental disorder (delay in rate)? In the latter case, it must always be determined by comparison to same-age peers. Although the DSM criteria imply that ADHD is a developmental disorder (symptoms must be developmentally inappropriate), it also treats the disorder as a relatively static category by using fixed symptom cutoff scores across all age groups. Available research indicates that ADHD is most likely a dimensional disorder (Levy & Hay, 2001), representing an extreme of or delay in normal traits, and so is akin to other developmental disorders (e.g., mental retardation). If so, then, like all developmental disorders, ADHD reflects a delay in the *rate* at which a normal trait is developing—not an absolute loss of function, failure to develop, or pathological state. It needs to be diagnosed as a developmentally relative deficit, such as the 93rd or 98th percentile in severity of symptoms for age (DuPaul, Power, et al., 1998).

This notion of changing symptom thresholds with age raises another critical issue for developing diagnostic criteria for ADHD, and this is the appropriateness of the content of the item set for different developmental periods. Inspection of the item lists suggests that the items for inattention may have a wider developmental applicability across the school-age range of childhood, and even into adolescence and young adulthood. Those for hyperactive–impulsive behavior, in contrast, seem much more applicable to young children and less appropriate or not at all to older teens and adults. As noted above (Hart et al., 1995), the symptoms of inattention remain stable across middle childhood into early adolescence, whereas those for hyperactive–impulsive behavior decline significantly over this same course. Although this may represent a true developmental decline in the severity of the latter symptoms, and possibly in the severity and prevalence of ADHD itself, it could also represent an illusory developmental trend. That is, it might be an artifact of using more preschool-focused items for hyperactivity and more school-age-focused items for inattention.

An analogy using mental retardation may be instructive. Consider the following items that might be chosen to assess developmental level in preschool-age children: being toilet-trained, recognizing colors, counting to 10, repeating 5 digits, buttoning snaps on clothing, recognizing simple geometric shapes, and using a vocabulary repertoire of at least 50 words. Evaluating whether or not a child is able to do these things may prove to be very useful in distinguishing mental retardation in preschoolers. However, if one continued to use this same item set to assess children with mental retardation as they grew older, one would find a decline in the severity of the retardation in such children as progressively more items were achieved with age. One would also find that the prevalence of retardation would decline markedly with age as many formerly delayed children "outgrew" these problems. But we know this would be illusory, because mental retardation represents a developmentally relative deficit in the achievement of mental and adaptive milestones.

To return to the diagnosis of ADHD, if the same developmentally restricted item sets are applied throughout development with no attempt to adjust either the thresholds or, more importantly, the types of items developmentally appropriate for different periods, we might see the same results as with the analogy to mental retardation described here. Similar results are found in ADHD (see below), which should give one pause before interpreting the observed decline in symptom severity (and even the observed decline in apparent prevalence!) as being accurate.

As it now stands, ADHD is being defined mainly by one of its earliest developmental manifestations (hyperactivity) and one of its later (school-age) yet secondary sequelae (deficient goal-directed persistence), and only minimally by its central features (deficits in inhibition and executive functioning).

Also of concern is the absence of any requirement in the DSM for the symptoms to be corroborated by someone who has known the patient well, such as a parent, sibling, long-time friend, or partner. Most likely, this arises from the focus on children throughout much of the history of the ADHD diagnostic category. Children routinely come to professionals with people who know them well (parents). But, in the case of adults who are self-referred to professionals, this oversight could prove potentially problematic. For instance, available evidence suggests that children with ADHD (Henry, Moffitt, Caspi, Langley, & Silva, 1994) and teens with the disorder (Edwards, Barkley, Laneri, Fletcher, & Metevia, 2001; Fischer et al., 1993b; Mannuzza & Gittelman, 1986; Romano, Tremblay, Vitaro, Zoccolillo, & Pagani, 2001) significantly underreport the severity of their symptoms, relative to the reports of parents. If this occurs in adults with ADHD as well, it would mean that self-referred patients might underestimate the severity of their disorder, resulting in a sizable number of false-negative decisions being made by clinicians. There are good reasons why self-awareness might be limited by this disorder. Neuropsychological research indicates that self-awareness is relatively localized to the prefrontal lobes, and that disorders affecting this region (such as Alzheimer's disease) markedly reduce self-awareness (Fuster, 1997; Stuss & Benson, 1986). As evidence reviewed below suggests, underactivity and underdevelopment in these same regions of the brain are likely to be involved in ADHD, and so the disorder ought to restrict self-awareness.

These issues are not merely academic. My colleagues and I have been involved in follow-up research on children with ADHD into their adulthood and have been impressed at the chronicity of impairments created by the disorder, despite an apparent decline in the percentage of cases continuing to meet diagnostic criteria and an apparent decline in the severity of the symptoms used in these criteria (Barkley, Fischer, Edelbrock, & Smallish, 1990; Barkley, Fischer, Fletcher, & Smallish, 2002; Fischer et al., 1993a). Recently, we found that if these children, who are now adults, were interviewed using the DSM criteria, just 5% of them reported sufficient symptoms to receive the diagnosis (Barkley, Fischer, Fletcher, & Smallish, 2002)—a figure nearly identical to that for the New York longitudinal studies (Mannuzza, Klein, Bessler, Malloy, & LaPadula, 1993, 1998). If instead the parents were interviewed, this figure rose to 46%—a ninefold difference in persistence of disorder as a function of reporting source. If instead of the recommended DSM symptom threshold, one were to substitute a developmentally referenced criterion (the 98th percentile) based on same-age control adults, then 12% of the probands would now have the disorder as adults based on self-reports, while the figure would climb to 66% based on parental reports. Whose reports of current functioning were more valid? We addressed this by examining the relationship of self-reports and parent reports to various domains of major life activities and outcomes (education, occupational functioning, friendships, crime, etc.). Parent reports made a substantially larger contribution to nearly all outcome domains and did so for more such domains than did self-reports, suggesting that the parent reports probably had greater validity. The higher rates of disorder parents reported at outcome were thus probably the more accurate ones. Such adjustments for age and source of reporting, however, do not correct for the potentially increasing inappropriateness of the item sets for this agng sample, and so it is difficult to say how many of those not meeting these adjusted criteria may still have had the disorder.

A different issue pertains to whether or not the criteria should be adjusted for the gender of the children being diagnosed. Research evaluating these and similar item sets demonstrates that male youngsters display more of these items, and do so to a more severe degree, than do female youngsters in the general population (Achenbach, 1991; DuPaul, Power, et al., 1998). Given that the majority of children in the DSM-IV field trial were boys (Lahey et al., 1994), the symptom threshold chosen in the DSM-IV is more appropriate to males. This results in girls' having to meet a higher threshold relative to other girls to be diagnosed as having ADHD than do boys relative to other boys. Gender-adjusted thresholds would seem to be in order to address this problem; yet this would evaporate the currently disproportionate male-to-female ratio of 3:1 found across studies (see below).

The DSM-IV requirement of an age of onset for ADHD symptoms (7 years) in the diagnostic criteria has also come under attack from its own field trial (Applegate et al., 1997); a longitudinal study (McGee, Williams, & Feehan, 1992); and a review of this criterion from historical, empirical, and pragmatic perspectives (Barkley & Biederman, 1997). Such a criterion for age of onset suggests that there may be qualitative differences between those who meet the criterion (early-onset) and those who do not (late-onset). Some results do suggest that those with an onset before age 6 years may have more severe and persistent conditions, and more problems with reading and school performance generally (McGee et al., 1992). But these were matters of degree and not kind in this study. The DSM-IV field trial also was not able to show any clear discontinuities in degree of ADHD or in the types of impairments it examined between those meeting and those not meeting the 7-year age of onset. It remains unclear at this time just how specific an age of onset may need to be for distinguishing ADHD from other disorders. Suffice it to say that no other mental disorder in the DSM-IV has so precise an age of onset; this suggests that ADHD should not as well.

A related potential problem for these criteria occurs in their failure to stipulate a lower-bound age group for giving the diagnosis, below which no diagnosis should be made. This is important because research on preschool children has shown that a separate dimension of hyperactive–impulsive behavior from aggression or defiant behavior does not seem to emerge until about 3 years of age (Achenbach & Edelbrock, 1987; Campbell, 1990). Below this age, these behaviors cluster together to form what has been called "behavioral immaturity," "externalizing problems," or an "undercontrolled pattern of conduct." This implies that the symptoms of ADHD may be difficult to distinguish from other early behavioral disorders until at least 3 years of age, and so this age might serve as a lower bound for diagnostic applications.

Similarly, research implies that a lower bound of IQ might also be important (IQ > 50), below which the nature of ADHD may be quite different. Minimal research seems to exist that speaks to the issue of a discontinuity or qualitative shift in the nature of ADHD in individuals with IQs below 50. Some indirect evidence implies that this may occur, however. Rutter and colleagues (Rutter, Bolton, et al., 1990; Rutter, Macdonald, et al., 1990) have concluded that children who fall below this level of IQ may have a qualitatively different form of mental retardation. This is inferred from findings that this group is overrepresented for its position along a normal distribution, and from findings that genetic defects contribute more heavily to this subgroup. Given this shift in the prevalence and causes of mental retardation below this level of IQ, a similar state of affairs might exist for the form of ADHD associated with it, necessitating its distinction from the type of ADHD that occurs in individuals above this IQ level. Consistent with such a view have been findings that the percentage of those responding positively to stimulant medication falls off sharply below this threshold of IQ (Demb, 1991).

Another issue pertinent to this discussion is the problem of the duration requirement's being set at 6 months. This has been chosen mainly out of tradition (because earlier DSMs have done this), with no research support for selecting this particular length of time for symptom presence. It is undoubtedly important that the symptoms be relatively persistent if we are to view this disorder as a developmental disability, rather than as a problem arising purely from context or out of a transient, normal developmental stage. Yet specifying a precise duration is difficult in the absence of much research to guide the issue. Research on preschool-age children may prove helpful here, however. Such research has shown that many children aged 3 years (or younger) may have parents or preschool teachers who report concerns about the activity level or attention of the children; yet these concerns have a high likelihood of remission within 12 months (Beitchman, Wekerle, & Hood, 1987; Campbell, 1990; Lerner, Inui, Trupin, & Douglas, 1985; Palfrey, Levine, Walker, & Sullivan, 1985). It would seem for preschoolers that the 6-month duration specified in the DSM-IV may be too brief, resulting in overidentification of children with ADHD at this age (false positives). However, this same body of research found that for those children whose problems lasted at least 12 months or beyond age 4 years, the behavior problems were highly persistent and predictive of continuance into the school-age range. Such research suggests that the duration of symptoms be set at 12 months or more.

The DSM-IV requirement that the symptoms be demonstrated in at least two of three environments, so as to establish pervasiveness of symptoms, is new to this edition and problematic. The DSM-IV implies that two of three sources of information (parent, teacher, employer) must agree on the presence of the symptoms. This confounds settings with sources of information. The degree of agreement between parents and teacher for any dimension of child behavior is modest, often ranging between .30 and .50 (Achenbach, McConaughy, & Howell, 1987). This sets an upper limit on the extent to which parents and teachers are going to agree on the severity of ADHD symptoms, and thus on whether or not a child has the disorder in that setting. Such disagreements among sources certainly reflect differences in the child's behavior as a function of true differential demands of these settings. But they also reflect differences in the attitudes and judgments of different people. Insisting on such agreement may reduce the application of the diagnosis to some children unfairly as a result of such well-established differences between parent and teacher opinions. It may also create a confounding of the disorder with, or issues of comorbidity with, ODD (Costello, Loeber, & Stouthamer-Loeber, 1991). Parent-only-identified children with ADHD may have predominantly ODD with relatively milder ADHD, whereas teacher-only-identified children with ADHD may have chiefly ADHD and minimal or no ODD symptoms. Children identified by both parents and teachers as having ADHD may therefore carry a higher likelihood of having ODD. They may also simply have a more severe form of ADHD than do the home- or school-only cases, being different in degree rather than in kind. Research is clearly conflicting on the matter (Cohen & Minde, 1983; Rapoport, Donnelly, Zametkin, & Carrougher, 1986; Schachar, Rutter, & Smith, 1981; Taylor, Sandberg, Thorley, & Giles, 1991). Considering that teacher information on children is not always obtainable or convenient, that parents can convey the essence of that information to clinicians, and that diagnosis based on parents' reports will lead to a diagnosis based on teacher reports 90% of the time (Biederman, Keenan, & Faraone, 1990), all imply that parent reports may suffice for diagnostic purposes for now. However, more recent evidence suggests that the best discrimination of children with ADHD from other groups may be achieved by blending the reports of parents and teachers, such that one counts the number of different symptoms endorsed across *both* sources of information (Crystal, Ostrander, Chen, & August, 2001; Mitsis, McKay, Schulz, Newcorn, & Halperin, 2000).

Many of these problematic issues are likely to be addressed in future editions of the DSM. Even so, the present criteria are actually some of the best ever advanced for the disorder; they represent a vast improvement over the state of affairs that existed prior to 1980. The various editions of DSM also have spawned a large amount of research into ADHD—its symptoms, subtypes, criteria, and even etiologies—that probably would not have occurred had such criteria not been set forth for professional consumption and criticism. The most recent criteria provide clinicians with a set of guidelines more specific, more reliable, more empirically based or justifiable, and closer to the scientific literature on ADHD than earlier editions. With some attention to the issues described above, the DSM criteria could be made to be even more rigorous, valid, and useful.

Is ADHD a "Real" Disorder?

Social critics (Breggin, 1998; Kohn, 1989; Schrag & Divoky, 1975) have charged that professionals have been too quick to label energetic and exuberant children as having a mental disorder. They also assert that educators may be using these labels as an excuse for simply poor educational environments. In other words, children who are diagnosed with hyperactivity or ADHD are actually normal, but are being labeled as mentally disordered because of parent and teacher intolerance (Kohn, 1989) or lack of love at home (Breggin, 1998). If this were actually true, then we should find no differences of any cognitive, neurological, genetic, behavioral, or social significance between children so labeled and normal children. We should also find that the diagnosis of ADHD is not associated with any significant risks later in development for maladjustment within any domains of adaptive functioning, or for problems with social, occupational, or school performance. Furthermore, research on potential etiologies for the disorder should likewise come up empty-handed. This is hardly the case, as evidence reviewed in this chapter attests. Differences between children with ADHD and normal children are too numerous to take these assertions of normality seriously. As will be shown later, substantial developmental risks await children meeting clinical diagnostic criteria for the disorder, and certain potential etiological factors are becoming consistently noted in the research literature.

Conceding all of this, however, does not automatically entitle ADHD to be placed within the realm of valid ("real") disorders. Wakefield (1999) has argued that disorders must meet two criteria to be viewed as valid: They must (1) engender substantial harm to the individual or those around him or her, and (2) incur dysfunction of natural and universal mechanisms that have been selected in an evolutionary sense (i.e., have survival value). The latter criterion is based on the definition of an adaptation as used in evolutionary biology. Disorders are failures in adaptations that produce harm. In the case of psychology, these universal mechanisms are psychological ones possessed by all normally developing humans, regardless of culture. ADHD handily meets both criteria. Those with ADHD, as described in the theory above, have significant deficits in behavioral inhibition and inattention (the executive functions) that are critical for effective self-regulation. And those with ADHD experience numerous domains of impairment (risks of harm) over development, as will become evident below.

EPIDEMIOLOGY

Prevalence

The prevalence of ADHD varies across studies, at least in part due to different methods of selecting samples, the nature of the populations from which they are drawn (differing nationalities or ethnicities, urban vs. rural, community vs. primary care settings, etc.), the criteria used to define ADHD (DSM criteria vs. rating scale cutoff), and certainly the age range and sex composition of the samples. When only the endorsement of the presence of the behavior of hyperactivity (not the clinical disorder) is required from either parent or teacher rating scales, prevalence rates can run as high as 22–57% (Lapouse & Monk, 1958; McArdle, O'Brien, & Kolvin, 1995; Werry & Quay, 1971). This underscores the point made earlier that being described as inattentive or overactive by a parent or teacher does not in and of itself constitute a disorder in a child.

Szatmari (1992) reviewed the findings of six large epidemiological studies that identified cases of ADHD within these samples. The prevalences found in these studies ranged from a low of 2% to a high of 6.3%, with most falling within the range of 4.2% to 6.3%. Other studies have found similar prevalence rates in elementary school-age children (4–5.5% in Breton et al., 1999; 7.9% in Briggs-Gowan, Horwitz, Schwab-Stone, Leventhal, & Leaf, 2000; 5–6% in DuPaul, 1991; and 2.5–4% in Pelham, Gnagy, Greenslade, & Milich, 1992). Lower rates result from using complete DSM criteria and parent reports (2–6% in Breton et al., 1999), and higher ones if just a cutoff on teacher ratings is used (up to 23% in DuPaul, Power, et al., 1998; 15.8% in Nolan, Gadow, & Sprafkin, 2001; 14.3% in Trites, Dugas, Lynch, & Ferguson, 1979). Sex and age differences in prevalence are routinely found in research. For instance, prevalence rates may be 4% in girls and 8% in boys in the preschool age group (Nolan et al., 2001), yet fall to 2–4% in girls and 6–9% in boys during the 6- to 12-year-old age period based on parent reports (Breton et al., 1999; Szatmari, Offord, & Boyle, 1989). The prevalence decreases again to 0.9–2% in girls and 1–5.6% in boys by adolescence (Breton et al., 1999; Lewinsohn, Hops, Roberts, Seeley, & Andrews, 1993; McGee et al., 1990; Romano et al., 2001; Szatmari et al., 1989). Even then, if both a symptom threshold and the requirement for impairment are used, the prevalence may decrease by 20–60% from that figure based on symptom thresholds alone (Breton et al., 1999; Romano et al., 2001; Wolraich, Hannah, Baumgaertel, & Feurer, 1998). As noted above, prevalence rates are routinely higher (sometimes more than double) when teacher reports are used in comparison to parent reports (Breton et al., 1999; DuPaul, Power, et al., 1998; Nolan et al., 2001). Switching from DSM-III-R criteria (used before 1994) to DSM-IV (in use since that time) may have resulted in a near-doubling in prevalence, owing to the inclusion of the new inattentive subtype (ADHD-PI), which was not included in DSM-III-R (Wolraich, Hannah, Pinnock, Baumgaertel, & Brown, 1996). Some segments of the population may also have greater levels of ADHD than others. For instance, Jensen et al. (1995), using DSM-III-R criteria, found a prevalence of 12% for ADHD among the children of military personnel—a figure more than double that found in other studies using these same criteria with general population samples (Szatmari, 1992).

Szatmari et al. (1989) found that the prevalence of ADHD in a large sample of children from Ontario, Canada also varied as a function of young age, male gender, chronic health problems, family dysfunction, low socioeconomic status (SES), presence of a developmental impairment, and urban living. Others have found similar conditions associated with the risk for ADHD (Lavigne et al., 1996; Velez, Johnson, & Cohen, 1989). Important, however, was the additional finding in the Szatmari et al. (1989) study that when comorbidity with other disorders was statistically controlled for in the analyses, gender, family dysfunction, and low SES were no longer significantly associated with prevalence. Health problems, developmental impairment, young age, and urban living remained significantly associated with prevalence, however.

As noted above in the discussion of DSM-IV criteria, it may be that the declining prevalence of ADHD with age is partly artifactual. This could result from the use of items in the diagnostic symptom lists that are chiefly applicable to young children. This could create a situation where individuals remain impaired in the fundamental constructs of ADHD as they mature, while outgrowing the symptom list for the disorder, resulting in an illusory decline in prevalence (as was noted in my follow-up study discussed above). Until more age-appropriate symptoms are studied for adolescent and adult populations, this issue remains unresolved.

Sex Differences

As noted above, sex appears to play a significant role in determining prevalence of ADHD within a population. On average, male children are between 2.5 and 5.6 times more likely than female children to be diagnosed as having ADHD within epidemiological samples, with the average being roughly 3:1 (Breton et al., 1999; DuPaul, Power, et al., 1998; Lewinsohn et al., 1993; McGee et al., 1990; Szatmari, 1992). Within clinic-referred samples, the sex ratio can be considerably higher, suggesting that boys with ADHD are far more likely to be referred to clinics than girls. This is probably because boys are more likely to have comorbid ODD or CD. Szatmari's (1992) finding that sex differences were no longer associated with the occurrence of ADHD, once other comorbid conditions were controlled for in statistical analyses, implies that this may be the case. The sex ratio could also be an artifact of applying a set of diagnostic criteria developed primarily on males to females, as discussed above.

Studies of clinic-referred girls often find that they are as impaired as clinic-referred boys with ADHD, have as much comorbidity, and may even have greater deficits in intelligence, according to meta-analytic reviews of sex differences in ADHD (Gaub & Carlson, 1997; Gershon, 2001). Some studies suggest that these clinic-referred girls, at least as adolescents, may have more internalizing symptoms (e.g., depression, anxiety, and stress), greater problems with teacher relationships, and poorer verbal abilities (vocabulary) than boys with ADHD (Rucklidge & Tannock, 2001). Like the boys, girls with ADHD also manifest more CD, mood disorders, and anxiety disorders; have lower intelligence; and have greater academic achievement deficits than do control samples (Biederman, Faraone, et al., 1999; Rucklidge & Tannock, 2001). Males with ADHD had greater problems with cognitive processing speed than females in one study, but these differences were no longer significant after severity of ADHD was controlled for (Rucklidge & Tannock, 2001). No sex differences have been identified in executive functioning, with both sexes being more impaired than control samples on such measures (Castellanos et al., 2000; Murphy et al., 2001). In contrast, studies drawing their ADHD samples from the community find that girls are significantly less likely to have comorbid ODD and CD than boys with ADHD, and do not have greater intellectual deficits than these boys; however, they may be as socially and academically impaired as boys with the disorder (Carlson, Tamm, & Gaub, 1997; Gaub & Carlson, 1997; Gershon, 2001).

Socioeconomic Differences

Few studies have examined the relationship of ADHD to SES, and those that have are not especially consistent. Lambert, Sandoval, and Sassone (1978) found only slight differences in the prevalence of hyperactivity across SES when parent, teacher, and physician all agreed on the diagnosis. However, SES differences in prevalence did arise when only two of these three sources had to agree; in this instance, there were generally more children with ADHD from lower- than higher-SES backgrounds. For instance, when parent and teacher agreement (but not physician) was required, 18% of those identified as hyperactive were from high-SES, 36% from middle-SES, and 45% from low-SES backgrounds. Where only teachers' opinions were used, the percentages were 17%, 41%, and 41%, respectively. Trites (1979), and later Szatmari (1992), both found that rates of ADHD tended to increase with lower SES. However, in his own study Szatmari (Szatmari et al., 1989) found that low SES was no longer associated with rates of ADHD when other comorbid conditions, such as CD, were controlled for. For now, it is clear that

ADHD occurs across all socioeconomic levels. Variations across SES may be artifacts of the source used to define the disorder or of the comorbidity of ADHD with other disorders related to SES, such as ODD and CD.

Ethnic/Cultural/National Issues

Early studies of the prevalence of hyperactivity, relying principally on teacher ratings, found significant disparities across four countries (United States, Germany, Canada, and New Zealand)—ranging from 2% in girls and 9% in boys in the United States to 9% in girls and 22% in boys in New Zealand (Trites et al., 1979). Similarly, O'Leary, Vivian, and Nisi (1985), using this same teacher rating scale and cutoff score, found rates of hyperactivity to be 3% in girls and 20% in boys in Italy. However, this may have resulted from the use of a threshold established on norms collected in the United States across these other countries, where the distributions were quite different from those found in the United States.

Later studies, especially those using DSM criteria, have found the disorder across numerous countries. In a Japanese study (Kanbayashi, Nakata, Fujii, Kita, & Wada, 1994) using parent ratings of items from DSM-III-R, a prevalence rate of 7.7% of the sample was found. Baumgaertel (1994) used teacher ratings of DSM-III, DSM-III-R, and DSM-IV symptom lists in a large sample of German elementary school children and found rates of 4.8% for ADHD-C, 3.9% for ADHD-PHI, and 9% for ADHD-PI based on DSM-IV. In India, among over 1,000 children screened at a pediatric clinic, 5.2% of children ages 3–4 years were found to have ADHD by DSM-III-R criteria, whereas the rate rose to over 29% for ages 11–12 years (Bhatia, Nigam, Bohra, & Malik, 1991). This was not a true epidemiological sample, however. Differences in prevalence across ages could simply reflect cohort effects; children may be referred to this clinic for different reasons at different ages. Prevalence rates found in other countries more recently are as follows:

- 3.8% among 2,290 Dutch 6- to 8-year-olds in a study using parent-reported DSM criteria (Kroes et al., 2001).
- 5.3% among 2,936 Chinese 6- to 11-year-olds, falling to 3.9% for 1,694 Chinese 12- to 16-year-olds, in a study using teacher ratings (Liu et al., 2000).
- 5.8% among 1,013 Brazilian 12- to 14-year-olds, in a study using teacher ratings (Rhohde et al., 1999).
- 20% of boys and 12% of girls 4–17 years of age in 504 children randomly sampled from 80,000 Colombian children, in a study using just DSM-IV symptom thresholds with parent ratings (Pineda et al., 1999).
- 14.9% of 1,110 primary school children randomly chosen from more than 31,000 in the United Arab Emirates, in a study using teacher ratings (Bu-Haroon, Eapen, & Bener, 1999).
- 19.8% of 600 Ukrainian 10- to 12-year-old children, in a study using parent ratings of DSM-IV symptoms (Gadow et al., 2000).

Cultural differences in the interpretations given to symptoms of ADHD by teachers or parents and in expectations for child behavior undoubtedly exist and have probably contributed to the higher rates of disorder found in some of these countries compared to North American rates. Also, most of these studies used teacher or parent ratings rather than clinical diagnostic criteria. As already noted above, prevalence rates of hyperactivity or ADHD are typically higher when a threshold on a rating scale is the only criterion for establishing a case of the disorder. When clinical criteria are employed, rates are more conservative. Nevertheless, these studies together show that hyperactivity or ADHD is present in all countries studied to date. Although it may not receive the same diagnostic label in each, the behavior pattern constituting the disorder appears to be universal.

Differences among ethnic groups in rates of hyperactivity within the United States have been reported. Langsdorf, Anderson, Walchter, Madrigal, and Juarez (1979) reported that almost 25% of African American children and 8% of Hispanic American children met a cutoff score on a teacher rating scale commonly used to define hyperactivity, whereas Ullmann (cited in O'Leary et al., 1985) reported rates of 24% for African American children and 16% of European American children on a teacher rating scale. Lambert et al. (1978) found higher rates of hyperactivity among African American than European American children only when the teachers were the only ones reporting the diagnosis; Hispanic American children were not found to differ from European American children in this respect. Such differences, however, may arise in part because of socioeconomic factors that are differentially associated with these ethnic groups in the United States. Such psychosocial factors are strongly correlated with aggression and conduct problems. As noted above, those factors no longer make a significant contribution to the prevalence of ADHD when comorbidity for other disorders is controlled for (Szatmari, 1992). Doing the same within studies of ethnic differences might well reduce or eliminate these differences in prevalence among them. Thus it would seem that ADHD arises in all ethnic groups studied so far. Whether the differences in prevalence across these ethnic groups are real or are a function of the source of information about the symptoms of ADHD (and possibly socioeconomic factors) remains to be determined.

DEVELOPMENTAL COURSE AND ADULT OUTCOMES

Major follow-up studies of clinically referred hyperactive children have been ongoing during the last 25 years at five sites: (1) Montreal (Weiss & Hechtman, 1993), (2) New York City (Gittelman, Mannuzza, Shenker, & Bonagura, 1985; Mannuzza et al., 1993), (3) Iowa City (Loney, Kramer, & Milich, 1981), (4) Los Angeles (Satterfield, Hoppe, & Schell, 1982), and (5) Milwaukee (Barkley, Fischer, et al., 1990). Follow-up studies of children identified as hyperactive from a general population have also been conducted in the United States (Lambert, 1988), New Zealand (McGee, Williams, & Silva, 1984; Moffitt, 1990), and England (Taylor et al., 1991), among others.

But before I embark on a summary of their results, some cautionary notes are in order. First, the limited number of follow-up studies does not permit a great deal of certainty to be placed in the specificity of the types and degrees of outcomes likely to be associated with ADHD. Even so, more can likely be said about the outcomes of ADHD than about those of most other childhood mental disorders. Second, the discontinuities of measurement that exist in these follow-up studies between their different points of assessments of their subjects make straightforward conclusions about developmental course difficult. Third, the differing sources of children greatly affect the outcomes to be found, with children drawn from clinic-referred populations having two to three times the occurrence of some negative outcomes and more diverse negative outcomes than those drawn from population screens (e.g., Barkley, Fischer, et al., 1990, vs. Lambert, 1988). Fourth, the differing entry/diagnostic criteria across follow-up studies must be kept in mind in interpreting and cross-referencing their outcomes. Most studies selected for children known at the time as "hyperactive." Such children are most likely representative of the course of ADHD-C from the current DSM taxonomy. Even then, the degree of deviance of the samples on parent and teacher ratings of these symptoms was not established at the entry point in most of these studies. These studies also cannot be viewed as representing ADHD-PI, for which no follow-up information is currently available. The descriptions of clinic-referred children with ADHD who are of similar age groups to those in the follow-up studies, but who are not followed over time, may help us understand the risks associated with different points in development. However, these may also be contaminated by cohort effects at the time of referral and so can only be viewed as suggestive. Such cohort effects may be minor; that is, adolescents with ADHD referred to clinics seem to have types and degrees of impairment similar to those of children with ADHD followed up to adolescence (Barkley, Anastopoulos, Guevremont, & Fletcher, 1991 vs. Barkley, Fischer, et al., 1990). In painting the picture of the developmental outcome of ADHD, then, broad strokes are permissible, but the finer details await more and better-refined studies. I concentrate here on the course of the disorder itself, returning to the comorbid disorders and associated conditions likely to arise in the course of ADHD in a later section of this chapter ("Comorbid Psychiatric Disorders").

The average onset of ADHD symptoms, as noted earlier, is often in the preschool years, typically at ages 3–4 (Applegate et al., 1997; Loeber et al., 1992; Taylor et al., 1991) and more generally by entry into formal schooling. Yet onset is heavily dependent on the type of ADHD under study. First to arise is the pattern of hyperactive–impulsive behavior (and, in some cases, oppositional and aggressive conduct), giving that subtype the earliest age of onset. ADHD-C has an onset within the first few grades of primary school (ages 5–8; Hart et al., 1995), most likely due to the requirement that both hyperactivity and inattention be present to diagnose this subtype. ADHD-PI appears to emerge a few years later (ages 8–12) than the other types (Applegate et al., 1997).

Preschool-age children who are perceived as difficult and resistant to control, or who have inattentive and hyperactive behavior that persists for at least a year or more, are highly likely to have ADHD and to remain so into elementary school years (Beitchman et al., 1987; Campbell, 1990; Palfrey et al., 1985) and even adolescence (Olson, Bates, Sandy, & Lanthier, 2000). Persistent cases seem especially likely to occur where parent–child conflict, greater maternal directiveness and negativity, and greater child defiant behavior exist (Campbell, March, Pierce, Ewing, & Szumowski, 1991; Olson et al., 2000; Richman, Stevenson, & Graham, 1982). More negative temperament and greater emotional reactivity to events are also more common in preschool children with ADHD (Barkley, DuPaul, & McMurray, 1990; Campbell, 1990). It is little wonder that greater parenting stress is associated with having preschool children with ADHD, and such stress seems to be at its highest with preschoolers relative to later age groups (Mash & Johnston, 1983a, 1983b). Within the preschool setting, children with ADHD will be found to be more often out of their seats, wandering the classroom, being excessively talkative and vocally noisy, and disruptive of other children's activities (Campbell, Schleifer, & Weiss, 1978; Schleifer et al., 1975).

By the time children with ADHD move into the elementary school-age range of 6–12 years, the problems with hyperactive–impulsive behavior are likely to continue and to be joined now by difficulties with attention (executive functioning and goal-directed persistence). Difficulties with work completion and productivity, distraction, forgetfulness related to what needs doing, lack of planning, poor organization of work activities, trouble meeting time deadlines associated with home chores, school assignments, and social promises or commitments to peers are now combined with the impulsive, heedless, and disinhibited behavior typifying these children since preschool age. Problems with oppositional and socially aggressive behavior may emerge at this age in at least 40–70% of children with ADHD (Barkley, 1998; Loeber et al., 1992; Taylor et al., 1991).

By ages 8–12 years, these early forms of defiant and hostile behavior may evolve further into symptoms of CD in 25–45% or more of all children with ADHD (Barkley, Fischer, et al., 1990; Gittelman et al., 1985; Loeber et al., 1992; Mannuzza et al., 1993; Taylor et al., 1991). Certainly by late childhood, most or all of the deficits in the executive functions related to inhibition in the model presented earlier are likely to be arising and interfering with adequate self-regulation (Barkley, 1997b). Not surprisingly, the overall adaptive functioning (self-sufficiency) of many children with ADHD (Stein, Szumowski, et al., 1995) is significantly below their intellectual ability. This is also true of preschoolers with high levels of these externalizing symptoms (Barkley, Shelton, et al., 2002). The disparity between adaptive functioning and age-appropriate expectations (or IQ) may itself be a predictor of greater severity of ADHD, as well as risk for oppositional and conduct problems in later childhood (Shelton et al., 1998). The disorder takes its toll on self-care, personal responsibility, chore performance, trustworthiness, independence, and appropriate social skills, as well as doing tasks on time specifically and moral conduct generally (Barkley, 1998; Hinshaw et al., 1993).

If ADHD is present in clinic-referred children, the likelihood is that 50–80% will continue to have their disorder into adolescence, with most studies supporting the higher figure (August, Stewart, & Holmes, 1983; Claude & Firestone, 1995; Barkley, Fischer, et al., 1990; Gittelman et al., 1985; Mannuzza et al., 1993). Using the same parent rating scales at both the childhood and adolescent evaluation points, Fischer et al. (1993a) were able to show that inattention, hyperactive–impulsive behavior, and home conflicts declined by adolescence. The hyperactive group showed far more marked declines than the control group, mainly because the former were so far from the mean of the normative group to begin with in childhood. Nevertheless, even at adolescence, the groups remained significantly different in each domain, with the mean for the hyperactive group remaining two standard deviations or more above the mean for the controls. This emphasizes a point made earlier: Simply because severity levels of symptoms are declining over development, this does not mean that children with ADHD are necessarily outgrowing their disorder relative to normal children. Like mental retardation, ADHD may need to be defined as a developmentally relative deficiency, rather than an absolute one, that persists in most children over time.

The persistence of ADHD symptoms across childhood as well as into early adolescence appears, again, to be associated with initial degree of hyperactive–impulsive behavior in childhood; the coexistence of conduct problems or oppositional hostile behavior; poor family relations, specifically conflict in parent–child interactions; and maternal depression, as well as duration of maternal mental health interventions (Fischer et al., 1993b; Taylor et al., 1991). These predictors have also been associated with the development and persistence of ODD and CD into this age range (12–17 years; Fischer et al., 1993b; Loeber, 1990; Mannuzza & Klein, 1992; Taylor et al., 1991).

Studies following large samples of clinic-referred children with hyperactivity, or ADHD, into adulthood are few in number. Only four follow-up studies have retained 50% or more of their original samples into adulthood and reported on the persistence of symptoms to that time. These are the Montreal study by Weiss, Hechtman, and their colleagues (see Weiss & Hechtman, in press); the New York City study by Mannuzza, Klein, and colleagues (see Mannuzza et al., 1993, 1998); the Swedish study by Rasmussen and Gillberg (2001); and my research with Mariellen Fischer in Milwaukee (Barkley, Fischer, Fletcher, & Smallish, 2002; Barkley, Fischer, Smallish, & Fletcher, in press; Fischer et al., in press-a, in press-b). The results regarding the persistence of disorder into young adulthood (middle 20s) are mixed, but can be better understood as being a function of reporting source and the diagnostic criteria used (Barkley, Fisher, Fletcher, & Smallish, 2002).

The Montreal study (n = 103) found that two-thirds of the original sample (n = 64; mean age = 25 years) claimed to be troubled as adults by at least one or more disabling core symptoms of their original disorder (restlessness, impulsivity, or inattention), and that 34% had at least moderate to severe levels of hyperactive, impulsive, and inattentive symptoms (Weiss & Hechtman, 1993). In Sweden (n = 50), Rasmussen and Gillberg (2001) obtained similar results, with 49% of probands reporting marked symptoms of ADHD at age 22 years compared to 9% of controls. Formal diagnostic criteria for ADHD, such as those in DSM-III or later editions, were not employed at any of the outcome points in either study, however. In contrast, the New York study has followed two separate cohorts of hyperactive children, using DSM criteria to assess persistence of disorder. That study found that 31% of the initial cohort (n = 101) and 43% of the second cohort (n = 94) met DSM-III criteria for ADHD by ages 16–23 (mean age = 18.5 years) (Gittelman et al., 1985; Mannuzza et al., 1991). Eight years later (mean age = 26 years), however, these figures fell to 8% and 4%, respectively (with DSM-III-R criteria now being used) (Mannuzza et al., 1993, 1998). Those results might imply that the vast majority of hyperactive children no longer qualify for the diagnosis of ADHD by adulthood.

The interpretation of the relatively low rate of persistence of ADHD into adulthood, particularly for the New York study, is clouded by at least two issues apart from differences in selection criteria. One is that the source of information about the disorder changed in all of these studies from that used at the childhood and adolescent evaluations to that used at the adult outcome. At study entry and at adolescence, all studies used the reports of others (parents and typically teachers). By midadolescence, all found that the majority of hyperactive participants (50–80%) continued to manifest significant levels of the disorder (see above). In young adulthood (approximately age 26 years), both the New York and Montreal studies switched to self-reports of disorder.

The rather marked decline in persistence of ADHD from adolescence to adulthood could stem from this change in source of information. Indeed, the New York study found this to be likely when, at late adolescence (mean age of 18–19 years), both the teenagers and their parents were interviewed about the teens' psychiatric status (Mannuzza & Gittelman, 1986). There was a marked disparity between the reports of parents and teens concerning the presence of ADHD (11% vs. 27%; agreement = 74%, kappa = .19). Other research also suggests that the relationship between 11-year-old children's self-reports of externalizing symptoms, such as those involved in ADHD, and those of parents and teachers is quite low (r = .16–.32; Henry et al., 1994). Thus changing sources of reporting in longitudinal studies on behavioral disorders can be expected to lead to marked differences in estimates of persistence of those disorders.

The question obviously arises as to whose assessment of the probands is more accurate. This would depend on the purpose of the assessment, but the prediction of impairment in major life activities would seem to be an important one in research on psychiatric disorders. Our Milwaukee study examined these issues by interviewing both the participants and their parents about ADHD symptoms at the young adult follow-up (age 21 years). It then examined the relationship of each source's reports to significant outcomes in major life activities (education, occupation, social, etc.), after controlling for the contribution made by the other source. As noted earlier, another limitation in the earlier studies may reside in the DSM criteria, in that they grow less sensitive to the disorder with age. Using a developmentally referenced criterion (age comparison) to determine diagnosis may identify more cases than would the DSM approach. As discussed earlier, the Milwaukee study found that the persistence of ADHD into adulthood was heavily dependent on the source of the information (self or parent) and the diagnostic criteria (DSM or developmentally referenced). Self-report identified just 5–12% of probands as currently having ADHD (DSM-III-R), whereas parent reports placed this figure at 46–66%. Using the DSM resulted in lower rates of persistence (5% for proband reports and 46% for parents), whereas using a developmentally referenced cutoff (98th percentile) yielded higher rates of persistence (12% by self-reports and 66% by parent reports). The parent reports appeared to have greater validity, in view of their greater contribution to impairment and to more domains of current impairment, than did self-reported information (Barkley, Fischer, Fletcher, & Smallish, 2002). We have concluded that past follow-up studies grossly underestimated the persistence of ADHD into adulthood by relying solely on the self-reports of the probands.

COMORBID PSYCHIATRIC DISORDERS

Individuals diagnosed with ADHD are often found to have a number of other disorders besides their ADHD. What is known about comorbidity is largely confined to the ADHD-C subtype. In community-derived samples, up to 44% of children with ADHD have at least one other disorder, and 43% have at least two or more additional disorders (Szatmari et al., 1989). The figure is higher, of course, for children drawn from clinics. As many as 87% of children clinically diagnosed with ADHD may have at least one other disorder, and 67% have at least two other disorders (Kadesjo & Gillberg, 2001). The disorders likely to co-occur with ADHD are briefly described below.

Conduct Problems and Antisocial Disorders

The most common comorbid disorders with ADHD-C are ODD and, to a lesser extent, CD. Indeed, the presence of ADHD increases the odds of ODD/CD by 10.7-fold (95% confidence interval [CI] = 7.7–14.8) in general population studies (Angold, Costello, & Erkanli, 1999). Studies of clinic-referred children with ADHD find that between 54% and 67% will meet criteria for a diagnosis of ODD by 7 years of age or later. ODD is a frequent precursor to CD, a more severe and often (though not always) later-occurring stage of ODD (Loeber, Burke, Lahey, Winters, & Zera, 2000). The co-occurrence of CD with ADHD may be 20–50% in children and 44–50% in adolescence with ADHD (Barkley, 1998; Barkley, Fischer, et al., 1990; Biederman, Faraone, & Lapey, 1992; Lahey, McBurnett, & Loeber, 2000). By adulthood, up to 26% may continue to have CD, while 12–21% will qualify for a diagnosis of antisocial personality disorder (ASPD) (Biederman et al., 1992; Fischer, Barkley, Smallish, & Fletcher, in press; Mannuzza & Klein, 1992; Rasmussen & Gillberg, 2001; Weiss & Hechtman, 1993b). Similar or only slightly lower degrees of overlap are noted in studies using epidemiologically identified samples rather than those referred to clinics. ADHD therefore has a strong association with conduct problems and antisocial disorders, such as ODD, CD, and ASPD, and has been found to be one of the most reliable early predictors of these disorders (Fischer et al., 1993b; Hinshaw & Lee, Chapter 3, this volume; Lahey et al., 2000). Recent longitudinal research suggests that severity of early ADHD is actually a contributing factor to risk for later ODD, regardless of severity of early ODD (Burns & Walsh, 2002), perhaps due to the problems with poor emotion (anger) regulation in ADHD noted above. Familial associations among the disorders have also been consistently found, whether across boys and girls with ADHD or across European American and African American samples (Biederman et al., 1992; Faraone et al., 2000; Samuel t al., 1999). This suggests some underlying causal connection among these disorders. Evidence from twin studies indicates a shared or common genetic contribution to the three disorders, particularly between ADHD and ODD (Coolidge, Thede, & Young, 2000; Silberg et al., 1996). When CD occurs in conjunction with ADHD, it may represent simply a more severe form of ADHD having a greater family genetic loading for ADHD (Thapar, Harrington, & McGuffin, 2001). Other research, however, also suggests a shared environmental risk factor may also account for the overlap of ODD and CD with ADHD beyond their shared genetics (Burt, Krueger, McGue, & Iacono, 2001), that risk factor likely being family adversity generally and impaired parenting specifically (Patterson, Degarmo, & Knutson, 2000). To summarize, ODD and CD have a substantial likelihood of co-occuring with ADHD, with the risk for ODD/CD being mediated in large part by severity of ADHD and its family genetic loading and in part by adversity in the familial environment.

One of the strongest predictors of risk for substance use disorders (SUDs) among children with ADHD upon reaching adolescence and adulthood is prior or coexisting CD or ASPD (Burke et al., 2001; Chilcoat & Breslau, 1999; Molina & Pelham, 1999; White, Xie, Thompson, Loeber, & Stouthamer-Loeber, 2001). Given the heightened risk for ODD/CD/ASPD in ADHD children as they mature, one would naturally expect a greater risk for SUDs as well. Although an elevated risk for alcohol abuse has not been documented in follow-up studies, the risk for other SUDs among hyperactive children followed to adulthood ranges from 12% to 24% (Fischer et al., in press-b; Gittelman et al., 1985; Mannuzza et al., 1993, 1998; Rasmussen & Gillberg, 2001). One longitudinal study of hyperactive children suggested that childhood treatment with stimulant medication may predispose youths to develop SUDs (Lambert, in press; Lambert & Hartsough, 1998). Most longitudinal studies, however, find no such elevated risk, and in some cases even a protective effect if stimulant treatment is continued for a year or more or into adolescence (Barkley, Fischer, Smallish, & Fletcher, in press; Biederman, Wilens, Mick, Spencer, & Faraone, 1999; Chilcoat & Breslau, 1999; Loney, Kramer, & Salisbury, in press). The basis for the conflicting findings in the Lambert study was probably not examining or statistically controlling for severity of ADHD and CD at adolescence and young adulthood (Barkley, Fischer, Smallish, & Fletcher, in press).

Anxiety and Mood Disorders

The overlap of anxiety disorders with ADHD has been found to range from 10% to 40% in clinic-referred children, averaging to about 25% (see Biederman, Newcorn, & Sprich, 1991, and Tannock, 2000, for reviews). In longitudinal studies of children with ADHD, however, the risk of anxiety disorders is no greater than in control groups at either adolescence or young adulthood (Fischer et al., in press-b; Mannuzza et al., 1993, 1998; Russo & Beidel, 1994; Weiss & Hechtman, 1993). The disparity in findings is puzzling. Perhaps some of the overlap of ADHD with anxiety disorders in children is due to referral bias (Biederman et al., 1992; Tannock, 2000). General population studies of children, however, do suggest an elevated odds ratio of having an anxiety disorder in the presence of ADHD of 3.0 (95% CI = 2.1–4.3), with this relationship being significant even after controlls for comorbid ODD/CD (Angold et al., 1999). This implies that the two disorders may have some association apart from referral bias, at least in childhood. The co-occurrence of anxiety disorders with ADHD has been shown to reduce the degree of impulsiveness, relative to ADHD without comorbid anxiety disorders (Pliszka, 1992). Some research suggests that the disorders are transmitted independently in families and so are not linked to each other in any genetic way (Biederman, Newcorn, & Sprich, 1991; Last, Hersen, Kazdin, Orvaschel, & Perrin, 1991). This may not be the case for ADHD-PI: Higher rates of anxiety disorders have been noted in some studies of these children (see Milich et al., 2001, for a review; Russo & Beidel, 1994), though not always (Barkley, DuPaul, & McMurray, 1990), and in their first- and second-degree relatives (Barkley, DuPaul, & McMurray, 1990; Biederman et al., 1992), though again not always (Lahey & Carlson, 1992; Milich et al., 2001). Regrettably, research on the overlap of anxiety disorders with ADHD has generally chosen to consider the various anxiety disorders as a single group in evaluating this issue. Greater clarity and clinical utility from these findings might occur if the types of anxiety disorders present were to be examined separately.

The evidence for the co-occurrence of mood disorders, such as major depression or dysthymia (a milder form of depression), with ADHD is now fairly substantial (see Faraone & Biederman, 1997; Jensen, Martin, & Cantwell, 1997; Jensen, Shervette, Xenakis & Richters,

1993; and Spencer, Wilens, Biederman, Wozniak, & Harding-Crawford, 2000, for reviews). Between 15% and 75% of those with ADHD may have a mood disorder, though most studies place the association between 20% and 30% (Biederman et al., 1992; Cuffe et al., 2001; Fischer et al., in press-b). The odds ratio of having depression, given the presence of ADHD in general population samples, is 5.5 (95% CI = 3.5–8.4) (Angold et al., 1999). Some evidence also suggests that these disorders may be related to each other, in that familial risk for one disorder substantially increases the risk for the other (Biederman, Newcorn, & Sprich, 1991; Biederman et al., 1992; Faraone & Biederman, 1997), particularly in cases where ADHD is comorbid with CD. Similarly, a recent follow-up study (Fischer et al., in press-b) found a 26% risk of major depression among children with ADHD by young adulthood, but this risk was largely mediated by the co-occurrence of CD. Likewise, a meta-analysis of general population studies indicated that the link between ADHD and depression was entirely mediated by the linkage of both disorders to CD (Angold et al., 1999). In the absence of CD, ADHD was not more likely to be associated with depression.

The comorbidity of ADHD with bipolar (manic–depressive) disorder is controversial (Carlson, 1990; Geller & Luby, 1997). Some studies of ADHD children indicate that 10–20% may have bipolar disorder (Spencer et al., 2000; Wozniak et al., 1995)—a figure substantially higher than the 1% risk for the general population (Lewinsohn, Klein, & Seeley, 1995). Follow-up studies, have not documented any significant increase in risk of bipolar disorder in children with ADHD followed into adulthood (Fischer et al., in press-b; Mannuzza et al., 1993, 1998; Weiss & Hechtman, in press); however, that risk would have to exceed 7% for these studies to have sufficient power to detect any comorbidity. A 4-year follow-up of children with ADHD reported that 12% met criteria for bipolar disorder in adolescence (Biederman, Faraone, Milberger, et al., 1996). Children with ADHD but without bipolar disorder do not have an increased prevalence of bipolar disorder among their biological relatives (Biederman et al., 1992; Faraone, Biederman, & Monuteaux, 2001; Lahey et al., 1988), whereas children with both ADHD and bipolar disorder do (Faraone et al., 1997, 2001); this suggests that where the overlap occurs, it may represent a familially distinct subset of ADHD. Children and adolescents diagnosed with childhood bipolar disorder often have a significantly higher lifetime prevalence of ADHD, particularly in their earlier childhood years (Carlson, 1990; Geller & Luby, 1997). Where the two disorders coexist, the onset of bipolar disorder may be earlier than in bipolar disorder alone (Faraone et al., 1997, 2001; Sachs, Baldassano, Truman, & Guille, 2000). Some of this overlap with ADHD may be partly an artifact of similar symptoms in the symptom lists used for both diagnoses (hyperactivity, distractibility, poor judgment, etc.) (Geller & Luby, 1997). In any cse, the overlap of ADHD with bipolar disorder appears to be unidirectional: A diagnosis of ADHD seems not to increase the risk for bipolar disorder, whereas a diagnosis of childhood bipolar disorder seems to dramatically elevate the risk of a prior or concurrent diagnosis of ADHD (Geller & Luby, 1997; Spencer et al., 2000).

Tourette's Disorder and Other Tic Disorders

Up to 18% of children may develop a motor tic in childhood, but this declines to a base rate of about 2% by midadolescence and less than 1% by adulthood (Peterson, Pine, Cohen, & Brook, 2001). Tourette's disorder, a more severe disorder involving multiple motor and vocal tics, occurs in less than 0.4% of the population (Peterson et al., 2001). A diagnosis of ADHD does not necessarily appear to elevate these risks for a diagnosis of tics or Tourette's disorder, at least not in childhood or adolescence (Peterson et al., 2001). Among clinic-referred adults diagnosed with ADHD, there may be a slightly greater occurrence of tic disorders (12%; Spencer et al., 2001). In contrast, individuals with obsessive–compulsive disorder or Tourette's disorder have a marked elevation in risk for ADHD, averaging 48% or more (range = 35–71%; Comings, 2000). Complicating matters is the fact that the onset of ADHD often seems to precede that of Tourette's disorder in cases of comorbidity (Comings, 2000). Yet Pauls et al. (1986) have shown that Tourette's disorder and ADHD occur independently among relatives of those with each disorder; this suggests that a "Berkson's bias" (comorbidity with ADHD leads to clinic referral) may be operating in clinical referrals for Tourette's disorder such that comorbid cases are more likely to get referred.

ASSOCIATED DEVELOPMENTAL AND SOCIAL PROBLEMS

Apart from an increased risk for various psychiatric disorders, children and teens with ADHD-C are also more likely to experience a substantial array of developmental, social, and health risks; these are discussed in this and the next section. Far less is known about the extent to which these correlated problems are evident in ADHD-PI, particularly the subgroup having problems with sluggish cognitive tempo described above. The various types of problems most likely to occur in children with ADHD-C are briefly listed in Table 2.2.

Motor Incoordination

As a group, as many as 60% of children with ADHD, compared to up to 35% of normal children, may have poor motor coordination or developmental coordination disorder (Barkley, DuPaul, & McMurray, 1990; Hartsough & Lambert, 1985; Kadesjo & Gillberg, 2001; Szatmari et al., 1989; Stewart, Pitts, Craig, & Dieruf, 1966). Neurological examinations for "soft" signs related to motor coordination and motor overflow movements find children with ADHD to demonstrate more such signs (as well as generally sluggish gross motor movements) than control children, including those with "pure" learning disabilities (Carte, Nigg, & Hinshaw, 1996; Denckla & Rudel, 1978; Denckla, Rudel, Chapman, & Krieger, 1985; McMahon & Greenberg, 1977). These overflow movements have been interpreted as indicators of delayed development of motor inhibition (Denckla et al., 1985).

Studies using tests of fine motor coordination, such as balance assessment, tests of fine motor gestures, electronic or paper-and-pencil mazes, and pursuit tracking, often find children with ADHD to be less coordinated in these actions (Hoy, Weiss, Minde, & Cohen, 1978; Mariani & Barkley, 1997; McMahon & Greenberg, 1977; Moffitt, 1990; Shaywitz & Shaywitz, 1985; Ullman, Barkley, & Brown, 1978). Simple motor speed, as measured by finger-tapping rate or grooved pegboard tests, does not seem to be as affected in ADHD as is the execution of complex, coordinated sequences of motor movements (Barkley, Murphy, & Kwasnik, 1996a; Breen, 1989; Grodzinsky & Diamond, 1992; Mariani & Barkley, 1997; Marcotte & Stern, 1997; Seidman, Benedict, et al., 1995: Seidman, Biederman, et al., 1995). The bulk of the available evidence therefore supports the existence of deficits in motor control, particularly when motor sequences must be performed, in those with ADHD.

Impaired Academic Functioning

The vast majority of clinic-referred children with ADHD have difficulties with school performance, most often underproductivity. Such children frequently score lower than normal or control groups of children on standardized achievement tests (Barkley, DuPaul, & McMurray, 1990; Fischer, Barkley, Edelbrock, & Smallish, 1990; Hinshaw, 1992, 1994). These differences are likely to be found even in preschool-age children with ADHD (Barkley, Shelton, et al., 2002; Mariani & Barkley, 1997), suggesting that the disorder may take a toll on the acquisition of academic skills and knowledge even before entry into first grade. This makes sense, given that some of the executive functions believed to be disrupted by ADHD in the model presented earlier are also likely to be involved in some forms of academic achievement (e.g., working memory in mental arithmetic or spelling; internalized speech in reading comprehension; verbal fluency in oral narratives and written reports, etc.).

Between 19% and 26% of children with ADHD are likely to have any single type of learning disability, conservatively defined as a significant delay in reading, arithmetic, or spelling relative to intelligence and achievement in one of these three areas at or below the 7th percentile (Barkley, 1990). If a learning disability is defined as simply a significant discrepancy between intelligence and achievement, then up to 53% of hyperactive children could be said to have such a disability (Lambert & Sandoval, 1980). Or, if the criterion of simply two grades below grade level is used, then as many as 80% of children with ADHD in late childhood (age 11 years) may have learning disorders (Cantwell & Baker, 1992). Studies suggest that the risk for reading disorders among children with ADHD is 16–39%, while that for spelling disorders is 24–27% and for math disorders is 13–33% (August & Garfinkel, 1990; Barkley, 1990; Casey, Rourke, & Del Dotto, 1996; Frick et al., 1991; Semrud-Clikeman et al., 1992).

Although the finding that children with ADHD are more likely to have learning disabilities

TABLE 2.2. Summary of Impairments Likely to Be Associated with ADHD

Cognitive
Mild deficits in intelligence (approximately 7–10 points below average)
Deficient academic achievement skills (range of 10–30 standard score points below average)
Learning disabilities: Reading (8–39%), spelling (12–26%), math (12–33%), and handwriting (common but unstudied)
Poor sense of time; inaccurate time estimation and reproduction
Decreased nonverbal and verbal working memory
Impaired planning ability
Reduced sensitivity to errors
Possible impairment in goal-directed behavioral creativity (??)

Language
Delayed onset of language (up to 35%, but not consistent)
Speech impairments (10–54%)
Excessive conversational speech (commonplace); reduced speech to confrontation
Poor organization and inefficient expression of ideas
Impaired verbal problem solving
Co-existence of central auditory processing disorder (minority, but still uncertain)
Poor rule-governed behavior
Delayed internalization of speech (30+% delay)
Diminished development of moral reasoning

Adaptive functioning: 10–30 standard score points below normal

Motor development
Delayed motor coordination (up to 52%)
More neurological "soft" signs related to motor coordination and overflow movements
Sluggish gross motor movements

Emotion
Poor self-regulation of emotion
Greater problems with frustration tolerance
Underreactive arousal system

School performance
Disruptive classroom behavior (commonplace)
Underperforming in school relative to ability (commonplace)
Academic tutoring (up to 56%)
Repeating a grade (30% or more)
Placement in one or more special education programs (30–40%)
School suspensions (up to 46%)
School expulsions (10–20%)
Failure to graduate from high school (10–35%)

Task performance
Poor persistence of effort/motivation
Greater variability in responding
Decreased performance/productivity under delayed rewards
Greater problems when delays are imposed within the task and as they increase in duration
Decline in performance as reinforcement changes from being continuous to intermittent
Greater disruption when non-contingent consequences occur during the task

Medical/health risks
Greater proneness to accidental injuries (up to 57%)
Possible delay in growth during childhood
Difficulties surrounding sleeping (up to 30–60%)
Greater driving risks: Vehicular crashes and speeding tickets

Note. Adapted from Barkley (1998). Copyright 1998 by The Guilford Press. Adapted by permission.

(Gross-Tsur, Shalev, & Amir, 1991; Tannock & Brown, 2000) might imply a possible genetic link between the two disorders, more recent research (Doyle, Faraone, DuPre, & Biederman, 2001; Faraone et al., 1993; Gilger, Pennington, & DeFries, 1992) shows that the two sets of disorders are transmitted independently in families. Some subtypes of reading disorders associated with ADHD may share a common genetic etiology (Gilger et al., 1992). This may arise from the finding that early ADHD may predispose children toward certain types of reading problems, whereas early reading problems do not generally give rise to later symptoms of ADHD (Chadwick, Taylor, Taylor, Heptinstall, & Danckaerts, 1999; Rabiner et al., 2000; Velting & Whitehurst, 1997; Wood & Felton, 1994). The picture is less clear for spelling disorders; a common or shared genetic etiology to both ADHD and spelling disorder has been shown in a joint analysis of twin samples from London and Colorado (Stevenson, Pennington, Gilger, DeFries, & Gillis, 1993). This may result from the fact that early spelling ability seems to be linked to the integrity of working memory (Mariani & Barkley, 1997; Levy & Hobbes, 1989), which may be impaired in those with ADHD (see the discussion of the theoretical model, above). Writing disorders have not received as much attention in research on ADHD, though handwriting deficits are often found among children with ADHD, particularly those having ADHD-C (Marcotte & Stern, 1997).

Rapport, Scanlan, and Denney (1999) provide some evidence for a dual-pathway model of the link between ADHD and academic underachievement. Briefly, ADHD may predispose to academic underachievement through its contribution to a greater risk for ODD/CD and conduct problems in the classroom more generally, the net effect of which is an adverse impact on productivity and general school performance. But ADHD is associated with cognitive deficits not only in attention, but general intelligence (see below) and working memory (see above), all of which may have a direct and adverse impact on academic achievement. Supportive of this view as well are findings that the inattention dimension of ADHD is more closely associated with academic achievement problems than is the hyperactive–impulsive dimension (Faraone, Biederman, Weber, & Russell, 1998; Hynd, Lorys, et al. 1991; Marshall et al., 1997). According to this dual-pathway model, both pathways will require interventions if the marked association of ADHD with school underachievement is to be addressed.

A higher prevalence of speech and language disorders has also been documented in many studies of children with ADHD, typically ranging from 30% to 64% of the samples (Gross-Tsur et al., 1991; Hartsough & Lambert, 1985; Humphries, Koltun, Malone, & Roberts, 1994; Szatmari et al., 1989; Taylor et al., 1991). The converse is also true: Children with speech and language disorders have a higher than expected prevalence of ADHD (approximately 30–58%), among other psychiatric disorders (see Tannock & Brown, 2000, for a review on comorbidity with ADHD).

Reduced Intelligence

Clinic-referred children with ADHD often have lower scores on intelligence tests than control groups used in these same studies, particularly in verbal intelligence (Barkley, Karlsson, & Pollard, 1985; Mariani & Barkley, 1997; McGee et al., 1992; Moffitt, 1990; Stewart et al., 1966; Werry, Elkind, & Reeves, 1987). Differences in IQ have also been found between hyperactive boys and their normal siblings (Halperin & Gittelman, 1982; Tarver-Behring, Barkley, & Karlsson, 1985; Welner, Welner, Stewart, Palkes, & Wish, 1977). The differences found in these studies often range from 7 to 10 standard score points. Studies using both community samples (Hinshaw, Morrison, Carte, & Cornsweet, 1987; McGee et al., 1984; Peterson et al., 2001) and samples of children with behavior problems (Sonuga-Barke et al., 1994) also have found significant negative associations between degree of ADHD and intelligence (r's = −.25 – −.35). In contrast, associations between ratings of conduct problems and intelligence in children are often much smaller or even nonsignificant, particularly when hyperactive–impulsive behavior is partialed out of the relationship (Hinshaw et al., 1987; Lynam, Moffitt, & Stouthamer-Loeber, 1993; Sonuga-Barke et al., 1994). This implies that the relationship between IQ and ADHD is not likely to be a function of comorbid conduct problems (see Hinshaw, 1992, for a review).

Social Problems

ADHD is classified in DSM-IV as an "attention-deficit and disruptive behavior disorder" because of the significant difficulties it creates in social conduct and general social adjustment. The interpersonal behaviors of those with ADHD, as noted earlier, are often characterized as more impulsive, intrusive, excessive, disorganized, engaging, aggressive, intense, and emotional. And so they are "disruptive" of the smoothness of the ongoing stream of social interactions, reciprocity, and cooperation, which is an increasingly important part of the children's daily life with others (Whalen & Henker, 1992).

Research finds that ADHD affects the interactions of children with their parents, and hence the manner in which parents may respond to these children (Johnston & Mash, 2001). Those with ADHD are more talkative, negative and defiant; less compliant and cooperative; more demanding of assistance from others; and less able to play and work independently of their mothers (Barkley, 1985; Danforth et al., 1991; Gomez & Sanson, 1994; Johnston, 1996; Johnston & Mash, 2001). Their mothers are less responsive to the questions of their children, more negative and directive, and less rewarding of their children's behavior (Danforth et al., 1991; Johnston & Mash, 2001). Mothers of children with ADHD have been shown to give both more commands and more rewards to sons with ADHD than to daughters with the disorder (Barkley, 1989b; Befera & Barkley, 1984), but also to be more emotional and acrimonious in their interactions with sons (Buhrmester, Camparo, Christensen, Gonzalez, & Hinshaw, 1992; Taylor et al., 1991). Children and teens with ADHD seem to be nearly as problematic for their fathers as their mothers (Buhrmester et al., 1992; Edwards et al., 2001; Johnston, 1996; Tallmadge & Barkley, 1983). Contrary to what may be seen in normal mother–child interactions, the conflicts between children and teens with ADHD (especially boys) and their mothers may actually increase when fathers join the interactions (Buhrmester et al., 1992; Edwards et al., 2001). Such increased maternal negativity and acrimony toward sons in these interactions has been shown to predict greater noncompliance in classroom and play settings and greater covert stealing away from home, even when the level of the sons' own negativity and parental psychopathology are statistically controlled for in the analyses (Anderson et al., 1994). The negative parent–child interaction patterns also occur in the preschool age group (Cohen, Sullivan, Minde, Novak, & Keens, 1983; DuPaul, McGoey, Eckert, & VanBrakle, 2001) and may be even more negative and stressful (to the parents) in this age range (Mash & Johnston, 1982, 1990) than in later age groups. With increasing age, the degree of conflict in these interactions lessens, but remains deviant from normal into later childhood (Barkley, Karlsson, & Pollard, 1985; Mash & Johnston, 1982) and adolescence (Barkley, Anastopoulos, Guevremont, & Fletcher, 1992; Barkley, Fischer, Edelbrock, & Smallish, 1991; Edwards et al., 2001). In families of children with ADHD, negative parent–child interactions in childhood have been observed to be significantly predictive of continuing parent–teen conflicts 8–10 years later in adolescence (Barkley, Fischer, et al., 1991). Few differences are noted between mothers' interactions with their children who have ADHD and their interactions with the siblings of these children (Tarver-Behring et al., 1985).

The presence of comorbid ODD is associated with the highest levels of interaction conflicts between parents and their ADHD children and adolescents (Barkley, Anastopoulos, et al., 1992; Barkley, Fischer, et al., 1991; Edwards et al., 2001; Johnston, 1996). In a sequential analysis of these parent–teen interaction sequences, investigators have noted that the immediate or first lag in the sequence is most important in determining the behavior of the other member of the dyad (Fletcher, Fischer, Barkley, & Smallish, 1996). That is, the behavior of each member is determined mainly by the immediately preceding behavior of the other member, and not by earlier behaviors of either member in the chain of interactions. The interactions of the comorbid ADHD/ODD group reflected a strategy best characterized as "tit for tat," in that the type of behavior (positive, neutral, or negative) of each member was most influenced by the same type of behavior emitted immediately preceding it. Mothers of teens with ADHD only and of normal teens were more likely to utilize positive and neutral behaviors regardless of the immediately preceding behavior of their teens; this has been characterized as a "be nice and forgive" strategy, which is thought to be more mature and more socially successful for both parties in the long run (Fletcher et al., 1996). Even so, those with ADHD alone are still found to be deviant from normal in these interaction patterns, though less so than the comorbid ADHD/ODD group. The presence of comorbid ODD has also been shown to be associated with greater maternal stress and psychopathology, as well as parental marital/couple difficulties (Barkley, Anastopoulos, et al.,

1992; Barkley, Fischer, et al., 1991; Johnston & Mash, 2001).

These interaction conflicts in families of children with ADHD are not limited to parent–child interactions. Increased conflicts have been observed between children with ADHD and their siblings, relative to normal child–sibling dyads (Mash & Johnston, 1983a; Taylor et al., 1991). Research on the larger domain of family functioning has shown that families of children with ADHD experience more parenting stress and decreased sense of parenting competence (Fischer, 1990; Johnston & Mash, 2001; Mash & Johnston, 1990); increased alcohol consumption in parents (Cunningham, Benness, & Siegel, 1988; Pelham & Lang, 1993); decreased extended family contacts (Cunningham et al., 1988); and increased marital/couple conflict, separations, and divorce, as well as maternal depression (Befera & Barkley, 1984; Cunningham et al., 1988; Barkley, Fischer, et al., 1990; Johnston & Mash, 2001; Lahey et al., 1988; Taylor et al., 1991). Again, the comorbid association of ADHD with ODD or CD is linked to even greater degrees of parental psychopathology, marital/couple discord, and divorce than is ADHD only (Barkley, Fischer, et al., 1990, 1991; Lahey et al., 1988; Taylor et al., 1991). Interestingly, Pelham and Lang (1993) have shown that the increased alcohol consumption in these parents is in part a direct function of their stressful interactions with their children with ADHD.

Research has demonstrated that the primary direction of effects within these interactions is from child to parent (Danforth et al., 1991; Johnston & Mash, 2001; Mash & Johnston, 1990), rather than the reverse. That is, much of the disturbance in the interaction seems to stem from the effects of the child's excessive, impulsive, unruly, noncompliant, and emotional behavior on the parent, rather than from the effects of the parent's behavior on the child. This was documented primarily through studies that evaluated the effects of stimulant medication on the behavior of such children and their interaction patterns with their mothers. Such research found that medication improves the compliance of those with ADHD and reduces their negative, talkative, and generally excessive behavior, so that their parents reduce their levels of directive and negative behavior as well (Barkley & Cunningham, 1979b; Barkley, Karlsson, Pollard, & Murphy, 1985; Danforth et al., 1991; Humphries, Kinsbourne, & Swanson, 1978). These effects of medication are noted even in preschool-age children with ADHD (Barkley, 1988) as well as in those in late childhood (Barkley et al., 1985), and in children of both sexes (Barkley, 1989b). Besides a general reduction in the negative, disruptive, and conflictual interaction patterns between children with ADHD and their parents as a result of stimulant medication, general family functioning also seems to improve when these children are treated with stimulant medication (Schachar, Taylor, Weiselberg, Thorley, & Rutter, 1987). None of this is to say that parental reactions to disruptive child behavior, parental skill and competence in child management and daily rearing, and parental psychological impairment are unimportant influences on children with ADHD. Evidence certainly shows that parental management, child monitoring, parental antisocial activity, maternal depression, father absence, and other parent and family factors are exceptionally important in the development of ODD, CD, major depression, ad other disorders likely to be comorbid with ADHD (Johnson, Cohen, Kasen, Smailes, & Brook, 2001; Johnston & Mash, 2001; Pfiffner, McBurnett, & Rathouz, 2001; Patterson et al., 2000). But it must be emphasized, as the behavioral genetic studies described below strongly attest, that these are not the origins of the impulsive, hyperactive, and inattentive behaviors or the related deficits in executive functioning and self-regulation.

The patterns of disruptive, intrusive, excessive, negative, and emotional social interactions that have been found between children with ADHD and their parents have been found to occur in the children's interactions with teachers (Whalen, Henker, & Dotemoto, 1980) and peers (Clark, Cheyne, Cunningham, & Siegel, 1988; Cunningham & Siegel, 1987; DuPaul et al., 2001; Whalen, Henker, Collins, McAuliffe, & Vaux, 1979). It should come as no surprise, then, that those with ADHD receive more correction, punishment, censure, and criticism than other children from their teachers, as well as more school suspensions and expulsions, particularly if they have ODD/CD (Barkley, Fischer, et al., 1990; Whalen et al., 1980). In their social relationships, children with ADHD are less liked by other children, have fewer friends, and are overwhelmingly rejected as a consequence (Erhardt & Hinshaw, 1994), particularly if they have comorbid conduct problems (Gresham, MacMillan, Bocian, Ward, & Forness, 1998; Hinshaw & Melnick, 1995). Indeed, among such comorbid cases, up to 70%

may be rejected by peers and have no reciprocated friendships by fourth grade (Gresham et al., 1998). These peer relationship problems are the results not only of these children's more active, talkative, and impulsive actions, but also of their greater emotional, facial, tonal, and bodily expressiveness (particularly anger), more limited reciprocity in interactions, use of fewer positive social statements, more limited knowledge of social skills, and more negative physical behavior (Casey, 1996; Erhardt & Hinshaw, 1994; Grenel, Glass, & Katz, 1987; Madan-Swain & Zentall, 1990). Those with ODD/CD also prefer more sensation-seeking, fun-seeking, and trouble-seeking activities, which further serve to alienate their normal peers (Hinshaw & Melnick, 1995; Melnick & Hinshaw, 1996). Furthermore, children with ADHD seem to process social and emotional cues from others in a more limited and error-prone fashion, as if they were not paying as much attention to emotional information provided by othrs. Yet they do not differ in their capacity to understand the emotional expressions of other children (Casey, 1996). However, in those with comorbid ODD/CD, there may be a greater misperception of anger and a greater likelihood of responding with anger and aggression to peers than normal children (Cadesky, Mota, & Schachar, 2000; Casey, 1996; Matthys, Cuperus, & van Engeland, 1999). Little wonder, then, that children with ADHD perceive themselves as receiving less social support from peers (and teachers) than do normal children (Demaray & Elliot, 2001). The problems with aggression and poor emotion regulation are also evident in the sports behavior of these children with their peers (Johnson & Rosen, 2000). Once more, stimulant medication has been observed to decrease these negative and disruptive behaviors toward teachers (Whalen et al., 1980) and peers (Cunningham, Siegel, & Offord, 1985; Wallander, Schroeder, Michelli, & Gualtieri, 1987; Whalen et al., 1987), but it may not result in any increase in more prosocial or positive initiatives toward peers (Wallander et al., 1987).

HEALTH OUTCOMES

Once again, caution should be used in extending the findings below beyond the ADHD-C subtype, given that very little research exists on the health outcomes of ADHD-PI.

Physical Health

The postnatal course of those with hyperactivity has been shown to be subject to more stress and complications in several studies (Hartsough & Lambert, 1985; Stewart et al., 1966; Taylor et al., 1991). Chronic health problems, such as recurring upper respiratory infections, asthma, and allergies, have also been documented in the later preschool and childhood years of hyperactive children (Hartsough & Lambert, 1985; Mitchell, Aman, Turbott, & Manku, 1987; Szatmari et al., 1989). And children with atopic (allergic) disorders have been shown to have more symptoms of ADHD (Roth, Beyreiss, Schlenzka, & Beyer, 1991). Yet more careful research using better control groups, longitudinal samples, or analysis of the familial aggregation of disorders has not shown a specific association of these disorders with hyperactivity (Biederman, Milberger, Faraone, Guite, & Warburton, 1994; McGee, Stanton, & Sears, 1993; Mitchell et al., 1987; Taylor et al., 1991).

One study suggests that ADHD may be associated with growth deficits, particularly in height, during childhood and early adolescence (Spencer et al., 1996). These deficits did not exist in older adolescents, suggesting that the problem with growth is one of delayed maturation.

Accident-Proneness and Injury

In one of the first studies of the issue, Stewart et al. (1966) found that four times as many hyperactive children as control children (43% vs. 11%) were described by parents as accident-prone. Later studies have also identified such risks; up to 57% of children with hyperactivity or ADHD are said to be accident-prone by parents, relative to 11% or fewer of control children (Mitchell et al., 1987; Reebye, 1997). Interestingly, knowledge about safety does not appear to be lower in overactive, impulsive children than in control children. And so simply teaching more knowledge about safety may not suffice to reduce the accident risks of hyperactive children (Mori & Peterson, 1995).

Most studies find that children with ADHD experience more injuries of various sorts than control children. In one study, 16% of the hyperactive sample had at least four or more serious accidental injuries (broken bones, lacerations, head injuries, severe bruises, lost teeth, etc.), compared to just 5% of control children (Hartsough & Lambert, 1985). Jensen, Shervette, Xenakis, and Bain (1988) found that 68% of children with DSM-III ADD, compared to 39% of control children, had experienced physical trauma sufficient to warrant sutures, hospitalization, or extensive/painful procedures. Several other studies likewise found a greater frequency of accidental injuries than among control children (Taylor et al., 1991), as did I when I analyzed data from research Terri Shelton and I had done (Shelton et al., 1998) and found that more than four times as many children with ADHD as control children (28.4% vs. 6.4%) had an accident related to their impulsive behavior. One of my own studies, however, did not find a higher proportion of children with ADHD as having accidents (Barkley, DuPaul, & McMurray, 1990). Sample sizes in this study were small, however, and may not have been able to detect moderate to small effect sizes with adequate statistical power.

Head trauma is not overrepresented among children with hyperactivity or ADHD (Stewart et al., 1966; Szatmari et al., 1989). As for burns, only one study of children with ADHD has been done, and it did not find a significantly elevated incidence (2.0% vs. 2.4% for controls) (Szatmari et al., 1989). Bone fractures, in contrast, seem to be somewhat more common in children with ADHD than in control children (23.5% vs. 15.1%) (Szatmari et al., 1989). Children with ADHD may be two to three times more likely to experience accidental poisonings (21% vs. 8% in Stewart, Thach, & Friedin, 1970; 7% vs. 3% in Szatmari et al., 1989). Jensen et al. (1988) found that 13% of children with ADD and 8% of control children had ingested poisonous substances.

Driving Risks and Auto Accidents

The most extensively studied form of accidents occurring among those with hyperactivity or ADHD is motor vehicle crashes. Evidence emerged years ago that hyperactive teens as drivers had a higher frequency of vehicular crashes than control subjects (1.3 vs. 0.07; $p < .05$) (Weiss & Hechtman, 1993). Also noteworthy in their driving histories was a significantly greater frequency of citations for speeding.

Subsequently, my colleagues and I (Barkley, Guevremont, Anastopoulos, DuPaul, & Shelton, 1993) found that teens with ADHD had more crashes as drivers (1.5 vs. 0.4) than did control teens over their first few years of driving. Forty percent of the group with ADHD had experienced at least two or more such crashes, relative to just 6% of the control group. Four times more teens with ADHD were deemed to have been at fault in their crashes as drivers than controls (48.6% vs. 11.1%), and these teens were at fault more frequently than the controls (0.8 vs. 0.4). In keeping with the Weiss and Hechtman (1993) initial report, teens with ADHD were more likely to get speeding tickets (65.7% vs. 33.3%) and got them more often (means = 2.4 vs. 0.6). Two studies in New Zealand using community samples suggest a similarly strong relationship between ADHD and vehicular accident risk (Nada-Raja et al., 1997; Woodward, Fergusson, & Horwood, 2000). Adults diagnosed with ADHD also manifest more unsafe motor vehicle operation and crashes. More adults with ADHD in one study had their licenses suspended (24% vs. 4.0%) than in the control group, and reported having received more speeding tickets (means = 4.9 vs. 1.1) than control adults (Murphy & Barkley, 1996a). The difference in the frequency of vehicular crashes between the groups was only marginally significant (means = 2.8 vs. 1.8, $p < .06$), however.

Later, in a more thorough examination of driving (Barkley, Murphy, & Kwasnik, 1996b), we found that the group with ADHD reported having had more vehicular crashes than the control group (means = 2.7 vs. 1.6), and that a larger proportion of this group had been involved in more severe crashes (resulting in injuries) than the control subjects (60% vs. 17%). Again, speeding citations were overrepresented in the self-reports of the subjects with ADHD (100% vs. 56%) and occurred more frequently in this group than in the control group (means = 4.9 vs. 1.3).

The most thorough study to date of driving performance among young adults with ADHD (Barkley, Murphy, DuPaul, & Bush, 2002) used a multimethod, multisource battery of measures. More than twice as many young adults with ADHD as members of the control group (26% vs. 9%) had been involved in three or more vehicular crashes as drivers, and more had been held at fault in three or more such crashes (7% vs. 3%). The ADHD group had also been involved in more vehicular crashes overall than the control group (means = 1.9 vs. 1.2) and had been held to be at fault in more crashes (means = 1.8 vs. 0.9). The dollar damage caused in their first accidents was estimated to be more than twice as high in the ADHD group as in the control group (means = $4,221 vs. $1,665). As in the earlier studies, the group with ADHD reported a greater frequency of speeding citations (3.9 vs. 2.4), and a higher percentage had had their licenses suspended than in the control group (22%vs. 5%). Both the greater frequency of speeding citations and license suspensions were corroborated through the official state driving records for these young adults.

These studies leave little doubt that ADHD, or its symptoms of inattention and hyperactive–impulsive behavior, are associated with a higher risk for unsafe driving and motor vehicle accidents than in the normal population. In view of the substantial costs that must be associated with such a higher rate of adverse driving outcomes, prevention and intervention efforts are certainly called for to attempt to reduce the driving risks among those having ADHD.

Sleep Problems

Many studies have suggested an association between ADHD and sleep disturbances (Ball, Tiernan, Janusz, & Furr, 1997; Gruber, Sadeh, & Raviv, 2000; Kaplan, McNichol, Conte, & Moghadam, 1987; Stewart et al., 1966; Trommer, Hoeppner, Rosenberg, Armstrong, & Rothstein, 1988; Wilens, Biederman, & Spencer, 1994). The problems are mainly more behavioral problems at bedtime, a longer time to fall asleep, instability of sleep duration, tiredness at awakening, or frequent night waking. For instance, Stein (1999) compared 125 psychiatrically diagnosed children with 83 pediatric outpatient children and found moderate to severe sleep problems in 19% of those with ADHD, 13% of the psychiatric controls, and 6% of pediatric outpatients. Treatment with stimulant medication increased the proportion of children with ADHD and sleep problems to 29%—a not unexpected finding, given the well-known stimulant side effect of increased insomnia (see Barkley, 1998). Sleep electroencephalograms (EEGs) have typically not revealed differences in the quality of sleeping, however (Ball & Kolonian, 1995). Other research implies that the comorbid disorders (ODD, anxiety disorders, etc.) associated with ADHD may contribute to the increased risk for some of these sleep problems (Corkum, Beig, Tannock, & Moldofsky, 1997). Indeed, a later study by Corkum and associates (Corkum, Moldofsky, Hogg-Johnson, Humphries, & Tannock, 1999) found that sleep problems occurred twice as often in ADHD than in control children. These problems could be reduced to three general factors: (1) dyssomnias (bedtime resistance, sleep onset problems, or difficulty arising); (2) sleep-related involuntary movements (teeth grinding, sleeptalking, restless sleep, etc.); and (3) parasomnias (sleep walking, night wakings, sleep terrors). Dyssomnias were primarily related to comorbid ODD or treatment with stimulant medication, whereas parasomnias were not significantly different from the control group. However, involuntary movements were significantly elevated in children with ADHD-C.

Within normal populations, quantity of sleep is inversely associated with an increased risk for school behavioral problems (Aronen, Paavonen, Fjallnerg, Soinen, & Torronen, 2000), particularly daytime sleepiness and inattention rather than hyperactive–impulsive behavior (Fallone, Acebo, Arnedt, Seifer, & Carskadon, 2001). The direction of effect, then, between ADHD and sleep problems is unclear. It is possible that sleep difficulties increase ADHD symptoms during the daytime, as the research on normal children implies. Yet some research finds that the sleep problems of children with ADHD are not associated with the severity of their symptoms; this suggests that the disorder, not the impaired sleeping, is what contributes to impaired daytime alertness, inattention, and behavioral problems (Lecendreux, Konofal, Bouvard, Falissard, & Mouren-Simeoni, 2000).

ETIOLOGIES

Since the first edition of this text was published, considerable research has accumulated on various etiologies for ADHD. Notably, virtually all of this research pertains to the ADHD-C subtype, or what was previously considered hyperactivity in children. Readers should not extend these findings to the ADHD-PI subtype, especially the subset noted above to have sluggish cognitive tempo and (probably) a qualitatively different disorder. But for ADHD-C, there is even less doubt now among career investigators in this field that although the disorder may have multiple etiologies, neurological and genetic factors are likely to play the greatest role in causing it. These two areas, along with the associated field of the neuropsychology of ADHD, have witnessed enormous growth in the past decade, further refining our understanding of the neurogenetic basis of the disorder. Our knowledge of the final common neurological pathway through which these causes produce their effects on behavior has become clearer from converging lines of evidence employing a wide array of assessment tools, including neuropsychological tests sensitive to frontal lobe functioning; electrophysiological measures (EEG, quantitative EEG [QEEG], and evoked response potentials [ERPs); measures of cerebral blood flow; and neuroimaging studies using positron emission tomography (PET), magnetic resonance imaging (MRI), and functional MRI. Several recent studies have even identified specific protein abnormalities in specific brain regions that may be linked to possible neurochemical dysregulation in the disorder. Precise neurochemical abnormalities that may underlie this disorder have proven extremely difficult to document with any certainty over the past decade, but advancing psychopharmacological, neurological, and genetic evidence suggests involvement in at least two systems—the dopaminergic and noradrenergic systems. Neurological evidence is converging on a highly probable neurological network for ADHD, as discussed below. Nevertheless, most findings on etiologies are correlational in nature and do not provide direct, precise, immediate molecular evidence of primary causality. But then that is the case for all psychiatric disorders (and, indeed, many medical ones as well), so ADHD is in good company. In fact, our understanding of causal factors here may be far more advanced than is the case in most other psychopathologies of childhood.

Neurological Factors

Various neurological etiologies have been proposed for ADHD. Brain damage was initially proposed as an initial and chief cause of ADHD symptoms (Still, 1902), whether it occurred as a result of known brain infections, trauma, or other injuries or complications occurring during pregnancy or at the time of delivery (see Barkley, 1998, for more on the history of ADHD). Several studies show that brain damage, particularly hypoxic/anoxic types of insults, is associated with greater attention deficits and hyperactivity (Cruickshank, Eliason, & Merrifield, 1988; O'Dougherty, Nuechterlein, & Drew, 1984). ADHD symptoms also occur more often in children with seizure disorders (Holdsworth & Whitmore, 1974) that are clearly related to underlying neurological malfunction. However, most children with ADHD have no history of significant brain injuries or seizure disorders, and so brain damage is unlikely to account for the majority of children with ADHD (Rutter, 1977).

Throughout the century, investigators have repeatedly noted the similarities between symptoms of ADHD and those produced by lesions or injuries to the frontal lobes more generally and the prefrontal cortex specifically (Barkley, 1997b; Benton, 1991; Heilman et al., 1991; Levin, 1938; Mattes, 1980). Both children and adults suffering injuries to the prefrontal region demonstrate deficits in sustained attention, inhibition, regulation of emotion and motivation, and the capacity to organize behavior across time (Fuster, 1997; Grattan & Eslinger, 1991; Stuss & Benson, 1986).

Neuropsychological Studies

Much of the neuropsychological evidence pertaining to ADHD has been reviewed above in relation to the particular forms of cognitive impairment seen in ADHD, especially as regards the theory described earlier. A large number of studies have used neuropsychological tests of frontal lobe functions and have detected deficits on these tests, albeit inconsistently (Barkley, Edwards, et al., 2001; Conners & Wells, 1986; Chelune, Ferguson, Koon, & Dickey, 1986; Fischer et al., 1990; Heilman et al., 1991; Mariani & Barkley, 1997; Murphy et al., 2001; Seidman, Biederman, Faraone, et al., 1997). I have reviewed much of this literature up to 1997 (Barkley, 1997b), but it has nearly doubled in volume since that time. Where consistent, the results suggest that poor inhibition of behavioral responses, or what Nigg (2001) has called "executive inhibition," is solidly established as impaired in this disorder, at least the ADHD-C and ADHD-PHI types. As noted earlier, evidence has mounted for difficulties as well with nonverbal and verbal working memory, planning, verbal fluency, response perseveration, motor sequencing, sense of time, and other frontal lobe functions. Adults with ADHD have also been shown to display similar deficits on neuropsychological tests of executive functions (Barkley, Murphy, & Bush, 2001; Murphy et al., 2001; Seidman, Biederman, Faraone, et al., 1997). One recent study of adults found diminished olfactory identification in adults with ADHD—a finding predicted on the basis of the fact that both executive functions and olfactory identification are mediated by prefrontal regions (Murphy et al., 2001).

Moreover, recent research shows not only that do siblings of children with ADHD who also have ADHD show similar executive function deficits, but even that siblings who do not actually manifest ADHD themselves appear to have milder yet significant impairments in these same executive functions (Sedman, Biederman, Weber, Monuteaux, & Faraone, 1997). Such findings imply a possible genetically linked risk for executive function deficits in families of children with ADHD, even if symptoms of ADHD are not fully manifested in those family members. Supporting this implication is evidence that the executive deficits in ADHD arise from the same substantial shared genetic liability as do the ADHD symptoms themselves and as does the overlap of ADHD with ODD/CD (Coolidge et al., 2000). Important in recent studies in this area has been the demonstration that these inhibitory and executive deficits are not the result of comorbid disorders, such as ODD, CD, anxiety, or depression, thus giving greater confidence to their affiliation with ADHD itself (Barkley, Edwards, et al., 2001; Barkley, Murphy, & Bush, 2001; Bayliss & Roodenrys, 2000; Chang et al., 1999; Clark et al., 2000; Klorman et al., 1999; Murphy et al., 2001; Nigg et al., 1998; Oosterlaan et al., in press; Wiers et al., 1998). This is not to say that some other disorders, such as learning disabilities or autism, do not affect some executive function tasks, such as those of verbal working memory, perhaps owing to their associated deficits in language development; still, the pattern of deficits associated with ADHD is not typical of these other disorders (Pennington & Ozonoff, 1996). The totality of findings in the neuropsychology of ADHD is impressive in further suggesting that some dysfunction of the prefrontal lobes (inhibition and executive function deficits) is involved in this disorder.

Neurological Studies

Early research in the 1960s and 1970s focused on psychophysiological measures of nervous system (central and autonomic) electrical activity, variously measured (EEGs, galvanic skin responses, heart rate deceleration, etc.). These studies were inconsistent in demonstrating group differences between children with ADHD and control children in resting arousal. But where differences from normal were found, they were consistently in the direction of diminished reactivity to stimulation, or arousability, in those with ADHD (see Hastings & Barkley, 1978, for a review). Recent research continues to demonstrate differences in skin conductance and heart rate parameters in response to stimulation in those with ADHD (Borger & van der Meere, 2000), which may distinguish them from children with CD or those with comorbid ADHD and CD (Beauchaine et al., 2001; Herpertz et al., 2001).

Far more consistent have been the results of QEEG and ERP measures, sometimes taken in conjunction with vigilance tests (Frank, Lazar, & Seiden, 1992; Klorman, 1992; Klorman, Salzman, & Borgstedt, 1988; Rothenberger, 1995). Although results have varied substantially across these studies (see Tannock, 1998, for a review), the most consistent pattern for EEG research is increased slow-wave or theta activity, particularly in the frontal lobe, and excess beta activity, all indicative of a pattern of underarousal and underreactivity in ADHD (Baving, Laucht, & Schmidt, 1999; Chabot & Serfontein, 1996; Kuperman, Johnson, Arndt, Lindgren, & Wolraich, 1996; Monastra, Lubar, & Linden, 2001). Children with ADHD have been found to have smaller amplitudes in the late positive and negative components of their ERPs. These late components are believed to be a function of the prefrontal regions of the brain, are related to poorer performances on inhibition and vigilance tests, and are corrected by stimulant medication (Johnstone, Barry, & Anderson, 2001; Pliszka, Liotti, & Woldorff, 2000; Kuperman et al., 1996). Thus psychophysiological abnormalities related to sustained attention and inhibition indicate an underresponsiveness of children with ADHD to stimulation that is corrected by stimulant medication.

Several studies have also examined cerebral blood flow using single-photon emission computed tomography (SPECT) in children with ADHD and normal children (see Tannock, 1998, and Hendren, DeBacker, & Pandina, 2000, for reviews). They have consistently shown decreased blood flow to the prefrontal regions (most recently in the right frontal area), and to pathways connecting these regions with the limbic system via the striatum and specifically its anterior region known as the caudate, and with the cerebellum (Gustafsson, Thernlund, Ryding, Rosen, & Cederblad, 2000; Lou, Henriksen, & Bruhn, 1984; Lou, Henriksen, Bruhn, Borner, & Nielsen, 1989; Sieg, Gaffney, Preston, & Hellings, 1995). Degree of blood flow in the right frontal region has been correlated with behavioral severity of the disorder, while that in more posterior regions and the cerebellum seems related to degree of motor impairment (Gustafsson et al., 2000).

Within the last few years, a radioactive chemical ligand known as [I^{123}] Altropane has been developed that binds specifically to the dopamine transporter protein in the striatum of the brain, and thus can be used to indicate level of dopamine transporter activity within this region. Following intravenous injection of the ligand, SPECT is used to detect the binding activity of Altropane in the striatum. The dopamine transporter is responsible for the reuptake of extracellular dopamine from the synaptic cleft after neuronal release. Several pilot studies found that adults with ADHD had significantly increased binding potential of Altropane and thus greater dopamine transporter activity (Dougherty et al., 1999; Krause, Dresel, Krause, Kung, & Tatsch, 2000). A third pilot study replicated this difference in binding potential and found that degree of transporter activity was significantly associated with severity of ADHD symptoms, but not with comorbid anxiety or depression (Barkley et al., 2002). These findings are interesting because research suggests that the drug methylphenidate, which is often used to treat ADHD, has a substantial effect on activity in this brain region and may produce its therapeutic effect by slowing down this dopamine transporter activity (Krause et al., 2000; Volkow et al., 2001).

Studies using PET to assess cerebral glucose metabolism have found diminished metabolism in adults with ADHD, particularly in the frontal region (Schweitzer et al., 2000; Zametkin et al., 1990), and in adolescent females with ADHD (Ernst et al., 1994), but have proven negative in adolescent males with ADHD (Zametkin et al., 1993). An attempt to replicate the finding in adolescent females with ADHD in younger female children with ADHD failed to find such diminished metabolism (Ernst, Cohen, Liebenauer, Jons, & Zametkin, 1997). Such studies are plagued by their exceptionally small sample sizes, which result in very low power to detect group differences and considerable unreliability in replicating previous findings. However, significant correlations have been noted between diminished metabolic activity in the anterior frontal region and severity of ADHD symptoms in adolescents with ADHD (Zametkin et al., 1993). Also, using a radioactive tracer that indicates dopamine activity, Ernst et al. (1999) found abnormal dopamine activity in the right midbrain region of children with ADHD, and discovered that severity of symptoms was correlated with the degree of this abnormality. These demonstrations of an association between the metabolic activity of certain brain regions on the one hand, and symptoms of ADHD and associated executive deficits on the other, is critical to proving a connection between the findings pertaining to brain activation and the behaviors constituting ADHD.

More recent neuroimaging technologies offer a more fine-grained analysis of brain structures using the higher-resolution MRI devices. Studies employing this technology find differences in selected brain regions in those with ADHD relative to control groups. Much of the initial work was done by Hynd and his colleagues (see Tannock, 1998, for a review). Initial studies from this group examined the region of the left and right temporal lobes associated with auditory detection and analysis (planum temporale) in children with ADHD, children with reading disorders, and normal children. The first two groups were found to have smaller right-hemisphere plana temporale than the control group, but only the reading-disordered subjects had a smaller left plana temporale (Hynd, Semrud-Clikeman, Lorys, Novey, & Eliopulos, 1990). In the next study, the corpus callosum was examined in those with ADHD. This structure assists with the interhemispheric transfer of information. Those with ADHD were found to have a smaller callosum, particularly in the area of the genu and splenium and that region just anterior to the splenium (Hynd, Semrud-Clikeman, et al., 1991). An attempt to replicate this finding, however, failed to show any differences between children with ADHD and control children in the size or shape of the entire corpus callosum, with the exception of the region of the splenium (posterior portion), which again was significantly smaller in the subjects with ADHD (Semrud-Clikeman et al., 1994).

The various brain regions often implicated in ADHD in the most recent MRI research are illustrated in Figure 2.2. Here the right hemisphere of the brain is shown, but the left hemisphere has been cut away to expose the location of the striatum in relation to the prefrontal regions controlling movement specifically and behavior generally.

In a later study by Hynd and colleagues (Hynd et al., 1993), children with ADHD had a significantly smaller left caudate nucleus, creating a reversal of the normal pattern of left > right asym-

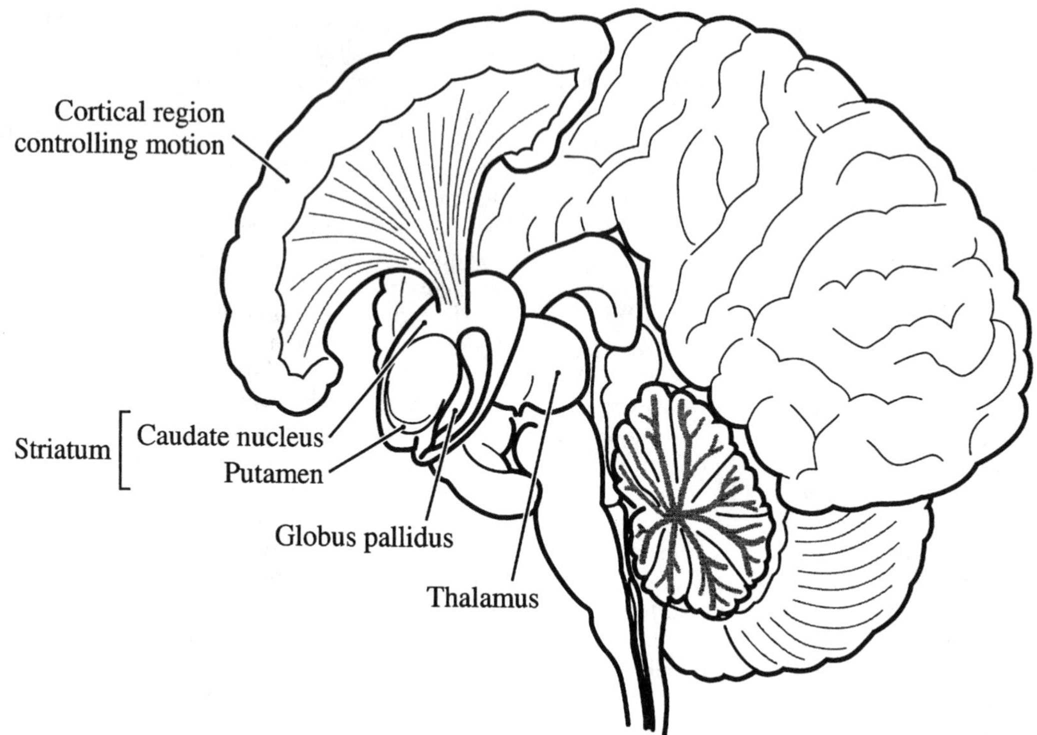

FIGURE 2.2. Diagram of the human brain showing the right hemisphere, and particularly the location of the striatum, globus pallidus, and thalamus. Most of the left hemisphere has been cut away up to the prefrontal lobes to reveal the striatum and other midbrain structures. Adapted from an illustration by Carol Donner in Youdin & Riederer (1997). Copyright 1997 by *Scientific American*. Adapted by permission.

metry of the caudate. This finding is consistent with the earlier blood flow studies of decreased activity in this brain region. Several more recent studies, using quantitative MRI technology, have used larger samples of subjects with ADHD and control subjects. These studies have indicated significantly smaller anterior right frontal regions, smaller size of the caudate nucleus, reversed asymmetry of the head of the caudate, and smaller globus pallidus regions in children with ADHD compared to control subjects (Aylward et al., 1996; Castellanos et al., 1994, 1996; Filipek et al., 1997; Singer et al., 1993). Important as well have been the findings that the size of some of these regions, particularly the structures in the basal ganglia and right frontal lobe, has been shown to correlate with the degree of impairment in inhibition and attention in the children with ADHD (Casey et al., 1997; Semrud-Clikeman et al., 2000). The putamen, however, has not been found to be smaller in children with ADHD (Aylward et al., 1996; Castellanos et al., 1996; Singer et al., 1993), or to be associated with behavioral inhibition deficits in these children (Casey et al., 1997).

Interestingly, the study by Castellanos et al. (1996) also found smaller cerebellar volume in those with ADHD. This would be consistent with recent views that the cerebellum plays a major role in executive functioning and the motor-presetting aspects of sensory perception that derive from planning and other executive actions (Diamond, 2000).

No differences between groups on MRI were found in the regions of the corpus callosum in either of the studies by Castellanos et al. (1994, 1996), as had been suggested in the small studies discussed above or as had been found in a prior study by this same research team (Giedd et al., 1994). However, the study by Filipek et al. (1997) did find smaller posterior volumes of white matter in both hemispheres in the regions of the parietal and occipital lobes, which might be consistent with the earlier studies showing smaller volumes of the corpus callosum in this same area. Castellanos et al. (1996) suggest that such differences in corpus callosal volume, particularly in the posterior regions, may be more closely related to learning disabilities (which are found in a large minority of children with ADHD) than to ADHD itself.

The results for the smaller size of the caudate nucleus are quite consistent across studies, but are inconsistent in indicating which side of the caudate may be smaller. The work by Hynd et al. (1993) discussed earlier found the left caudate to be smaller than normal in their subjects with ADHD. The more recent studies by Filipek et al. (1997) and Semrud-Clikeman et al. (2000) found the same result. However, Castellanos et al. (1996) also reported a smaller caudate, but found this to be on the right side of the caudate. The normal human brain demonstrates a relatively consistent asymmetry in volume, in favor of the right frontal cortical region's being larger than the left (Giedd et al., 1996). This led Castellanos et al. (1996) to conclude that a lack of frontal asymmetry (a smaller than normal right frontal region) probably mediates the expression of ADHD. However, whether this asymmetry of the caudate (right side > left side) is true in normal subjects is debatable, as other studies found the opposite pattern in their normal subjects (Filipek et al., 1997; Hynd et al., 1993). More consistent across these studies are the findings of smaller right prefrontal cortical regions, smaller caudate volume, and smaller regions of the cerebellar vermis (again, more likely on the right than on the left side).

With the advent of even more advanced MRI technology, researchers can now evaluate functional activity in various brain regions while administering psychological tests to subjects being scanned. These studies find children with ADHD to have abnormal patterns of activation during attention and inhibition tasks than do normal children, particularly in the right prefrontal region, the basal ganglia (striatum and putamen), and the cerebellum (Rubia et al., 1999; Teicher et al., 2000; Vaidya et al., 1998). Again, the demonstrated linkage of brain structure and function with psychological measures of ADHD symptoms and executive deficits is exceptionally important in such research, to permit causal inferences to be made about the role of these brain abnormalities in the cognitive and behavioral abnormalities constituting ADHD.

Neurotransmitter Deficiencies

Possible neurotransmitter dysfunction or imbalances have been proposed in ADHD for quite some time (see Pliszka, McCracken, & Maas, 1996, for a review). Initially, these rested chiefly on the responses of children with ADHD to differing drugs. These children respond remarkably well to stimulants, most of which act by increasing the availability of dopamine via various mechanisms, and by producing some effects on the noradrenergic pathways as well (DuPaul, Barkley, & Connor, 1998). These children also respond well to tricyclic antidepressants, giving further support to a possible noradrenergic basis to ADHD (Connor, 1998). Consequently, it seemed sensible to hypothesize that these two neurotransmitters might be involved in the disorder. The finding that normal children show a positive (albeit lesser) response to stimulants (Rapoport et al., 1978), however, partially undermines this logic. Other, more direct evidence comes from studies of cerebrospinal fluid in children with ADHD and normal children, which indicate decreased brain dopamine in the children with ADHD (Raskin, Shaywitz, Shaywitz, Anderson & Cohen, 1984). Similarly, other studies have used blood and urinary metabolites of brain neurotransmitters to infer deficiencies in ADHD, largely related to dopamine regulation. Early studies of this sort proved conflicting in their results (Shaywitz, Shaywitz, Cohen, & Young, 1983; Shaywitz et al., 1986; Zametkin & Rapoport, 1986). A subsequent study continued to find support for reduced noradrenergic activity in ADHD, as inferred from significantly lower levels of a metabolite of this neurotransmitter (Halperin et al., 1997). The limited evidence from this literature thus seems to point to a selective deficiency in the availability of both dopamine and norepinephrine, but this evidence cannot be considered conclusive at this time.

Pregnancy and Birth Complications

Some studies have not found a greater incidence of pregnancy or birth complications in children with ADHD compared to normal children (Barkley, DuPaul, & McMurray, 1990), whereas others have found a slightly higher prevalence of unusually short or long labor, fetal distress, low forceps delivery, and toxemia or eclampsia (Hartsough & Lambert, 1985; Minde, Webb, &

Sykes, 1968). Nevertheless, though children with ADHD may not experience greater pregnancy complications, prematurity, or lower birthweight as a group, children born prematurely or who have markedly lower birthweights are at high risk for later hyperactivity or ADHD (Breslau et al., 1996; Nichols & Chen, 1981; Schothorst & van Engeland, 1996; Sykes et al., 1997; Szatmari, Saigal, Rosenbaum, & Campbell, 1993). It is not merely low birthweight that seems to pose the risk for symptoms of ADHD or the disorder itself (among other psychiatric disorders), but the extent of white matter abnormalities due to birth injuries, such as parenchymal lesions and/or ventricular enlargement (Whittaker et al., 1997). These findings suggest that although certain pregnancy complications may not be the cause of most cases of ADHD, some cases may arise from such complications, especially prematurity associated with minor bleeding in the brain.

Several studies suggest that mothers of children with ADHD are younger when they conceive these children than are mothers of control children, and that such pregnancies may have a greater risk of adversity (Denson, Nanson, & McWatters, 1975; Hartsough & Lambert, 1985; Minde et al., 1968). Since pregnancy complications are more likely to occur among young mothers, mothers of children with ADHD may have a higher risk for such complications, which may act neurologically to predispose their children toward ADHD. However, the complications that have been noted to date are rather mild and hardly compelling evidence of pre- or perinatal brain damage as a cause of ADHD. Furthermore, large-scale epidemiological studies have generally not found a strong association between pre- or perinatal adversity (apart from prematurity as noted above) and symptoms of ADHD once other factors are taken into account—such as maternal smoking and alcohol use (see below) as well as socioeconomic disadvantage, all of which may predispose offspring to perinatal adversity and hyperactivity (Goodman & Stevenson, 1989; Nichols & Chen, 1981; Werner et al., 1971).

One study found that the season of a child's birth was significantly associated with risk for ADHD, at least among those subgroups of children who either also had a learning disability or did not have any psychiatric comorbidity (Mick, Biederman, & Faraone, 1996). Birth in September was overrepresented in this subgroup of children with ADHD. The authors conjecture that the season of birth may serve as a proxy for the timing of seasonally mediated viral infections to which these mothers and their fetuses may have been exposed, and that such infections may account for approximately 10% of cases of ADHD.

Genetic Factors

Evidence for a genetic basis to this disorders comes from three sources: family studies, twin studies, and (most recently) molecular genetic studies identifying individual candidate genes. Again, nearly all of this research applies to the ADHD-C subtype.

Family Aggregation Studies

For years, researchers have noted the higher prevalence of psychopathology in the parents and other relatives of children with ADHD. Between 10% and 35% of the immediate family members of children with ADHD are also likely to have the disorder, with the risk to siblings being approximately 32% (Biederman et al., 1992; Biederman, Faraone, Keenan, & Tsuang, 1991: Pauls, 1991; Welner et al., 1977). Even more striking is the finding that if a parent has ADHD, the risk to the offspring is 57% (Biederman et al., 1995). Thus, ADHD clusters significantly among the biological relatives of children or adults with the disorder, strongly implying a hereditary basis to this condition. Subsequently, these elevated rates of disorders have been noted in African American samples with ADHD (Samuel et al., 1999) as well as in girls with ADHD compared to boys (Faraone et al., 2000).

These studies of families further suggest that ADHD with CD may be a distinct familial subtype of ADHD. In research separating children with ADHD into those with and without CD, it has been shown that conduct problems, SUDs, and depression in the parents and other relatives are related more to the presence of CD in the children with ADHD than to ADHD itself (August & Stewart, 1983; Biederman, Faraone, Keenan, & Tsuang, 1991; Faraone, Biederman, et al., 1995; Faraone, Biederman, Mennin, Russell, & Tsuang, 1998; Lahey et al., 1988). Rates of hyperactivity or ADHD remain high even in relatives of children with ADHD but not CD (Biederman, Faraone, Keenan, & Tsuang, 1991); however, depression and antisocial spectrum disorders are most likely to appear in the comorbid group. Using sibling pairs in which both siblings had ADHD, Smalley et al. (2000) have also recently supported this view through findings that CD significantly clusters among the families of only those sibling pairs having CD.

Some research has also suggested that girls who manifest ADHD may need to have a greater genetic loading (higher family member prevalence) than do males with ADHD (Smalley et al., 2000). Faraone et al. (1995) also found some evidence in support of this view, in that male siblings from families with one affected child were more likely to have ADHD than were female siblings from these families. They also reported that the gender difference noted earlier for ADHD (a 3:1 male-to-female ratio) may apply primarily to children from families in which either an affected child or a parent has antisocial behavior.

Interestingly, research by Faraone and Biederman (1997) suggests that depression among family members of children with ADHD may be a nonspecific expression of the same genetic contribution that is related to ADHD. This is based on their findings that family members of children with ADHD are at increased risk for major depression, while individuals having major depression have first-degree relatives at increased risk for ADHD. Even so, as noted above, the risk for depression among family members is largely among those children having ADHD with CD.

Adoption Research

Another line of evidence for genetic involvement in ADHD has emerged from studies of adopted children. Cantwell (1975) and Morrison and Stewart (1973) both reported higher rates of hyperactivity in the biological parents of hyperactive children than in the adoptive parents of such children. Both studies suggest that hyperactive children are more likely to resemble their biological parents than their adoptive parents in their levels of hyperactivity. Yet both studies were retrospective, and both failed to study the biological parents of the adopted hyperactive children as a comparison group (Pauls, 1991). Cadoret and Stewart (1991) studied 283 male adoptees and found that if one of the biological parents had been judged delinquent or had an adult criminal conviction, the adopted-away sons had a higher likelihood of having ADHD. A later study (van den Oord, Boomsma, & Verhulst, 1994), using biologically related and unrelated pairs of international adoptees, identified a strong genetic component (47% of the variance) for high scores on the Attention Problems dimension of the Child Behavior Checklist, a rating scale commonly used in research on ADHD. More recently, a study of three groups of children (adopted children with ADHD, children with ADHD living with their biological parents, and a control group) and their families showed the same pattern of an elevated prevalence of ADHD among just the biological parents of the children with ADHD (6% vs. 18% vs. 3%, respectively) (Sprich, Biederman, Crawford, Mundy, & Faraone, 2000). Thus, like the family association studies discussed earlier, the adoption studies point to a strong possibility of a significant hereditary contribution to hyperactivity.

Twin Studies

Since the first edition of this text, the number of twin studies of ADHD and its underlying behavioral dimensions has increased markedly. More exciting has been the striking consistency across all of these studies. This research strategy provides a third avenue of evidence for a genetic contribution to ADHD. But it also provides a means of testing any competing environmental theories of the disorder (e.g., that ADHD is due to poor parenting, adverse family life, excessive TV viewing, etc.). This is because twin studies can not only compute the proportion of variance in a trait that is genetically influenced (heritability), but also the proportion that results from common or shared environment (things twins and siblings have in common growing up in the same family) and that which results from unique environment (all nongenetic factors or events that are unique or specific to one child and not to others in the family) (Plomin, Defries, McClearn, & Rutter, 1997).

Early research on ADHD using twins looked only at twin concordance (likelihood of twins' sharing the same disorder) and did not compute these estimates of heritability, shared environment, and unique environment. These early studies demonstrated a greater agreement (concordance) for symptoms of hyperactivity and inattention between monozygotic (MZ) twins than between dizygotic (DZ) twins (O'Connor, Foch, Sherry, & Plomin, 1980; Willerman, 1973). Studies of very small samples of twins (Heffron, Martin, & Welsh, 1984; Lopez, 1965) found complete (100%) concordance for MZ twins for hyperactivity, and far less agreement for DZ twins. Gilger et al. (1992) found that if one twin was diagnosed as having ADHD, the concordance for the disorder was 81% in MZ twins and 29% in DZ twins. Sherman, McGue, and Iacono (1997) found that the concordance for MZ twins having ADHD (mother-identified) was 67%, as opposed to 0% for DZ twins.

Later research has computed heritability and environmental contributions to ADHD. One such study of a large sample of twins (570) found that approximately 50% of the variance in hyperactivity and inattention in this sample was due to heredity, while 0–30% may have been environmental (Goodman & Stevenson, 1989). The relatively limited number of items assessing these two behavioral dimensions, however, may have reduced the sensitivity of the study to genetic effects. Later and even larger twin studies have found an even higher degree of heritability for ADHD, ranging from .75 to .97 (see Levy & Hay, 2001, and Thapar, 1999, for reviews) (Burt et al., 2001; Coolidge et al., 2000; Gjone, Stevenson, & Sundet, 1996; Gjone, Stevenson, Sundet, & Eilertsen, 1996; Levy, Hay, McStephen, Wood, & Waldman, 1997; Rhee, Waldman, Hay, & Levy, 1999; Sherman, Iacono, & McGue, 1997; Sherman, McGue, & Iacono, 1997; Silberg et al., 1996; Thapar et al., 2001; Thapar, Hervas, & McGuffin, 1995; van den Oord, Verhulst, & Boomsma, 1996). Thus twin studies indicate that the average heritability of ADHD is at least .80, being nearly that for human height (.80–.91) and higher than that found for intelligence (.55–.70). These studies consistently find little if any effect of shared (rearing) environment on the traits of ADHD, while sometimes finding a small significant contribution for unique environmental events. In their totality, shared environmental factors seem to account for 0–6% of individual differences in the behavioral trait(s) related to ADHD. This is why I have stated at the opening of this section that little attention is given here to discussing purely environmental or social factors as involved in the causation of ADHD.

The twin studies cited above have also been able to indicate the extent to which individual differences in ADHD symptoms are the result of nonshared environmental factors. Such factors include not only those typically thought of as involving the social environment, but also all biological factors that are nongenetic in origin. Factors in the nonshared environment are those events or conditions that will have uniquely affected only one twin and not the other. Besides biological hazards or neurologically injurious events that may have befallen only one member of a twin pair, the nonshared environment also includes those differences in the manner in which parents may have treated each child. Parents do not interact with all of their children in an identical fashion, and such unique parent–child interactions are believed to make more of a contribution to individual differences among siblings than do those factors about the home and child rearing that are common to all children in the family. Twin studies to date have suggested that approximately 9–20% of the variance in hyperactive–impulsive–inattentive behavior or ADHD symptoms can be attributed to such nonshared environmental (nongenetic) factors (Levy et al., 1997; Sherman, Iacono, & McGue 1997; Silberg et al., 1996). A portion of this variance, however, must be attributed to the error of the measure used to assess the symptoms. Research suggests that the nonshared environmental factors also contribute disproportionately more to individual differences in other forms of child psychopathology than do factors in the shared environment (Pike & Plomin, 1996). Thus, if researchers are interested in identifying environmental contributors to ADHD, these studies suggest that such research should focus on those biological and social experiences that are specific and unique to the individual and are not part of the common environment to which other siblings have been exposed.

Molecular Genetic Research

Although a quantitative genetic analysis of the large sample of families studied in Boston by Biederman and his colleagues suggested that a single gene may account for the expression of the disorder (Faraone et al., 1992), most investigators suspect multiple genes, given the complexity of the traits underlying ADHD and their dimensional nature. The focus of research was initially on the dopamine type 2 gene, given findings of its increased association with alcoholism, Tourette's disorder, and ADHD (Blum, Cull, Braverman, & Comings, 1996; Comings et al., 1991), but others have failed to replicate this finding (Gelernter et al., 1991; Kelsoe et al., 1989). More recently, the dopamine transporter gene (DAT1) has been implicated in two studies of children with ADHD (Cook et al., 1995; Cook, Stein, & Leventhal, 1997; Gill, Daly, Heron, Hawi, & Fitzgerald, 1997). Again, however, other laboratories have not been able to replicate this association (Swanson et al., 1997).

Another gene related to dopamine, the DRD4 (repeater gene), has been the most reliably found in samples of children with ADHD (Faraone et al., 1999). It is the seven-repeat form of this gene that has been found to be overrepresented in children with ADHD (Lahoste et al., 1996). Such a finding is quite interesting, because this gene has previously been associated with the personality trait of high novelty-seeking behavior; because this variant of the gene affects pharmacological responsiveness; and because the gene's impact on postsynaptic sensitivity is primarily found in frontal and prefrontal cortical regions believed to be associated with executive functions and attention (Swanson et al., 1997). The finding of an overrepresentation of the seven-repeat DRD4 gene has now been replicated in a number of other studies—not only of children with ADHD, but also of adolescents and adults with the disorder (Faraone et al., 1999).

Thyroid Disorder

Resistance to thyroid hormone (RTH) represents a variable tissue hyposensitivity to thyroid hormone. It is inherited as an autosomal dominant characteristic in most cases. It has been associated with mutations in the thyroid hormone beta receptor gene; thus a single gene for the disorder has been identified. One study (Hauser et al., 1993) found that 70% of individuals with RTH had ADHD. Other research has suggested that 64% of patients with RTH display hyperactivity or learning disabilities (Refetoff, Weiss, & Usala, 1993). A later study was not able to corroborate a link between RTH and ADHD, however (Weiss et al., 1993). In a subsequent study, Stein, Weiss, and Refetoff (1995) did find that half of their children with RTH met clinical diagnostic criteria for ADHD. Even so, the degree of ADHD in patients with RTH is believed to be milder than that seen in clinic-referred and diagnosed cases of ADHD. The patients with RTH often have more learning difficulties and cognitive impairments than do the children with ADHD but without RTH. Given that RTH is exceptionally rare in children with ADHD (prevalence of 1:2,500) (Elia et al., 1994), then thyroid dysfunction is unlikely to be a major cause of ADHD in the population. An interesting recent finding is that children with both RTH and ADHD may show a positive behavioral response to liothyronine, with decreased impulsiveness, than do children with ADHD who do not have RTH (Stein, Weiss, & Refetoff, 1995).

Environmental Toxins

As the twin and quantitative genetic studies have suggested, unique environmental events may play some role in individual differences in symptoms of ADHD. This should not be taken to mean only those influences within the realm of psychosocial or family influences. As noted above, variance in the expression of ADHD that may be due to "environmental sources" means all nongenetic sources more generally. These include pre-, peri, and postnatal complications, as well as malnutrition, diseases, trauma, toxin exposure, and other neurologically compromising events that may occur during the development of the nervous system before and after birth. Among these various biologically compromising events, several have been repeatedly linked to risks for inattention and hyperactive behavior.

One such factor is exposure to environmental toxins, specifically lead. Elevated body lead burden has been shown to have a small but consistent and statistically significant relationship to the symptoms of ADHD (Baloh, Sturm, Green, & Gleser, 1975; David, 1974; de la Burde & Choate, 1972, 1974; Needleman et al., 1979; Needleman, Schell, Bellinger, Leviton, & Alfred, 1990). However, even at relatively high levels of lead, fewer than 38% of children in one study were rated as having the behavior of hyperactivity on a teacher rating scale (Needleman et al., 1979), implying that most lead-poisoned children do not develop symptoms of ADHD. And most children with ADHD likewise, do not have significantly elevated lead burdens, although one study indicates that their lead levels may be higher than those of control subjects (Gittelman & Eskinazi, 1983). Studies that have controlled for the presence of potentially confounding factors in this relationship have found the association between body lead (in blood or dentition) and symptoms of ADHD to be .10–.19; the more factors are controlled for, the more likely the relationship is to fall below .10 (Fergusson, Fergusson, Horwood, & Kinzett, 1988; Silva, Hughes, Williams, & Faed, 1988; Thomson et al., 1989). Only 4% or less of the variance in the expression of these symptoms in children with elevated lead is explained by lead levels. Moreover, two serious methodological issues plague even the better-conducted studies in this area: (1) None of the studies have used clinical criteria for a diagnosis of ADHD to determine precisely what percentage of lead-burdened children actually have the disorder (all have simply used behavior ratings comprising only a small number of items of inattention or hyperactivity); and (2) none of the studies have assessed for the presence of ADHD in the parents and controlled its contribution to the relationship. Given the high heritability of ADHD, this factor alone could attenuate the already small correlation between lead and symptoms of ADHD by as much as a third to a half of its present leels.

Other types of environmental toxins found to have some relationship to inattention and hyperactivity are prenatal exposure to alcohol and tobacco smoke (Bennett, Wolin, & Reiss, 1988; Denson et al., 1975; Milberger, Biederman, Faraone, Chen, & Jones, 1996a; Nichols & Chen, 1981; Shaywitz, Cohen, & Shaywitz, 1980; Streissguth et al., 1984; Streissguth, Bookstein, Sampson, & Barr, 1995). It has also been shown that mothers of children with ADHD do consume more alcohol and smoke more tobacco than control groups even when they are not pregnant (Cunningham et al., 1988; Denson et al., 1975). Thus it is reasonable for research to continue to pursue the possibility that these environmental toxins may be causally related to ADHD. However, most research in this area suffers from the same two serious methodological limitations as the lead studies discussed above: the failure to utilize clinical diagnostic criteria to determine rates of ADHD in exposed children, and the failure to evaluate and control for the presence of ADHD in the parents. Until these steps are taken in future research, the relationships demonstrated so far between these toxins and ADHD must be viewed with some caution. In the area of maternal smoking during pregnancy, at least, such improvements in methodology were used in a recent study, which found the relationship between maternal smoking during pregnancy and ADHD to remain significant even after symptoms of ADHD in the mothers were controlled for (Milberger et al., 1996a).

Psychosocial Factors

A few environmental theories of ADHD were proposed over 20 years ago (Block, 1977; Willis & Lovaas, 1977), but they have not received much support in the available literature since then. Willis and Lovaas (1977) claimed that hyperactive behavior was the result of poor stimulus control by maternal commands and that this poor regulation of behavior arose from poor parental management of the children. Others have also conjectured that ADHD results from difficulties in the parents' overstimulating approach to caring for and managing the children, as well as parental psychological problems (Carlson, Jacobvitz, & Sroufe, 1995; Jacobvitz & Sroufe, 1987; Silverman & Ragusa, 1992). But these conjectures have not articulated just how the deficits in behavioral inhibition, executive functioning, and other cognitive deficits commonly associated with clinically diagnosed ADHD as described above could arise purely from such social factors. Moreover, many of these studies proclaiming to have evidence of parental characteristics as potentially causative of ADHD have not used clinical diagnostic criteria to identify children as having ADHD; instead, they have relied merely on elevated parental ratings of hyperactivity or laboratory demonstrations of distractibility to classify the children as having ADHD (Carlson et al., 1995; Silverman & Ragusa, 1992). Nor have these purely social theories received much support in the available literature that has studied clinically diagnosed children with ADHD (see Danforth et al., 1991; Johnston & Mash, 2001).

In view of the twin studies discussed above, which show minimal, nonsignificant contributions of the common or shared environment to the expression of symptoms of ADHD, theories based entirely on social explanations of the origins of ADHD are difficult to take seriously any longer. This is not to say that the family and larger social environment do not matter, for they surely do. Despite the large role heredity seems to play in ADHD symptoms, they remain malleable to unique environmental influences and nonshared social learning. The actual severity of the symptoms within a particular context, the continuity of those symptoms over development, the types of comorbid disorders that will develop, the peer relationship problems that may arise, and various outcome domains of the disorder are likely to be related in varying degrees to parental, familial, and larger environmental factors (Johnson et al., 2001; Johnston & Mash, 2001; Milberger, 1997; Pfiffner et al., 2001; van den Oord & Rowe, 1997). Yet even here, care must be taken in interpreting these findings as evidence of a purely social contribution to ADHD. This is because many measures of family functioning and adversity also show a strong heritable contribution to them, largely owing to the presence of the same or similar symptoms and disorders (and genes!) in the parents as in the children (Pike & Plomin, 1996; Plomin, 1995). Thus there is a genetic con-

. young men.[150] Even when women
en, they may gain less relative muscle
e mass is presumed to be mediated by
ecause of the well known effect of
reported sex-related differences in the
unt for the sex difference in muscle

visited: Is It a By-Product?

ggests some explanations for the odd
. Many physiological sex differences
echanisms, including the testosterone
Perhaps only few sex differentiated
, while the others are by-products of
aits. This hypothesis is supported by
ensions of intelligence.[154] On each
ability, such as spatial rotation, while
rent ability, such as some aspect of
ensions exhibit a trade-off: individuals
ension tend to be low in ability at the
rotation abilities tend to be low in the

typically female, while intensive
cannot be explained by a purel
would suggest a large female ro
and not dangerous. Indeed, int
and is in that respect more com
males appears to result from th
particular importance in plow ag

Functional explanations
patterns. For example, female
rearing and their dominanc
complementarity to child reari
have both environmental and
swing activities is important e
The sexual division of labor
environmental circumstances.
activities are relatively product
some of their activity to cha
However, they also often reall
high levels of male-male viole
this response provides some
contradicts a version of gene
dominate subsistence activitie

tribution to the family environment—a fact that often goes overlooked in studies of family and social factors involved in ADHD.

Summary

It should be evident from the research reviewed here that ADHD arises from multiple factors, and that neurological and genetic factors are substantial contributors. Like Taylor (1999), I envision ADHD as having a heterogeneous etiology, with various developmental pathways leading to this behavioral syndrome. These various pathways, however, may give rise to the disorder through disturbances in a final common pathway in the nervous system. That pathway appears to be the integrity of the prefrontal cortical–striatal network. It now appears that hereditary factors play the largest role in the occurrence of ADHD symptoms in children. It may be that what is transmitted genetically is a tendency toward a smaller and less active prefrontal–striatal–cerebellar network. The condition can also be caused or exacerbated by pregnancy complications, exposure to toxins, or neurological disease. Social factors alone cannot be supported as causal of this disorder, but such factors may exacerbate the condition, contribute to its persistence, and (more likely) contribute to the forms of comorbid disorders associated with ADHD. Cases of ADHD can also arise without a genetic predisposition to the disorder, provided that children are exposed to significant disruption of or injury to this final common neurological pathway, but this would seem to account for only a small minority of children with ADHD. In general, then, research conducted since the first edition of this text was published has further strengthened the evidence for genetic and developmental neurological factors as likely causal of this disorder while greatly reducing the support for purely social or environmental factors as having a role. Even so, environmental factors involving family and social adversity may still serve as both exacerbating factors, determinants of comorbidity, and contributors to persistence of disorder over development.

THE INATTENTIVE SUBTYPE

Mounting research on the predominantly inattentive subtype of ADHD (ADHD-PI) suggests that it differs in many important respects from the combined subtype (ADHD-C) of the disorder. Children with the ADHD-C manifest more oppositional and aggressive symptoms, a greater likelihood of having ODD and CD, and more peer rejection than children with ADHD-PI (Crystal et al., 2001; Milich et al., 2001; Willcutt, Pennington, Chhabildas, Friedman, & Alexander, 1999). Those with ADHD-PI also may have a qualitatively different impairment in attention (selective attention and speed of information processing) (see Milich et al., 2001, for a thorough review). More than twice as many children with ADHD-C as with ADHD-PI were diagnosed as having ODD (41% vs. 19%) in a study using DSM-III-R criteria, and more than three times as many were diagnosed as having CD (21% vs. 6%) (Barkley, DuPaul, & McMurray, 1990). The children with ADHD-C may also be more likely to have speech and language problems (Cantwell & Baker, 1992). Children with ADHD-C are described as more noisy, disruptive, messy, irresponsible, and immature; in contrast, children with ADHD-PI are characterized as more daydreamy, hypoactive, passive, apathetic, lethargic, confused, withdrawn, and sluggish (Edelbrock, Costello, & Kessler, 1984; Lahey, Shaughency, Strauss, & Frame, 1984; Lahey, Schaughency, Hynd, Carlson, & Nieves, 1987; McBurnett, Pfiffner, & Frick, 2001; Milich et al., 2001). Research suggests that these symptoms of sluggish cognitive tempo in ADHD-PI form a separate dimension of inattention from that in the DSM-IV (McBurnett et al., 2001), which may have resulted in their being prematurely discarded from the DSM-IV inattention list (Milich et al., 2001). A recent study by Carlson and Mann (2002) indicates that if the subset of children with ADHD-PI characterized by sluggish cognitive tempo are separated from children with this subtype who are not so characterized, then greater problems with anxiety/depression, social withdrawal, and general unhappiness and fewer problems with externalizing symptoms may be more evident in this former subset.

Social passivity and withdrawal have been reported in other studies of children with ADHD-PI as well, when parent and teacher ratings of social adjustment are used (Maedgen & Carlson, 2000; Milich et al., 2001). Direct observations of the peer interactions of these subtypes tend to corroborate these ratings, finding that children with ADHD-C are more prone to fighting and arguing, whereas children with ADHD-PI are more shy (Hodgens, Cole, & Boldizar, 2000).

Research using objective tests and other lab measures has met with mixed results in identifying consistent distinctions between these subtypes. When measures of academic achievement and neuropsychological functions have been used, most studies have found no important differences between the groups (Carlson, Lahey, & Neeper, 1986; Casey et al., 1996; Lamminmaki, Aohen, Narhi, Lyytinen, & Todd de Barra, 1995); both groups have been found to be more impaired in academic skills and in some cognitive areas than normal control children. A more recent study suggests that children with ADHD-C are more impaired in response inhibition (Nigg, Blaskey, Huang-Pollack, & Rappley, 2002), but otherwise manifest comparable deficits on executive function tasks. As in many studies of this issue, however, sample sizes were low, so that statistical power may have compromised the sensitivity of the study to all but large effect sizes. Hynd and colleagues (Hynd, Lorys, et al., 1991; Morgan, Hynd, Riccio, & Hall, 1996) found greater academic underachievement, particularly in math, and a higher percentage of learning disabilities (60%) in their samples of children with ADHD-PI compared to children with ADHD-C. My colleagues and I, however, were not able to find any differences between the subtypes on measures of achievement or in rates of learning disabilities (Barkley, 1990). Nor were Casey et al. (1996) able to find such differences in achievement or rates of learning disabilities, using the same means to define the subtypes and to classify children as learning-disabled. Both groups of children with ADHD were impaired in their academic achievement. Our own study also found both subtypes to have been retained in grade (32% in each group), and placed in special education considerably more often than our normal control children (45% vs. 53%). We did find that children with ADHD-C were more likely to have been placed in special classes for behavior-disordered children (emotionally disturbed) than children with ADHD-PI (12% vs. 0%), whereas the children with ADHD-PI were more likely to be in classes for learning-disabled children than the children with ADHD-C (53% vs. 34%). Others have also found that children with ADHD-PI needed more remedial assistance in school than children with ADHD-C (Faraone, Biederman, Weber, & Russell, 1998). We have found that both groups seem to have equivalent rates of learning disabilities, but that the additional problems with conduct and antisocial behavior are likely to result in the children with ADHD-C being assigned to the programs for behavioral disturbance rather than the programs for learning disabilities. Only one study has examined handwriting problems among subtypes of children with ADHD (Marcotte & Stern, 1997); these were found to be greatest in children with ADHD-C, but present to some extent in children with ADHD-PI compared to control children.

Unfortunately, few of these studies have directly addressed the issue of whether these subtypes differ in the components of attention they disrupt. This would require a more comprehensive and objective assessment of different components of attention in both groups. But the results of some studies suggest that their attentional disturbances are not identical (see Milich et al., 2001). Children with ADHD-PI may have more deficits on tests of selective or focused attention (such as the Coding subtest of the Wechsler Intelligence Scale for Children—Revised), problems in the consistent retrieval of verbal information from memory, and even more visual–spatial deficits than children with ADHD-C (Barkley, DuPaul, & McMurray, 1990; Garcia-Sanchez, Estevez-Gonzalez, Suarez-Romero, & Junque, 1997; Johnson, Altmaier, & Richman, 1999). Children with ADHD-C, in contrast, have more problems with motor inhibition, sequencing, and planning (Barkley, Grodzinsky, & DuPaul, 1992; Marcotte & Stern, 1997; Nigg et al., 2002). These findings intimate a qualitative difference in the attention deficits of children with ADHD-PI, which may fall more in the realms of perceptual–motor speed and central cognitive processing speed.

Studies of family psychiatric disorders are also limited and inconsistent. Some have found children with ADHD-C to have families with greater discord between their parents, and more maternal psychiatric disorders generally (Cantwell & Baker, 1992). We found a greater history of ADHD among the paternal relatives and of SUDs among the maternal relatives of children with ADHD-C (Barkley, DuPaul, & McMurray, 1990). In contrast, Frank and BenNun (1988) did not find such differences in family histories. Moreover, we noted a significantly greater prevalence of anxiety disorders among the maternal relatives of children with ADHD-PI, which was not reported by the Frank and BenNun study. That finding, however, also was not replicated in another study of family history (Lahey & Carlson, 1992), suggesting that anxiety disorders may not be more common among the relatives of children with ADHD-PI.

In general, these results suggest that children with ADHD-PI and those with ADHD-C have considerably different patterns of psychiatric comorbidity. Children with ADHD-C are at significantly greater risk for ODD and CD, academic placement in programs for behaviorally disturbed children, school suspensions, and psychotherapeutic interventions than are children with ADHD-PI. The research also appears to indicate that children with ADHD-PI can be distinguished in a number of domains of social adjustment from those with ADHD-C. Cognitive differences are less consistently noted, but this may have to do with sample selection procedures in which the children with ADHD-PI are chosen solely on the basis of the DSM inattention list, rather than focusing more on symptoms of sluggish cognitive tempo (which are not represented in that list). *Based on the evidence available to date, I concur with Milich et al. (2001) that we should begin considering these two subtypes as actually separate and unique childhood psychiatric disorders, and not as subtypes of an identical attention disturbance.*

A survey (Szatmari et al., 1989) indicates that the prevalence of these two disorders within the general population is different, especially in the childhood years (6–11 years of age). ADHD-PI appeared to be considerably less prevalent than ADHD-C in this epidemiological study. Only 1.4% of boys and 1.3% of girls had ADHD-PI, whearas 9.4% of boys and 2.8% of girls had ADHD-C. These figures changed considerably in the adolescent age groups, where 1.4% of males and 1% of females had ADHD-PI, while 2.9% of males and 1.4% of females had ADHD-C. In other words, the rates of ADHD-PI remained relatively stable across these developmental age groupings, whereas ADHD-C (especially in males) showed a considerable decline in prevalence with age. Among all children with either type, about 78% of boys and 63% of girls had ADHD-C. Baumgaertel, Wolraich, and Dietrich (1995) found a considerably higher prevalence rate for ADHD-PI among German school children. According to the DSM-III definitions for these subtypes, 3.2% had ADD without hyperactivity (corresponding to ADHD-PI), while 6.4% had ADD with hyperactivity (corresponding to ADHD-C). In contrast, when the more recent DSM-IV criteria for subtyping were employed, 9% percent of the children met criteria for ADHD-PI, while 8.8% fell into the ADHD-PHI and ADHD-C categories. The differences in these studies are difficult to reconcile, as both employed rating scales to define their subtypes. However, the Szatmari et al. (1989) study did not use DSM symptom lists but constructed their subtypes based on rating scale items, whereas Baumgaertel et al. (1995) employed symptom lists from the past three versions of the DSM.

It remains to be seen just how stable ADHD-PI is over development. No follow-up studies have focused on this subtype of ADHD, and so the long-term risks associated with it remain unknown.

FUTURE DIRECTIONS

A number of the issues raised in this chapter point the way to potentially fruitful research. The theoretical model discussed above, alone, suggests numerous possibilities for studying working memory; time and its influence over behavior; the internalization of language; creativity and fluency; the self-regulation of affect and motivation; and motor fluency in those with ADHD. Such research will not only be theory-driven, but should have the laudable outcome of linking studies of a child psychopathological condition with the larger literature of developmental psychology, developmental neuropsychology, information processing, and behavior analysis—linkages already being examined in a general way for commonalities among their paradigms and findings (Lyon, 1995).

Certainly, the diagnostic criteria developed to date, even though the most rigorous and empirical ever provided, may still suffer from problems. The fact that such criteria are not theory-driven and developmentally referenced, despite being empirically derived, risks creating several difficulties for understanding the disorder and clinically applying these criteria. Among these are the following: (1) Apparent developmental declines in the disorder and its symptoms may be more illusion than fact; (2) subtypes of a disorder are created that may simply be developmental stages of the same disorder (ADHD-PHI and ADHD-C) or are different disorders entirely (ADHD-PI); (3) female subjects may be underidentified, given that current criteria were developed predominantly from male populations; and (4) a criterion for pervasiveness that confounds the source of information with its setting may be resulting in overly restrictive criteria. These are just a few of the difficulties.

Important in future research will be efforts to understand the nature of the attentional problems in ADHD, given that extant research seriously questions whether these problems are actually within the realm of attention at all, and that the subtypes of ADHD may have qualitatively different attentional disturbances. Most studies point to impairment within the motor or output systems of the brain rather than the sensory processing systems in ADHD-C; this is not as evident in ADHD-PI. The theoretical model presented here hypothesizes that even this supposed problem with sustained attention represents a deficiency in a more complex, developmentally later form of goal-directed persistence associated with working memory and executive functioning. It arises out of poor self-regulation, rather than representing a disturbance in the more basic and traditional form of sustained responding that is contingency-shaped and maintained. Our understanding of the very nature of the disorder of ADHD is at stake in how research comes to resolve these issues.

That the field of behavioral and especially molecular genetics offers exciting prospects for future research on ADHD goes without saying. Evidence available to date shows a strong hereditary influence in the behavior patterns constituting ADHD, as well as the clinical disorder itself. As of this writing, the race seems to be on to identify the very genes that give rise to it. Such exciting prospects also exist within the domain of neurobiological and neuroimaging studies, in view of present (albeit limited) evidence that diminished metabolic activity and even minute structural differences in brain morphology within highly specific regions of the prefrontal and midbrain systems may be associated with this disorder. The increasing availability, economy, safety, and sensitivity of modern neuroimaging devices should result in a plethora of new studies on ADHD, given the promising starts to date.

Key to understanding ADHD may be the notion that it is actually a disorder of performance, rather than skill; of how one's intelligence is applied in everyday effective adaptive functioning, rather than intelligence itself; of doing what you know, rather than knowing what to do; and of when, rather than how, in the performance of behavior generally. The concept of time, how it is sensed, and particularly how one uses it in self-regulation may come to be critical elements in our understanding of ADHD, as they are coming to be in our understanding of the unique role of the prefrontal cortex more generally (Fuster, 1997). Likewise, the study of how events are mentally represented and prolonged in working memory, and of how private thought arises out of initially public behavior through the developmental process of internalization, are likely to hold important pieces of information for the understanding of ADHD itself. And as the evolutionary (adaptive) purposes of the prefrontal lobes and the executive functions they mediate come to be better understood (Barkley, 2001c), it is highly likely that these findings will yield a rich vein of insights into the sorts of adaptive deficits caused by ADHD.

ACKNOWLEDGMENTS

During the preparation of this chapter, I was supported in part by a grant from the National Institute for Child Health and Human Development (No. HD28171).

REFERENCES

Accardo, P. J., Blondis, T. A., Whitman, B. Y., & Stein, M. A. (2000). *Attention deficits and hyperactivity in children and adults*. New York: Dekker.

Achenbach, T. M. (1991). *Manual for the Revised Child Behavior Profile and Child Behavior Checklist*. Burlington: University of Vermont, Department of Psychiatry.

Achenbach, T. M., & Edelbrock, C. S. (1983). *Manual for the Child Behavior Profile and Child Behavior Checklist*. Burlington: University of Vermont, Department of Psychiatry.

Achenbach, T. M., & Edelbrock, C. S. (1987). Empirically based assessment of the behavioral/emotional problems of 2- and 3-year-old children. *Journal of Abnormal Child Psychology, 15*, 629–650.

Achenbach, T. M., McConaughy, S. H., & Howell, C. T. (1987). Child/adolescent behavioral and emotional problems: Implications of cross-informant correlations for situational specificity. *Psychological Bulletin, 101*, 213–232.

Altepeter, T. S., & Breen, M. J. (1992). Situational variation in problem behavior at home and school in attention deficit disorder with hyperactivity: A factor analytic study. *Journal of Child Psychology and Psychiatry, 33*, 741–748.

American Psychiatric Association. (1968). *Diagnostic and statistical manual of mental disorders* (2nd ed.). Washington, DC: Author.

American Psychiatric Association. (1980). *Diagnostic and statistical manual of mental disorders* (3rd ed.). Washington, DC: Author.

American Psychiatric Association. (1987). *Diagnostic and statistical manual of mental disorders* (3rd ed., rev.). Washington, DC: Author.

American Psychiatric Association. (1994). *Diagnostic and statistical manual of mental disorders* (4th ed.). Washington, DC: Author.

Anderson, C. A., Hinshaw, S. P., & Simmel, C. (1994). Mother–child interactions in ADHD and comparison boys: Relationships with overt and covert externalizing behavior. *Journal of Abnormal Child Psychology, 22*, 247–265.

Angold, A., Costello, E. J., & Erkanli, A. (1999). Comorbidity. *Journal of Child Psychology and Psychiatry, 40*, 57–88.

Antrop, I., Roeyers, H., Van Oost, P., & Buysse, A. (2000). Stimulant seeking and hyperactivity in children with ADHD. *Journal of Child Psychology and Psychiatry, 41*, 225–231.

Applegate, B., Lahey, B. B., Hart, E. L., Waldman, I., Biederman, J., Hynd, G. W., Barkley, R. A., Ollendick, T., Frick, P. J., Greenhill, L., McBurnett, K., Newcorn, J., Kerdyk, L., Garfinkel, B., & Shaffer, D. (1997). Validity of the age-of-onset criterion for ADHD: A report of the DSM-IV field trials. *Journal of American Academy of Child and Adolescent Psychiatry, 36*, 1211–1221.

Aronen, E. T., Paavonen, J., Fjallberg, M., Soininen, M., & Torronen, J. (2000). Sleep and psychiatric symptoms in school-age children. *Journal of the American Academy of Child and Adolescent Psychiatry, 39*, 502–508.

August, G. J., & Garfinkel, B. D. (1990). Comorbidity of ADHD and reading disability among clinic-referred children. *Journal of Abnormal Child Psychology, 18*, 29–45.

August, G. J., & Stewart, M. A. (1983). Family subtypes of childhood hyperactivity. *Journal of Nervous and Mental Disease, 171*, 362–368.

August, G. J., Stewart, M. A., & Holmes, C. S. (1983). A four-year follow-up of hyperactive boys with and without conduct disorder. *British Journal of Psychiatry, 143*, 192–198.

Aylward, E. H., Reiss, A. L., Reader, M. J., Singer, H. S., Brown, J. E., & Denckla, M. B. (1996). Basal ganglia volumes in children with attention-deficit hyperactivity disorder. *Journal of Child Neurology, 11*, 112–115.

Babinski, L. M., Hartsough, C. S., & Lambert, N. M. (1999). Childhood conduct problems, hyperactivity–impulsivity, and inattention as predictors of adult criminal activity. *Journal of Child Psychology and Psychiatry, 40*, 347–355.

Ball, J. D., & Kolonian, B. (1995). Sleep patterns among ADHD children. *Clinical Psychology Review, 15*, 681–691.

Ball, J. D., Tiernan, M., Janusz, J., & Furr, A. (1997). Sleep patterns among children with attention-deficit hyperactivity disorder: A reexamination of parent perceptions. *Journal of Pediatric Psychology, 22*, 389–398.

Baloh, R., Sturm, R., Green, B., & Gleser, G. (1975). Neuropsychological effects of chronic asymptomatic increased lead absorption. *Archives of Neurology, 32*, 326–330.

Barkley, R. A. (1981). *Hyperactive children: A handbook for diagnosis and treatment.* New York: Guilford Press.

Barkley, R. A. (1985). The social interactions of hyperactive children: Developmental changes, drug effects, and situational variation. In R. McMahon & R. Peters (Eds.), *Childhood disorders: Behavioral–developmental approaches* (pp. 218–243). New York: Brunner/Mazel.

Barkley, R. A. (1988). The effects of methylphenidate on the interactions of preschool ADHD children with their mothers. *Journal of the American Academy of Child and Adolescent Psychiatry, 27*, 336–341.

Barkley, R. A. (1989a). The problem of stimulus control and rule-governed behavior in children with attention deficit disorder with hyperactivity. In J. Swanson & L. Bloomingdale (Eds.), *Attention deficit disorders* (pp. 203–234). New York: Pergamon Press.

Barkley, R. A. (1989b). Hyperactive girls and boys: Stimulant drug effects on mother–child interactions. *Journal of Child Psychology and Psychiatry, 30*, 379–390.

Barkley, R. A. (1990). *Attention-deficit hyperactivity disorder: A handbook for diagnosis and treatment*. New York: Guilford Press.

Barkley, R. A. (1994). Impaired delayed responding: A unified theory of attention deficit hyperactivity disorder. In D. K. Routh (Ed.), *Disruptive behavior disorders: Essays in honor of Herbert Quay* (pp. 11–57). New York: Plenum Press.

Barkley, R. A. (1997a). Behavioral inhibition, sustained attention, and executive functions: Constructing a unifying theory of ADHD. *Psychological Bulletin, 121*, 65–94.

Barkley, R. A. (1997b). *ADHD and the nature of self-control*. New York: Guilford Press.

Barkley, R. A. (1998). *Attention-deficit hyperactivity disorder: A handbook for diagnosis and treatment* (2nd ed.). New York: Guilford Press.

Barkley, R. A. (1999a). Response inhibition in attention deficit hyperactivity disorder. *Mental Retardation and Developmental Disabilities Research Reviews, 5*, 177–184.

Barkley, R. A. (1999b). Theories of attention-deficit/hyperactivity disorder. In H. Quay & A. Hogan (Eds.), *Handbook of disruptive behavior disorders* (pp. 295–316). New York: Plenum Press.

Barkley, R. A. (2001a). The inattentive type of ADHD as a distinct disorder: What remains to be done. *Clinical Psychology: Science and Practice, 8*, 489–493.

Barkley, R. A. (2001b). Genetics of childhood disorders: XVII. ADHD, Part I: The executive functions and ADHD. *Journal of the American Academy of Child and Adolescent Psychiatry, 39*, 1064–1068.

Barkley, R. A. (2001c). The executive functions and self-regulation: An evolutionary neuropsychological perspective. *Neuropsychology Review, 11*, 1–29.

Barkley, R. A., Anastopoulos, A. D., Guevremont, D. G., & Fletcher, K. F. (1991). Adolescents with attention deficit hyperactivity disorder: Patterns of behavioral adjustment, academic functioning, and treatment utilization. *Journal of the American Academy of Child and Adolescent Psychiatry, 30*, 752–761.

Barkley, R. A., Anastopoulos, A. D., Guevremont, D. G., & Fletcher, K. F. (1992). Adolescents with attention deficit hyperactivity disorder: Mother–adolescent interactions, family beliefs and conflicts, and maternal psychopathology. *Journal of Abnormal Child Psychology, 20*, 263–288.

Barkley, R. A., & Biederman, J. (1997). Towards a broader definition of the age of onset criterion for attention deficit hyperactivity disorder. *Journal of the American Academy of Child and Adolescent Psychiatry, 36*, 1204–1210.

Barkley, R. A., & Cunningham, C. E. (1979a). Stimulant drugs and activity level in hyperactive children. *American Journal of Orthopsychiatry, 49*, 491–499.

Barkley, R. A., & Cunningham, C. E. (1979b). The effects of methylphenidate on the mother–child interactions of hyperactive children. *Archives of General Psychiatry, 36*, 201–208.

Barkley, R., Cunningham, C., & Karlsson, J. (1983). The speech of hyperactive children and their mothers: Comparisons with normal children and stimulant drug effects. *Journal of Learning Disabilities, 16*, 105–110.

Barkley, R. A., DuPaul, G. J., & McMurray, M.B. (1990). A comprehensive evaluation of attention deficit disorder with and without hyperactivity. *Journal of Consulting and Clinical Psychology, 58*, 775–789.

Barkley, R. A., & Edelbrock, C. S. (1987). Assessing situational variation in children's behavior problems: The Home and School Situations Questionnaires. In R. Prinz (Ed.), *Advances in behavioral assessment of children and families* (Vol. 3, pp. 157–176). Greenwich, CT: JAI Press.

Barkley, R. A., Edwards, G., Laneri, M., Fletcher, K., & Metevia, L. (2001). Executive functioning, temporal discounting, and sense of time in adolescents with attention deficit hyperactivity disorder and oppositional defiant disorder. *Journal of Abnormal Child Psychology, 29*, 541–556.

Barkley, R. A., Fischer, M., Edelbrock, C. S., & Smallish, L. (1990). The adolescent outcome of hyperactive children diagnosed by research criteria: I. An 8 year prospective follow-up study. *Journal of the American Academy of Child and Adolescent Psychiatry, 29*, 546–557.

Barkley, R. A., Fischer, M., Edelbrock, C. S., & Smallish, L. (1991). The adolescent outcome of hyperactive children diagnosed by research criteria: III. Mother–child interactions, family conflicts, and maternal psychopathology. *Journal of Child Psychology and Psychiatry, 32*, 233–256.

Barkley, R. A., Fischer, M., Smallish, L, & Fletcher, K. (2002). Persistence of attention deficit hyperactivity disorder into adulthood as a function of reporting source and definition of disorder. *Journal of Abnormal Psychology, 111*, 269–289.

Barkley, R. A., Fischer, M., Smallish, L., & Fletcher, K. (in press). Does the treatment of ADHD with stimulant medication contribute to illicit drug use and abuse in adulthood?: Results from a 15-year prospective study. *Pediatrics*.

Barkley, R. A., Grodzinsky, G., & DuPaul, G. (1992). Frontal lobe functions in attention deficit disorder with and without hyperactivity: A review and research report. *Journal of Abnormal Child Psychology, 20*, 163–188.

Barkley, R. A., Guevremont, D. G., Anastopoulos, A. D., DuPaul, G. J., & Shelton, T. L. (1993). Driving-related risks and outcomes of attention deficit hyperactivity disorder in adolescents and young adults: A 3–5 year follow-up survey. *Pediatrics, 92*, 212–218.

Barkley, R. A., Karlsson, J., & Pollard, S. (1985). Effects of age on the mother–child interactions of hyperactive children. *Journal of Abnormal Child Psychology, 13*, 631–638.

Barkley, R. A., Karlsson, J., Pollard, S., & Murphy, J. V. (1985). Developmental changes in the mother–child interactions of hyperactive boys: Effects of two dose levels of Ritalin. *Journal of Child Psychology and Psychiatry and Allied Disciplines, 26*, 705–715.

Barkley, R. A., Licho, R., McGough, J. J., Tuite, P., Feifel, D., Mishkin, F., Sullivan, M., Williams, B., Murphy, K., McCracken, J., Corbett, B., Hoh, C., Bush, B., Schacherer, R., Kawamoto, B., Fischman, A., Trout, J. R., Lanser, M., & Spencer, T. (2002). *Excessive dopamine transporter density in adults with attention deficit hyperactivity disorder assessed by SPECT with [^{123}I] altropane*. Unpublished manuscript, University of Massachusetts Medical School, Worcester.

Barkley, R. A., Murphy, K. R., & Bush, T. (2001). Time perception and reproduction in young adults with attention deficit hyperactivity disorder (ADHD). *Neuropsychology, 15*, 351–360.

Barkley, R. A., Murphy, K. R., DuPaul, G. R., & Bush, T. (in press). Driving in young adults with attention deficit hyperactivity disorder: Knowledge, performance, adverse outcomes and the role of executive functions. *Journal of the International Neuropsychological Society*.

Barkley, R. A., Murphy, K. R., & Kwasnik, D. (1996a). Psychological functioning and adaptive impairments in young adults with ADHD. *Journal of Attention Disorders, 1*, 41–54.

Barkley, R. A., Murphy, K. R., & Kwasnik, D. (1996b). Motor vehicle driving competencies and risks in teens and young adults with attention deficit hyperactivity disorder. *Pediatrics, 98*, 1089–1095.

Barkley, R. A., Shelton, T. L., Crosswait, C., Moorehouse, M., Fletcher, K., Barrett, S., Jenkins, L., & Metevia, L. (2002). Preschool children with high levels of disruptive behavior: Three-year outcomes as a function of adaptive disability. *Development and Psychopathology, 14*, 45–68.

Barkley, R. A., & Ullman, D. G. (1975). A comparison of objective measures of activity level and distractibility in hyperactive and nonhyperactive children. *Journal of Abnormal Child Psychology, 3*, 213–244.

Bate, A. J., Mathias, J. L., & Crawford, J. R. (2001). Performance of the Test of Everyday Attention and standard tests of attention following severe traumatic brain injury. *Clinical Neuropsychologist, 15*, 405–422.

Baumgaertel, A. (1994, June). *Assessment of German school children using DSM criteria based on teacher report*. Paper presented at the meeting of the Society for Research in Child and Adolescent Psychopathology, London.

Baumgaertel, A., Wolraich, M. L., & Dietrich, M. (1995). Comparison of diagnostic criteria for attention deficit disorders in a German elementary school sample. *Journal of the American Academy of Child and Adolescent Psychiatry, 34*, 629–638.

Baving, L., Laucht, M., & Schmidt, M. H. (1999). Atypical frontal brain activation in ADHD: Preschool and elementary school boys and girls. *Journal of the American Academy of Child and Adolescent Psychiatry, 38*, 1363–1371.

Bayliss, D. M., & Roodenrys, S. (2000). Executive processing and attention deficit hyperactivity disorder: An application of the supervisory attentional system. *Developmental Neuropsychology, 17*, 161–180.

Beauchaine, T. P., Katkin, E. S., Strassberg, Z., & Snarr, J. (2001). Disinhibitory psychopathology in male adolescents: Discriminating conduct disorder from attention-deficit/hyperactivity disorder through concurrent assessment of multiple autonomic states. *Journal of Abnormal Psychology, 110*, 610–624.

Befera, M., & Barkley, R. A. (1984). Hyperactive and normal girls and boys: Mother–child interactions, parent psychiatric status, and child psychopathology. *Journal of Child Psychology and Psychiatry, 26*, 439–452.

Beiser, M., Dion, R., & Gotowiec, A. (2000). The structure of attention-deficit and hyperactivity symptoms among Native and non-Native elementary school children. *Journal of Abnormal Child Psychology, 28*, 425–537.

Beitchman, J. H., Wekerle, C., & Hood, J. (1987). Diagnostic continuity from preschool to middle childhood. *Journal of the American Academy of Child and Adolescent Psychiatry, 26*, 694–699.

Bennett, L. A., Wolin, S. J., & Reiss, D. (1988). Cognitive, behavioral, and emotional problems among school-age children of alcoholic parents. *American Journal of Psychiatry, 145*, 185–190.

Benton, A. (1991). Prefrontal injury and behavior in children. *Developmental Neuropsychology*, *7*, 275–282.

Berk, L. E., & Potts, M. K. (1991). Development and functional significance of private speech among attention-deficit hyperactivity disorder and normal boys. *Journal of Abnormal Child Psychology*, *19*, 357–377.

Bhatia, M. S., Nigam, V. R., Bohra, N., & Malik, S. C. (1991). Attention deficit disorder with hyperactivity among paediatric outpatients. *Journal of Child Psychology and Psychiatry*, *32*, 297–306.

Biederman, J., Faraone, S. V., Keenan, K., & Tsuang, M. T. (1991). Evidence of a familial association between attention deficit disorder and major affective disorders. *Archives of General Psychiatry*, *48*, 633–642.

Biederman, J., Faraone, S. V., & Lapey, K. (1992). Comorbidity of diagnosis in attention-deficit hyperactivity disorder. *Child and Adolescent Psychiatric Clinics of North America*, *1*(2), 335–360.

Biederman, J., Faraone, S. V., Mick, E., Spencer, T., Wilens, T., Kiely, K., Guite, J., Ablon, J. S., Reed, E., & Warburton, R. (1995). High risk for attention deficit hyperactivity disorder among children of parents with childhood onset of the disorder: A pilot study. *American Journal of Psychiatry*, *152*, 431–435.

Biederman, J., Faraone, S., Mick, E., Wozniak, J., Chen, L., Ouellette, C., Marrs, A., Moore, P., Garcia, J., Mennin, D., & Lelon, E. (1996). Attention-deficit hyperactivity disorder and juvenile mania: An overlooked comorbidity? *Journal of the American Academy of Child and Adolescent Psychiatry*, *35*, 997–1008.

Biederman, J., Faraone, S. V., Mick, E., Williamson, S., Wilens, T. E., Spencer, T. J., Weber, W., Jetton, J., Kraus, I., Pert, J., & Zallen, B. (1999). Clinical correlates of ADHD in females: Findings from a large group of girls ascertained from pediatric and psychiatric referral sources. *Journal of the American Academy of Child and Adolescent Psychiatry*, *38*, 966–975.

Biederman, J., Faraone, S., Milberger, S., Curtis, S., Chen, L., Marrs, A., Ouellette, C., Moore, P., & Spencer, T. (1996). Predictors of persistence and remission of ADHD into adolescence: Results from a four-year prospective follow-up study. *Journal of the American Academy of Child and Adolescent Psychiatry*, *35*, 343–351.

Biederman, J., Keenan, K., & Faraone, S. V. (1990). Parent-based diagnosis of attention deficit disorder predicts a diagnosis based on teacher report. *American Journal of Child and Adolescent Psychiatry*, *29*, 698–701.

Biederman, J., Milberger, S., Faraone, S. V., Guite, J., & Warburton, R. (1994). Associations between childhood asthma and ADHD: Issues of psychiatric comorbidity and familiality. *Journal of the American Academy of Child and Adolescent Psychiatry*, *33*, 842–848.

Biederman, J., Newcorn, J., & Sprich, S. (1991). Comorbidity of attention deficit hyperactivity disorder with conduct, depressive, anxiety, and other disorders. *American Journal of Psychiatry*, *148*, 564–577.

Biederman, J., Wilens, T., Mick, E., Spencer, T., & Faraone, S. V. (1999). Pharmacotherapy of attention-deficit/hyperactivity disorder reduces risk for substance use disorder. *Pediatrics*, *104*(2), e20.

Block, G. H. (1977) Hyperactivity: A cultural perspective. *Journal of Learning Disabilities*, *110*, 236–240.

Blum, K., Cull, J. G., Braverman, E. R., & Comings, D. E. (1996). Reward deficiency syndrome. *American Scientist*, *84*, 132–145.

Borger, N., & van der Meere, J. (2000). Visual behaviour of ADHD children during an attention test: An almost forgotten variable. *Journal of Child Psychology and Psychiatry*, *41*, 525–532.

Braaten, E. B., & Rosen, L. A. (2000). Self-regulation of affect in attention deficit–hyperactivity disorder (ADHD) and non-ADHD boys: Differences in empathic responding. *Journal of Consulting and Clinical Psychology*, *68*, 313–321.

Breen, M. J. (1989). Cognitive and behavioral differences in ADHD boys and girls. *Journal of Child Psychology and Psychiatry*, *30*, 711–716.

Breggin, P. (1998). *Talking back to Ritalin*. Monroe, ME: Common Courage Press.

Breslau, N., Brown, G. G., DelDotto, J. E., Kumar, S., Exhuthachan, S., Andreski, P., & Hufnagle, K. G. (1996). Psychiatric sequelae of low birth weight at 6 years of age. *Journal of Abnormal Child Psychology*, *24*, 385–400.

Breton, J., Bergeron, L., Valla, J. P., Berthiaume, C., Gaudet, N., Lambert, J., St. Georges, M., Houde, L., & Lepine, S. (1999). Quebec Children Mental Health Survey: Prevalence of DSM-III-R mental health disorders. *Journal of Child Psychology and Psychiatry*, *40*, 375–384.

Briggs-Gowan, M. J., Horwitz, S. M., Schwab-Stone, M. E., Leventhal, J. M., & Leaf, P. J. (2000). Mental health in pediatric settings: Distribution of disorders and factors related to service use. *Journal of the American Academy of Child and Adolescent Psychiatry*, *39*, 841–849.

Bronowski, J. (1977). *A sense of the future*. Cambridge, MA: MIT Press.

Bu-Haroon, A., Eapen, V., & Bener, A. (1999). The prevalence of hyperactivity symptoms in the United Arab Emirates. *Nordic Journal of Psychiatry*, *53*, 439–442.

Buhrmester, D., Camparo, L., Christensen, A., Gonzalez, L. S., & Hinshaw, S. P. (1992). Mothers and fathers interacting in dyads and triads with normal and hyperactive sons. *Developmental Psychology*, *28*, 500–509.

Burke, J. D., Loeber, R., & Lahey, B. B. (2001). Which aspects of ADHD are associated with tobacco use in early adolescence? *Journal of Child Psychology and Psychiatry*, 493–502.

Burks, H. (1960). The hyperkinetic child. *Exceptional Children*, *27*, 18–28.

Burns, G. L., Boe, B., Walsh, J. A., Sommers-Flannagan, R., & Teegarden, L. A. (2001). A confirmatory factor analysis on the DSM-IV ADHD and ODD symptoms: What is the best model for the organization of these symptoms? *Journal of Abnormal Child Psychology*, *29*, 339–349.

Burns, G. L., & Walsh, J. A. (2002). The influence of ADHD-hyperactivity/impulsivity symptoms on the development of oppositional defiant disorder symptoms in a two-year longitudinal study. *Journal of Abnormal Child Psychology*, *30*, 245–256.

Burt, S. A., Krueger, R. F., McGue, M., & Iacono, W. G. (2001). Sources of covariation among attention-deficit hyperactivity disorder, oppositional defiant disorder, and conduct disorder: The importance of shared environment. *Journal of Abnormal Psychology*, *110*, 516–525.

Cadesky, E. B., Mota, V. L., & Schachar, R. J. (2000). Beyond words: How do children with ADHD and/or conduct problems process nonverbal information about affect? *Journal of the American Academy of Child and Adolescent Psychiatry*, *39*, 1160–1167.

Cadoret, R. J., & Stewart, M. A. (1991). An adoption study of attention deficit/hyperactivity/aggression and their relationship to adult antisocial personality. *Comprehensive Psychiatry*, *32*, 73–82.

Campbell, S. B. (1990). *Behavior problems in preschool children*. New York: Guilford Press.

Campbell, S. B., March, C. L., Pierce, E. W., Ewing, L. J., & Szumowski, E. K. (1991). Hard-to-manage preschool boys: Family context and the stability of externalizing behavior. *Journal of Abnormal Child Psychology, 19*, 301–318.

Campbell, S. B., Schleifer, M., & Weiss, G. (1978). Continuities in maternal reports and child behaviors over time in hyperactive and comparison groups. *Journal of Abnormal Child Psychology, 6*, 33–45.

Cantwell, D. P. (1975). *The hyperactive child*. New York: Spectrum.

Cantwell, D. P., & Baker, L. (1992). Association between attention deficit-hyperactivity disorder and learning disorders. In S. E. Shaywitz & B. A. Shaywitz (Eds.), *Attention deficit disorder comes of age: Toward the twenty-first century* (pp. 145–164). Austin, TX: Pro-Ed.

Carlson, C. L., Lahey, B. B., & Neeper, R. (1986). Direct assessment of the cognitive correlates of attention deficit disorders with and without hyperactivity. *Journal of Behavioral Assessment and Psychopathology, 8*, 69–86.

Carlson, C. L., & Mann, M. (2002). Sluggish cognitive tempo predicts a different pattern of impairment in the attention deficit hyperactivity disorder, predominantly inattentive type. *Journal of Clinical Child and Adolescent Psychology, 31*, 123–129.

Carlson, C. L., & Tamm, L. (2000). Responsiveness of children with attention deficit-hyperactivity disorder to reward and response cost: Differential impact on performance and motivation. *Journal of Consulting and Clinical Psychology, 68*, 73–83.

Carlson, C. L., Tamm, L., & Gaub, M. (1997). Gender differences in children with ADHD, ODD, and co-occurring ADHD/ODD identified in a school population. *Journal of the American Academy of Child and Adolescent Psychiatry, 36*, 1706–1714.

Carlson, E. A., Jacobvitz, D., & Sroufe, L. A. (1995). A developmental investigation of inattentiveness and hyperactivity. *Child Development, 66*, 37–54.

Carlson, G. A. (1990). Child and adolescent mania: Diagnostic considerations. *Journal of Child Psychology and Psychiatry, 31*, 331–342.

Carte, E. T., Nigg, J. T., & Hinshaw, S. P. (1996). Neuropsychological functioning, motor speed, and language processing in boys with and without ADHD. *Journal of Abnormal Child Psychology, 24*, 481–498.

Casey, B. J., Castellanos, F. X., Giedd, J. N., Marsh, W. L., Hamburger, S. D., Schubert, A. B., Vauss, Y. C., Vaituzis, A. C., Dickstein, D. P., Sarfatti, S. E., & Rapoport, J. L. (1997). Implication of right frontstriatal circuitry in response inhibition and attention-deficit/hyperactivity disorder. *Journal of the American Acdemy of Child and Adolescent Psychiatry, 36*, 374–383.

Casey, J. E., Rourke, B. P., & Del Dotto, J. E. (1996). Learning disabilities in children with attention deficit disorder with and without hyperactivity. *Child Neuropsychology, 2*, 83–98.

Casey, R. J. (1996). Emotional competence in children with externalizing and internalizing disorders. In M. Lewis & M. W. Sullivan (Eds.), *Emotional development in atypical children* (pp. 161–183). Mahwah, NJ: Erlbaum.

Castellanos, F. X., Giedd, J. N., Eckburg, P., Marsh, W. L., Vaituzis, C., Kaysen, D., Hamburger, S. D., & Rapoport, J. L. (1994). Quantitative morphology of the caudate nucleus in attention deficit hyperactivity disorder. *American Journal of Psychiatry, 151*, 1791–1796.

Castellanos, F. X., Giedd, J. N., Marsh, W. L., Hamburger, S. D., Vaituzis, A. C., Dickstein, D. P., Sarfatti, S. E., Vauss, Y. C., Snell, J. W., Lange, N., Kaysen, D., Krain, A. L., Ritchhie, G. F., Rajapakse, J. C., & Rapoport, J. L. (1996). Quantitative brain magnetic resonance imaging in attention-deficit hyperactivity disorder. *Archives of General Psychiatry, 53*, 607–616.

Castellanos, F. X., Marvasti, F. F., Ducharme, J. L., Walter, J. M., Israel, M. E., Krain, A., Pavlovsky, C., & Hommer, D. W. (2000). Executive function oculomotor tasks in girls with ADHD. *Journal of the American Academy of Child and Adolescent Psychiatry, 39*, 644–650.

Chadwick, O., Taylor, E., Taylor, A., Heptinstall, E., & Danckaerts, M. (1999). Hyperactivity and reading disability: A longitudinal study of the nature of the association. *Journal of Child Psychology and Psychiatry, 40*, 1039–1050.

Chang, H. T., Klorman, R., Shaywitz, S. E., Fletcher, J. M., Marchione, K. E., Holahan, J. M., Stuebing, K. K., Brumaghim, J. T., & Shaywitz, B. A. (1999). Paired-associate learning in attention-deficit/hyperactivity disorder as a function of hyperactivity–impulsivity and oppositional defiant disorder. *Journal of Abnormal Child Psychology, 27*, 237–245.

Chee, P., Logan, G., Schachar, R., Lindsay, P., & Wachsmuth, R. (1989). Effects of event rate and display time on sustained attention in hyperactive, normal, and control children. *Journal of Abnormal Child Psychology, 17*, 371–391.

Chess, S. (1960). Diagnosis and treatment of the hyperactive child. *New York State Journal of Medicine, 60*, 2379–2385.

Chilcoat, H. D., & Breslau, N. (1999).Pathways from ADHD to early drug use. *Journal of the American Academy of Child and Adolescent Psychiatry. 38*, 1347–1354.

Chabot, R. J., & Serfontein, G. (1996). Quantitative electroencephalographic profiles of children with attention deficit disorder. *Biological Psychiatry, 40*, 951–963.

Chelune, G. J., Ferguson, W., Koon, R., & Dickey, T. O. (1986). Frontal lobe disinhibition in attention deficit disorder. *Child Psychiatry and Human Development, 16*, 221–234.

Clark, C., Prior, M., & Kinsella, G. J. (2000). Do executive function deficits differentiate between adolescents with ADHD and oppositional defiant/conduct disorder?: A neuropsychological study using the Six Elements Test and Hayling Sentence Completion Test. *Journal of Abnormal Child Psychology, 28*, 405–414.

Clark, M. L., Cheyne, J. A., Cunningham, C. E., & Siegel, L. S. (1988). Dyadic peer interaction and task orientation in attention-deficit-disordered children. *Journal of Abnormal Child Psychology, 16*, 1–15.

Claude, D., & Firestone, P. (1995). The development of ADHD boys: A 12–year follow-up. *Canadian Journal of Behavioural Science, 27*, 226–249.

Cohen, N. J., & Minde, K. (1983). The "hyperactive syndrome" in kindergarten children: Comparison of children with pervasive and situational symptoms. *Journal of Child Psychology and Psychiatry, 24*, 443–455.

Cohen, N. J., Sullivan, J., Minde, K., Novak, C., & Keens, S. (1983). Mother–child interaction in hyperactive and normal kindergarten-aged children and the effect of treatment. *Child Psychiatry and Human Development, 13*, 213–224.

Cohen, N. J., Vallance, D. D., Barwick, M., Im, N., Menna, R., Horodezky, N. B., & Isaacson, L. (2000). The interface between ADHD and language impairment: An examination of language, achievement, and cognitive processing. *Journal of Child Psychology and Psychiatry, 41*, 353–362.

Comings, D. E. (2000). Attention deficit hyperactivity disorder with Tourette syndrome. In T. E. Brown (Ed.), *Attention-deficit disorders and comorbidities in children, adolescents, and adults* (pp. 363–392). Washington, DC: American Psychiatric Press.

Comings, D. E., Comings, B. G., Muhleman, D., Dietz, G., Shahbahrami, B., Tast, D., Knell, E., Kocsis, P., Baumgarten, R., Kovacs, B. W., Levy, D. L., Smith, M., Borison, R. L., Evans, D. D., Klein, D. N., MacMurray, J., Tosk, J. M., Sverd, J., Gysin, R., & Flanagan, S. D. (1991). The dopamine D_2 receptor locus as a modifying gene in neuropsychiatric disorders. *Journal of the American Medical Association, 266*, 1793–1800.

Conners, C. K., & Wells, K. (1986). *Hyperactive children: A neuropsychological approach*. Beverly Hills, CA: Sage.

Connor, D. F. (1998). Other medications in the treatment of child and adolescent ADHD. In R. A. Barkley, *Attention deficit hyperactivity disorder: A handbook for diagnosis and treatment* (2nd ed., pp. 564–581). New York: Guilford Press.

Cook, E. H., Stein, M. A., Krasowski, M. D., Cox, N. J., Olkon, D. M., Kieffer, J. E., & Leventhal, B. L. (1995). Association of attention deficit disorder and the dopamine transporter gene. *American Journal of Human Genetics, 56*, 993–998.

Cook, E. H., Stein, M. A., & Leventhal, D. L. (1997). Family-based association of attention-deficit/hyperactivity disorder and the dopamine transporter. In K. Blum & E. P. Noble (Eds.), *Handbook of psychiatric genetics* (pp. 297–310). Boca Raton, FL: CRC Press.

Coolidge, F. L., Thede, L. L., & Young, S. E. (2000). Heritability and the comorbidity of atetntion deficit hyperactivity disorder with behavioral disorders and executive function deficits: A preliminary investigation. *Developmental Neuropsychology, 17*, 273–287.

Copeland, A. P. (1979). Types of private speech produced by hyperactive and nonhyperactive boys. *Journal of Abnormal Child Psychology, 7*, 169–177.

Corkum, P. V., Beig, S., Tannock, R., & Moldofsky, H. (1997, October). *Comorbidity: The potential link between attention-deficit/hyperactivity disorder and sleep problems*. Paper presented at the annual meeting of the American Academy of Child and Adolescent Psychiatry, Toronto.

Corkum, P., Moldofsky, H., Hogg-Johnson, S., Humphries, T., & Tannock, R. (1999). Sleep problems in children with attention-deficit/hyperactivity disorder: Impact of subtype, comorbidity, and stimulant medication. *Journal of the American Academy of Child and Adolescent Psychiatry, 38*, 1285–1293.

Costello, E. J., Loeber, R., & Stouthamer-Loeber, M. (1991). Pervasive and situational hyperactivity—Confounding effect of informant: A research note. *Journal of Child Psychology and Psychiatry, 32*, 367–376.

Cruickshank, B. M., Eliason, M., & Merrifield, B. (1988). Long-term sequelae of water near-drowning. *Journal of Pediatric Psychology, 13*, 379–388.

Crystal, D. S., Ostrander, R., Chen, R. S., & August, G. J. (2001). Multimethod assessment of psychopathology among DSM-IV subtypes of children with attention-deficit/hyperactivity disorder: Self-, parent, and teacher reports. *Journal of Abnormal Child Psychology, 29*, 189–205.

Cuffe, S. P., McKeown, R. E., Jackson, K. L., Addy, C. L., Abramson, R., & Garrison, C. Z. (2001). Prevalence of attention-deficit/hyperactivity disorder in a community sample of older adolescents. *Journal of the American Academy of Child and Adolescent Psychiatry, 40*, 1037–1044.

Cunningham, C. E., Benness, B. B., & Siegel, L. S. (1988). Family functioning, time allocation, and parental depression in the families of normal and ADDH children. *Journal of Clinical Child Psychology, 17*, 169–177.

Cunningham, C. E., & Siegel, L. S. (1987). Peer interactions of normal and attention-deficit disordered boys during free-play, cooperative task, and simulated classroom situations. *Journal of Abnormal Child Psychology, 15*, 247–268.

Cunningham, C. E., Siegel, L. S., & Offord, D. R. (1985). A developmental dose response analysis of the effects of methylphenidate on the peer interactions of attention deficit disordered boys. *Journal of Child Psychology and Psychiatry, 26*, 955–971.

Dane, A. V., Schachar, R. J., & Tannock, R. (2000). Does actigraphy differentiate ADHD subtypes in a clinical research setting? *Journal of the American Academy of Child and Adolescent Psychiatry, 39*, 752–760.

Danforth, J. S., Barkley, R. A., & Stokes, T. F. (1991). Observations of parent–child interactions with hyperactive children: Research and clinical implications. *Clinical Psychology Review, 11*, 703–727.

Daugherty, T. K., & Quay, H. C. (1991). Response perseveration and delayed responding in childhood behavior disorders. *Journal of Child Psychology and Psychiatry, 32*, 453–461.

David, O. J. (1974). Association between lower level lead concentrations and hyperactivity. *Environmental Health Perspective, 7*, 17–25.

de la Burde, B., & Choate, M. (1972). Does asymptomatic lead exposure in children have latent sequelae? *Journal of Pediatrics, 81*, 1088–1091.

de la Burde, B., & Choate, M. (1974). Early asymptomatic lead exposure and development at school age. *Journal of Pediatrics, 87*, 638–642.

Demaray, M. K., & Elliot, S. N. (2001). Perceived social support by children with characteristics of attention-deficit/hyperactivity disorder. *School Psychology Quarterly, 16*, 68–90.

Demb, H. B. (1991). Use of Ritalin in the treatment of children with mental retardation. In L. L. Greenhill & B. B. Osmon (Eds.), *Ritalin: Theory and patient management* (pp. 155–170). New York: Mary Ann Liebert.

Denckla, M. B. (1994). Measurement of executive function. In G. R. Lyon (Ed.), *Frames of reference for the assessment of learning disabilities: New views on measurement issues* (pp. 117–142). Baltimore: Brookes.

Denckla, M. B., & Rudel, R. G. (1978). Anomalies of motor development in hyperactive boys. *Annals of Neurology, 3*, 231–233.

Denckla, M. B., Rudel, R. G., Chapman, C., & Krieger, J. (1985). Motor proficiency in dyslexic children with and without attentional disorders. *Archives of Neurology, 42*, 228–231.

Denson, R., Nanson, J. L., & McWatters, M. A. (1975). Hyperkinesis and maternal smoking. *Canadian Psychiatric Association Journal, 20*, 183–187.

Diamond, A. (1990). The development and neural bases of memory functions as indexed by the AB and delayed response task in human infants and infant monkeys. *Annals of the New York Academy of Sciences, 608*, 276–317.

Diamond, A. (2000). Close interrelation of motor development and cognitive development and of the cerebellum and prefrontal cortex. *Developmental Psychology, 71*, 44–56.

Diamond, A., Cruttenden, L., & Niederman, D. (1994). AB with multiple wells: 1. Why are multiple wells sometimes easier than two wells? 2. Memory or memory + inhibition? *Developmental Psychology, 30*, 192–205.

Diaz, R. M., & Berk, L. E. (Eds.). (1992). *Private speech: From social interaction to self-regulation*. Hillsdale, NJ: Erlbaum.

Dolphin, J. E., & Cruickshank, W. M. (1951). Pathology of concept formation in children with cerebral palsy. *American Journal of Mental Deficiency, 56*, 386–392.

Dougherty, D. D., Bonab, A. A., Spencer, T. J., Rauch, S. L., Madras, B. K., & Fischman, A. J. (1999). Dopamine transporter density in patients with attention deficit hyperactivity disorder. *Lancet, 354*, 2132–2133.

Douglas, V. I. (1972). Stop, look, and listen: The problem of sustained attention and impulse control in hyperactive and normal children. *Canadian Journal of Behavioural Science, 4*, 259–282.

Douglas, V. I. (1980). Higher mental processes in hyperactive children: Implications for training. In R. Knights & D. Bakker (Eds.), *Treatment of hyperactive and learning disordered children* (pp. 65–92). Baltimore: University Park Press.

Douglas, V. I. (1983). Attention and cognitive problems. In M. Rutter (Ed.), *Developmental neuropsychiatry* (pp. 280–329). New York: Guilford Press.

Douglas, V. I. (1999). Cognitive control processes in attention-deficit/hyperactivity disorder. In H. C. Quay & A. Horgan (Eds.), *Handbook of disruptive behavior disorders* (pp. 105–138). New York: Plenum Press.

Douglas, V. I., & Parry, P. A. (1983). Effects of reward on delayed reaction time task performance of hyperactive children. *Journal of Abnormal Child Psychology, 11*, 313–326.

Douglas, V. I., & Parry, P. A. (1994). Effects of reward and non-reward on attention and frustration in attention deficit disorder. *Journal of Abnormal Child Psychology, 22*, 281–302.

Douglas, V. I., & Peters, K. G. (1978). Toward a clearer definition of the attentional deficit of hyperactive children. In G. A. Hale & M. Lewis (Eds.), *Attention and the development of cognitive skills* (pp. 173–248). New York: Plenum Press.

Doyle, A. E., Faraone, S. V., DuPre, E. P., & Biederman, J. (2001). Separating attention deficit hyperactivity disorder and learning disabilities in girls: A familial risk analysis. *American Journal of Psychiatry, 158*, 1666–1672.

Draeger, S., Prior, M., & Sanson, A. (1986). Visual and auditory attention performance in hyperactive children: Competence or compliance. *Journal of Abnormal Child Psychology, 14*, 411–424.

DuPaul, G. J. (1991). Parent and teacher ratings of ADHD symptoms: Psychometric properties in a community-based sample. *Journal of Clinical Child Psychology, 20*, 245–253.

DuPaul, G. J., & Barkley, R. A. (1992). Situational variability of attention problems: Psychometric properties of the Revised Home and School Situations Questionnaires. *Journal of Clinical Child Psychology, 21*, 178–188.

DuPaul, G. J., Barkley, R. A., & Connor, D. F. (1998). Stimulants. In R. A. Barkley, *Attention deficit hyperactivity disorder: A handbook for diagnosis and treatment* (2nd ed., pp. 510–551). New York: Guilford.

DuPaul, G. J., McGoey, K. E., Eckert, T. L., & VanBrakle, J. (2001). Preschool children with attention-deficit/hyperactivity disorder: impairments in behavioral, social, and school functioning. *Journal of the American Academy of Child and Adolescent Psychiatry, 40*, 508–515.

DuPaul, G. J., Power, T. J., Anastopoulos, A. D., & Reid, R. (1998). *ADHD Rating Scale-IV: Checklists, norms, and clinical interpretation*. New York: Guilford Press.

Ebaugh, F. G. (1923). Neuropsychiatric sequelae of acute epidemic encephalitis in children. *American Journal of Diseases of Children, 25*, 89–97.

Edelbrock, C. S., Costello, A., & Kessler, M. D. (1984). Empirical corroboration of attention deficit disorder. *Journal of the American Academy of Child and Adolescent Psychiatry, 23*, 285–290.

Edwards, F., Barkley, R., Laneri, M., Fletcher, K., & Metevia, L. (2001). Parent–adolescent conflict in teenagers with ADHD and ODD. *Journal of Abnormal Child Psychology, 29*, 557–572.

Elia, J., Gullotta, C., Rose, J. R., Marin, G., & Rapoport, J. L. (1994). Thyroid function in attention deficit hyperactivity disorder. *Journal of the American Academy of Child and Adolescent Psychiatry, 33*, 169–172.

Erhardt, D., & Hinshaw, S. P. (1994). Initial sociometric impressions of attention-deficit hyperactivity disorder and comparison boys: Predictions from social behaviors and from nonbehavioral variables. *Journal of Consulting and Clinical Psychology, 62*, 833–842.

Ernst, M., Cohen, R. M., Liebenauer, L. L., Jons, P. H. & Zametkin, A. J. (1997). Cerebral glucose metabolism in adolescent girls with attention-deficit/hyperactivity disorder. *Journal of the American Academy of Child and Adolescent Psychiatry, 36*, 1399–1406.

Ernst, M., Liebenauer, L. L., King, A. C., Fitzgerald, G. A., Cohen, R. M., & Zametkin, A. J. (1994). Reduced brain metabolism in hyperactive girls. *Journal of the American Academy of Child and Adolescent Psychiatry, 33*, 858–868.

Ernst, M., Zametkin, A. J., Matochik, J. A., Pascualvaca, D., Jons, P. H., & Cohen, R. M. (1999). High midbrain [^{18}F]DOPA accumulation in children with attention deficit hyperactivity disorder. *American Journal of Psychiatry, 156*, 1209–1215.

Fallone, G., Acebo, C., Arnedt, J. T., Seifer, R., & Carskadon, M. A. (2001). Effects of acute sleep restriction on behavior, sustained attention, and response inhibition in children. *Perceptual and Motor Skills, 93*, 213–229.

Faraone, S. V., & Biederman, J. (1997). Do attention deficit hyperactivity disorder and major depression share familial risk factors? *Journal of Nervous and Mental Disease, 185*, 533–541.

Faraone, S. V., Biederman, J., Chen, W. J., Krifcher, B., Keenan, K., Moore, C., Sprich, S., & Tsuang, M. T. (1992). Segregation analysis of attention deficit hyperactivity disorder. *Psychiatric Genetics, 2*, 257–275.

Faraone, S. V., Biederman, J., Lehman, B., Keenan, K., Norman, D., Seidman, L. J., Kolodny, R., Kraus, I., Perrin, J., & Chen, W. (1993). Evidence for the independent familial transmission of attention deficit hyperactivity disorder and learning disabilities: Results from a family genetic study. *American Journal of Psychiatry, 150*, 891–895.

Faraone, S. V., Biederman, J., Mennin, D., Russell, R., & Tsuang, M. T. (1998). Familial subtypes of attention deficit hyperactivity disorder: A 4–year follow-up study of children from antisocial–ADHD families. *Journal of Child Psychology and Psychiatry, 39*, 1045–1053.

Faraone, S. V., Biederman, J., Mick, E., Williamson, S., Wilens, T., Spencer, T., Weber, W., Jetton, J., Kraus, I., Pert, J., & Zallen, B. (2000). Family study of girls with attention deficit hyperactivity disorder. *American Journal of Psychiatry, 157*, 1077–1083.

Faraone, S. V., Biederman, J., & Monuteaux, M. C. (2001). Attention deficit hyperactivity disorder with bipolar disorder in girls: Further evidence for a familial subtype? *Journal of Affective Disorders, 64*, 19–26.

Faraone, S. V., Biederman, J., Weber, W., & Russell, R. L. (1998). Psychiatric, neuropsychological, and psychosocial features of DSM-IV subtypes of attention-deficit/hyperactivity disorder: Results from a clinically referred sample. *Journal of the American Academy of Child and Adolescent Psychiatry, 37*, 185–193.

Faraone, S. V., Biederman, J., Weiffenbach, B., Keith, T., Chu, M. P., Weaver, A., Spencer, T. J., Wilens, T. E., Frazier, J., Cleves, M., & Sakai, J. (1999). Dopamine D4 gene 7-repeat allele and attention deficit hyperactivity disorder. *American Journal of Psychiatry, 156*, 768–770.

Faraone, S. V., Biederman, J., Wozniak, J., Mundy, E., Mennin, D., & O'Donnell, D. (1997). Is comorbidity with ADHD a marker for juvenile-onset mania? *Journal of the American Academy of Child and Adolescent Psychiatry, 36*, 1046–1055.

Fergusson, D. M., Fergusson, I. E., Horwood, L. J., & Kinzett, N. G. (1988). A longitudinal study of dentine lead levels, intelligence, school performance, and behaviour. *Journal of Child Psychology and Psychiatry, 29*, 811–824.

Filipek, P. A., Semrud-Clikeman, M., Steingard, R. J., Renshaw, P. F., Kennedy, D. N., & Biederman, J. (1997). Volumetric MRI analysis comparing subjects having attention-deficit hyperactivity disorder with normal controls. *Neurology, 48*, 589–601.

Fischer, M. (1990). Parenting stress and the child with attention deficit hyperactivity disorder. *Journal of Clinical Child Psychology, 19*, 337–346.

Fischer, M., Barkley, R. A., Edelbrock, C. S., & Smallish, L. (1990). The adolescent outcome of hyperactive children diagnosed by research criteria: II. Academic, attentional, and neuropsychological status. *Journal of Consulting and Clinical Psychology, 58*, 580–588.

Fischer, M., Barkley, R. A., Fletcher, K. & Smallish, L. (1993a). The stability of dimensions of behavior in ADHD and normal children over an 8 year period. *Journal of Abnormal Child Psychology, 21*, 315–337.

Fischer, M., Barkley, R. A., Fletcher, K., & Smallish, L. (1993b). The adolescent outcome of hyperactive children diagnosed by research criteria: V. Predictors of outcome. *Journal of the American Academy of Child and Adolescent Psychiatry, 32*, 324–332.

Fischer, M., Barkley, R. A., Smallish, L., & Fletcher, K. R. (in press-a). Hyperactive children as young adults: Deficits in attention, inhibition, and response perseveration and their relationship to severity of childhood and current ADHD and conduct disorder. *Journal of Abnormal Psychology*.

Fischer, M., Barkley, R. A., Smallish, L., & Fletcher, K. R. (in press-b). Young adult outcome of hyperactive children as a function of severity of childhood conduct problems: Comorbid psychiatric disorders and interim mental health treatment. *Journal of Abnormal Child Psychology*.

Flavell, J. H. (1970). Developmental studies of mediated memory. In H. W. Reese & L. P. Lipsett (Eds.), *Advances in child development and behavior* (pp. 181–211). New York: Academic Press.

Fletcher, K., Fischer, M., Barkley, R. A., & Smallish, L. (1996). A sequential analysis of the mother–adolescent interactions of ADHD, ADHD/ODD, and normal teenagers during neutral and conflict discussions. *Journal of Abnormal Child Psychology, 24*, 271–298.

Frank, Y., & Ben-Nun, Y. (1988). Toward a clinical subgrouping of hyperactive and nonhyperactive attention deficit disorder; Results of a comprehensive neurological and neuropsychological assessment. *American Journal of Diseases of Children, 142*, 153–155.

Frank, Y., Lazar, J. W., & Seiden, J. A. (1992). Cognitive event-related potentials in learning-disabled children with or without attention-deficit hyperactivity disorder [abstract]. *Annals of Neurology, 32*, 478.

Frick, P. J., Kamphaus, R. W., Lahey, B. B., Loeber, R., Christ, M. A. G., Hart, E. L., & Tannenbaum, L. E. (1991). Academic underachievement and the disruptive behavior disorders. *Journal of Consulting and Clinical Psychology, 59*, 289–294.

Fuster, J. M. (1997). *The prefrontal cortex* (3rd ed.). New York: Raven Press.

Gadow, K. D., Nolan, E. E., Litcher, L., Carlson, G. A., Panina, N., Golovakha, E., Sprafkin, J., & Bromet, E. J. (2000). Comparison of attention-deficit/hyperactivity disorder symptom subtypes in Ukrainian schoolchildren. *Journal of the American Academy of Child and Adolescent Psychiatry, 39*, 1520–1527.

Garcia-Sanchez, C., Estevez-Gonzalez, A., Suarez-Romero, E., & Junque, C. (1997). Right hemisphere dysfunction in subjecst with attention-deficit disorder with and without hyperactivity. *Journal of Child Neurology, 12*, 107–115.

Gaub, M., & Carlson, C. L. (1997). Gender differences in ADHD: A meta-analysis and critical review. *Journal of the American Academy of Child and Adolescent Psychiatry, 36*, 1036–1045.

Gelernter, J. O., O'Malley, S., Risch, N., Kranzler, H. R., Krystal, J., Merikangas, K., Kennedy, J. L., et al. (1991). No association between an allele at the D_2 dopamine receptor gene (DRD_2) and alcoholism. *Journal of the American Medical Association, 266*, 1801–1807.

Geller, B., & Luby, J. (1997). Child and adolescent bipolar disorder: A review of the past 10 years. *Journal of the American Academy of Child and Adolescent Psychiatry, 36*, 1168–1176.

Gershon, J. (2002). A meta-analytic review of gender differences in ADHD. *Journal of Attention Disorders, 5*(3), 143–154.

Giedd, J. N., Castellanos, F. X., Casey, B. J., Kozuch, P., King, A. C., Hamburger, S. D., & Rapoport, J. L. (1994). Quantitative morphology of the corpus callosum in attention deficit hyperactivity disorder. *American Journal of Psychiatry, 151*, 665–669.

Giedd, J. N., Snell, J. W., Lange, N., Rajapakse, J. C., Casey, B. J., Kozuch, P. L., Vaituzis, A. C., Vauss, Y. C., Hamburger, S. D., Kaysen, D., & Rapoport, J. L. (1996). Quantitative magnetic resonance imaging of human brain development: Ages 4–18. *Cerebral Cortex, 6*, 551–560.

Gilger, J. W., Pennington, B. F., & DeFries, J. C. (1992). A twin study of the etiology of comorbidity: Attention-deficit hyperactivity disorder and dyslexia. *Journal of the American Academy of Child and Adolescent Psychiatry, 31*, 343–348.

Gill, M., Daly, G., Heron, S., Hawi, Z., & Fitzgerald, M. (1997). Confirmation of association between attention deficit hyperactivity disorder and a dopamine transporter polymorphism. *Molecular Psychiatry, 2*, 311–313.

Gittelman, R., & Eskinazi, B. (1983). Lead and hyperactivity revisited. *Archives of General Psychiatry, 40*, 827–833.

Gittelman, R., Mannuzza, S., Shenker, R., & Bonagura, N. (1985). Hyperactive boys almost grown up: I. Psychiatric status. *Archives of General Psychiatry, 42*, 937–947.

Gjone, H., Stevenson, J., & Sundet, J. M. (1996). Genetic influence on parent-reported attention-related problems in a Norwegian general population twin sample. *Journal of the American Academy of Child and Adolescent Psychiatry, 35*, 588–596.

Gjone, H., Stevenson, J., Sundet, J. M., & Eilertsen, D. E. (1996). Changes in heritability across increasing levels of behavior problems in young twins. *Behavior Genetics, 26*, 419–426.

Glow, P. H., & Glow, R. A. (1979). Hyperkinetic impulse disorder: A developmental defect of motivation. *Genetic Psychological Monographs, 100*, 159–231.

Goldman-Rakic, P. S. (1987). Development of cortical circuitry and cognitive function. *Child Development, 58*, 601–622.

Gomez, R., & Sanson, A. V. (1994). Mother–child interactions and noncompliance in hyperactive boys with and without conduct problems. *Journal of Child Psychology and Psychiatry, 35*, 477–490.

Goodman, J. R., & Stevenson, J. (1989). A twin study of hyperactivity: II. The aetiological role of genes, family relationships, and perinatal adversity. *Journal of Child Psychology and Psychiatry, 30*, 691–709.

Goyette, C. H., Conners, C. K., & Ulrich, R. F. (1978). Normative data on revised Conners Parent and Teacher Rating Scales. *Journal of Abnormal Child Psychology, 6*, 221–236.

Grattan, L. M., & Eslinger, P. J. (1991). Frontal lobe damage in children and adults: A comparative review. *Developmental Neuropsychology, 7*, 283–326.

Gray, J. A. (1982). *The neuropsychology of anxiety*. New York: Oxford University Press.

Green, L., Fry, A. F., & Meyerson, J. (1994). Discounting of delayed rewards: A life-span comparison. *Psychological Science, 5*, 33–36.

Grenell, M. M., Glass, C. R., & Katz, K. S. (1987). Hyperactive children and peer interaction: Knowledge and performance of social skills. *Journal of Abnormal Child Psychology, 15*, 1–13.

Gresham, F. M., MacMillan, D. L., Bocian, K. M., Ward, S. L., & Forness, S. R. (1998). Comorbidity of hyperactivity–impulsivity–inattention and conduct problems: Risk factors in social, affective, and academic domains. *Journal of Abnormal Child Psychology, 26*, 393–406.

Grodzinsky, G. M., & Diamond, R. (1992). Frontal lobe functioning in boys with attention-deficit hyperactivity disorder. *Developmental Neuropsychology, 8*, 427–445.

Gross-Tsur, V., Shalev, R. S., & Amir, N. (1991). Attention deficit disorder: Association with familial–genetic factors. *Pediatric Neurology, 7*, 258–261.

Gruber, R., Sadeh, A., & Raviv, A. (2000). Instability of sleep patterns in children with attention-deficit/hyperactivity disorder. *Journal of the American Academy of Child and Adolescent Psychiatry, 39*, 495–501.

Gustafsson, P., Thernlund, G., Ryding, E., Rosen, I., & Cederblad, M. (2000). Associations between cerebral blood-flow measured by single photon emission computed tomorgraphy (SPECT), electro-encephalogram (EEG), behavior symptoms, cognition and neurological soft signs in children with attention-deficit hyperactivity disorder (ADHD). *Acta Paediatrica, 89*, 830–835.

Haenlein, M., & Caul, W. F. (1987). Attention deficit disorder with hyperactivity: A specific hypothesis of reward dysfunction. *Journal of the American Academy of Child and Adolescent Psychiatry, 26*, 356–362.

Halperin, J. M., & Gittelman, R. (1982). Do hyperactive children and their siblings differ in IQ and academic achievement? *Psychiatry Research, 6*, 253–258.

Halperin, J. M., Matier, K., Bedi, G., Sharma, V., & Newcorn, J. H. (1992). Specificity of inattention, impulsivity, and hyperactivity to the diagnosis of attention-deficit hyperactivity disorder. *Journal of the American Academy of Child and Adolescent Psychiatry, 31*, 190–196.

Halperin, J. M., Newcorn, J. H., Koda, V. H., Pick, L., McKay, K. E., & Knott, P. (1997). Noradrenergic mechaisms in ADHD children with and without reading disabilities: A replication and extension. *Journal of the American Academy of Child and Adolescent Psychiatry, 36*, 1688–1697.

Hamlett, K. W., Pellegrini, D. S., & Conners, C. K. (1987). An investigation of executive processes in the problem solving of attention deficit disorder-hyperactive children. *Journal of Pediatric Psychology, 12*, 227–240.

Hart, E. L., Lahey, B. B., Loeber, R., Applegate, B., & Frick, P. J. (1995). Developmental changes in attention-deficit hyperactivity disorder in boys: A four-year longitudinal study. *Journal of Abnormal Child Psychology, 23*, 729–750.

Hartsough, C. S., & Lambert, N. M. (1985). Medical factors in hyperactive and normal children: Prenatal, developmental, and health history findings. *American Journal of Orthopsychiatry, 55*, 190–210.

Harvey, W. J., & Reid, G. (1997). Motor performance of children with attention-deficit hyperactivity disorder: A preliminary investigation. *Adapted Physical Activity Quarterly, 14*, 189–202.

Hastings, J., & Barkley, R. A. (1978). A review of psychophysiological research with hyperactive children. *Journal of Abnormal Child Psychology, 7*, 413–337.

Hauser, P., Zametkin, A. J., Martinez, P., Vitiello, B., Matochik, J., Mixson, A., & Weintraub, B. (1993). Attention deficit hyperactivity disorder in people with generalized resistance to thyroid hormone. *New England Journal of Medicine, 328*, 997–1001.

Heffron, W. A., Martin, C. A., & Welsh, R. J. (1984). Attention deficit disorder in three pairs of monozygotic twins: A case report. *Journal of the American Academy of Child Psychiatry, 23*, 299–301.

Heilman, K. M., Voeller, K. K. S., & Nadeau, S. E. (1991). A possible pathophysiological substrate of attention deficit hyperactivity disorder. *Journal of Child Neurology, 6*, 74–79.

Hendren, R. L., De Backer, I., & Pandina, G. J. (2000). Review of neuroimaging studies of child and adolescent psychiatric disorders from the past 10 years. *Journal of the American Academy of Child and Adolescnt Psychiatry, 39*, 815–828.

Henry, B., Moffitt, T. E., Caspi A., Langley, J., & Silva, P. A. (1994). On the "remembrance of things past": A longitudinal evaluation of the retrospective method. *Psychological Assessment, 6*, 92–101.

Herpertz, S. C., Wenning, B., Mueller, B., Qunaibi, M., Sass, H., & Herpetz-Dahlmann, B. (2001). Psychological responses in ADHD boys with and without conduct disorder: Implications for adult antisocial behavior. *Journal of the American Academy of Child and Adolescent Psychiatry, 40*, 1222–1230.

Hinshaw, S. P. (1992). Externalizing behavior problems and academic underachievement in childhood and adolescence: Causal relationships and underlying mechanisms. *Psychological Bulletin, 111*, 127–155.

Hinshaw, S. P. (1994). *Attention deficits and hyperactivity in children*. Thousand Oaks, CA: Sage.

Hinshaw, S. P. (2001). Is the inattentive type of ADHD a separate disorder? *Clinical Psychology: Science and Practice, 8*, 498–501.

Hinshaw, S. P., Buhrmeister, D., & Heller, T. (1989). Anger control in response to verbal provocation: Effects of stimulant medication for boys with ADHD. *Journal of Abnormal Child Psychology, 17*, 393–408.

Hinshaw, S. P., Herbsman, C., Melnick, S., Nigg, J., & Simmel, C. (1993, February). *Psychological and familial processes in ADHD: Continuous or discontinuous with those in normal comparison children?* Paper presented at the Society for Research in Child and Adolescent Psychopathology, Santa Fe, NM.

Hinshaw, S. P., & Melnick, S. M. (1995). Peer relationships in boys with attention-deficit hyperactivity disorder with and without comorbid aggression. *Development and Psychopathology, 7*, 627–647.

Hinshaw, S. P., Morrison, D. C., Carte, E. T., & Cornsweet, C. (1987). Factorial dimensions of the Revised Behavior Problem Checklist: Replication and validation within a kindergarten sample. *Journal of Abnormal Child Psychology, 15*, 309–327.

Hodgens, J. B., Cole, J., & Boldizar, J. (2000). Peer-based differences among boys with ADHD. *Journal of Clinical Child Psychology, 29*, 443–452.

Hohman, L. B. (1922). Post-encephalitic behavior disorders in children. *Johns Hopkins Hospital Bulletin, 33*, 372–375.

Holdsworth, L., & Whitmore, K. (1974). A study of children with epilepsy attending ordinary schools: I. Their seizure patterns, progress, and behaviour in school. *Developmental Medicine and Child Neurology, 16*, 746–758.

Hoy, E., Weiss, G., Minde, K., & Cohen, N. (1978). The hyperactive child at adolescence: Cognitive, emotional, and social functioning. *Journal of Abnormal Child Psychology, 6*, 311–324.

Hoza, B., Pelham, W. E., Waschbusch, D. A., Kipp, H., & Owens, J. S. (2001). Academic task performance of normally achieving ADHD and control boys: Performance, self-evaluations, and attributions. *Journal of Consulting and Clinical Psychology, 69*, 271–283.

Humphries, T., Kinsbourne, M., & Swanson, J. (1978). Stimulant effects on cooperation and social interaction between hyperactive children and their mothers. *Journal of Child Psychology and Psychiatry, 19*, 13–22.

Humphries, T., Koltun, H., Malone, M., & Roberts, W. (1994). Teacher-identified oral language difficulties among boys with attention problems. *Developmental and Behavioral Pediatrics, 15*, 92–98.

Hynd, G. W., Hern, K. L., Novey, E. S., Eliopulos, D., Marshall, R., Gonzalez, J. J., & Voeller, K. K. (1993). Attention-deficit hyperactivity disorder and asymmetry of the caudate nucleus. *Journal of Child Neurology, 8*, 339–347.

Hynd, G. W., Lorys, A. R., Semrud-Clikeman, M., Nieves, N., Huettner, M. I. S., & Lahey, B. B. (1991). Attention deficit disorder without hyperactivity: A distinct behavioral and neurocognitive syndrome. *Journal of Child Neurology, 6*, S37–S43.

Hynd, G. W., Semrud-Clikeman, M., Lorys, A. R., Novey, E. S., & Eliopulos, D. (1990). Brain morphology in developmental dyslexia and attention deficit disorder/hyperactivity. *Archives of Neurology, 47*, 919–926.

Hynd, G. W., Semrud-Clikeman, M., Lorys, A. R., Novey, E. S., Eliopulos, D., & Lyytinen, H. (1991). Corpus callosum morphology in attention deficit-hyperactivity disorder: Morphometric analysis of MRI. *Journal of Learning Disabilities, 24*, 141–146.

Jacobvitz, D., & Sroufe, L. A. (1987). The early caregiver–child relationship and attention-deficit disorder with hyperactivity in kindergarten: A prospective study. *Child Development, 58*, 1488–1495.

James, W. (1950). *The principles of psychology*. New York: Dover. (Original work published 1890)

Jensen, P. S., Martin, D., & Cantwell, D. P. (1997). Comorbidity in ADHD: Implications for research, practice, and DSM-V. *Journal of the American Academy of Child and Adolescent Psychiatry, 36*, 1065–1079.

Jensen, P. S., Shervette, R. E., Xenakis, S. N., & Bain, M. W. (1988). Psychosocial and medical histories of stimulant-treated children. *Journal of the American Academy of Child and Adolescent Psychiatry, 27*, 798–801.

Jensen, P. S., Shervette, R. E. III, Xenakis, S. N., & Richters, J. (1993). Anxiety and depressive disorders in attention deficit disorder with hyperactivity: New findings. *American Journal of Psychiatry, 150*, 1203–1209.

Jensen, P. S., Watanabe, H. K., Richters, J. E., Cortes, R., Roper, M., & Liu, S. (1995). Prevalence of mental disorder in military children and adolescents: Findings from a two-stage community survey. *Journal of the American Academy of Child and Adolescent Psychiatry, 34*, 1514–1524.

Johnson, B. D., Altmaier, E. M., & Richman, L. C. (1999). Attention deficits and reading disabilities: Are immediate memory defects additive? *Developmental Neuropsychology, 15*, 213–226.

Johnson, J. G., Cohen, P., Kasen, S., Smailes, E., & Brook, J. S. (2001). Association of maladaptive parental behavior with psychiatric disorder among parents and their offspring. *Archives of General Psychiatry, 58*, 453–460.

Johnson, R. C., & Rosen, L. A. (2000). Sports behavior of ADHD children. *Journal of Attention Disorders, 4*, 150–160.

Johnston, C. (1996). Parent characteristics and parent–child interactions in families of nonproblem children and ADHD children with higher and lower levels of oppositional-defiant disorder. *Journal of Abnormal Child Psychology, 24*, 85–104.

Johnston, C., & Mash, E. J. (2001). Families of children with attention-deficit/hyperactivity disorder: Review and recommendations for future research. *Clinical Child and Family Psychology Review, 4*, 183–207.

Johnstone, S. J., Barry, R. J., & Anderson, J. W. (2001). Topographic distribution and developmental timecourse of auditory event-related potentials in two subtypes of attention-deficit hyperactivity disorder. *International Journal of Psychophysiology, 42*, 73–94.

Kadesjo, B., & Gillberg, C. (2001). The comorbidity of ADHD in the general population of Swedish school-age children. *Journal of Child Psychology and Psychiatry, 42*, 487–492.

Kanbayashi, Y., Nakata, Y., Fujii, K., Kita, M., & Wada, K. (1994). ADHD-related behavior among non-referred children: Parents' ratings of DSM-III-R symptoms. *Child Psychiatry and Human Development*, *25*, 13–29.

Kanfer, F. H., & Karoly, P. (1972). Self-control: A behavioristic excursion into the lion's den. *Behavior Therapy*, *3*, 398–416.

Kaplan, B. J., McNichol, J., Conte, R. A., & Moghadam, H. K. (1987). Sleep disturbance in preschool-aged hyperactive and nonhyperactive children. *Pediatrics*, *80*, 839–844.

Keenan, K. (2000). Emotion dysregulation as a risk factor for child psychopathology. *Clinical Psychology: Science and Practice*, *7*, 418–434.

Kelsoe, J. R., Ginns, E. I., Egeland, J. A., Gerhard, D. S., Goldstein, A. M., Bale, S. J., Pauls, D. L., et al. (1989). Re-evaluation of the linkage relationship between chromosome 11p loci and the gene for bipolar affective disorder in the Old Order Amish. *Nature*, *342*, 238–243.

Kessler, J. W. (1980). History of minimal brain dysfunction. In H. Rie & E. Rie (Eds.), *Handbook of minimal brain dysfunctions: A critical view* (pp. 18–52). New York: Wiley.

Klorman, R. (1992). Cognitive event-related potentials in attention deficit disorder. In S. E. Shaywitz & B. A. Shaywitz (Eds.), *Attention deficit disorder comes of age: Toward the twenty-first century* (pp. 221–244). Austin, TX: Pro-Ed.

Klorman, R., Salzman, L. F., & Borgstedt, A. D. (1988). Brain event-related potentials in evaluation of cognitive deficits in attention deficit disorder and outcome of stimulant therapy. In L. Bloomingdale (Ed.), *Attention deficit disorder* (Vol. 3, pp. 49–80). New York: Pergamon Press.

Klorman, R., Hazel-Fernandez, H., Shaywitz, S. E., Fletcher, J. M., Marchione, K. E., Holahan, J. M., Stuebing, K. K., & Shaywitz, B. A. (1999). Executive functioning deficits in attention-deficit/hyperactivity disorder are independent of oppositional defiant or reading disorder. *Journal of the American Academy of Child and Adolescent Psychiatry*, *38*, 1148–1155.

Knobel, M., Wolman, M. B., & Mason, E. (1959). Hyperkinesis and organicity in children. *Archives of General Psychiatry*, *1*, 310–321.

Kohn, A. (1989, November). Suffer the restless children. *The Atlantic Monthly*, pp. 90–100.

Kopp, C. B. (1982). Antecedents of self-regulation: A developmental perspective. *Developmental Psychology*, *18*, 199–214.

Krause, K., Dresel, S. H., Krause, J., Kung, H. F., & Tatsch, K. (2000). Increased striatal dopamine transporter in adult patients with attention deficit hyperactivity disorder: Effects of methylphenidate as masured by single photon emission computed tomography. *Neuroscience Letters*, *285*, 107–110.

Kroes, M., Kalff, A. C., Kessels, A. G. H., Steyaert, J., Feron, F., van Someren, A., Hurks, P., Hendriksen, J., van Zeban, T., Rozendaal, N., Crolla, I., Troost, J., Jolles, J., & Vles, J. (2001). Child psychiatric diagnoses in a population of Dutch schoolchildren aged 6 to 8 years. *Journal of the American Academy of Child and Adolescent Psychiatry*, *40*, 1401–1409.

Kuntsi, J., Oosterlaan, J., & Stevenson, J. (2001). Psychological mechanisms in hyperactivity: I. Response inhibition deficit, working memory impairment, delay aversion, or something else? *Journal of Child Psychology and Psychiatry*, *42*, 199–210.

Kuperman, S., Johnson, B., Arndt, S., Lindgren, S., & Wolraich, M. (1996). Quantitative EEG differences in a nonclinical sample of children with ADHD and undifferentiated ADD. *Journal of the American Academy of Child and Adolescent Psychiatry*, *35*, 1009–1017.

Lahey, B. B. (2001). Should the combined and predominantly inattentive types of ADHD be considered distinct and unrelated disorders?: Not now, at least. *Clinical Psychology: Science and Practice*, *8*, 494–497.

Lahey, B. B., Applegate, B., McBurnett, K., Biederman, J., Greenhill, L., Hynd, G. W., et al. (1994). DSM-IV field trials for attention deficit/hyperactivity disorder in children and adolescents. *American Journal of Psychiatry*, *151*, 1673–1685.

Lahey, B. B., & Carlson, C. L. (1992). Validity of the diagnostic category of attention deficit disorder without hyperactivity: A review of the literature. In S. E. Shaywitz & B. A. Shaywitz (Eds.), *Attention deficit disorder comes of age: Toward the twenty-first century* (pp. 119–144). Austin, TX: Pro-Ed.

Lahey, B. B., McBurnett, K., & Loeber, R. (2000). Are attention-deficit/hyperactivity disorder and oppositional defiant disorder developmental precursors to conduct disorder? In A. J. Sameroff, M. Lewis, & S. M. Miller (Eds.), *Handbook of developmental psychopathology* (2nd ed., pp. 431–446.). New York: Kluwer Academic Plenum.

Lahey, B. B., Pelham, W. E., Schaughency, E. A., Atkins, M. S., Murphy, H. A., Hynd, G. W., Russo, M., Hartdagen, S., & Lorys-Vernon, A. (1988). Dimensions and types of attention deficit disorder with hyperactivity in children: A factor and cluster-analytic approach. *Journal of the American Academy of Child and Adolescent Psychiatry*, *27*, 330–335.

Lahey, B. B., Schaughency, E., Hynd, G., Carlson, C., & Nieves, N. (1987). Attention deficit disorder with and without hyperactivity: Comparison of behavioral characteristics of clinic-referred children. *Journal of the American Academy of Child Psychiatry*, *26*, 718–723.

Lahey, B. B., Schaughency, E., Strauss, C., & Frame, C. (1984). Are attention deficit disorders with and without hyperactivity similar or dissimilar disorders? *Journal of the American Academy of Child Psychiatry*, *23*, 302–309.

Lahoste, G. J., Swanson, J. M., Wigal, S. B., Glabe, C., Wigal, T., King, N., & Kennedy, J. L. (1996). Dopamine D4 receptor gene polymorphism is associated with attention deficit hyperactivity disorder. *Molecular Psychiatry*, *1*, 121–124.

Lambert, N. M. (1988). Adolescent outcomes for hyperactive children. *American Psychologist*, *43*, 786–799.

Lambert, N. M. (in press) Stimulant treatment as a risk factor for nicotine use and substance abuse. In P. S. Jensen & J. R. Cooper (Eds.), *Diagnosis and treatment of attention deficit hyperactivity disorder: An evidence-based approach*. New York: American Medical Association Press.

Lambert, N. M., & Hartsough, C. S. (1998). Prospective study of tobacco smoking and substance dependencies among samples of ADHD and non-ADHD participants. *Journal of Learning Disabilities*, *31*, 533–544

Lambert, N. M., & Sandoval, J. (1980). The prevalence of learning disabilities in a sample of children considered hyperactive. *Journal of Abnormal Child Psychology*, *8*, 33–50.

Lambert, N. M., Sandoval, J., & Sassone, D. (1978). Prevalence of hyperactivity in elementary school children as a function of social system definers. *American Journal of Orthopsychiatry*, *48*, 446–463.

Lamminmaki, T., Ahonen, T., Narhi, V., Lyytinent, H., & Todd de Barra, H. (1995). Attention deficit hyperactivity disorder subtypes: Are there differences in academic problems? *Developmental Neuropsychology, 11,* 297–310.

Landau, S., Berk, L. E., & Mangione, C. (1996, March). *Private speech as a problem-solving strategy in the face of academic challenge: The failure of impulsive children to get their act together.* Paper presented at the meeting of the National Association of School Psychologists, Atlanta, GA.

Lang, P. (1995). The emotion probe. *American Psychologist, 50,* 372–385.

Langsdorf, R., Anderson, R. F., Walchter, D., Madrigal, J. F., & Juarez, L. J. (1979). Ethnicity, social class, and perception of hyperactivity. *Psychology in the Schools, 16,* 293–298.

Lapouse, R., & Monk, M. (1958). An epidemiological study of behavior characteristics in children. *American Journal of Public Health, 48,* 1134–1144.

Last, C. G., Hersen, M., Kazdin, A., Orvaschel, H., & Perrin, S. (1991). Anxiety disorders in children and their families. *Archives of General Psychiatry, 48,* 928–934.

Laufer, M., Denhoff, E., & Solomons, G. (1957). Hyperkinetic impulse disorder in children's behavior problems. *Psychosomatic Medicine, 19,* 38–49.

Lavigne, J. V., Gibbons, R. D., Christoffel, . K., Arend, R., Rosenbaum, D., Binns, H., Dawson, N., Sobel, H., & Isaacs, C. (1996). Prevalence ratse and correlates of psychiatric disorders among preschool children. *Journal of the American Academy of Child and Adolescent Psychiatry, 35,* 204–214.

Lecendreux, M., Konofal, E., Bouvard, M., Falissard, B., & Mouren-Simeoni, M. (2000). Sleep and alertness in children with ADHD. *Journal of Child Psychology and Psychiatry, 41,* 803–812.

Lerner, J. A., Inui, T. S., Trupin, E. W., & Douglas, E. (1985). Preschool behavior can predict future psychiatric disorders. *Journal of the American Academy of Child Psychiatry, 24,* 42–48.

Levin, P. M. (1938). Restlessness in children. *Archives of Neurology and Psychiatry, 39,* 764–770.

Levy, F., & Hay, D. A. (2001). *Attention, genes, and ADHD.* Philadelphia: Brunner-Routledge.

Levy, F., Hay, D. A., McStephen, M., Wood, C., & Waldman, I. (1997). Attention-deficit hyperactivity disorder: A category or a continuum? Genetic analysis of a large-scale twin study. *Journal of the American Academy of Child and Adolescent Psychiatry, 36,* 737–744.

Levy, F., & Hobbes, G. (1989). Reading, spelling, and vigilance in attention deficit and conduct disorder. *Journal of Abnormal Child Psychology, 17,* 291–298.

Lewinsohn, P. M., Hops, H., Roberts, R. E., Seeley, J. R., & Andrews, J. A. (1993). Adolescent psychopathology: I. Prevalence and incidence of depression and other DSM-III-R disorders in high school students. *Journal of Abnormal Psychology, 102,* 133–144.

Lewinsohn, P. M., Klein, D. N., & Seeley, J. R. (1995). Bipolar disorders in a community sample of older adolescents: Prevalence, phenomenology, comorbidity, and course. *Journal of the American Academy of Child and Adolescent Psychiatry, 34,* 454–463.

Liu, X., Kurita, H., Guo, C., Tachimori, H., Ze, J., & Okawa, M. (2000). Behavioral and emotional problems in Chinese children: Teacher reports for ages 6 to 11. *Journal of Child Psychology and Psychiatry, 41,* 253–260.

Loeber, R. (1990). Development and risk factors of juvenile antisocial behavior and delinquency. *Clinical Psychology Review, 10,* 1–42.

Loeber, R., Burke, J. D., Lahey, B. B., Winters, A., & Zera, M. (2000). Oppositional defiant and conduct disorder: A review of the past 10 years, Part I. *Journal of the American Academy of Child and Adolescent Psychiatry, 39,* 1468–1484.

Loeber, R., Green, S. M., Lahey, B. B., Christ, M. A. G., & Frick, P. J. (1992). Developmental sequences in the age of onset of disruptive child behaviors. *Journal of Child and Family Studies, 1,* 21–41.

Loney, J., Kramer, J., & Milich, R. (1981). The hyperkinetic child grows up: Predictors of symptoms, delinquency, and achievement at follow-up. In K. Gadow & J. Loney (Eds.), *Psychosocial aspects of drug treatment for hyperactivity.* (pp. 381–415). Boulder, CO: Westview Press.

Loney, J., Kramer, J. R., & Salisbury, H. (in press). Medicated versus unmedicated ADHD children: Adult involvement with legal and illegal drugs. In P. S. Jensen & J. R. Cooper (Eds.), *Diagnosis and treatment of attention deficit hyperactivity disorder: An evidence-based approach.* New York: American Medical Association Press.

Lopez, R. (1965). Hyperactivity in twins. *Canadian Psychiatric Association Journal, 10,* 421.

Lorch, E. P., Milich, M., Sanchez, R. P., van den Broek, P., Baer, S., Hooks, K., Hartung, C., & Welsh, R. (2000). Comprehension of televised stories in boys with attention deficit/hyperactivity disorder and nonreferred boys. *Journal of Abnormal Psychology, 109,* 321–330.

Losier, B. J., McGrath, P. J., & Klein, R. M. (1996). Error patterns on the continuous performance test in non-medication and medicated samples of children with and without ADHD: A meta-analysis. *Journal of Child Psychology and Psychiatry, 37,* 971–987.

Lou, H. C., Henriksen, L., & Bruhn, P. (1984). Focal cerebral hypoperfusion in children with dysphasia and/or attention deficit disorder. *Archives of Neurology, 41,* 825–829.

Lou, H. C., Henriksen, L., Bruhn, P., Borner, H., & Nielsen, J. B. (1989). Striatal dysfunction in attention deficit and hyperkinetic disorder. *Archives of Neurology, 46,* 48–52.

Luk, S. (1985). Direct observations studies of hyperactive behaviors. *Journal of the American Academy of Child and Adolescent Psychiatry, 24,* 338–344.

Lynam, D., Moffitt, T., & Stouthamer-Loeber, M. (1993). Explaining the relation between IQ and delinquency: Class, race, test motivation, school failure, or self-control? *Journal of Abnormal Psychology, 102,* 187–196.

Lyon, G. R. (1995). *Attention, memory, and executive functions.* Baltimore: Brookes.

Madan-Swain, A., & Zentall, S. S. (1990). Behavioral comparisons of liked and disliked hyperactive children in play contexts and the behavioral accommodations by teir classmates. *Journal of Consulting and Clinical Psychology, 58,* 197–209.

Maedgen, J. W., & Carlson, C. L. (2000). Social functioning and emotional regulation in the attention deficit hyperactivity disorder subtypes. *Journal of Clinical Child Psychology, 29,* 30–42.

Malone, M. A., & Swanson, J. M. (1993). Effects of methylphenidate on impulsive responding in children with attention deficit hyperactivity disorder. *Journal of Child Neurology, 8,* 157–163.

Mannuzza, S., & Gittelman, R. (1986). Informant variance in the diagnostic assessment of hyperactive children as young adults. In J. E. Barrett & R. M. Rose (Eds.), *Mental disorders in the community* (pp. 243–254). New York: Guilford Press.

Mannuzza, S., & Klein, R. G. (1992). Predictors of outcome of children with attention-deficit hyperactivity disorder. *Child and Adolescent Psychiatric Clinics of North America, 1*(2), 567–578.

Mannuzza, S., Klein, R., G., Bessler, A., Malloy, P., & LaPadula, M. (1993). Adult outcome of hyperactive boys: Educational achievement, occupational rank, and psychiatric status. *Archives of General Psychiatry, 50*, 565–576.

Mannuzza, S., Klein, R., G., Bessler, A., Malloy, P., & LaPadula, M. (1998). Adult psychiatric status of hyperactive boys grown up. *American Journal of Psychiatry, 155*, 493–498.

Mannuzza, S., Klein, R. G., Bonagura, N., Malloy, P., Giampino, H., & Addalli, K. A. (1991). Hyperactive boys almost grown up: Replication of psychiatric status. *Archives of General Psychiatry, 48*, 77–83.

Marcotte, A. C., & Stern, C. (1997). Qualitative analysis of graphomotor output in children with attentional disorders. *Child Neuropsychology, 3*, 147–153.

Mariani, M., & Barkley, R. A. (1997). Neuropsychological and academic functioning in preschool children with attention deficit hyperactivity disorder. *Developmental Neuropsychology, 13*, 111–129.

Marshall, R. M., Hynd, G. W., Handwerk, M. J., et al. (1997). Academic underachievement in ADHD subtypes. *Journal of Learning Disabilities, 30*, 635–642.

Mash, E. J., & Johnston, C. (1982). A comparison of mother–child interactions of younger and older hyperactive and normal children. *Child Development, 53*, 1371–1381.

Mash, E. J., & Johnston, C. (1983a). Sibling interactions of hyperactive and normal children and their relationship to reports of maternal stress and self-esteem. *Journal of Clinical Child Psychology, 12*, 91–99.

Mash, E. J., & Johnston, C. (1983b). The prediction of mothers' behavior with their hyperactive children during play and task situations. *Child and Family Behavior Therapy, 5*, 1–14.

Mash, E. J., & Johnston, C. (1990). Determinants of parenting stress: Illustrations from families of hyperactive children and families of physically abused children. *Journal of Clinical Child Psychology, 19*, 313–328.

Mattes, J. A. (1980). The role of frontal lobe dysfunction in childhood hyperkinesis. *Comprehensive Psychiatry, 21*, 358–369.

Matthys, W., Cuperus, J. M., & van Engeland, H. (1999). Deficient social problem-solving in boys with ODD/CD, with ADHD, and with both disorders. *Journal of the American Academy of Child and Adolescent Psychiatry, 38*, 311–321.

Matthys, W., van Goozen, S. H. M., de Vries, H., Cohen-Kettenis, P. T., & van Engeland, H. (1998). The dominance of behavioural activation over behavioural inhibition in conduct disordered boys with or without attention deficit hyperactivity disorder. *Journal of Child Psychology and Psychiatry, 39*, 643–651.

McArdle, P., O'Brien, G., & Kolvin, I. (1995). Hyperactivity: Prevalence and relationship with conduct disorder. *Journal of Child Psychology and Psychiatry, 36*, 279–303.

McBurnett, K., Pfiffner, L. J., & Frick, P. J. (2001). Symptom properties as a function of ADHD type: An argument for continued study of sluggish cognitive tempo. *Journal of Abnormal Child Psychology, 29*, 207–213.

McGee, R., Feehan, M., Williams, S., Partridge, F., Silva, P. A., & Kelly, J. (1990). DSM-III disorders in a large sample of adolescents. *Journal of the American Academy of Child and Adolescent Psychiatry, 29*, 611–619.

McGee, R., Stanton, W. R., & Sears, M. R. (1993). Allergic disorders and attention deficit disorder in children. *Journal of Abnormal Child Psychology, 21*, 79–88.

McGee, R., Williams, S., & Feehan, M. (1992). Attention deficit disorder and age of onset of problem behaviors. *Journal of Abnormal Child Psychology, 20*, 487–502.

McGee, R., Williams, S., & Silva, P. A. (1984). Behavioral and developmental characteristics of aggressive, hyperactive, and aggressive–hyperactive boys. *Journal of the American Academy of Child Psychiatry, 23*, 270–279.

McMahon, S. A., & Greenberg, L. M. (1977). Serial neurologic examination of hyperactive children. *Pediatrics, 59*, 584–587.

Melnick, S. M., & Hinshaw, S. P. (1996). What they want and what they get: The social goals of boys with ADHD and comparison boys. *Journal of Abnormal Child Psychology, 24*, 169–185.

Melnick, S. M., & Hinshaw, S. P. (2000). Emotion regulation and parenting in AD/HD and comparison boys: Linkages with social behaviors and peer preference. *Journal of Abnormal Child Psychology, 28*, 73–86.

Michon, J. (1985). Introduction. In J. Michon & T. Jackson (Eds.), *Time, mind, and behavior* (pp. 1–11). Berlin: Springer-Verlag.

Mick, E., Biederman, J., & Faraone, S. V. (1996). Is season of birth a risk factor for attention-deficit hyperactivity disorder? *Journal of the American Academy of Child and Adolescent Psychiatry, 35*, 1470–1476.

Milberger, S. (1997, October). *Impact of adversity on functioning and comorbidity in girls with ADHD*. Paper presented at the annual meeting of the American Academy of Child and Adolescent Psychiatry, Toronto.

Milberger, S., Biederman, J., Faraone, S. V., Chen, L., & Jones, J. (1996). Is maternal smoking during pregnancy a risk factor for attention deficit hyperactivity disorder in children? *American Journal of Psychiatry, 153*, 1138–1142.

Milich, R., Hartung, C. M., Matrin, C. A., & Haigler, E. D. (1994). Behavioral disinhibition and underlying processes in adolescents with disruptive behavior disorders. In D. K. Routh (Ed.), *Disruptive behavior disorders in childhood* (pp. 109–138). New York: Plenum Press.

Milich, R., Balentine, A. C., & Lynam, D. R. (2001). ADHD combined type and ADHD predominantly inattentive type are distinct and unrelated disorders. *Clinical Psychology: Science and Practice, 8*, 463–488.

Minde, K., Webb, G., & Sykes, D. (1968). Studies on the hyperactive child: VI. Prenatal and perinatal factors associated with hyperactivity. *Developmental Medicine and Child Neurology, 10*, 355–363.

Mirsky, A. F. (1996). Disorders of attention: A neuropsychological perspective. In R. G. Lyon & N. A. Krasnegor (Eds.), *Attention, memory, and executive function* (pp. 71–96). Baltimore: Brookes.

Mitchell, E. A., Aman, M. G., Turbott, S. H., & Manku, M. (1987). Clinical characteristics and serum essential fatty acid levels in hyperactive children. *Clinical Pediatrics, 26*, 406–411.

Mitsis, E. M., McKay, K. E., Schulz, K. P., Newcorn, J. H., & Halperin, J. M. (2000). Parent–teacher concordance in DSM-IV attention-deficit/hyperactivity disorder in a clinic-referred sample. *Journal of the American Academy of Child and Adolescent Psychiatry, 39*, 308–313.

Moffitt, T. E. (1990). Juvenile delinquency and attention deficit disorder: Boys' developmental trajectories from age 3 to 15. *Child Development, 61*, 893–910.

Molina, B. S. G., & Pelham, W. E. (2001). Substance use, substance abuse, and LD among adolescents with a childhood history of ADHD. *Journal of Learning Disabilities*, *34*, 333–342.

Molina, B. S. G., Smith, B. H., & Pelham, W. E. (1999). Interactive effects of attention deficit hyperactivity disorder and conduct disorder on early adolescent substance use. *Psychology of Addictive Behavior*, *13*, 348–358.

Monastra, V. J., Lubar, J. F., & Linden, M. (2001). The development of a quantitative electroencephalographic scanning process for attention deficit-hyperactivity disorder: Reliability and validity studies. *Neuropsychology*, *15*, 136–144.

Mori, L., & Peterson, L. (1995). Knowledge of safety of high and low active–impulsive boys: Implications for child injury prevention. *Journal of Clinical Child Psychology*, *24*, 370–376.

Morgan, A. E., Hynd, G. W., Riccio, C. A., & Hall, J. (1996). Validity of DSM-IV predominantly inattentive and combined types: relationship to previous DSM diagnoses/subtype differences. *Journal of the American Academy of Child and Adolescent Psychiatry*, *35*, 325–333.

Morrison, J., & Stewart, M. (1973). The psychiatric status of the legal families of adopted hyperactive children. *Archives of General Psychiatry*, *28*, 888–891.

Murphy, K. R., & Barkley, R. A. (1996a). Prevalence of DSM-IV symptoms of ADHD in adult licensed drivers: Implications for clinical diagnosis. *Journal of Attention Disorders*, *1*, 147–161.

Murphy, K. R., & Barkley, R. A. (1996b). Attention deficit hyperactivity disorder in adults: Comorbidities and adaptive impairments. *Comprehensive Psychiatry*, *37*, 393–401.

Murphy, K. R., Barkley, R. A., & Bush, T. (2001). Executive functioning and olfactory identification in young adults with attention deficit hyperactivity disorder. *Neuropsychology*, *15*, 211–220.

Nada-Raja, S., Langley, J. D., McGee, R., Williams, S. M., Begg, D. J., & Reeder, A. I. (1997). Inattentive and hyperactive behaviors and driving offenses in adolescence. *Journal of the American Academy of Child and Adolescent Psychiatry*, *36*, 515–522.

Needleman, H. L., Gunnoe, C., Leviton, A., Reed, R., Peresie, H., Maher, C., & Barrett, P. (1979). Deficits in psychologic and classroom performance of children with elevated dentine lead levels. *New England Journal of Medicine*, *300*, 689–695.

Needleman, H. L., Schell, A., Bellinger, D. C., Leviton, L., & Alfred, E. D. (1990). The long-term effects of exposure to low doses of lead in childhood: An 11-year follow-up report. *New England Journal of Medicine*, *322*, 83–88.

Newcorn, J. H., Halperin, J. M., Jensen, P. S., Abikoff, H. B., Arnold, L. E., Cantwell, D. P., Conners, C. K., Elliott, G. R., Epstein, J. N., Greenhill, L. L., Hechtman, L., Hinshaw, S. P., Hoza, B., Kraemer, H. C., Pelham, W. E., Severe, J. B., Swanson, J. M., Wells, K. C., Wigal, T., & Vitiello, B. (2001). Symptom profiles in children with ADHD: Comorbidity and gender. *Journal of the American Academy of Child and Adolescent Psychiatry*, *40*, 137–146.

Nichols, P. L., & Chen, T. C. (1981). *Minimal brain dysfunction: A prospective study*. Hillsdale, NJ: Erlbaum.

Nigg, J. T. (1999). The ADHD response-inhibition deficit as measured by the stop task: Replication with DSM-IV combined type, extension, and qualification. *Journal of Abnormal Child Psychology*, *27*, 393–402.

Nigg, J. T. (2000). On inhibition/disinhibition in developmental psychopathology: Views from cognitive and personality psychology and a working inhibition taxonomy. *Psychological Bulletin*, *126*, 220–246.

Nigg, J. T. (2001). Is ADHD an inhibitory disorder? *Psychological Bulletin*, *125*, 571–596.

Nigg, J. T., Blaskey, L. G., Huang-Pollock, C. L., & Rappley, M. D. (2002). Neuropsychological executive functions in DSM-IV ADHD subtypes. *Journal of the American Academy of Child and Adolescent Psychiatry*, *41*, 59–66.

Nigg, J. T., Hinshaw, S. P., Carte, E. T., & Treuting, J. J. (1998). Neuropsychological correlates of childhood attention-deficit/hyperactivity disorder: Explainable by comorbid disruptive behavior or reading problems? *Journal of Abnormal Psychology*, *107*, 468–480.

Nolan, E. E., Gadow, K. D., & Sprafkin, J. (2001). Teacher reports of DSM-IV ADHD, ODD, and CD symptoms in schoolchildren. *Journal of the American Academy of Child and Adolescent Psychiatry*, *40*, 241–249.

Nucci, L. P., & Herman, S. (1982). Behavioral disordered children's conceptions of moral, conventional, and personal issues. *Journal of Abnormal Child Psychology*, *10*, 411–426.

O'Connor, M., Foch, T., Sherry, T., & Plomin, R. (1980). A twin study of specific behavioral problems of socialization as viewed by parents. *Journal of Abnormal Child Psychology*, *8*, 189–199.

O'Dougherty, M., Nuechterlein, K. H., & Drew, B. (1984). Hyperactive and hypoxic children: Signal detection, sustained attention, and behavior. *Journal of Abnormal Psychology*, *93*, 178–191.

O'Leary, K. D., Vivian, D., & Nisi, A. (1985). Hyperactivity in Italy. *Journal of Abnormal Child Psychology*, *13*, 485–500.

Olson, S. L., Bates, J. E., Sandy, J. M., & Lanthier, R. (2000). Early developmental precursors of externalizing behavior in middle childhood and adolescence. *Journal of Abnormal Child Psychology*, *28*, 119–133.

Olson, S. L., Schilling, E. M., & Bates, J. E. (1999). Measurement of impulsivity: Construct coherence, longitudinal stability, and relationship with externalizing problems in middle childhood and adolescence. *Journal of Abnormal Child Psychology*, *27*, 151–165.

Oosterlaan, J., Logan, G. D., & Sergeant, J. A. (1998). Response inhibition in AD/HD, CD, comorbid AD/HD + CD, anxious, and control children: A meta-analysis of studies with the stop task. *Journal of Child Psychology and Psychiatry*, *39*, 411–425.

Oosterlaan, J., Scheres, A., & Sergeant, J. A. (in press). Verbal fluency, working memory, and planning in children with ADHD, ODD/CD, and comorbid ADHD + ODD/CD: Specificity of executive functioning deficits. *Journal of Abnormal Psychology*.

Palfrey, J. S., Levine, M. D., Walker, D. K., & Sullivan, M. (1985). The emergence of attention deficits in early childhood: A prospective study. *Journal of Developmental and Behavioral Pediatrics*, *6*, 339–348.

Parry, P. A., & Douglas, V. I. (1983). Effects of reinforcement on concept identification in hyperactive children. *Journal of Abnormal Child Psychology*, *11*, 327–340.

Patterson, G. R., Degarmo, D. S., & Knutson, N. (2000). Hyperactive and antisocial behaviors: Comorbid or two points in the same process. *Development and Psychopathology*, *12*, 91–106.

Pauls, D. L. (1991). Genetic factors in the expression of attention-deficit hyperactivity disorder. *Journal of Child and Adolescent Psychopharmacology*, *1*, 353–360.

Pauls, D. L., Hurst, C. R., Kidd, K. K., Kruger, S. D., Leckman, J. F., & Cohen, D. J. (1986). Tourette syndrome and attention deficit disorder: Evidence against a genetic relationship. *Archives of General Psychiatry, 43*, 1177–1179.

Pelham, W. E., Jr. (2001). Are ADHD/I and ADHD/C the same or different? Does it matter? *Clinical Psychology: Science and Practice, 8*, 502–506.

Pelham, W. E., Gnagy, E. M., Greenslade, K. E., & Milich, R. (1992). Teacher ratings of DSM-III-R symptoms for the disruptive behavior disorders. *Journal of the American Academy of Child and Adolescent Psychiatry, 31*, 210–218.

Pelham, W. E., & Lang, A. R. (1993). Parental alcohol consumption and deviant child behavior: Laboratory studies of reciprocal effects. *Clinical Psychology Review, 13*, 763–784.

Pennington, B. F., & Ozonoff, S. (1996). Executive functions and developmental psychopathology. *Journal of Child Psychology and Psychiatry, 37*, 51–87.

Peterson, B. S., Pine, D. S., Cohen, P., & Brook, J. S. (2001). Prospective, longitudinal study of tic, obsessive–compulsive, and attention-deficit/hyperactivity disorders in an epidemiological sample. *Journal of the American Academy of Child and Adolescent Psychiatry, 40*, 685–695.

Pfiffner, L. J., McBurnett, K., & Rathouz, P. J. (2001). Father absence and familial antisocial characteristics. *Journal of Abnormal Child Psychology, 29*, 357–367.

Pike, A., & Plomin, R. (1996). Importance of nonshared environmental factors for childhood and adolescent psychopathology. *Journal of the American Academy of Child and Adolescent Psychiatry, 35*, 560–570.

Pillow, D. R., Pelham, W. E., Jr., Hoza, B., Molina, B. S. G., & Stultz, C. H. (1998). Confirmatory factor analyses examining attention deficit hyperactivity disorder symptoms and other childhood disruptive behaviors. *Journal of Abnormal Child Psychology, 26*, 293–309.

Pineda, D., Ardila, A., Rosselli, M., Arias, B. E., Henao, G. C., Gomex, L. F., Mejia, S. E., & Miranda, M. L. (1999). Prevalence of attention-deficit/hyperactivity disorder symptoms in 4- to 17-year old children in the general population. *Journal of Abnormal Child Psychology, 27*, 455–462.

Pliszka, S. R. (1992). Comorbidity of attention-deficit hyperactivity disorder and overanxious disorder. *Journal of the American Academy of Child and Adolescent Psychiatry, 31*, 197–203.

Pliszka, S. R., Liotti, M., & Woldorff, M. G. (2000). Inhibitory control in children with attention-deficit/hyperactivity disorder: Event-related potentials identify the processing component and timing of an impaired right-frontal response-inhibition mechanism. *Biological Psychiatry, 48*, 238–246.

Pliszka, S. R., McCracken, J. T., & Maas, J. W. (1996). Catecholamines in attention deficit hyperactivity disorder: Current perspectives. *Journal of the American Academy of Child and Adolescent Psychiatry, 35*, 264–272.

Plomin, R. (1995). Genetics and children's experiences in the family. *Journal of Child Psychology and Psychiatry, 36*, 33–68.

Plomin, R., DeFries, J. C., McClearn, G. E., & Rutter, M. (1997). *Behavioral genetics* (3rd ed.). New York: Freeman.

Porrino, L. J., Rapoport, J. L., Behar, D., Sceery, W., Ismond, D. R., & Bunney, W. E., Jr. (1983). A naturalistic assessment of the motor activity of hyperactive boys. *Archives of General Psychiatry, 40*, 681–687.

Purvis, K. L., & Tannock, R. (1997). Language abilities in children with attention deficit hyperactivity disorder, reading disabilities, and normal controls. *Journal of Abnormal Child Psychology, 25*, 133–144.

Quay, H. C. (1997). Inhibition and attention deficit hyperactivity disorder. *Journal of Abnormal Child Psychology, 25*, 7–13.

Rabiner, D., Coie, J. D., & the Conduct Problems Prevention Research Group. (2000). Early attention problems and children's reading achievement: A longitudinal investigation. *Journal of the American Academy of Child and Adolescent Psychiatry, 39*, 859–867.

Rapoport, J. L., Buchsbaum, M. S., Zahn, T. P., Weingarten, H., Ludlow, C., & Mikkelsen, E. J. (1978). Dextroamphetamine: Cognitive and behavioral effects in normal prepubertal boys. *Science, 199*, 560–563.

Rapoport, J. L., Donnelly, M., Zametkin, A., & Carrougher, J. (1986). "Situational hyperactivity" in a U.S. clinical setting. *Journal of Child Psychology and Psychiatry, 27*, 639–646.

Rapport, M. D., Scanlan, S. W., & Denney, C. B. (1999). Attention-deficit/hyperactivity disorder and scholastic achievement: A model of dual developmental pathways. *Journal of Child Psychology and Psychiatry, 40*, 1169–1183.

Rapport, M. D., Tucker, S. B., DuPaul, G. J., Merlo, M., & Stoner, G. (1986). Hyperactivity and frustration: The influence of control over and size of rewards in delaying gratification. *Journal of Abnormal Child Psychology, 14*, 181–204.

Raskin, L. A., Shaywitz, S. E., Shaywitz, B. A., Anderson, G. M., & Cohen, D. J. (1984). Neurochemical correlates of attention deficit disorder. *Pediatric Clinics of North America, 31*, 387–396.

Rasmussen, P., & Gillberg, C. (2001). Natural outcome of ADHD with developmental coordination disorder at age 22 years: A controlled, longitudinal, community-based study. *Journal of the American Academy of Child and Adolescent Psychiatry, 39*, 1424–1431.

Reebye, P. N. (1997, October), *Diagnosis and treatment of ADHD in preschoolers*. Paper presented at the annual meeting of the American Academy of Child and Adolescent Psychiatry, Toronto.

Refetoff, S., Weiss, R. W., & Usala, S. J. (1993). The syndromes of resistance to thyroid hormone. *Endocrine Research, 14*, 348–399.

Rhee, S. H., Waldman, I. D., Hay, D. A., & Levy, F. (1999). Sex differences in genetic and environmental influences on DSM-III-R attention-deficit hyperactivity disorder (ADHD). *Journal of Abnormal Psychology, 108*, 24–41.

Richman, N., Stevenson, J., & Graham, P. (1982). *Preschool to school: A behavioural study*. New York: Academic Press.

Roberts, M. A. (1990). A behavioral observation method for differentiating hyperactive and aggressive boys. *Journal of Abnormal Child Psychology, 18*, 131–142.

Rohde, L. A., Biederman, J., Busnello, E. A., Zimmermann, H., Schmitz, M., Martins, S., & Tramontina, S. (1999). ADHD in a school sample of Brazilian adolescents: A study of prevalence, comorbid conditions, and impairments. *Journal of the American Academy of Child and Adolescent Psychiatry, 38*, 716–722.

Roizen, N. J., Blondis, T. A., Irwin, M., & Stein, M. (1994). Adaptive functioning in children with attention-deficit hyperactivity disorder. *Archives of Pediatric and Adolescent Medicine, 148*, 1137–1142.

Romano, E., Tremblay, R. E., Vitaro, F., Zoccolillo, M., & Pagani, L. (2001). Prevalene of psychiatric diagnoses and the role of perceived impairment: Findings from an adolescent community sample. *Journal of Child Psychology and Psychiatry*, *42*, 451–462.

Roth, N., Beyreiss, J., Schlenzka, K., & Beyer, H. (1991). Coincidence of attention deficit disorder and atopic disorders in children: Empirical findings and hypothetical background. *Journal of Abnormal Child Psychology*, *19*, 1–13.

Rothenberger, A. (1995). Electrical brain activity in children with hyperkinetic syndrome: Evidence of a frontal cortical dysfunction. In J. A. Sergeant (Ed.), *Eunethydis: European approaches to hyperkinetic disorder* (pp. 255–270). Amsterdam: Author.

Routh, D. K., & Schroeder, C. S. (1976). Standardized playroom measures as indices of hyperactivity. *Journal of Abnormal Child Psychology*, *4*, 199–207.

Rubia, K., Overmeyer, S., Taylor, E., Brammer, M., Williams, S. C. R., Simmons, A., & Bullmore, E. T. (1999). Hypofrontality in attention deficit hyperactivity disorder during higher-order motor control: A study with functional MRI. *American Journal of Psychiatry*, *156*, 891–896.

Rucklidge, J. J., & Tannock, R. (2001). Psychiatric, psychosocial, and cognitive functioning of female adolescents with ADHD. *Journal of the American Academy of Child and Adolescent Psychiatry*, *40*, 530–540.

Russo, M. F., & Beidel, D. C. (1994). Comorbidity of childhood anxiety and externalizing disorders: Prevalence, associated characteristics, and validation issues. *Clinical Psychology Review*, *14*, 199–221.

Rutter, M. (1977). Brain damage syndromes in childhood: Concepts and findings. *Journal of Child Psychology and Psychiatry*, *18*, 1–21.

Rutter, M., Bolton, P., Harrington, R., LeCouteur, A., Macdonald, H., & Simonoff, E. (1990). Genetic factors in child psychiatric disorders: I. A review of research strategies. *Journal of Child Psychology and Psychiatry*, *31*, 3–37.

Rutter, M., Macdonald, H., LeCouteur, A., Harrington, R., Bolton, P., & Bailey, P. (1990). Genetic factors in child psychiatric disorders: II. Empirical findings. *Journal of Child Psychology and Psychiatry*, *31*, 39–83.

Sachs, G. S., Baldassano, C. F., Truman, C. J., & Guille, C. (2000). Comorbidity of attention deficit hyperactivity disorder with early- and late-onset bipolar disorder. *American Journal of Psychiatry*, *157*, 466–468.

Samuel, V. J., George, P., Thornell, A., Curtis, S., Taylor, A., Brome, D., Mick, E., Faraone, S. V., & Biederman, J. (1999). A pilot controlled family study of DSM-III-R and DSM-IV ADHD in African-American children. *Journal of the American Academy of Child and Adolescent Psychiatry*, *38*, 34–39.

Sanchez, R. P., Lorch, E. P., Milich, R., & Welsh, R. (1999). Comprehension of televised stories in preschool children with ADHD. *Journal of Clinical Child Psychology*, *28*, 376–385.

Satterfield, J. H., Hoppe, C. M., & Schell, A. M. (1982). A prospective study of delinquency in 110 adolescent boys with attention deficit disorder and 88 normal adolescent boys. *American Journal of Psychiatry*, *139*, 795–798.

Schachar, R. J., & Logan, G. D. (1990). Impulsivity and inhibitory control in normal development and childhood psychopathology. *Developmental Psychology*, *26*, 710–720.

Schachar, R., Rutter, M., & Smith, A. (1981). The characteristics of situationally and pervasively hyperactive children: Implications for syndrome definition. *Journal of Child Psychology and Psychiatry*, *22*, 375–392.

Schachar, R. J., Tannock, R., & Logan, G. (1993). Inhibitory control, impulsiveness, and attention deficit hyperactivity disorder. *Clinical Psychology Review*, *13*, 721–740.

Schachar, R., Taylor, E., Weiselberg, M., Thorley, G., & Rutter, M. (1987). Changes in family function and relationships in children who respond to methylphenidate. *Journal of the American Academy of Child and Adolescent Psychiatry*, *26*, 728–732.

Scheres, A., Oosterlaan, J., & Sergeant, J. A. (2001). Response execution and inhibition in children with AD/HD and other disruptive disorders: The role of behavioural activation. *Journal of Child Psychology and Psychiatry*, *42*, 347–357.

Schleifer, M., Weiss, G., Cohen, N. J., Elman, M., Cvejic, H., & Kruger, E. (1975). Hyperactivity in preschoolers and the effect of methylphenidate. *American Journal of Orthopsychiatry*, *45*, 38–50.

Schothorst, P. F., & van Engeland, H. (1996). Long-term behavioral sequelae of prematurity. *Journal of the American Academy of Child and Adolescent Psychiatry*, *35*, 175–183.

Schrag, P., & Divoky, D. (1975). *The myth of the hyperactive child*. New York: Pantheon.

Schweitzer, J. B., Faber, T. L., Grafton, S. T., Tune, L. E., Hoffman, J. M., & Kilts, C. D. (2000). Alterations in the functional anatomy of working memory in adult attention deficit hyperactivity disorder. *American Journal of Psychiatry*, *157*, 278–280.

Seidman, L. J., Benedict, K. B., Biederman, J., Bernstein, J. H., Seiverd, K., Milberger, S., Norman, D., Mick, E., & Faraone, S. V. (1995). Performance of children with ADHD on the Rey–Osterrieth Complex Figure: A pilot neuropsychological study. *Journal of Child Psychology and Psychiatry*, *36*, 1459–1473.

Seidman, L. J., Biederman, J., Faraone, S. V., Milberger, S., Norman, D., Seiverd, K., Benedict, K., Guite, J., Mick, E., & Kiely, K. (1995). Effects of family history and comorbidity on the neuropsychological performance of children with ADHD: Preliminary findings. *Journal of the American Academy of Child and Adolescent Psychiatry*, *34*, 1015–1024.

Seidman, L. J., Biederman, J., Faraone, S. V., Weber, W., & Ouellette, C. (1997). Toward defining a neuropsychology of attention deficit-hyperactivity disorder: Performance of children and adolescence from a large clinically referred sample. *Journal of Consulting and Clinical Psychology*, *65*, 150–160.

Seguin, J. R., Boulerice, B., Harden, P. W., Tremblay, R. E., & Pihl, R. O. (1999). Executive functions and physical aggression after controlling for attention deficit hyperactivity disorder, general memory, and IQ. *Journal of Child Psychology and Psychiatry*, *40*, 1197–1208.

Semrud-Clikeman, M., Biederman, J., Sprich-Buckminster, S., Lehman, B. K., Faraone, S. V., & Norman, D. (1992). Comorbidity between ADDH and learning disability: A review and report in a clinically referred sample. *Journal of the American Academy of Child and Adolescent Psychiatry*, *31*, 439–448.

Semrud-Clikeman, M., Filipek, P. A., Biederman, J., Steingard, R., Kennedy, D., Renshaw, P., & Bekken, K. (1994). Attention–deficit hyperactivity disorder: Magnetic resonance imaging morphometric analysis of the corpus callosum. *Journal of the American Academy of Child and Adolescent Psychiatry, 33*, 875–881.

Semrud-Clikeman, M., Steingard, R. J., Filipek, P., Biederman, J., Bekken, K., & Renshaw, P. F. (2000). Using MRI to examine brain–behavior relationships in males with attention deficit disorder with hyperactivity. *Journal of the American Acdemy of Child and Adolescent Psychiatry, 39*, 477–484.

Sergeant, J. (1988). From DSM-III attentional deficit disorder to functional defects. In L. Bloomingdale & J. Sergeant (Eds.), *Attention deficit disorder: Criteria, cognition, and intervention* (pp. 183–198). New York: Pergamon Press.

Sergeant, J., & Scholten, C. A. (1985a). On data limitations in hyperactivity. *Journal of Child Psychology and Psychiatry, 26*, 111–124.

Sergeant, J., & Scholten, C. A. (1985b). On resource strategy limitations in hyperactivity: Cognitive impulsivity reconsidered. *Journal of Child Psychology and Psychiatry, 26*, 97–109.

Sergeant, J., & van der Meere, J. P. (1994). Toward an empirical child psychopathology. In D. K. Routh (Ed.), *Disruptive behavior disorders in children* (pp. 59–86). New York: Plenum Press.

Shaywitz, S. E., Cohen, D. J., & Shaywitz, B. E. (1980). Behavior and learning difficulties in children of normal intelligence born to alcoholic mothers. *Journal of Pediatrics, 96*, 978–982.

Shaywitz, S. E., Shaywitz, B. A., Cohen, D. J., & Young, J. G. (1983). Monoaminergic mechanisms in hyperactivity. In M. Rutter (Ed.), *Developmental neuropsychiatry* (pp. 330–347). New York: Guilford Press.

Shaywitz, S. E., Shaywitz, B. A., Jatlow, P. R., Sebrechts, M., Anderson, G. M., & Cohen, D. J. (1986). Biological differentiation of attention deficit disorder with and without hyperactivity: A preliminary report. *Annals of Neurology, 21*, 363.

Shelton, T. L., Barkley, R. A., Crosswait, C., Moorehouse, M., Fletcher, K., Barrett, S., Jenkins, L., & Metevia, L. (1998). Psychiatric and psychological morbidity as a function of adaptive disability in preschool children with high levels of aggressive and hyperactive–impulsive–inattentive behavior. *Journal of Abnormal Child Psychology, 26*, 475–494.

Sherman, D. K., Iacono, W. G., & McGue, M. K. (1997). Attention-deficit hyperactivity disorder dimensions: A twin study of inattention and impulsivity–hyperactivity. *Journal of the American Academy of Child and Adolescent Psychiatry, 36*, 745–753.

Sherman, D. K., McGue, M. K., & Iacono, W. G. (1997). Twin concordance for attention deficit hyperactivity disorder: A comparison of teachers' and mothers' reports. *American Journal of Psychiatry, 154*, 532–535.

Sieg, K. G., Gaffney, G. R., Preston, D. F., & Hellings, J. A. (1995). SPECT brain imaging abnormalities in attention deficit hyperactivity disorder. *Clinical Nuclear Medicine, 20*, 55–60.

Silberg, J., Rutter, M., Meyer, J., Maes, H., Hewitt, J., Simonoff, E., Pickles, A., Loeber, R., & Eaves, L. (1996). Genetic and environmental influences on the covariation between hyperactivity and conduct disturbance in juvenile twins. *Journal of Child Psychology and Psychiatry, 37*, 803–816.

Silva, P. A., Hughes, P., Williams, S., & Faed, J. M. (1988). Blood lead, intelligence, reading attainment, and behaviour in eleven year old children in Dunedin, New Zealand. *Journal of Child Psychology and Psychiatry, 29*, 43–52.

Silverman, I. W., & Ragusa, D. M. (1992). Child and maternal correlates of impulse control in 24–month old children. *Genetic, Social, and General Psychology Monographs, 116*, 435–473.

Simmell, C., & Hinshaw, S. P. (1993, March). *Moral reasoning and antisocial behavior in boys with ADHD.* Poster presented at the biennial meeting of the Society for Research in Child Development, New Orleans, LA.

Singer, H. S., Reiss, A. L., Brown, J. E., Aylward, E. H., Shih, B., Chee, E., Harris, E. L., Reader, M. J., Chase, G. A., Bryan, R. N., & Denckla, M. B. (1993). Volumetric MRI changes in basal ganglia of children with Tourette's syndrome. *Neurology, 43*, 950–956.

Slusarek, M., Velling, S., Bunk, D., & Eggers, C. (2001). Motivational effects on inhibitory control in children with ADHD. *Journal of the American Academy of Child and Adolescent Psychiatry, 40*, 355–363.

Smalley, S. L., McGough, J. J., Del'Homme, M., NewDelman, J., Gordon, E., Kim, T., Liu, A., & McCracken, J. T. (2000). Familial clustering of symptoms and disruptive behaviors in multiplex families with attention-deficit/hyperactivity disorder. *Journal of the American Academy of Child and Adolescent Psychiatry, 39*, 1135–1143.

Solanto, M. V., Abikoff, H., Sonuga-Barke, E., Schachar, R., Logan, G. D., Wigal, T., Hechtman, L., Hinshaw, S., & Turkel, E. (2001). The ecological validity of delay aversion and response inhibition as measures of impulsivity in AD/HD: A supplement to the NIMH Multimodal Treatment Study of ADHD. *Journal of Abnormal Child Psychology, 29*, 215–228.

Sonuga-Barke, E. J., Lamparelli, M., Stevenson, J., Thompson, M., & Henry, A. (1994). Behaviour problems and pre-school intellectual attainment: The associations of hyperactivity and conduct problems. *Journal of Child Psychology and Psychiatry, 35*, 949–960.

SonugaBarke, E. J. S., Taylor, E., & Heptinstall, E. (1992). Hyperactivity and delay aversion: II. The effect of self versus externally imposed stimulus presentation periods on memory. *Journal of Child Psychology and Psychiatry, 33*, 399–409.

Southam-Gerow, M. A., & Kendall, P. C. (2002). Emotion regulation and understanding: Impliations for child psychopathology and therapy. *Clinical Psychology Review, 22*, 189–222.

Spencer, T. J., Biederman, J., Faraone, S., Mick, E., Coffey, B., Geller, D., Kagan, J., Bearman, S. K., & Wilens, T. (2001). Impact of tic disorders on ADHD outcome across the life cycle: Findings from a large group of adults with and without ADHD. *American Journal of Psychiatry, 158*, 611–617.

Spencer, T. J., Biederman, J., Harding, M., O'Donnell, D., Faraone, S. V., & Wilens, T. E. (1996). Growth deficits in ADHD children revisited: Evidence for disorder-associated growth delays? *Journal of the American Academy of Child and Adolescent Psychiatry, 35*, 1460–1469.

Spencer, T., Wilens, T., Biederman, J., Wozniak, J., & Harding-Crawford, M. (2000). Attention-deficit/hyperactivity disorder with mood disorders. In T. E. Brown (Ed.), *Attention deficit disorders and comorbidities in children, adolescents, and adults* (pp. 79–124). Washington, DC: American Psychiatric Press.

Sprich, S., Biederman, J., Crawford, M. H., Mundy, E., & Faraone, S. V. (2000). Adoptive and biological families of children and adolescents with ADHD. *Journal of the American Academy of Child and Adolesent Psychiatry, 39*, 1432–1437.

Stein, M. A. (1999). Unravelling sleep problems in treated and untreated children with ADHD. *Journal of Child and Adolescent Psychopharmacology, 9*, 157–168.

Stein, M. A., Szumowski, E., Blondis, T. A., & Roizen, N. J. (1995). Adaptive skills dysfunction in ADD and ADHD children. *Journal of Child Psychology and Psychiatry, 36*, 663–670.

Stein, M. A., Weiss, R. E., & Refetoff, S. (1995). Neurocognitive characteristics of individuals with resistance to thyroid hormone: Comparisons with individuals with attention-deficit hyperactivity disorder. *Journal of Developmental and Behavioral Pediatrics, 16*, 406–411.

Stevenson, J., Pennington, B. F., Gilger, J. W., DeFries, J. C., & Gilies, J. J. (1993). Hyperactivity and spelling disability: Testing for shared genetic aetiology. *Journal of Child Psychology and Psychiatry, 34*, 1137–1152.

Stewart, M. A. (1970). Hyperactive children. *Scientific American, 222*, 94–98.

Stewart, M. A., Pitts, F. N., Craig, A. G., & Dieruf, W. (1966). The hyperactive child syndrome. *American Journal of Orthopsychiatry, 36*, 861–867.

Stewart, M. A., Thach, B. T., & Friedin, M. R. (1970). Accidental poisoning and the hyperactive child syndrome. *Diseases of the Nervous System, 31*, 403–407.

Still, G. F. (1902). Some abnormal psychical conditions in children. *Lancet, i*, 1008–1012, 1077–1082, 1163–1168.

Strauss, A. A., & Kephardt, N. C. (1955). *Psychopathology and education of the brain-injured child: Vol. 2. Progress in theory and clinic*. New York: Grune & Stratton.

Strauss, A. A., & Lehtinen, L. E. (1947). *Psychopathology and education of the brain-injured child*. New York: Grune & Stratton.

Strauss, M. E., Thompson, P., Adams, N. L., Redline, S., & Burant, C. (2000). Evaluation of a model of attention with confirmatory factor analysis. *Neuropsycholoy, 14*, 201–208.

Streissguth, A. P., Bookstein, F. L., Sampson, P. D., & Barr, H. M. (1995). Attention: Prenatal alcohol and continuities of vigilance and attentional problems from 4 through 14 years. *Development and Psychopathology, 7*, 419–446.

Streissguth, A. P., Martin, D. C., Barr, H. M., Sandman, B. M., Kirchner, G. L., & Darby, B. L. (1984). Intrauterine alcohol and nicotine exposure: Attention and reaction time in 4-year-old children. *Developmental Psychology, 20*, 533–541.

Stryker, S. (1925). Encephalitis lethargica—The behavior residuals. *Training School Bulletin, 22*, 152–157.

Stuss, D. T., & Benson, D. F. (1986). *The frontal lobes*. New York: Raven Press.

Swaab-Barneveld, H., DeSonneville, L., Cohen-Kettenis, P., Gielen, A., Buitelaar, J., & van Engeland, H. (2000). Visual sustained attention in a child psychiatric population. *Journal of the American Academy of Child and Adolescent Psychiatry, 39*, 651–659.

Swanson, J. M., Sunohara, G. A., Kennedy, J. L., Regino, R., Fineberg, E., Wigal, E., LaHoste, G. J., & Wigal, S. (1997). *Association of the dopamine receptor D4 (DRD4) gene with a refined phenotype of attention deficit hyperactivity disorder (ADHD): A family-based approach*. Manuscript submitted for publication.

Sykes, D. H., Hoy, E. A., Bill, J. M., McClure, B. G., Halliday, H. L., & Reid, M. M. (1997). Behavioural adjustment in school of very low birthweight children. *Journal of Child Psychology and Psychiatry, 38*, 315–325.

Szatmari, P. (1992). The epidemiology of attention-deficit hyperactivity disorders. *Child and Adolescent Psychiatric Clinics of North America, 1*(2), 361–372).

Szatmari, P., Offord, D. R., & Boyle, M. H. (1989). Correlates, associated impairments, and patterns of service utilization of children with attention deficit disorders: Findings from the Ontario Child Health Study. *Journal of Child Psychology and Psychiatry, 30*, 205–217.

Szatmari, P., Saigal, S., Rosenbaum, P. & Campbell, D. (1993). Psychopathology and adaptive functioning among extremely low birthweight children at eight years of age. *Development and Psychopathology, 5*, 345–357.

Tallmadge, J., & Barkley, R. A. (1983). The interactions of hyperactive and normal boys with their mothers and fathers. *Journal of Abnormal Child Psychology, 11*, 565–579.

Tannock, R. (1998). Attention deficit hyperactivity disorder: Advances in cognitive, neurobiological, and genetic research. *Journal of Child Psychology and Psychiatry, 39*, 65–100.

Tannock, R. (2000). Attention-deficit/hyperactivity disorder with anxiety disorders. In T. E. Brown (Ed.), *Attention deficit disorders and comorbidities in children, adolescents, and adults* (pp. 125–170). Washington, DC: American Psychiatric Press.

Tannock, R., & Brown, T. E. (2000). Attention-deficit disorders with learning disorders in children and adolescents. In T. E. Brown (Ed.), *Attention deficit disorders and comorbidities in children, adolescents, and adults* (pp. 231–296). Washington, DC: American Psychiatric Press.

Tannock, R., Martinussen, R., & Frijters, J. (2000). Naming speed performance and stimulant effects indicate effortful, semantic processing deficits in attention-deficit/hyperactivity disorder. *Journal of Abnormal Child Psychology, 28*, 237–252.

Tarver-Behring, S., Barkley, R. A., & Karlsson, J. (1985). The mother–child interactions of hyperactive boys and their normal siblings. *American Journal of Orthopsychiatry, 55*, 202–209.

Taylor, E. (1999). Developmental neuropsychology of attention deficit and impulsiveness. *Development and Psychopathology, 11*, 607–628.

Taylor, E., Sandberg, S., Thorley, G., & Giles, S. (1991). *The epidemiology of childhood hyperactivity*. Oxford: Oxford University Press.

Teicher, M. H., Anderson, C. M., Polcari, A., Glod, C. A., Maas, L. C., & Renshaw, P. F. (2000). Functional deficits in basal ganglia of children with attention-deficit/hyperactivity disorder shown with functional magnetic resonance imaging relaxometry. *Nature Medicine, 6*, 470–473.

Thapar, A. J. (1999). Genetic basis of attention deficit and hyperactivity. *Briisht Journal of Psychiatry, 174*, 105–111.

Thapar, A. J., Hervas, A., & McGuffin, P. (1995). Childhood hyperactivity scores are highly heritable and show sibling competition effects: Twin study evidence. *Behavior Genetics, 25*, 537–544.

Thapar, A., Harrington, R., & McGuffin, P. (2001). Examining the comorbidity of ADHD-related behaviours and conduct problems using a twin study design. *British Journal of Psychiatry, 179*, 224–229.

Thomson, G. O. B., Raab, G. M., Hepburn, W. S., Hunter, R., Fulton, M., & Laxen, D. P. H. (1989). Blood-lead levels and children's behaviour: Results from the Edinburgh lead study. *Journal of Child Psychology and Psychiatry, 30*, 515–528.

Torgesen, J. K. (1994). Issues in the assessment of of executive function: An information-processing perspective. In

G. R. Lyon (Ed.), *Frames of reference for the assessment of learning disabilities: New views on measurement issues* (pp. 143–162). Baltimore: Brookes.

Tripp, G., & Alsop, B. (1999). Sensitivity to reward frequency in boys with attention deficit hyperactivity disorder. *Journal of Clinical Child Psychology, 28,* 366–375.

Tripp, G., & Alsop, B. (2001). Sensitivity to reward delay in children with attention deficit hyperactivity disorder (ADHD). *Journal of Child Psychology and Psychiatry, 42,* 691–698.

Trites, R. L. (1979). *Hyperactivity in children: Etiology, measurement, and treatment implications.* Baltimore: University Park Press.

Trites, R. L., Dugas, F., Lynch, G., & Ferguson, B. (1979). Incidence of hyperactivity. *Journal of Pediatric Psychology, 4,* 179–188.

Trommer, B. L., Hoeppner, J. B., Rosenberg, R. S., Armstrong, K. J., & Rothstein, J. A. (1988). Sleep disturbances in children with attention deficit disorder. *Annals of Neurology, 24,* 325.

Ullman, D. G., Barkley, R. A., & Brown, H. W. (1978). The behavioral symptoms of hyperkinetic children who successfully responded to stimulant drug treatment. *American Journal of Orthopsychiatry, 48,* 425–437.

Vaidya, C. J., Austin, G., Kirkorian, G., Ridlehuber, H. W., Desmond, J. E., Glover, G. H., Gabrieli, J. D. E. (1998). Selective effects ofmethylphenidate in attention deficit hyperactivity disorder: A functional magnetic resonance study. *Proceedings of the National Academy of Sciences USA, 95,* 14494–14499.

van den Oord, E. J. C. G., Boomsma, D. I., & Verhulst, F. C. (1994). A study of problem behaviors in 10- to 15-year-old biologically related and unrelated international adoptees. *Behavior Genetics, 24,* 193–205.

van den Oord, E. J. C., & Rowe, D. C. (1997). Continuity and change in children's social maladjustment: A developmental behavior genetic study. *Developmental Psychology, 33,* 319–332.

van den Oord, E. J. C. G., Verhulst, F. C., & Boomsma, D. I. (1996). A genetic study of maternal and paternal ratings of problem behaviors in 3-year-old twins. *Journal of Abnormal Psychology, 105,* 349–357.

Velez, C. N., Johnson, J., & Cohen, P. (1989). A longitudinal analysis of selected risk factors for childhood psychopathology. *Journal of the American Academy of Child and Adolescent Psychiatry, 28,* 861–864.

Velting, O. N., & Whitehurst, G. J. (1997). Inattention–hyperactivity and reading achievement in children from low-income families: A longitudinal model. *Journal of Abnormal Child Psychology, 25,* 321–331.

Voelker, S. L., Carter, R. A., Sprague, D. J., Gdowski, C. L., & Lachar, D. (1989). Developmental trends in memory and metamemory in children with attention deficit disorder. *Journal of Pediatric Psychology, 14,* 75–88.

Volkow, N. D., Wang, G. J., Fowler, J. S., Logan, J., Gerasimov, M., Maynard, L., Ding, Y., Gatley, S. J., Gifford, A., & Franceschi, D. (2001). Therapeutic doses of oral methylphenidate significantly increase extracelluar dopamine in the human brain. *Journal of Neuroscience, 21,* 1–5.

Vygotsky, L. S. (1978). *Mind in society.* Cambridge, MA: Harvard University Press.

Vygotsky, L. S. (1987). Thinking and speech. In R. W. Rieber & A. S. Carton (Eds.) & N. Minick (Trans.), *The collected works of L. S. Vygotsky: Vol. 1. Problems in general psychology* (pp. 37–285). New York: Plenum Press. (Original work published 1966)

Wakefield, J. C. (1999). Evolutionary versus prototype analyses of the concept of disorder. *Journal of Abnormal Psychology, 108,* 374–399.

Wallander, J. L., Schroeder, S. R., Michelli, J. A., & Gualtieri, C. T. (1987). Classroom social interactions of attention deficit disorder with hyperactivity children as a function of stimulant medication. *Journal of Pediatric Psychology, 12,* 61–76.

Weiss, G., & Hechtman, L. (1993). *Hyperactive children grown up* (2nd ed.). New York: Guilford Press.

Weiss, R. E., Stein, M. A., Trommer, B., et al. (1993). Attention-deficit hyperactivity disorder and thyroid function. *Journal of Pediatrics, 123,* 539–545.

Welner, Z., Welner, A., Stewart, M., Palkes, H., & Wish, E. (1977). A controlled study of siblings of hyperactive children. *Journal of Nervous and Mental Disease, 165,* 110–117.

Welsh, M. C., & Pennington, B. F. (1988). Assessing frontal lobe functioning in children: Views from developmental psychology. *Developmental Neuropsychology, 4,* 199–230.

Werner, E. E., Bierman, J. M., French, F. W., Simonian, K., Connor, A., Smith, R. S., & Campbell, M. (1971). Reproductive and environmental casualties: A report on the 10–year follow-up of the children of the Kauai pregnancy study. *Pediatrics, 42,* 112–127.

Werry, J. S., Elkind, G. S., & Reeves, J. S. (1987). Attention deficit, conduct, oppositional, and anxiety disorders in children: III. Laboratory differences. *Journal of Abnormal Child Psychology, 15,* 409–428.

Werry, J. S., & Quay, H. C. (1971). The prevalence of behavior symptoms in younger elementary school children. *American Journal of Orthopsychiatry, 41,* 136–143.

Whalen, C. K., & Henker, B. (1992). The social profile of attention-deficit hyperactivity disorder: Five fundamental facets. *Child and Adolescent Psychiatric Clinics of North America, 1,* 395–410.

Whalen, C. K., Henker, B., Collins, B. E., McAuliffe, S., & Vaux, A. (1979). Peer interaction in structured communication task: Comparisons of normal and hyperactive boys and of methylphenidate (Ritalin) and placebo effects. *Child Development, 50,* 388–401.

Whalen, C. K., Henker, B., & Dotemoto, S. (1980). Methylphenidate and hyperactivity: Effects on teacher behaviors. *Science, 208,* 1280–1282.

Whalen, C. K., Henker, B., Swanson, J. M., Granger, D., Kliewer, W., & Spencer, J. (1987). Natural social behaviors in hyperactive children: Dose effects of methylphenidate. *Journal of Consulting and Clinical Psychology, 55,* 187–193.

White, H. R., Xie, M., Thompson, W., Loeber, R., & Stouthamer-Loeber, M. (2001). Psychopathology as a predictor of adolescent drug use trajectories. *Psychology of Addictive Behavior, 15,* 210–218.

Whittaker, A. H., Van Rossem, R., Feldman, J. F., Schonfeld, I. S., Pinto-Martin, J. A., Torre, C., Shaffer, D., & Paneth, N. (1997). Psychiatric outcomes in low-birth-weight children at age 6 years: Relation to neonatal cranial ultrasound abnormalities. *Archives of General Psychiatry, 54,* 847–856.

Wiers, R. W., Gunning, W. B., & Sergeant, J. A. (1998). Is a mild deficit in executive functions in boys related to childhood ADHD or to parental multigenerational alcoholism. *Journal of Abnormal Child Psychology, 26,* 415–430.

Wilens, T. E., Biederman, J., & Spencer, T. (1994). Clonidine for sleep disturbances associated with attention-deficit hyperactivity disorder. *Journal of the American Academy of Child and Adolescent Psychiatry, 33,* 424–426.

Willcutt, E. G., Pennington, B. F., Boada, R., Ogline, J. S., Tunick, R. A., Chhabildas, N. A., & Olson, R. K. (2001). A comparison of the cognitive deficits in reading disability and attention-deficit/hyperactivity disorder. *Journal of Abnormal Psychology, 110,* 157–172.

Willcutt, E. G., Pennington, B. F., Chhabildas, N. A., Friedman, M. C., & Alexander, J. (1999). Psychiatric comorbidity associated with DSM-IV ADHD in a nonreferred sample of twins. *Journal of the American Academy of Child and Adolescent Psychiatry, 38,* 1355–1362.

Willerman, L. (1973). Activity level and hyperactivity in twins. *Child Development, 44,* 288–293.

Willis, T. J., & Lovaas, I. (1977). A behavioral approach to treating hyperactive children: The parent's role. In J. B. Millichap (Ed.), *Learning disabilities and related disorders* (pp. 119–140). Chicago: Year Book Medical.

Winsler, A. (1998). Parent–child interaction and private speech in boys with ADHD. *Applied Developmental Science, 2,* 17–39.

Winsler, A., Diaz, R. M., Atencio, D. J., McCarthy, E. M., & Chabay, L. A. (2000). Verbal self-regulation over time in preschool children at risk for attention and behavior problems. *Journal of Child Psychology and Psychiatry, 41,* 875–886.

Wolraich, M. L., Hannah, J. N., Baumgaertel, A., & Feurer, I. D. (1998). Examination of DSM-IV criteria for attention deficit/hyperactivity disorder in a county-wide sample. *Journal of Developmental and Behavioral Pediatrics, 19,* 162–168.

Wolraich, M . L., Hannah, J. N., Pinnock, T. Y., Baumgaertel, A., & Brown, J. (1996). Comparison of diagnostic criteria for attention-deficit hyperactivity disorder in a country-wide sample. *Journal of the American Academy of Child and Adolescent Psychiatry, 35,* 319–324.

Wood, F. B., & Felton, R. H. (1994). Separate linguistic and attentional factors in the development of reading. *Topics in Language Disorders, 14,* 52–57.

Woodward, L. J., Fergusson, D. M., & Horwood, L. J. (2000). Driving outcomes of young people with attentional difficulties in adolescence. *Journal of the American Academy of Child and Adolescent Psychiatry, 39,* 627–634.

World Health Organization. (1993). *The ICD-10 classification of mental and behavioural disorders: Diagnostic criteria for research.* Geneva: Author.

Wozniak, J., Biederman, J., Kiely, K., Ablon, S., Faraone, S. V., Mundy, E., & Mennin, D. (1995). Mania-like symptoms suggestive of childhood-onset bipolar disorder in clinically referred children. *Journal of the American Academy of Child and Adolescent Psychiatry, 34,* 867–876.

Youdin, M. B. H., & Riederer, P. (1997). Understanding Parkinson's disease. *Scientific American, 276,* 52–59.

Zagar, R., & Bowers, N. D. (1983). The effect of time of day on problem-solving and classroom behavior. *Psychology in the Schools, 20,* 337–345.

Zametkin, A. J., Liebenauer, L. L., Fitzgerald, G. A., King, A. C., Minkunas, D. V., Herscovitch, P., Yamada, E. M., & Cohen, R. M. (1993). Brain metabolism in teenagers with attention-deficit hyperactivity disorder. *Archives of General Psychiatry, 50,* 333–340.

Zametkin, A. J., Nordahl, T. E., Gross, M., King, A. C., Semple, W. E., Rumsey, J., Hamburger, S., & Cohen, R. M. (1990). Cerebral glucose metabolism in adults with hyperactivity of childhood onset. *New England Journal of Medicine, 323,* 1361–1366.

Zametkin, A. J., & Rapoport, J. L. (1986). The pathophysiology of attention deficit disorder with hyperactivity: A review. In B. B. Lahey & A. E. Kazdin (Eds.), *Advances in clinical child psychology* (Vol. 9, pp. 177–216). New York: Plenum Press.

Zentall, S. S. (1985). A context for hyperactivity. In K. Gadow & I. Bialer (Eds.), *Advances in learning and behavioral disabilities* (Vol. 4, pp. 273–343). Greenwich, CT: JAI Press.

Zentall, S. S. (1988). Production deficiencies in elicited language but not in the spontaneous verbalizations of hyperactive children. *Journal of Abnormal Child Psychology, 16,* 657–673.

Zentall, S. S., & Smith, Y. S. (1993). Mathematical performance and behaviour of children with hyperactivity with and without coexisting aggression. *Behaviour Research and Therapy, 31,* 701–710.

CHAPTER THREE

Conduct and Oppositional Defiant Disorders

Stephen P. Hinshaw
Steve S. Lee

Problems related to delinquency and youth violence in our nation are entwined in a complex web of public concern, community fear and outrage, media attention, concerted research efforts, and multifaceted prevention and intervention programs. Even though official rates of antisocial behavior (ASB) among children, adolescents, and adults in the United States showed evidence of a leveling off or slight decline during the 1990s, following decades of steady increases (Snyder & Sickmund, 1995; Zimring, 1998; Fingerhut & Kleinman, 1990), few would contend that aggression and ASB have receded as salient, impairing, disturbing, and even (in some instances) lethal problems. Indeed, notorious instances of youth violence in middle-class, suburban settings in recent years have propelled national interest in the alarmingly high rates of aggression, acting out, and even murder among young people—rates that have long been salient in impoverished, urban neighborhoods. Furthermore, levels of violence in the United States continue to surpass those in other industrialized nations (Loeber & Hay, 1997: Rutter, Giller, & Hagell, 1998). Among youths in general, the highest rates of referral for mental health services involve aggressive, acting-out, and disruptive behavior patterns, which have shown a detectable increase over the period of time from the 1960s through the 1990s (Achenbach & Howell, 1993). In addition, the threat—or reality—of violence continues to create climates of fear, intimidation, and deprivation in many communities (Richters & Martinez, 1993). Overall, despite the ever-increasing amounts of research on this topic, the need for sound scientific efforts directed toward understanding the roots, classification, underlying mechanisms, and treatment of ASB has never been greater.

Although we base much of the organizational scheme of this chapter on the contents of the parallel chapter in the first edition of this volume (Hinshaw & Anderson, 1996), we not only update the huge literature in the field but also pursue several expanded directions. First, we pay even greater attention to the multiple causal pathways that may portend clinically significant oppositionality and aggression among children and adolescents, incorporating the constructs of equifinality (the presence of divergent etiological roots that lead to phenotypically similar behavior patterns) and multifinality (the developmental diversity of outcomes from similar initial states) (Cicchetti & Rogosch, 1996). It is clear that the behavior patterns under consideration are the products of influences at multiple levels (e.g., genetic, temperamental, family systemic, socioeconomic, school-related, community-wide), which interact and transact in complex ways. Second, given the maturation of several important prospective, longitudinal samples into adulthood, we present additional information on the extended developmental outcomes of children with both early-onset and adolescent-onset manifestations of aggression and ASB. Third, we more explicitly feature what is known (and unknown) about female manifestations of such behavioral patterns. Accordingly, we note the increasing recognition given to a less overt and less violent form of antisocial activities—indirect or relational aggression—which appear to be particularly salient among girls. Fourth, we present a preliminary conceptual model regarding the development and maintenance of ASB patterns, recognizing that any overarching theories must recognize the considerable heterogeneity among (1) types of externalizing behavior, (2) subtypes of youths at risk for such behavior, and (3) developmental pathways or trajectories that characterize youngsters with such tendencies.

At the outset, we make clear that our chapter does not focus on species-wide influences on aggression (Coie & Dodge, 1998). Rather, we deal with influences on individual differences in aggression and ASB, through a strongly developmental perspective. In addition, given the huge literature on this topic, we direct the reader to key review articles, chapters, and books that have appeared since the first edition of this volume was published. Such works include the masterful historical, conceptual, and developmental review of Coie and Dodge (1998); key reviews of developmental issues by Loeber and Hay (1997), Loeber and Stouthamer-Loeber (1998), Maughan and Rutter (1998), and Tremblay (2000); the comprehensive edited volumes of Hill and Maughan (2001), Loeber and Farrington (1998, 2001), Quay and Hogan (1999), and Stoff, Breiling, and Maser (1997), each of which contains a large number of seminal chapters; the lucid and comprehensive book-length account of Rutter et al. (1998), and the data-rich volume on ASB plus other mental health problems by Loeber, Farrington, Stouthamer-Loeber, and Van Kammen (1998); the recent work on female manifestations of ASB by Moffitt, Caspi, Rutter, and Silva (2001); the review of the diagnostic categories of oppositional defiant disorder (ODD) and conduct disorder (CD) by Loeber, Burke, Lahey, Winters, and Zera (2000); the syntheses of young children's risk for ASB by Keenan and Shaw (1997), Campbell, Shaw, and Gilliom (2000), and Loeber and Farrington (2000); and the integrative causal model of Lahey, Waldman, and McBurnett (1999). Note that this list is far from exhaustive; our entire reference section is, of necessity, limited to selected citations.

As highlighted in the first edition (Hinshaw & Anderson, 1996), considerable theoretical controversy still surrounds the field. At the most general level, there is dispute regarding the proper disciplines that should investigate antisocial activity and the optimal perspectives from which to view such behavior patterns. Indeed, because of the differing definitions of normative behavior across cultures, perhaps anthropological or sociological perspectives on antisocial functioning should receive primacy (e.g., Hirschi, 1969). Although our focus herein is directed more toward individual, familial, and social-contextual influences than toward the role of culture per se, the ascription of ASB exclusively to intraindividual causes is a real danger. Throughout this work, we develop the argument that only a subset of individuals displaying ASB patterns fall under the umbrella of mental disorder or impairment (Richters & Cicchetti, 1993), given the age- and sex-normative nature of a wide range of aggression and ASB during adolescence. On the other hand, just because a large proportion of antisocial youths appear to be those with adolescent onset, without long histories of multiple childhood impairments, does not imply that such youths are not in need of intervention (Moffitt, Caspi, Harrington, & Milne, 2002). In other words, the diagnoses of ODD and CD do not "cover the map" with respect to the personal and societal impact of aggression and violence.

Along this line, a salient theme throughout the chapter is that antisocial patterns, whether considered as dimensions of behavior or as distinct categorical entities, are heterogeneous with respect to constituent behaviors, causation, developmental mechanisms, and long-term course. Phrased alternatively, antisocial actions that appear similar at a given point in time may betray fundamentally disparate subtypes when viewed longitudinally (Loeber, 1988; Moffitt, 1993; Rutter et al., 1998). Any theories of such actions must actively consider the divergent underlying patterns and differing developmental trajectories relevant for distinct subgroups of youngsters.

Our main goals are to present current perspectives on the extensive literature surrounding patterns of aggression and ASB in childhood and adolescence (including brief coverage of the adult construct of psychopathy), and to illuminate current thinking about definitions, conceptualization, prevalence, comorbidity, and models of risk and etiology. Although we focus on the psychiatric disorders of ODD and CD, we go well beyond these categorical conceptions to consider dimensional features of aggression and ASB in childhood and adolescence, and alternative means of categorizing such behavioral manifestations. We emphasize throughout that ASB develops in relation to multiple influences, including biological and psychobiological risk variables, parent–child interactions, familial traits, school settings, neighborhood characteristics, peer networks, social service agencies and mental health services, and subcultural and societal norms; we also highlight that patterns of interaction and transaction across such influences is the rule rather than the exception in terms of the development of significant aggression and violence (Campbell, in press; Rutter et al., 1998). That is, underlying predispositions are translated into antisocial and violent behavior only through complex patterns of active engagement with the environment (Lahey, Waldman, & McBurnett, 1999). We hope that readers will come to appreciate the complexity of the issues surrounding this salient and troublesome type of behavioral disturbance, as well as the necessity of considering developmental perspectives on their etiology, maintenance, and outcome.

We begin by defining several key terms in the field and by discussing a number of core conceptual issues regarding aggression and ASB (see parallel consideration by Maughan & Rutter, 1998). We next provide a brief historical account of conceptions of ASB, covering current diagnostic criteria and related issues. After a discussion of prevalence and developmental progressions, we highlight the themes of comorbidity as well as risk and etiological factors, with emphasis on integrated, transactional models related to the development of ASB. We then provide an expanded section on sex differences, and conclude with an attempt at an integrated theoretical model of the development of aggression and ASB. Page limitations necessitate our neglecting almost entirely the topics of assessment and of prevention/intervention (for recent perspectives on these topics, see Hinshaw & Zupan, 1997; Hinshaw & Nigg, 1999; relevant chapters in Quay & Hogan, 1999; Rutter et al., 1998, Chs. 11 and 12; and McMahon & Wells, 1998, among many other sources).

TERMINOLOGICAL AND CONCEPTUAL ISSUES

Defining the Domain

Judges and juvenile justice workers, research investigators, clinicians, and societal commentators have utilized a host of terms to describe ASB in children, adolescents, and adults, yielding a sometimes chaotic level of imprecision and confusion in the field at large. Even basic definitions of ASB and aggression are problematic (see the lucid discussion in Coie & Dodge, 1998). For example, must harmful intent be present for an act to be considered aggressive? If so, key problems in defining intentionality come into play. In addition, can ASB patterns be considered in any way universal, or are judgments of such actions always constrained by cultural norms? Expanded consideration of such definitional and philosophical issues can be found in Coie and Dodge (1998), Parke and Slaby (1983), and Rutter et al. (1998).

First, from a legal perspective, child and adolescent manifestations of ASB are termed "delinquent," and adult manifestations are called "criminal." Indeed, with rates of imprisonment at unprecedented levels in the United States, legal definitions of antisocial activity are salient. These types of definitions have limitations for psychological analysis, however, including the usual necessity of apprehension in allowing their usage; this means that relevant investigations may index the correlates of "being caught" or of police targeting (such as ethnic discrimination or selective reporting), rather than of ASB per se. In addition, most studies of delinquency neglect of the aggressive or antisocial activities of young children, whose early, "predelinquent" behavioral patterns may be the most likely routes for investigations of risk and causal factors and of preventive intervention. Note also that delinquency may be defined by a single act rather than a pattern of related behaviors, contributing to disparate estimates of its prevalence. We point out that many investigators distinguish between "official" delinquency and "self-reported" delinquency, with the latter indexed by children's or adolescents' self-report disclosures of various illegal activities. Readers are cautioned to make note of the particular measurement strategy in use in any particular investigation of delinquency.

Second, empirical psychological investigations often distinguish so-called "externalizing" behavior patterns—those marked by impulsive, overactive, aggressive, and antisocial actions—from "internalizing" (e.g., anxious, dysphoric, withdrawn, thought-disordered, somaticizing) features (Achenbach, 1991). Indeed, a long tradition of research posits fundamental distinctions between these two domains with respect to underlying behavioral components, risk and etiological factors, and long-term course (e.g., Quay, 1986). Clearly, the subject matter of interest for this chapter lies in the externalizing domain. On the other hand, we highlight at the outset that overlap between externalizing and internalizing patterns is strong. We also point out that externalizing and internalizing behavior patterns are clearly dimensional in nature, ranging from normative levels to the extreme ends of their respective continua. Whether dimensional or categorical conceptualizations of ASB better fit the underlying nature of the constituent problems is a thorny and long-standing problem, as we take up subsequently.

It is essential to recognize that within the externalizing domain—also termed "acting-out," "disruptive," or undercontrolled"[1]—a fundamental distinction exists between aggression and ASB on the one hand, and the spectrum of inattentive/impulsive/overactive symptoms, which are the constituent behavior patterns of attention-deficit/hyperactivity disorder (ADHD), on the other (Fergusson, Horwood, & Lloyd, 1991; Loney, 1987). Whereas these types of behavior frequently co-occur—as witnessed by their loading together on higher-order externalizing dimensions (Achenbach, 1991), and by the diagnostic overlap of categories reflecting oppositional or aggressive actions with disorders of attention and impulse control (Biederman, Newcorn, & Sprich, 1991)—the distinction has been validated in many investigations (see Hinshaw, 1987; Jensen, Martin, & Cantwell, 1997).[2] Because the overlap or comorbidity between aggressive/antisocial actions and the constituent behaviors of ADHD is quite important for the development of long-term antisocial patterns (e.g., Loeber et al., 1998; Moffitt, 1990; Rutter et al., 1998), we scrutinize this association later in the chapter.

Third, in the psychiatric tradition of forming diagnostic categories, CD and ODD are the constituent disorders of the "disruptive behavior disorders" category in the *Diagnostic and Statistical Manual of Mental Disorders*, Fourth edition (DSM-IV; American Psychiatric Association, 1994). ODD is denoted by the age-inappropriate and persistent display of angry, defiant, irritable, and oppositional behaviors; CD includes a far more severe list of aggressive and antisocial actions that involve the infliction of pain (e.g., initiating fights, fire setting), denial of the rights of others (e.g., stealing, breaking and entering), as well as status offenses such as running away from home (American Psychiatric Association, 1994). The intention behind these diagnostic categories is to include youngsters whose patterns of defiance or ASB are persistent and clearly impairing. Thus, whereas most youngsters diagnosed with CD will by definition display delinquent behavior patterns, only a minority of delinquent adolescents would qualify for a diagnosis of CD, given the transitory and relatively nonimpaired nature of much delinquency during adolescence (Hinshaw, Lahey, & Hart, 1993; Moffitt, 1993). Elaboration of the diagnostic criteria for ODD and CD, and appraisal of their validity and viability, are central topics of this chapter.

Fourth, the diagnostic category for adults with the persistent display of ASB is antisocial personality disorder (ASPD), found on Axis II of the DSM-IV nosology (American Psychiatric Association, 1994). As we highlight later, conceptions of ASPD in recent decades have emphasized the repetitive display of multiple illegal behaviors, with the necessity of a history of CD before adulthood. Such a behaviorally based definition can be differentiated from an alternative conception of "psychopathy," which emphasizes a callous, manipulative, impulsive, and remorseless psychological and interpersonal profile (Cleckley, 1976; Hart & Hare, 1997; Sutker, 1994), over and above antisocial and socially deviant actions per se. Importantly, careful empirical research supports the viability of psychopathy as a separable taxon, whereas repetitive criminality is best conceived as dimensional in nature (Harris, Rice, & Quinsey, 1994).

Fifth, in order to bring in a needed developmental perspective on the roots of psychopathic behavior and functioning, investigators have begun to identify traits among children termed "callous/unemotional" (Barry, Frick, DeShazo, & McCoy, 2000), which may be downward extensions of the affective/interpersonal factor of psychopathy noted in the preceding paragraph. The objective is to identify those psychological features (rather than oppositional or aggressive behaviors per se) that could identify those youths at the highest risk for displaying subsequent psychopathy. Recent investigations have been promising in this regard, although ultimate validation awaits prospective research into adulthood.

In sum, the various terms for depicting the domain under consideration often hamper clear communication in the field. Although our primary focus herein is on the diagnostic categories of ODD and CD in childhood and adolescence, the heated debate in the field as to the utility of such categorical conceptions, the considerable research on dimensional approaches to aggression and ASB, and the voluminous literature on delinquency all necessitate our explicitly considering alternate frameworks in the sections that follow. Note also that our clear focus is on childhood and adolescence; we consider adult ASPD and psychopathy as potential outcomes of earlier ASB, but we do not have room to take up the extensive literature on adult psychopathic behavior and crime.

Subtypes of Aggression and ASB

Key reviews of the development of aggression (Feschbach, 1970; Parke & Slaby, 1983; Coie & Dodge, 1998) emphasize the importance of subdividing this class of behaviors into theoretically and empirically distinguishable subcategories. Brief descriptions of several dichotomized distinctions may help to convey such diversity. Although a contrasting view is that there is an overarching, underlying "antisocial trait" or propensity that subsumes most if not all of the distinctions below (e.g., Jessor & Jessor, 1977), the subtypes of aggression and ASB we discuss have received considerable external validation. In short, investigators, clinicians, and all interested parties must pay close attention to precise definitions of the behavior patterns they are studying and treating.

1. Interpersonal aggression may be *verbal* (taunting, threatening, name calling, swearing) versus *physical* (bullying, fighting, assaulting). This distinction is evidenced not only descriptively but developmentally: Physical aggression emerges rather early in development, with peak levels during the preschool years, whereas verbal aggression shows a later onset (Parke & Slaby, 1983). Thus the persistence of high levels of physical aggression into middle childhood may signal the need for clinical attention, as may the early onset of noteworthy verbal aggression during the preschool years. In addition, as development progresses, physical aggression may become *violent*, marked by assaultive behavior, injury, and (frequently) the use of weapons. Such violence is, of course, of extreme interest to scientists, clinicians, and society at large.

2. Aggression can be categorized as *instrumental* (goal-directed) versus *hostile* (Feschbach, 1970); for the latter type, the infliction of pain is characterized as the intent of the behavior. Some levels of instrumental aggression are clearly normative for toddlers, whose cries of "mine" as they grab toys may signal a consolidating sense of self. On the other hand, extreme levels of hostile aggression demand further assessment at any age

3. Relatedly (but not identically), aggressive behavior may be *proactive* (bullying, threatening) versus *reactive* (retaliatory). In a systematic program of research, Dodge and colleagues (e.g., Dodge, 1991; Dodge, Lochman, Harnisch, & Bates, 1997) have shown that these two subtypes of aggression are marked by different kinds of social-cognitive information-processing deficits and distortions. That is, whereas children with a propensity for reactive aggression underutilize cues in reaching interpersonal decisions and show a propensity to attribute hostile intent to others in ambiguous social situations, those with a tendency toward proactive aggression tend to hold strong expectations that aggressive actions will help them obtain desired ends. Thus, in terms of the multistage social-cognitive information-processing model of Crick and Dodge (1994, 1996), reactive aggression involves "early" problems in encoding and interpretation of cues, whereas proactive aggression is associated with "late" expectancies regarding the value of aggressive behavior. Overall, despite the moderate to strong empirical associations between these forms of aggression, this distinction appears to have important theoretical and empirical underpinnings.

4. Another important distinction pertains to aggression that is *direct* (see the verbal and physical manifestations noted above) versus *indirect* or *relational* ("getting even" by having a third party retaliate; degrading another's reputation by spreading rumors; excluding a peer from activities). Such indirect aggression may pertain to girls more than to boys (Bjorkqvist, Lagerspitz, & Kaukianiinen, 1992); its consideration may illuminate (and mitigate) the often-cited sex differences in rates of aggression and ASB (see Goodman & Kohlsdorf, 1994). Indeed, a growing literature on relational aggression in girls (e.g., Crick & Grotpeter, 1995: Crick & Bigbee, 1998) highlights the impairing nature of such means of excluding or harming the reputations of others. We elaborate on relevant research subsequently, when discussing sex differences in aggression. Note that the terms "indirect" and "relational" are not interchangeable, as certain forms of socially and relationally excluding agemates may be quite direct (delivered to a peer's face), whereas

others may be surreptitious and performed via third parties (see Coie & Dodge, 1998).

5. At a broader level of categorization, ASB can be defined as *overt* (exemplified by most of the types of physically aggressive actions noted in the preceding paragraphs) versus *covert*, clandestine, or nonaggressive, with the latter subcategory characterized by such actions as lying, stealing, destroying property, abusing substances, being truant, and firesetting. On the widely used and well-validated Child Behavior Checklist (CBCL; Achenbach, 1991), the overt–covert distinction is evidenced by separate narrow-band scales of Aggressive Behavior versus Delinquent Behavior. Although many severely antisocial youths display both types of antisocial activity, the overt–covert distinction is empirically robust (Loeber & Schmaling, 1985), with growing evidence for divergent external correlates and causal factors. For instance, the Aggression Behavior scale of the CBCL displays substantial heritability, but the Delinquent Behavior scale (covering covert behaviors) yields lower heritability estimates (Edelbrock, Rende, Plomin, & Thompson, 1995). These two domains are also marked by somewhat different familial childrearing styles (Patterson & Stouthamer-Loeber, 1984) and disparate developmental trajectories (Loeber, Wung, et al., 1993; Loeber & Hay, 1997). Importantly, because the DSM-IV diagnosis of CD includes an admixture of overt and covert behavioral criteria—for example, assault and forced sexual activity as well as lying, shoplifting, and truancy—the CD diagnosis incorporates, by definition, disparate subtypes of antisocial youths (Achenbach, 1993). We return to this point in our subsequent discussion of diagnostic criteria.

Overall, even at the level of description of the constituent actions, the realm of aggression/ASB is complex and variegated. Much of the literature on aggression, antisocial activity, and delinquency confounds multiple subcategories of this domain, leading to difficulty in comparing investigations from different laboratories or from different time periods and inconsistencies in reports of the correlates of or risk factors for such externalizing behavior. Given that precision in terminology is of critical importance for the field, we again highlight the careful attention that must be paid to the definitions of ASB and to the subtypes of antisocial youths in research and clinical endeavors.

Dimensions or Categories?

A key issue for the field of psychopathology in general and ASB in particular pertains to the conception of deviance as dimensional or continuous on the one hand, versus discrete or categorical on the other (see Eysenck, 1986, for a seminal discussion). For our purposes, the question may be posed as follows: Is ASB in children and adolescents best conceived as lying on a continuum, with quantitative (but not qualitative) differences between youngsters in the levels of their constituent behaviors? Or do actual categories, diagnostic entities, or taxa (e.g., ODD or CD) exist—constructs that are qualitatively distinct from other forms of psychopathology? In other words, are there cutoff points for the underlying behavioral features (or for correlates of the symptom patterns) that reflect true discontinuities in the population? This deceptively simple dichotomy between dimensional and categorical perspectives is quite pertinent to any discussion of ASB.

In the first place, current nosologies (e.g., DSM-IV) are presented largely in a Kraepelinian framework, in which distinct disorders—defined by inclusionary and exclusionary criteria—are held to be present versus absent and to be distinct from other diagnoses (see Achenbach, 1993). As argued elsewhere (Hinshaw et al., 1993), however, categorical approaches must reflect actual discontinuities in the underlying distributions of the constituent behavior patterns if they are to be viable. If such discontinuities are not found, the chief advantages of categorical approaches would be convenience or the maintenance of tradition. Although few data explicitly address this issue regarding ASB, the empirical report of Robins and McEvoy (1990) is heuristic. Here the question was whether the overt and covert symptoms of CD in childhood, assessed retrospectively by American adults who participated in the landmark Epidemiologic Catchment Area study (Robins & Regier, 1991), could predict adolescent and adult patterns of substance abuse. Specifically, would the prediction be linear, with each successive number of aggressive/antisocial symptoms incrementing the predictive power in stepwise fashion, or would it increase precipitously when a certain diagnostic threshold was reached? The prediction function was in fact entirely linear: Each successively higher number of childhood CD symptoms incremented the prediction to later substance abuse, with no evidence for a "jump" in predictive power above any given cutoff. Overall, despite the limitations of this example, a conception of CD as continuous or dimensional appeared optimal.

In addition, it may well be the case that criteria other than levels of the constituent behaviors may define distinct categories. In fact, as we discuss in considerable detail, early age of onset plus the presence of ADHD symptoms, neuropsychological dysfunction, family discord, peer rejection, and academic failure appear to be joint markers of fundamentally divergent taxa of ASB: (1) an early-onset type, with youngsters manifesting clear psychopathology and showing strong evidence for considerable persistence of ASB across the life span; and (2) an adolescent-onset type, with youngsters failing to show most indicators of psychological disturbance, and demonstrating instead an age-expected tendency to violate social norms during the extended "gap" between physical and social maturity in Western societies (Moffitt, 1993). Importantly, both subgroups display similar rates of offending during adolescence (except for the higher rates of physical violence in the group with early-onset/persistent ASB), highlighting the need to transcend symptoms in forming this typology or categorization.

Dimensional and categorical approaches to psychopathology can be complementary and supplementary, rather than mutually exclusive (Achenbach, 1993; Pickles & Angold, in press; Rutter et al., 1998). For instance, subgroups of individuals with discrete psychopathology may emerge when cluster-analytic approaches are applied to dimensional measures of behavioral disturbance (e.g., Nagin & Tremblay, 1999). In other words, empirically derived typologies may emerge from quantitative, dimensional data, but the crucial criteria for validating such taxa must emanate from measures (e.g., risk factors, biological or environmental correlates, long-term course, treatment response) that are external to the defining symptoms themselves. Along this line, investigators who examine the predictive relations between dimensional measures of ASB on the one hand, and external correlates on the other, should carefully examine whether the associations that are found hold up at all points along the ASB continuum, especially the extreme scores that could potentially define a distinctive subgroup. Alternatively, those who study existing categories of ASB (e.g., ODD or CD) should examine whether group differences in mean levels of the dependent measures of interest might be better predicted from the dimensionalized symptom scores than from the diagnostic groups themselves (see Fergusson & Horwood, 1995). We hasten to point out, however, that categorical definitions may yield great practical advantages. For example, clinical or placement decisions (e.g., should a child receive special education services or be placed outside the home?) are far more easily made via yes–no designations, even if those involve dichotomizing an underlying dimension. Furthermore, the often-cited statistical dictum that dimensional scores always yield more statistical power than categorical indicators may not always be the case, as ably discussed by Farrington and Loeber (2000).

A related point bears mention. Particularly within the realm of ASB, for which multiple socioeconomic, familial, peer-related, neighborhood, and societal influences are salient, it may be that classification of youths into discrete categories—especially those with a psychiatric, intraindividual orientation—may render relevant parties (e.g., clinicians, families, policy makers) insensitive to the very real social influences on these troublesome behavior patterns. That is, a child may be seen as the sole locus of the "disorder." Indeed, because treatment decisions are quite likely to follow from conceptions regarding the source of the problem, classification of a child as psychopathological or mentally disordered could well steer clinicians or practitioners toward individual rather than systemic prevention or treatment strategies. (Note, in this regard, that recent high-quality prevention programs blend efforts directed toward individual, school, family, and wider community levels; see Conduct Problems Prevention Research Group, 2002). In sum, despite the scientific and practical benefits that may accrue to accurate classification, real dangers exist when labeling unjustly or unthinkingly ascribes the underlying problem to psychopathology or to a mental disorder (Richters & Cicchetti, 1993). On the other hand, if viable categories are found to exist, and if certain youngsters with ASB are found to evidence clear psychopathology, the resultant precision could aid in the mounting of therapeutic efforts (Moffitt, 1993; Rutter et al., 1998).

DSM-IV DEFINITIONAL CRITERIA

We begin this section with a short history of categorical psychiatric classification of externalizing or disruptive behavior disorders, and then proceed to a review of the DSM-IV definitional criteria for ODD, CD, and ASPD. We also raise the issue of how to decide whether patterns of aberrant emotion and behavior lie properly in the domain of psychopathology or mental disorder, with particular emphasis on juvenile aggressive and antisocial patterns, which present difficult problems with respect to such decisions.

Brief Historical Overview

Children and Adolescents

Some of the earliest applications of multivariate statistical analysis to child psychopathology helped to establish the psychometric viability of aggressive and ASB patterns in children and adolescents as key dimensions (e.g., Hewitt & Jenkins, 1946). This work also began the tradition of subtyping this domain, as youngsters' social bonds and types of antisocial activities formed the basis of two discrete dimensions: (1) "undersocialized," marked by assaultive, aggressive behaviors that were typically committed alone; and (2) "socialized" or "group-delinquent," characterized by the presence of social connections and by covert as well as overt antisocial activity. This empirical distinction has continued to receive internal and external validation. Indeed, so-called "socialized" delinquency—which may be evidenced by gang membership—is typically marked by fewer indicators of psychopathological functioning and a better long-term course than the "undersocialized" variant (Quay, 1987). Accordingly, much of the psychological and psychiatric literature on aggression in childhood and adolescence has focused on youngsters who display an undersocialized pattern of ASB. Indeed, as we discuss later, the undersocialized group is similar in most respects to subgroups defined by early age of onset.

In the landmark 1980 publication of DSM-III (American Psychiatric Association, 1980), which revolutionized psychiatric nosology in the United States through its neo-Kraepelinian orientation, CD received "operational" criteria for the first time, which incorporated a number of severe overt and covert manifestations of ASB. Because only one constituent action, displayed over long time periods, was necessary for a diagnosis, inflated prevalence rates were a potential problem. DSM-III also listed four subcategories of CD, corresponding to the cells of a 2 × 2 matrix of (1) socialized versus undersocialized and (2) aggressive versus nonaggressive dimensions. The reliability of classification into these subtypes was poor, however, largely because of the confounding of the two components (e.g., few undersocialized–nonaggressive youngsters were found).

In DSM-III-R (American Psychiatric Association, 1987), the number of symptoms required for a diagnosis of CD was increased to 3 (from a list of 13), with each needing to be displayed for at least 6 months. This raising of the threshold reflected the established finding that the diversity (rather than any particular form) of antisocial activity—committed at early ages—best predicts chronic antisocial functioning and recidivism in adolescence and adulthood (e.g., Robins, 1966; Stattin & Magnusson, 1989). Furthermore, the subtyping scheme was simplified to the following: (1) a group (or socialized) type; (2) a solitary, aggressive subcategory; and (3) an undifferentiated type with mixed features.

With regard to milder forms of ASB, DSM-III included, for the first time, a variant of CD termed "oppositional disorder." The intention behind this category was to capture early manifestations of aggression/ASB that are exhibited in early to middle childhood. The constituent symptoms were irritable, stubborn, and defiant behavioral features, displayed at rates considered deviant developmentally. Because of the ubiquity of such behavioral features in young children, however, along with marginal reliabilities in empirical investigations, considerable doubt was raised as to the viability of this category (Rey et al., 1988). The revision in DSM-III-R—with the name changed to ODD—included nine behavioral symptoms, five of which were necessary for diagnosis. In our consideration of developmental trajectories related to ASB, we consider whether ODD constitutes a valid diagnostic category (e.g., Achenbach, 1993; Loeber, Lahey, & Thomas, 1991).

Adults

Regarding adult manifestations of chronic ASB, a sizable literature has appeared over the years with respect to so-called "psychopathy" or "sociopathy," signified by a manipulative, exploitive, predatory lifestyle (see Cleckley, 1976; Hart & Hare, 1997). Psychopathy has been the subject of considerable research regarding its psychodynamic, familial, and psychobiological underpinnings, with early socialization practices as well as the potential for impaired avoidance conditioning and diminished response to punishment implicated as key mechanisms for this disorder (see the review by Sutker, 1994).

In DSM-III (American Psychiatric Association, 1980), Axis II personality disorders were presented for the first time, with the goal of operationalizing chronic, maladaptive traits that yield substantial impairment. Reflecting the DSM's adherence to non-etiology-oriented operational criteria, the new category of ASPD borrowed heavily from the formulations of Robins (1966, 1978), who eschewed inferences of internal psychological processes and instead advocated a set of behavioral indicators of chronic antisocial functioning in adulthood. Many of the psychological and interpersonal hallmarks of psychopathy per se (e.g., callousness, manipulativeness, charm, deceitfulness, superficiality) were ignored in favor of multiple indicators of a persistent antisocial lifestyle (e.g., inconsistent work behavior, lack of monogamous relationships, aggression, multiple offenses). In addition, the diagnosis of ASPD in DSM-III and DSM-III-R has mandated the presence of CD in childhood or adolescence. Thus, by definition, the display of antisocial patterns beginning early in development is considered a necessary precondition for ASPD. This requirement has continued in DSM-IV, as discussed below.

The exclusively behavioral focus of the ASPD criteria was criticized by Hare, Hart, and Harpur (1991), who contend that psychopathy comprises key psychological and interpersonal features (e.g., callousness and manipulation as well as shallow, nonempathic affect). Indeed, their position is that ASPD definitions run the risk of labeling repetitive criminality as a form of personality disorder, with pertinent psychological and interpersonal features ignored in the diagnostic criteria. In defense of their position, psychopathy per se has been found to constitute a discrete taxon, as noted above, whereas repetitive criminality in adulthood appears to fit a dimensional characterization (Harris et al., 1994). Investigation of the developmental roots of adult antisocial functioning, however characterized, is crucial.

TABLE 3.1. DSM-IV Diagnostic Criteria for Oppositional Defiant Disorder (ODD)

A. A pattern of negativistic, hostile, and defiant behavior lasting at least 6 months, during which four (or more) of the following are present:

(1) often loses temper
(2) often argues with adults
(3) often actively defies or refuses to comply with adults' requests or rules
(4) often deliberately annoys people
(5) often blames others for his or her mistakes or misbehavior
(6) is often touchy or easily annoyed by others
(7) is often angry or resentful
(8) is often spiteful or vindictive

Note. Consider a criterion met only if the behavior occurs more frequently than is typically observed in individuals of comparable age and developmental level.

B. The disturbance in behavior causes significant impairment in social, academic, or occupational functioning.

C. The behaviors do not occur exclusively during the course of a Psychotic or Mood Disorder.

D. Criteria are not met for Conduct Disorder and, if the individual is age 18 years or older, criteria are not met for Antisocial Personality Disorder.

Note. From American Psychiatric Association (1994, pp. 93–94).

Current Definitions of ODD and CD

The DSM-IV definitional criteria for ODD are presented in Table 3.1, and the criteria for CD are listed in Table 3.2. As can be seen, ODD requires four of eight indicators of hostile, defiant, negativistic, and irritable behaviors for a duration of at least 6 months, which must be present at levels considered developmentally extreme and impairing. A diagnosis of CD mandates 3 of 15 examples of more serious overt and covert antisocial behaviors, with personal and social impairment required. Thus, compared to DSM-III-R, the symptom list was decreased by one for ODD and increased by two for CD. Several themes and issues regarding the definitions of these taxa bear discussion.

Developmental Norms

As reviewed by Coie and Dodge (1998), oppositional and defiant symptoms are relatively common during the preschool years; this means that it would take an extremely high level (and severity) of such patterns, in comparison with age and sex norms, to warrant diagnosis. The typical developmental course, in fact, is for such difficul-

TABLE 3.2. DSM-IV Criteria for Conduct Disorder (CD)

A. A repetitive and persistent pattern of behavior in which the basic rights of others or major age-appropriate societal norms or rules are violated, as manifested by the presence of three (or more) of the following criteria in the past 12 months, with at least one criterion present in the past 6 months:

Aggression to people and animals

(1) often bullies, threatens, or intimidates others
(2) often initiates physical fights
(3) has used a weapon that can cause serious physical harm to others (e.g., a bat, brick, broken bottle, knife, gun)
(4) has been physically cruel to people
(5) has been physically cruel to animals
(6) has stolen while confronting a victim (e.g., mugging, purse snatching, extortion, armed robbery)
(7) has forced someone into sexual activity

Destruction of property

(8) has deliberately engaged in fire setting with the intention of causing serious damage
(9) has deliberately destroyed others' property (other than by fire setting)

Deceitfulness or theft

(10) has broken into someone else's house, building, or car
(11) often lies to obtain goods or favors or to avoid obligations (i.e., "cons" others)
(12) has stolen items of nontrivial value without confronting a victim (e.g., shoplifting, but without breaking and entering; forgery)

Serious violations of rules

(13) often stays out at night despite parental prohibitions, beginning before age 13 years
(14) has run away from home overnight at least twice while living in parental or parental surrogate home (or once without returning for a lengthy period)
(15) often truant from school, beginning before age 13 years

B. The disturbance in behavior causes clinically significant impairment in social, academic, or occupational functioning.

C. If the individual is age 18 years or older, criteria are not met for Antisocial Personality Disorder.

Specify type based on age at onset:

Childhood-Onset Type: onset of at least one criterion characteristic of Conduct Disorder prior to age 10 years

Adolescent-Onset Type: absence of any criteria characteristic of Conduct Disorder prior to age 10 years

Specify severity:

Mild: few if any conduct problems in excess of those required to make the diagnosis and conduct problems cause only minor harm to others

Moderate: number of conduct problems and effect on others intermediate between "mild" and "severe"

Severe: many conduct problems in excess of those required to make the diagnosis or conduct problems cause considerable harm to others

Note. From American Psychiatric Association (1994, pp. 90–91). Copyright 1994 by the American Psychiatric Association. Reprinted by permission.

ties with stubbornness, tantrums, defiance, and the like to attenuate by middle childhood. For those children who do not display the usual age-related declines, and particularly for the subgroup who "diversify" into more frankly aggressive behavior as well, the ODD diagnostic category appears warranted.

As for CD, the types of seriously aggressive and antisocial actions in the symptom list are not normative during childhood. Preadolescents who begin to display such actions are therefore a group for whom clinical concern is deserved. Yet sharp increases in the prevalence of multiple forms of delinquent activity can be observed in early to middle adolescence (see review in Coie & Dodge, 1998), with a particularly steep rise for girls. Furthermore, the covert actions from the CD symptom list show clear increases, even in normative samples, through adolescence (Loeber & Hay, 1997).

Viability of the Categories

A key means of appraising the validity of ODD and CD is to appraise their distinctiveness from other behavioral syndromes. As discussed earlier, ODD and CD display such divergent validity from ADHD, whether the domains are considered dimensionally or categorically (e.g., Fergusson et al., 1991; Hinshaw, 1987; Jensen et al., 1997). In brief, ADHD is frequently associated with "individual" risk factors (difficult temperament, cognitive deficits), whereas aggressive-spectrum disorders are embedded in environmental/contextual risks such as discordant family interactions, harsh or inconsistent discipline, and impoverished neighborhoods (e.g., Hinshaw, 1992; Patterson, Reid, & Dishion, 1992). Yet these behavioral patterns frequently overlap, as do some of their risk factors (Hinshaw, 1987; Jensen et al., 1997; Waschbusch, 2002), and the theoretical and empirical importance of their co-occurrence bears much closer scrutiny in the subsequent section on comorbidity. With respect to predictive validity, it is clear that diverse aggressive and antisocial activities with an early onset strongly predict persistent ASB as well as myriad adjustment difficulties (e.g., Robins, 1966; Stattin & Magnusson, 1989; Zoccolillo, Pickles, Quinton, & Rutter, 1992; Rutter et al., 1998).

Another means of validation is to examine whether clear impairment accrues to the behavioral symptomatology. That is, we may ask (1) whether the constituent behavioral features of ODD and CD yield clear evidence of dysfunction in school, at home, and in interpersonal relationships; and (2) whether any evidence exists for discontinuous levels of such impairment above the diagnostic thresholds. In regard to point 1, the disruption, pain, and even tragedy resulting from CD-like behavior patterns are clear, as violence and property destruction may take a considerable toll on individuals, families, and communities at large. Furthermore, nonaggressive aspects of CD (e.g., theft, truancy) can yield considerable harm to the self and to others as well. Indeed, youths with CD are at substantial risk for peer rejection, academic failure, and a persistent course, attesting to the virulence of the syndrome (Rutter et al., 1998; Patterson et al., 1992). As for point 2, however, whereas the field trials for DSM-IV confirmed that three or more constituent symptoms of CD are associated with marked impairment, it is not clear that a true discontinuity with respect to external criteria exists at or above any given threshold of the defining behaviors (e.g., Robins & McEvoy, 1990). In short, the viability of categorical notions of CD that are based on the number of constituent symptoms is not at all assured, whereas the subdivision of this category on the basis of age of onset has more potential to yield a qualitative distinction (see subsequent discussion).

To an even greater extent, the validity of ODD as a diagnostic entity is an unresolved issue (see Loeber et al., 2000). Unlike most of the actions subsumed under the CD criteria, which involve severe manifestations of overt and covert behaviors, the constituent symptoms of ODD are clearly in the realm of normal developmental actions, particularly for children of preschool ages and again during adolescence (Coie & Dodge, 1998; Loeber et al., 2000). Furthermore, as we take pains to elaborate in the subsequent section on developmental progressions, the majority of youngsters reliably diagnosed with ODD in childhood will *not* progress to the more serious manifestations of CD. Yet, if a child's initial diagnosis must await display of the severe list of CD symptoms, intervention efforts may be unduly delayed (Loeber et al., 1991), particularly given evidence that the pathways to serious ASB often involve high levels of opposition and defiance earlier in development (Loeber, Wung, et al., 1993). As a result, debate regarding the appropriateness of this category in formal nosologies has continued for well over a decade (Achenbach, 1993; Loeber, Keenan, Lahey, Green, & Thomas, 1993; Lahey, Loeber, Quay, Frick, & Grimm, 1997). Lahey et al. (1997) concluded that ODD might well be considered a developmental precursor to CD—in other words, that ODD is basically a less severe variant of CD—but ODD does not inevitably portend CD, and some cases of CD do not originate with ODD patterns, constraining such a classification. We note, as well, that popular-press critiques of diagnostic systems like DSM-IV have featured ODD as a prime example of the overmedicalization of normal-range behavior (e.g., Kirk & Hutchins, 1994). Resolution of this issue will not come easily.

In sum, the coherence and distinctiveness of ASB patterns have been recognized for decades in the field of child psychopathology. The divergent validity of these patterns from ADHD has clearly been established, despite considerable overlap or comorbidity in actual samples; and diverse forms of ASB emerging early in development are highly predictive of a persistent course. It is still unclear, however, whether current symptom cutoff scores yield truly discontinuous categories, and the viability of ODD in particular is hotly debated. We turn now to additional issues raised by the categories of ODD and CD.

Admixture of Overt and Covert Symptomatology

Examination of Table 3.2 reveals clearly that a combination of overt and covert features is included in the diagnostic criteria for CD. Indeed, the subheadings for the criterion list highlight the disparate symptomatology among the 15 behavioral indicators of this category. As noted by Achenbach (1993), as well as other investigators, this diverse listing—combined with the requirement of only 3 of the 15 symptoms for diagnosis—means that some youngsters with CD will have exclusively covert problems, some others will show only overt aggression, and still others will have mixed symptomatology. This state of affairs guarantees the heterogeneity of the diagnosis; indeed, samples of youngsters diagnosed with CD may well contain fundamentally disparate subgroups in terms of symptom presentation. Because of the separability and discriminant validity of overt and covert dimensions, we reiterate a point made in the first edition of this chapter (Hinshaw & Anderson, 1996) that the field would be well served by investigations that identify the explicit types of behavioral symptoms characterizing CD samples.

Social/Environmental Context

In psychiatric nosologies, the locus of deviant behavior is by definition intraindividual. As a result, the clear roles of poverty, traumatic stress, and violent communities in fostering ASB may be greatly underappreciated. To counter the overascription of all aggressive/antisocial activity to individual psychopathology, DSM-IV has incorporated the following wording regarding the diagnosis of CD (American Psychiatric Association, 1994, p. 88):

> Concerns have been raised that the Conduct Disorder diagnosis may at times be misapplied to individuals in settings where patterns of undesirable behavior are sometimes viewed as protective (e.g., threatening, impoverished, high-crime) . . . the Conduct Disorder diagnosis should be applied only when the behavior in question is symptomatic of an underlying dysfunction within the individual and not simply a reaction to the immediate social context. Moreover, immigrant youth from war-ravaged countries who have a history of aggressive behaviors that may have been necessary for their survival in that context would not necessarily warrant a diagnosis of Conduct Disorder. It may be helpful for the clinician to consider the social and economic context in which the undesirable behaviors have occurred.

Although these words convey a crucial point, we hasten to add that the clinical realities of severe ASB are complex, without clear demarcations of contextual versus intraindividual locus of the behavior patterns. Who can determine, for example, that an aggressive or antisocial lifestyle fostered by exposure to violence-prone environments is purely a "reaction" to such settings, as opposed to an internalized, pervasive way of life that now threatens others? Or that some children exposed to violent neighborhoods have not also suffered from a host of individual and family risk factors as well? Or that genetic mediation could explain some (but certainly not all) of the prediction to later ASB among children who live with abusive parents? A pointed example of the ambiguity inherent in the "environmental reaction" versus "intraindividual pathology" perspectives is found in the provocative portrayal of mob boss John Gotti by Richters and Cicchetti (1993). Although Gotti developed and acted in a subculture that clearly sanctioned extremes of aggression and violence, he appeared to display severe psychopathy as well, with a long history of brutality that transcended even his prescribed and chosen environment. Deviant behavior is multidetermined and transactional, with no clear separation of cultural, environmental, or intraindividual causal factors at the level of the individual case.

Mental Dysfunction or Disorder?

Along this line, what are the criteria that should be invoked to decide that a certain individual suffers from psychopathology or a mental disorder? This issue has received close scrutiny by nosologists and critics alike. The perspective of Wakefield (1992, 1999) has been heuristic for the field. Not satisfied with the often-utilized criteria of social deviance, personal distress, psychological handicap, and the like for defining mental disorder—standards that are too prone to cultural variation and that may not reflect actual psychopathology—Wakefield has invoked the dual-criterion set of "harmful dysfunction" to characterize mental disorder per se. First, the deviant behavioral or emotional pattern must yield actual harm, in the form of meaningful suffering or impairment. Clearly, this criterion is admittedly context-dependent, as "harm" may be variously defined across cultures or subcultures. Second, however, the pattern must also be dysfunctional, in the sense of exemplifying aberrations in the abilities of mental mechanisms to perform natural functions, with the latter defined as having been selected by evolution for the good of the species. Through this latter criterion, Wakefield (1992, 1999) is attempting to transcend arbitrary, cultural definitions of deviance and posit underlying dysfunction in evolutionary terminology.

Few would doubt the clear harm yielded by conduct-disordered behavior patterns (and by severe manifestations of oppositional defiant patterns), at least as defined by most cultures. As noted earlier, physical and sexual assault, property destruction, fire setting, and stealing are inherently harmful, engendering understandable fear. Yet what of the dysfunction criterion? The evidence, in fact, suggests rather strongly that the majority of ASB is committed by individuals during adolescence, who lack childhood histories of cognitive dysfunction, ADHD symptoms, or serious family discord that would indicate intra-individual dysfunction (e.g., Moffitt, 1993). Only a relatively rare type of antisocial youngster—marked by early aggression and, nearly always, by severely impulsive and hyperactive behavior patterns and neuropsychological deficits early in development—may actually display the kinds of dysfunctions of mental mechanisms that would yield evidence for mental disorder. But even here, can it be unequivocally asserted that such early childhood problems (e.g., somewhat subaverage cognitive abilities, mild neuropsychological deficits, patterns of insecure attachments) are actually dysfunctional in the sense of reflecting aberrations in mental processes selected by evolutionary forces (Lilienfeld & Marino, 1999)? Or are such patterns perhaps reflective of a poor fit with current environmental contingencies, which differ substantially from those in the environment of evolutionary adaptation? In other words, the use of naturally selected mechanisms as the key criterion for defining mental disorder leads to difficult and probably untestable scientific problems, and the lack of consensus regarding these issues casts doubt on the viability of Wakefield's authoritative guide for deciding what is and what is not mental disorder (e.g., Richters & Hinshaw, 1999).

Despite the thorny philosophical, scientific, and evolutionary issues involved in deciding on the boundaries of mental disorder, consensus has emerged that defining subtypes of CD on the basis of age of onset (and persistence of symptomatology) may reveal fundamentally disparate types of youngsters. The importance of the age-of-onset variable mandates specific discussion of this means of subdividing the diagnosis. Indeed, the only officially recognized subcategorizaton of CD in DSM-IV is made on the basis of the timing of the onset of core symptomatology.

Subtypes of CD Defined by Age of Onset

The DSM-IV criteria include childhood-onset and adolescent-onset subtypes of CD, with the difference relating to the presence of at least one constituent symptom prior to the age of 10 years. The rationale for this bifurcation can be traced in large measure to the work of Moffitt (1993), Loeber (1988), and Patterson (1993; Patterson, DeBaryshe, & Ramsey, 1989), all of whom have formulated parallel conceptions of early-onset or "early-starter" models of ASB and CD.

To present a capsule perspective, we cite Moffitt's (1993) description of the puzzling nature of the literature on ASB and delinquency—in particular, the troubling inconsistency in findings related to causal factors, correlates, underlying mechanisms, and response to intervention. Her key contention is that such confusion stems largely from the confounding of two subgroups in most cross-sectional investigations of adolescent functioning: (1) a relatively small subgroup of youngsters (predominantly boys) with onset of aggressive behavior in childhood, who are at high risk for display of a persistent course of antisocial activity that unfolds and expands with development; and (2) a far larger category of youths (including a far higher proportion of girls) for whom forays into antisocial activity begin in adolescence and are relatively time-limited. Importantly, the former group is characterized by several features that suggest chronic psychopathology: high levels of ADHD symptoms, neuropsychological deficits, problems with academic underachievement, family members within the antisocial spectrum, discordant family interaction patterns (including histories of insecure attachment as well as overly punitive parenting practices), and a high likelihood of escalation into physically aggressive and violent actions. Because this group with early-onset ASB accounts for a disproportionate percentage of illegal antisocial acts and is quite likely to persist in ASB across the life span, Moffitt's term for this subgroup is "life-course-persistent." Note, however, that in the research of Moffitt and colleagues, this subgroup is predefined as having not only early onset but also persistence of ASB throughout childhood, and in some reports into adolescence (e.g., Moffitt & Caspi, 2001; Moffitt et al., 2002; Moffitt, Caspi, Dickson, Silva, & Stanton, 1996). In practice, of course, a clinician or investigator needs to make a diagnosis immediately, without the luxury of waiting for longitudinal follow-up. A key question, then, is whether all early-onset antisocial activity (plus the additional intraindividual and familial risk factors that presumably go along with such early onset) will escalate into violence and continuing ASB.

Youngsters with adolescent-onset ASB, on the other hand, do not evidence the signs of psychopathology characteristic of their peers with the early-onset type (Moffitt & Caspi, 2001). Crucially, although they display significant rates of antisocial activity during adolescence, their behavioral profiles are not nearly so likely to include violent offending. Moffitt (1993) invokes the concept of social mimicry to explain the onset of ASB in such otherwise "normal" youths. That is, because of the ever-increasing gap between biological maturity and the opportunity for full psychological and educational independence in modern society, with puberty emerging earlier but the need for higher education becoming more important than previously, many adolescents mimic the antisocial actions of early-onset youngsters in an attempt to gain prestige and desired commodities (e.g., sexual partners, money, status).

The upshot is that unless investigators and policy makers differentiate these subgroups, little progress will be made in efforts to understand, predict, and treat juvenile ASB, because youngsters with two fundamentally different types of ASB will be lumped together. Several other points are salient:

1. The specific age-of-onset criterion in DSM-IV (i.e., one CD symptom prior to the age of 10 years) is arbitrary, often difficult to discern from retrospective accounts, and of unknown validity for females with aggressive behavior patterns (see the later section on sex differences)

2. To the extent that the age-of-onset variable is valid, it may well be a more parsimonious subtyping scheme than the socialized–undersocialized and aggressive–nonaggressive designations from DSM-III, in that the clear majority of early-onset CD is both undersocialized and aggressive (Hinshaw et al., 1993). Thus the current DSM-IV subtyping algorithm may be a viable, and simpler, replacement for the prior subcategorizations.

3. Empirical data from the past few years provide a rather complex picture of the validity of these two key subgroups. Indeed, investigations suggest strongly that (a) early onset of ASB does not always portend life course persistence (i.e., a relatively high percentage of those with early-onset ASB may desist later; see Nagin & Tremblay, 1999; Rutter et al., 1998); (b) youths with adolescent-onset ASB may still display noteworthy difficulties in young adulthood (see Moffitt et al., 2002); and (c) a small subgroup of individuals do not display noteworthy ASB until young adulthood. Furthermore, the viability of the age-of-onset distinction may depend on the clinic-referred versus community nature of the samples under investigation (Lahey et al., 1998). In our subsequent discussion of developmental progressions, we take up such evidence in detail.

We note, in passing, that the 10th revision of the *International Classification of Diseases* (ICD-10; World Health Organization, 1992) has attempted reconciliation of its CD diagnosis with the DSM classification system; it includes a childhood- versus adolescent-onset subcategorization, similar to that of DSM-IV. Several additional subtypes are also listed: CD confined to the family context, unsocialized CD, socialized CD, and ODD.

Current Definition of ASPD

Although our focus herein is on child and adolescent ASB patterns, we mention briefly the DSM-IV (American Psychiatric Association, 1994) definition of ASPD. In contrast to the preceding editions of the American nosology (DSM-III and DSM-III-R; American Psychiatric Association, 1980, 1987), which defined ASPD almost exclusively in terms of ASB patterns (see earlier discussion), the DSM-IV definition began haltingly to integrate conceptions of psychopathy (Cleckley, 1976; Sutker, 1994) and psychopathic personality disorder (see Hare et al., 1991) with the behavioral indicators of antisocial activity (see Table 3.3). As can be seen, several indicators of psychological and interpersonal features are now displayed in the symptom list (e.g., deceitfulness, lack of remorse, impulsivity), supplementing the patterns of ASB, nonconformity, and aggression that predominated in the DSM-III and DSM-III-R conceptions of ASPD. DSM-IV marks a step toward integration of the personological/interpersonal and the more behavioral definitions that have competed in recent decades, although without the explicit separation of these two subdomains, as is done in the two-factor model of Hare and colleagues. Accordingly, this category guarantees that there will be confounding of interpersonal and affective symptoms with those of a more behavioral/antisocial nature in the DSM-IV nosology.

TABLE 3.3. DSM-IV Diagnostic Criteria for Antisocial Personality Disorder (ASPD)

A. There is a pervasive pattern of disregard for and violation of the rights of others occurring since age 15 years, as indicated by three (or more) of the following:
   (1) failure to conform to social norms with respect to lawful behaviors as indicated by repeatedly performing acts that are grounds for arrest
   (2) deceitfulness, as indicated by repeated lying, use of aliases, or conning others for personal profit or pleasure
   (3) impulsivity or failure to plan ahead
   (4) irritability and aggressiveness, as indicated by repeated physical fights and assaults
   (5) reckless disregard for safety of self or others
   (6) consistent irresponsibility, as indicated by repeated failure to sustain consistent work behavior or honor financial obligations
   (7) lack of remorse, as indicated by being indifferent to or rationalizing having hurt, mistreated, or stolen from another

B. The individual is at least age 18 years.

C. There is evidence of Conduct Disorder with onset before age 15 years.

D. The occurrence of antisocial behavior is not exclusively during the course of Schizophrenia or a Manic Episode.

Note. From American Psychiatric Association (1994, pp. 649–650).

PREVALENCE

Consideration of prevalence estimates for ODD and CD must immediately be qualified by several important considerations. First, definitions of these disorders have changed at a fast rate over the past two decades. Indeed, as discussed earlier, oppositional disorder was first introduced as a diagnostic category in 1980 (DSM-III), with its name changed to ODD and other changes made in 1987 (DSM-III-R), and the diagnosis further modified in 1994 (DSM-IV); the definition of CD was made significantly more stringent in DSM-III-R, with additional modifications in DSM-IV. Not only are American epidemiological data with respect to the current definitional criteria relatively sparse, given that a national-level investigation of the incidence and prevalence of child mental disorders has not been undertaken, but estimates of prevalence are highly dependent on the particular definitional criteria and particular samples that are utilized (Lahey, Miller, Gordon, & Riley, 1999). Second, given developmental progressions with and between ODD and CD (see the next section), the rates of adolescents meeting diagnostic criteria in any single cross-sectional evaluation may be misleading. Along this line, it is crucial to specify the ages of onset in samples or populations of aggressive or conduct-disordered youths. Yet, in the absence of prospective investigations of representative samples that begin at early ages, reports that rely on retrospective recall of the age of onset are bound to be suspect. Third, as highlighted in our earlier discussion, categorical definitions of aggressive and ASB patterns may reflect rather arbitrary numbers of constituent symptoms. Thus, unless considerable efforts are made to index impairment that accrues to the disruptive behavior patterns, prevalence estimates may be misguided.

Overall, estimates of the prevalence of ODD have ranged widely—from under 1% to more than 20%, with a median prevalence estimate of about 3% (Lahey, Miller, et al., 1999). Prevalence estimates of CD among children and adolescents also range widely, from less than 1% to slightly over 10% (see, e.g., Lahey, Miller, et al., 1999; Zoccolillo, 1993). The DSM-IV cites rates of

6–16% for males and 2–9% for females (American Psychiatric Association, 1994), although developmental differences in prevalence are not emphasized. Indeed, varying definitional criteria and sampling methods heavily influence results. The well-executed investigation of Offord and colleagues in Canada uncovered an overall rate among children and adolescents aged 4–16 of 5.5% (8.1% for boys and 2.8% for girls), with DSM-III criteria defined by CBCL items serving as the operationalization of CD (Offord, Alder, & Boyle, 1986). Importantly, a majority of the youths diagnosed with CD had at least one additional psychiatric diagnosis, highlighting the widespread nature and the importance of comorbidity for this disorder. Substantial impairment characterizes most youngsters meeting criteria for CD, in peer-related, academic, family, and personal/psychological domains.

Key intraindividual and systemic factors appear to influence prevalence of CD. For instance, most reports find substantially lower rates in females than in males, particularly for children; yet by adolescence, the gender disparity abates markedly (Zoccolillo, 1993). Furthermore, inner-city life and its attendant insults to families and children (e.g., impoverishment) clearly increase the risk for CD (e.g., Rutter et al., 1974, 1998). In all, epidemiologists would do well to heed the advice of Costello and Angold (1993) regarding the importance of developmental perspectives on the epidemiology of disruptive behavior disorders. Clearly, CD is not a static clinical entity, as the next section details; the field must begin to incorporate notions of flux and of developmental pathways into future nosological efforts.

DEVELOPMENTAL PROGRESSIONS

Heterotypic Continuity

Students of the development of aggression and ASB must come to terms with two competing facts: (1) measures of these behaviors show considerable stability across the life span, with correlations across lengthy intervals approaching those for IQ (e.g., Olweus, 1979; Loeber, 1982; Farrington, 1992; Frick & Loney, 1999); but (2) the composition of antisocial activity changes markedly over the years (see, e.g., Cairns, Cairns, Neckerman, Ferguson, & Gariepy, 1989; Coie & Dodge, 1998). How can these seemingly disparate findings be reconciled?

Increasingly, developmental psychopathologists recognize that predictability and congruence across development are not necessarily synonymous with simple consistency or similarity. That is, developmental precursors may be related in systematic and meaningful ways to subsequent outcomes, even though the topographic patterns of behavior shift markedly with development. ASB or antisocial traits may therefore show moderate to strong stability over the course of development, but the surface manifestations of the underlying propensity will shift with growth, typically in terms of the accretion of new and more virulent forms of the behavior patterns across time. Patterson (1993) uses the term "chimera" to describe this phenomenon in relation to ASB, analogizing to the mythical creatures that grow new appendages on the core underlying frame. In short, the constituent behavior patterns change with development, but appear to do so in predictable and lawful ways (Patterson, Forgatch, Yoerger, & Stoolmiller, 1998). Such so-called "heterotypic continuity" is an important concept for the topic at hand.

More specifically, in individuals with strong antisocial tendencies, the argumentative and defiant behaviors of preschool and early childhood predate physical aggression and stealing in middle and late childhood and sexual assault, substance abuse, and/or concentrated property destruction in adolescence. Extending the developmental span, infant and toddler behavioral patterns of irritability, overactivity, and fussiness may be part of the same continuum, as may the chronic criminality and interpersonal callousness (as well as patterns of spousal or partner abuse) of antisocial adults. At a statistical level, the field can explore predictability: What is the magnitude of such relationships, in terms of correlating earlier patterns with later ones, if we assume that all are manifestations of an underlying antisocial propensity? Note that correlation coefficients, the usual means of portraying stability, describe the preservation of rank order of ASB across time; they index interindividual continuity (see Cairns, 1979, for a masterful analysis of the various definitions of the construct of continuity). But such correlations do not begin to tell the whole story. First, the rank order may be preserved, when at the same time the mean levels of ASB are decreasing with development (as is usually the case with overt aggression) or, in contrast, increasing (as may be the case with covert ASB or violence through adolescence). Second, most correlation coefficients are not corrected for measurement error in either the early or later markers of ASB; when they are, estimates of overall stability rise (see commentary in Moffitt & Caspi, 2001). Third, and crucially, there may well be individual differences in stability. In fact, the most stably aggressive persons tend to be those with the highest or the lowest baseline levels of aggression (Loeber & Hay, 1997). Omnibus correlations may mask these individual differences, which are of crucial importance for deciding which individual profiles of youthful ASB are likely to escalate or diminish (for additional information on person-centered approaches to psychopathology, see Bergman & Magnusson, 1997).

In addition, other concepts may help to illuminate developmental progressions. "Pathways"—defined as within-individual changes in the patterns of ASB—were initially explored by Loeber (1988). The first developmental pathway defined by Loeber was an Exclusive Substance Use path, involving progression from more accessible to "harder" substances, but not including aggression or covert activities other than drug use. The onset of substance use for youths following this trajectory is typically rather late, beyond childhood. Another path was a Nonaggressive (or covert) trajectory; a third was a pernicious Aggressive/Versatile pathway, involving early onset and linkages with ADHD, as well as escalation into increasing violence. It is noteworthy that all three paths were found to contribute to adolescent substance abuse, exemplifying "equifinality"—the presence of similar outcomes from disparate paths (Cicchetti & Rogosch, 1996).

Loeber, Wung, et al. (1993) have since proposed expanded versions of such pathways, with origins earlier in development. First, the Authority Conflict trajectory typically pertains to defiant, oppositional patterns that progress to more serious conflict with adults; the Overt path progresses from early fighting and overt aggression to assault; and the Covert pathway focuses on links between shoplifting and property defacement at earlier stages and more serious property crime later in development. Most pertinent to the ongoing discussion is that many antisocial youngsters do not stay in any one path, but tend to "expand" into multiple trajectories over time (see also Patterson, 1993). Furthermore, the validity and viability of pathway conceptualizations may well depend on subclassfications of youths with ASB. That is, the three-pathway model appears to be more valid for children and adolescents defined as persistent in their ASB than for those with more transient forays into such behavior patterns (Loeber, Keenan, & Zhang, 1997). In our subsequent discussion of etiological factors, we return to the complex ways in which developmental predictability, continuity, and discontinuity may be shaped by interactive and transactional processes (for discussion, see Campbell et al., 2000; Lahey, Waldman, & McBurnett, 1999; Maughan & Rutter, 1998; Rutter et al., 1998).

At this point, we first discuss the linkage between ODD in early to middle childhood and CD in late childhood and early adolescence. Evidence regarding such predictability is crucial for validating both the diagnostic category of ODD and the concept of a childhood-onset variant of CD. Second, we note briefly extant evidence for linkages between syndromes of ASB in childhood/adolescence and adult ASPD. We highlight, in addition, evidence for the predictability of ASB patterns from extremely early precursors in infancy or toddlerhood. In light of the rather descriptive focus of this discussion, we highlight that the material presented later on (1) comorbidity with other childhood emotional and behavioral disturbance and (2) risk factors and etiological formulations is necessary for a full understanding of developmental processes.

Developmental Trajectories: Progression from ODD to CD

We have noted earlier the ongoing debate regarding the viability of ODD as a diagnostic category. In the first place, important meta-analytic findings provide some corroboration of the ODD symptom complex (Frick et al., 1993; see also Loeber et al., 1991). As shown in Figure 3.1, the overt–covert continuum, described earlier in the section on definitions of ASB, is supplemented by an orthogonal destructive–nondestructive dimension. When these two dimensions of ASB are crossed, four quadrants of constituent behaviors emerge; the region defined by overt, nondestructive behaviors corresponds quite closely to the ODD symptom pattern in DSM-IV (e.g., argumentative, stubborn, defiant, angry). In terms of separability from other forms of ASB, then, and at least from a cross-situational perspective, the ODD behavioral complex has coherence.

Next, with regard to developmental timing, the behaviors characteristic of ODD emerge 2–3 years earlier than do CD symptoms (Loeber, Green, Lahey, Christ, & Frick, 1992; Lahey et al., 1997;

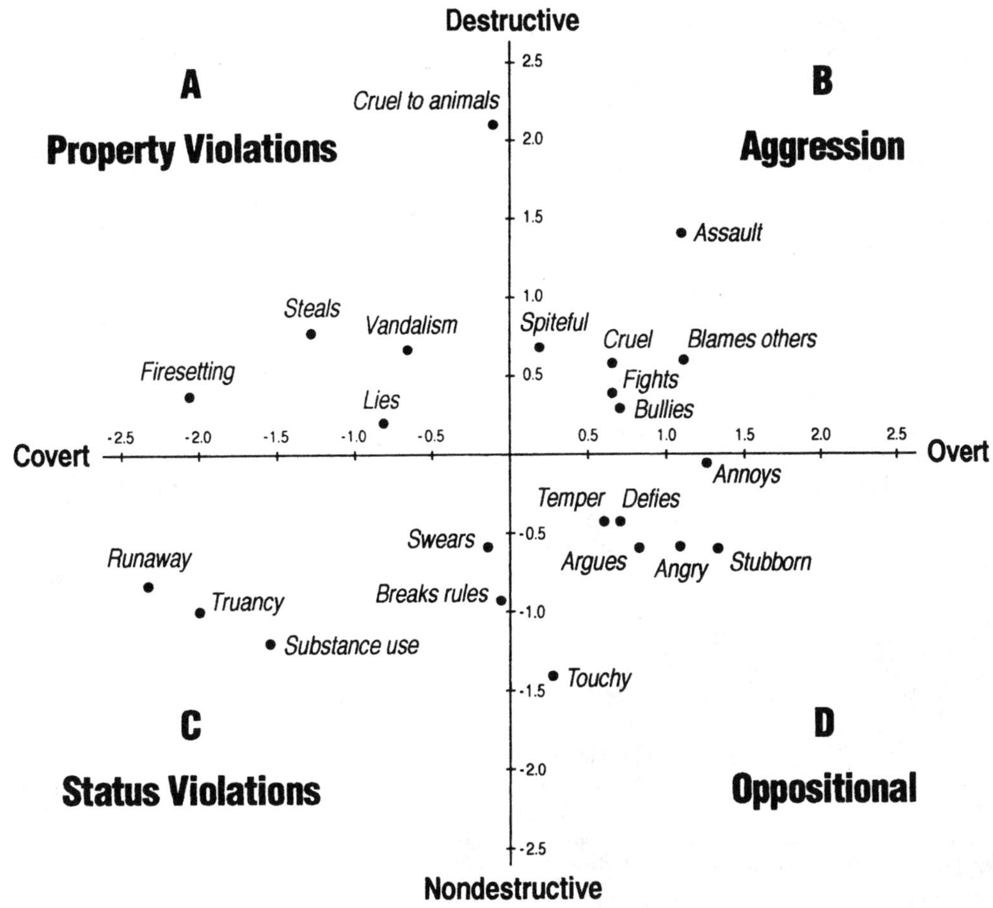

FIGURE 3.1. Results of meta-analysis of factor analyses of disruptive child behavior (see Frick et al., 1993). Copyright by Benjamin B. Lahey. Reprinted by permission.

Loeber & Farrington, 2000): The average age of onset for the former is approximately 6 years, compared to 9 years for CD behaviors. This finding provides circumstantial evidence that the ODD pattern could serve as a developmental precursor to CD (Loeber et al., 1991). Also, key risk factors (e.g., poverty, family history of antisocial activity) appear salient for the development of both ODD and CD, but the magnitude of association between such factors and these behavioral repertoires is stronger for CD than for ODD (Lahey et al., 1997; Loeber et al., 2000). The suggestion, once again, is that ODD serves as a milder (and presumably earlier) variant of CD.

All of this evidence, however, does not pertain directly to the predictive relationship between early ODD and subsequent CD. The Developmental Trends Study of Loeber, Lahey, and colleagues provides an important data base regarding this issue (e.g., Loeber, Keenan, et al., 1993). In this two-site sample of approximately 175 clinic-referred boys initially aged 7–12 years—recruited to reflect large proportions of disruptive and attention deficit disorders—newly developing cases of CD over the initial 3-year longitudinal interval were almost always preceded by ODD patterns earlier in development (Lahey, Loeber, Quay, Frick, & Grimm, 1992). In addition, children with the severe behavioral profile constituting CD typically "retained" many of the features of ODD that had emerged earlier in development. (Note that in DSM-IV, a diagnosis of CD supersedes a diagnosis of ODD in the diagnostic algorithm.) It therefore appears that a developmental sequence exists linking ODD in middle childhood with CD in late childhood or early adolescence. Yet the sensitivity of a measure or construct (the proportion of cases with the prior marker) is not equivalent to "positive predictive power" (PPP; the proportion of individuals with the predictor or marker who later become cases). Indeed, despite the strong sensitivity of the prediction to CD from ODD—that is, over 90% of youths with CD have previously met (and still retain) ODD criteria—the majority of youngsters with ODD do *not* appear to progress to the more severe constellation of ASB characterizing CD. That is, false-positive predictions predominate, lowering the PPP. In the Developmental Trends Study, for example, only about a quarter of the boys with ODD had developed CD by the initial 3-year follow-up interval, whereas approximately one-half maintained this diagnosis over the 3-year period but without progressing to CD, and a final quarter desisted from diagnostic criteria for ODD (see Hinshaw et al., 1993). Overall, the clear developmental progression from ODD to CD exists only for a minority of children with ODD—and this rate may actually be smaller in community than in clinical samples. Still unresolved, however, is the question of what other forms of diagnosis or impairment may pertain to those youngsters with early ODD who do not progress to CD.

Different scientists have formed divergent conclusions regarding such findings. Loeber et al. (1991) contend that such predictive validity signifies the importance of the ODD taxon; without this category, they claim, early manifestations of later CD would be missed, depriving the child, family, and community of important early intervention strategies. Waiting for a child to display the severe symptom constellation characterizing CD may well overlook, in early childhood, the oppositional defiant patterns that serve as a sensitive predictor. Yet, with a PPP of well under 50%, it is apparent that most youngsters with ODD will not develop CD; which indicates that early identification and/or treatment may be misguided, particularly if it leads to labeling of a child as inevitably "delinquent" or "criminal." This cautionary note would apply even more to designations of young children based on ODD symptoms.

In all, whereas CD is nearly universally preceded by ODD, in only a minority of cases does the latter symptom pattern predict the former. For a subgroup of youngsters, then, ODD appears to have heterotypic continuity with subsequent antisocial activity—signifying clear harm and possible dysfunction, in terms of the criterion set of Wakefield (1992, 1999). In most instances, however, ODD may signify an extreme of normal developmental variation, linked with important triggering factors (e.g., family discord, extremes of temperament), but transitory in nature and not portending escalation to a "toxic" course. Also salient is the age-normative rise in prevalence of ODD in adolescence, a period often marked by authority conflict and testing of limits. Highly needed is precise specification of those risk factors that propel certain cases of ODD toward a continuing antisocial trajectory (see Loeber, Green, Keenan, & Lahey, 1995; see also Caspi & Moffitt, 1995), as well as of the protective factors that aid in desistance (for theoretical accounts of risk and resilience, see Luthar, Cicchetti, & Becker, 2000). Finally, we note in passing that nearly all of the evidence cited in this section pertains to males. For females, it is possible that different predictive relationships hold across development (see the subsequent section on sex differences).

Progression to Adult ASPD

A parallel set of findings to those presented immediately above for relationships between ODD and CD appears to hold regarding the linkage between CD in childhood or adolescence and ASPD in adulthood. That is, (1) adults with ASPD have almost always met criteria for CD earlier in their development, signifying the extremely high sensitivity of the link between CD and ASPD; but (2) only a minority of youths with CD go on to develop the chronic ASB patterns characteristic of ASPD, highlighting the rather low PPP of the predictive relationship (see the reviews by Hinshaw, 1994, and Robins, 1978). The PPP ranges from about 25% to 40% (Robins, 1966; Zoccolillo et al., 1992). Importantly, if the adult outcome is broadened to include exclusive substance use, the predictive power increases significantly (Robins, 1991).

Several additional findings supplement these descriptive statistics. First, several variables increment the predictability of adult ASPD from childhood manifestations, including early onset of diverse aggressive and antisocial behaviors and persistence of symptomatology in childhood (Robins, 1978, 1991). A host of additional factors (academic underachievement, family variables, poverty, association with deviant peers) will receive additional attention subsequently. Second, the predictive relationship with the adult disorder appears to differ in females as opposed to males, as CD in girls is a strong predictor of later *internalizing* disorders and features as well as antisocial tendencies (Robins, 1986). Third, despite the rather low PPP statistics for predicting ASPD from CD, the clear majority of youths displaying CD will show substantial social and personal impairment in adulthood, even if full diagnostic criteria for ASPD are not met (Rutter et al., 1988; Zoccolillo et al., 1992). In other words, the lack of perfect prediction to adult ASPD should not lead to the conclusion that CD has a benign outcome in most cases. Fourth, the predictive relationships to adult antisocial personality dysfunction have been obtained almost exclusively with respect to the more behavioral conceptions of ASPD rather than to the psychological/interpersonal features of psychopathy, meaning that far less is known about the developmental roots of psychopathy per se. A growing literature has taken on the identification of the "fledgling psychopath" (Lynam, 1998), but no prospective data into adulthood are yet available on the predictive power of such childhood characteristics.

In sum, nearly all individuals meeting criteria for adult ASPD will have begun their antisocial activity earlier in development. Indeed, a requirement for the DSM-IV ASPD diagnosis is that the person must have met criteria for CD before the age of 15. Yet the predictive validity—like that for ODD-CD links—is far lower, on the order of one-third. Spanning the years from early childhood to adulthood, then, only a tenth or fewer of youngsters (calculated by multiplying the approximate rate of the ODD-CD linkage by the CD-ASPD progression rate) with ODD will progress to persistent adult manifestations of ASPD; those who do will almost inevitably have displayed the symptomatology of CD "en route." Also, there is a dearth of literature prospectively linking CD in childhood with ASPD or psychopathy in adulthood; prospective data are critically needed to help elucidate mechanisms underlying developmental links. Finally, although Robins (1978) has contended that the emergence of serious ASB de novo in adulthood is extremely rare (and is linked when it happens with the emergence of psychosis or other extremely severe psychopathology), there may be a small but important subgroup of adults who engage in antisocial activities without noteworthy childhood precursors (see Kratzer & Hodgins, 1999). Our childhood focus in this chapter precludes discussion of this important contention.

Viability of the Childhood-Onset and Adolescent-Onset Subtypes in Light of Recent Evidence

We have discussed earlier the crucial addition, in DSM-IV, of age of onset as a subtyping variable for the CD diagnosis, and the linkages of this subcategorization to the by now substantial empirical work of Moffitt (1993; Moffitt & Caspi, 2001), Loeber (1988; Loeber, Wung, et al., 1993), and Patterson (1993; Patterson et al., 1992). At this point, sufficient longitudinal data have been accumulated to provide initial evidence regarding the viability of this classification, with particular focus on two key questions: (1) Is the childhood-onset subtype truly psychopathological and/or "life-course persistent," and (2) is the adolescent-onset subtype truly "adolescence-limited"?

We have space for only a brief review. First, in terms of the Dunedin data base that provided the impetus for Moffitt's (1993) formulation, Moffitt and Caspi (2001) have demonstrated that the backgrounds of the subgroup whose ASB has been defined as childhood-onset and persistent through adolescence are substantially different from those of a subgroup defined in terms of adolescent onset of ASB. Specifically, neuropsychological, neurocognitive, familial, and temperamental variables are clearly more extreme in the former than in the latter, which typically does not show deviance compared with population norms. Crucially, such findings have been shown to be robust across several different cultures and nations (see review in Moffitt & Caspi, 2001). Thus, in terms of multiple indicators of serious psychopathology, the subgroup whose ASB has been defined as both early-onset and persistent with respect to aggression (the so-called "life-course-persistent" group) appears clearly impaired, whereas the subgroup with adolescent-onset ASB is not.

Second, and crucially, there should be no automatic assumption that children (especially boys, who are overrepresented in such groups) with early onset of aggression will automatically "progress" to a life-course-persistent path. Note that the life-course-persistent subtype of Moffitt and colleagues is defined on the basis of both early *and* persisting aggression and ASB; when ASB is defined solely on the basis of early onset, a substantial proportion of children desist by adolescence (Rutter et al., 1998). Indeed, even in the Dunedin sample, a group of "desisters" (tentatively called "recoveries") were identified by Moffitt et al. (1996), although further analyses revealed that the recovery in these cases was far from complete (see Moffitt et al., 2002). Furthermore, the careful, typological work of Nagin and Tremblay (1999) revealed that the *majority* of boys displaying high rates of physical aggression at age 6 "desisted" across the next decade of life. Although this group's rates of aggression at age 6 were high, the relatively small group of "persisters" (under 5% of the total population screened during kindergarten) had demonstrated even more severe levels of physical aggression during the initial assessment. It is almost certainly the case as well that looking beyond aggression per se in early childhood—to the constellation of neurobiological/neurocognitive, familial, and socioeconomic factors posited by Moffitt (1993; Moffitt & Caspi, 2001) to be linked specifically to a propensity toward life course persistence—will help to enhance the predictability from childhood through adolescence or adulthood. Indeed, Gorman-Smith, Tolan, Loeber, and Henry (1998) distinguished serious and chronic offenders from other subgroups of youths with ASB on the basis of multiple family problems and extreme deviance of family values and attitudes.

In addition, within several important population cohorts, a small subgroup of "low-level chronic" offenders has been noted. These individuals are defined on the basis of persistent, but low-base-rate, ASB from adolescence to adulthood (Nagin, Farrington, & Moffitt, 1995) or even from childhood onward (Fergusson, Horwood, & Nagin, 2000). The initial levels of ASB are low enough, however, that the children were not "flagged" as having early-onset ASB on the basis of severity alone.

Thus, given the presence of at least three subtypes of children (nearly exclusively boys) with early signs of ASB—"persisters," "desisters," and "low-level chronics," the typology of children displaying impairing aggression at an early age appears variegated. As we discuss later in the section on sex differences, extremely few girls with early-onset ASB have emerged in existing research. In addition, recent large-scale population data suggest that there may well be more "adult-starter" individuals with ASB and criminality (Kratzer & Hodgins, 1999) than was suggested by the widely cited formulations of Robins (1978).

As for the group with adolescent-onset ASB, the recent investigation by Moffitt et al. (2002), reporting on the progress of the Dunedin male population investigation up to age 26, is essential reading. Those participants defined as having adolescent-onset ASB (who were, it should be noted, matched with the early-onset/life-course-persistent group in terms of rates of offending during adolescence) were predicted to desist from ASB in early adulthood (see Moffitt, 1993), in keeping with their designation as adolescence-limited. However, in their mid-20s, this subgroup showed elevations (compared to the norm) on impulsivity, substance abuse and dependence, property crime, and mental health variables in addition to financial difficulties. Such findings challenge the use of the term "adolescence-limited" as applied to this subgroup. We hasten to reiterate that the subgroup with life-course-persistent ASB, defined as both early-onset and persistent through adolescence, had a far more virulent pattern of poor education, partner and child abuse, fighting and violence, psychopathic tendencies, and general life difficulties than did those with adolescent-onset ASB. Yet the current findings challenge the assumption that the life course of those with adolescent-onset ASB will be benign, given their continuing criminality (chiefly property crimes), mental health problems, poor employment histories, and substance use problems. As stated by Moffitt et al. (2002, p. 199), "Despite all this promise [referring to their nonpathological childhood histories], the [adolescence-limited] men at 26 were still in trouble" (see also Aguilar, Sroufe, Egeland, & Carlson, 2000; Kratzer & Hodgins, 1999; Rutter et al., 1998). It may be that offending in adolescence leads to "snares" and losses of opportunity that accumulate to yield serious consequences (see Caspi & Moffitt, 1995, and Moffitt, 1993, for elaboration of the sequelae of aggressive behavior that may propel a continuing course, even in the absence of early indicators of psychopathology). It is also possible, as articulated by Moffitt et al. (2002) that the poorer-than-expected outcomes of this subgroup at age 26 can be traced to the extended "maturity gap" present in modern Western societies (e.g., delays in ages of becoming parents), particularly in a nation like New Zealand with high unemployment. Only further follow-up will tell whether the participants with onset of ASB in adolescence finally desist in earnest by their early to mid-30s. In all, even without a virulent childhood history of psychopathology and early ASB, youths initiating delinquent actions in adolescence may have difficulty in suddenly desisting at the close of the teenage years.

(For additional reading on the timing of adolescent-onset delinquency in urban youths, see Tolan, Gorman-Smith, & Loeber, 2000.)

Additional Issues

Although we have been discussing the predictability of persistent ASB from childhood manifestations, it is also important to ask whether ASB can be predicted with any confidence from even earlier behavioral manifestations or risk tendencies. Although indices of difficult temperament in infancy appear to be only weakly correlated with later behavioral manifestations, and although sex differences in early temperament are not noteworthy (see the subsequent section on sex differences), Campbell and Ewing (1990) and White, Moffitt, Earls, Robins, and Silva (1990) have shown that extremes of early childhood problems can predict later hyperactive and antisocial tendencies at rates far above chance levels. Furthermore, Caspi, Henry, McGee, Moffitt, and Silva (1995) showed that temperamental features at age 3—particularly a dimension called "lack of control"—were a significant predictor of later antisocial tendencies (see also Henry, Caspi, Moffitt, & Silva, 1996; for a lucid summation of more general research on temperamental links to adult outcome, see Caspi, 2000). Although some might contend that temperament measured at age 3 is confounded with behavioral styles that are similar to the outcomes of interest, or in other words that the boundaries between "temperament" and "behavior" are fluid, the point is that predictability is an established fact (see Tremblay, Pihl, Vitaro, & Dobkin, 1994). At the level of individual cases, however, the predictability from early temperamental patterns is far from certain. As we highlight in the upcoming section on risk factors and etiological formulations, such developmental pathways typically involve multiple risks, including socioeconomic disadvantage, family adversity, victimization by abuse, achievement problems, neuropsychological deficits, and (later in development) a peer network that supports antisocial activity. Thus pathways to extremes of ASB are quite likely to include a multiplicity of interacting and transacting variables (Campbell, in press; Moffitt, 1993; Capaldi & Patterson, 1994), and there is no inevitability of high risk for ASB from early temperamental patterns.

Along this line, we encourage readers to examine three important research programs: (1) the studies by Shaw and colleagues (e.g., Shaw, Bell, & Gilliom, 2000; Shaw, Owens, Giovannelli, & Winslow, 2001), which pertain to very young children's risk for developing ASB; (2) the research of Campbell (e.g., Campbell, in press), which involves the investigation of 3- and 4-year-olds with severe ADHD and oppositionality; and (3) the studies by Speltz, DeKlyen, and Greenberg (e.g., Speltz, DeKlyen, & Greenberg, 1999; Speltz, Greenberg, & DeKlyen, 1990; DeKlyen & Speltz, 2001), which pertain to preschoolers with oppositional patterns. All three of these programs have examined the influences of multiple, interacting factors in relation to oppositional, aggressive, and hyperactive behavior patterns across development. With findings too numerous to recount herein, these research programs suggest strongly that the presence and interaction of intraindividual risk factors, including difficult temperament; family disharmony, incorporating insecure attachment and discordant parent–child interactions; and sociocultural risk, involving poverty and low social support, are most likely to propel the continuation, intensification, and chronicity of early aggressive behavior patterns into later childhood and adolescence.

Finally, what about the predictability of psychopathic traits and features from childhood indicators? The work of Lynam (e.g., 1998) suggests that the "fledgling psychopath" is likely to be a child (a boy, in most instances) with the constellation of ADHD symptomatology and early aggressive tendencies. Frick and colleagues, however (see Barry et al., 2000; Frick, Bodin, & Barry, 2000), contend that only the subset of such children who also display the constellation of emotional, interpersonal, and personality-related features termed "callous/unemotional" are at elevated risk for subsequent psychopathy. Wootton, Frick, Shelton, and Silverthorn (1997), for example, found that whereas most aggressive boys showed the expected associations between negative parenting practices and the severity of their ASB, the subgroup high on callous/unemotional traits actually showed *no* association between parenting practices and severity; these findings suggest that this subset of boys is relatively impervious to conditioning from parents. As noted earlier, however, only prospective follow-up of youths with such configurations of predictor variables in childhood into adulthood can confirm the predictability of psychopathic traits and functioning.

Conclusions

Although serious ASB is almost always preceded by earlier manifestations of aggression or oppositionality, only a minority of oppositional, defiant, and aggressive youths progress to diagnosable CD in adolescence. Similarly, despite the continuing interpersonal, academic, and personal adjustment problems of adolescents with CD, only a minority of youths with this disorder develop the adult manifestations of ASPD. Such information highlights the importance of identifying a subgroup of youngsters with early-onset ASB (who will also tend to display a constellation of individual, family, and neighborhood variables indicative of psychopathology), but prediction across development from such a group is plagued by overprediction to subsequent ASB. Nonetheless, adolescents and young adults with the most violent and virulent forms of ASB will have had histories from childhood; this relatively small subgroup (5% or fewer of the population) commits a highly disproportionate level of criminal acts. Despite the far larger numbers of youths with adolescent-onset ASB, and their typical absence of childhood indicators of psychopathology, recent longitudinal evidence suggests strongly that their difficulties may well extend beyond the adolescent period. Current perspectives point to the interaction of multiple risk factors in predicting extremes of antisocial activity later in life; a subgroup of children with (1) indicators of early ADHD and aggression plus (2) callous/unemotional traits may be at particular risk for psychopathic outcomes later in life. Finally, nearly all of the information presented in this section regarding developmental trajectories is available for male samples only; of crucial importance is examination of females with extremes of aggression and ASB (see the subsequent discussion of sex differences). Indeed, females with CD and delinquent tendencies appear to be at risk for a broad spectrum of internalizing as well as externalizing problems in adulthood.

COMORBIDITY

Although we have highlighted that the group of children at highest risk for persistent ASB appears to display both aggressive behavior and the symptoms of ADHD early in development, it would be wise to frame such associations in terms of the more general topic of "comorbidity." This term refers to a greater-than-chance rate of overlap between two or more independent disorders. Such overlap between conditions (or, dimensionally, this association between behavioral syndromes or dimensions) is receiving considerable attention in the field—in part because of evidence for widespread comorbidity across multiple childhood behavioral/emotional disorders, and in part because of the theoretical importance of such cross-domain linkages (Angold, Costello, & Erkanli, 1999; Caron & Rutter, 1991; Hinshaw et al., 1993; Jensen et al., 1997). Whereas a great deal of so-called comorbidity in child psychopathology may relate to (1) poor or ambiguous definitions of mental disorders[3] or (2) conflation of what are actually developmental progressions into the overlap of two independent conditions (Caron & Rutter, 1991; Lahey et al., 1997; Rutter et al., 1998), true comorbidity challenges univariate conceptions of the genesis of disorders, and investigation of comorbidity may help to uncover relevant developmental mechanisms of psychopathology. In the interests of space, we restrict our discussion of comorbidity to ADHD, academic underachievement/learning disabilities, and key internalizing disorders. Unfortunately, space limitations dictate that we bypass the important domain of comorbidity between conduct problems/CD and substance abuse/dependence, a key concern during adolescence. We highlight that recent reviews demonstrate reciprocal effects regarding this comorbidity, with aggressive behavior fueling substance abuse and dependence, as well as the converse (e.g., White, Loeber, Stouthamer-Loeber, & Farrington, 1999). Please refer also to Chassin, Ritter, Trim, and King, Chapter 4, this volume.

Before discussing substantive issues regarding comorbidity, we note briefly that any discussions of this topic are tied in with the clinic-referred versus representative nature of the samples involved. That is, with clinical samples, rates of comorbidity are spuriously inflated (Angold et al., 1999; Berkson, 1946; Caron & Rutter, 1991). The clear implication is that community samples are a prerequisite for accurate estimates of true comorbidity.

Attention-Deficit/Hyperactivity Disorder

When ADHD is considered dimensionally, scales of its constituent symptoms correlate significantly and at least moderately with counterpart dimensions of overt and covert antisocial actions

(Hinshaw, 1987; Quay, 1986). In particular, the hyperactivity–impulsivity subdimension of ADHD is more strongly associated with aggression and ASB than is the inattention dimension. When ADHD is viewed categorically, substantial overlap between it and either ODD or CD is apparent. Such association and degrees of overlap are not complete, however, and as noted earlier, there is clear evidence for a differential pattern of external correlates of these two domains (Hinshaw, 1987; Waschbush, 2002). Thus the preponderance of evidence supports the contention that ADHD and conduct problems/aggression are partially independent aspects of child and adolescent psychopathology.

Yet the association between these two areas of externalizing behavior is quite important for consideration of developmental patterns. First, the overlapping subgroup with conduct problems and ADHD displays a far more pernicious form of psychopathology than does either single-diagnosis category. Indeed, youngsters with both CD and ADHD display greater amounts of physical aggression, a greater range and greater persistence of antisocial activity, more severe academic underachievement, and higher rates of peer rejection (see Hinshaw, 1999). In addition, they tend to have parents with not only ADHD-related symptomatology but also high rates of maternal depression, paternal ASB, and substance abuse and dependence. Not surprisingly, the parent–child interactions in such family configurations are marked by coercion and discord (Patterson, DeGarmo, & Knutson, 2000). All of these factors have been shown to be strong predictors of negative outcomes in later life. Importantly, as demonstrated by Walker, Lahey, Hynd, and Frame (1987), such greater impairment accrues specifically to the comorbidity of CD with ADHD, and not to the overlap of CD with other symptom patterns.

Second, the conjoint presence of ADHD serves to propel an earlier onset of CD symptomatology (Hinshaw et al., 1993; Loeber et al., 1995; Rutter et al., 1998). In terms of mechanisms, one key possibility is that the strongly heritable, temperamentally difficult emotional and behavior patterns associated with ADHD (e.g., irritability, impulsivity, high activity level, sensation seeking) elicit negative reactions from the environment, with aggressive behavior highly likely to result from the resultant coercion and stress (Lahey et al., 1999; Patterson et al., 2000). Whatever the mechanism or mechanisms, the early onset of serious aggression continues to be the strongest predictor of the subsequent development of antisocial patterns in adolescence and adulthood, as emphasized repeatedly above. Indeed, Robins (1991) has shown that age at onset of CD symptomatology remains an independent predictor of APD in adulthood, even when the number and diversity of CD symptoms in childhood are controlled for statistically. Thus comorbidity of early aggression with ADHD is strongly associated with early onset of conduct problems, setting in motion a chain of interactions likely to lead to escalation and persistence.

Third, a crucial question is whether ADHD symptomatology is an independent predictor of subsequent ASB, or whether its apparent predictability is tied in chiefly with its high likelihood of association with aggression and conduct problems during childhood. The literature on this point is voluminous as well as contentious. Some of the first systematic follow-up investigations of "hyperactivity" (e.g., Satterfield, Hoppe, & Schell, 1982) contained evidence that this syndrome was a strong predictor of adolescent delinquency. Such reports did not, however, account for the potential overlap or comorbidity between ADHD-related symptomatology and aggression during childhood. With this confound accounted for, careful reviews concluded that childhood aggression and conduct problems were stronger predictors of later antisocial tendencies than were ADHD symptoms per se (Lilienfeld & Waldman, 1990). On the other hand, two key European investigations (Farrington, Loeber, & Van Kammen, 1990; Magnusson, 1987) demonstrated that dimensions of hyperactivity, impulsivity, and inattentiveness in childhood independently predicted antisocial outcomes in adulthood. In addition, with the Dunedin sample, Moffitt (1990) found that ADHD-related behavior patterns contributed independent variance to the prediction of adolescent delinquency, with early aggression partialed out. Furthermore, the American longitudinal investigation of Mannuzza et al. (1991) concluded that ADHD in childhood, in the absence of CD, still yielded a strong risk for substance abuse and antisocial disorders in young adulthood. It is conceivable, however, that this latter sample could have displayed ODD (or other forerunners of CD) in preadolescence and that the oppositional behavior patterns, rather than the attention deficits, presaged the later ASB. In fact, in a further follow-up of the Satterfield sample, it was found that that whereas childhood ADHD symptoms somewhat increased the later risk for delinquency, the childhood combination of ADHD and aggression yielded the strongest risk (Satterfield, Swanson, Schell, & Lee, 1994). A key recent review contends that ADHD is a risk factor largely, if not exclusively, through its association with early ODD in boys, but that ADHD could be an independent risk marker in girls (Lahey, McBurnett, & Loeber, 2000).

Whether ADHD in and of itself is a predictor, early ADHD in conjunction with early aggression is clearly a risk factor for a persistent, problem-laden course of ASB. Indeed, the bulk of recent research has pointed clearly to the conclusion that early ADHD features constitute a risk factor for such a negative course largely through their fueling of an early onset of conduct problems (see, e.g., Nagin & Tremblay, 1999; Loeber et al., 2000). Conceptually, it is unclear which aspect or aspects of ADHD symptomatology (inattention vs. overactivity, restlessness, impulsivity) constitute the risk mechanism, although impulse control problems and hyperactivity appear to be stronger candidates than inattention (Coie & Dodge, 1998). Regardless, the genetic, familial, peer-related, academic, cognitive, neuropsychological, and socioeconomic backgrounds of this comorbid subgroup set the stage for complex, interactional, and transactional models related to their high risk for later psychopathology. In terms of assessment, we note that because the externalizing behaviors are relatively difficult to disentangle during the preschool years, clinicians and investigators must use instruments that can separate ADHD from oppositional and aggressive symptoms early in development (see Hinshaw & Nigg, 1999; Hinshaw & Zupan, 1997).

Academic Underachievement/Learning Disabilities

Another important comorbid condition or associated dimension pertains to the domain of academic failure. For years, linkages between aggressive/delinquent behavior patterns and underachievement have been noted, but only in the past decade did key developmental manifestations of this important comorbidity become clarified. At the outset, we must note that many forms of academic failure and underachievement exist. Indeed, because such variables as grade retention, placement in special education, and suspension or expulsion follow rather directly from acting-out behavior patterns, we focus our attention on academic underachievement per se.

Hinshaw (1992) has presented an integrated account of the association between ASB and academic underachievement; in the interests of space, we highlight only the key conclusions herein (see also the thorough consideration of Maguin & Loeber, 1996). First, developmental shifts in this relationship are salient. In early to middle childhood, the specific association pertains to underachievment and ADHD, as opposed to underachievement and ODD or CD. Indeed, the apparent link between aggressive-spectrum disorders and learning failure before adolescence relates to the comorbidity of such disorders and ADHD (see Frick et al., 1991, for a clear empirical demonstration). By the teenage years, however, underachievement is clearly and specifically associated with delinquency and ASB patterns, signaling a developmental shift in the causal linkages. Second, unilateral, "main effect" models that aspire to account for the relationship between externalizing behavior problems and underachievement are usually oversimplifications. Whereas in some individuals early underachievement may predict later ASB (via demoralization, frustration, and the like), and whereas in others early aggression and defiance may precipitate learning failure (via poor classroom behavior, oppositional attitudes, etc.), the association between inattentive and aggressive behavior patterns on the one hand, and risk for school failure on the other, often appears quite early in development, prior to the start of formal schooling. This state of affairs strongly suggests that underlying "third variables"—for example, language deficits, socioeconomic disadvantage, or neurodevelopmental delay—require further exploration as mechanisms underlying the subsequent comorbidity (Hinshaw, 1992; Maguin & Loeber, 1996). In other words, the association between academic failure and ASB, is marked by a complex developmental trajectory, with an array of intraindividual and familial variables predating the formal comorbidity, and with ADHD-related symptomatology playing a key role in middle childhood.

Thus the effects of underachievement and ASB are likely to be reciprocally deterministic, "snowballing" across development. A child with subtle language deficits may have difficulty with the phonological processes necessary for mastery of reading; he or she may also have trouble comprehending parental requests, fueling the development of contentious relationships with caregivers and peers. In addition, ADHD symptomatology will interact negatively with both academic readiness and behavioral regulation. Over time, the early adolescent with poor academic preparation is increasingly likely to lose motivation for schooling and to form bonds with deviant, antisocial peers, intensifying his or her own aggression and ASB patterns. Recall, however, that differential trajectories appear salient for different subgroups: For some underachieving children, ASB may follow from learning failure without childhood signs of aggression (Maughan, Gray, & Rutter, 1985), whereas in most youths the comorbid pattern is evident early in development. Overall, in adolescence, virulent ASB is all too often associated with school failure and early termination from formal education, yielding another "snare" that may compromise ultimate adjustment. Appraising the academic aptitudes and skills of youths on the trajectory toward ASB is important clinically as well as conceptually.

Internalizing Disorders

Although internalizing conditions like anxiety disorders and depression may appear at first glance to be diametric opposites of such prototypically externalizing difficulties as ODD and CD, dimensional and categorical investigations reveal substantially above-chance rates of overlap for these two domains (see reviews of Rutter et al., 1998; Loeber & Keenan, 1994; and Zoccolillo, 1992). In the interests of space, we summarize recent directions.

First, with respect to anxiety disorders, contradictory findings have been evident regarding their linkages with ASB. As reviewed in the first edition of this chapter (Hinshaw & Anderson, 1996), data from the Developmental Trends Study revealed a puzzling finding—namely, that whereas the comorbidity of conduct problems with anxiety disorders appeared to predict a less intense and assaultive type of CD during initial assessments, over time the comorbid subgroup appeared to become more aggressive than youths with CD but without anxiety disorders (see also Hinshaw et al., 1993). Other investigations have been puzzling as well: In some, anxiety disorders appeared to serve as a protective factor with respect to outcomes for children with externalizing disorders, whereas in others, anxiety-related problems appeared to heighten the risk (see review in Rutter et al., 1998). Some resolution may be found in the important distinction within anxiety-related symptomatology between inhibition and fear on the one hand, and social withdrawal on the other. The former appears to be a protective factor with regard to both the presence of assaultive behavior and the intensification of ASB, whereas the presence of social isolation and withdrawal predicts severity of aggression as well as a worse course. This area of research promises to be an important one, given the linkages between anxiety and such crucial (and heterogeneous) constructs as behavioral inhibition (Nigg, 2000).

Second, the other major type of internalizing problem encompasses depressive symptoms and syndromes. Importantly, CD and depressive syndromes display comorbidity at significant levels (see Kovacs, Paulauskas, Gatsonis, & Richards, 1988; Loeber & Keenan, 1994; for a meta-analytic review, see Angold et al., 1999). At present, it is indeterminate whether (1) major depression precipitates acting-out behavior; (2) CD and its associated impairment lead to demoralization and dysphoria; or (3) similar "third variables" or underlying causal factors—psychological, familial, or psychobiological—trigger the joint display of such symptomatology (for empirical data related to this issue, see Patterson et al., 1992). It is likely that each of these causal scenarios applies to certain subgroups. The comorbidity between these domains is important theoretically. Depression is believed to emanate from loss events, with aggressive impulses introjected and displayed against the self. Thus the dynamic boundary between self-directed and other-directed aggression may be a narrow one. This relationship is also demonstrated by the increased likelihood of suicidal behavior among youths with features of both CD and depression (e.g., Shaffi, Carrigan, Whittinghill, & Derrick, 1985). Indeed, adolescent aggression alone is a significant risk factor for suicidal behavior (Cairns, Peterson, & Neckerman, 1988; Loeber & Farrington, 2000). Psychobiologically, decreased serotonergic activity is associated with both (1) dimensions of impulsivity and aggression and (2) suicidal behavior (Brown & van Praag, 1991; see review in Lahey, Hart, Pliszka, Applegate, & McBurnett, 1993). In all, research strategies that focus on groups with CD, depression, and both disorders will be necessary to uncover important relationships between these domains (for exemplary research, see Capaldi, 1991).

Finally, in terms of a broader construct of internalizing symptoms (depression, shyness/withdrawal, and anxiety), Loeber, Stouthamer-Loeber, and White (1999) showed that pathways to persistent substance use and delinquency during adolescence were predicted by oppositionality during early childhood, followed by persistent internalizing problems in middle to late childhood. Such prospective investigations reveal fascinating linkages between externalizing and internalizing symptoms and syndromes, and indicate the complex ways in which comorbidity with internalizing problems may influence the serious problems of conjoint delinquency and substance abuse in adolescence.

Summary

It is an exception for child disorders to occur in isolation; indeed, comorbidity is the typical state of affairs for clinical samples and even for representative samples. Although it is essential to differentiate artifactual from "true" comorbidity, the latter clearly exists in child psychopathology. For youth with ODD or CD, overlap with ADHD occurs in approximately 50% of cases. Such comorbidity is clearly associated with an early onset of aggression and with substantial impairment in personal, interpersonal, and family domains. In particular, the impulse control problems pertinent to youngsters with joint attention deficits and aggression appear to propel a negative course. Next, academic underachievement often appears in youngsters with early-onset conduct problems and in delinquent adolescents; in childhood, learning failure is linked specifically with ADHD, but over time ASB and underachievement become more clearly associated, with reciprocally deterministic modes of interplay likely. Understanding the unfolding transactions between and among cognitive, academic, and behavioral factors in aggression and CD will be important clinically and conceptually. Finally, internalizing disorders (anxiety disorders, depression) also appear alongside aggression and ASB at above-chance rates. Subtypes of anxiety-related features may show different types of association with aggressive behavior patterns, with fearful inhibition serving as a protective factor but social withdrawal acting as an intensifier. Importantly, understanding of comorbidity with depression may also help to uncover causal pathways to suicidality as well as to certain forms of violence. In sum, all relevant research must include information on the phenomenon of comorbidity; without it, mistaken attributions regarding the etiology of ODD and CD are likely to be made.

RISK FACTORS AND ETIOLOGICAL FORMULATIONS

Any comprehensive attempt to account for the etiology of disruptive behavior disorders and ASB would easily encompass book length (for an exemplary work, see Rutter et al., 1998; see also the edited volumes of Quay & Hogan, 1999, and Stoff et al., 1997). We cannot do justice to the huge literature on risk and causal factors herein but instead attempt to provide a heuristic (though far from complete) guide to intraindividual, familial, cognitive, peer-related, and wider community influences. Four key points bear mention at the outset. First, as before, we do not feature discussion of influences that shape species-wide aggressive responding, such as crowding, perception of threat, and the like (for a lucid account of such factors, see Coie & Dodge, 1998). Rather, our focus is on those individual, social, and community factors that relate to individual differences in the display and development of clinically significant aggression and ASB. Second, as perceptively discussed by Kraemer et al. (1997), risk factors—those variables associated with a higher-than-expected rate of an outcome of interest—range from variables that show statistical correlations with such outcomes (whether or not they are independent of confounds or third variables) to those that display independent contribution and those that may in fact be implicated in the causal chain. Given the near-impossibility of performing experimental research on most risk or causal influences regarding aggressive behavior disorders, the attribution of causal or etiological influence to a variable (or set of variables) known to yield risk for ASB is an effort made at the peril of the investigator, clinician, or consumer. Nonetheless, although we begin this section with a table of empirically established risk and etiological influences on aggression and ASB, we wish to move this section beyond a mere listing of the many known risk factors to an account of possible causal influences.

Third, we point out that the act of subdividing this section into subsections on different classes of risk and causal factors belies the actual state of affairs in the field—namely, that causal mechanisms are multifaceted and transactional. Indeed, as emphasized throughout this chapter, combinations of risk factors, interacting and transacting in chain-like fashion, are crucial for the development of persistent aggression and ASB (Caspi & Moffitt, 1995; Patterson et al., 1998;

Rutter et al., 1998). Given the ascendancy of models that integrate psychobiological, personological, familial, neighborhood, and socioeconomic causal factors, and that attempt explanation in terms of moderation and mediation (e.g., Campbell, in press; Capaldi & Patterson, 1994; Hinshaw & Park, 1999; Rutter et al., 1998), our subdivision should not be read as an attempt to compartmentalize risk and etiological influences into neatly demarcated domains or to posit univariate, "main effect" models. Although it should go without saying at this point in the history of relevant research endeavors, we feel compelled to say it again: Biology influences behavior at the same time that behavior influences biological mechanisms; persons both shape and are shaped by the environment (e.g., Coie & Dodge, 1998; Lahey et al., 1993; Richters & Cicchetti, 1993; Rutter et al., 1998).

Fourth, the organization of this section into separate subsections related to various classes of causal factors betrays a "variable-centered" approach to the problem at hand. That is, we examine whether certain variables of interest, singly or in combination, predict dimensions of ASB or differentiate diagnostic categories of interest (e.g., CD vs. other disorders). From a different perspective (see Bergman & Magnusson, 1997), we could be distinguishing homogeneous subgroups of children or adolescents who display similar background characteristics or trajectories. Such "person-centered" research has the potential for painting a clearer picture, as variable-centered models typically assume that a risk or causal factor operates homogeneously across subgroups of the population (see, e.g., Greenberg, Speltz, DeKlyen, & Jones, 2001). In fact, however, recent research efforts in the field are taking important steps toward an integration of variable- and person-centered approaches (see, e.g., the subtype models of Moffitt, 1993, and Loeber, Wung, et al., 1993; see also Nagin & Tremblay, 2001, who utilize a person-centered approach to defining different trajectories of antisocial actions across development and then attempt to discern intraindividual and family factors that can distinguish these subgroups). As summarized by Hinshaw and Park (1999), the field will be best served at present by research strategies that bridge the strengths and delimit the shortcomings of each approach.

We open this section with a reproduction of a table of empirically validated risk factors for childhood aggression and delinquency from Loeber and Farrington (2000); see Table 3.4. Even though this table is far from exhaustive, note the sheer numbers of risk factors involved, as well as the multiple levels at which they occur—from intraindividual to family, school, peer, and neighborhood. No such listing, however, can give any kind of explanatory story regarding how such factors may fit together in a coherent fashion, or can describe which variable may be relevant for which particular types of aggressive behavior or which subcategories of children with ASB. In addition, such a listing does not distinguish those factors that may directly influence aggression and violence from those that are indirect risks, mediated by other factors or combinations of factors. Following our truncated accounting of several classes of risk and etiological factors, we attempt an integrated model (see subsequent section).

Intraindividual Factors

Genetic influences

Are aggression and ASB heritable? Although "crime genes" do not, of course, exist (Raine, 1993; Rutter et al., 1998), any discussion of genetic influences on this domain of behavior is laden with ethical and policy implications. We believe that further knowledge of genetic effects can be used to empower and enhance treatment rather than discriminate and stigmatize, but only if the relationship between genes and behavior becomes more thoroughly known (e.g., Plomin & Crabbe, 2000). For instance, it must be remembered that "heritability" refers to genetic influences on individual differences across a population of interest and that even for conditions or traits that are strongly heritable, environmental influences are quite salient at the level of the individual (Hinshaw, 1999). Furthermore, estimates of genetic (and environmental) influences on any behavior patterns will be influenced significantly by the types of twin or adoptive samples under investigation. As such, extant investigations in the field, particularly those of adoptees, are highly likely to underestimate environmental influences because of the restricted range of adoptive families (for a lucid discussion, see Rutter et al., 1998).

In the first place, genetic effects differ for different classes of ASB. Across the externalizing spectrum in childhood, heritability is strongest (and of considerable magnitude) for ADHD symptomatology, of moderate strength for overt

TABLE 3.4. Childhood Risk Factors for Child Delinquency and Later Serious and Violent Juvenile Offending

Child factors	Single parenthood
Difficult temperament	Large family
Hyperactivity (but only when co-occurring with conduct disorder)	High turnover of caretakers
Impulsivity	Low SES of family
Substance use	Unemployed parent
Aggression	Poorly educated mother
Early-onset disruptive behavior	Family members' carelessness in allowing children access to weapons, especially guns
Withdrawn behavior	
Low intelligence	School factors
Lead toxicity	Poor academic performance
	Old for grade
Family factors	Weak bonding to school
Parental antisocial or delinquent behavior	Low educational aspirations
Parental substance abuse	Low school motivation
	Poorly organized and functioning schools
Parents' poor child-rearing practices	
Poor supervision	Peer factors
Physical punishment	Associations with deviant/delinquent siblings/peers
Poor communication	Rejection by peers
Poor parent–child relations	
Parental neglect	Neighborhood factors
Maternal depression	Neighborhood disadvantage and poverty
Mother's smoking during pregnancy	Disorganized neighborhoods
Teenage motherhood	Availability of weapons
Parents disagree on child discipline	Media portrayal of violence

Note. From Loeber and Farrington (2000, p. 749). Copyright 2000 by Cambridge University Press. Reprinted by permission.

ASB, but relatively small for covert forms of ASB (e.g., Edelbrock et al., 1995). Indeed, for the latter, shared environmental influences are considerable. It is noteworthy as well that the comorbidity of ASB with ADHD symptomatology is itself quite heritable (Silberg et al., 1996), although recent evidence points to large contributions from shared environmental facters to covariation between ADHD, ODD, and CD (Burt, Truger, McGue & Iacono, 2001). In addition, and provocatively, recent evidence suggests stronger heritability for childhood-onset than for adolescent-onset forms of aggression and ASB (Taylor, Iacono, & McGue, 2000), again bespeaking the need to subtype accurately the domains under consideration. Also, stronger heritabilities have emerged by adulthood for property crimes than for violent crimes (Rutter et al., 1998).

Second, the heritability of ASB appears to increase with development (Jacobson, Prescott, & Kendler, 2002). That is, genetic contributions to children's aggression are relatively small, but these influences appear to increase with age, demonstrating the dynamic influences of genes on behavior and belying the notion that genetic effects are static and immutable (Jacobson et al., 2002).

Third, and crucially, the heritability of violence per se is not strong (Rutter et al., 1998). Thus society-wide cultural and legal norms (e.g., access to guns in the United States vs. other nations) and exclusively psychosocial socialization processes (e.g., Athens, 1997; Rhodes, 1999) appear to exert considerable influence on rates of violence. Along this line, it must be remembered that that Moffitt's (1993) and Patterson's (Patterson et al., 1992) models of life-course-persistent ASB, although starting with (presumably heritable) temperamental, neurospsychological, and neurophysiological influences early in development, are transactional in nature; they posit that the child's early biologically based difficulties will both evoke and be influenced by aberrant family socialization, peer rejection, and academic failure. Indeed, gene–environment interactions and correlations are undoubtedly the rule with regard to the development of severe ASB (Lahey, Waldman, & McBurnett, 1999; Rutter et al., 1998). Genes appear to exert their influence on temperamental irritability, lack of inhibition (i.e., high impulsivity), or sensation seeking; these tendencies in turn (1) are likely to be met by similar tendencies in biological parents, and (2) serve to elicit maladaptive parent–child interaction patterns. Furthermore, (3) children with biological parents with severe psychopathology may be more "susceptible" to punitive or inconsistent relations. In all, genetic influences are therefore likely to be indirect in relation to the development of ASB (Lahey, Waldman, & McBurnett, 1999); it is impossible to consider one category of causal influence (e.g., genes) without invoking others (e.g., parenting). For essential, current thinking on the need to transcend simple genetic determinism with respect to behavior, see Gottlieb (1995, 1998) and Maccoby (2000).

Psychobiological Influences

The first edition of this chapter highlighted the review of Lahey et al. (1993) regarding psychobiological influences on aggression and ASB. We cannot recapitulate such evidence herein, and we point out that interest in this area has continued (e.g., Lahey, McBurnett, Loeber, & Hart, 1995; Raine, 1993; Raine & Liu, 1998; see in particular the section on "Biology of Antisocial Behavior" in Stoff et al., 1997, containing nine excellent chapters). The area is far too complex for a reasonable synthesis herein. We feature brief highlights, but we point out that nearly all psychobiologically oriented investigators of ASB have commented on the need to incorporate biosocial or integrated environmental–biological accounts (see Coie & Dodge, 1998; Raine, 1997). Indeed, we note the contention of Lahey et al. (1993) that investigation of biological variables—whether they be neurotransmitter systems, skin conductance, event-related potentials, or hormonal influences—does not rule out important roles for psychosocial factors in the genesis or maintenance of antisocial behavior: Lahey et al. state "that a socioenvironmental event (e.g., abnormal infant experience) could be one of the *causes* of aggression, but that the effect of this experience on aggression is *mediated* by alterations in neurotransmitter activity" (1993, p. 142; emphasis in original). "Either–or" characterizations of biology versus environment, attachment versus temperament, and the like, will not facilitate progress in the field.

A key theoretical milestone in the field was the integration and synthesis by Quay (1993) of the complex neurobiological and neuroanatomical work of Jeffrey Gray, who posited a behavioral activation (or reward) system, a behavioral inhibition system, and a generalized arousal (fight–flight) system, with each comprising distinct neuroanatomical regions and neurotransmitter pathways. Several lines of research have indicated that youths diagnosed with CD who display (1) early onset, (2) aggressive features, and (3) "undersocialized" symptom patterns demonstrate low psychophysiological or cortical arousal and low autonomic reactivity on a variety of relevant indices. Such findings are strongly reminiscent of findings with adult samples composed of psychopathic individuals (see Fowles & Missel, 1994). Note that the opposite pattern is found in youths with nonaggressive, socialized, and/or late-onset CD, who often display arousal and reactivity responses that are elevated above those not only of the aforementioned CD subgroups, but of normal comparison samples as well (see McBurnett & Lahey, 1994; Lahey et al., 1995). The assumption is that the low arousal and low reactivity associated with early-onset CD reduce the potential for avoidance conditioning to socialization stimuli, fueling poor response to punishment. Related findings have been interpreted in terms of an imbalance favoring the behavioral activation/reward system over the behavioral inhibition system in youths with undersocialized, aggressive CD (Quay, 1993; see also Kruesi et al., 1990).

Research on hormonal influences is less conclusive, with inconsistent findings pertinent to testosterone levels (see Coie & Dodge, 1998), but with recent evidence that low cortisol levels may characterize boys at risk for persistent ASB (McBurnett, Lahey, Rathouz, & Loeber, 1999). This latter finding is based on a prospective investigation—a crucial methodological issue when the goal is to ascribe causal status to biological variables with respect to the development or maintenance of ASB. As for other biological influences, several reports have demonstrated a linkage between perinatal factors and later propensity for ASB (e.g., Brennan, Mednick, & Raine, 1997). Of crucial importance for these variables are patterns of interaction with early parental rejection (see the subsection on interactional and transactional processes). As for prenatal exposure to teratogenic substances, several reports have linked maternal smoking during pregnancy with the offspring's subsequent risk for ASB (e.g., Brennan, Grekin, & Mednick, 1999; Wakschlag et al., 1997). Such effects appear to hold up when related variables (e.g., low maternal age, socioeconomic status [SES]) are controlled for. Furthermore, Arsenault, Tremblay, Boulerice, Seguin, and Saucier (2000) recently documented that the total number of minor physical anomalies (particularly those around the mouth area, appraised in adolescence) was associated with violent delinquency, even when childhood rates of physical aggression and an index of family adversity were partialed out. Whether this finding reflects neurological injury, the likelihood of early feeding problems, and/or a risk for difficult socialization requires prospective investigation from infancy onward. On the other hand, Hodgins, Kratzer, and McNeil (2001) found that inadequate parenting, rather than early obstetrical complications, was the stronger predictor of later criminal behavior.

Overall, the range of potential psychobiological influences on ASB is wide, and replication of predictive findings is crucial. Research on female samples is urgently needed in the field. Interactions of neurophysiological and neuropsychological risk with pathogenic environmental circumstances are strongly implicated in the genesis and maintenance of ASB patterns (see Raine, Brennan, & Mednick, 1997; see also the subsection on interactive and transactional effects, below).

Familial Factors

Parental Psychopathology

At the outset, we alert the reader to the obvious but often overlooked point that in biological families, familial influences on child development may be psychological in nature, may be genetically mediated, or may result from correlated (or interacting) joint influences of genes and environment. Given our prior discussion of the heritability of ASB—and the arbitrary designation of our placement of genetic influences in the subsection on intraindividual as opposed to familial influences, highlighting the artificiality of the classes of risk and causal factors herein and elsewhere—we briefly take up the kinds of family configurations in which individuals with ASB are raised and then discuss more explicitly family socialization and interaction, noting once again the strong potential for gene–environment correlation and interaction.

Intergenerational linkages with respect to criminal behavior have been demonstrated for some time, with mounting evidence that certain types of parental psychopathology are associated with child aggression and ASB. Parental ASPD is strongly and specifically related to child CD (Faraone, Biederman, Keenan, & Tsuang, 1991; Lahey, Piacentini, et al., 1988). This association is particularly clear for fathers (Frick et al., 1992), as are the links of (1) paternal substance use disorders and (2) maternal histrionic personality configurations with child ASB patterns (Lahey, Piacentini, et al., 1988). Intriguingly, children's aggression is also associated with their parents' childhood aggression when they were the same age as the children (Huesmann, Eron, Lefkowitz, & Walder, 1984). Maternal depression has also been implicated in linkages to child aggression, with an association found in some investigations but not in others. One explanation for such inconsistency is that maternal depression is a nonspecific risk factor for child maladjustment, predicting a wide range of psychopathology (Downey & Coyne, 1990; Goodman & Gotlib, 1999).[4]

Family Structure

ASB in children is associated with single-parent status, with family dissolution (particularly parental divorce), with large family size (i.e., large number of children), and with young age of mothers. Each of these seemingly straightforward risk factors actually signals a complex story. First, all of these family structural features are associated with poverty, which is itself a risk factor for ASB (see the subsequent subsection on wider contextual influences). The effects of poverty, however, as well as those of these structural variables, appear to be indirect in terms of their influence on ASB—mediated largely if not exclusively by parenting practices and parent–child interactions, which we discuss in the next subsection (Capaldi & Patterson, 1994; Coie & Dodge, 1998; McLoyd, 1990; Rutter et al., 1998). Second, we take up each family structural variable in turn:

1. Single-parent status is associated with a host of strains and stresses on parents (the modal case applies to single mothers); these strains negatively affect a mother's ability to provide authoritative parenting.
2. Death of a parent is not typically a risk factor for ADHD, whereas family divorce is, particularly for boys (Rutter et al., 1998). Yet careful longitudinal work reveals that the marital conflict and the discordant parent–child interactions often both precede and postdate the divorce; moreover, preexisting behavior patterns in the child, rather than the dissolution per se, are the risk factors for

the offspring's aggression and antisocial activities (Amato & Keith, 1991). Furthermore, Lahey, Hartdagen, et al. (1988) discovered that the effects of divorce on boys' conduct problems were reduced dramatically when diagnoses of ASPD in the parents were statistically controlled for.

3. Large family size is associated with poverty; it appears to exert its etiological influence on ASB through poor parental monitoring of the index child or adolescent and/or modeling of aggressive actions by older siblings.

4. Young age of motherhood, especially teenage parenthood, is clearly associated with ASB in the offspring (Rutter et al., 1998). Genetic mediation could play a role here—the same sorts of impulsive tendencies in the mother leading to early pregnancy could be passed on to the children—as could "assortative mating," the tendency for antisocial girls/young women to procreate with similarly antisocial males. Furthermore, in an important investigation, Wakschlag et al. (2000) found that young maternal age was confounded with maternal history of problem behavior in predicting the ASB of the offspring. Thus the compromised parenting skills of teenage mothers are embedded in a wider historical net of influences (see Jaffe, Moffitt, Caspi, Belsky, & Silva, 2001).

In all, complex causal chains appear to be the rule in relation to the effects of family structure on ASB.

Family Functioning and Parent–Child Interaction

Several features of parent–child interaction display moderate to strong relationships with children's aggression and ASB (for an earlier synthesis, see Loeber & Stouthamer-Loeber, 1986): (1) low levels of parental involvement in children's activities, (2) poor supervision of offspring, and (3) harsh and inconsistent discipline practices. The most comprehensive model in the field is the coercion theory of Patterson (1982; Patterson et al., 1992), which is supported by microanalyses of in-home observations of family interaction.[5] What emerges is a pattern of harsh, ultimately unsuccessful interchanges between parents and child, leading to the development and intensification of ASB. In brief, by backing down from requests and adhering to the child's escalating demands, parents negatively reinforce the child's increasingly defiant and aggressive behavior patterns; similarly, harsh and abusive discipline practices, displayed when the child escalates to severe misbehavior, are rewarded by the child's temporary capitulation (see Patterson, 1982; see also the cogent summary in Coie & Dodge, 1998). Such mutual training in aversive responding fuels both aggressive child behavior and greater levels of harsh, nonresponsive parenting. (Note that in Wahler's alternative formulation, the child's misbehavior serves to reduce the uncertainty associated with inconsistent parental responses.) Aversive interchanges serve to intensify aggressive behavior outside the home and to precipitate a widening array of negative consequences for the child and family, including risk for academic underachievement and peer rejection by the child, depressed mood in family members, and a strong likelihood of persisting ASB (Patterson et al., 1992). Thus discordant parent–child interactions propel in motion a cascade of additional risk factors and impairments associated with ASB.

Research on family socialization related to aggression increasingly recognizes bidirectional influences, in which child behavior influences parent behavior as well as the converse (Lytton, 1990). It is conceivable, in fact, that negative parenting is largely a reaction to the difficult, oppositional, and aggressive behaviors displayed by the child with developing CD. Anderson, Lytton, and Romney (1986) performed an intriguing experimental study involving mothers of boys with CD and comparison boys, in which each mother interacted with (1) her own son, (2) an unrelated boy with a diagnosis of CD, and (3) an unrelated comparison boy. Mothers in both groups displayed more negativity toward and made more requests of the youngsters with CD, strongly supporting child-to-parent effects in eliciting coercive interchange. Importantly, however, mothers of the youngsters with CD responded with the most negativity to their own boys, suggesting that a history of negative interactions plays an important role. Indeed, research with clinical samples demonstrates that maternal negativity during parent–child interactions predicts the independently observed noncompliance and covert ASB of children with ADHD, over and above the effects of the children's negativity during the interaction and maternal indices of psychopathology (Anderson, Hinshaw, & Simmel, 1994). Understanding the "ultimate" cause (parent- vs. child-related) of the escalating behavior patterns is probably futile; reciprocal determinism is likely to paint the most accurate picture. It is also clear that the negative interchanges in at-risk families begin quite early in children's development (Campbell, in press; Shaw et al., 2001), leading Tremblay (2000) to conclude that subsequent investigations of risk for ASB must begin with recruitment of families during pregnancy! Finally, we reiterate that interactional and transactional models and those that consider subtypes of aggressive behavior are the rule rather than the exception with respect to parenting practices and parent–child iteractions (e.g., Coon, Carey, Corley, & Fulker, 1992; Coie & Dodge, 1998). For example, O'Connor, Deater-Deckard, Fulker, Ruttter, and Plomin (1998) uncovered evidence for gene–environment correlations regarding linkages between coercive parenting and ASB. In addition, as noted earlier, Gorman-Smith et al. (1998) found that multiple family problems, including severely deviant parental attitudes and patterns of interchange that could be considered neglectful, characterized only a subgroup of their inner-city sample defined as serious, chronic offenders. Once again, transactional models and specificity of effects are essential to consider.

The most conclusive evidence for the causal role of parenting practices in promoting ASB would emanate from experimental investigations with interventions designed to reduce coercive interchange. In fact, Dishion, Patterson, and Kavanagh (1992) demonstrated that in families randomly assigned to receive intensive behavioral intervention, the risk for child ASB was markedly reduced, with indices of parenting skill following treatment serving as predictors of teacher-reported ASB patterns. Similarly, in a large sample of children with ADHD, many of whom displayed comorbid ODD or CD, Hinshaw et al. (2000) discovered that reduction of negative and ineffective discipline practices mediated the effects of combined medication plus behavioral intervention on children's social skill and disruptive behavior at school. Thus, despite the potential for genetic mediation or for bidirectional effects, ineffective parenting practices appear to play a causal role in the genesis of ASB.

Are there variables that moderate the relation between parenting practices and ASB? First, as noted above, Wootton et al. (1997) found that aggressive boys scoring high on callous/unemotional behavioral traits did not show the expected association between negative parenting and rates of aggressive/externalizing behavior, suggesting that males with this "prepsychopathic" personality configuration were less responsive to parental socialization influences (and presumably that their proclivity toward ASB was more biologically mediated). Second, Deater-Deckard and Dodge (1997) discovered that whereas European American children assessed during the preschool years showed the expected correlation between harsh, authoritarian parental practices and risk for aggression and conduct problems several years later, African American children did not show such predictability at all. (Importantly, however, children from both ethnic backgrounds showed strong associations between actual abusive parenting and later aggression.) This provocative finding of an ethnic moderator effect requires explanation: Is there a different cultural meaning related to authoritarian parenting in different cultural subgroups? What are the implications for parenting interventions across ethnic and other subcultural groups? Clearly, the search for moderator variables is necessary to qualify any generic theories of the development of aggression and ASB.

Abuse

With respect to effects of abuse and family violence, physical abuse is a strong and consistently replicated risk factor (and, quite probably, etiological factor) for later aggression and violence in the child (see Coie & Dodge, 1998). Dodge, Bates, and Pettit (1990) discovered that early physical abuse was a clear risk factor for later aggressive behavior reported in school settings, even with statistical control of family ecological variables and child temperament. Indeed, intergenerational effects of abuse are empirically validated (Widom, 1989, 1997), strongly supporting the need for prevention and early intervention efforts in this area. Such effects could of course be genetically mediated, but evidence for psychosocial mechanisms in transmission is compelling (Coie & Dodge, 1998). Intriguingly, the effects of familial abuse on children's antisocial tendencies appear to be mediated in part by social-cognitive information-processing variables that emanate from the abuse experience and that appear related to reactive, retaliatory aggression (Dodge, 1991; Dodge, Pettit, Bates, & Valente, 1995; see also subsequent section). Furthermore, for girls sexual abuse may be a salient risk factor (Chesney-Lind & Shelden, 1992), albeit one that has diffuse and nonspecific effects on a host of behavioral and psychological facets of later functioning.

Along this line, we highlight that, given the low heritabilities of violent behavior per se (see earlier section), abusive psychosocial influences (beyond those pertinent to child abuse per se) may be strongly implicated in the causal pathways to violent interactions. A provocative perspective on this issue is provided by the sociologist Athens (1997; see description in Rhodes, 1999), who posits an exclusively psychosocial pathway termed "violentization." In brief, this formulation claims that a necessary and sufficient explanation of extreme violence encompasses a process of brutalization (often from abusive parents, but potentially from other sources), which includes violent subjugation, personal horrification, and "coaching" in violence—all of which lead to dramatic alterations in self-perception and interpersonal judgment, and which then proceed through stages toward belligerence, violent acts, and in some cases virulence. It is tempting to posit that such experiences are more likely to occur in families and individuals with biological proclivities toward impulse control problems and aggression, but Athens insists that the process can be entirely psychosocial. Furthermore, it can pertain to females as well as males (though the latter are more likely to receive training in violentization). Readers are encouraged to discover this fascinating, alternative perspective on the socialization of violence.

Attachment and Multiple Family Risk Factors

A different approach to the development of conduct problems has been taken by theorists and investigators within the attachment tradition, with primary focus on the development of problem behavior early in life. Attachment theory focuses on the quality of parent–child relationships (not only in infancy but across the life span) to explain the development of psychopathology; behavior problems in children are often seen as strategies for receiving attention or gaining proximity to caregivers who may not respond to other approach signals (see the seminal formulation of Greenberg & Speltz, 1988).

Empirical studies of attachment security have found that some of the behaviors differentiating securely from insecurely attached children are identical to symptoms of early disruptive behavior disorders (Greenberg, Speltz, & DeKlyen, 1993). Furthermore, investigations linking infant attachment status with behavior problems in the preschool years have yielded provocative (but inconsistent) findings: The avoidant pattern of insecure attachment is prospectively linked to oppositional defiant problems in the preschool years, and the disorganized/disoriented classification at 18 months predicts subsequent behavior problems of a hostile nature (Lyons-Ruth, Alpern, & Repacholi, 1993). Negative findings have also been reported, however (see Coie & Dodge, 1998).

Current formulations (DeKlyen & Speltz, 2001; Greenberg, Speltz, & DeKlyen, 1993) synthesize extant results by concluding that main effects from insecure attachment to child ASB have not been found but rather that attachment relationships interact with the child's sex, with biological/temperamental aspects of the child, family ecological variables, and parent management practices to precipitate ASB. Indeed, the most supportive evidence comes from high-risk samples, which by definition include additional risk factors. Thus, as noted at the outset of the section on etiology, multivariate, transactional causal pathways are gaining ascendancy in the field. In addition, the meaning of and predictability from different attachment classifications may differ across cultures.

Cognitive and Social-Cognitive Variables

IQ and Neuropsychological Functioning

With regard to neuropsychological variables, we highlight the important synthesis of Moffitt and Lynam (1994), as well as the more recent integrative model of Lynam and Henry (2001). Their initial contention was that the often-cited IQ deficit (approaching half a standard deviation) in antisocial and delinquent samples is actually far greater (over a full standard deviation) in youth with early-onset CD and is not explicable on the basis of such factors as official detection of delinquency, motivation, racial status, SES, or school failure (Lynam, Moffitt, & Stouthamer-Loeber, 1993; Moffitt & Silva, 1988). Moving to more specific types of neuropsychological dysfunction, Moffitt and Lynam (1994) posited that deficits in (1) verbal reasoning and (2) "executive" functioning characterize the profiles of youngsters with early-onset, aggressive ASB and comorbid ADHD. Such deficits, which appear at quite early ages, yield cumulative effects on ASB over the course of development, by promoting impulsive responding, facilitating disruption of early caretaker–child relationships, precipitating harsh or inconsistent parenting, and presaging academic underachievement. This framework thus holds that even subtle neuropsychological deficits will interact with a host of other variables—including parental socialization influences—to produce indirect and distal effects on the development and intensification of ASB. Indeed, one contention is that neuropsychological difficulties may increase vulnerability to pathological environmental circumstances (Moffitt & Lynam, 1994; see also Lahey, Waldman, & McBurnett, 1999).

We point out several additional considerations. First, recent research has highlighted that executive deficits as typically measured in neuropsychological batteries are specific to ADHD and not to ODD or CD (Nigg, Hinshaw, Carte, & Treuting, 1998; Hinshaw, Carte, Sami, Treuting, & Zupan, 2002). Still, the early comorbidity of aggression and ADHD is a clear risk factor for persistent conduct problems, as noted earlier; the executive dysfunction related to this comorbidity may well be implicated in the causal chain. In addition, for severe and violent criminality, Raine and Liu (1998) clearly implicate the role of frontal lobe/executive dysfunction. Furthermore, a long history of research implicates verbal deficits in the causal pathway to early-onset ASB and delinquency (Lynam & Henry, 2001). Second, Aguilar et al. (2000) have challenged the contention that early neuropsychological and biological indicators are the key components of early-onset ASB, proposing instead that family relational factors are the key. For a lively debate on the primacy of psychobiological versus environmental variables, see the rejoinders of Mofftt and Caspi (2001) and Moffitt et al. (2002). Third, neurospsychological effects are typically of small magnitude in relation to the risk for persistent ASB. Yet, as noted, their key influence may be in interaction and transaction with environmental factors. Fourth, despite the strong attention paid to deficits in verbal skills as related to CD and ASB, recent evidence suggests that early in development, spatial and perceptual forms of cognitive processing may set the stage for the development of aggression and ASB (Raine, Yaralian, Reynolds, Venables, & Mednick, 2002). More research with a developmental focus is sorely needed in this area.

Social-Cognitive Information Processing

One mechanism by which both psychobiological and familial factors may exert effects on ASB patterns is through a child's means of perceiving, construing, and evaluating the social world. Because this area has received extensive attention in the cogent reviews of Crick and Dodge (1994) and Coie and Dodge (1998), we present only headlines herein. Spanning developmental, cognitive, and clinical child psychology, this work has proven heuristic for the study of aggressive behavior.

In the most detailed formulation of this model (Crick & Dodge, 1994), a dynamic, transactional network of cognitive processes is held to mediate children's interpersonal responses and ultimate social adjustment. These processes include, at early stages of information processing, the encoding and interpretation of social cues and the clarification of social goals; at intermediate stages, response access/construction and response decision; and finally, behavioral enactment, with consequent evaluation and response. Interrelationships among these stages are believed to be fluid and nonlinear, with continual interplay among biological predispositions, environmental cues, information-processing variables per se, and feedback from the interpersonal behavior and peer response.

A programmatic series of investigations has revealed that aggressive youngsters display deficits and distortions at various levels of this information-processing model. At an overview level, such children and adolescents (in comparison with nonaggressive youths) underutilize pertinent social cues, misattribute hostile intent to ambiguous peer provocations, generate fewer assertive solutions to social problems, and expect that aggressive responses will lead to reward (e.g., Dodge & Frame, 1982; Dodge, Price, Bachorowski, & Newman, 1990; see review in Crick & Dodge, 1994). Importantly, such effects are found in both community and clinical samples of aggressive youths, including severely violent offenders (Lochman & Dodge, 1994). More specific examination of subgroups, however, reveals that such "early-stage" deficits as cue underutilization and attributional distortions pertain specifically to the subgroup of aggressive youngsters with comorbid ADHD (Milich & Dodge, 1984) and/or to the earlier-noted subtype displaying reactive aggression (see Dodge, 1991). Presumably, the impulsive cognitive style displayed by these children limits a full scanning of pertinent social cues before behavioral decisions are made, and ambiguous interpersonal situations are (mis)construed as threats to the self. In contrast, proactively aggressive children, whose aggression subserves instrumental goals, may show their primary information-processing differences at later stages of the model that incorporate the expectation of positive outcomes from aggressive acts (Dodge, 1991). In short, the model has allowed for specificity with respect to subcategories of aggressive youths.

As highlighted throughout the chapter, interplay among causal factors and underlying mechanisms is increasingly recognized as critical for accurate formulation of aggressive behavior patterns. It is certainly conceivable, for example, that certain temperamental styles, including those characterized by suboptimal attention, may relate to impulsive cognitive processing. Furthermore, as discussed earlier regarding familial influences, punitive and abusive parenting practices appear to influence aggressive behavior through their instigation of early-stage information-processing deficits and distortions (Dodge, Bates, & Pettit, 1990; Dodge et al., 1995). In other words, a child exposed to a harsh, abusive upbringing may begin to attribute malevolent intent to others, fueling negative and aggressive interchanges that reinforce the biased attribution. In passing, we must point out that despite the elegance of the social-cognitive information-processing model, large effect sizes are the exception rather than the rule (Coie & Dodge, 1998); social-cognitive factors are not sufficient in providing a full explanation of persistent ASB. Thus, once again, it is necessary to invoke multivariate models that can predict and explain, with greater precision, the complex interrelationships among causal and risk factors.

Although space does not permit a separate heading, we wish to highlight that the variables of lack of inhibition (i.e., impulsivity), social-cognitive information-processing deficits, and compromised verbal abilities all point to the potential for youths at risk for ASB (particularly reactive forms of aggression and persistent ASB) to suffer from emotion dysregulation. Even defining this construct is laden with pitfalls, but theoretical and empirical accounts of the role of excesses in emotional reactivity and deficits in emotion regulation regarding the development of child psychopathology are beginning to appear (e.g., Keenan, 2000). Interested readers are advised to keep abreast of developments in this potentially fruitful area of investigation.

Peer Influences

In our truncated review, we make a key distinction—that between (1) peer rejection in childhood and (2) association with deviant (i.e., antisocial) peers in preadolescence and adolescence. Each is related to the development of ASB and delinquency, yet perhaps in different ways, and apparently for different subgroups of youths with aggression and conduct problems.

First, peer rejection in childhood is strongly related to early onset of both aggressive behavior and ADHD-related symptomatology, and particularly to their combination (Hinshaw & Melnick, 1995). Indeed, whereas ADHD is clearly associated with peer rejection, aggression in the absence of ADHD (particularly, proactive aggression) may be related to "controversial" sociometric status (e.g., Milich & Landau, 1988). Yet children with comorbid ADHD and aggressive behavior patterns receive extremes of peer rejection (Hinshaw & Melnick, 1995). Importantly, considerable evidence (especially from the programmatic research of Coie and colleagues) demonstrates that peer rejection in childhood is a significant, incremental predictor of ASB and delinquent behavior during adolescence, even when baseline levels of aggression are controlled for (Coie, Terry, Lenox, Lochman, & Hyman, 1995; see review in Coie & Dodge, 1998). Thus, whereas peer rejection may be a marker during childhood of externalizing, intrusive, and insensitive behavior patterns, it also appears to be a causal factor in and of itself for the persistence and escalation of antisocial patterns. Mechanisms responsible for this predictive relationship could include a child's exclusion from opportunities for peer socialization, modeling of aggressive behavior by other rejected children, or demoralization in response to the self-perception of peer rejection (see the discussion in Laird, Jordan, Dodge, Pettit, & Bates, 2001). Coie and Lenox (1994) provide a view from the microanalytic level as to the processes by which aggressive children who are also rejected by their peers display a qualitatively distinct pattern of peer interactions that promotes further escalation of aggressive behavior.

Second, even for children without a history of aggression and ASB during childhood, association with deviant, antisocial peers during early adolescence clearly appears to be a direct causal influence on the propensity for delinquent behavior (see Capaldi & Patterson, 1994). Two perspectives are important in this regard: One is "selection," whereby youngsters with marginal social skills or subclinical aggressive tendencies select deviant peer networks; the other is "facilitation," in which associations with antisocial peers propel and escalate a pattern of antisocial behaviors via conversational dynamics, modeling, and provision of opportunity for delinquent involvement. The work of Dishion and his research group (e.g., Dishion, Andrews, & Crosby, 1995) provides a heuristic perspective on the types of peer processes that are salient in this regard.

In a recent longitudinal, multivariate model, Laird et al. (2001) showed that both processes may operate to pave the way for adolescent ASB, but that peer rejection may be more salient for early-onset ASB, whereas deviant peer association pertains selectively to those with later-onset ASB. (Laird et al. also found that the continuity of aggressive behavior mediated the relationship between early peer rejection and later association with deviant peers.) Indeed, the review of Capaldi and Patterson (1994) suggests strongly that involvement with antisocial peers is a direct influence on delinquent behavior patterns in adolescent-onset ASB. At the same time, both peer rejection and association with deviant peers do not occur in a vacuum; multiple levels of influence appear operative.

Wider Contextual Factors

For many years, investigators have noted a clear link between measures of psychosocial adversity—including impoverishment, high rates of crime in the neighborhood, family crowding, and related factors—and children's risk for ASB (see review in Coie & Dodge, 1998). Indeed, the risk for antisocial activity is far higher in crowded, poverty-stricken, inner-city areas than in rural settings (Rutter et al., 1974)—a factor of considerable influence for the large numbers of impoverished, urban youths (often of ethnic minority status). Whereas anything more than a cursory review of the long history of research regarding social/cultural influences on ASB and delinquency is beyond the scope of this chapter, a key issue is whether such socioeconomic and neighborhood factors contribute directly to ASB patterns or whether their effects are mediated by more specific variables, such as parent–child interactions or social-cognitive processes.

We again cite the masterful synthesis of Capaldi and Patterson (1994), who examined a wide array of contextual factors for their predictive relationships to ASB patterns for males, testing for direct versus indirect effects of such factors. The research program is provocative, in that Patterson and colleagues are conceptualizing a far broader network for the development of aggression and CD than microsocial parent–child interactions per se. First, high levels of family adversity and several related contextual factors (multiple family transitions, unemployment, and low SES) were shown to relate specifically to early-onset (but not adolescent-onset) CD. This list of factors adds to those proposed by Moffitt (1993) for childhood-onset ASB, which include neuropsychological dysfunction and attention deficits as well as discordant family interchange. Early-onset, persistent ASB patterns are clearly overdetermined.

Second, as indicated above, evidence supported the direct (as opposed to mediated) effects on ASB of the contextual factor of exposure to a deviant peer group, particularly for boys *without* a childhood onset of ASB. High rates of such association strongly influence delinquency (Sampson & Groves, 1989). This finding once again underscores the importance of subtyping aggression and ASB; direct effects of deviant peer groups pertain chiefly to the adolescent-onset subtype. Third, the effects of several important contextual factors on ASB were reduced or rendered nonsignificant when parenting variables were added to the predictive equations of Capaldi and Patterson (1994). The direct effects of low SES in particular were erased when parent management variables were included (see also Dodge, Pettit, & Bates, 1994); the roles of family transitions, stress, and unemployment also appeared to be indirect. Fourth, community and other contextual variables related to antisocial outcomes in a "chain reaction" fashion (Capaldi & Patterson, 1994), whereby unemployment (for example) predicted greater levels of stress and greater numbers of family transitions, which in turn reduced family involvement and monitoring and predicted higher levels of coercive parenting.

We point out that neighborhood effects on child psychopathology have recently been found, in a genetically sensitive design, to be separable from genetic effects or genetic mediation and to be of substantive importance (Caspi, Taylor, Moffitt, & Plomin, 2000). Thus it is not just the case that neighborhood influences reflect "selection" (the tendencies of persons with antisocial histories to aggregate in disenfranchised locations); they also appear to exert causal influence on the risk for dysfunction and impairment. But again, interactive and protective factors are operative. For example, Richters and Martinez (1993) examined the role of children's exposure to community violence in predicting maladjustment. Whereas such exposure predicted youths' self-reported symptomatology, the effects were mitigated when indices of family stability were controlled statistically. In this instance, family-level variables served as a protective factor against the risk incurred by high-frequency encounters with significant violence in the neighborhood and community.

School-based violence has been in the news considerably during the past several years. Mulvey and Cauffman (2001) provide a thoughtful perspective on (1) the difficulties involved in predicting extremely low-base-rate phenomena like school violence, and (2) the kinds of environmental changes that are most likely to be preventive. They note, as well, the contextual interrelatedness of school violence in neighborhood and family factors (see Laub & Lauritsen, 1998). Finally, we note that the lack of direct effects for many wider contextual variables does not reduce their importance in explaining ASB. Indeed, researchers and policy makers must be aware of the economic and community-level factors that predispose certain families to provide markedly poor socialization for their offspring. ASB patterns are not only intergenerational, but are intertwined with important economic, community, and family ecological factors.

Additional Data on Interaction and Transaction

We now present several additional examples of research findings regarding the development of ASB that exemplify interaction and transaction across risk and etiological factors. Our purpose here is to illustrate the kinds of results, and the kinds of models, that are most likely to portray how risk and etiological factors work in combination to yield the patterns of aggression and ASB likely to come to clinical attention.

First, as indicated in the first edition of this chapter (Hinshaw & Anderson, 1996), in a study that paved the way for her conceptualization of subtypes of ASB, Moffitt (1990) examined predictive relations between early (age 5) measures of aggressive and ADHD-related symptomatology and early adolescent indicators of delinquency. Whereas the strongest predictor of delinquent functioning incorporated early indicators of aggressive behavior, measures of ADHD behaviors at age 5 significantly incremented the prediction; that is, they accounted for significant variance, even when baseline aggression was controlled for. Crucially, however, the effects of early behavior patterns in predicting adolescent ASB were moderated by (1) a composite measure of family adversity and (2) child IQ, such that the highest-risk youths were those displaying high rates of externalizing behavior patterns at an early age, but only if they also had either subaverage IQ scores or multiple indicators of family adversity. Hence intraindividual behavioral factors, intraindividual cognitive/neuropsychological factors, and several indices of family-level factors (e.g., parental distress, family discord) worked interactively to increase the risk for early adolescent ASB.

Next, Raine and colleagues (Raine, Brennan, & Mednick, 1994; Raine et al., 1997) have embarked on systematic research with respect to the "biosocial" interactive effects of (1) birth complications (defined as presence of any of the variables of forceps extraction, breech delivery, umbilical cord prolapse, pre-eclampsia at delivery, and/or long duration of the birth process) with (2) early maternal rejection of child (defined as public institutional care of infant, attempt to abort fetus, and/or unwanted pregnancy). Utilizing a large Danish birth cohort, they found that with respect to outcomes measured at ages 17–19 (Raine et al., 1994) and age 34 (Raine, Brennan, Mednick, & Mednick, 1996), interactions between these two factors attained significance with respect to the prediction of violent crime (as opposed to nonviolent offending) and to the prediction of early-onset (but not late-onset) ASB. Raine et al. (1996) discovered that the same interaction patterns held with respect to prediction of academic problems as well. For most outcomes, the interaction pattern was provocative, such that neither single-risk group displayed elevated rates of violence, whereas the "biosocial" (i.e., dual-risk) participants showed rates far above those of any other subgroup. Raine et al. (1997) found that the presence of maternal psychiatric history in the prediction equations did not mediate the core results, and that the key maternal rejection variables "carrying" the interactions were institutional placement and the attempt to abort the fetus. Although the viability of these findings has been challenged by Rutter et al. (1998)—who questioned, for example, the mechanism whereby birth complications would specifically influence risk for violence—the overall pattern strongly suggests that interactive effects of early biological and early environmental variables are influential.

Third, and briefly, Lynam et al. (2000) found a provocative interaction between neighborhood characteristics and an intraindividual child variable, impulsivity, in predicting risk for adolescent offending. The pattern of findings was such that the expected predictive power from children's impulsivity was amplified when the children lived in more impoverished neighborhoods. Hence, in this report, both within-child and broad contextual factors were implicated in the highest risk for ASB.

Fourth, although it does not exemplify interactive effects per se, we highlight the recent research of Nagin and Tremblay (2001), who combined person-centered and variable-centered research strategies in an attempt to understand mechanisms responsible for persistence of ASB (in this case, physical aggression) from childhood through midadolescence. They first utilized their own typology (Nagin & Tremblay, 1999), which comprised four classifications of a Canadian, high-risk, kindergarten-defined, male sample: (1) chronic physical aggression (4% of the sample)—high aggression throughout the 9-year time span; (2) high-level declining trajectory (28%)—high aggression in kindergarten that subsequently declined; (3) moderate-level declining trajectory (52%)—modest rates in kindergarten that subsequently decreased to near zero; and (4) low trajectory (17%)—rare displays of physical aggression throughout development. (Recall our earlier discussion of Nagin & Tremblay's [1999] work, when we made the case that the majority of boys with early onset of ASB do not persist in it.) The goal of Nagin and Tremblay (2001) was to appraise which intraindividual and parental/family factors best distinguished the trajectory groups. In brief, child-level factors distinguished groups 1 and 2, those with high initial rates of physical aggression, from 3 and 4, those low on initial aggression. The specific factors were the presence of hyperactivity and oppositionality in kindergarten. On the other hand, family-level factors separated group 1 from group 2: Teenage status of mothers and their low educational attainment distinguished the small, but virulent, subgroup displaying physical aggression that persisted from age 6 through age 15 from the children showing high aggression in kindergarten that subsequently declined. Thus factors responsible for the onset of aggressive behavior patterns may differ from those predicting persistence.

Space does not permit additional examples (e.g., as noted above, O'Connor et al. [1998] present data on gene–environment correlations in relation to ASB). After discussing sex differences in aggression and ASB, we return to such interactive and person-centered models as we attempt an integrated theoretical statement regarding the development of these behavior patterns.

SEX DIFFERENCES

Readers may have noticed that the vast majority of the literature reviewed herein pertains largely or exclusively to males. In fact, key reviews in the last decade have called for focused attention on the crucial topic of sex differences regarding ODD, CD, and ASB in general (e.g., Coie & Dodge, 1998; Keenan, Loeber, & Green, 1999; Rutter et al., 1998). We have deferred our discussion of this issue until now, so that the reader may be able to appraise information on sex differences in light of the prior evidence regarding definitional issues, background information, prevalence, developmental progressions, and etiological influences. For recent, essential reading on this domain, see Moffitt et al. (2001).

We note at the outset that among all the risk factors for conduct problems and ASB, male sex has been considered by some experts as the most important (see Robins, 1991). Yet increasing awareness of the growing problems of ASB among girls and women is clearly evident (Keenan et al., 1999), with recognition that female manifestations of disruptive behavior disorders and aggression are quite real and quite prevalent. Note, however, that investigations of sex differences in a particular form of psychopathology (or investigations of other kinds of group differences, including ethnic or socioeconomic) often begin and end with description of mean levels of the amounts of psychopathological functioning in the relevant subgroups (e.g., boys vs. girls). A key point in this regard is that similar mean levels in different subgroups may belie fundamentally different patterns of risk processes, just as divergent levels across subgroups may be undergirded by similar underlying causal processes. The essential goal is explanation, not just documentation of rates and sex differences in such rates.

Rates of Aggression, ASB, and Disruptive Behavior Disorders

Crucially, recent investigations of aggression among females, utilizing such objective data collection efforts as videotaped observations during laboratory assessments, yield remarkably consistent findings regarding baseline rates of externalizing behavior in early development. That is, during the initial years of life, there are virtually no sex differences in activity level, noncompliance, other problem behaviors, and the temperament-related variables of "difficult" temperament or behavioral disinhibition (see reviews by Keenan & Shaw, 1997; Keenan et al., 1999). The exception here may relate to boys' greater likelihood of angry expressions during infancy, though data are not clear in this regard. By the preschool years and certainly by the start of elementary school, however, sex differences are apparent and are robust until adolescence. That is, male predominance is evident across different forms of aggression, both physical and verbal, with samples spanning community, epidemiological, and clinic-referred ascertainment procedures (see review in Coie & Dodge, 1998). For a theoretically rich account of putative reasons why males begin to "outperform" females with respect to the display of aggressive behavior patterns during childhood, the synthetic review of Keenan and Shaw (1997) is essential reading. In brief, they note that girls' earlier development of basic psychobiological, cognitive, and emotion-regulating capacities promote socialization patterns that funnel girls into internalizing, rather than externalizing, manifestations.

How strong are the sex differences in childhood regarding externalizing behavior patterns? With respect to categorical definitions, rates of ODD in early childhood appear similar between girls and boys, but by the late preschool and early elementary years, males predominate (Keenan et al., 1999). On the other hand, as do boys, girls display increases in rates of oppositionality and defiance in adolescence (McDermott, 1996; Rutter et al., 1998). With regard to CD, boys greatly outnumber girls in childhood and preadolescence, with ratios of 4:1 commonly reported (e.g., Zoccolillo, 1993). By adolescence, however, girls appear to show a precipitous rise in rates of disruptive behavior disorders and ASB, with the clear exception that rates of physical aggression, particularly violence, continue to be substantially elevated in males. Still, although males outnumber females in terms of CD diagnoses during adolescence, the sex ratio is closer to even. Thus CD constitutes a major mental health problem for girls during the teenage years.

We note, in passing, that research methods may be partly responsible for the overarching conclusion that males are more aggressive than females during childhood. For example, Webster-Stratton (1996) utilized home observations by objective staffers and found no significant sex differences among a sample of boys and girls (ages 4–7) on scores of total externalizing behaviors, verbal deviance, noncompliance, and positive affect. On the whole, however, a plethora of research has found that beyond infancy and toddlerhood, male and female rates of aggressive behavior patterns begin to diverge (Coie & Dodge, 1998; Keenan & Shaw, 1997). One consequence of this general conclusion is that girls with early conduct problems are behaviorally more deviant relative to same-sex peers than are boys with conduct problems; as a result, girls suffer from more negative peer regard related to behavioral acting-out than do boys (e.g., Carlson, Tamm, & Gaub, 1997; Lancelotta & Vaughan, 1989). Furthermore, in terms of comorbidity, a gender paradox may be salient, whereby the sex (in this case, females) with *lower* base rates of the disorder in question tends to show *higher* rates of comorbidity with other disorders (see, e.g., Loeber & Keenan, 1994).

A notable exception to the male predominance in aggressive behavior patterns is the subdomain of indirect or relational aggression. Broadly defined (see also the earlier section on subtypes of aggressive behavior), "relational aggression" is an attempt to inflict harm upon another person by manipulating and damaging social relationships (Crick & Grotpeter, 1995). Relevant behaviors include efforts at ostracizing another student, encouraging retaliation by others, exclusionary play, and generating rumors. Among school-age children, girls show significantly higher rates of these acts than do boys; importantly, peer-nominated relational aggression predicts such negative outcomes as loneliness, social isolation, depression, and sociometric rejection (Crick & Grotpeter, 1995; Crick & Bigbee, 1998). Thus relational aggression appears to be an important variant of ASB in girls, with the potential for significant psychological distress. Most investigations appear to have underestimated the prevalence of aggression among girls, given the assumption that their behaviors would be identical to those exemplified by males.

Considerable controversy exists about the inclusion of other behavior patterns, which are not part of the current diagnostic classification systems, as relevant to disruptive behavior disorders. Substance use/abuse and sexual promiscuity are prime examples; although they lie outside the parameters of CD per se (American Psychiatric

Association, 1994), they may be important indicators of current or future psychopathology (and can certainly be impairing) for both sexes. Other investigators have suggested that somatization may be a constituent feature of the antisocial spectrum for girls (Lilienfeld, 1992), despite its lack of inclusion in formal diagnostic criteria. Discussion about potential changes in diagnostic thresholds (sex-specific vs. universal) has been an important debate in the field (see Zoccolillo, 1993; Zahn-Waxler, 1993). In brief, Zoccolillo (1993; see also Zoccolillo, Tremblay, & Vitaro, 1996) has contended that (1) addition of additional, pertinent behavioral features and (2) sex-specific norms would more fully capture the real range of ASB in females, whereas Zahn-Waxler (1993) has contended that "watering down" the criterion levels of behavioral deviance and including a range of nonviolent and nonharmful actions in the nosological systems would conflate nonharmful behavior patterns with diagnosable disorders in females. These and other issues underscore the points that current estimates of prevalence may reflect flawed assumptions about the manifestation of aggression and ASB in girls, and that classification and diagnostic systems must restrict diagnosis to individuals with significant impairment. Along this line, we once again call attention to the importance of recognizing the heterogeneity and subtypes of aggression and ASB, particularly when investigators are describing and discussing sex differences and positing developmental models for females.

Developmental Trajectories

A clear finding is that boys clearly outnumber girls in terms of early-onset variants of ASB and/or CD. Indeed, in the entire Dunedin sample (described earlier), only 6 girls out of over 500 qualified for the life-course-persistent subcategory, defined on the basis of early-onset and persistent aggression and ASB (Moffitt & Caspi, 2001). Note in this regard that boys also greatly outnumber girls with respect to key risk factors for and correlates of ASB, including ADHD, language delays, and neuropsychological deficits. Intriguingly, some evidence suggests that the construct of "difficult" temperament during toddlerhood may predict to later internalizing problems in girls as opposed to externalizing problems in boys (Fagot & Leve, 1998). In any event, by the late preschool years, boys outpace girls in terms of externalizing behavior problems.

Adolescence is a significant developmental transition that marks the onset of important changes with respect to rates of aggression, ASB, and CD. Whether measured dimensionally or categorically, the overall gender discrepancy appears to diminish beyond childhood. Findings from the Dunedin birth cohort in New Zealand reveal substantially increased rates of nonaggressive ASB in adolescent females (McGee, Feehan, Williams, & Anderson, 1992), and adolescent girls in other samples have shown an increase in their overall rates of CD (Offord, Boyle, & Racine, 1991), which collectively account for a significant portion of this narrowing gap. Thus girls show substantial increases in covert or status offenses, such as truancy, theft, substance use/abuse, and frequent lying, in the transition to adolescence. Overall, girls lag behind boys in the propensity to display physical aggression, especially violence; yet the peak age of offending among girls is during the period of early adolescence, whereas for boys the peak age is at the end of adolescence (Rutter et al., 1998). Thus girls—perhaps because their onset of puberty is earlier than that of boys —show particular risk for ASB during the early adolescent period (see below for potential mechanisms).

Whereas female rates of aggression and CD (at least the nonaggressive subtype) begin to approach those of males in adolescence, the underlying mechanisms and processes governing such relationships may be different. Despite the extensive impact of Moffitt's (1993) typology, which features age of onset as a key subclassification variable, the applicability of these typologies to female aggression and ASB is still questionable. In fact, Silverthorn and Frick (1999) have hypothesized that a dual-pathway model may not be appropriate for severely antisocial girls. Specifically, they contend (1) that girls with significant levels of ASB show the same types of cognitive, neuropsychological, and familial risk factors as do boys with early-onset ASB, but (2) that such girls' initiation of aggression and antisocial responding is "delayed" by several years into early adolescence. Furthermore, Kratzer and Hodgins (1999) found that a considerable amount of female criminal behavior in early adulthood was accounted for by adolescent-onset and even "adult-starter" subtypes, rather than the early-starter subtype, as was the case for boys. In all, according to this viewpoint, early age of onset per se may yield less robust predictions to persistent antisocial behavior for girls than it has for boys.

Yet at least some evidence exists that girls and boys with conduct problems have comparable ages at onset of problem behavior (see review in Keenan et al., 1999). Furthermore, recent data from the ongoing birth cohort study in Dunedin (Moffitt & Caspi, 2001) challenge the viability of the "delayed-onset" concept: Despite extremely low cell sizes for females on the life-course-persistent path, these girls demonstrated a pattern of early childhood risk factors (temperament, family adversity and ineffective parenting, and neurocognitive dysfunction) identical to that of the early-onset boys. In addition, the adolescent-onset boys and girls (*n*'s = 122 and 78 youths, respectively, showing a relative "catch-up" of girls with late-onset conduct problems) both displayed extremely high rates of contact with deviant peers, consistent with the "adolescent-limited" typology. Overall, examination of sex differences in pathways and mechanisms may also be facilitated by examination of other large samples (Aguilar et al., 2000; Fergusson et al., 2000; Kratzer & Hodgins, 1999). At present, the applicability of pathway notions developed for males to females is not assured.

Adult Outcomes: Evidence for Multi- and Equifinality

Although the stability of aggression and ASB is as stable over short time periods in female as it is in males, female stability appears lower than male stability over longer assessment intervals (Frick & Loney, 1999). In fact, a reliable conclusion from multiple investigations is that the adult outcomes of girls with severe externalizing behavior patterns reveal impairment across numerous psychological and functional domains (Robins, 1991; Woodward & Fergusson, 1999; Bardone, Moffitt, Caspi, Dickson, & Silva, 1996; Werner & Smith, 1992). Although such negative outcomes are frequently antisocial in nature—indeed, females may show the same rates of predictability of antisocial patterns in adulthood as do males (Keenan et al., 1999)—outcomes appear to be more highly dispersed in females than in males. Early pregnancy, suicide, physical partner violence, earlier marriage and earlier divorce, lower educational attainment, psychiatric distress (particularly internalizing conditions), difficult parent–child relationships, and higher rates of service utilization have all shown some association with childhood or adolescent aggression and ASB in girls (see reviews by Keenan et al., 1999, and Pajer, 1998). These findings suggest that multifinality (the display of diverging outcomes from similar initial conditions) pertains more to girls than to boys with ASB. Such results should be viewed with some caution, however, as highly divergent methods, sample characteristics, and experimental designs make direct sex comparisons impossible. In addition, as we have emphasized throughout, a key priority for developmental psychopathologists is to elucidate the relevant mechanisms governing these relationships. For example, Woodward and Fergusson (1999) showed that predictions to adolescent pregnancy from early conduct problems were partially mediated by sociodemographic factors, family functioning, and "risk taking."

On the basis of these preliminary results, it appears that females with externalizing disorders (many of whom have onsets of these disorders during adolescence) show more evidence than do males of multifinality, as evidenced by a wider range of outcomes (especially in the internalizing domain) that emanate from their early aggression. A requirement for future research efforts, however, is the inclusion of multiple clinical or psychiatric groups, allowing for comparisons of developmental trajectories across such groups, with the potential for finding equifinality between or among disorders. For example, in an important investigation, Bardone et al. (1996) showed that whereas CD versus depression in females showed several distinct outcomes at age 21, there were also similar outcomes, including comorbid anxiety disorders, multiple drug use, early school departure, and early childbearing. In addition, Kratzer and Hodgins (1997) discovered that the risk ratios related to the prediction of adult criminality and mental health problems from child conduct problems were *higher* for girls than for boys, once initial baseline differences in childhood conduct problems (higher in boys, as would be expected) were controlled for. Interestingly, for these girls, the adult criminal outcomes were limited nearly exclusively to substance use disorders, again suggesting that more specific predictions to aggression and violence occur in males.

Mechanisms of Differentiation

In the spirit of supplementing general models of development with work on specific, interactive mechanisms that may drive predictive outcomes, we review two domains that offer potential insight into the differentiation of sex-related ASB patterns: the influence of social groups and pubertal development.

Maccoby's (1998) review examining sex differences of young children's play styles and play groups underscores several key lessons. First, she suggests that the characteristics of the groups in which children play are as salient for development as is temperament or personality. Among boys, play styles are generally more physical and active, involving greater risks. Thus developmentally extreme boys may miss important socialization from the peer group about "normative" levels and types of aggression. Given that levels of activity are generally lower among female groups, aggressive girls risk even more ostracism and loss of friendship (and consequently a key source of socialization). Put another way, the social sanctions against acting-out behaviors may contribute to lower base rates of aggression in girls than in boys; however, they may also explain the finding that girls who exhibit severe conduct problems despite such sanctions tend to show even greater impairment than boys with comparable behavior problems (Coie & Dodge, 1998).

Late childhood and early adolescence mark an important transition in the social groups of children, as individuals no longer participate in groups that are almost universally same-sex (Maccoby, 1998). As they enter adolescence, males and females begin to interact more consistently, perhaps with the effect of introducing females to certain ASB patterns that were previously the domain of boys. Such interactions are particularly salient among girls undergoing early puberty, to which we now direct attention.

Early menarche has been shown to be a reliable precursor to behavior problems among female adolescents (Caspi, Lynam, Moffitt, & Silva, 1993; Garber, Lewinsohn, Seeley, & Brooks, 1997; Ge, Conger, & Elder, 1996). However, such main effects disguise otherwise rich and complex relations, including the role of prior problem behavior in accentuating the effects of early puberty (Moffitt, Caspi, Belsky, & Silva, 1992); the moderating role of same-sex versus different-sex schools (Caspi et al., 1993); and the mediating roles of association with older and deviant male peers, as well as explicit sexual pressure (Ge et al., 1996). Thus early puberty appears to be a risk factor for ASB in girls only if the girls attend coeducational schools, where they experience boys with early-onset ASB as models, instigators, and provocateurs (Caspi et al., 1993). Furthermore, although hormonal influences may be associated with mood and behavior problems in girls, such factors are likely to interact with other variables, such as the developmental stage of the endocrine system. Similarly, the direct impact of hormones is apt to influence related systems, such as excitability and emotionality, with indirect effects on psychopathology per se (Brooks-Gunn & Warren, 1989). Finally, the social context appears essential for expression of such propensities in terms of ASB. In summary, physiological development and maturation, particularly with an early onset, may represent a generative mechanism of behavior problems (or of accentuating existing distress) that transacts with the environment to elicit significant levels of ASB in females.

In closing this section, we note briefly the strong likelihood that conduct problems and CD predict risky sexual behavior and early pregnancy in girls (see Keenan et al., 1999). With this point in mind, recall that (1) a key risk factor for children's ASB (and particularly for persistent ASB) is being born to a teenage mother; and (2) the risk of teenage parenting in predicting offspring's conduct problems is accentuated by a history of acting-out behavior in the mother (see the subsection on family structure in "Risk Factors and Etiological Formulations"). It is likely, therefore, that conduct problems in the mother, if resulting in teenage pregnancy and birth, may precipitate an intergenerational cycle of conduct problems in the offspring, abetted by socioeconomic disadvantage and mediated via problematic parenting skills. If so, this would demonstrate reciprocal influences related to developmental trajectories span generations. The gravity and persistence of such multigenerational influences are sobering, in terms of how far the field needs to travel to make a significant difference in the trajectories pertaining to serious ASB.

THEORETICAL SYNTHESIS

In this final section, we attempt to amalgamate the extensive information reported above into a synthetic account of the development of ODD, CD, and persistent ASB. Of course, given the salience of such constructs as divergent developmental pathways, multfinality, and equifinality, no single unifying theory is adequate to the task. Rather, we incorporate a multipronged model. Critics will be able to detect many gaps in our brief synthesis, which is intended to be heuristic rather than comprehensive, and which strains the page limits for our already long chapter.

Developmental Models

First, although our account reflects the considerable empirical data base supporting the notion that ASB has extensive intraindividual and familial risk factors, wide cultural factors are no doubt responsible for (1) the increases in aggression and violence across recent generations, and (2) the widely diverging rates across cultures and nations (Rutter et al., 1998). Indeed, variables and processes that promote and maintain individual differences in aggressive and antisocial tendencies need not overlap with those that promote cohort or area differences. For example, although the role of genetic vulnerability has now been shown to contribute substantially to the risk for early-onset ASB (Taylor et al., 2000), perhaps through its linkage with comorbid hyperactivity or impulsivity (Silberg et al., 1996; see also White et al., 1994), genetic factors have little if anything to do with the huge surplus of homicide in the United States (particularly among young people), which clearly relates more to the ready access to guns and other violent weaponry in our nation (Loeber, Delamatre, et al., 1999; Rutter et al., 1998). Furthermore, at the level of individuals, factors that promote initiation of aggressive and violent behavior are not necessarily the same as those that maintain such actions. Recall the relevant research of Nagin and Tremblay (2001): Child variables predicted early initiation of physical aggression, but family factors (teenage parenting, low parental educational attainment) predicted its persistence. (Note, however, that such parenting factors may themselves be subject to genetic mediation, raising yet again the interconnectedness of levels of causation.) Thus the strong evidence for multifactorial and interactive models of the development and maintenance of aggression and ASB makes it difficult to put forth an explanatory model in linear fashion.

We begin at the earliest stages of development, at which time (1) heritabilities for temperamental factors related to later aggression are not strong, and (2) sex differences in such emotional and behavioral patterns are minimal. By the preschool years, however, traits of impulsivity and sensation seeking become salient and more heritable, as are sex differences in aggressive interchanges, perhaps fueled by caregiver patterns of response to individual differences in difficult temperament or to early neurocognitive and language deficits. Indeed, caregivers of young children with such intraindividual tendencies are likely to be young, poorly educated parents with problems of impulse control and emotion regulation themselves. Furthermore, surprisingly early in development (and particularly by the preschool years), boys' and girls' peer socialization patterns have become substantially separate, accentuating externalizing tendencies among boys and internalizing patterns among girls (Keenan & Shaw, 1997; Maccoby, 1998). Thus, even before the onset of formal schooling, a web of gene–environment correlations and interactions is being spun, such that youngsters with high ADHD-related symptomatology (particularly impulsivity) and low verbal abilities (and perhaps executive functions) tend to elicit chains of negative, coercive interaction from families and peers, (Snyder & Patterson, 1995; see also the model of Moffitt, 1993). Note in this regard that the cognitive and behavioral patterns characteristic of ADHD are strongly heritable; when they occur in combination with early oppositionality and aggression, they tend to fuel the onset of a pernicious pattern of escalating coercion at home (often preceded by insecure attachment during infancy), academic failure at school, and peer rejection from agemates, all of which predict continuation of externalizing behavior patterns (e.g., Campbell, in press; Hinshaw, 1992, 1999; Parker & Asher, 1987; Patterson et al., 1992). If physical abuse is added to the mix, the risk of ensuing aggression—mediated by social-cognitive information-processing biases and failures of empathic responding—is even stronger (Coie & Dodge, 1998).

Many of the risk factors identified in Table 3.4, in fact, pertain to such "early starters," who are highly likely to be male and who are at far higher than average risk for continuation of aggression and ASB beyond childhood. Note that in the cases with the worst prognosis, individual and parenting risks are embedded in a matrix of family structural variables, neighborhood disenfranchisement, poverty, and unresponsive schooling. Such variables do not appear to have large direct effects on emerging ASB patterns, but rather appear to be mediated on the whole by discordant, harsh, and unresponsive parent–child interactions (Capaldi & Patterson, 1994).

We hasten to point out, however, three essential points. First, far from all boys with early signs of aggressive, hyperactive, and impulsive behavior will show an escalating, "life-course-persistent" pathway; in fact, desistance is normative. Second, it may well take examination of factors present well before the preschool years to ascertain just which "early starters" show the highest rates of persistence and escalation. Indeed, those with actual risk may need to be tracked from infancy or even earlier (e.g., Tremblay, 2000). The flip side, of course, is that the earlier the time period of the prediction, the more likely it is that false-positive predictions will occur, given current knowledge; this state of affairs presents an empirical and ethical conundrum for the field. Third, those children most likely to show the greatest risk for intensification of ASB are those with combinations of etiological influences (Rutter et al., 1974; Greenberg et al., 1993). That is, risks from insecure attachment, difficult temperament, discordant parent–child interactions after infancy and toddlerhood, neuropsychological deficits, unfavorable family structural factors, and socioeconomic adversity are far more pernicious in combination than when present singly or dually.

Thus, regarding the development of forms of ODD that are likely to escalate into CD, important patterns of transaction with the environment during the preschool years are essential contributing forces. In some cases, extremes of temperament; extremes of parental psychopathology/antisocial activities; extremes of heritable risk for ADHD; extremes of exposure to violent neighborhoods; and/or extremes of harsh, inconsistent, and unresponsive parenting may be sufficient in and of themselves to demarcate a trajectory heading toward aggression and delinquency. In most cases, however, the interaction and transaction of such risks are likely to yield higher probabilities of early initiation and persistence of ASB. Moreover, continued developmental influences via inconsistent and harsh families, unresponsive and chaotic schools, and deviant peer groups are undoubtedly necessary to maintain and fuel escalation to serious aggression and violence. Recall that early age at onset of diverse manifestations of antisocial activities is what best predicts persistent conduct problems. The developmental models of Lahey, Loeber, and colleagues are heuristic in this regard (see Hinshaw et al., 1993): When early ADHD symptoms and oppostionality are followed by physical fighting, stealing at home, and persistent lying by the start of elementary school, the pernicious problems of physical and sexual assault, serious burglary, initiation of substance abuse, and repetitive delinquency are likely by adolescence. Furthermore, the constellation of callous/unemotional traits may betray a psychophysiological pattern of poor conditionability and poor response to threatened punishment, which sets in motion the precursors to adult psychopathy (Frick et al., 2000).

It must be recalled that it is normative for physical aggression to decrease throughout childhood and adolescence. Thus, from this perspective, perhaps the field should be examining not so much what propels increases in ASB across development as what factors attenuate the age-expected decrease in vulnerable individuals. In addition, we reiterate that heritabilities for violence are low, leaving open the possibility that psychosocial influences are strong determinants of the propensity for violent behavior patterns. Interested readers are again referred to the provocative work of Athens (1997) and Rhodes (1999) for an account of the psychosocial, social-cognitive, and developmental construct of violentization.

We have not adequately emphasized, throughout this chapter, the strong likelihood that aggressive offenders have a high rate of being victimized as well as of victimizing. They are also, as noted earlier, far more likely than the norm to attempt suicide (Cairns et al., 1988). Thus added risks of aggression and ASB include serious injury or death (Loeber & Farrington, 2000).

A different pathway to adolescent ASB and offending is seen in the "adolescent-limited" subtype of Moffitt (1993), comprising relatively (and, in some investigations, absolutely) large numbers of adolescents who engage in nonaggressive forms of conduct problems but without the complex psychopathological histories of those with early-onset ASB. Social and historical factors, especially the "maturity gap" in many Western societies, may contribute to the protracted adolescence of large numbers of youths, who seek power and status otherwise unavailable to them through antisocial actions. Association with delinquent and otherwise deviant peers is a direct socialization influence on such adolescents. Thus youths with early-onset ASB may provide negative models for a far larger subset of teens. Recent data suggest, as well, that the depiction of such individuals as rapidly desisting from ASB at the end of the teenage years may be overstated (Kratzer & Hodgins, 1999; Moffitt et al., 2002). Indeed, engagement in an antisocial lifestyle during adolescence may set in motion a host of roadblocks or snares to the types of educational, vocational, and social experiences needed for optimal development.

Recent media attention to horrific acts of middle-class violence (e.g., the U.S. school massacres of the late 1990s) has suggested a different pathway to lethal violence—one marked by extreme peer victimization and scapegoating during childhood and adolescence, leading to vengeance when supported by (1) portrayals of violent models in the mass media (including the Internet) and (2) ready access to lethal weapons. Linkages between victimization, shame, and depression on the one hand, and uncontrolled rage on the other, require the serious attention of investigators and clinicians.

In all, our brief synthesis has emphasized the nature of interactive and transactional processes that begin early in life for a small subgroup of at-risk children, facilitating their development of threatening, aggressive, and antisocial patterns that constitute a major mental health and social problem for many years of their subsequent development. These youths are, in all likelihood, the "models" of antisocial responding for the far greater numbers of youth who begin to display delinquent behavior patterns in adolescence. Early intervention, and the search for factors that can promote desistance and resilience, are key goals for the field.

Closing Themes

We reiterate several central themes that have been the focus of our chapter. First, important subtypes and subcategories of the domain of ASB exist, and their recognition is essential for progress in the field. Second, these behavior patterns are multidetermined and multigenerational; breaking the cycles of aggression mediated by abuse, poverty, despair, and cultural acceptance of violence is a daunting goal. Third, causal pathways are complex and transactional: The interplay of psychobiological, psychological, familial, social-cognitive, socioeconomic, and sociocultural factors in shaping different types of ASB in different individuals is intriguing and challenging. Fourth, enhanced understanding of underlying mechanisms and of effective preventive intervention strategies is essential for individual and societal well-being.

For the future, at the level of developmental science, investigations are needed that span multiple levels of analysis (e.g., genes and behavior; social-cognitive processes and peer/family socialization) and that span the entire life course (Tremblay, 2000). In addition, person-centered strategies should supplement variable-centered risk research paradigms, given the importance of identifying risk and protective mechanisms within validated subtypes. Intervention and prevention trials must be recognized not only for their clinical importance, but also for their ability to yield causal inferences about underlying psychopathological mechanisms (Hinshaw, in press). In all, ideological rancor must give way to informed, multidisciplinary efforts aimed at understanding, reducing, and channeling aggression and antisocial activity.

We note, in closing, that many historic issues pertinent to psychopathology tend to be cyclic in nature. For example, patterns of use and abuse of different substances have ebbed and flowed in recent years, as a function of availability, cost, shifting legal strictures, and the like. It is therefore conceivable that rates of violence and antisocial activity, which have precipitously increased in recent decades but which have leveled off and even declined during the 1990s, will again increase as the new millennium opens with a failing economy and the threat (and reality) of worldwide terrorism. Along this line, the ever-growing portrayal of violence in the public media, the increasing rates of blended families, and still-easy access to dangerous weapons in our society may also portend an increase in violence. Furthermore, following Moffitt's (1993) analysis, the disparity between biological and psychosocial maturity in our culture is likely to widen rather than narrow in future years, as a function of earlier physical maturity in an increasingly technological age. Such trends presage continuing escalations in adolescent-onset antisocial activity, particularly in societies with ever-widening gaps between the wealthiest and poorest segments of the population, and particularly as the earth's population reaches critical levels. It is also conceivable that the constellation of teratogenic and perinatal factors, disrupted attachments, and poor educational preparation that accrue to ever-escalating numbers of stressed, impoverished families will also propel an increase in multiproblem youths with early-onset ASB. Overall, to reiterate our closing words in 1996, it is not the time to rest on the laurels of the field's quite real scientific gains of recent decades, but rather to redouble scientific and policy-related efforts.

ACKNOWLEDGMENT

Work on this chapter was supported by National Institute of Mental Health Grants No. R01 MH45064 and No. U01 MH50461.

NOTES

1. The term "undercontrolled" may be a misnomer, in the view of Block and Gjerde (1986), who contend that a disruptive, aggressive behavioral style may be associated with either an undercontrolled (impulsive) or an overcontrolled (planful, psychopathic) cognitive structure.

2. In addition, regarding the realm of attention deficits/hyperactivity, research has converged on the finding of a fundamental distinction between inattentive–disorganized and impulsive–hyperactive behaviors (see also Barkley, Chapter 2, this volume).

3. In adult psychopathology, for example, the ambiguously defined nature of Axis II personality disorders leads to extremely high rates of "comorbidity," signified by the ascription of multiple personality disorders to the same individual. Such overlap of disorders may in part be an artifact of a lack of coherence of the definitional criteria.

4. Richters (1992) provides thoughtful commentary on the nature of the association between mothers' depression and their often-noted tendency to rate their own children at high levels on scales measuring externalizing tendencies. Whereas definitive results await better-designed investigations, it appears that, rather than reflecting distorted or biased ratings, the linkage may well reflect accurate detection by mothers of independently corroborated acting-out behavior.

5. Space permits only brief mention of another seminal set of works regarding parent socialization and child aggression—namely, those by Wahler and colleagues. Over many years Wahler has emphasized the roles of maternal coercion and maternal attention/neglect in shaping aggressive behavior (e.g., Wahler & Dumas, 1987), with important consideration of such social-ecological variables as maternal isolation/insularity and family stress (e.g., Wahler & Hann, 1987; Wahler & Dumas, 1989). Wahler's work provides an important counterpoint to the seminal model of Patterson.

REFERENCES

Achenbach, T. M. (1991). *Manual for the Child Behavior Checklist/4–18 and 1991 Profile*. Burlington: University of Vermont, Department of Psychiatry.

Achenbach, T. M. (1993). Taxonomy and comorbidity of conduct problems: Evidence from empirically based approaches. *Development and Psychopathology, 5*, 51–64.

Achenbach, T. M., & Howell, C. T. (1993). Are American children's problems getting worse?: A 13-year comparison. *Journal of the American Academy of Child and Adolescent Psychiatry, 32*, 1145–1154.

Aguilar, B., Sroufe, L. A., Egeland, B., & Carlson, E. (2000). Distinguishing the early-onset persistent and adolescent-onset antisocial behavioral types: From birth to 16 years. *Development and Psychopathology, 12*, 109–132.

Amato, P. R., & Keith, B. (1991). Parental divorce and the well-being of children: A meta-analysis. *Psychological Bulletin, 110*, 26–46.

American Psychiatric Association. (1980). *Diagnostic and statistical manual of mental disorders* (3rd ed.). Washington, DC: Author.

American Psychiatric Association. (1987). *Diagnostic and statistical manual of mental disorders* (3rd ed., rev.). Washington, DC: Author.

American Psychiatric Association. (1994). *Diagnostic and statistical manual of mental disorders* (4th ed.). Washington, DC: Author.

Anderson, C. A., Hinshaw, S. P., & Simmel, C. (1994). Mother–child interactions in ADHD and comparison boys: Relationships to overt and covert externalizing behavior. *Journal of Abnormal Child Psychology, 22*, 247–265.

Anderson, K. E., Lytton, H., & Romney, D. M. (1986). Mothers' interactions with normal and conduct-disordered boys: Who affects whom? *Developmental Psychology, 22*, 604–609.

Angold, A., Costello, E. J., & Erkanli, A. (1999). Comorbidity. *Journal of Child Psychology and Psychiatry, 40*, 57–87.

Arsenault, L., Tremblay, R. E., Boulerice, B., Seguin, J., & Saucier, J. (2000). Minor physical anomalies and family adversity as risk factors for violent delinquency in adolescence. *American Journal of Psychiatry, 157*, 917–923.

Athens, L. (1997). *Violent criminal acts and actors revisited.* Urbana: University of Illinois Press.

Bardone, A. M., Moffitt, T. E., Caspi, A., Dickson, N., & Silva, P. A. (1996). Adult mental health and social outcomes of adolescent girls with depression and conduct disorder. *Development and Psychopathology, 8*, 811–829.

Barry, C. T., Frick, P. J., DeShazo, T. M., & McCoy, M. (2000). The importance of callous–unemotional traits for extending the concept of psychopathy to children. *Journal of Abnormal Psychology, 109*, 335–340.

Bergman, L. M., & Magnusson, D. (1997). A person-oriented approach in research on developmental psychopathology. *Development and Psychopathology, 9*, 291–319.

Berkson, J. (1946). Limitations on the applications of fourfold table analysis to hospital data. *Biometrics, 2*, 47–53.

Biederman, J., Newcorn, J., & Sprich, S. E. (1991). Comorbidity of attention deficit hyperactivity disorder with conduct, depressive, anxiety, and other disorders. *American Journal of Psychiatry, 148*, 564–577.

Bjorkqvist, K., Osterman, K., & Kaukianinen, A. (1992). The development of direct and indirect aggressive strategies in males and females. In K. Bjorkqvist & P. Niemala (Eds.), *Of mice and women: Aspects of female aggression* (pp. 51–64). New York: Academic Press.

Block, J., & Gjerde, P. (1986). Distinguishing between antisocial behavior and undercontrol. In D. Olweus, J. Block, & M. Radke-Yarrow (Eds.), *Development of antisocial and prosocial behavior: Research, theories, and issues* (pp. 177–206). Orlando, FL: Academic Press.

Brennan, P. A., Grekin, E. R., & Mednick, S. A. (1999). Maternal smoking during pregnancy and adult male criminal outcomes. *Archives of General Psychiatry, 56*, 215–219.

Brennan, P. A., Mednick, S. A., & Raine, A. (1997). Biosocial interactions and violence. In A. Raine (Ed.), *Biosocial bases of violence* (pp. 163–174). New York: Plenum Press.

Brooks-Gunn, J., & Warren, M. P. (1989). Biological and social contributions to negative affect in young adolescent girls. *Child Development, 60*, 40–55.

Brown, S., & van Praag, H. M. (Eds.). (1991). *The role of serotonin in psychiatric disorders*. New York: Brunner/Mazel.

Burt, S. A., Truger, R. F., McGue, M., & Iacono, W. G. (2001). Sources of covariation among attention deficit / hyperactivity disorder, oppositional defiant disorder, and conduct disorder: The importance of shared environment. *Journal of Abnormal Psychology, 110*, 516–525.

Cairns, R. B. (1979). *Social development: The origins and plasticity of interchanges*. San Francisco: Freeman.

Cairns, R. B., Cairns, B. D., Neckerman, H. J., Ferguson, L. L., & Gariepy, J. (1989). Growth and aggression: I. Childhood to early adolescence. *Developmental Psychology, 25*, 320–330.

Cairns, R. B., Peterson, G., & Neckerman, H. J. (1988). Suicidal behavior in aggressive adolescents. *Journal of Clinical Child Psychology, 27*, 298–309.

Campbell, S. B. (in press). *Behavior problems in preschool children: Clinical and developmental issues* (2nd ed.). New York: Guilford Press.

Campbell, S. B., & Ewing, L. J. (1990). Follow-up of hard-to-manage preschoolers: Adjustment at age 9 and predictors of continuing symptoms. *Journal of Child Psychology and Psychiatry, 31*, 871–889.

Campbell, S. B., Shaw, D. S., & Gilliom, M. (2000). Early externalizing behavior problems: Toddlers and preschoolers at risk for later maladjustment. *Development and Psychopathology, 12*, 467–488.

Capaldi, D. M. (1991). Co-occurrence of conduct problems and depressive symptoms in early adolescent boys: I. Familial factors and general adjustment in grade 6. *Development and Psychopathology, 3*, 277–300.

Capaldi, D. M., & Patterson, G. R. (1994). Interrelated influences of contextual factors on antisocial behavior in childhood and adolescence for males. In D. C. Fowles, P. Sutker, & S. H. Goodman (Eds.), *Progress in experimental personality and psychopathology research* (pp. 165–198). New York: Springer.

Caron, C., & Rutter, M. (1991). Comorbidity in child psychopathology: Concepts, issues, and research strategies. *Journal of Child Psychology and Psychiatry, 32*, 1063–1080.

Carlson, C. L., Tamm, L., & Gaub, M. (1997). Gender differences in children with ADHD, ODD, and co-occurring ADHD/ODD identified in a school population. *Journal of the American Academy of Child and Adolescent Psychiatry, 36*, 1706–1714.

Caspi, A. (2000). The child is father of the man: Personality continuities from childhood to adulthood. *Journal of Personality and Social Psychology, 78*, 158–172.

Caspi, A., Henry, B., McGee, R. O., Moffitt, T. E., & Silva, P. A. (1995). Temperamental origins of child and adolescent behavior problems: From age three to age fifteen. *Child Development, 66*, 55–68.

Caspi, A., Lynam, D., Moffitt, T. E., & Silva, P. A. (1993). Unraveling girls' delinquency: Biological, dispositional, and contextual contributions to adolescent misbehavior. *Developmental Psychology, 29*, 19–30.

Caspi, A., & Moffitt, T. E. (1995). The continuity of maladaptive behavior: From description to understanding in the study of antisocial behavior. In D. Cicchetti & D. Cohen (Eds.), *Developmental psychopathology* (Vol. 2, pp. 472–511). New York: Wiley.

Caspi, A., Taylor, A., Moffitt, T. E., & Plomin, R. (2000). Neighborhood deprivation affects children's mental health: Environmental risks identified in a genetic design. *Psychological Science, 11*, 338–342.

Chesney-Lind, M., & Shelden, R. G. (Eds.). (1992). *Girls: Delinquency and juvenile justice*. Pacific Grove, CA: Brooks/Cole.

Cicchetti, D., & Rogosch, F. (1996). Equifinality and multifinality in developmental psychopathology. *Development and Psychopathology, 8*, 597–600.

Cleckley, H. (1976). *The mask of sanity* (5th ed.). St. Louis, MO: Mosby.

Coie, J. D., & Dodge, K. A. (1998). Aggression and antisocial behavior. In W. Damon (Series Ed.) & N. Eisenberg (Vol. Ed.), *Handbook of child psychology: Vol. 3. Social, emotional, and personality development* (5th ed., pp. 779–862). New York: Wiley.

Coie, J. D., & Lenox, K. F. (1994). The development of antisocial individuals. In D. C. Fowles, P. Sutker, & S. H. Goodman (Eds.), *Progress in experimental personality and psychopathology research* (pp. 45–72). New York: Springer.

Coie, J. D., Terry, R., Lenox, K., Lochman, J. E., & Hyman, C. (1995). Childhood peer rejection and aggression as predictors of stable patterns of adolescent disorder. *Development and Psychopathology, 7*, 697–713.

Conduct Problems Prevention Research Group. (2002). The implementation of the Fast Track program: An example of a large-scale prevention science efficacy trial. *Journal of Abnormal Child Psychology, 30*, 1–17.

Coon, H., Carey, G., Corley, R., & Fulker, D. W. (1992). Identifying children in the Colorado Adoption Project at risk for conduct disorder. *Journal of the American Academy of Child and Adolescent Psychiatry, 31*, 503–511.

Costello, E. J., & Angold, A. (1993). Toward a developmental epidemiology of the disruptive behavior disorders. *Development and Psychopathology, 5*, 91–101.

Crick, N. R., & Bigbee, M. A. (1998). Relational and overt forms of peer victimization: A multi-informant approach. *Journal of Consulting and Clinical Psychology, 66*, 337–347.

Crick, N. R., & Dodge, K. A. (1994). A review and reformulation of social information processing mechanisms in children's social adjustment. *Psychological Bulletin, 115*, 74–101.

Crick, N. R., & Dodge, K. A. (1996). Social information-processing mechanisms in reactive and proactive aggression. *Child Development, 67*, 993–1002.

Crick, N. R., & Grotpeter, J. K. (1995). Relational aggression, gender, and social-psychological adjustment. *Child Development, 66*, 710–722.

Deater-Deckard, K., & Dodge, K. A. (1997). Externalizing behavior problems and discipline revisited: Nonlinear effects and variation by culture, context, and gender. *Psychological Inquiry, 8*, 161–175.

DeKlyen, M., & Speltz, M. L. (2001). Attachment and conduct disorder. In J. Hill & B. Maughan (Eds.), *Conduct disorders in childhood and adolescence* (pp. 320–345). New York: Cambridge University Press.

Dishion, T. J., Andrews, D. W., & Crosby, L. (1995). Antisocial boys and their friends in early adolescence: Relationship characteristics, quality, and interactional process. *Child Development, 66*, 139–151.

Dishion, T. J., Patterson, G. R., & Kavanagh, K. (1992). An experimental test of the coercion model: Linking theory, measurement, and intervention. In J. McCord & R. Tremblay (Eds.)., *The interaction of theory and practice: Experimental studies of interventions* (pp. 253–282). New York: Guilford Press.

Dodge, K. A. (1991). The structure and function of reactive and proactive aggression. In D. Pepler & K. Rubin (Eds.), *The development and treatment of childhood aggression* (pp. 201–218). Hillsdale, NJ: Erlbaum.

Dodge, K. A., Bates, J., & Pettit, G. S. (1990). Mechanisms in the cycle of violence. *Science, 250*, 1678–1683.

Dodge, K. A., & Frame, C. L. (1982). Social cognitive biases and deficits in aggressive boys. *Child Development, 53*, 629–635.

Dodge, K. A., Lochman, J. E., Harnish, J. D., & Bates, J. E. (1997). Reactive and proactive aggression in school children and psychiatrically impaired chronically assaultive youth. *Journal of Abnormal Psychology, 106*, 37–51.

Dodge, K. A., Pettit, G. S., & Bates, J. E. (1994). Socialization mediators of the relation between socioeconomic status and child conduct problems. *Child Development, 65*, 649–665.

Dodge, K. A., Pettit, G. S., Bates, J. E., & Valente, E. (1995). Social information-processing patterns partially mediate the effect of early physical abuse on later conduct problems. *Journal of Abnormal Psychology, 104*, 632–643.

Dodge, K. A., Price, J. M., Bachorowski, J., & Newman, J. M. (1990). Hostile attributional biases in severely aggressive adolescents. *Journal of Abnormal Psychology, 99*, 385–392.

Downey, G., & Coyne, J. C. (1990). Children of depressed parents: An integrative review. *Psychological Bulletin, 108*, 50–76.

Edelbrock, C., Rende, R., Plomin, R., & Thompson, L. A. (1995). A twin study of competence and problem behavior in childhood and early adolescence. *Journal of Child Psychology and Psychiatry, 36*, 775–785.

Eysenck, H. J. (1986). A critique of classification and diagnosis. In T. Millon & G. L. Klerman (Eds.), *Contemporary directions in psychopathology* (pp. 73–98). New York: Guilford Press.

Fagot, B. I., & Leve, L. D. (1998). Teacher ratings of externalizing behavior at school entry for boys and girls: Similar early predictors and different correlates. *Journal of Child Psychology and Psychiatry, 39*, 555–566.

Faraone, S. V., Biederman, J., Keenan, K., & Tsuang, M. T. (1991). Separation of DSM-III attention deficit disorder and conduct disorder: Evidence from a family genetic study of American child psychiatry patients. *Psychological Medicine, 21*, 109–121.

Farrington, D. P. (1992). Explaining the beginning, progress, and ending of antisocial behavior from birth to adulthood. In J. McCord (Ed.), *Advances in criminological theory* (pp. 253–286). New Brunswick, NJ: Transaction.

Farrington, D. P., & Loeber, R. (2000). Some benefits of dichotomization in psychiatric and criminological research. *Criminal Behavior and Mental Health, 10*, 100–122.

Farrington, D. P., Loeber, R., & Van Kammen, W. B. (1990). Long-term criminal outcomes of hyperactivity–impulsivity–attention deficit and conduct problems in childhood. In L. N. Robins & M. Rutter (Eds.), *Straight and devious pathways from childhood to adulthood* (pp. 62–81). Cambridge, England: Cambridge University Press.

Fergusson, D. M., & Horwood, L. J. (1995). Predictive validity of categorically and dimensionally scored measures of disruptive childhood behaviors. *Journal of the American Academy of Child and Adolescent Psychiatry, 34*, 477–485.

Fergusson, D. M., Horwood, L. J., & Lloyd, M. (1991). Confirmatory factor analysis of attention deficit and conduct disorder. *Journal of Child Psychology and Psychiatry, 32*, 257–274.

Fergusson, D. M., Horwood, L. J., & Nagin, D. S. (2000). Offending trajectories in a New Zealand birth cohort. *Criminology, 38*, 525–552.

Feschbach, S. (1970). Aggression. In P. H. Mussen (Ed.), *Carmichael's manual of child psychology* (pp. 159–259). New York: Wiley.

Fingerhut, L. A., & Kleinman, J. C. (1990). International and interstate comparisons of homicide among young males. *Journal of the American Medical Association, 263*, 3292–3295.

Fowles, D. C., & Missel, K. A. (1994). Electrodermal hyporeactivity, motivation, and psychopathy: Theoretical issues. In D. C. Fowles, P. Sutker, & S. H. Goodman (Eds.), *Progress in experimental personality and psychopathology research* (pp. 263–283). New York: Springer.

Frick, P. J., Bodin, S. D., & Barry, C. T. (2000). Psychopathic traits and conduct problems in community and clinic-referred samples of children: Further development of the PSD. *Psychological Assessment, 12*, 352–363.

Frick, P. J., Kamphaus, R. W., Lahey, B. B., Christ, M. A. G., Hart, E. L., & Tannenbaum, T. E. (1991). Academic underachievement and the disruptive behavior disorders. *Journal of Consulting and Clinical Psychology, 59*, 289–294.

Frick, P. J., Lahey, B. B., Loeber, R., Stouthamer-Loeber, M., Christ, M.A.G., & Hanson, K. (1992). Familial risk factors to oppositional defiant disorder and conduct disorder: Parental psychopathology and maternal parenting. *Journal of Consulting and Clinical Psychology, 60*, 49–55.

Frick, P. J., Lahey, B. B., Loeber, R., Tannenbaum, L., Van Horn, Y., Christ, M. A. G., Hart, E. L., & Hanson, K. (1993). Oppositional defiant disorder and conduct disorder: A meta-analytic review of factor analyses and cross-validation in a clinic sample. *Clinical Psychology Review, 13*, 319–340.

Frick, P. J., & Loney, B. (1999). Outcomes of children and adolescents with oppositional defiant disorder and conduct disorder. In H. C. Quay & A. E. Hogan (Eds.), *Handbook of disruptive behavior disorders* (pp. 507–524). New York: Plenum Press.

Garber, J. A., Lewinsohn, P.M., Seeley, J. R., & Brooks, J. (1997). Is psychopathology associated with the timing of pubertal development? *Journal of the American Academy of Child and Adolescent Psychiatry, 36*, 1768–1776.

Ge, X., Conger, R. D., & Elder, G.H. (1996). Coming of age too early: Pubertal influences on girls' vulnerability to psychological distress. *Child Development, 67*, 3386–3400.

Goodman, S. H., & Gotlib, I. H. (1999). Risk for psychopathology in the children of depressed mothers: A developmental model for understanding mechanisms of transmission. *Psychological Review, 106*, 458–490.

Goodman, S. H., & Kohlsdorf, B. (1994). The developmental psychopathology of conduct problems: Gender issues. In D. D. Fowles, P. Sutker, & S. H. Goodman (Eds.), *Progress in experimental personality and psychopathology research* (pp. 121–161). New York: Springer.

Gorman-Smith, D., Tolan, P. H., Loeber, R., & Henry, D. (1998). The relation of family problems to patterns of delinquency involvement among urban youth. *Journal of Abnormal Child Psychology, 26*, 319–333.

Gottlieb, G. (1995). Some conceptual deficiencies in 'developmental' behavioral genetics. *Human Development*, *38*, 131–141.

Gottlieb, G. (1998). Normally occurring environmental and behavioral influences on gene activity: From central dogma to probabilistic epigenesis. *Psychological Review*, *105*, 792–802.

Greenberg, M. T., & Speltz, M. L. (1988). Attachment and the ontogeny of conduct problems. In J. Belsky & T. Nezworski (Eds.), *Clinical implications of attachment* (pp. 177–218). Hillsdale, NJ: Erlbaum.

Greenberg, M. T., Speltz, M. L., & DeKlyen, M. (1993). The role of attachment in the early development of disruptive behavior problems. *Development and Psychopathology*, *5*, 191–213.

Greenberg, M. T., Speltz, M. L., DeKlyen, M., & Jones, K. (2001). Correlates of clinic referral for early conduct problems: Variable- and person-centered approaches. *Development and Psychopathology*, *13*, 255–276.

Hare. R. D., Hart, S. D., & Harpur, T. J. (1991). Psychopathy and the DSM-IV criteria for antisocial personality disorder. *Journal of Abnormal Psychology*, *100*, 391–398.

Harris, G. T., Rice, M. E., & Quinsey, V. L. (1994). Psychopathy as a taxon: Evidence that psychopaths are a discrete class. *Journal of Consulting and Clinical Psychology*, *62*, 387–397.

Hart, S. D., & Hare, R. D. (1997). Psychopathy: Assessment and association with criminal conduct. In D. M. Stoff, J. Breiling, & J. D. Maser (Eds.), *Handbook of antisocial behavior* (pp. 22–35). New York: Wiley.

Henry, B., Caspi, A., Moffitt, T. E., & Silva, P. A. (1996). Temperamental and familial predictors of violent and nonviolent criminal convictions: Age 3 to age 18. *Developmental Psychology*, *32*, 614–623.

Hewitt, L. E., & Jenkins, R. L. (1946). *Fundamental patterns of maladjustment: The dynamics of their origin*. Springfield: State of Illinois.

Hill, J., & Maughan, B. (Eds.). (2001). *Conduct disorders in childhood and adolescence*. New York: Cambridge University Press.

Hinshaw, S. P. (1987). On the distinction between attentional deficits/hyperactivity and conduct problems/aggression in child psychopathology. *Psychological Bulletin*, *101*, 443–463.

Hinshaw, S. P. (1992). Externalizing behavior problems and academic underachievement in childhood and adolescence: Causal relationships and underlying mechanisms. *Psychological Bulletin*, *111*, 127–155.

Hinshaw, S. P. (1994). Conduct disorder in childhood: Conceptualization, diagnosis, comorbidity, and risk status for antisocial functioning in adulthood. In D. C. Fowles, P. Sutker, & S. H. Goodman (Eds.), *Progress in experimental personality and psychopathology research* (pp. 3–44). New York: Springer.

Hinshaw, S. P. (1999). Psychosocial intervention for childhood ADHD: Etiologic and developmental themes, comorbidity, and integration with pharmacotherapy. In D. Cicchetti & S. L. Toth (Eds.), *Rochester Symposium on Developmental Psychopathology: Vol. 9. Developmental approaches to prevention and intervention* (pp. 221–270). Rochester, NY: University of Rochester Press.

Hinshaw, S. P. (in press). Intervention research, theoretical mechanisms, and causal processes related to externalizing behavior patterns. *Development and Psychopathology*.

Hinshaw, S. P., & Anderson, C. A. (1996). Conduct and oppositional defiant disorders. In E. J. Mash & R. A. Barkley (Eds.), *Child psychopathology* (pp. 108–148). New York: Guilford Press.

Hinshaw, S. P., Carte, E. T., Sami, N., Treuting., J. J., & Zupan, B. A. (2002). Preadolescent girls with attention-deficit/hyperactivity disorder: II. Neuropsychological performance in relation to subtypes and individual classification. *Journal of Consulting and Clinical Psychology*, *70*, 1099–1111.

Hinshaw, S. P., Lahey, B. B., & Hart, E. L. (1993). Issues of taxonomy and comorbidity in the development of conduct disorder. *Development and Psychopathology*, *5*, 31–49.

Hinshaw, S. P., & Melnick, S. M. (1995). Peer relationships in children with attention-deficit hyperactivity disorder with and without comorbid aggression. *Development and Psychopathology*, *7*, 627–647.

Hinshaw, S. P., & Nigg, J. T. (1999). Behavior rating scales in the assessment of disruptive behavior problems in childhood. In D. Shaffer, C. Lucas, & J. E. Richters (Eds.), *Diagnostic assessment in child and adolescent psychopathology* (pp. 91–126). New York: Guilford Press.

Hinshaw, S. P., Owens, E. B., Wells, K. C., Kraemer, H. C., Abikoff, H. B., Arnold, L. E., Conners, C. K., Elliott, G., Greenhill, L. L., Hechtman, L., Hoza, B., Jensen, P. S., March, J. S., Newcorn, J., Pelham, W. E., Swanson, J. M., Vitiello, B., & Wigal, T. (2000). Family processes and treatment outcome in the MTA: Negative/ineffective parenting practices in relation to multimodal treatment. *Journal of Abnormal Child Psychology*, *28*, 555–568.

Hinshaw, S. P., & Park, T. (1999). Research issues and problems: Toward a more definitive science of disruptive behavior disorders. In H. C. Quay & A. E. Hogan (Eds.), *Handbook of disruptive behavior disorders* (pp. 593–620). New York: Plenum Press.

Hinshaw, S. P., & Zupan, B. A. (1997). Assessment of antisocial behavior and conduct disorder in children. In D. Stoff, J. Breiling, & J. D. Maser (Eds.), *Handbook of antisocial behavior* (pp. 36–50). New York: Wiley.

Hirschi, T. (1969). *Causes of delinquency*. Berkeley: University of California Press.

Hodgins, S., Kratzer, L., & McNeil, T. F. (2001). Obstetrical complications, parenting, and risk of criminal behavior. *Archives of General Psychiatry*, *58*, 746–752.

Huesmann, L. R., Eron, L. D., Lefkowitz, M. M., & Walder, L. O. (1984). Stability of aggression over time and generations. *Developmental Psychology*, *20*, 1120–1134.

Jacobson, K. C., Prescott, C. A., & Kendler, K. S. (2002). Sex differences in the genetic and environmental influences on the development of antisocial behavior. *Development and Psychopathology*, *14*, 395–416.

Jaffe, S., Moffitt, T. E., Caspi, A., Belsky, J., & Silva, P. A. (2001). Why are children of teen mothers at risk? *Development and Psychopathology*, *13*, 377–397.

Jensen, P. S., Martin, D., & Cantwell, D. P. (1997). Comorbidity in ADHD: Implications for research, practice, and DSM-V. *Journal of the American Academy of Child and Adolescent Psychiatry*, *36*, 1065–1079.

Jessor, R., & Jessor, S. L. (1977). *Problem behavior and psychosocial development: A longitudinal study of youth*. New York: Academic Press.

Keenan, K. (2000). Emotion dysregulation as a risk factor for child psychopathology. *Clinical Psychology: Science and Practice*, *7*, 418–434.

Keenan, K., Loeber, R., & Green, S. (1999). Conduct disorder in girls: A review of the literature. *Clinical Child and Family Psychology Review*, *2*, 3–19.

Keenan, K., & Shaw, D. S. (1997). Developmental and social influences on young girls' early problem behavior. *Psychological Bulletin, 121*, 95–113.

Kirk, S. A., & Hutchins, H. (1994, June 20). Is bad writing a mental disorder? *The New York Times*.

Kovacs, M., Paulauskas, S., Gatsonis, C., & Richards, C. (1988). Depressive disorders in childhood: A longitudinal study of comorbidity with and risk for conduct disorders. *Journal of Affective Disorders, 15*, 205–217.

Kraemer, H. C., Kazdin, A. E., Offord, D. R., Kessler, R. C., Jensen, P. S., & Kupfer, D. J. (1997). Coming to terms with the terms of risk. *Archives of General Psychiatry, 54*, 337–343.

Kratzer, L., & Hodgins, S. (1997). Adult outcomes of child conduct problems: A cohort study. *Journal of Abnormal Child Psychology, 25*, 65–81.

Kratzer, L., & Hodgins, S. (1999). A typology of offenders: A test of Moffitt's theory among males and females from childhood to age 30. *Criminal Behaviour and Mental Health, 9*, 57–73.

Kruesi, M. J. P., Rapoport, J. L., Hamburger, S., Hibbs, E., Potter, W. Z., Lenane, M., & Brown, G. L. (1990). Cerebrospinal fluid monoamine metabolites, aggression, and impulsivity in disruptive behavior disorders of children and adolescents. *Archives of General Psychiatry, 47*, 419–426.

Lahey, B. B., Hart, E. L., Pliszka, S., Applegate, B., & McBurnett, K. (1993). Neurophysiological correlates of conduct disorder: A rationale and review of current research. *Journal of Clinical Child Psychology, 22*, 141–153.

Lahey, B. B., Hartdagen, S. E., Frick, P. J., McBurnett, K., Connor, R., & Hynd, G. W. (1988). Conduct disorder: Parsing the confounded relationship between parental divorce and antisocial personality. *Journal of Abnormal Psychology, 97*, 334–337.

Lahey, B. B., Loeber, R., Quay, H. C., Frick, P. J., & Grimm, S. (1992). Oppositional defiant and conduct disorders: Issues to be resolved for DSM-IV. *Journal of the American Academy of Child and Adolescent Psychiatry, 31*, 539–546.

Lahey, B. B., Loeber, R., Quay, H. C., Applegate, B., Shaffer, D., Waldman, I., Hart, E. L., McBurnett, K., Frick, P. J., Jensen, P., Dulcan, M., Canino, G., & Bird, H. (1998). Validity of DSM-IV subtypes of conduct disorder based on age of onset. *Journal of the American Academy of Child and Adolescent Psychiatry, 37*, 435–442.

Lahey, B. B., Loeber, R., Quay, H. C., Frick, P. J., & Grimm, J. (1997). Oppositional defiant disorder and conduct disorder. In T. A. Widiger, A. J. Frances, H. A. Pincus, R. Ross, M. B. First, & W. Davis (Eds.), *DSM-IV sourcebook* (Vol. 3, pp. 189–209). Washington, DC: American Psychiatric Press.

Lahey, B. B., McBurnett, K., & Loeber, R. (2000). Are attention-deficit/hyperactivity disorder and oppositional defiant disorder developmental precursors to conduct disorder? In A. J. Sameroff, M. Lewis, & S. M. Miller (Eds.), *Handbook of developmental psychopathology* (2nd ed., pp. 431–446). New York: Kluwer Academic/Plenum.

Lahey, B. B., McBurnett, K., Loeber, R., & Hart, E. L. (1995). Psychobiology of conduct disorder. In G. P. Sholevar (Ed.), *Conduct disorders in children and adolescents: Assessments and interventions* (pp. 27–44). Washington, DC: American Psychiatric Press.

Lahey, B. B., Miller, T. L., Gordon, R. A., & Riley, A. W. (1999). Developmental epidemiology of the disruptive behavior disorders. In H. C. Quay & A. E. Hogan (Eds.), *Handbook of disruptive behavior disorders* (pp. 23–48). New York: Plenum Press.

Lahey, B. B., Piacentini, J. C., McBurnett, K., Stone, P., Hartdagen, S., & Hynd, G. (1988). Psychopathology and antisocial behavior in the parents of children with conduct disorder and hyperactivity. *Journal of the American Academy of Child and Adolescent Psychiatry, 27*, 163–170.

Lahey, B. B., Waldman, I. D., & McBurnett, K. (1999). The development of antisocial behavior: An integrative causal model. *Journal of Child Psychology and Psychiatry, 40*, 669–682.

Laird, R. D., Jordan, K. Y., Dodge, K. A., Pettit, G. S., & Bates, J. E. (2001). Peer rejection in childhood, involvement with antisocial peers in early adolescence, and the development of externalizing behavior problems. *Development and Psychopathology, 13*, 337–354.

Lancelotta, G. X., & Vaughn, S. (1989). Relation between types of aggression and sociometric status: Peer and teacher perceptions. *Journal of Educational Psychology, 81*, 86–90.

Laub, J., & Lauritsen, J. (1998). The interdependence of school violence with neighborhood and family conditions. In D. Elliott, B. Hamburg, & K. Williams (Eds.), *Violence in American schools* (pp. 55–93). New York: Cambridge University Press.

Lilienfeld, S. O. (1992). The association between antisocial personality and somatization disorders: A review and integration of theoretical models. *Clinical Psychology Review, 12*, 641–662.

Lilienfeld, S. O., & Marino, L. (1999). Essentialism revisited: Evolutionary theory and the concept of mental disorder. *Journal of Abnormal Psychology, 108*, 400–411.

Lilienfeld, S. O., & Waldman, I. D. (1990). The relation between childhood attention-deficit hyperactivity disorder and adult antisocial behavior reexamined: The problem of heterogeneity. *Clinical Psychology Review, 10*, 699–725.

Lochman, J. E., & Dodge, K. A. (1994). Social-cognitive processes of severely violent, moderately aggressive, and nonaggressive boys. *Journal of Consulting and Clinical Psychology, 62*, 366–374.

Loeber, R. (1982). The stability of antisocial and delinquent child behavior: A review. *Child Development, 53*, 1431–1446.

Loeber, R. (1988). Natural histories of conduct problems, delinquency, and associated substance use: Evidence for developmental progressions. In B. B. Lahey & A. E. Kazdin (Eds.), *Advances in clinical child psychology* (pp. 73–124). New York: Plenum Press.

Loeber, R., Burke, J. D., Lahey, B. B., Winters, A., & Zera, M. (2000). Oppositional defiant and conduct disorder: A review of the last 10 years, part I. *Journal of the American Academy of Child and Adolescent Psychiatry, 39*, 1468–1484.

Loeber, R., DeLamatre, M., Tita, G., Cohen, J., Stouthamer-Loeber, M., & Farrington, D. P. (1999). Gun injury and mortality: The delinquent backgrounds of juvenile victims. *Violence and Victims, 14*, 339–352.

Loeber, R., & Farrington, D. P. (Eds.). (1998). *Serious and violent juvenile offenders: Risk factors and successful interventions*. Thousand Oaks, CA: Sage.

Loeber, R., & Farrington, D. P. (2000). Young children who commit crime: Epidemiology, developmental origins, risk factors, early interventions, and policy implications. *Development and Psychopathology, 12*, 737–762.

Loeber, R., & Farrington, D. P. (Eds.). (2001). *Child delinquents: Development, intervention, and service needs.* Thousand Oaks, CA: Sage.

Loeber, R., Farrington, D. P., Stouthamer-Loeber, M., & Van Kammen, W. B. (1998). *Antisocial behavior and mental health problems: Explanatory factors in childhood and adolescence*. Mahwah, NJ: Erlbaum.

Loeber, R., Green, S. M., Keenan, K., & Lahey, B. B. (1995). Which boys will fare worse?: Early predictors of the onset of conduct disorder in a six-year longitudinal study. *Journal of the American Academy of Child and Adolescent Psychiatry, 34*, 499–509.

Loeber, R., Green, S. M., Lahey, B. B., Christ, M. A. G., & Frick, P. J. (1992). Developmental sequences in the age of onset of disruptive child behaviors. *Journal of Child and Family Studies, 1*, 21–41.

Loeber, R., & Hay, D. (1997). Key issues in the development of aggression and violence from childhood to early adulthood. *Annual Review of Psychology, 48*, 371–410.

Loeber, R., & Keenan, K. (1994). Interaction between conduct disorder and its comorbid conditions: Effects of age and gender. *Clinical Psychology Review, 14*, 497–523.

Loeber, R., Keenan, K., Lahey, B. B., Green, S. M., & Thomas, C. (1993). Evidence for developmentally based diagnoses of oppositional defiant disorder and conduct disorder. *Journal of Abnormal Child Psychology, 21*, 377–410.

Loeber, R., Keenan, K., & Zhang, Q. (1997). Boys' experimentation and persistence in developmental pathways toward serious delinquency. *Journal of Child and Family Studies, 6*, 321–357.

Loeber, R., Lahey, B. B., & Thomas, C. (1991). Diagnostic conundrum of oppositional defiant disorder and conduct disorder. *Journal of Abnormal Psychology, 100*, 379–390.

Loeber, R., & Schmaling, K. B. (1985). Empirical evidence for overt and covert patterns of antisocial conduct problems: A meta-analysis. *Journal of Abnormal Child Psychology, 13*, 337–352.

Loeber, R., & Stouthamer-Loeber, M. (1986). Family factors as correlates and predictors of juvenile conduct problems and delinquency. In M. Tonry & N. Morris (Eds.), *Crime and justice* (Vol. 17, pp. 29–149). Chicago: University of Chicago Press.

Loeber, R., & Stouthamer-Loeber, M. (1998). Development of juvenile aggression and violence: Some common misconceptions and controversies. *American Psychologist, 53*, 242–259.

Loeber, R., Stouthamer-Loeber, M., & White, H. R. (1999). Developmental aspects of delinquency and internalizing problems and their association with persistent juvenile substance abuse between ages 7 and 18. *Journal of Clinical Child Psychology, 28*, 322–332.

Loeber, R., Wung, P., Keenan, K., Giroux, B., Stouthamer-Loeber, M., Van Kammen, W. B., & Maughan, B. (1993). Developmental pathways in disruptive child behavior. *Development and Psychopathology, 5*, 103–133.

Loney, J. (1987). Hyperactivity and aggression in the diagnosis of attention deficit disorder. In B. B. Lahey & A. E. Kazdin (Eds.), *Advances in clinical child psychology* (Vol. 10, pp. 99–135). New York: Plenum Press.

Luthar, S., Cicchetti, D., & Becker, B. (2000). The construct of resilience: A critical evaluation and guidelines for work. *Child Development, 71*, 543–562.

Lynam, D. R. (1998). Early identification of the fledgling psychopath: Locating the psychopathic child in the current nomenclature. *Journal of Abnormal Psychology, 107*, 566–575.

Lynam, D. R., Caspi, A., Moffitt, T., Wikstrom, P.-O., Loeber, R., & Novak, S. (2000). The interaction between impulsivity and neighborhood context on offending: The effects of impulsivity are stronger in poorer neighborhoods. *Journal of Abnormal Psychology, 109*, 563–574.

Lynam, D. R., & Henry, B. (2001). The role of neuropsychological deficits in conduct disorders. In J. Hill & B. Maughan (Eds.), *Conduct disorders in childhood and adolescence* (pp. 235–263). New York: Cambridge University Press.

Lynam, D., R., Moffitt, T. E., & Stouthamer-Loeber, M. (1993). Explaining the relationship between IQ and delinquency: Class, race, test motivation, school failure, or self-control? *Journal of Abnormal Psychology, 102*, 187–196.

Lyons-Ruth, K., Alpern, L., & Repacholi, B. (1993). Disorganized infant attachment classification and maternal psychosocial problems as predictors of hostile–aggressive behavior in the preschool classroom. *Child Development, 64*, 572–585.

Lytton, H. (1990). Child and parent effects in boys' conduct disorder: A reinterpretation. *Developmental Psychology, 26*, 683–697.

Maccoby, E. E. (1998). *The two sexes: Growing up apart, coming together*. Cambridge, MA: Harvard University Press.

Maccoby, E. E. (2000). Parenting and its effects on children: On reading and misreading behavior genetics. *Annual Review of Psychology, 51*, 1–27.

Magnusson, D. (1987). Adult delinquency in the light of conduct and physiology at an early age: A longitudinal study. In D. Magnusson & A. Ohman (Eds.), *Psychopathology: An interactional perspective* (pp. 221–234). Orlando, FL: Academic Press.

Maguin, E., & Loeber, R. (1996). Academic performance and delinquency. In M. Tonry (Ed.), *Crime and justice* (Vol. 20, pp. 145–264). Chicago: University of Chicago Press.

Mannuzza, S., Klein, R. G., Bonagura, N., Malloy, P., Giampino, T. L., & Addalli, K. A. (1991). Hyperactive boys almost grown up: V. Replication of psychiatric status. *Archives of General Psychiatry, 48*, 77–83.

Maughan, B., Gray, G., & Rutter, M. (1985). Reading retardation and antisocial behavior: A follow-up into employment. *Journal of Child Psychology and Psychiatry, 26*, 741–758.

Maughan, B., & Rutter, M. (1998). Continuities and discontinuities in antisocial behavior from childhood to adult life. In T. H. Ollendick & R. J. Prinz (Eds.), *Advances in clinical child psychology* (Vol. 20, pp. 1–47). New York: Plenum Press.

McBurnett, K., & Lahey, B. B. (1994). Neuropsychological and neuroendocrine correlates of conduct disorder and antisocial behavior in children and adolescents. In D. C. Fowles, P. Sutker, & S. H. Goodman (Eds.), *Progress in experimental personality and psychopathology research* (pp. 199–231). New York: Springer.

McBurnett, K., Lahey, B. B., Rathouz, P. J., & Loeber, R. (1999). Low salivary cortisol and persistent aggression in boys referred for disruptive behavior. *Archives of General Psychiatry, 57*, 38–43.

McDermott, P. A. (1996). A nationwide study of developmental and gender prevalence for psychopathology in childhood and adolescence. *Journal of Abnormal Child Psychology, 24*, 53–66.

McGee, R., Feehan, M., Williams, S., & Anderson, J. (1992). DSM-III disorders from age 11 to age 15 years. *Journal of the American Academy of Child and Adolescent Psychiatry, 31*, 50–59.

McLoyd, V. (1990). The impact of economic hardship on black families and children: Psychological distress, parenting, and socioemotional development. *Child Development*, *61*, 311–346.

McMahon, R. J., & Wells, K. C. (1998). Conduct problems. In E. J. Mash & R. A. Barkley (Eds.), *Treatment of childhood disorders* (2nd ed., pp. 111–207). New York: Guilford Press.

Milich, R., & Dodge, K. A. (1984). Social information processing deficits in child psychiatry populations. *Journal of Abnormal Child Psychology*, *12*, 471–489.

Milich, R., & Landau, S. (1988). The role of social status variables in differentiating subgroups of hyperactive children. In L. M. Bloomingdale & J. M. Swanson (Eds.), *Attention deficit disorder* (Vol. 4, pp. 1–16). Oxford: Pergamon Press.

Moffitt, T. E. (1990). Juvenile delinquency and attention deficit disorder: Boys' developmental trajectories from age 3 to age 15. *Child Development*, *61*, 893–910.

Moffitt, T. E. (1993). "Life-course persistent" and "adolescence-limited" antisocial behavior: A developmental taxonomy. *Psychological Review*, 674–701.

Moffitt, T. E., & Caspi, A. (2001). Childhood predictors differentiate life-course persistent and adolescence-limited antisocial pathways among males and females. *Development and Psychopathology*, *13*, 355–375.

Moffitt, T. E., Caspi, A., Belsky, J., & Silva, P. A. (1992). Childhood experience and the onset of menarche: A test of a sociobiological model. *Child Development*, *63*, 47–58.

Moffitt, T. E., Caspi, A., Dickson, N., Silva, P. A., & Stanton, W. (1996). Childhood-onset vs. adolescence-limited antisocial conduct in males: Natural history from age 3 to 18. *Development and Psychopathology*, *8*, 399–424.

Moffitt, T. E, Caspi, A., Harrington, H., & Milne, B. J. (2002). Males on the life-course persistent and adolescence-limited antisocial pathways: Follow-up at age 26 years. *Development and Psychopathology*, *14*, 179–207.

Moffitt, T. E., Caspi, A., Rutter, M., & Silva, P. A. (2001). *Sex differences in antisocial behaviour: Conduct disorder, delinquency, and violence in the Dunedin longitudinal study*. Cambridge, England: Cambridge University Press.

Moffitt, T. E., & Lynam, D. (1994). The neuropsychology of conduct disorder and delinquency: Implications for understanding antisocial behavior. In D. C. Fowles, P. Sutker, & S. H. Goodman (Eds.), *Progress in experimental personality and psychopathology research* (pp. 233–262). New York: Springer.

Moffitt, T. E., & Silva, P. A. (1988). IQ and delinquency: A direct test of the differential detection hypothesis. *Journal of Abnormal Psychology*, *97*, 330–333.

Mulvey, E. P., & Cauffman, E. (2001). The inherent limits of predicting school violence. *American Psychologist*, *56*, 797–802.

Nagin, D. S., Farrington, D. P., & Moffitt, T. E. (1995). Life-course trajectories of different types of offenders. *Criminology*, *33*, 111–139.

Nagin, D. S., & Tremblay, R. E. (1999). Trajectories of boys' physical aggression, opposition, and hyperactivity on the path to physically violent and nonviolent juvenile delinquency. *Child Development*, *70*, 1181–1196.

Nagin, D. S., & Tremblay, R. E. (2001). Parental and early childhood predictors of persistent physical aggression in boys from kindergarten to high school. *Archives of General Psychiatry*, *58*, 389–394.

Nigg, J. T. (2000). On inhibition/disinhibition in developmental psychopathology: Views from cognitive and personality psychology and a working inhibition taxonomy. *Psychological Bulletin*, *126*, 220–246.

Nigg, J. T., Hinshaw, S. P., Carte, E. T., & Treuting, J. (1998). Neuropsychological correlates of childhood attention deficit hyperactivity disorder: Explainable by comorbid disruptive behavior or reading problems? *Journal of Abnormal Psychology*, *107*, 468–480.

O'Connor, T. G., Deater-Deckard, K., Fulker, D., Rutter, M., & Plomin, R. (1998). Genotype–environment correlations in late childhood and early adolescence: Antisocial behavior problems and coercive parenting. *Developmental Psychology*, *34*, 970–981.

Offord, D. R., Alder, R. J., & Boyle, M. H. (1986). Prevalence and sociodemographic correlates of conduct disorder. *American Journal of Social Psychiatry*, *4*, 272–278.

Offord, D. R., Boyle, M. H., & Racine, Y. A. (1991). The epidemiology of antisocial behavior in childhood and adolescence. In D. J. Pepler & K. H. Rubin (Eds.), *The development and treatment of childhood aggression* (pp. 31–54). Hillsdale, NJ: Erlbaum.

Olweus, D. (1979). Stability of aggressive reaction patterns in males: A review. *Psychological Bulletin*, *86*, 852–875.

Pajer, K. A. (1998). What happens to "bad" girls?: A review of the adult outcomes of antisocial adolescent girls. *American Journal of Psychiatry*, *155*, 862–870.

Parke, R. D., & Slaby, R. G. (1983). The development of aggression. In P. Mussen (Series Ed.) & E. M. Hetherington (Vol. Ed.), *Handbook of child psychology: Vol. 4. Socialization, personality, and social development* (4th ed., pp. 547–641). New York: Wiley.

Parker, J. G., & Asher, S. R. (1987). Peer relations and later personal adjustment: Are low accepted children at risk? *Psychological Bulletin*, *102*, 357–389.

Patterson, G. R. (1982). *Coercive family process*. Eugene, OR: Castalia.

Patterson, G. R. (1993). Orderly change in a stable world: The antisocial trait as a chimera. *Journal of Consulting and Clinical Psychology*, *61*, 911–919.

Patterson, G. R., DeBaryshe, B. D., & Ramsey, E. (1989). A developmental perspective on antisocial behavior. *American Psychologist*, *44*, 329–335.

Patterson, G. R., DeGarmo, D. S., & Knutson, N. (2000). Hyperactive and antisocial behaviors: Comorbid or two points in the same process? *Development and Psychopathology*, *12*, 91–106.

Patterson, G. R., Forgatch, M. S., Yoerger, K. L., & Stoolmiller, M. (1998). Variables that initiate and maintain an early-onset trajectory for juvenile offending. *Development and Psychopathology*, *10*, 531–547.

Patterson, G. R., Reid, J. B., & Dishion, T. J. (1992). *Antisocial boys*. Eugene, OR: Castalia.

Patterson, G. R., & Stouthamer-Loeber, M. (1984). The correlation of family management practices and delinquency. *Child Development*, *55*, 1299–1307.

Pickles, A., & Angold, A. (in press). Natural categories or fundamental dimensions: On carving nature at the joints and the re-articulation of psychopathology. *Development and Psychopathology*.

Plomin, R., & Crabbe, J. (2000). DNA. *Psychological Bulletin*, *126*, 806–828.

Quay, H. C. (1986). Conduct disorders. In H. C. Quay & J. S. Werry (Eds.), *Psychopathological disorders of childhood* (3rd ed., pp. 35–72). New York: Wiley.

Quay, H. C. (1987). Patterns of delinquent behavior. In H. C. Quay (Ed.), *Handbook of juvenile delinquency* (pp. 118–138). New York: Wiley.

Quay, H. C. (1993). The psychobiology of undersocialized aggressive conduct disorder: A theoretical perspective. *Development and Psychopathology, 5,* 165–180.

Quay, H. C., & Hogan, A. E. (Eds.). (1999). *Handbook of disruptive behavior disorders.* New York: Plenum Press.

Raine, A. (1993). *The psychopathology of crime: Criminal behavior as a clinical disorder.* San Diego, CA: Academic Press.

Raine, A. (1997). Antisocial behavior and psychophysiology: A biosocial perspective and a prefrontal dysfunction hypothesis. In D. Stoff, J. Breiling, & J. D. Maser (Eds.), *Handbook of antisocial behavior* (pp. 289–304). New York: Wiley.

Raine, A., Brennan, P., & Mednick, S. A. (1994). Birth complications combined with early maternal rejection at age 1 predispose to violent crime at age 18 years. *Archives of General Psychiatry, 51,* 984–988.

Raine, A., Brennan, P., & Mednick, S. A. (1997). Interaction between birth complications and early maternal rejection in predisposing individuals to adult violence: Specificity to serious, early-onset violence. *American Journal of Psychiatry, 154,* 1265–1271.

Raine, A., Brennan, P., Mednick, B., & Mednick, S. A. (1996). High rates of violence, crime, academic problems, and behavioral problems in males with both early neuromotor deficits and unstable early environments. *Archives of General Psychiatry, 53,* 544–549.

Raine, A., & Liu, J.-H. (1998). Biological predispositions to violence and their implications for biosocial treatment and prevention. *Psychology, Crime and Law, 4,* 107–125.

Raine, A., Yaralian, P. S., Reynolds, C. Venables, P. H., & Mednick, S. (2002). Spatial but not verbal cognitive deficits at age 3 years in persistently antisocial individuals. *Development and Psychopathology, 14,* 25–44.

Rey, J. M., Bashir, M. R., Schwarz, M., Richards, I. N., Plapp, J. M., & Stewart, G. W. (1988). Oppositional disorder: Fact or fiction? *Journal of the American Academy of Child and Adolescent Psychiatry, 27,* 157–162.

Rhodes, R. (1999). *Why they kill: The discoveries of a maverick criminologist.* New York: Vintage Books.

Richters, J. E. (1992). Depressed mothers as informants about their children: A critical review of the evidence for distortion. *Psychological Bulletin, 112,* 485–499.

Richters, J. E., & Cicchetti, D. (1993). Mark Twain meets DSM-III-R: Conduct disorder, development, and the concept of harmful dysfunction. *Development and Psychopathology, 5,* 5–29.

Richters, J. E., & Hinshaw, S. P. (1999). The abduction of disorder in psychiatry. *Journal of Abnormal Psychology, 105,* 438–445.

Richters, J. E., & Martinez, P. E. (1993). Violent communities, family choices, and children's chances: An algorithm for improving the odds. *Development and Psychopathology, 5,* 609–627.

Robins, L. N. (1966). *Deviant children grown up: A sociological and psychiatric study of sociopathic personality.* Baltimore: Williams & Wilkins.

Robins, L. N. (1978). Aetiological implications in studies of childhood histories relating to antisocial personality. In R. D. Hare & D. Schalling (Eds.), *Psychopathic behaviour: Approaches to research* (pp. 255–271). Chichester, England: Wiley.

Robins, L. N. (1986). The consequences of conduct disorder in girls. In D. Olweus, J. Block, & M. Radke-Yarrow (Eds.), *The development of antisocial and prosocial behavior: Research, theories, and issues* (pp. 385–414). Orlando, FL: Academic Press.

Robins, L. N. (1991). Conduct disorder. *Journal of Child Psychology and Psychiatry, 32,* 193–212.

Robins, L. N., & McEvoy, L. (1990). Conduct problems as predictors of substance abuse. In L. N. Robins & M. Rutter (Eds.), *Straight and devious pathways from childhood to adulthood* (pp. 182–204). Cambridge, England: Cambridge University Press.

Robins, L. N., & Regier, D. A. (1991). *Psychiatric disorders in America: The Epidemiologic Catchment Area study.* New York: Free Press.

Rutter, M., Giller, H., & Hagell, A. (1998). *Antisocial behavior by young people.* Cambridge, England: Cambridge University Press.

Rutter, M., Yule, B., Quinton, D., Rowlands, O., Yule, W., & Berger, M. (1974). Attainment and adjustment in two geographical areas: III. Some factors accounting for area differences. *British Journal of Psychiatry, 125,* 520–533.

Sampson, R. J., & Groves, W. B. (1989). Community structure and crime: Testing social-disorganization theory. *American Journal of Sociology, 94,* 774–802.

Satterfield, J. H., Hoppe, C. M., & Schell, A. M. (1982). A prospective study of delinquency in 110 adolescent boys with attention deficit disorder and 88 normal adolescent boys. *American Journal of Psychiatry, 139,* 795–798.

Satterfield, J. H., Swanson, J., Schell, A. M., & Lee, F. (1994). Prediction of antisocial behavior in attention deficit hyperactivity disorder boys from aggression/defiance scores. *Journal of the American Academy of Child and Adolescent Psychiatry, 33,* 185–190.

Shaffi, N., Carrigan, S., Whittinghill, J. R., & Derrick, A. (1985). Psychological autopsy of completed suicide of children and adolescents. *American Journal of Psychiatry, 142,* 1061–1064.

Shaw, D. S., Bell, R. Q., & Gilliom, M. (2000). A truly early starter model of antisocial behavior revisited. *Clinical Child and Family Psychology Review, 3,* 158–172.

Shaw, D. S., Owens, E. B., Giovannelli, J., & Winslow, E. B. (2001). Infant and toddler pathways leading to early externalizing disorders. *Journal of the American Academy of Child and Adolescent Psychiatry, 40,* 36–43.

Silberg, J., Meyer, J., Rutter, M., Simonoff, E., Hewitt, J., Loeber, R., Pickles, A., Maes, H., & Eaves, L. (1996). Genetic and environmental influences on the covariation between hyperactivity and conduct disturbance in juvenile twins. *Journal of Child Psychology and Psychiatry, 37,* 803–816.

Silverthorn, P., & Frick, P. J. (1999). Developmental pathways to antisocial behavior: The delayed-onset pathway in girls. *Development and Psychopathology, 11,* 101–126.

Snyder, J. J., & Patterson, G. R. (1995). Individual differences in social aggression: A test of a reinforcement model of socialization in the natural environment. *Behavior Therapy, 26,* 371–391.

Snyder, H. N., & Sickmund, M. (1995). *Juvenile offenders and victims: A national report.* Washington, DC: Office for Juvenile Justice and Delinquency Prevention.

Speltz, M. L., DeKlyen, M., & Greenberg, M. T. (1999). Attachment in boys with early-onset conduct problems. *Development and Psychopathology, 11,* 269–285.

Speltz, M. L., Greenberg, M. T., & DeKlyen, M. (1990). Attachment in preschoolers with disruptive behavior: A comparison of clinic-referred and nonproblem children. *Development and Psychopathology, 2,* 31–46.

Stattin, H., & Magnusson, D. (1989). The role of early aggressive behavior in the frequency, seriousness, and types

of later crime. *Journal of Consulting and Clinical Psychology, 57*, 710–718.
Stoff, D. M., Breiling, J., & Maser, J. D. (Eds.). (1997). *Handbook of antisocial behavior*. New York: Wiley.
Sutker, P. B. (1994). Psychopathy: Traditional and clinical antisocial concepts. In D. C. Fowles, P. Sutker, & S. H. Goodman (Eds.), *Progress in experimental personality and psychopathology research* (pp. 73–120). New York: Springer.
Taylor, J., Iacono, W. G., & McGue, M. (2000). Evidence for a genetic etiology of early-onset delinquency. *Journal of Abnormal Psychology, 109*, 634–643.
Tolan, P. H., Gorman-Smith, D., & Loeber, R. (2000). Developmental timing of onsets of disruptive behaviors and later delinquency of inner-city youth. *Journal of Child and Family Studies, 9*, 203–230.
Tremblay, R. E. (2000). The development of aggressive behavior during childhood: What have we learned in the past century? *International Journal of Behavioral Development, 24*, 129–141.
Tremblay, R. E., Pihl, R. O., Vitaro, F., & Dobkin, P. L. (1994). Predicting early onset of male antisocial behavior from preschool behavior. *Archives of General Psychiatry, 51*, 732–738.
Wahler, R. G., & Dumas, J. E. (1987). Family factors in childhood psychopathology: Toward a coercion–neglect model. In T. Jacob (Ed.), *Family interaction and psychopathology: Theories, methods, and findings* (pp. 581–627). New York: Plenum Press.
Wahler, R. G., & Dumas, J. E. (1989). Attentional problems in dysfunctional mother–child interactions: An interbehavioral model. *Psychological Bulletin, 105*, 116–130.
Wahler, R. G., & Hann, D. M. (1987). An interbehavioral approach to clinical child psychology: Toward an understanding of troubled families. In D. H. Ruben & D. J. Delprato (Eds.), *New ideas in therapy: Introduction to an interdisciplinary approach* (pp. 53–78). New York: Greenwood Press.
Wakefield, J. C. (1992). The concept of mental disorder: On the boundary between biological facts and social values. *American Psychologist, 47*, 373–388.
Wakefield, J. C. (1999). Evolutionary versus prototype analyses of the concept of disorder. *Journal of Abnormal Psychology, 108*, 374–399.
Wakschlag, L. S., Gordon, R. A., Lahey, B. B., Loeber, R., Green, S. M., & Leventhal, B. N. (2000). Maternal age at first birth and boys' risk for conduct disorder. *Journal of Research on Adolescence, 10*, 417–441.
Wakschlag, L. S., Lahey, B. B., Loeber, R., Green, S. M., Gordon, R. A., & Leventhal, B. L. (1997). Maternal smoking during pregnancy and the risk of conduct disorder in boys. *Archives of General Psychiatry, 54*, 670–676.
Walker, J. L., Lahey, B. B., Hynd, G. W., & Frame, C. L. (1987). Comparison of specific patterns of antisocial behavior in children with conduct disorder with or without coexisting hyperactivity. *Journal of Consulting and Clinical Psychology, 55*, 910–913.
Waschbusch, D. (2002). A meta-analytic examination of comorbid hyperative–impulsive-attention problems and conduct problems. *Psychological Bulletin, 128*, 118–150.
Webster-Stratton, C. (1996). Early-onset conduct problems: Does gender make a difference? *Journal of Consulting and Clinical Psychology, 64*, 540–551.
Werner, E. E., & Smith, R. S. (1992). *Overcoming the odds: High risk children from birth to adulthood*. Ithaca, NY: Cornell University Press.
White, H. R., Loeber, R., Stouthamer-Loeber, M., & Farrington, D. P. (1999). Developmental associations between substance use and violence. *Development and Psychopathology, 11*, 785–803.
White, J., L., Moffitt, T. E., Earls, F., Robins, L., & Silva, P. (1990). How early can we tell?: Predictors of childhood conduct disorder and adolescent delinquency. *Criminology, 28*, 507–528.
White, J. L., Moffitt, T. E., Caspi, A., Jeglum-Bartusch, D., Needles, D. J., & Stouthamer-Loeber, M. (1994). Measuring impulsivity and examining its relation to delinquency. *Journal of Abnormal Psychology, 103*, 192–205.
Widom, K. S. (1989). Intergenerational transmission of child abuse. *Science, 244*, 160–166.
Widom, K. S. (1997). Child abuse, neglect, and witnessing violence. In D. M. Stoff, J. Breiling, & J. D. Maser (Eds.), *Handbook of antisocial behavior* (pp. 159–170). New York: Wiley.
Woodward, L. J., & Fergusson, D. M. (1999). Early conduct problems and later risk of teenage pregnancy in girls. *Development and Psychopathology, 11*, 127–141.
Wootton, J. M., Frick, P. J., Shelton, K. K., & Silverthorn, P. (1997). Ineffective parenting and childhood conduct problems: The moderating role of callous-unemotional traits. *Journal of Consulting and Clinical Psychology, 65*, 301–308.
World Health Organization. (1992). *International classification of diseases* (10th ed.). Geneva: Author.
Zahn-Waxler, C. (1993). Warriors and worriers: Gender and psychopathology. *Development and Psychopathology, 5*, 79–89.
Zimring, F. E. (1998). *American youth violence*. New York: Oxford University Press.
Zoccolillo, M. (1992). Co-occurrence of conduct disorder and its adult outcomes with depressive and anxiety disorders: A review. *Journal of the American Academy of Child and Adolescent Psychiatry, 31*, 547–556.
Zoccolillo, M. (1993). Gender and the development of conduct disorder. *Development and Psychopathology, 5*, 65–78.
Zoccolillo, M., Pickles, A., Quinton, D., & Rutter, M. (1992). The outcome of conduct disorder: Implications for defining adult personality disorder and conduct disorder. *Psychological Medicine, 22*, 971–986.
Zoccolillo, M., Tremblay, R., & Vitaro, F. (1996). DSM-III-R and DSM-III criteria for conduct disorder in preadolescent girls: Specific but insensitive. *Journal of the American Academy of Child and Adolescent Psychiatry, 35*, 461–470.

CHAPTER
FOUR

Adolescent Substance Use Disorders

Laurie Chassin
Jennifer Ritter
Ryan S. Trim
Kevin M. King

Adolescent substance use and substance use disorders are topics of important clinical and public health concern because of their prevalence and associated negative consequences. Considering all age groups, recent estimates suggest that the use and misuse of alcohol, nicotine, and illegal drugs cost the United States approximately $257 billion per year—exceeding the costs associated with heart disease or cancer (Institute of Medicine, 1994a). Although many adolescents experiment with substance use without experiencing adverse consequences, the risks associated with substance use include mortality and morbidity as the result of impaired driving, increased risk for HIV infection, and risk for smoking-related disease (Institute of Medicine, 1994a; National Institute on Alcohol Abuse and Alcoholism, 1997). Frequent and prolonged consumption among adolescents not only increases their risk for developing a substance use disorder, but can also impair emerging developmental competence and psychosocial functioning (Baumrind & Moselle, 1985; Chassin, Pitts, & DeLucia, 1999; see Newcomb & Bentler, 1988, for a review).

This chapter describes the features and epidemiology of adolescent substance use and substance use disorders, and examines etiological factors with an emphasis on recent evidence. The chapter is not intended to be comprehensive; for example, we do not consider issues of treatment or prevention (see Deas & Thomas, 2001; Hser et al., 2001; and Ozechowski & Liddle, 2000, for discussions of treatment, and Bukoski, 1997; Substance Abuse and Mental Health Services Administration, 1999; and U.S. Department of Health and Human Services [DHHS], 2000a, for discussions of prevention). Moreover, because many empirical studies consider only substance use, we include coverage of adolescent substance use as well as the substance use disorders, while noting the distinctions among them. Finally, our discussion spans developmental periods ranging from early childhood precursors of adolescent substance use disorders to the period of "emerging adulthood" (ages 18–25), when substance use disorders reach their peak.

HISTORICAL CONTEXT

The use and misuse of alcohol and other substances date to antiquity. The medical use of marijuana, and the use of beer and wine, were documented as early as 1600 B.C. in Egypt, Greece, and Rome (Schultes, 1970). There are also historical references to concerns about substance use among young people. For example, while sailing from Britain to North America aboard a Puritan ship, the *Arabella*, in 1630, Puritan elders noted that some youths were "prone to drink hot waters very immoderately" (Lender & Martin, 1987, p. 22).

A historical perspective on adolescent substance use/misuse must be placed within the broader context of historical changes in the definitions of adolescence. Prior to the 19th century, the transition from childhood to adulthood was short, and after puberty children often gained many of the freedoms and responsibilities of adulthood, including substance use (Lender & Martin, 1987). However, as the American economy changed in the 19th century, adult occupations required greater training and maturity. Adolescence began to be viewed as a period that required moral instruction, as well as preparation for the economic and social demands of adulthood. As adolescence became more strongly differentiated from adulthood, societal attitudes to adolescent substance use shifted toward a more restrictive view (Lender & Martin, 1987).

Coincident with increasing societal restrictiveness on adolescent substance use in 19th-century America was a rise in alcohol temperance movements, which later peaked with Prohibition (1919–1933). Since then, movements against psychoactive substances have included laws against opiate use in the early 20th century, a fervor over marijuana in the 1920s, concerns over narcotics in the 1950s, and fears over the use of cocaine and crack in the 1980s and 1990s (Bukstein, 1995).

Modern attention to adolescent substance use in the United States, and the origins of the current "war on drugs," can be tied to the rise of the counterculture of the late 1950s and 1960s. This brought increases in the use and social acceptance of many psychoactive drugs, particularly marijuana and lysergic acid diethylamide (LSD). As substance use became more common among middle-class American college students, the 1960s also saw increased societal concern about drug use and increased antidrug legislation. Most notably, the Drug Abuse Control Amendment of 1965 and the Controlled Substances Act of 1970 brought hallucinogens, stimulants, and depressants under the regulatory control of the federal government, whereas before only narcotics had been treated as controlled substances (Maisto, Galizio, & Connors, 1999). In the 1970s, national epidemiological studies were undertaken to monitor trends in adolescent substance use (e.g., the Monitoring the Future Study [MTF], which is discussed later in more detail, was begun in 1975). The "war on drugs" under Presidents Reagan and G. H. Bush saw increases in federal funding of nearly 700% for federal drug programs, the appointment of a federal "drug czar,"and increased military activity to counteract drug supply (Humphreys & Rappaport, 1993). Currently, societal conceptualizations of and attitudes toward adolescent substance use continue to evolve, with recent trends including increases in the legal drinking age, a reconceptualization of tobacco use as an addictive behavior, and concomitant increased regulation of youths' access to tobacco (Institute of Medicine, 1994b; U.S. DHHS, 1988, 2000b).

DEFINITIONAL AND DIAGNOSTIC ISSUES

Diagnostic Systems

In the United States, the most commonly used diagnostic system at present is the *Diagnostic and Statistical Manual of Mental Disorders*, fourth edition (DSM-IV; American Psychiatric Association, 1994), which recognizes two classes of substance-related disorders: substance use disorders and substance-induced disorders. Substance-induced disorders are those that result from ingestion of or exposure to substances (e.g., substance-induced delirium, substance-induced persisting dementia, substance-induced psychotic disorder). More germane to the current chapter are the DSM-IV substance use disorders, which include substance dependence and substance abuse. These disorders relate to the maladaptive use of alcohol and other drugs.

DSM-IV diagnoses of substance abuse and dependence may be applied to 11 different drug types, including alcohol, amphetamine, caffeine, cannabis, cocaine, hallucinogens, inhalants, nicotine, opioids, phencyclidine (PCP), and sedatives (including hypnotics and anxiolytics). Adolescent substance dependence and abuse are diagnosed using the same DSM-IV criteria that are applied to adults; these criteria are displayed in Tables 4.1 and 4.2, respectively. The specific symptoms vary slightly with different drugs, but the essential features remain constant.

TABLE 4.1. DSM-IV Criteria for Substance Dependence

A maladaptive pattern of substance use, leading to clinically significant impairment or distress, as manifested by three (or more) of the following, occurring at any time in the same 12-month period:

(1) tolerance, as defined by either of the following:
  (a) a need for markedly increased amounts of the substance to achieve intoxication or desired effect
  (b) markedly diminished effect with continued use of the same amount of the substance

(2) withdrawal, as manifested by either of the following:
  (a) the characteristic withdrawal syndrome for the substance . . .
  (b) the same (or a closely related) substance is taken to relieve or avoid withdrawal symptoms

(3) the substance is often taken in larger amounts or over a longer period than was intended

(4) there is a persistent desire or unsuccessful efforts to cut down or control substance use

(5) a great deal of time is spent in activities necessary to obtain the substance (e.g., visiting multiple doctors or driving long distances) use the substance (e.g., chain-smoking), or recover from its effects

(6) important social, occupational, or recreational activities are given up or reduced because of substance use

(7) the substance use is continued despite knowledge of having a persistent or recurrent physical or psychological problem that is likely to have been caused or exacerbated by the substance (e.g., current cocaine use despite recognition of cocaine-induced depression, or continued drinking despite recognition that an ulcer was made worse by alcohol consumption)

Specify if:
  With Physiological Dependence: evidence of tolerance or withdrawal (i.e., either Item 1 or 2 is present)
  Without Physiological Dependence: no evidence of tolerance or withdrawal (i.e., neither Item 1 nor 2 is present)

Course specifiers (see [DSM-IV] text for definitions):
  Early Full Remission
  Early Partial Remission
  Sustained Full Remission
  Sustained Partial Remission
  On Agonist Therapy
  In a Controlled Environment

Note. From American Psychiatric Association (1994, p. 181). Copyright 1994 by the American Psychiatric Association. Reprinted by permission.

TABLE 4.2. DSM-IV Criteria for Substance Abuse

A. A maladaptive pattern of substance use leading to clinically significant impairment or distress, as manifested by one (or more) of the following, occurring within a 12-month period:
  (1) recurrent substance use resulting in a failure to fulfill major role obligations at work, school, or home (e.g., repeated absences or poor work performance related to substance use; substance-related absences, suspensions, or expulsions from school; neglect of children or household)
  (2) recurrent substance use in situations in which it is physically hazardous (e.g., driving an automobile or operating a machine when impaired by substance use)
  (3) recurrent substance-related legal problems (e.g., arrests for substance-related disorderly conduct)
  (4) continued substance use despite having persistent or recurrent social or interpersonal problems caused or exacerbated by the effects of the substance (e.g., arguments with spouse about consequences of intoxication, physical fights)

B. The symptoms have never met the criteris for Substance Dependence for this class of substance.

Note. From American Psychiatric Association (1994, pp. 182–183). Copyright 1994 by the American Psychiatric Association. Reprinted by permission.

The hallmark of substance dependence is a maladaptive pattern of substance use that continues for at least 12 months, despite three or more cognitive, behavioral, and/or physiological symptoms. The DSM-IV criteria for substance dependence include tolerance (needing increased amounts of the substance in order to achieve intoxication, or experiencing reduced effects from the same amount of consumption); withdrawal (cognitive and physiological changes upon discontinuation of the substance); and several indices of compulsive use reflecting psychological dependence (see Table 4.1). Substance dependence may be diagnosed in the absence of physiological dependence (i.e., in the absence of tolerance and withdrawal), given the presence of at least three psychological symptoms.

By contrast, DSM-IV substance abuse involves one or more harmful and repeated negative consequences of substance use (see Table 4.2), which must recur during a 12-month period; however, the individual must not meet criteria for dependence. (If an individual meets criteria for substance dependence, a diagnosis of substance abuse is preempted, given the presumed greater severity of substance dependence.) Given their lesser severity, diagnoses of substance abuse tend to be more prevalent than diagnoses of substance dependence.

Although it is the most commonly used, the DSM-IV is not the only diagnostic system, and others yield differing rates of diagnoses when used with adolescent populations. For example, Pollock, Martin, and Lagenbucher (2000) examined concordance for diagnoses of adolescent alcohol abuse and dependence among the DSM-IV; the two earlier versions of the DSM (DSM-III and DSM-III-R); and the *International Classification of Diseases*, 10th revision (ICD-10). Agreement among the various diagnostic systems was fair to high for diagnoses of alcohol dependence (kappa = .51 to .83), but was quite low for diagnoses of alcohol abuse (kappa = .10 to. 23), suggesting that the concept and definition of alcohol abuse vary greatly across the different systems as applied to adolescents. Similarly, Fulkerson, Harrison, and Beebe (1999) compared a one-factor to a two-factor model of adolescent substance use problems, and found that a one-factor model was a better fit to the data. They suggest that separate diagnoses of substance abuse and dependence may not reflect the nature of substance use problems in adolescence. These findings suggest a need for further refinement of diagnostic classifications when they are used with adolescents.

The adequacy of the definitions of adolescent substance use disorders has also been questioned when adolescents' symptoms have been compared to those of adults. Although identical criteria are used to diagnose adolescents and adults, only one of seven research sites for the DSM-IV contributed data from adolescents (Cottler et al., 1995), and the pattern of symptoms in DSM-IV may not reflect the unique features of adolescent substance use involvement. Several studies have reported a group of "diagnostic orphans" (i.e., adolescents who endorse one or two dependence symptoms but no abuse symptoms, and thus do not qualify for a substance-related diagnosis despite problematic use). Rates of these "diagnostic orphans" are substantial. For example, in studies of adolescents who regularly use alcohol, these rates have ranged from 13% to 30% (Harrison, Fulkerson, & Beebe, 1998; Lewinsohn, Rohde, & Seeley, 1996; Pollock & Martin, 1999).

There are several reasons why current diagnostic criteria may be inadequate for adolescents, and these can be illustrated in recent studies of adolescent alcohol use disorders. (Fewer studies have examined the adequacy of diagnostic criteria for adolescent drug use disorders, and since adolescent drug and alcohol disorders often co-occur, similar diagnostic issues arise.) First, the developmental status of adolescents decreases the likelihood that they will exhibit impairment in occupational and romantic functioning (Vik, Brown, & Meyers, 1997). Furthermore, several studies report that alcohol-dependent teens are less likely than are adults to experience physiological dependence, including symptoms such as tolerance, withdrawal, and medical complications (Martin, Kaczynski, Maisto, Bukstein, & Moss, 1995; Stewart & Brown, 1995); adolescents, particularly girls, are also less likely than are adults to experience legal problems as a result of their alcohol use (Lewinsohn et al., 1996). Instead, some of the more common alcohol dependence symptoms seen in youths include affective symptoms, blackouts, reduced activity level, risky sexual behavior, and cravings (Martin et al., 1995; Stewart & Brown, 1995). It should be noted, however, that not all investigators concur with these findings. Deas, Riggs, Langenbucher, Goldman, and Brown (2000) found that alcohol-abusing adolescents acquired symptoms of physiological dependence within 7 months after the onset of their drinking (compared to a period of 3 years for adults), and that adolescent drinkers met criteria for dependence within 1.5 years of drinking onset (compared to an average of 3 years for adults). In general, the degree to which criteria for substance use disorders capture the unique features of adolescents versus adults is the subject of a new and rapidly developing literature, which suggests that some modifications to adult classification systems may be necessary (see Colby, Tiffany, Shiffman, & Niaura, 2000, for a discussion of nicotine dependence in adolescents,and Mikulich, Hall, Whitemore, & Crowley, 2001, and Winters, Latimer, & Stinchfield, 1999, for a discussion of drug dependence diagnoses in adolescents).

Related Symptoms and Disorders

Adolescent substance use problems are typically accompanied by a number of related symptoms, both clinical and subclinical. Most notably, adolescents with a substance use disorder are highly likely to show polydrug use. Typically, adolescent substance use begins with the use of so-called "gateway" drugs (alcohol and nicotine), followed by marijuana and subsequently by other illegal drugs (Kandel, Yamaguchi, & Chen, 1992). Recent evidence suggests that the majority of adolescents who are diagnosed with alcohol abuse or dependence use multiple drugs, with the most common combination being alcohol and marijuana, followed by alcohol and hallucinogens (Deas et al., 2000; Martin, Kaczynski, Maisto, & Tarter, 1996). Substance-abusing or substance-dependent adolescents are further characterized by functional impairment in numerous domains. They exhibit poorer academic achievement and higher rates of academic failure relative to youths without substance use disorders (Moss, Kirisci, Gordon, & Tarter, 1994; Tarter, Mezzich, Hsieh, & Parks, 1995). Adolescents with substance use disorders also tend to associate with deviant peer groups, to engage in delinquent behaviors (Blackson et al., 1999; Hawkins, Catalano, & Miller, 1992), and to experience frequent negative interactions with their parents (Kuperman et al., 2001; Mezzich et al., 1997).

Given the characteristics associated with adolescent substance use disorders, it is not surprising that there are high rates of comorbidity between adolescent substance abuse and dependence and other disorders. Because most studies of comorbidity are cross-sectional, they are not designed to examine causal pathways, and the significance of this comorbidity for the etiology of substance use disorders remains unclear. However, consistent patterns emerge across studies that link substance use disorders to other forms of child and adolescent psychopathology (see Weinberg, Rahdert, Colliver, & Glantz, 1998, for a review).

Perhaps the most consistent finding is that adolescent substance use disorders are commonly comorbid with the attention-defict and disruptive behavior disorders (i.e., oppositional defiant disorder, conduct disorder, and attention-deficit/hyperactivity disorder [ADHD]). For example, Cohen et al. (1993) found that half of adolescents ages 10–20 with a substance use disorder were also diagnosed with one of these three behavior disorders. Among those with diagnosed substance use disorders, odds ratios for diagnoses of these behavior disorders have been reported from 5.6 (Lewinsohn, Hops, Roberts, Seeley, & Andrews, 1993) to 9.8 (Fergusson, Horwood, & Lynskey, 1993). Although the relations between substance use disorders and conduct problems appear unique, the link between ADHD and substance use disorders is more controversial, and may be produced by the presence of co-occurring conduct disorder (Costello, Erkanli, Federman, & Angold, 1999; Weinberg et al., 1998). Indeed, because adolescent substance use problems rarely occur in the absence of other problem behaviors, heavy adolescent substance use is often considered a specific manifestation of a more broad-based behavior problem (Donovan & Jessor, 1985). Developmentally, many researchers consider adolescent substance use disorders as the culmination of a deviant trajectory, manifested in childhood and early adolescence by behavioral undercontrol and oppositional behavior (Tarter & Vanyukov, 1994).

The relation between substance use disorders and mood and anxiety disorders is less clear. Costello and colleagues (Costello et al., 1999; Kaplow, Curran, Angold, & Costello, 2001) found that depression and generalized anxiety disorder, but not separation anxiety disorder, were related to the onset of adolescent substance use. Other studies have found that both depression and anxiety are comorbid with adolescent substance use disorders, but that relations with depression are stronger (Fergusson et al., 1993; Kandel et al., 1997; Lewinsohn et al., 1993). Because these latter studies examined somewhat older samples, the associations between substance use disorders and emotional disorders may strengthen with age, and emotional disorders may be the result of continued substance use. Moreover, some studies suggest that associations between emotional disorders and substance use disorders are stronger for females than for males (e.g., Bukstein, Glancy, & Kaminer, 1992; Federman, Costello, Angold, Farmer, & Erkanli, 1997; Tarter, Kirisci, & Mezzich, 1997; Whitmore et al., 1997).

EPIDEMIOLOGY

Prevalence Rates

Given the public health importance of adolescent substance use, several large-scale national epidemiological studies were launched in the 1970s to monitor trends over time in adolescent substance use prevalence. The Monitoring the Future Study (MTF) was begun in 1975 as a school-based survey of substance use among the nation's high school seniors, and is currently administered annually to over 45,000 students in 8th, 10th, and 12th grades in 435 schools nationwide (Johnston, O(Malley, & Bachman, 2000). The National Household Survey on Drug Abuse (NHSDA) has been conducted since 1971, and obtains information from over 70,000 civilians aged 12 and older across the nation in face-to-face interviews (U.S. DHHS, 2000a). Although neither sample is completely representative (i.e., the MTF excludes adolescents who are not in school, and the NHSDA excludes military personnel, prisoners, and homeless persons), they provide valuable information about substance use prevalence over time.

Epidemiological studies and most other research on adolescent alcohol and drug use rely on adolescents(self-reports, because parents are likely to be unaware of their adolescents' substance use. Indeed, parent and adolescent reports show low levels of agreement (Cantwell, Lewinsohn, Rohde, & Seeley, 1997). Although it is beyond the scope of this chapter, a large literature has addressed the validity (and threats to validity) of these adolescent self-reports, including their validation with biological measures (e.g., Dolcini, Adler, & Ginsberg, 1996; Murray, O(Connell, Schmid, & Perry, 1987). In general, these data suggest that self-reports can be valid if they are obtained under conditions of anonymity and privacy, and if there is little motivation to distort responses. For example, data from a 1990 NHSDA field test sample suggested that self-administered questionnaires substantially improved reporting, compared to interviewer-style questioning (Rogers, Miller, & Turner, 1998).

Some illustrative data from the MTF are provided in Table 4.3. As these data show, adolescent substance use is relatively common by the end of the high school years. For example, the MTF data from 2000 showed that approximately 54% of 12th-graders had used some illegal drug in their lifetimes, with 24.9% using in the past month (a common definition of "current" use). Marijuana was the most frequently used illegal drug, with 48.8% of 12th-graders reporting some lifetime use and 6% using daily in 2000 (Johnston, O(Malley, & Bachman, 2001). The use of substances that are legal for adults (i.e., alcohol and tobacco) was even more common, with 73.2% of high school seniors reporting drinking in the past year and 50% reporting drinking in the past month (Johnston et al., 2001); 62.5% of high school seniors reported some experience with cigarette smoking, and 20% were daily smokers (Johnston et al., 2001). The use of different drugs is highly interrelated in both epidemiological and clinical samples of adolescents (Clayton, 1992; Johnston et al., 2001; Kandel, Davies, Karus, & Yamaguchi, 1986; Single, Kandel, & Faust, 1974). For example, the 1985 NHSDA data show that 24% of those who reported some illicit drug use had used multiple drugs simultaneously within the past year, and 43% had used alcohol in conjunction with an illicit drug (Clayton, 1992).

The MTF data also reveal interesting patterns of change over time (see Table 4.4 for examples). In general, adolescent substance use involvement reached a peak in the mid-1970s and early 1980s and then declined. Substance use rose again in the early 1990s but has since leveled off. Specific drugs show marked increases and decreases in use over time. For example, cocaine use among 12th-graders peaked in the late 1970s, showed dramatic declines between 1986 and 1992 (to about one-fourth the rate), but then began to increase again until 2000. At the time of this writ-

TABLE 4.3. Use Rates for Various Drugs for 8th-, 10th-, and 12th-Graders in 2000

	Lifetime use			Annual use			Past-month use		
	8th	10th	12th	8th	10th	12th	8th	10th	12th
Alcohol	51.7	71.4	80.3	43.1	65.3	73.2	22.4	41.0	50.0
Cigarettes	40.5	55.1	62.5	N/A	N/A	N/A	14.6	23.9	31.4
Marijuana/hashish	20.3	40.3	48.8	15.6	32.2	36.5	9.1	19.7	21.6
Amphetamines	9.9	15.7	15.6	6.5	11.1	10.5	3.4	5.4	5.0
Cocaine	4.5	6.9	8.6	2.6	4.4	5.0	1.2	1.8	2.1
Heroin	1.9	2.2	2.4	1.1	1.4	1.5	0.5	0.5	0.7
Any illicit drug	26.8	45.6	54.0	19.5	36.4	40.9	11.9	22.5	24.9
Any illicit drug other than marijuana	15.8	23.1	29.0	10.2	16.7	20.4	5.6	8.5	10.4

Note. From Johnston, O'Malley and Bachman (2001).

TABLE 4.4. Long-Term Trends in Past-Month Use of Various Drugs for 12th-Graders

	1976	1979	1982	1985	1988	1991	1994	1997	2000
Alcohol	68.3	71.8	69.7	65.9	63.9	54.0	50.1	52.7	50.0
Cigarettes	38.8	34.4	30.0	30.1	28.7	28.3	31.2	36.5	31.4
Marijuana/hashish	32.2	36.5	28.5	25.7	18.0	13.8	19.0	23.7	21.6
Amphetamines	7.7	9.9	10.7	6.8	4.6	3.2	4.0	4.8	5.0
Cocaine	2.0	5.7	5.0	6.7	3.4	1.4	1.5	2.3	2.1
Heroin	0.2	0.2	0.2	0.3	0.2	0.2	0.3	0.5	0.7
Any illicit drug	34.2	38.9	32.5	29.7	21.3	16.4	21.9	26.2	24.9
Any illicit drug other than marijuana	13.9	16.8	17.0	14.9	10.0	7.1	8.8	10.7	10.4

Note. From Johnston, O'Malley, and Bachman (2001).

ing, there are declining trends for inhalants and cigarettes, but increasing trends for "ecstasy," heroin, and steroids. Johnston et al. (2001) note that as older drugs wane in popularity, new drugs replace them. For example, PCP showed a rapid rise in the 1970s, crack and cocaine in the 1980s, and rophynol and ecstasy in the 1990s. Interestingly, the popularity of specific drugs often revives after a period of low use. Johnston et al. (2001) suggest that the use of particular drugs may make such a "comeback," because knowledge of their risks and negative effects gets lost from the adolescent culture after a period of nonuse. They refer to this phenomenon as "generational forgetting."

Substantial numbers of adolescents who use alcohol or drugs also report some problem associated with their substance use. For example, in a community sample of adolescents, Zoccolillo, Vitaro, and Tremblay (1999) found that of those using alcohol more than five times, 70% of boys and 53% of girls reported experiencing at least one alcohol-related problem (e.g., going to school "high"), and 20% of boys and 11% of girls reported three or more problems. Of those who had used drugs more than five times, 94% of boys and 85% of girls reported at least one drug-related problem, and 68% of boys and 52% of girls reported three or more problems. However, the prevalence of diagnosable substance use disorders among adolescents is substantially lower, with point prevalences of 3–4% for alcohol use disorders and 2–3% for drug use disorders among younger adolescents (13–16 years of age). For example, Fergusson et al. (1993) found that 5.5% of their New Zealand birth cohort of 15-year-olds could be diagnosed with a substance use disorder, with 1.7% meeting lifetime criteria for drug abuse or dependence, and 3.5% meeting lifetime criteria for alcohol abuse or dependence. Warner, Kessler, Hughes, Anthony, and Nelson (1995) found that among 15- to 24-year-olds, 3.3% met criteria for drug abuse or dependence. In a school-based sample of high school students, Lewinsohn et al. (1993) found lifetime prevalence rates of 4.6% for alcohol abuse or dependence and 6.3% for drug abuse or dependence. In an older sample aged 17–20, Cohen et al. (1993) found that 14.9% of the sample met criteria for alcohol abuse or dependence, and 4% met criteria for drug abuse or dependence. Taken together, these studies suggest that rates of drug use disorders rise only slightly throughout adolescence, whereas rates of alcohol use disorders rise more substantially.

Demographic Correlates

Gender

Numerous studies have documented gender differences in substance use prevalence, such that girls use fewer types of drugs and use them with less frequency than do boys (Johnston et al., 2000). For example, the 2000 MTF data showed that 12th-grade males reported substantially higher prevalence rates (at least 1.5 times as much as females) in the annual use of heroin, LSD, steroids, and smokeless tobacco, as well as in the daily use of marijuana and alcohol. At younger grades, however, males and females showed similar rates for many drugs, and females even had higher rates of annual use of inhalants, tranquilizers, and amphetamines in 8th grade (Johnston et al., 2001). This pattern may reflect a developmental phenomenon (with accentuating gender differences emerging over the course of adolescence) or a cohort effect (with gender differences decreasing among more recent cohorts of adolescents). Similar accentuation of gender differences at older ages has been reported for diagnosable substance use disorders. For example, Cohen et al. (1993) found few gender differences for younger adolescents, but found that males aged 17–20 were more likely to be diagnosed with alcohol abuse or dependence than were females.

In addition to differential prevalence rates, males and females may use drugs for different reasons. For example, males report higher levels of social and mood enhancement motives for drinking than do females (Cooper, 1994). Younger females report higher levels of coping and conformity motives for drinking than do males, although this gender difference reverses at older ages (Cooper, 1994). Studies of tobacco use have found that females report stronger weight regulation and anxiety reduction motives than do males (Grunberg, Winders, & Wewers, 1991; Rose, Chassin, Presson, & Sherman, 1996; see also Amaro, Blake, Schwartz, & Flinchbaugh, 2001, for a review of drug use among adolescent girls, and White & Huselid, 1997, for a review of gender differences in adolescent alcohol use).

Socioeconomic Status

Adolescent drug use has also been associated with socioeconomic status (SES). In the MTF data, an association between parental education as a measure of SES and drug use appears in the middle school years but not in the high school years (Johnston et al, 2000). For example, among 8th-graders in the MTF in 2000, 20.9% in the lowest-SES category had used an illicit drug in the past month, compared to 9.3% for those in the highest-SES category of SES. However, these differences became negligible among 12th-graders, for whom there was little relationship between family SES and the use of most substances (less than 2% variation among all five SES categories) (Johnston et al., 2001). These diminished SES differences may reflect differential school dropout as a function of parental education or substance use, or a developmental phenomenon (with use becoming equally common across SES levels by the end of adolescence). They may also reflect a cohort effect, such that substance use is becoming more concentrated in less educated subgroups among more recent cohorts (as has been argued for cigarette smoking; Fiore, Newcomb, & McBride, 1993). Only minimal relations have been reported between adolescent substance use and other indicators of SES, including family income (Parker, Calhoun, & Weaver, 2000) and subjective ratings of familial social class (Fawzy, Combs, Simon, & Bowman-Terrell, 1987). It has also been suggested that SES increases risk for adolescent substance use only when poverty is extreme and occurs with childhood behavior problems (Hawkins et al., 1992); this might explain the overall weak relations between SES and adolescent use. Moreover, the relation between adolescent substance use and SES may also vary with different drugs. For example, with the rise in prevalence of crack cocaine in the early 1980s, lower-SES populations exhibited increases in cocaine use, while their higher-SES counterparts showed declining use. Although this trend ceased in 1985, it illustrates how social and economic factors—namely, the increased opportunity to acquire this cheaper form of cocaine—can influence the SES distribution for a specific drug.

Ethnicity

In terms of ethnic correlates of use, the MTF data show that African American high school seniors have lower prevalence rates (lifetime, annual, monthly, and daily) for all drugs than do European American and Hispanic American seniors. In 6th and 8th grades, Hispanic students report more use than do non-Hispanic European Americans, but this difference reverses at 12th grade. Possible reasons for this crossover are the comparatively high dropout rate of Hispanics, which may diminish initial ethnic differences, and/or the fact that European Americans start using drugs later in adolescence and eventually overtake the prevalence rates of Hispanic Americans (Johnston et al., 2000). Native American adolescents also show high rates of use (Plunkett & Mitchell, 2000), although their levels of use vary by geographic location. Ethnic differences also appear in diagnosed adolescent substance use disorders. For example, Costello, Farmer, Angold, Burns, and Erkanli (1997) found that Native American adolescents had significantly higher odds of receiving a substance use disorder diagnosis than did European American adolescents, and results from another large-scale study (Kandel et al., 1997) showed that European American and African American adolescents were more likely to be diagnosed with a substance use disorder than were Hispanic American adolescents (see Barrera,

Castro, & Biglan, 1999, and Kandel, 1995, for reviews of ethnic differences in drug use).

It has also been suggested that what appears as ethnic differences in substance use may actually reflect ethnic differences in reporting bias. For example, Bauman and Ennett (1994) found that when self-reports were validated against a biological measure of tobacco use, African American adolescents underreported their smoking, whereas European American adolescents overreported their smoking. However, more recent studies that used larger and more ethnically heterogeneous samples have suggested that the validity of self-reports is comparable across ethnic groups (e.g., Wills & Cleary, 1997).

As these data illustrate, rates of adolescent substance use vary with gender, SES, and ethnicity. However, these conclusions may oversimplify a more complex picture, in that prevalence rates may vary as a function of complex interactions among gender and ethnicity (Griesler & Kandel, 1998), and the correlated effects of ethnicity and SES are difficult to disaggregate. Moreover, the mechanisms underlying these demographic differences have not been well articulated, and methodological artifacts (such as sampling biases and reporter biases) can influence findings.

DEVELOPMENTAL COURSE AND PROGNOSIS

Both substance use and substance use disorders show systematic age-related patterns from adolescence to adulthood, which have led some researchers to view substance abuse and dependence as "developmental disorders" (Sher & Gotham, 1999; Tarter & Vanyukov, 1994). Substance use is typically initiated in adolescence. For example, the MTF data suggest that the typical time for alcohol use onset as well as for first intoxication is between 7th and 10th grades (Johnston et al., 2000). Adolescent substance use typically begins with the use of legal drugs (tobacco and alcohol), and rates of illegal drug use onset peak in the high school years (Johnston et al., 2000; Kandel, 1975). As noted earlier, some type of substance use during adolescence is developmentally and statistically normative. Thus, for researchers and clinicians interested in developmental psychopathology, an important feature of adolescent substance use is its heterogeneity, and it is necessary to distinguish trajectories of substance use that are relatively benign from those that result in clinical impairment or diagnosable substance use disorders.

Several studies have suggested that an early age of substance use onset is one predictor of subsequent course and of clinical impairment. For example, Grant and Dawson (1997) found that alcohol use initiation before age 14 was associated with elevated risk for the development of alcohol abuse or dependence. Similarly, Robins and Pryzbeck (1985) reported that early onset of illegal drug use (before age 15) was associated with increased likelihood of later drug abuse or dependence.

Recent developments in "mixture modeling" (Muthen & Shedden, 1999; Nagin, 1999) have allowed researchers to empirically identify multiple developmental trajectories of substance use within longitudinal studies. The few studies that have used this method have identified a subtype in which early age of onset is associated with a steeply escalating course of use and with the most problematic outcomes (including diagnosed abuse or dependence). This has been found both for cigarette smoking (Chassin, Presson, Pitts, & Sherman, 2000) and for heavy drinking (Chassin, Pitts, & Prost, 2002; K. Hill, White, Chung, Hawkins, & Catalano, 2000). Moreover, studies of this "early-escalating" subtype have shown it to be associated with a family history of use, abuse, or dependence, as well as with high levels of conduct problems (Chassin et al., 2002; Costello et al., 1999; S. Hill, Shen, Lowers, & Locke, 2000; Loeber, Stouthamer-Loeber, & White, 1999). In these characteristics, the early-escalating subtype of substance use resembles a subtype of early-onset alcoholism (onset of disorder before age 25) that has been identified in the adult literature as associated with strong family history risk and high levels of antisociality (Cloninger, 1987; Zucker, 1987).

Conversely, longitudinal studies of adolescents have also identified a "late-onset" subtype (at least late in the adolescent age period), in which smoking or heavy drinking does not begin until after the high school years (Chassin et al., 2000, 2002). For these adolescents, substance use initiation may be associated with decreases in parental supervision, perhaps during the transition out of the parental home. Adolescent substance use that begins after the high school years has been relatively neglected by researchers, and most prevention programs have been targeted at younger age groups. Thus relatively little is known about this subtype of substance use, and it represents an important target for future research. In any case, because substance use initiation typically begins in adolescence, it has been associated with hallmarks of this developmental period, such as increasing autonomy and independence from parental supervision.

Over the adolescent years, alcohol use and drug use increase in quantity and frequency to reach a peak in the age period that Arnett (2000) has referred to as "emerging adulthood" (i.e., 18–25 years of age). Moreover, the prevalence of diagnosed abuse and dependence also peaks in this age period (e.g., Grant et al., 1994). Then, in the middle to late 20s, the consumption of alcohol and illegal drugs begins to decline—perhaps in response to the demands of newly acquired adult roles, such as marriage, work, and parenthood (Bachman, Wadsworth, O(Malley, Johnston, & Schulenberg, 1997; Yamaguchi & Kandel, 1985). Transition to adult roles at these ages also reduces risk for developing a substance use disorder (Chilcoat & Breslau, 1996). Substance use disorders that decline in young adulthood have been referred to as "developmentally limited" (Zucker, 1987).

These age-related declines suggest that adolescent substance use, abuse, and dependence are not necessarily persistent throughout the life course, and that there is recovery in the young adult years. However, empirical evidence concerning prognosis for adolescents with substance use disorders is not extensive. Some studies of adolescent drug treatment programs suggest that substantial relapse is associated with any one particular treatment attempt. For example, Spears, Ciesla, and Skala (1999) reported a relapse rate of 61.1% within 12 months of treatment, and Winters, Stinchfield, Opland, Weller, and Latimer (2000) reported that 53% of a treated group was abstinent at 12-month follow-up. As with adults, repeated attempts may be necessary to produce long-term abstinence in the treatment of adolescent substance use disorders.

RISK FACTORS AND ETIOLOGICAL MODELS

Risk factors for adolescent substance use and misuse have been identified on multiple levels ranging from intrapersonal to macroenvironmental (see Hawkins et al., 1992) and have also been integrated into biopsychosocial theoretical models of etiology (see, e.g., Sher, 1991). Given the heterogeneity of substance abuse and dependence, it is unlikely that any one factor or etiological pathway could explain the development of substance use disorders. For example, theory and research in alcoholism has suggested subtypes of alcoholism that may have different etiological antecedents. In particular, researchers have distinguished between early-onset alcoholism (which has a higher prevalence in males, typically begins in adolescence, and is strongly associated with antisociality) and later-onset alcoholism (which is more strongly associated with neuroticism and negative affectivity) (Cloninger, 1987).

Here we review some of the major risk factors and etiological models, with an emphasis on recent empirical evidence. These models suggest that the antecedents of and etiological pathways into adolescent substance abuse and dependence have their roots in earlier stages of development. In regard to the etiology of substance use disorders, it is important to remember that they represent only a segment of a larger series of stages in substance use progression. These stages include initiation, experimental or occasional use, regular or escalating use, and "problem" use, as well as cycles of cessation and relapse (Flay, d'Avernas, Best, Kersell, & Ryan, 1983; Glantz & Pickens, 1992). As such, it is likely that movement across the different stages has different etiological determinants. However, existing empirical studies have often blurred these distinctions, and much of the existing data refer to predictors of adolescent substance use rather than clinical substance abuse or dependence. Thus the existing data base makes it difficult to specify etiological models of transition that are unique to different stages of substance use behavior.

Family History of Substance Abuse or Dependence

A robust finding in the literature is that adults whose parents have a history of alcohol or drug abuse or dependence are at elevated risk for substance use and substance use disorders (McGue, 1994; Russell, 1990), although the magnitude of the risk varies substantially across samples. For example, parental alcoholism raises risk for offspring alcoholism anywhere from a risk ratio of 2–3 in community samples to a risk ratio of 9 in severely alcohol-dependent and antisocial samples (McGue, 1994; Russell, 1990). There is also elevated risk (as high as eightfold) for drug disorders among relatives of probands with drug disorders (Merikangas et al., 1998)

Family history risk is also associated with adolescent substance use—both with an early adolescent onset of substance use (Chassin et al., 2000; Costello et al., 1999) and with the persistence of substance use over time (Chassin et al., 2000). Twin studies suggest that this family history risk for substance use and misuse in adolescence has both heritable and environmental mediators, and that the importance of environmental influences may vary for different substances (Merikangas & Avenevoli, 2000). For example, in a study of 17-year-old twins, McGue, Elkins, and Iacono (2000) found that heritability of use and abuse for illegal drugs was 25% or less, whereas heritability for tobacco use and dependence was more powerful (40–60%). Similarly, Han, McGue, and Iacono (1999) reported varying magnitudes of heritability estimates for tobacco use (59%), alcohol use (60%), and drug use (33%) in male adolescents, again suggesting that the importance of genetic and environmental influences may vary by the type of substance used. On the other hand, because there was also significant covariation among these heritability estimates, some aspects of susceptibility to adolescent substance use may be common across different forms of use. Human and animal studies of the molecular genetics of substance abuse and dependence have proposed multiple possibilities for candidate genes that influence vulnerability to substance use disorders. Although a review of this literature is beyond the scope of this chapter, recent reviews of the molecular genetic literature can be found in Nestler (2000), Reich, Hinrichs, Culverhouse, and Bierut (1999), and Uhl (1999).

Adult data has suggested that heritability may be stronger for males than for females (see McGue, 1999, for a review). However, these findings may be influenced by the lower base rates of disorders for females than for males, limiting the power to detect genetic influences for women (Heath et al., 1997). Moreover, some recent studies of adolescents conclude that gender differences in heritability are not statistically significant, and that gender-invariant models are better-fitting than those that model heritability for substance use separately as a function of gender (Han et al., 1999; Heath & Martin, 1988; Iacono, Carlson, Taylor, Elkins, & McGue, 1999); some data have even found stronger genetic influences for women than for men (Russell, Cooper, & Frone, 1990). In general, the question of gender differences in heritability for substance use disorders is in need of additional research.

Although twin and adoption studies indicate significant heritability for substance use and abuse in adolescence, family history risk can also exert influence through fetal exposure mechanisms. For example, Baer, Barr, Bookstein, Sampson, and Streissguth (1998) found that prenatal exposure to alcohol raised risk for adolescent alcohol use and use-related negative consequences above and beyond the risk linked with a family history of alcoholism alone. Similarly, Cornelius, Leech, Goldschmidt, and Day (2000) found that prenatal tobacco exposure raised risk for offspring tobacco use in childhood, although other data suggest that this effect varies with different measures of prenatal tobacco exposure (Kandel & Udry, 1999). It has been suggested that prenatal exposure may raise risk for adolescent substance use either through its effect on receptors (which then make the child more biologically sensitive to the effects of the substance) or by raising risk for temperamental underregulation and conduct problems (which are themselves risk factors for adolescent substance use) (Cornelius et al., 2000).

Given that a family history of substance abuse or dependence is a well-established and robust risk factor for adolescent substance use and misuse, an important goal for research is to understand how this risk is mediated. As described above, results of twin and adoption studies have demonstrated that there are both genetic and environmental components to the intergenerational transmission of risk. Risk may be mediated through personality and temperamental characteristics (e.g., propensities for negative affectivity, poor self-regulation, and sensation seeking), through individual differences in the pharmacological effects and reinforcement value of substances, and through the effects of risky environments. Given the complexity of these processes, researchers have postulated multiple and interrelated pathways of risk that are biopsychosocial in nature. A heuristic model of such pathways has been offered by Sher (1991) and provides the guiding framework for the current review. Sher (1991) hypothesizes that vulnerability to substance use disorders can be described by three submodels or pathways: a deviance-proneness pathway, a pathway that emphasizes stress and negative affect, and a pathway that focuses on substance use effects (the enhanced reinforcement pathway). These pathways are not meant to be mutually exclusive, and indeed, the same factors can contribute to more than one pathway. Although Sher's model was originally proposed to explain the effects of familial alcoholism on vulnerability to alcoholism, the same pathways can be examined with respect to substance use disorders more broadly. We also briefly discuss the macro-level influences of schools and neighborhoods, which are not explicitly included in Sher's model but may be relevant to all three pathways.

THE DEVIANCE-PRONENESS SUBMODEL

Sher's (1991) deviance-proneness submodel is depicted in Figure 4.1 (with the exception of contributions from negative affect, which are considered within the stress and negative affect submodel). In general, the deviance-proneness submodel suggests that the development of substance abuse or dependence occurs within a broader context of the development of conduct problems and antisociality. Adolescents at risk for substance abuse or dependence are thought to be temperamentally "difficult," and prone to cognitive deficits (including verbal skill deficits) and executive functioning deficits that contribute to a lack of self-regulation. In addition, high-risk children are thought to receive poor parenting, and this combination of temperamental, cognitive, and environmental risk factors sets the stage for failure at school and ejection from the mainstream peer group. This results in affiliation with deviant peers, who provide opportunities, models, and approval for alcohol and drug use. Because this submodel considers substance use within the broader context of antisocial behavior, it is quite similar to theories that attempt to explain the etiology of aggression and conduct problems more generally (see, e.g,, Patterson, 1986). Empirical evidence for each of these links is reviewed below.

Temperament and Personality

A host of studies report that temperamental and personality traits reflecting behavioral undercontrol and poor self-regulation are associated with adolescent substance use problems. For instance, in two reviews, the personality characteristics most consistently associated with adolescent substance use included unconventionality, low

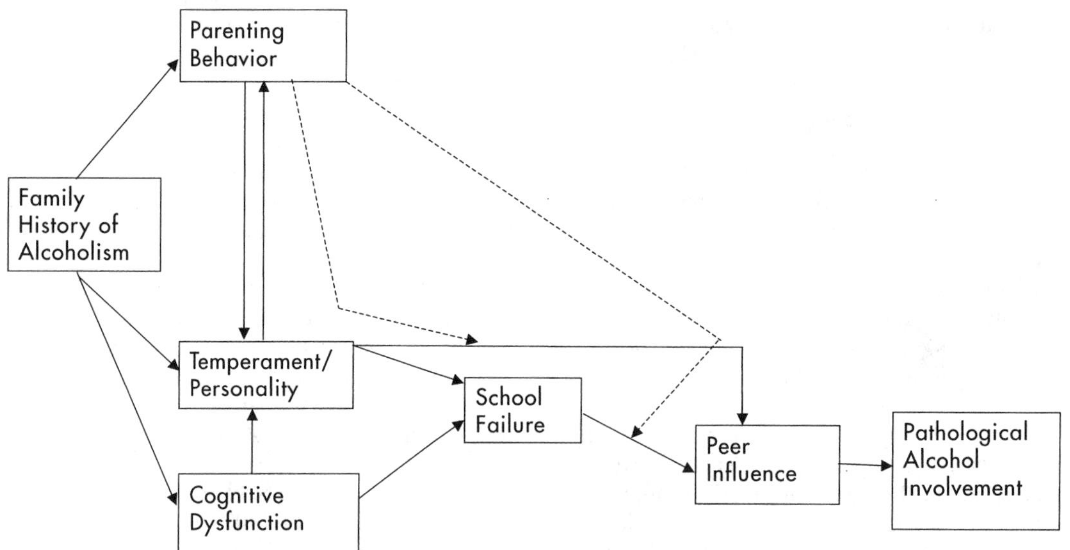

FIGURE 4.1. Schematic diagram of Sher's (1991) deviance-proneness submodel. Mediating paths are indicated by solid lines; moderating paths are indicated by dashed lines. The effects of emotional distress (depicted in Sher's original model) are omitted here and depicted in the stress and negative affect submodel (Figure 4.2). Adapted from Sher (1991). Copyright 1991 by University of Chicago Press. Adapted by permission.

ego control, sensation seeking, aggression, impulsivity, and an inability to delay gratification (Bates, 1993; Hawkins et al., 1992).

Longitudinal research has demonstrated that childhood temperamental characteristics reflecting undercontrolled behavior are longitudinally predictive of later substance use problems in adolescence and young adulthood. For instance, Block and colleagues (Block, Block, & Keyes, 1988; Shedler & Block, 1990) found that adolescents who used marijuana at least weekly were characterized as children by heightened levels of behavioral undercontrol and interpersonal alienation, and that these traits were observable as early as 3–4 years of age. Similarly, Caspi, Moffitt, Newman, and Silva (1996) found that 3-year-old boys described by others as impulsive, restless, and distractible were at increased risk for a diagnosis of drug dependence by age 21. Lerner and Vicary (1984) found that 5-year-old children with "difficult" temperamental profiles, including high levels of behavioral reactivity and emotionality, and slow adaptability were more likely than non-"difficult" children to use substances in adolescence and young adulthood. Brook, Whiteman, Cohen, Shapiro, and Balka (1995) found that childhood characteristics of unconventionality and poor control of emotions were associated with increased levels of drug use in adolescence and young adulthood. Such findings suggest that poor self-regulation and undercontrolled behavior are not simply correlates of problematic substance use, but that they prospectively predict future adolescent drug and alcohol problems (although causal mechanisms are not known).

Several biobehavioral markers of behavioral undercontrol, and consequent risk for adolescent substance use problems, have been identified. One is a diminished P3 component in event-related potentials (ERPs). P3 components of ERPs occur approximately 300 milliseconds after the presentation of a novel or task relevant stimulus. Reductions in P3 amplitude have been reported for several forms of undercontrolled behaviors, including antisocial personality disorder, ADHD, and aggression, as well as substance use disorders (Begleiter & Porjesz, 1999; Iacono et al., 1999; Klorman, 1992). Moreover, young children of alcoholic parents also show reduced P3 amplitude even before the onset of drinking (Begleiter & Porjesz, 1999), and reduced P3 amplitude predicts drinking onset in this population (S. Hill et al., 2000; Iacono et al., 1999). Given these data, reductions in P3 amplitude have been viewed as a potential marker for behavioral undercontrol as a diathesis for early-onset substance use. Other candidate biobehavioral markers for behavioral undercontrol and risk for substance use include neurochemical and neuroendocrine responses and the ability to modulate autonomic nervous system reactivity (Iacono et al., 1999; see Tarter et al., 1999, for a review).

Additional data suggest that the intergenerational transmission of adolescent substance use problems may be mediated by a predisposition toward behavioral undercontrol. For instance, research has consistently found that children of alcoholic parents (a population at heightened risk for the development of alcohol problems) show high levels of impulsivity, aggression, and high levels of motor activity (e.g., Blackson, 1994; Jansen, Fitzgerald, Ham, & Zucker, 1995; Martin et al., 1994; Tarter, Alterman, & Edwards, 1985), and that these traits are observed in their alcoholic parents as well (e.g., Blackson, 1994). Data from twin studies further suggest that indicators of behavioral undercontrol have substantial heritability, and may serve to increase risk for substance use problems in adolescents, particularly in the context of familial alcoholism. Ongoing longitudinal data from the Minnesota Family Twin Study (Iacono et al., 1999) have shown substantial heritability for various indices of undercontrol, including reduced constraint, poor psychophysiological modulation in response to stress, and high levels of externalizing behavior. These traits were also more likely to characterize children with a family history of alcoholism. Specifically, sons of "undersocialized" alcoholic parents (i.e., alcoholic adults with comorbid externalizing disorders) were more likely than sons of "socialized" alcoholic parents (i.e., adults without comorbid externalizing disorders) or sons of nonalcoholic parents to meet diagnostic criteria for ADHD, conduct disorder, or antisocial peersonality disorder; to have had contact with the police; and to have a personality style typified by low constraint. In turn, these risk factors were strongly associated with a diagnosis of adolescent substance dependence, even after controls for effects of paternal alcoholism. Taken together, these findings support a genetic diathesis model for adolescent substance use problems, with the diathesis consisting of heritable individual differences in behavioral undercontrol.

Although temperament is presumed to reflect a relatively stable behavioral style, the effects of temperament on developmental outcomes is also presumed to be modified by the environment—particularly by parenting and family environments. In studies of adolescent externalizing behavior, it has been reported that poor parenting is particularly detrimental when adolescents show high levels of temperamental reactivity or deficient regulation (e.g., Bates, Pettit, Dodge, & Ridge, 1998; Stice & Gonzales, 1998). Similar results have been reported with respect to adolescent substance use. Specifically, Wills, Sandy, Yaeger, and Shinar (2001) examined moderating effects of temperament and parenting on adolescent substance use (including alcohol, tobacco, and marijuana use), and found that parental risk factors (i.e., substance use, conflict) differentially exacerbated risk for substance use among adolescents with high activity levels and high levels of negative emotionality. Such findings suggest that despite their heritable bases, the effects of temperamental characteristics on substance use outcomes may be either exacerbated or buffered by the type of parenting that adolescents receive. However, there have been relatively few studies to examine this moderation hypothesis in the area of adolescent substance use, and this is an important direction for future research.

Cognitive Functioning

Additional evidence for deficient self-regulation as a risk factor for adolescent substance use and misuse may be found at the level of cognitive functioning. Specifically, adolescents with substance use problems are characterized by lower levels of executive functioning. "Executive functioning" is a multidimensional construct encompassing a variety of related higher-order cognitive processes that allow for future goal-oriented behavior. A myriad of different processes have been included in this construct, including planning, organizational skills, selective attention, hypothesis generation, cognitive flexibility, maintenance of cognitive set, decision making, judgment, inhibitory control, and self-regulation (Lezak, 1995; Spreen & Strauss, 1998).

The role of executive functioning and its relation to behavioral undercontrol and externalizing behavior problems has been receiving increasing attention in the field of child psychopathology. For instance, in his recent taxonomy of inhibitory processes within the cognitive and personality literatures, Nigg (2000) has recognized a conceptual overlap between cognitive aspects of executive control and temperamental aspects of behavioral regulation, and suggested that these two aspects of self-regulation have joint influences in ADHD and conduct disorder. In a recent conceptual model of ADHD, Barkley (1997; see also Chapter 2, this volume) has proposed that deficits in response inhibition lead to deficits in executive functions, which in turn result in decreased control over motor behavior and ADHD symptoms. Thus there appears to be an interplay between cognitive and behavioral aspects of self-regulation as they pertain to risk for child psychopathology.

From the point of view of risk for adolescent substance use/misuse, a common theme is that deficits in executive cognitive functions make it difficult for children both to create strategic and goal-oriented responses to environmental stimuli, and to use feedback to modify behavior in response to environmental events (Peterson & Pihl, 1990). Such cognitive difficulties in creating goal-directed responses to environmental stimuli then produce heightened levels of behavioral undercontrol, such as impulsive and externalizing behavior, which raise risk for substance use and substance use disorders (Peterson & Pihl, 1990).

Deficits in cognitive functioning have been well documented in studies of adults with substance use disorders, particularly among alcoholic adults (see Rourke & Loberg, 1996, for a recent review), and emerging research suggests that these findings may also apply to adolescents with substance use problems. For example, Brown and colleagues reported that relative to youths without alcohol problems, alcohol-dependent adolescents were characterized by poorer retention of verbal and nonverbal information, poorer attentional capacities, and deficits in visual–spatial planning (Brown, Tapert, Granholm, & Delis, 2000; Tapert & Brown, 1999). Moreover, substance-dependent adolescents with poor cognitive skills and poor coping skills were also more likely to continue using alcohol and drugs over time (Tapert, Brown, Myers, & Granholm, 1999). Similarly, Giancola, Mezzich, and Tarter (1998) found that adolescent girls with a substance use disorder exhibited poorer executive functioning than controls did. Thus adolescents with drug and alcohol problems show deficits in a variety of cognitive functions, and these deficits may contribute to more extensive and prolonged substance use problems.

Additional research with community samples suggests that deficits in executive functioning are associated with alcohol use in late adolescence. For example, Deckel, Bauer, and Hesselbrock (1995) found that lower levels of executive functioning were associated with earlier drinking onset, greater frequency of drinking to get drunk, and higher scores on the Michigan Alcoholism Screening Test in a sample of young adults. Research with college students has yielded similar findings. Giancola, Zeichner, Yarnell, and Dickson (1996) found that lower levels of executive functioning were associated with more adverse consequences of drinking, even after absolute levels of alcohol consumption were controlled for. Sher, Martin, Wood, and Rutledge (1997) found that first-year undergraduates with diagnoses of alcohol abuse or dependence performed more poorly than did non-problem-drinking students on measures of visual–spatial ability, motor skill, and attention. Although these studies were cross-sectional in design (and thus could not speak to the directionality of effects), their findings suggest that lower levels of executive functioning are associated with higher levels of drinking, and may thus increase risk for the development of alcohol problems.

Several studies have also suggested that executive functioning deficits are found in children of alcoholic parents, even at early ages, before alcohol problems have developed (e.g., Corral, Holguin, & Cadaveira, 1999; Drejer, Theilgard, Teasdale, Schulsinger, & Goodwin, 1985; Giancola, Martin, Tarter, Pelham, & Moss, 1996; Harden & Pihl, 1995; Peterson, Finn, & Pihl, 1992; Poon, Ellis, Fitzgerald, & Zucker, 2000). These data suggest that executive functioning may be an antecedent risk factor rather than a result of alcohol consumption in this population. Similarly, Deckel and Hesselbrock (1996) found that children of alcoholic parents with poorer executive functioning showed greater increases in alcohol consumption over a 3-year period than did children of alcoholic parents with higher levels of executive functioning; this finding suggests that executive functioning may be a prospective predictor of substance use among high-risk adolescents. In a separate longitudinal investigation, Atyaclar, Tarter, Kirisci, and Lu (1999) reported significant independent effects of paternal substance abuse and executive functioning on several measures of adolescent drug use, including the lifetime number of drugs used, lifetime exposure to cannabis and tobacco, and severity of consequences resulting from drug use.

Although these findings suggest that executive functioning impairments play an important role in the pathogenesis of substance use, particularly among those at high risk because of parental alcoholism, it is important to note that not all studies have replicated these findings. Many investigators have not found differences in cognitive functioning between children of alcoholic parents and controls (e.g., Bates & Pandina, 1992; Wiers, Gunning, & Sargeant, 1998), and at least one review of the literature has concluded that evidence for executive functioning deficits in children of alcoholic parents is weak and inconsistent across studies (Hesselbrock, Bauer, Hesselbrock, & Gillen, 1991). Moreover, executive function deficits have been well documented in children with conduct problems (e.g., Moffitt, 1993), and several investigations have reported that executive functioning deficits among substance-abusing adolescents may be related to externalizing symptomatology rather than being specific to substance use (Giancola & Mezzich, 2000; Giancola et al., 1998). Children with ADHD (who are characterized by deficits in executive functioning; Barkley, 1997) do not appear to be at increased risk for substance use unless they suffer from comorbid conduct disorder symptoms (Molina, Smith, & Pelham, 1999). Given these findings, it may be conduct disorder symptoms rather than executive functioning deficits that raise risk for adolescent substance use, abuse, and dependence.

Overall, few studies have prospectively tested associations between deficits in executive functioning and later alcohol or drug problems in adolescents. Studies are needed to test mediational models of the processes through which executive functioning deficits increase risk for substance use disorders, and to clarify the role of conduct problems in those processes.

Parenting and Socialization

Parenting that combines high levels of nurturance with consistent discipline— in other words, what Baumrind (1991) has termed "authoritative" parenting—has been associated with a lowered risk of adolescent substance use (see Hawkins et al., 1992, for a review). Stice and Barrera (1995) found that low levels of parental social support and discipline prospectively predicted increases in adolescent substance use over time. Similarly, low levels of parental monitoring have been shown to prospectively predict the onset both of substance use and of heavy drinking in adolescence (Reifman, Barnes, Dintcheff, Farrell, & Uhteg, 1998; Steinberg, Fletcher, & Darling, 1994). Finally, high levels of family conflict (Webb & Baer, 1995) and parental divorce and single-parent families (T. E. Duncan, Duncan, & Hops, 1998) have been associated with higher levels of adolescent substance use, although it is unclear whether the single-parent family structure or correlated processes (such as elevated conflict and disrupted parent–adolescent relationships) are more important risk factors (Brody & Forehand, 1993).

Not only is adolescent substance use related to general parenting style, family climate, and parent–adolescent relationships, but data also suggest that adolescent substance use may be related to parents(specific socialization about the use of substances. That is, parents set not only general rules and expectations for adolescent behavior, but also rules and policies about the use of tobacco, alcohol, and other drugs; they may discuss reasons not to use these substances; and they may punish substance use behavior. Cross-sectional studies have suggested that these forms of socialization specific to substance use may also deter adolescents' substance use behavior (Chassin, Presson, Todd, Rose, & Sherman, 1998; Jackson & Henriksen, 1997).

Thus available data suggest that parent socialization—either in the form of general parenting and parent–adolescent relationships, or in the form of specific attempts to deter substance use—may influence the development of adolescent substance use behavior. Moreover, although data are not extensive, several investigators suggest that the effects of parenting on adolescent substance use may be mediated through the effects of parenting on affiliations with deviant peer networks (Chassin, Curran, Hussong, & Colder, 1996; Dishion, Patterson, & Reid, 1988). However, there are also limitations to these data that should be acknowledged. First, most of these studies examine adolescent substance use rather than abuse or dependence, and the importance of parenting in the development of clinical substance use disorders is not as well studied. Second, the relation between parenting and adolescent substance use may be explained by other characteristics of the adolescents. That is, adolescents who are rebellious, externalizing, and poorly regulated may be difficult to monitor and discipline, and they may also evoke parental rejection (Ge et al., 1996); it may be these adolescent characteristics that raise risk for substance abuse and dependence, rather than the parenting behavior per se. Third, because parents provide both genetic and environmental influences, the correlations between parenting and adolescent substance use that are reported in the literature may inflate the magnitude of what appears to be environmental influence. For example, McGue, Sharma, and Benson (1996) reported only relatively small correlations between adolescent alcohol involvement and family functioning in adoptive families compared to biological families, suggesting that the magnitude of family environmental influences on adolescent alcohol use may be relatively modest. Finally, it is not known how the role of parenting and family environment factors may differentially affect adolescent substance abuse and dependence across different ethnic or cultural groups. Although evidence for generalizability of familial influences across ethnic groups has been produced (Barrera et al., 1999), other investigators have also reported differential magnitudes of correlations between parenting and substance use across ethnicity (e.g., Griesler & Kandel, 1998, for tobacco use), or have speculated that the relations between authoritative parenting and adolescent deviance-proneness may vary as a function of ethnicity and community context (Lamborn, Dornbusch, & Steinberg, 1996).

School Failure and Academic Aspirations

Children who are temperamentally poorly regulated; who receive poor parental nurturance and involvement, as well as deficient parental monitoring and discipline; and who have cognitive deficits in executive and verbal functioning are at heightened risk for school failure (Patterson, 1986). Moreover, school failure itself may further elevate risk for the onset of adolescent substance use through several mechanisms. First, school failure is a source of stress and negative affect, which can raise risk for substance use to regulate that affect. Second, school failure can weaken school attachment (e.g., aspirations for higher education, values placed on academic success, participation in mainstream school activities). Many theories of adolescent substance use and deviant behavior—including social control theory (Elliott, Huizinga, & Ageton, 1985), the social development model (Catalano, Kosterman, Hawkins, Newcomb, & Abbott, 1996), and problem behavior theory (Jessor & Jessor, 1977)—

suggest that estrangement from conventional mainstream social institutions makes adolescents more vulnerable to engaging in problem behaviors, including drug use, because they feel less bound by conventional social norms and values. Moreover, adolescents who are not committed to academic success will experience less role conflict between the demands of academic roles and the impairment produced by alcohol and drug use, so that they have less reason to refrain from substance use. Third, school failure can increase risk for adolescent drug use because it raises risk for adolescents' ejection from a mainstream peer group, particularly if the school failure is associated with aggressive or underregulated behavior (Dishion, Patterson, Stoolmiller, & Skinner, 1991; Flicek, 1992). Adolescents who are ejected from a mainstream peer group are more likely to affiliate with deviant peers, who model and approve of substance use behavior. Consistent with these mechanisms, available empirical evidence suggests that adolescents with poor grades (S. C. Duncan, Duncan, Biglan, & Ary, 1998; Kandel, 1978; Luthar & D'Avanzo, 1999), low educational aspirations (e.g., Paulson, Combs, & Richardson, 1990), and low value and expectations for attaining educational success (Jessor & Jessor, 1977) are more likely to use alcohol or drugs. However, it is important to note that these data refer to substance use rather than clinical abuse or dependence outcomes. Moreover, some studies examining the relation between early school achievement and later delinquency suggest that the relation is due to correlated risk factors (IQ and early disruptive behavior) rather than the causal influence of school failure per se (Fergusson & Horwood, 1995).

Peer Influences

A widely replicated finding is that adolescents' alcohol and drug use can be predicted from the alcohol and drug use behavior of their friends (Hawkins et al., 1992; Kandel, 1978). Affiliation with a drug-using peer group elevates risk for adolescent substance use by providing models and opportunities for engaging in drug use, as well as norms that approve of drug use behavior (Oetting & Donnermeyer, 1998). Indeed, peer drug use is an extremely robust predictor of adolescents' own use, and this includes the influence both of close friends and of larger friendship groups (Urberg, Degirmencioglu, & Pilgrim, 1997). Moreover, siblings can constitute an important source of peer influence on adolescent drug use (Brook, Nomura, & Cohen, 1989) and significant correlations have been found between adolescent alcohol use and sibling alcohol use in both biological and adoptive sibling pairs, suggesting an environmental transmission mechanism (McGue et al., 1996). Finally, drug use is also related to membership in different adolescent "cliques" (e.g., "preppies," "jocks," etc.; Sussman, Dent, & McCullar, 2000), and drug use may serve to communicate particular social images that are characteristic of these social groups (Barton, Chassin, Presson, & Sherman, 1982). However, even though peer use is typically the strongest predictor of adolescent substance use, researchers have also questioned the interpretation of this relation. Because most studies use adolescents' reports on both their own use and the behavior of their friends, the magnitude of the correlation between peer use and adolescent use is inflated, because adolescents who themselves use drugs systematically overestimate their friends' use (Bauman & Ennett, 1996). Correlations between adolescent and friends' drug use are lower (although still significant) when peers are surveyed directly (Kandel, 1978). Moreover, cross-sectional correlations reflect the contribution of two different processes: peer selection (in which drug-using adolescents seek out similar friends) and peer influence (in which drug-using peers influence adolescents' behavior). The contribution of peer selection further inflates the magnitude of the association between peer use and adolescent use (Bauman & Ennett, 1996), although longitudinal data suggest that both peer selection and peer influence processes are operative (Curran, Stice, & Chassin, 1997; Kandel, 1978).

Childhood Conduct Problems

A central assumption of the deviance-proneness submodel is that adolescent substance use disorders are related to the broader development of conduct problems and antisociality, and this assumption has widespread empirical support (Hawkins et al., 1992). Conduct problems and aggression predict adolescent substance use (Henry et al., 1993; Kellam, Brown, Rubin, & Ensminger, 1983), escalations in use over time (K. Hill et al., 2000; Hussong, Curran, & Chassin, 1998) and later substance abuse and dependence diagnoses (Chassin, Pitts, DeLucia, & Todd, 1999). Moreover, conduct disorder is a strong risk factor for adolescent substance use disorders (Clark, Parker, & Lynch, 1999; Costello et al., 1999; Disney, Elkins, McGue, & Iacono, 1999; Weinberg & Glantz, 1999), and conduct problems have been found to predict substance abuse and dependence for both boys and girls (Chassin et al., 1999; Costello et al., 1999; Disney et al., 1999). Interestingly, the relation has been somewhat specific to conduct problems rather than all externalizing disorders in general. For example, although ADHD is associated with substance abuse and dependence, these associations seem largely mediated by the development of associated conduct disorder rather than specific to ADHD per se (Costello et al., 1999; Disney et al., 1999; Lynsky & Fergusson, 1995; Molina et al., 1999). An exception to this pattern occurs for tobacco dependence, which has been linked to ADHD even in the absence of conduct disorder (Disney et al., 1999; McMahon, 1999).

THE STRESS AND NEGATIVE AFFECT SUBMODEL

The stress and negative affect submodel hypothesizes that adolescents who are at high risk for substance abuse or dependence experience a high level of environmental stress and resulting negative affect, and use alcohol or drugs as a way to decrease this negative affect (i.e., as a form of self-medication). Sher's (1991) elaboration of this submodel is depicted in Figure 4.2. However, although this submodel is intuitively appealing, it has not enjoyed widespread empirical support and remains controversial in the adolescent literature. Here we review the evidence for each link in this hypothesized mediational chain (although we will not repeat our discussion of temperamental and cognitive variables, considered in connection with the deviance-proneness submodel above).

Environmental Stress

Multiple studies have reported consistent findings that adolescents who experience high levels of environmental stress are more likely to use alcohol or drugs, and to escalate the quantity and frequency of their use over time (Aseltine & Gore, 2000; Chassin et al., 1996; Hoffman, Cerbone, & Su, 2000; Wills, Vaccaro, McNamara, & Hirky, 1996). However, the literature on the relationship of stress to substance use in adolescence may also overestimate the effects of stress, because some measures of stress include items that may reflect the adolescents' behavioral undercontrol and conduct problems. For example, studies that include

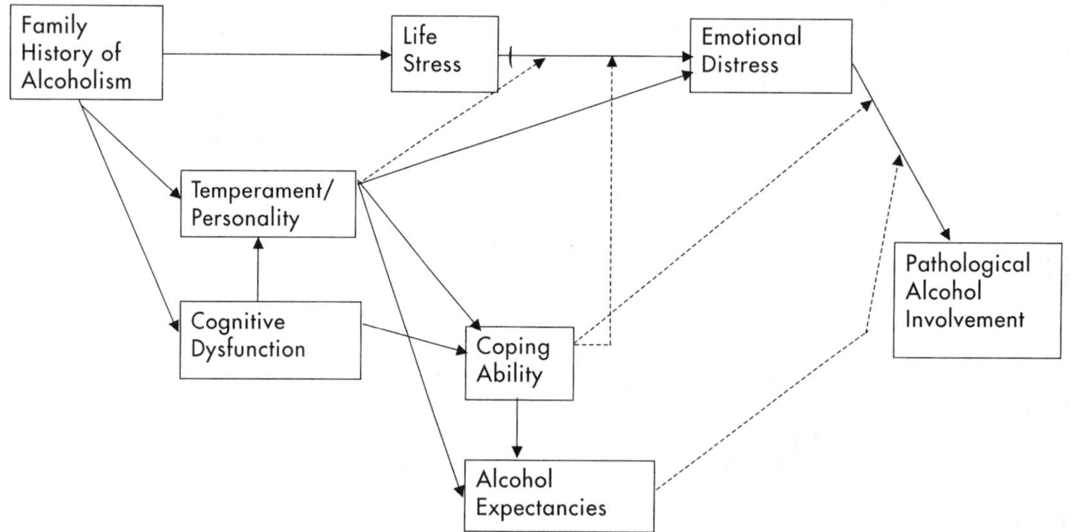

FIGURE 4.2. Schematic diagram of Sher's (1991) stress and negative affect submodel. Mediating paths are indicated by solid lines; moderating paths are indicated by dashed lines. Adapted from Sher (1991). Copyright 1991 by University of Chicago Press. Adapted by permission.

"conflicts with teachers" or "school problems" as stress items may confound the effects of environmental stress with the effects of such undercontrol and conduct problems. Nevertheless, even studies that restrict their stress measures to include only uncontrollable life events still report significant relations between negative life events and adolescent substance use (e.g., Chassin et al., 1996; Newcomb & Harlow, 1986).

Adolescents who are at risk for substance use may be not only exposed to heightened levels of environmental stress, but also characterized by abnormal stress responses. Adult children of alcoholic parents have been reported to exhibit elevated psychophysiological responses to stress in the laboratory, compared to those without parental alcoholism (Conrod, Pihl, & Ditto, 1995). Similar findings have been obtained with a small sample of young boys (mean age = 12 years) whose families had multiple alcoholic members (Harden & Pihl, 1995). These young boys showed greater heart rate increases and peripheral vasoconstriction during a mental arithmetic task than did boys without a family history of alcoholism. These researchers suggest that hyperreactivity to stress may produce risk for substance use, because substance use provides a way to regulate stress response. In contrast, however, Moss, Vanyukov, Yao, and Irillova (1999) found that sons whose fathers had a substance use disorder had a decreased salivary cortisol response to an anticipated stressor, and that those boys with lower cortisol responses also showed more marijuana use. Moss et al. (1999) suggest that hyporeactivity in these boys may represent an adaptation to chronic exposure to high levels of environmental stress. Finally, Iacono et al. (1999) suggest that adolescents at risk for substance use problems show poor modulation of stress responses, as reflected in an ability to control psychophysiological arousal in predictable versus unpredictable exposures to a laboratory stressor. The possibility that high-risk children and adolescents show abnormalities in stress response (coupled with the possibility, described later, that they show heightened stress-response-dampening effects of substance use) represents an important etiological factor in the development of substance abuse and dependence. However, because there have been very few empirical studies of stress response in high-risk children or adolescents (particularly in young girls), conclusions must reman preliminary at this point.

The Role of Emotional Distress

The relation of emotional distress to adolescent substance use and substance use disorders has been less consistently upheld. Many studies have reported cross-sectional correlations between negative affect and adolescent substance use (Chassin, Pillow, Curran, Molina, & Barrera, 1993; Cooper, Frone, Russell, & Mudar, 1995), as well as substantial comorbidity between clinically diagnosed depression and adolescent nicotine dependence (Fergusson, Lynsky, & Horwood, 1996), alcoholism (Rohde, Lewinsohn, & Seeley, 1996), and drug abuse or dependence (Deykin, Buka, & Zeena, 1992). However, other researchers have argued that emotional distress or negative affect has only weak and indirect relations to adolescent substance use, compared to such factors as peer affiliations (Swaim, Oetting, & Beauvais, 1989). Moreover, studies considering the role of negative affect have often failed to consider the effects of externalizing symptoms and conduct problems. Because there is considerable covariation between internalizing and externalizing symptoms, it has not been clearly established that negative affect has a unique relation to adolescent substance use (above and beyond co-occurring conduct problems).

Perhaps most important, longitudinal studies have not consistently confirmed that negative affect prospectively predicts the onset or escalation of adolescent substance use or the development of substance abuse and dependence. For example, Hussong et al. (1998) found that internalizing symptoms did not prospectively predict growth over time in alcohol use, and K. Hill et al. (2000) found that internalizing symptoms did not prospectively predict trajectories of heavy drinking from adolescence to young adulthood. Hansell and White (1991) failed to find a prospective effect of psychological distress on later adolescent drug use. In fact, anxiety has been associated with delayed onset of "gateway" drug use, such as cigarette smoking (Costello et al., 1999). In terms of clinical substance use disorders, Chassin, Pitts, DeLucia, and Todd (1999) found that adolescent internalizing symptoms did not prospectively predict young adult alcohol and drug diagnoses, and Rohde et al. (1996) did not find that depressive disorders preceded the development of adolescent alcohol abuse and dependence. This pattern of cross-sectional but not prospective relations between negative affect and adolescent substance use and substance use disorders has suggested that negative affect may be a result rather than a cause of adolescent substance use and related problems (Hansell & White, 1991).

Nevertheless, despite the inconsistent prospective findings, it may be premature to dismiss the role of negative affect in the development of adolescent substance use disorders, for several reasons. First, some studies have found prospective effects. For example, Windle and Windle (2001) found that persistent and severe depressive symptoms prospectively predicted persistent and heavy cigarette smoking in a large, school-based adolescent sample (although this prospective prediction was confined to regression analyses and did not appear in growth modeling). Moreover, the time lag of effect in these longitudinal studies (often a year or more between measurements) is not optimal for detecting self-medication effects, which should occur much more proximally to the occurrence of negative affect or a life stress event. More microanalytic techniques, such as experience-sampling methods, might reveal different patterns of findings (Hussong, Hicks, Levy & Curran, 2001).

In addition, conflicting findings may be due to variation in the type of negative affect assessed. Support has been stronger for depression, irritability, and anger as prospective predictors of adolescent substance use than for anxiety (Block et al., 1988; Swaim et al., 1989). For example, Swaim et al. (1989) found that among different forms of emotional distress, only anger had a unique direct effect on adolescent substance use. Hussong and Chassin (1994) found that depression, but not anxiety, mediated the relation between stress and adolescent alcohol use. Perhaps anxiety lowers risk for adolescent substance use, because anxious adolescents are less likely to select (or to be selected into) peer contexts that promote substance use. However, because other researchers suggest that clinically diagnosed social phobia increases risk for substance use (Merikangas & Avenevoli, 2000), further studies of social phobia are warranted before the role of anxiety in adolescent substance use can be determined. In short, variations in both the type of negative affect (depression, anger, and irritability vs. anxiety) and the severity of the distress (e.g., measures of symptomatology versus actual clinical diagnosis) may produce differing findings in terms of risk for adolescent substance use and abuse.

Related to the distinction between the roles of anxiety and depression as etiological factors is the role that may be played by positive affect. Recent theoretical conceptualizations of the distinction between anxiety and depression suggest that one difference between these two affective states is that anxiety may co-occur with positive affect, whereas depression is more likely to be correlated with low levels of positive affect (Watson, Clark, & Carey, 1988). Indeed, a motivation to use substances in order to increase positive affect has also been posited within affect regulation models (Cooper et al., 1995), although it has not been as widely studied as the motivation to reduce negative affect. Some researchers have suggested that positive and negative affect regulation may be associated with different levels of adolescent substance use. That is, adolescents who use substances to maintain or enhance positive affect may use them at moderate levels of quantity and frequency, whereas those who use substances to relieve negative affect may show higher consumption (Labouvie, Pandina, White, & Johnson, 1990). Data also suggest that low levels of positive affect are particularly associated with adolescent substance use for those adolescents who are also highly impulsive (Colder & Chassin, 1997). Thus future studies of the role of affect regulation in adolescent substance use should consider theoretical models that include depression, anxiety, general distress, and positive affect (Watson et al., 1988).

Finally, the lack of consistent relations between negative affect and adolescent substance use may reflect the presence of moderator variables, such that negative affect produces risk for substance use, abuse, or dependence under only certain circumstances. In Sher's (1991) submodel, one important potential moderator variable is coping strategies. Theoretically, adolescents should not react to life stress or emotional distress by turning to substance use if other, more adaptive coping mechanisms are available to them. Some data suggest that behavioral coping (e.g., "Make a plan and follow it") may serve such an adaptive function (Wills, 1986), but that "disengagement coping" (e.g., coping through anger, hanging out with friends) may actually amplify the effects of life stress events on increases over time in adolescent substance use (Wills, Sandy, Yaeger, Cleary, & Shinar, 2001). Thus coping may serve either to buffer or to exacerbate the relation between life stress and adolescent substance use, depending on the type of coping strategy that is employed. Similarly, Sher's (1991) submodel suggests that the relation between stress or emotional distress and substance use should be stronger for those who expect substance use to relieve their emotional distress, and this hypothesis has received some empirical support (Cooper, Russell, Skinner, Frone, & Mudar, 1992; Kushner, Sher, Wood, & Wood, 1994).

Individual differences may also moderate the relation between negative affect and adolescent substance use. For example, research in social development has suggested that low levels of temperamental self-regulation will amplify the relation between reactivity (a propensity to experience intense affective states) and conduct problems (Eisenberg et al., 2000). Thus adolescents who are highly emotionally reactive may show particularly heightened risk for substance use, abuse, or dependence when they also show low levels of temperamental self-regulation. Interestingly, some laboratory data also suggest that individuals who are temperamentally "underregulated" may derive the strongest psychophysiological stress-response-dampening benefits from consuming alcohol (Levenson, Oyama, & Meek, 1987; see below for a review). If behaviorally undercontrolled individuals derive greater stress-response-dampening effects from consuming alcohol and drugs, then this would be consistent with stronger links between stress or negative affect and substance use for individuals who are low in self-regulation. This notion of self-regulation as a moderator variable in the relation between negative affect and substance use can serve to bridge the deviance-proneness submodel and the stress and negative affect submodel of adolescent substance use. Although these two submodels have typically been conceptualized and studied in isolation from each other, the relation between these two pathways is worthy of future study. Finally, both gender and age may moderate the relation between negative affect and substance use disorders. Data on subtypes of alcoholism suggest that negative affect and self-medication motives may be more strongly linked to substance abuse and dependence that has a late onset (later in adulthood) and among females (Babor et al., 1992; Cloninger, 1987).

THE SUBSTANCE USE EFFECTS SUBMODEL

The discussion above of the deviance-proneness submodel and the stress and negative affect submodel of adolescent substance use serves to illustrate the importance of considering some of the functions that substance use may serve for adolescents. The deviance-proneness submodel highlights the fact that adolescent substance use occurs in a broader social context of low behavioral constraint and drug-use-promoting peer networks. Within these peer social networks, adolescent substance use may serve to communicate a social image of toughness and precocity, and to express an adolescent's actual or ideal self-concept (Barton et al., 1982; Jessor & Jessor, 1977; Sussman et al., 2000). The stress and negative affect submodel highlights the affect-regulating functions that alcohol and drug use may serve for adolescents. As such, it is important to remember that alcohol and drug consumption involves reinforcing pharmacological effects, and to consider these effects within any etiological model of adolescent substance use and abuse. Sher's (1991) alcohol effects submodel (which, again, we extrapolate to substance use effects in general) is depicted in Figure 4.3. In this submodel, a family history of alcoholism is thought to be associated with individual differences in sensitivity to the pharmacological effects of alcohol and other drugs (as well as with temperamental and cognitive variables discussed earlier). As people experience different effects of their alcohol and drug use, these experiences then influence their expectancies about the effects of future consumption. These expectancies, in turn, influence the likelihood of future substance use involvement.

In terms of substance use effects, a large literature has examined the impact of alcohol and drug self-administration in both human and animal laboratory studies; this literature is beyond the scope of the current chapter. Moreover, for ethical reasons, laboratory studies of alcohol or drug administration have been confined to adult participants, so that little is known about the relation between alcohol or drug effects in the laboratory and adolescent alcohol or drug use in the natural environment. Rather, researchers who are interested in child and adolescent populations have focused on their beliefs or expectancies about substance use effects. These expectancies can be measured in young children even before substance use begins, and they become increasingly complex and more positive in adolescence (Dunn & Goldman, 1996). Moreover, adolescents' expectancies about substance use effects are systematically related to their consumption. For example, adolescents' expectancies that alcohol

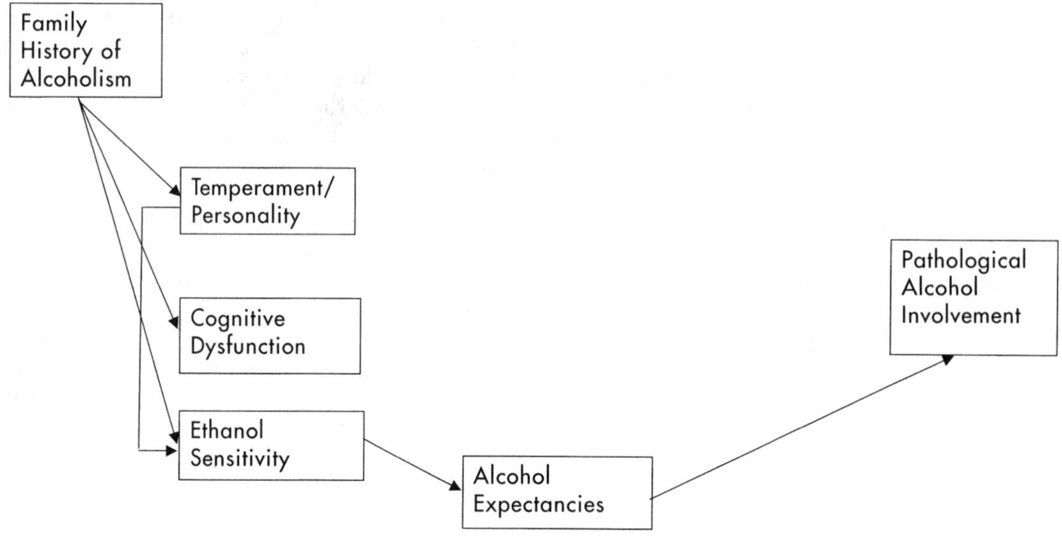

FIGURE 4.3. Schematic diagram of Sher's (1991) alcohol effects submodel. Adapted from Sher (1991). Copyright 1991 by University of Chicago Press. Adapted by permission.

has positive effects prospectively predict their drinking behavior (Smith, Goldman, Greenbaum, & Christiansen, 1995; Stacy, Newcomb, & Bentler, 1991), and expectancies concerning the effects of marijuana and stimulants are also associated with adolescent drug preferences and drug use (Aarons, Brown, Stice, & Coe, 2001).

Although laboratory studies of substance use effects have been confined to adult samples, they are certainly important for etiological theories of substance use and substance use disorders. To illustrate the laboratory data, we briefly highlight some findings concerning individual differences in alcohol effects that have been related to risk for alcoholism in adults.

In general, this literature has suggested that men who are at high risk because of multigenerational family histories of alcoholism experience either enhanced reinforcement effects or weaker punishing effects of alcohol consumption than do their low-risk peers. Specifically, these high-risk men derive greater cardiovascular stress-response-dampening benefits from consuming alcohol in anticipation of a laboratory stressor (e.g., Levenson et al., 1987, see Greeley & Oei, 1999, for a review). Although it is unclear whether this benefit takes the form of specific dampening of stress response or more general attenuation of arousal to both positive and negative stimuli (Stritzke, Patrick, & Lang, 1995), and although the data have been criticized on methodological grounds (see Sayette, 1993), the findings suggest that high-risk men derive more reinforcement from drinking than do their low-risk peers. Moreover, these high-risk men have also been reported to show greater increases in resting heart rate after consuming alcohol, and these data have been interpreted as reflecting greater reinforcement from the "psychostimulant" effects of alcohol (Conrod, Peterson, & Pihl, 1997). If high-risk individuals derive enhanced reinforcement benefits from consuming alcohol, then this might explain their greater alcohol consumption and consequent risk for alcohol abuse and dependence. Similarly, it has been demonstrated that high-risk men experience less negative impact of alcohol consumption than do their low-risk peers (e.g., less body sway and less perceived intoxication), and that a lowered response to the negative effects of alcohol prospectively predicts the development of an alcohol use disorder 15 years later (Schuckit & Smith, 2000). Individuals who experience little negative impact of drinking will have little reason to curtail their intake, thus raising their risk for high levels of consumption and subsequent alcohol use disorders. Taken together, these data suggest that high-risk individuals experience either heighteed reinforcement or lowered punishment as a result of their substance use, and that these pharmacological effects help to explain their risk of developing a substance use disorder.

MACRO-LEVEL INFLUENCES: NEIGHBORHOODS AND SCHOOLS

Sher's (1991) deviance-proneness, stress and negative affect, and substance use effects submodels do not explicitly focus on the effects of social influences that are broader than peer and family environments. However, researchers have become increasingly interested in ways in which such macro-level environments as neighborhoods and schools may influence adolescent substance use and substance use disorders (mirroring broader trends in the study of macro-level influences on developmental psychopathology). Conceptually, these macro-level influences may be important across all of Sher's three etiological pathways. That is, schools and neighborhoods may influence risk for substance use and misuse by providing social norms about the relative acceptability of use, by providing different ease of access to different substances, and by providing different degrees of punishment or sanctions for use. Theoretically, these factors would influence the prevalence of use for adolescents in all three pathways.

In terms of neighborhoods, the most commonly assessed aspects have been SES, ethnic composition, and residential mobility (Leventhal & Brooks-Gunn, 2000). Surprisingly, although indicators of neighborhood social disadvantage have been shown to be related to adolescent conduct problems and delinquency (Leventhal & Brooks-Gunn, 2000), the opposite has been true for adolescent substance use. For example, higher rates of adolescent substance use have been reported for neighborhoods with higher SES (Skager & Fisher, 1989); low rates of residential instability, high neighborhood attachment, and low population density (Ennett, Flewelling, Lindrooth, & Norton, 1997); and higher prevalences of residents with professional or managerial occupations (Luthar & Cushing, 1999). Perhaps poverty and social disadvantage are more strongly associated with problematic substance use than with normal adolescent experimentation (Brook et al., 1989), or perhaps only extremes of social disadvantage are associated with increased use. More research is necessary to identify the mechanisms underlying these neighborhood effects, and also to examine ways in which they interrelate with other etiological factors, such as personality characteristics and family environment. For example, although some research suggests that neighborhood influences serve to moderate the effects of personality characteristics on juvenile offending (Lynam et al., 2000) and that neighborhood influences on adolescent problem behaviors are mediated through family environment effects (Simons, Johnson, Beamans, Conger, & Whitbeck, 1996), these types of analyses have not been applied to studies of adolescent substance use or substance use disorders as specific outcomes. Finally, some data suggest that these neighborhood effects are stronger for boys than for girls (e.g., Luthar & Cushing, 1999; Simons et al., 1996), and the reasons for such gender differences are worthy of further study.

In addition to such factors as SES and social disadvantage, researchers have suggested that schools and neighborhoods in which norms are more favorable toward substance use, and in which there are greater availability of and easier access to substances, are associated with higher use rates. For example, school norms have been related to adolescent substance use (Allison et al., 1999), and density of alcohol outlets has been related to alcohol use at the community level (Scribner, Cohen, & Fisher, 2000). For legal drugs such as alcohol and tobacco, findings such as these have been used to support public policies that aim to decrease adolescents(access to substances and change community norms (e.g., raising drinking ages, reducing sales to minors, increasing tobacco taxes, restricting advertising) as ways of reducing adolescent substance use (see, e.g., Institute of Medicine, 1994b, for a review). These broader community-level interventions are potentially important avenues for adolescent substance use prevention, and may be useful additions to programs that target individual-level risk factors or high-risk subgroups.

CONCLUSIONS AND FUTURE DIRECTIONS

As illustrated by the discussion above, much is known about the nature of adolescent substance use and substance use disorders, as well as about etiological factors; moreover, much effort has already gone into the development of empirically evaluated treatment and prevention programs. For example, a large and diverse literature has produced a consensus across studies that a family history of substance misuse, childhood conduct problems, temperament or personality traits reflecting "behavioral undercontrol," and affiliations with drug-using peer networks all raise risk for substance use and adolescent substance use disorders.

However, there are also many unanswered questions and areas for future research. First, the adequacy of existing diagnostic criteria as they are applied to adolescents must be clarified. In particular, more studies are needed of drug diagnoses (where few data exist compared to alcohol diagnoses), and the question of whether it is useful to maintain the distinction between abuse and dependence as separate diagnoses must be examined further. In terms of etiology, although the role of family history risk is well established, much less is known about the mechanisms underlying the intergenerational transmission of risk, or about the protective factors that might buffer this risk. Moreover, the pathway from stress and negative affect to adolescent substance use disorders is particularly controversial and in need of further study. In this regard, further research is needed to clarify the roles of different types of negative affect (i.e., anxiety vs. depression vs. anger), and particularly the importance of moderating variables such as coping or behavioral undercontrol. That is, instead of considering the affect regulation pathway and the deviance-proneness pathway in isolation, it may be more useful to focus on behavioral undercontrol and underregulation as moderators of the relation between environmental stress or negative affect and subsequent substance use outcomes. In terms of the deviance-proneness pathway, more research is needed on the specificity of effects in order to identify variables that are related specifically to substance use outcomes rather than to conduct problems in general.

Across all the etiological models, data are lacking on ways in which our existing findings might vary across particular gender and ethnic subgroups. Moreover, this topic is in need of stronger theory development that would help guide our interpretations of why particular risk or protective factors might operate in particular ways within certain gender or ethnic subgroups. Beyond questions of gender and ethnic variation, the examination of macro-level societal and cultural factors (such as neighborhood effects, school effects, and effects of social policies like taxation) has often been conducted in isolation from more individual-level factors. Research is needed to study the effects of neighborhood, school, and social policy influences as they interact with individual, family, and peer factors.

Finally, as is evident from our review, it is unlikely that a single etiological pathway will be capable of explaining the development of adolescent substance use disorders. Thus we are in need of studies and methods capable of differentiating among multiple pathways that may underlie different trajectories of substance use. To accomplish these ambitious goals requires studies that are multilevel and multidisciplinary, and that embed studies of substance use disorders within a broader developmental perspective. Given the clinical and public health importance of adolescent substance use and substance use disorders, it is likely that the field will continue to expand in these future directions.

ACKNOWLEDGMENT

Preparation of this chapter was supported by Grant No. DA05227 from the National Institute on Drug Abuse.

REFERENCES

Aarons, G., Brown, S., Stice, E., & Coe, M. (2001). Psychometric evaluation of the marijuana and stimulant effect expectancy questionnaires for adolescents. *Addictive Behaviors*, *26*, 219–236.

Allison, K. W., Crawford, I., Leone, P., Trickett, E., Perez-Febles, A., Burton, L., & Le Blanc, R. (1999). Adolescent substance use: Preliminary examinations of school and neighborhood context. *American Journal of Community Psychology*, *27*, 111–141.

Amaro, H., Blake. S., Schwartz, P., & Flinchbaugh, L. (2001). Developing theory-based substance abuse prevention programs for young adolescent girls. *Journal of Early Adolescence*, *21*, 256–293.

American Psychiatric Association. (1994). *Diagnostic and statistical manual of mental disorders* (4th ed.). Washington, DC: Author.

Arnett, J. J. (2000). A theory of development from the late teens through the twenties. *American Psychologist*, *55*, 469–480.

Aseltine, R. H., & Gore, S. L. (2000). The variable effects of stress on alcohol use from adolescence to adulthood. *Substance Use and Misuse*, *35*, 643–668.

Atyaclar, S., Tarter, R. E., Kirisci, L., & Lu, S. (1999). Association between hyperactivity and executive cognitive functioning in childhood and substance use in early adolescence. *Journal of the American Academy of Child and Adolescent Psychiatry*, *38*, 172–178.

Babor, T., Hoffmann, M., DelBoca, F., Hesselbrock, V., Meyer, R., Dolinski, A., & Rounsaville, B. (1992). Types of alcoholics: I. Evidence for an empirically derived typology based on indicators of vulnerability and severity. *Archives of General Psychiatry*, *49*, 599–608.

Bachman, J. G., Wadsworth, K., O'Malley, P., Johnston, L., & Schulenberg, J. (1997). *Smoking, drinking, and drug use in young adulthood: The impact of new freedoms and new responsibilities*. Mahwah, NJ: Erlbaum.

Baer, J. S., Barr, H., Bookstein, F., Sampson, P., & Streissguth, A. (1998). Prenatal alcohol exposure and family history of alcoholism in the etiology of adolescent alcohol problems. *Journal of Studies on Alcohol, 59*, 533–543.

Barkley, R. A. (1997). Behavioral inhibition, sustained attention, and executive functions: Constructing a unifying theory of ADHD. *Psychological Bulletin, 121*, 65–94.

Barrera, M. B., Castro, F. G., & Biglan, A. (1999). Ethnicity, substance use, and development: Exemplars for exploring group differences and similarities. *Development and Psychopathology, 11*, 805–822.

Barton, J., Chassin, L., Presson, C., & Sherman, S. J. (1982). Social image factors as motivators of smoking initiation in early and middle adolescents. *Child Development, 53*, 1499–1511.

Bates, J. E., Pettit, G. S., Dodge, K. A., & Ridge, B. (1998). Interaction of temperamental resistance to control and restrictive parenting in the development of externalizing behavior. *Developmental Psychology, 34*, 982–995.

Bates, M. (1993). Psychology. In M. Galanter (Ed.), *Recent developments in alcoholism: Vol. 11. Ten years of progress* (pp. 45–72). New York: Plenum Press.

Bates, M., & Pandina, R. (1992). Familial alcoholism and premorbid cognitive deficit: A failure to replicate subtype differences. *Journal of Studies on Alcohol, 53*, 320–327.

Bauman, K. E., & Ennett, S. T. (1994). Tobacco use by black and white adolescents: The validity of self-reports. *American Journal of Public Health, 84*, 394–398.

Bauman, K. E., & Ennett, S. T. (1996). On the importance of peer influence for adolescent drug use: Commonly neglected considerations. *Addiction, 91*, 185–198.

Baumrind, D. (1991). The influence of parenting style on adolescent competence and substance use. *Journal of Early Adolescence, 11*, 56–95.

Baumrind, D., & Moselle, K. (1985). A developmental perspective on adolescent drug abuse. *Advances in Alcohol and Substance Abuse, 4*, 41–67.

Begleiter, H., & Porjesz, B. (1999). What is inherited in the predisposition toward alcoholism: A proposed model. *Alcoholism: Clinical and Experimental Research, 23*, 1125–1135.

Blackson, T. C. (1994). Temperament: A salient correlate of risk factors for alcohol and drug abuse. *Drug and Alcohol Dependence, 36*, 205–214.

Blackson, T. C., Butler, T., Belsky, J., Ammerman, R. T., Shaw, D. S., & Tarter, R. E. (1999). Individual traits and family contexts predict sons(externalizing behavior and preliminary relative risk ratios for conduct disorder and substance use disorder outcomes. *Drug and Alcohol Dependence, 56*, 115–131.

Block, J., Block, H., & Keyes, S. (1988). Longitudinally foretelling drug usage in adolescence: Early childhood personality and environmental precursors. *Child Development, 59*, 336–355.

Brody, G. H., & Forehand, R. (1993). Prospective associations among family form, family processes, and adolescents' alcohol and drug use. *Behaviour Research and Therapy, 31*, 587–593.

Brook, J. S., Nomura, C., & Cohen, P. (1989). A network of influences on adolescent drug involvement: Neighborhood, school, peer, and family. *Genetic, Social and General Psychology Monographs, 115*, 125–145.

Brook, J. S., Whiteman, M., Cohen, P., Shapiro, J., & Balka, E. (1995). Longitudinally predicting late adolescent and young adult drug use: Childhood and adolescent precursors. *Journal of the American Academy of Child and Adolescent Psychiatry, 34*, 1230–1238.

Brown, S. A., Tapert, S. F., Granholm, E., & Delis, D. C. (2000). Neurocognitive functioning of adolescents: Effects of protracted alcohol use. *Alcoholism: Clinical and Experimental Research, 24*, 164–171.

Bukoski, N. (1997). *Meta-analysis of drug abuse prevention programs* (NIDA Research Monograph No. 170). Washington, DC: U. S. Government Printing Office.

Bukstein, O. G. (1995). *Adolescent substance abuse: Assessment, prevention, and treatment.* New York: Wiley.

Bukstein, O. G., Glancy, L. J., & Kaminer, Y. (1992). Patterns of affective comorbidity in a clinical population of dually diagnosed adolescent substance abusers. *Journal of the American Academy of Child and Adolescent Psychiatry, 31*, 1041–1045.

Cantwell, D., Lewinsohn, P., Rohde, P., & Seeley, J. R. (1997). Correspondence between adolescent report and parent report of psychiatric diagnostic data. *Journal of the American Academy of Child and Adolescent Psychiatry, 36*, 610–619.

Caspi, A., Moffitt, T., Newman, D., & Silva, P. (1996). Behavioral observations at age 3 predict adult psychiatric disorders. *Archives of General Psychiatry, 53*, 1033–1039.

Catalano, R., Kosterman, R., Hawkins, J. D., Newcomb, M., & Abbott, R. (1996). Modeling the etiology of adolescent substance use: A test of the social development model. *Journal of Drug Issues, 26*, 429–455.

Chassin, L., Curran, P. J., Hussong, A. M., & Colder, C. R. (1996). The relation of parent alcoholism to adolescent substance use: A longitudinal follow-up study. *Journal of Abnormal Psychology, 105*, 70–80.

Chassin, L., Pillow, D. R., Curran, P. J., Molina, B. S. G., & Barrera, M., Jr. (1993). Relation of parental alcoholism to early adolescent substance use: A test of three mediating mechanisms. *Journal of Abnormal Psychology, 102*, 3–19.

Chassin, L., Pitts, S., & DeLucia, C. (1999). The relation of adolescent substance use to young adult autonomy, positive activity involvement, and perceived competence. *Development and Psychopathology, 11*, 915–932.

Chassin, L., Pitts, S., DeLucia, C., & Todd, M. (1999). A longitudinal study of children of alcoholics: Predicting young adult substance use disorders, anxiety and depression. *Journal of Abnormal Psychology, 108*, 106–119.

Chassin, L., Pitts, S., & Prost, J. (2002). Heavy drinking trajectories from adolescence to young adulthood in a high risk sample: Predictors and substance abuse outcomes. *Journal of Consulting and Clinical Psychology, 70*, 67–78.

Chassin, L., Presson, C. C., Pitts, S., & Sherman, S. J. (2000). The natural history of cigarette smoking from adolescence to adulthood in a Midwestern community sample: Multiple trajectories and their psychosocial correlates. *Health Psychology, 19*, 223–231.

Chassin, L., Presson, C. C., Todd, M., Rose, J., & Sherman, S. J. (1998). Maternal socialization of adolescent smoking: The intergenerational transmission of parenting and smoking. *Developmental Psychology, 34*, 1189–1201.

Chilcoat, H. D., & Breslau, N. (1996). Alcohol disorders in young adulthood: Effects of transitions into adult roles. *Journal of Health and Social Behavior, 37*, 339–349.

Clark, D. B., Parker, A. M., & Lynch, K. G. (1999). Psychopathology and substance-related problems during early adolescence: A survival analysis. *Journal of Clinical Child Psychology, 28*, 333–341.

Clayton, R. (1992). Transitions in drug use: Risk and protective factors. In M. Glantz & R. Pickens (Eds.), *Vulnerability to drug abuse* (pp. 15–51). Washington, DC: American Psychological Association.

Cloninger, C. R. (1987). Neurogenetic adaptive mechanisms in alcoholism. *Science, 236*, 410–416.

Cohen, P., Cohen, J., Kassen, S., Velez, C., Hartmark, C., Johnson, J., Rojas, M., Bropk, J., & Streuning, E. (1993). An epidemiologic study of disorders in late childhood and adolescence: I. Age-specific and gender-specific prevalence. *Journal of Child Psychology and Psychiatry, 34*, 851–867.

Colby, S., Tiffany, S., Shiffman, S., & Niaura, R. (2000). Measuring nicotine dependence among youth: A review of available approaches and instruments. *Drug and Alcohol Dependence, 59*, S23–S39.

Colder, C., & Chassin, L. (1997). Affectivity and impulsivity: Temperament risk for adolescent alcohol involvement. *Psychology of Addictive Behaviors, 11*, 83–97.

Conrod, P., Pihl, R., & Ditto, B. (1995). Autonomic reactivity and alcohol-induced dampening in men at risk for alcoholism and men at risk for hypertension. *Alcoholism: Clinical and Experimental Research, 19*, 482–489.

Conrod, P., Petersen, J., & Pihl, R. O. (1997). Disinhibited personality and sensitivity to alcohol reinforcement: Independent correlates of drinking behavior in sons of alcoholics. *Alcoholism: Clinical and Experimental Research, 21*, 1320–1332.

Cooper, M. L. (1994). Motivations for alcohol use among adolescents: Development and validation of a four-factor model. *Psychological Assessment, 6*, 117–128.

Cooper, M. L., Frone, M. R., Russell, M., & Mudar, P. (1995). Drinking to regulate positive and negative emotions: A motivational model of alcohol use. *Journal of Personality and Social Psychology, 69*, 990–1005.

Cooper, M. L., Russell, M., Skinner, J., Frone, M. R., & Mudar, P. (1992). Stress and alcohol use: Moderating effects of gender, coping, and alcohol expectancies. *Journal of Abnormal Psychology, 101*, 139–152.

Cornelius, M., Leech, S., Goldschmidt,. L., & Day, N. (2000). Prenatal tobacco exposure: Is it a risk factor for early tobacco experimentation? *Nicotine and Tobacco Research, 2*, 45–52.

Corral, M. M., Holguin, S. R., & Cadaveira, F. (1999). Neuropsychological characteristics in children of alcoholics: Familial density. *Journal of Studies on Alcohol, 60*, 509–513.

Costello, E. J., Erkanli, A., Federman, E., & Angold, A. (1999). Development of psychiatric comorbidity with substance abuse in adolescents: Effects of timing and sex. *Journal of Clinical Child Psychology, 28*, 298–311.

Costello, E. J., Farmer, E. M. Z., Angold, A., Burns, B. J., & Erkanli, A. (1997). Psychiatric disorders among American Indian and white youth in Appalachia: The Great Smoky Mountains Study. *American Journal of Public Health, 87*, 827–832.

Cottler, L., Schuckit, M., Helzer, J., Crowley, T., Woody, G., Nathan, P., & Hughes, J. (1995). The DSM-IV field trial for substance use disorders: Major results. *Drug and Alcohol Dependence, 38*, 59–68.

Curran, P. J., Stice, E., & Chassin, L. (1997). The relation between adolescent alcohol use and peer alcohol use: A longitudinal random coefficients model. *Journal of Consulting and Clinical Psychology, 65*, 130–140.

Deas, D., Riggs, P., Langenbucher, J., Goldman, M., & Brown, S. (2000). Adolescents are not adults: Developmental considerations in alcohol users. *Alcoholism: Clinical and Experimental Research, 24*, 232–237.

Deas, D., & Thomas, S. (2001). An overview of controlled studies of adolescent substance abuse treatment. *American Journal on Addictions, 10*, 178–189.

Deckel, A. W., Bauer, L., & Hesselbrock, V. (1995). Anterior brain dysfunction as a risk factor in alcoholic behaviors. *Addiction, 90*, 1323–1334.

Deckel, A. W. & Hesselbrock, V. (1996). Behavioral and cognitive measurements predict scores on the MAST: A 3-year prospective study. *Alcoholism: Clinical and Experimental Research, 20*, 1173–1178.

Deykin, E., Buka, S., & Zeena, T. (1992). Depressive illness among chemically dependent adolescents. *American Journal of Psychiatry, 149*, 1341–1347.

Dishion, T., Patterson, G. R., & Reid, J. R. (1988). Parent and peer factors associated with drug sampling in early adolescence: Implications for treatment. In E. R. Rehdert & J. Grabowski (Eds.), *Adolescent drug abuse: Analyses of treatment* research (NIDA Research Monograph No. 77, pp. 69–93). Washington, DC: U.S. Government Printing Office.

Dishion, T., Patterson, G. R., Stoolmiller, M., & Skinner, M. (1991). Family, school, and behavioral antecedents to early adolescent involvement with antisocial peers. *Developmental Psychology, 27*, 127–180.

Disney, E., Elkins, I., McGue, M., & Iacono, W. (1999). Effects of ADHD, conduct disorder, and gender on substance use and abuse in adolescence. *American Journal of Psychiatry, 156*, 1515–1521.

Dolcini, M., Adler, N., & Ginsberg, D. (1996). Factors influencing agreement between self-reports and biological measures of smoking among adolescents. *Journal of Research on Adolescence, 6*, 515–542.

Donovan, J., & Jessor, R. (1985). Structure of problem behavior in adolescence and young adulthood. *Journal of Consulting and Clinical Psychology, 53*, 890–904.

Drejer, K., Theilgard, A., Teasdale, T. W., Schulsinger, F., & Goodwin, D. W. (1985). A prospective study of young men at high risk for alcoholism: Neuropsychological assessment. *Alcoholism: Clinical and Experimental Research, 9*, 498–502.

Duncan, S. C., Duncan, T. E., Biglan, A., & Ary, D. (1998). Contributions of the social context to the development of adolescent substance use: A multivariate latent growth modeling approach. *Drug and Alcohol Dependence, 50*, 57–71.

Duncan, T. E., Duncan, S. C., & Hops, H. (1998). Latent variable modeling of longitudinal and multilevel alcohol use data. *Journal of Studies on Alcohol, 59*, 399–408.

Dunn, M., & Goldman, M. (1996). Empirical modeling of an alcohol expectancy network in elementary-school children as a function of grade. *Experimental and Clinical Psychopharmacology, 4*, 209–217.

Eisenberg, N., Guthrie, I., Fabes, S., Shepard, S., Losoya, S., Murphy, B., Jones, S., Poulin, R., & Reiser, M. (2000). Prediction of elementary school childrens(externalizing problem behaviors from attentional and behavioral regulation and negative emotionality. *Child Development, 71*, 1367–1382.

Elliott, D. S., Huizinga, D., & Ageton, S. (1985). *Explaining delinquency and drug use*. Beverly Hills, CA: Sage.

Ennett, S., Flewelling, R., Lindrooth, R., & Norton, E. (1997). School and neighborhood characteristics associated with school rates of alcohol, cigarette, and marijuana use. *Journal of Health and Social Behavior*, *38*, 55–71.

Fawzy, F., Combs, R., Simon, J., & Bowman-Terrell, M. (1987). Family composition, socioeconomic status, and adolescent substance use. *Addictive Behaviors*, *12*, 79–83.

Federman, E. B., Costello, E. J., Angold, A., Farmer, E. M. Z., & Erkanli, A. (1997). Development of substance use and psychiatric comorbidity in an epidemiologic study of white and American Indian young adolescents: The Great Smoky Mountains Study. *Drug and Alcohol Dependence*, *44*, 69–78.

Fergusson, D. M., & Horwood, L. J. (1995). Early disruptive behavior, IQ, and later school achievement and delinquent behavior. *Journal of Abnormal Child Psychology*, *23*, 183–199.

Fergusson, D. M., Horwood, L. J., & Lynskey, M. T. (1993). Prevalence and comorbidity of DSM-III-R diagnoses in a birth cohort of 15 year olds. *Journal of the American Academy of Child and Adolescent Psychiatry*, *32*, 1127–1134.

Fergusson, D. M., Lynsky, M., & Horwood, L. J. (1996). Comorbidity between depressive disorders and nicotine dependence in a cohort of 16 year olds. *Archives of General Psychiatry*, *53*, 1043–1047.

Fiore, M., Newcomb, P., & McBride, P. (1993). Natural history and epidemiology of tobacco use and addiction. In C. T. Orleans & J. D. Slade (Eds.), *Nicotine addiction: Principles and management* (pp. 89–104). New York: Oxford University Press.

Flay, B., d(Avernas, J., Best, J. A., Kersell, M., & Ryan, K. (1983). Cigarette smoking: Why young people do it and ways of preventing it. In P. McGrath & P. Firestone (Eds.), *Pediatric and adolescent behavioral medicine* (pp. 132–183). New York: Springer.

Flicek, M. (1992). Social status of boys with both academic problems and attention-deficit hyperactivity disorder. *Journal of Abnormal Child Psychology*, *20*, 353–366.

Fulkerson, J. A., Harrison, P. A., & Beebe, T. J. (1999). DSM-IV substance abuse and dependence: Are there really two dimensions of substance use problems in adolescents? *Addiction*, *94*, 495–506.

Ge, X., Conger, R., Cadoret, R., Neiderheiser, J., Yates, W., Troughton, E., & Stewart, M. (1996). The developmental interface between nature and nurture: A mutual influence model of child antisocial behavior and parent behavior. *Developmental Psychology*, *32*, 574–589.

Giancola, P. R., Martin, C. S., Tarter, R. E., Pelham, W., & Moss, H. B. (1996). Executive cognitive functioning and aggressive behavior in preadolescent boys at high risk for substance abuse/dependence. *Journal of Studies on Alcohol*, *57*, 352–359.

Giancola, P. R., & Mezzich, A. C. (2000). Neuropsychological deficits in female adolescents with a substance use disorder: Better accounted for by conduct disorder. *Journal of Studies on Alcohol*, *61*, 809–817.

Giancola, P. R., Mezzich, A. C., & Tarter, R. E. (1998). Disruptive, delinquent, and aggressive behavior in adolescents with a psychoactive substance use disorder: Relation to executive cognitive functioning. *Journal of Studies on Alcohol*, *59*, 560–567.

Giancola, P. R., Zeichner, A., Yarnell, J. E., & Dickson, K. E. (1996). Relation between executive cognitive functioning and the adverse consequences of alcohol use in social drinkers. *Alcoholism: Clinical and Experimental Research*, *20*, 1094–1098.

Glantz, M., & Pickens, R. (1992). *Vulnerability to drug abuse*. Washington, DC: American Psychological Association.

Grant, B. F., & Dawson, D. A. (1997). Age at onset of alcohol use and its association with DSM-IV alcohol abuse and dependence: Results from the National Longitudinal Epidemiologic Survey. *Journal of Substance Abuse*, *9*, 103–110.

Grant, B. F., Harford, T., Dawson, D. A., Chou, P. Dufour, M., & Pickering, K. (1994). Prevalence of DSM-IV alcohol abuse and dependence. *Alcohol Health and Research World*, *18*, 243–248.

Greeley, J., & Oei, T. (1999). Alcohol and tension reduction. In K. E. Leonard & H. T. Blane (Eds.), *Psychological theories of drinking and alcoholism* (2nd ed., pp. 14–53). New York: Guilford Press.

Griesler, P. C., & Kandel, D. B. (1998). Ethnic differences in the correlates of adolescent cigarette smoking. *Journal of Adolescent Health*, *23*, 167–180.

Grunberg, N., Winders, S., & Wewers, M. (1991). Gender differences in tobacco use. *Health Psychology*, *10*, 143–153.

Han, C., McGue, M., & Iacono, W. (1999). Lifetime tobacco, alcohol, and other substance use in adolescent Minnesota twins: Univariate and multivariate behavior genetic analyses. *Addiction*, *94*, 981–983.

Hansell, S., & White, H. R. (1991). Adolescent drug use, psychological distress, and physical symptoms. *Journal of Health and Social Behavior*, *32*, 288–301.

Harden, P., & Pihl, R. (1995). Cognitive function, cardiovascular reactivity, and behavior in boys at high risk for alcoholism. *Journal of Abnormal Psychology*, *104*, 94–103.

Harrison, P., Fulkerson, J., & Beebe, T. (1998). DSM-IV substance use disorder criteria for adolescents: A critical examination based on a statewide school survey. *American Journal of Psychiatry*, *155*, 486–492.

Hawkins, J. D., Catalano, R., & Miller, J. (1992). Risk and protective factors for alcohol and other drug problems in adolescence and early adulthood: Implications for substance abuse prevention. *Psychological Bulletin*, *112*, 64–105.

Heath, A. C., Bucholz, K. K., Madden, P. A. F., Dinwiddie, S. H., Slutske, W. S., Bierut, L. J., Statham, D. J., Dunne, M. P., Whitfield, J. B., & Martin, N. G. (1997). Genetic and environmental contributions to alcohol dependence in a national twin sample: Consistency of findings in women and men. *Psychological Medicine*, *27*, 1381–1396.

Heath, A. C. & Martin, N. G. (1988). Teenage alcohol use in the Australian twin register: Genetic and social determinants of starting to drink. *Alcoholism: Clinical and Experimental Research*, *12*, 735–741.

Henry, B., Feehan, M., McGee, R., Stanton, W., Moffitt, T., & Silva, P. (1993). The importance of conduct problems and depressive symptoms in predicting adolescent substance use. *Journal of Abnormal Child Psychology*, *21*, 469–480.

Hesselbrock, V., Bauer, L. O., Hesselbrock, M. N., & Gillen, R. (1991). Neuropsychological factors in individuals at high risk for alcoholism. In M. Galanter & H. Begleiter (Eds.), *Recent developments in alcoholism* (Vol. 9, pp. 21–40). New York: Plenum Press.

Hill, K., White, H. R., Chung, I.-J., Hawkins, J. D., & Catalano, R. F. (2000). Early adult outcomes of adolescent binge drinking: Person- and variable-centered analyses of binge drinking trajectories. *Alcoholism: Clinical and Experimental Research*, *24*, 892–901.

Hill, S., Shen, S., Lowers, L., & Locke, J. (2000). Factors predicting the onset of adolescent drinking in families at high risk for developing alcoholism. *Biological Psychiatry, 48*, 265–275.

Hoffman, J., Cerbone, F., & Su, S. (2000). A growth curve analysis of stress and adolescent drug use. *Substance Use* and Misuse, 35, 687–716.

Hser, Y., Grella, C., Hubbard, R., Hsieh, S., Fletcher, B., Brown, B., & Anglin, D. (2001). An evaluation of drug treatments for adolescents in four US cities. *Archives of General Psychiatry, 58*, 689–695.

Humphreys, K., & Rappaport, J. (1993). From the community mental health movement to the war on drugs: A study in the definition of social problems. *American Psychologist, 48*, 892–901.

Hussong, A., & Chassin, L. (1994). The stress–negative affect model of adolescent alcohol use: Disaggregating negative affect. *Journal of Studies on Alcohol, 55*, 707–718.

Hussong, A., Curran, P., & Chassin, L. (1998). Pathways of risk for accelerated heavy alcohol use among adolescent children of alcoholic parents. *Journal of Abnormal Child Psychology, 26*, 453–466.

Hussong, A., Hicks, R., Levy, S., & Curran, P. (2001). Specifying the relations between affect and heavy alcohol use among young adults. *Journal of Abnormal Psychology, 110*, 449–461.

Iacono, W. G., Carlson, S. R., Taylor, J., Elkins, I. J., & McGue, M. (1999). Behavioral disinhibition and the development of substance-use disorders: Findings from the Minnesota Twin Family Study. *Development and Psychopathology, 11*, 869–900.

Institute of Medicine. (1994a). *Pathways of addiction: Opportunities in drug abuse research*. Washington, DC: National Academy Press.

Institute of Medicine. (1994b). *Growing up tobacco free: Preventing nicotine addiction in children and youths* (B. Lynch & R. Bonnie, Eds.). Washington, DC: National Academy Press.

Jackson, C., & Henriksen, L. (1997). Do as I say: Parent smoking, antismoking socialization, and smoking onset among children. *Addictive Behaviors, 22*, 107–114.

Jansen, R. E., Fitzgerald, H. E., Ham, H. P., & Zucker, R. E. (1995). Pathways to risk: Temperament and behavior problems in three- to five-year-old sons of alcoholics. *Alcoholism: Clinical and Experimental Research, 19*, 501–509.

Jessor, R., & Jessor, S. (1977). *Problem behavior and psychosocial development: A longitudinal study of youth*. New York: Academic Press.

Johnston, L., O'Malley, P., & Bachman, J. (2000). *Monitoring the Future: National survey results on drug use, 1975–1999* (NIH Publication No. 00-4802). Bethesda, MD: National Institute on Drug Abuse.

Johnston, L., O'Malley, P., & Bachman, J. (2001). *Monitoring the Future: National results on adolescent drug use. Overview of key findings, 2000* (NIH Publication No. 01-4923). Bethesda, MD: National Institute on Drug Abuse.

Kandel, D. B. (1975). Stages in adolescent involvement in drug use. *Science, 165*, 912–914.

Kandel, D. B. (1978). Convergences in prospective longitudinal surveys of drug use in normal populations. In D. B. Kandel (Ed.), *Longitudinal research on drug use: Empirical findings and methodological issues* (pp. 3–40). New York: Wiley.

Kandel, D. B. (1995). Ethnic differences in drug use: Patterns and paradoxes. In G. J. Botvin, S. Schinke, & M. Orlandi (Eds.), *Drug abuse prevention with multiethnic youth* (pp. 81–104). Thousand Oaks, CA: Sage.

Kandel, D. B., Davies, M., Karus, D., & Yamaguchi, K. (1986). The consequences in young adulthood of adolescent drug involvement. *Archives of General Psychiatry, 43*, 746–754.

Kandel, D. B., Johnson, J. G., Bird, H. R., Canino, G., Goodman, S., Lahey, B., Regier, D., & Schwab Stone, M. (1997). Psychiatric disorders associated with substance use among children and adolescents: Findings from the Methods for the Epidemiology of Child and Adolescent Mental Disorders (MECA) study. *Journal of Abnormal Child Psychology, 25*, 121–132.

Kandel, D. B., & Udry, J. (1999). Prenatal effect of maternal smoking on daughters(smoking: Nicotine or testosterone exposure? *American Journal of Public Health, 89*, 1377–1383.

Kandel, D., Yamaguchi, K., & Chen, K. (1992). Stages of progression in drug use involvement from adolescence to adulthood: Further evidence for the gateway theory. *Journal of Studies on Alcohol, 53*, 447–457.

Kaplow, J. B., Curran, P. J., Angold, A., & Costello, E. J. (2001). The prospective relation between dimensions of anxiety and the initiation of adolescent alcohol use. *Journal of Clinical Child Psychology, 30*, 316–326.

Kellam, S., Brown, C., Rubin, B., & Ensminger, M. (1983). Paths leading to teenage psychiatric symptoms and substance use: Developmental epidemiological studies in Woodlawn. In S. B. Guze, J. Earls, & J. Barrett (Eds.), *Childhood psychopathology and development* (pp. 17–52), New York: Norton.

Klorman, R. (1992). Cognitive event-related potentials in attention deficit disorder. In S. E. Shaywitz & B. A. Shaywitz (Eds.), *Attention deficit disorder comes of age: Toward the twenty-first century* (pp. 221–244). New York: Wiley.

Kuperman, S., Schlosser, S. S., Kramer, J. R., Bucholz, K., Hesselbrock, V., Reich, T., & Reich, W. (2001). Risk domains associated with an adolescent alcohol dependence diagnosis. *Addiction, 96*, 629–636.

Kushner, M., Sher, K. J., Wood, M., & Wood, P. (1994). Anxiety and drinking behavior: Moderating effects of tension-reduction expectancies. *Alcoholism: Clinical and Experimental Research, 18*, 852–860.

Labouvie, E., Pandina, R. J., White, J. R., & Johnson, V. (1990). Risk factors of adolescent drug use: An affect-based interpretation. *Journal of Substance Abuse, 2*, 262–285.

Lamborn, S. D., Dornbusch, S. M., & Steinberg, L. (1996). Ethnicity and community context as moderators of the relations between family decision-making and adolescent adjustment. *Child Development, 67*, 283–301.

Lender, M. E., & Martin, J. K. (1987). *Drinking in America: A history*. New York: Free Press.

Lerner, J. V., & Vicary, J. R. (1984). Difficult temperament and drug use: Analyses from the New York Longitudinal Study. *Journal of Drug Education, 14*, 1–8.

Levenson, R., Oyama, O., & Meek, P. (1987). Greater reinforcement from alcohol for those at risk: Parental risk, personality risk, and sex. *Journal of Abnormal Psychology, 96*, 247–253.

Leventhal, T., & Brooks-Gunn, J. (2000). The neighborhoods they live in: The effects of neighborhood residence on child and adolescent outcomes. *Psychological Bulletin, 126*, 309–337.

Lewinsohn, P., Hops, H., Roberts, R., Seeley, J., & Andrews, J. (1993). Adolescent psychopathology I: Prevalence and incidence of depression and other DSM-III-R disorders in high school students. *Journal of Abnormal Psychology, 102*, 133–144.

Lewinsohn, P., Rohde, P., & Seeley, J. (1996). Alcohol consumption in high school adolescents: Frequency of use and dimensional structure of associated problems. *Addiction, 91*, 375–390.

Lezak, M. D. (1995). *Neuropsychological assessment* (3rd ed.). New York: Oxford University Press.

Loeber, R., Stouthamer-Loeber, M., & White, H. R. (1999). Developmental aspects of delinquency and internalizing problems and their association with persistent juvenile substance use between ages 7 and 18. *Journal of Clinical Child Psychology. 28*, 322–332.

Luthar, S. S., & Cushing, G. (1999). Neighborhood influences and child development: A prospective study of substance abusers(offspring. *Development and Psychopathology, 11*, 763–784.

Luthar, S. S., & D'Avanzo, K. (1999). Contextual factors in substance use: A study of suburban and inner city adolescents. *Development and Psychopathology, 11*, 845–867.

Lynam, D., Caspi, A., Moffitt, T., Wikstrom, P.-O., Loeber, R., & Novak, S. (2000). The interaction between impulsivity and neighborhood context on offending: The effects of impulsivity are stronger in poorer neighborhoods. *Journal of Abnormal Psychology, 109*, 563–574.

Lynsky, M. T., & Fergusson, D. M. (1995). Childhood conduct problems, attention deficit behaviors, and adolescent alcohol, tobacco and illicit drug use. *Journal of Abnormal Child Psychology, 23*, 281–302.

Maisto, S. A., Galzio, M., & Connors, G. J. (1999). *Drug use and abuse* (3rd ed.). Orlando, FL: Harcourt Brace.

Martin, C. S., Earleywine, M., Blackson, T. C., Vanyukov, M., Moss, H. B., & Tarter, R. E. (1994). Aggressivity, inattention, hyperactivity, and impulsivity in boys and high and low risk for substance abuse. *Journal of Abnormal Child Psychology, 22*, 177–203.

Martin, C. S., Kaczynski, N. A., Maisto, S. A., Bukstein, O. M., & Moss, H. B. (1995). Patterns of DSM-IV alcohol abuse and dependence in adolescent drinkers. *Journal of Studies on Alcohol, 56*, 672–680.

Martin, C. S., Kaczynski, N. A., Maisto, S. A., & Tarter, R. E. (1996). Polydrug use in adolescent drinkers with and without DSM-IV alcohol abuse and dependence. *Alcoholism: Clinical and Experimental Research, 20*, 1099–1108.

McGue, M. (1994). Genes, environment, and the etiology of alcoholism. In R. Zucker, G. Boyd, & J. Howard (Eds.), *The development of alcohol problems: Exploring the biopsychosocial matrix of risk* (NIAAA Research Monograph No. 26, pp. 1–40). Washington, DC: U.S. Government Printing Office.

McGue, M. (1999). Behavioral genetic models of alcoholism and drinking. In K. E. Leonard & H. T. Blane (Eds.), *Psychological theories of drinking and alcoholism* (2nd ed., pp. 372–421). New York: Guilford Press.

McGue, M., Elkins, I., & Iacono, W. (2000). Genetic and environmental influences on adolescent substance use and abuse. *American Journal of Medical Genetics, 96*, 671–677.

McGue, M., Sharma, A., & Benson, P. (1996). Parent and sibling influences on adolescent alcohol use and misuse: Evidence from a U.S. adoption cohort. *Journal of Studies on Alcohol, 57*, 8–18.

McMahon, R. J. (1999). Child and adolescent psychopathology as risk factors for subsequent tobacco use. *Nicotine and Tobacco Research, 1*, S45–S50.

Merikangas, K., & Avenevoli, S. (2000). Implications of genetic epidemiology for the prevention of substance use disorders. *Addictive Behaviors, 25*, 807–820.

Merikangas, K., Stolar, M., Stevens, D., Goulet, J., Preisign, M., Fenton, B., O'Malley, S., & Rounsaville, B. (1998). Familial transmission of substance use disorders. *Archives of General Psychiatry, 55*, 973–979.

Mezzich, A. C., Giancola, P. R., Tarter, R. E., Lu, S., Parks, S. M., & Barrett, C. M. (1997). Violence, suicidality, and alcohol/drug use involvement in adolescent females with a psychoactive substance use disorder and controls. *Alcoholism: Clinical and Experimental Research, 21*, 1300–1307.

Mikulich, S. K., Hall, S. K., Whitmore, E. A., & Crowley, T. J. (2001). Concordance between DSM-III-R and DSM-IV diagnoses of substance use disorders in adolescents. *Drug and Alcohol Dependence, 61*, 237–248.

Moffitt, T. E. (1993). Adolescence-limited and life-course-persistent antisocial behavior: a developmental taxonomy. *Psychological Review, 100*, 674–701.

Molina, B. S. G., Smith, B. H., & Pelham, W. E. (1999). Interactive effects of attention-deficit hyperactivity disorder and conduct disorder on early adolescent substance use. *Psychology of Addictive Behaviors, 13*, 348–358.

Moss, H. B., Kirisci, L., Gordon, H., & Tarter, R. (1994). A neuropsychologic profile of adolescent alcoholics. *Alcoholism: Clinical and Experimental Research, 18*, 159–163.

Moss, H. B., Vanyukov, M., Yao, J., & Irillova, G. (1999). Salivary cortisol responses in prepubertal boys: The effects of parental substance abuse and association with drug use behavior during adolescence. *Biological Psychiatry, 45*, 1293–1299.

Murray, D., O'Connell, C., Schmid, L., & Perry, C. (1987). The validity of smoking self-reports by adolescents: A reexamination of the bogus pipeline procedure. *Addictive Behaviors, 12*, 7–15.

Muthen, B., & Shedden, K. (1999). Finite mixture modeling with mixture outcomes using the EM algorithm. *Biometrics, 55*, 463–469.

Nagin, D. (1999). Analyzing developmental trajectories: A semi-parametric group-based approach. *Psychological Methods, 4*, 139–157.

National Institute on Alcohol Abuse and Alcoholism. (1997). *Youth drinking: Risk factors and consequences.* Rockville, MD: Author.

Nestler, E. (2000). Genes and addiction. *Nature Genetics, 26*, 277–281.

Newcomb, M., & Bentler, P. (1988). *Consequences of adolescent drug use: Impact on the lives of young adults.* Newbury Park, CA: Sage.

Newcomb, M., & Harlow, L. (1986). Life events and substance use among adolescents: Mediating effects of perceived loss of control and meaninglessness in life. *Journal of Personality and Social Psychology, 51*, 564–577.

Nigg, J. T. (2000). On inhibition/disinhibition in developmental psychology: Views from cognitive and personality psychology and a working inhibition taxonomy. *Psychological Bulletin, 126*, 220–246.

Oetting, E. R., & Donnermeyer, J. F. (1998). Primary socialization theory: The etiology of drug use and deviance. *Substance Use and Misuse, 33*, 995–1026.

Ozechowski, T., & Liddle, H. (2000). Family-based therapy for adolescent drug abuse: Knowns and unknowns. *Clinical Child and Family Psychology Review, 3*, 269–298.

Parker, K., Calhoun, T., & Weaver, G. (2000). Variables associated with adolescent alcohol use: A multiethnic comparison. *Journal of Social Psychology, 140*, 51–62.

Patterson, G. R. (1986). Performance models for antisocial boys. *American Psychologist, 41*, 432–444.

Paulson, M., Combs, R., & Richardson, M. (1990). School performance, educational aspirations, and drug use among children and adolescents. *Journal of Drug Education, 20*, 289–303.

Peterson, J. B., Finn, P. R., & Pihl, R. O. (1992). Cognitive dysfunction and the inherited predisposition to alcoholism. *Journal of Studies on Alcohol, 53*, 154–160.

Peterson, J. B., & Pihl, R. O. (1990). Information processing, neuropsychological function, and the inherited predisposition to alcoholism. *Neuropsychological Review, 1*, 343–369.

Plunkett, M., & Mitchell, C. (2000). Substance use rates among American Indian adolescents: Regional comparisons with Monitoring the Future high school seniors. *Journal of Drug Issues, 30*, 593–620.

Pollock, N. K., & Martin, C. S. (1999). Diagnostic orphans: Adolescents with alcohol symptoms who do not qualify for DSM-IV abuse or dependence diagnoses. *American Journal of Psychiatry, 156*, 897–901.

Pollock, N. K., Martin, C. S., & Langenbucher, J. W. (2000). Diagnostic concordance of DSM-III, DSM-III-R, DSM-IV, and ICD-10 alcohol diagnoses in adolescents. *Journal of Studies on Alcohol, 61*, 439–446.

Poon, E., Ellis, D. E., Fitzgerald, H. E., & Zucker, R. E. (2000). Intellectual, cognitive, and academic performance among sons of alcoholics during the early school years: Differences related to subtypes of familial alcoholism. *Alcoholism: Clinical and Experimental Research, 24*, 1020–1027.

Reich, T., Hinrichs, A., Culverhouse, R., & Bierut, L. (1999). Genetic studies of alcoholism and substance dependence. *American Journal of Human Genetics, 65*, 599–605.

Reifman, A., Barnes, G. M., Dintcheff, B. A., Farrell, M. P., & Uhteg, L. (1998). Parental and peer influences on the onset of heavier drinking among adolescents. *Journal of Studies on Alcohol, 59*, 311–317.

Robins, L. N., & Pryzbeck, T. R. (1985). Age of onset of drug use as a factor in drug and other disorders. In C. L. Jones & R. J. Battjes (Eds.), *Etiology of drug abuse: Implications for prevention* (NIDA Research Monograph No. 56, pp. 178–192). Washington, DC: U. S. Government Printing Office.

Rogers, S., Miller, H., & Turner, C. (1998). Effects of interview mode on bias in survey measurement of drug use: Do respondent characteristics make a difference? *Substance Use and Misuse, 33*, 2179–2220.

Rohde, P., Lewinsohn, P., & Seeley, J. (1996). Psychiatric comorbidity with problematic alcohol use in high school students. *Journal of the American Academy of Child and Adolescent Psychiatry, 35*, 101–109.

Rose, J., Chassin, L., Presson, C., & Sherman, S. J. (1996). Demographic factors in adult smoking status: Mediating and moderating influences. *Psychology of Addictive Behaviors, 10*, 28–37.

Rourke, S. B., & Loberg, T. (1996). Neurobehavioral correlates of alcoholism. In I. Grant & K. M. Adams (Eds.), *Neuropsychological assessment of neuropsychiatric disorders* (2nd ed., pp. 423–485). New York: Oxford University Press.

Russell, M. (1990). Prevalence of alcoholism among children of alcoholics. In M. Windle & J. Searles (Eds.), *Children of alcoholics: Critical perspectives* (pp. 9–38). New York: Guilford Press.

Russell, M., Cooper, M. L., & Frone, M. (1990). The influence of sociodemographic characteristics on familial alcohol problems: Data from a community sample. *Alcoholism: Clinical and Experimental Research, 14*, 221–226.

Sayette, M. (1993). Heart rate as an index of stress response in alcohol administration research: A critical review. *Alcoholism: Clinical and Experimental Research, 17*, 802–809.

Schuckit, M. A., & Smith, T. L. (2000). The relationships of a family history of alcohol dependence, a low level of response to alcohol and six domains of life functioning to the development of alcohol use disorders. *Journal of Studies on Alcohol, 61*, 827–835.

Schultes, R. E. (1970). Botanical and chemical distribution of hallucinogens. *Annual Review of Plant Physiology, 21*, 571–598.

Scribner, R., Cohen, D., & Fisher, W. (2000). Evidence of a structural effect for alcohol outlet density: A multilevel analysis. *Alcoholism: Clinical and Experimental Research, 24*, 188–196.

Shedler, J., & Block, J. (1990). Adolescent drug use and psychological health: A longitudinal inquiry. *Psychological Bulletin, 45*, 612–630.

Sher, K. J. (1991). *Children of alcoholics: A critical appraisal of theory and research.* Chicago: University of Chicago Press.

Sher, K. J., & Gotham, J. J. (1999). Pathological alcohol involvement: A developmental disorder of young adulthood. *Development and Psychopathology, 11*, 933–956.

Sher, K. J., Martin, E. D., Wood, P. K., & Rutledge, P. C. (1997). Alcohol use disorders and neuropsychological functioning in first-year undergraduates. *Experimental and Clinical Psychopharmacology, 5*, 304–315.

Simons, R., Johnson, C., Beamans, J., Conger, R., & Whitbeck, L. (1996). Parents and peer group as mediators of the effect of community structure on adolescent problem behavior. *American Journal of Community Psychology, 24*, 145–171.

Single, E., Kandel, D. B., & Faust, R. (1974). Patterns of multiple drug use in high school. *Journal of Health and Social Behavior, 15*, 344–357.

Skager, R., & Fisher, D. (1989). Substance use among high schoolers in relation to school characteristics. *Addictive Behaviors, 14*, 129–138.

Smith, G. T., Goldman, M. S., Greenbaum, P. E., & Christiansen, B. A. (1995). Expectancy for social facilitation from drinking: The divergent paths of high-expectancy and low-expectancy adolescents. *Journal of Abnormal Psychology, 104*, 32–40.

Spears, S. F., Ciesla, J. R., & Skala, S. Y. (1999). Relapse patterns among adolescents treated for chemical dependency. *Substance Use and Misuse, 34*, 1795–1815.

Spreen, O., & Strauss, E. (1998). *A compendium of neuropsychological tests: Administration, norms, commentary.* New York: Oxford University Press.

Stacy, A., Newcomb, M., & Bentler, P. (1991). Cognitive motivation and problem drug use: A 9 year longitudinal study. *Journal of Abnormal Psychology, 100*, 502–515.

Steinberg, L., Fletcher, A., & Darling, N. (1994). Parental monitoring and peer influences on adolescent substance use. *Pediatrics, 93*, 1060–1064.

Stewart, D. G., & Brown, S. A. (1995). Withdrawal and dependency symptoms among adolescent alcohol and drug abusers. *Addiction, 90*, 627–635.

Stice, E., & Barrera, M. (1995). A longitudinal examination of the reciprocal relations between perceived parenting and adolescents(substance use and externalizing behaviors. *Developmental Psychology, 33*, 322–334.

Stice, E., & Gonzales, N. (1998). Adolescent temperament moderates the relationship of parenting to antisocial behavior. *Journal of Adolescent Research, 13*, 5–31.

Stritzke, W., Patrick, C. J., & Lang, A. R. (1995). Alcohol and human emotion: A multidimensional analysis incorporating startle probe methodology. *Journal of Abnormal Psychology, 104*, 114–122.

Substance Abuse and Mental Health Services Administration. (1999). *Understanding substance abuse prevention: Toward the 21st century. A primer on effective programs* (DHHS Publication No. SMA 99-3301). Washington, DC: U. S. Government Printing Office.

Sussman, S., Dent, C., & McCullar, W. (2000). Group self-identification as a prospective predictor of drug use and violence in high-risk youth. *Psychology of Addictive Behaviors, 14*, 192–196.

Swaim, R., Oetting, E., & Beauvais, F. (1989). Links from emotional distress to adolescent drug use: A path model. *Journal of Consulting and Clinical Psychology, 57*, 227–231.

Tapert, S. F., & Brown, S. A. (1999). Neuropsychological correlates of adolescent substance use: Four-year outcomes. *Journal of the International Neuropsychological Society, 5*, 481–493.

Tapert, S. F., Brown, S. A., Myers, M. G., & Granholm, E. (1999). The role of neurocognitive abilities in coping with adolescent relapse to alcohol and drug use. *Journal of Studies on Alcohol, 60*, 500–508.

Tarter, R. E., Alterman, A. I., & Edwards, K. L. (1985). Vulnerability to alcoholism in men: A behavior-genetic perspective. *Journal of Studies on Alcohol, 46*, 329–356.

Tarter, R. E., Kirisci, L., & Mezzich, A. (1997). Multivariate typology of adolescents with alcohol use disorder. *American Journal on Addictions, 6*, 150–158.

Tarter, R. E., Mezzich, A. C., Hsieh, Y. C., & Parks, S. M. (1995). Cognitive capacity in female adolescent substance abusers. *Drug and Alcohol Dependence, 39*, 15–21.

Tarter, R. E., & Vanyukov, M. (1994). Alcoholism: A developmental disorder. *Journal of Consulting and Clinical Psychology, 62*, 1096–2007.

Tarter, R. E., Vanyukov, M., Giancola, P., Dawes, M., Blackson, T., Mezzich, A. C., & Clark, D. (1999). Etiology of early age onset substance use disorder: A maturational perspective. *Development and Psychopathology, 11*, 657–683.

Uhl, G. R. (1999). Molecular genetics of substance abuse vulnerability: A current approach. *Neuropsychopharmacology, 20*, 3–9.

Urberg, K. A., Degirmencioglu, S. M., & Pilgrim, C. (1997). Close friend and group influence on adolescent cigarette smoking and alcohol use. *Developmental Psychology, 33*, 834–844.

U.S. Department of Health and Human Services (DHHS). (1988). *The health consequences of smoking: Nicotine addiction. A report of the Surgeon General* (DHHS Publication No. CDC 88–8406. Washington, DC: U.S. Government Printing Office.

U.S. Department of Health and Human Services (DHHS). (2000a). *National Household Survey on Drug Abuse: Main findings, 1999*. Washington, DC: U.S. Government Printing Office.

U.S. Department of Health and Human Services (DHHS). (2000b). *Reducing tobacco use: A report of the Surgeon General.* Washington, DC: U.S. Government Printing Office.

Vik, P. W., Brown, S. A., & Meyers, M. G. (1997). Adolescent substance use problems. In E. J. Mash & L. G. Terdal (Eds.), *Assessment of childhood disorders* (3rd ed. pp. 717–748). New York: Guilford Press.

Warner, L., Kessler, R., Hughes, M., Anthony, J., & Nelson, C. (1995). Prevalence and correlates of drug use and drug dependence in the United States: Results from the National Comorbidity Survey. *Archives of General Psychiatry, 52*, 219–229.

Watson, D., Clark, L. A., & Carey, G. (1988). Positive and negative affectivity and their relation to anxiety and depressive disorders. *Journal of Abnormal Psychology, 97*, 346–353.

Webb, J. A., & Baer, P. E. (1995). Influence of family disharmony and parental alcohol use on adolescent social skills, self-efficacy and alcohol use. *Addictive Behaviors, 20*, 127–135.

Weinberg, N., & Glantz, M. (1999). Child psychopathology risk factors for drug abuse: overview. *Journal of Clinical Child Psychology, 28*, 290–297.

Weinberg, N., Rahdert, E., Colliver, J., & Glantz, M. (1998). Adolescent substance abuse: A review of the past ten years. *Journal of the American Academy of Child and Adolescent Psychiatry, 37*, 252–261.

White, H. R., & Huselid, R. F. (1997). Gender differences in alcohol use during adolescence. In R. W. Wilsnack & S. C. Wilsnack (Eds.), *Gender and alcohol: Individual and social perspectives* (pp. 176–198). New Brunswick, NJ: Rutgers Center for Alcohol Studies.

Whitmore, E. A., Mikulich, S. K., Thompson, L. L., Riggs, P. D., Aarons, G. A., & Crowley, T. J. (1997). Influences on adolescent substance dependence: Conduct disorder, depression, attention deficit hyperactivity disorder, and gender. *Drug and Alcohol Dependence, 47*, 87–97.

Wiers, R. W., Gunning, W. B., & Sergeant, J. A. (1998). Is a mild deficit in executive function in boys related to childhood ADHD or to parental multigenerational alcoholism? *Journal of Abnormal Child Psychology, 26*, 415–430.

Wills, T. A. (1986). Stress and coping in early adolescence: Relationships to substance use in urban school samples. *Health Psychology, 5*, 503–529.

Wills, T. A., & Cleary, S. (1997). The validity of self-reports of smoking: Analyses by race/ethnicity in a school sample of urban adolescents. *American Journal of Public Health, 87*, 56–61.

Wills, T. A., Sandy, J. M., Yaeger, A., Cleary, S., & Shinar, O. (2001). Coping dimensions, life stress, and adolescent substance use: A latent growth analysis. *Journal of Abnormal Psychology, 110*, 309–323.

Wills, T. A., Sandy, J. M., Yaeger, A., & Shinar, O. (2001). Family risk factors and adolescent substance use: Moderation effects for temperament dimensions. *Developmental Psychology, 37*, 283–297.

Wills, T. A., Vaccaro, D., McNamara, G., & Hirky, A. (1996). Escalated substance use: A longitudinal grouping analysis from early to middle adolescence. *Journal of Abnormal Psychology, 105*, 166–180.

Windle, M., & Windle, R. (2001). Depressive symptoms and cigarette smoking among middle adolescents: Prospective associations and intrapersonal and interpersonal influences. *Journal of Consulting and Clinical Psychology, 69,* 215–226.

Winters, K. C., Latimer, W., & Stinchfield, R. D. (1999). The DSM-IV criteria for adolescent alcohol and cannabis use disorders. *Journal of Studies on Alcohol, 60,* 337–344.

Winters, K. C., Stinchfield, R. D., Opland, E., Weller, C., & Latimer, W. W. (2000). The effectiveness of the Minnesota model approach in the treatment of adolescent drug abusers. *Addiction, 95,* 601–612.

Yamaguchi, K., & Kandel, D. B. (1985). On the resolution of role incompatibility: A life event history analysis of family roles and marijuana use. *American Journal of Sociology, 90,* 1284–1325.

Zoccolillo, M., Vitaro, F., & Tremblay, R. (1999). Problem drug and alcohol use in a community sample of adolescents. *Journal of the American Academy of Child and Adolescent Psychiatry, 38,* 900–907.

Zucker, R. A. (1987). The four alcoholisms: A developmental account of the etiologic process. In P. C. Rivers (Ed.), *Nebraska Symposium on Motivation: Vol. 34. Alcohol and addictive behavior* (pp. 27–83). Lincoln: University of Nebraska Press.

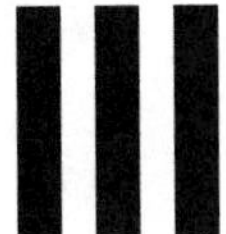

EMOTIONAL AND SOCIAL DISORDERS

CHAPTER FIVE

Childhood Mood Disorders

Constance Hammen
Karen D. Rudolph

In the first edition of this volume, we noted the emergence of a large body of research on child and adolescent depression, based on the relatively recent "discovery" that children sometimes suffered from the same depressive syndromes as defined for adults in standard diagnostic systems. In only the few years since the chapter was written, the field has grown enormously yet again. There have been significant new developments in our understanding of mood disorders in youngsters. In the present chapter, therefore, we update the state of the field, adding a section on bipolar disorders to reflect expanding interest despite diagnostic controversies. We note that unipolar depression is increasingly viewed as a disorder of childhood or adolescent onset with a chronic or recurrent course, and we include expanded coverage of genetic and neurobiological aspects of depressive disorders, as well as recent research reflecting increased interest in family and interpersonal aspects of juvenile depression. As in the first edition, we highlight methodological issues and empirical gaps, and present an integrative model of depressive disorders in children and adolescents.

DEFINING CHILDHOOD DEPRESSION

Joey is a 10-year-old boy whose mother and teacher have shared their concerns about his irritability and temper tantrums displayed both at home and at school. With little provocation, he bursts into tears, yells, and throws objects. In class, he seems to have difficulty concentrating and seems easily distracted. Increasingly shunned by his peers, he plays by himself at recess—and, at home, spends most of his time in his room watching TV. His mother notes that he has been sleeping poorly and has gained 10 pounds over the past couple of months from constant snacking. A consultation with the school psychologist has ruled out learning disabilities or attention-deficit/hyperactivity disorder (ADHD); instead, she says, Joey is a deeply unhappy child who expresses feelings of worthlessness and hopelessness—and even a wish that he would die. These experiences probably began about 6 months ago when his father (divorced from the mother for several years) remarried and moved to another town, where he spends far less time with Joey.

Diagnostic Criteria

The case of Joey is intended to illustrate three keys issues about the diagnosis of depression in youngsters. First, the same criteria used for adults can be applied, and the essential features of the depression syndrome are as recognizable in children as in adults (Carlson & Cantwell, 1980; Mitchell, McCauley, Burke, & Moss, 1988). Second, because children's externalizing or disruptive behaviors attract more attention or are more readily expressed than their internal, subjective suffering is, depression is sometimes overlooked. It may not be recognized, or it may not be assessed. As we note in a later section, "Definitional and Diagnostic Issues," the high level of comorbidity in childhood depression—especially that involving conduct and other disruptive behaviors—gave rise to the erroneous belief that depression is "masked." Third, a few features of the syndrome of depression (e.g., irritable mood) are more likely to be typical of children than of adults, leading to age-specific modifications of the diagnostic criteria. In addition, as we discuss below, certain features of depression are more typical at different ages.

Depressive disorders in children and adolescents are diagnosed with the same criteria as adults. The *Diagnostic and Statistical Manual of Mental Disorders*, fourth edition (DSM-IV; American Psychiatric Association, 1994) gives criteria for major depressive episode that are to be used for both adults and children, as shown in Table 5.1. Dysthymic disorder, presented in Table 5.2, is a diagnosis of persistent, chronic depressive symptoms, with a duration of at least 1 year (in adults, duration is at least 2 years). According to a study of dysthymic disorder in children, it differs from major depression primarily in the emphasis on gloomy thoughts and negative affect, with fewer symptoms such as anhedonia, social withdrawal, fatigue, reduced sleep, and poor appetite (Kovacs, Akiskal, Gatsonis, & Parrone, 1994).

The discriminant validity of separate diagnoses of dysthymic disorder and major depressive dis-

TABLE 5.1. DSM-IV Diagnostic Criteria For Major Depressive Episode

A. Five (or more) of the following symptoms have been present during the same 2-week period; at least one of the symptoms is either (1) depressed mood or (2) loss of interest or pleasure.

Note: Do not include symptoms that are clearly due to a general medical condition, or mood-incongruent delusions or hallucinations.

(1) depressed mood most of the day, nearly every day, as indicated by either subjective report (e.g., feels sad or empty) or observation made by others (e.g., appears tearful). **Note**: In children and adolescents, can be irritable mood.
(2) markedly diminished interest or pleasure in all or almost all activities most of the day, nearly every day (as indicated either by subjective account or observation made by others)
(3) significant weight loss when not dieting or weight gain (e.g., a change of more than 5% of body weight in a month), or decrease or increase in appetite nearly every day. **Note**: In children consider failure to make expected weight gains.
(4) insomnia or hypersomnia nearly every day
(5) psychomotor agitation or retardation nearly every day (observable by others, not merely subjective feelings of restlessness or being slowed down)
(6) fatigue or loss of energy nearly every day
(7) feelings of worthlessness or excessive or inappropriate guilt (which may be delusional) nearly every day (not merely self-reproach or guilt about being sick)
(8) diminished ability to think or concentrate, or indecisiveness, nearly every day (either by subjective account or as observed by others)
(9) recurrent thoughts of death (not just fear of dying), recurrent suicidal ideation without a specific plan, or a suicide attempt or a specific plan for committing suicide

B. The symptoms do not meet criteria for a Mixed Episode.

C. The symptoms cause clinically significant distress or impairment in social, occupational, or other important areas of functioning.

D. The symptoms are not due to the direct physiological effects of a substance (e.g., a drug of abuse, a medication) or a general medical condition (e.g., hypothyroidism).

E. The symptoms are not better accounted for by Bereavement, i.e., after the loss of a loved one, the symptoms persist for longer than 2 months or are characterized by marked functional impairment, morbid preoccupation with worthlessness, suicidal ideation, psychotic symptoms, or psychomotor retardation.

Note. A Major depressive episode (unipolar) can be further specified as mild, moderate, or severe (based on functional impairment and severity of symptoms); with or without psychotic, catatonic, melancholic, or atypical features; and single-episode or recurrent. From American Psychiatric Association (1994, p. 327).

TABLE 5.2. DSM-IV Diagnostic Criteria for Dysthymic Disorder

A. Depressed mood for most of the day, for more days than not, as indicated either by subjective account or observation by others, for at least 2 years. **Note**: In children and adolescents, mood can be irritable and duration must be at least 1 year.

B. Presence, while depressed, of two (or more) of the following:

(1) poor appetite or overeating
(2) insomnia or hypersomnia
(3) low energy or fatigue
(4) low self-esteem
(5) poor concentration or difficulty making decisions
(6) feelings of hopelessness

C. During the 2-year period (1 year for children or adolescents) of the disturbance, the person has never been without the symptoms in Criteria A and B for more than 2 months at a time.

D. No Major Depressive Episode . . . has been present during the first 2 years of the disturbance (1 year for children and adolescents); i.e., the disturbance is not better accounted for by chronic Major Depressive Disorder, or Major Depressive Disorder, In Partial Remission.

Note: there may have been a previous Major Depressive Episode provided there was a full Remission (no significant signs or symptoms for 2 months) before development of the Dysthymic Disorder. In addition, after the initial 2 years (1 year in children or adolescents) of Dysthymic Disorder, there may be superimposed episodes of Major Depressive Disorder, in which case both diagnoses may be given when the criteria are met for a Major Depressive Episode.

E. There has never been a Manic Episode, a Mixed Episode, or a Hypomanic Episode, and criteria have never been met for Cyclothymic Disorder.

F. The disturbance does not occur exclusively during the course of a chronic Psychotic Disorder, such as Schizophrenia or Delusional Disorder.

G. The symptoms are not due to the direct physiological effects of a substance (e.g., a drug of abuse, a medication) or a general medical condition (e.g., hypothyroidism).

H. The symptoms cause clinically significant distress or impairment in social, occupational, or other important areas of functioning.

Specify if:
Early Onset: if onset is before age 21 years
Late Onset: if onset is age 21 years or older

Specify (for most recent 2 years of Dysthymic Disorder):
With Atypical Features . . .

Note. From American Psychiatric Association (1994, p. 349). Copyright 1994 by the American Psychiatric Association. Reprinted by permission.

order has been raised in recent years. Several studies indicated little evidence of differences in clinical features and sociodemographic correlates of these disorders. Analyses from the Methods for the Epidemiology of Child and Adolescent Mental Disorders (MECA) study found few differences in clinical course, impairment, and sociodemographic factors between children with major depressive disorder only and those with dysthymic disorder only, other than earlier age of onset for the dysthymic children (Goodman, Schwab-Stone, Lahey, Shaffer, & Jensen, 2000). Therefore, the investigators have questioned whether a meaningful distinction can be made between the two diagnoses, and whether different treatments are warranted. On the other hand, the data clearly indicated that youngsters who had the combined or "double-depression" profile of both major depression and dysthymia were significantly more impaired and lacking in competence than those in the other categories (Goodman et al., 2000). The combination of severe and chronic depression appears to predict disruption of important developmental achievements, and warrants an emphasis on early detection and effective treatment to mitigate the long-term effects of clinical condition.

Phenomenology and Developmental Features

The only formal modification of adult criteria involves recognition by DSM-IV that irritability may be a significant feature of child and adolescent depression, and that irritable mood may be substituted for depressed mood. This adjustment to the diagnostic criteria recognizes that irritability is a common expression of distress in depressed youngsters, as shown in the case of Joey (e.g., Goodyer & Cooper, 1993; Ryan et al., 1987). In general, specific symptoms of the DSM criteria for major depression are similar in clinic-referred child and adolescent samples (Mitchell et al., 1988; Ryan et al., 1987). The exception is that depressed adolescents may have significantly higher rates of hypersomnia than do depressed children (e.g., for a review, see Kovacs, 1996).

Apart from formal diagnostic criteria, there may be other developmental differences in the expression of depression. Young depressed children, especially preschoolers and preadolescents, are unlikely to report subjective dysphoria and hopelessness (e.g., Ryan et al., 1987); instead, they show depressed appearance (e.g., Carlson & Kashani, 1988). Also, younger depressed children are more likely to have physically unjustified or exaggerated somatic complaints (Kashani, Rosenberg, & Reid, 1989; Ryan et al., 1987). Younger children, as noted earlier, also show more irritability, uncooperativeness, apathy, and disinterest (Kashani, Holcomb, & Orvaschel, 1986). It is possible that additional research on developmental expressions of depression will suggest further age-appropriate modifications of the diagnostic criteria.

In addition to comparisons of depressed children and adolescents, two studies compared the symptoms of depressed youngsters and adults. Overall, several symptoms increase with age, including anhedonia, psychomotor retardation, and diurnal variation, whereas several decrease with age, including depressed appearance, somatic complaints, and poor self-esteem (Carlson & Kashani, 1988). Comparing combined child–adolescent groups with a sample of adults, Mitchell et al. (1988) found similar differences for self-esteem, somatic complaints, and diurnal variation, and also found that adult depressed patients reported less guilt and more early morning awakening and weight loss than depressed youngsters did. The increased presence of vegetative, melancholic symptoms in adults could have been due to more severe depression in the adult (inpatient) sample than in the child–adolescent samples, which included a mixture of inpatients and outpatients.

Complementing studies that have examined developmental differences at the symptom level, other studies have examined age-related differences in the *syndrome* of depression—namely, which symptoms tend to cluster together. Findings are somewhat consistent with those from studies of symptom expression. For example, factor analyses of self-reported depressive symptoms (e.g., measured with the Children's Depression Inventory [CDI]; Kovacs, 1980) reveal that vegetative symptoms loaded with negative affect in adolescence but not in childhood (Weiss et al., 1991a, 1991b).

In addition to presentation of depressive symptoms, patterns of comorbid disorders are likely to be somewhat different at different ages. For instance, depressed children and young adolescents are more likely than depressed older adolescents to display separation anxiety disorder, whereas adolescents report more eating disorders and substance use disorders (e.g., Fleming & Offord, 1990). Other kinds of anxiety disorders, and attention-deficit and disruptive behavior disorders, appear to coexist with depression for both children and adolescents. We explore the issue of comorbidity more fully in later sections.

Additional Diagnostic Features

Like adult depression, childhood depression sometimes includes psychotic symptoms and endogenous (melancholic) features. Hallucinations, especially auditory ones, were observed in one-third to nearly one-half of preadolescent depressed patients (Chambers, Puig-Antich, Tabrizi, & Davies, 1982; Mitchell et al., 1988). Also, 31% of the Strober, Lampert, Schmidt, and Morrell (1993) sample of adolescent depressed inpatients were diagnosed as psychotic. These rates are higher than those typically reported for adult depressed patients. Delusions among depressed children and adolescents are less common (e.g., 7% in Chambers et al., 1982), although investigators note the difficulty in obtaining accurate information from children.

With respect to endogenous symptomatology, Ryan et al. (1987) reported that about half of both their prepubertal and adolescent samples had such symptoms as lack of reactivity, distinct quality of mood, diurnal variation, and the like. Presence of the endogenous type of depression may predict a worse course with shorter time to relapse (McCauley et al., 1993). In addition, a certain number of depressed youngsters display—or are seen to experience during follow-up—manic or hypomanic symptoms suggestive of a bipolar disorder. As noted in a later section, a significant proportion of youngsters who first present with apparently unipolar depressive disorders "switch" to a bipolar presentation over time. This switch may be even more likely for psychotically depressed children and adolescents (e.g., Strober et al., 1993).

Suicidal thoughts and attempts are among the diagnostic criteria for major depression. Suicidal ideation is quite common, and has been reported in more than 60% of depressed preschoolers, preadolescents, and adolescents (Kashani & Carlson, 1987; Mitchell et al., 1988; Ryan et al., 1987). Actual suicidal attempts also may occur, at rates that appear to be higher among depressed youngsters than among depressed adults (e.g., Mitchell et al., 1988). Suicidality among youths is not restricted to those with depression, however. It often occurs among those with substance use disorders and impulsive behavior disorders, and may be greatly affected by social-environmental factors (such as a friend's or a publicized suicide), as well as by depression itself (e.g., Lewinsohn, Rohde, & Seeley, 1994). Indeed, the correlates and predictors of childhood and adolescent suicidality represent an extensive body of work beyond the scope of this chapter (see Berman & Jobes, 1991; Pfeffer, 2001).

In addition to the specific diagnostic criteria for depressive disorders, several other symptoms are frequently seen in children and adolescents. For example, social withdrawal is common (Goodyer & Cooper, 1993; Kashani et al., 1989; Mitchell et al., 1988). Somatic symptoms and bodily complaints, as well as distress over negative body image in adolescent girls, are also commonly associated symptoms of depression (e.g., Allgood-Merten, Lewinsohn, & Hops, 1990; Petersen, Sarigiani, & Kennedy, 1991).

DEFINITIONAL AND DIAGNOSTIC ISSUES IN CHILDHOOD DEPRESSION

Confusion sometimes arises in the childhood depression field, as it does with adult depression, because of different usages of the term "depression" and associated differences in methods of assessment. For example, in studies of childhood and adolescent depression, the term is variously used to identify depressed mood, a constellation of mood and other symptoms forming a syndrome, or a set of symptoms meeting official diagnostic criteria for a depressive disorder. This distinction among mood, syndrome, and disorder has been discussed extensively elsewhere (e.g., Compas, Ey, & Grant, 1993). Each view of depression represents somewhat different assumptions and assessment procedures. For instance, mood measures refer to depression as a symptom indicating the presence of sad mood or unhappiness, which is typically rated by self-report on scales. Depression as a syndrome (or, more accurately, an anxious/depressed syndrome) has emerged from the multivariate statistical methods of assessing childhood emotional and behavioral problems (e.g., Achenbach, 1991). Each constellation of symptoms occurs together as a recognizable and statistically coherent pattern, and the anxious/depressed cluster may be rated by the child or adolescent, parents, and teachers on the Child Behavior Checklist, Youth Self-Report, or Teacher Report Form (Achenbach, 1991; Achenbach & Edelbrock, 1978). The items that cluster together in the anxious/depressed syndrome include the following: "lonely," "cries a lot," "fears impulses," "perfectionistic," "feels unloved," "feels persecuted," "feels worthless," "nervous," "fearful," "guilty," "self-conscious," "suspicious," "unhappy," and "worries." This definition of depression is an empirical one, and it makes no assumptions about a particular model of cause. Depression as defined by the third approach, diagnosis of a disorder, refers to the presence of a set of currently agreed-upon indicators of a disease embodied in a categorical diagnostic system such as DSM-IV (American Psychiatric Association, 1994) or the *International Classification of Diseases*, 10th revision (ICD-10; World Health Organization, 1993). This model assumes that there are specific disorders with relatively distinct boundaries.

One question that arises from different uses of the term "depression" (and the associated assessment methods) is whether depression is better construed as a dimension or a category. As we note later, the finding of high levels of comorbidity of childhood depression may be in part an artifact of a categorical method of defining disorders. If depression is viewed as a dimension, then individuals differ mainly by degree, regardless of whether or not they might also have other symptoms. Thus occurrence of depressive symptoms along with other disorders would not be unexpected in a dimensional perspective. Whether or not depression defined as a symptom or as a syndrome reflects the same construct and underlying disorder is in part an empirical issue, as discussed later.

Continuity of Depression Severity

A key issue that emerges in childhood depression studies using the various definitions and indicators of depression is whether they are measuring the same thing but at different levels of severity and specificity. There are two overlapping issues: (1) whether self-report scales and diagnoses yield similar samples, and (2) whether subsyndromal and syndromal depressions represent different populations and implications. Thus, when we present studies based on self-reports on questionnaires such as the CDI (Kovacs, 1980) or the Center for Epidemiologic Studies Depression Scale (CES-D; Radloff, 1977), are those results applicable to the phenomena of depression that are studied in a clinically diagnosed community or treatment sample?

One approach to this issue has been detailed by Compas et al. (1993) with respect to adolescent depressive phenomena. They reviewed studies of the correspondence among measures of symptom, syndrome, and disorder, and developed a sequential and hierarchical model of the interrelations among them. They argued that the symptom of depressed mood is the broadest and most nonspecific indicator, with a point prevalence of 15–40% in adolescents; most of these youngsters do not display a depressive syndrome, but a subset (approximately 5–6% of the total population) are classified as high scorers on the anxious/depressed syndrome of the Achenbach taxonomic approach. A further subset of these individuals (maybe 1–3% of the total population) meet diagnostic criteria for a depressive disorder. The three conditions share negative affect but differ in their symptom constellations, with the anxious/depressed syndrome including anxiety symptoms that are not part of a purely depressed mood, whereas depressive disorders include somatic and vegetative symptoms that are not included in the mood or syndrome definitions of depression (Compas et al., 1993). These authors have further argued that the transition from depressed mood to a depressive syndrome is mediated by dysregulation of biological, stress, and/or coping processes. In short, these authors emphasize both continuity and discontinuity in the different experiences of depression; they urge further research that includes all three levels of assessment, longitudinal analysis of the unfolding of the hypothesized sequence, and analyses of the implications of different levels of symptom expression.

A related issue is the validity of a clear distinction between subsyndromal and syndromal depression. Adult research has increasingly shown that so-called "subsyndromal" depression is associated with significant impairment, and may be highly predictive of later diagnosis (e.g., Hays, Wells, Sherbourne, Rogers, Spritzer, 1995; Judd et al., 1998). Similarly, high scores on self-report measures may portend significant clinical and functional impairment even if a person is not diagnosed (e.g., Gotlib, Lewinsohn, & Seeley, 1995).

Thus elevated symptoms of depression in children and adolescents should be regarded seriously; their clinical status is likely to be especially significant to the extent that they reflect symptoms persisting over time. This may especially be the case in childhood and early adolescent depression, where even moderate symptoms may disrupt normal developmental processes and contribute to impairment of functioning, and where syndromes are less distinct and boundaries less clear. Therefore, even somewhat elevated scores for children—if they indicate protracted distress and are accompanied by impaired functioning—may be on the same continuum as clinical cases.

Sources of Information in Defining Depression

An issue that arises above and beyond the question of the different meanings of the term "depression" is the matter of informants for depression. It is well known that in general, subjects themselves, parents, peers, and teachers may give discrepant reports of symptomatology (Achenbach, McConaughy, & Howell, 1987). This complication gives rise to two important issues. One is how to obtain the most valid picture of the existence of depression, and the other is whether mothers who are themselves depressed give negatively biased reports of their children's symptomatology.

The first question of valid diagnosis is typically resolved by using multiple informants and methods (e.g., Puig-Antich, Chambers, & Tabrizi, 1983; Rutter, 1986). Most diagnostic methods of assessing depression, such as the clinician-administered Schedule for Affective Disorders and Schizophrenia for School-Aged Children (K-SADS; Ambrosini, 2000) or the lay-administered Diagnostic Interview Schedule for Children (DISC; Shaffer, Fisher, Lucas, Dulcan, & Schwab-Stone, 2000), prescribe separate interviews for the child and parent. The manner of combining the information may differ from method to method or from project to project. The DISC, for example, is a highly structured interview administered by trained laypersons rather than clinicians, and it frequently uses a computer-based scoring algorithm for combining information about diagnostic criteria. The K-SADS, administered by clinicians, commonly uses a "best clinical estimate" method, combining information from the child and the parent but weighted by the type of information given, according to clinicians' judgment. Internal symptoms such as depressed feelings and negative thoughts, for example, cannot readily be detected by parents, and therefore the child's report of such symptoms may be given greater weight in a diagnosis of depression.

The other issue concerning informants is whether there might be systematic biases in the reports of certain informants. Specifically, some research has suggested that relatively depressed women might distort or exaggerate reports of their children's behavior as more negative than it actually is. However, a review of 22 studies by Richters (1992) found that such claims were based largely on inadequate designs, including simple associations between mothers' and children's symptoms that could be accurate, given the common finding of disorders in offspring of depressed women. Only a small number of studies were located that were appropriate to test the question (i.e., they included objective measures of children's behaviors from comparable perspectives, and they compared depressed and nondepressed women). Of those studies, none supported the idea that depressed women perceive more problem behaviors than actually exist—and two of the studies found that depressed women were *more* accurate in detecting true disorders in their children than were nondepressed women (Conrad & Hammen, 1989; Weissman et al., 1987). Subsequent studies have used sophisticated methods, such as covariance structure analysis with latent variables formed from different informants. Such studies have supported the hypothesis that depressed mothers may display reporting errors, but also have shown that because maternal depression truly is associated with more child disorder, the conclusion of "bias" is unclear (Boyle & Pickles, 1997; Fergusson, Lynskey, & Horwood, 1993). Boyle and Pickles (1997) and Renouf and Kovacs (1994) evaluated parent–child concordance over time and suggested that maternal bias, if any, may be more pronounced for younger than for older children.

Comorbidity

The co-occurrence of other disorders with depression in children and adolescents has been a focus of considerable discussion and research in the past decade. Initially relatively ignored, comorbidity has now become widely recognized as the rule rather than the exception with depressed youngsters. Depression co-occurs commonly with anxiety disorders of all forms, as well as with attention-deficit and disruptive behavior disorders, substance use disorders, and eating disorders. Angold, Costello, and Erkanli (1999) presented a meta-analysis of comorbidity in community studies of youngsters that employed standard diagnostic criteria. Community studies permit the best test of rates of comorbidity, inasmuch as clinical populations may be biased, because treatment seeking is more common among those with multiple and more severe conditions. The meta-analysis reported a median odds ratio (degree of association) of 8.2 for depression and anxiety disorders, 6.6 for depression and conduct disorder/oppositional defiant disorder, and 5.5 for depression and ADHD (Angold, Costello, & Erkanli, 1999). The frequency with which comorbidity occurs in depression has raised a number of conceptual, methodological, and etiological questions for further study. Comorbidity in depression also encourages caution in interpreting the results of studies in which depression, characteristics and correlates may have been erroneously attributed to the depression, when in fact concurrent disorders may have played a role.

It has been argued that comorbidity may reflect methodological and diagnostic shortcomings, including, for example, overlap between syndromes due to shared symptoms, or artifacts of referral or sample bias. Addressing the possible meaning of comorbidity, Angold, Costello, and Erkanli (1999) concluded, based on a review of studies, that methodological and sampling problems cannot account for the high rates of comorbidity seen in community samples. They argued that nosological deficiencies may contribute to (but probably do not account for) the magnitude of the problem, and they emphasized the need for more research exploring the development and features of comorbid conditions. More likely explanations than diagnostic artifact, according to Angold, Costello, and Erkanli (1999) and other investigators, are that etiological factors may be shared by co-occurring disorders (common-cause hypothesis), or that risk factors are correlated. Furthermore, in some instances there may be a functional relation between one disorder and a subsequent one (causal hypothesis). However, research that specifically investigates common-cause, correlated risk factors, or causal hypotheses is relatively rare; a few specific studies are noted below.

Concurrent comorbid depression and anxiety disorders and symptoms have been a particular focus of attention, and in the adult field have led to considerable research on their shared and unique aspects (e.g., the tripartite model of Clark & Watson, 1991). Kovacs (1990) reviewed studies of depressed youngsters and concluded that 30–75% had diagnosable anxiety disorders, including separation anxiety disorder, overanxious (generalized anxiety) disorder, severe phobias, or obsessive–compulsive disorder. Kovacs speculated that sometimes anxiety and depression are actually a single disorder, although in other cases they are distinct but mark a particularly pernicious course and prognosis. So common is the co-occurrence that Achenbach (1991) failed to find a "pure" depression syndrome emerging from principal-components analyses of reports by youths, parents, and teachers. Instead, depressive symptoms loaded on a factor that also included anxiety symptoms. Recent research on co-occurring depression and anxiety symptoms in children and adolescents has revealed shared and specific anxiety and depression components that are similar to those of adults (for a review, see Laurent & Ettelson, 2001), although they may differ in some ways (Rudolph, Lambert, Osborne, Gathright, & Kumar, 2001). Cole, Truglio, and Peeke (1997) have suggested that younger children are more likely to show a unified factor of depression and anxiety symptoms, whereas older children may show patterns more consistent with the tripartite model.

In addition to concurrent comorbidity between anxiety and depression, investigations of temporal sequencing have provided evidence of successive comorbidity. Many studies have reported that anxiety disorders occur earlier, followed by depressive disorders (e.g., Avenevoli, Stolar, Li, Dierker, & Ma, 2001; Kovacs, Gatsonis, Paulauskas, & Richards, 1989; Lewinsohn, Zinbarg, Seeley, Lewinsohn, & Sack, 1997; Pine, Cohen, Gurley, Brook, & Ma, 1998; Wickramaratne & Weissman, 1998). These patterns of concurrent and successive comorbidity have led some investigators to speculate that anxiety and depression may have correlated or common etiological factors. Several twin studies, for example, reported that the overlap was accounted for largely by genetic liability (Kendler, Neale, Kessler, Heath, & Eaves, 1992; Thapar & McGuffin, 1997; see also Silberg, Rutter, & Eaves, 2001). Overall, the association between anxiety and depressive disorders is substantial, especially for girls. It has been speculated that early anxiety disorders are a risk factor for later depression (e.g., Cole, Peeke, Martin, Truglio, & Seroczynski, 1998; Kovacs et al., 1989).

Depression also coexists commonly with the so-called "externalizing" disorders, including conduct disorder, oppositional defiant disorder, ADHD, and substance use disorders. The frequency of such combinations initially created the confusion of "masked" depression. Among specific studies, for example, Rohde, Lewinsohn, and Seeley (1991) reported a lifetime comorbidity rate of 12.1% for conduct disorder in the depressed group (compared with just 6% in nondepressed subjects). Clinical samples of depressed youngsters are especially likely to include coexisting conduct disorder, with rates ranging between 14% and 36% (e.g., Kovacs, Paulauskas, Gatsonis, & Richards, 1988; Mitchell et al., 1988; Puig-Antich, 1982; Ryan et al., 1987). Both community and treatment-referred sample studies also report elevations in rates of comorbid substance use disorders and ADHD (for a review, see Angold, Costello, & Erkanli, 1999). Faraone and Biederman (1997) reviewed family studies, and argued that ADHD and depression share a genetic predisposition. Studies of nondiagnosed depressions in community samples using self- and other-reported symptom scales similarly show covariation of depression and behavior disorder symptoms (e.g., Achenbach, 1991; Cole & Carpentieri, 1990).

Unsurprisingly, there are gender differences in patterns of comorbidity. Depressed girls, for instance, have higher rates of anxiety disorders, whereas depressed boys are more likely than girls to have higher rates of attention-deficit and disruptive behavior disorders (Kessler, Avenevoli, & Merikangas, 2001). The temporal order of depression and behavior disorders generally is similar to that of anxiety comorbidity: Depression usually follows onset of a behavior disorder (e.g., Rohde et al., 1991). Relatively little research has been conducted on the mechanisms that link depression and behavior disorders, although several hypotheses have been suggested. One is that depression comorbidity is a nonspecific reflection of greater psychopathology, indicating generally elevated symptoms of emotional and behavioral dysregulation. Another is that depression is a consequence of the stressful disruptions in family, school, and social circumstances that are created by behavior disorders. A third hypothesis is that depression and behavior disorders share correlated risk factors, such as parental depression, parental marital/couple conflict, assortative mating of depressed women and antisocial or substance-abusing men, and genetic liability. Considerably more work is needed to explore these options and to clarify the meaning and source of comorbidity (e.g., Angold, Costello, & Erkanli, 1999).

In summary, the issues of defining child depression, measuring it, and exploring its developmental pathways present unique challenges that would seem to call for more than merely downward extensions of how we measure and define adult depression. The fact that we can employ adult criteria has resulted in greater study of this important topic, but at the same time, it may have misled us into believing that the phenomena are the same and have similar consequences in children and adults.

EPIDEMIOLOGY OF CHILDHOOD DEPRESSION

Prevalence/Incidence

Only in recent years have investigators mounted methodologically sound epidemiological surveys of childhood disorders. Despite the advantage of large and reasonably representative samples, the studies have tended to use somewhat different methods of assessment and case identification processes. Specifically, they have differed in whether standard diagnostic instruments are used, who serves as the informants, whether data are represented by age groups and gender, and other aspects, all of which limit comparison across studies. These issues and other methodological shortcomings are discussed in Roberts, Attkisson, and Rosenblatt (1998) and Kessler et al. (2001).

Studies that report prevalence rates of DSM or ICD diagnoses in preadolescent children in large community surveys are relatively rare, because rates are not reported separately for younger children in samples that include both children and adolescents. In general, preadolescent school-age children have very low lifetime rates of depressive disorders, generally less than 3% (e.g., Cohen et al., 1993; Fleming & Offord, 1990). The largest U.S. study of children (ages, 9, 11, and 13) was conducted by Costello et al. (1996) in the Great Smoky Mountains Study of Youth; they reported a 3-month prevalence rate of 0.03% for major depressive episode and 0.13% for dysthymia (plus 1.45% depression not otherwise specified), for a total of 1.52% depressive disorders (see also Fombonne, 1994, in a French sample; Polaino-Lorente & Domenech, 1993, in a Spanish sample). Depression in preschool children is apparently rare, occurring in less than 1% (Kashani & Carlson, 1987); however, data in this age group are sparse, and children younger than about 7 years typically are not included in large-scale community surveys.

Rates of diagnosed depression among adolescents are comparable to those of adults. The National Comorbidity Study (NCS) is the only U.S. nationally representative community epidemiological survey that included adolescents (age 15 and above). Lifetime prevalence of major depression in the 15 to 18-year-olds was 14%, with an additional 11% reporting minor depression (Kessler & Walters, 1998; see also Lewinson, Hops, Roberts, Seeley, & Andrews, 1993). These rates are relatively comparable to those of smaller community surveys of adolescents (e.g., Cohen et al., 1993; Fergusson, Horwood, & Lynskey, 1993; McGee et al., 1990).

Even when diagnostic criteria are not met, subsyndromal depressive symptoms may indicate high levels of distress. For instance, Cooper and Goodyer (1993) reported that 20.7% of their female sample of 11- to 16-year-olds had significant symptoms but fell short of diagnostic criteria. Moreover, when self-report symptom scores, rather than diagnoses, are used to indicate depressive experiences, approximately 10–30% of adolescents exceed cutoffs for high levels (e.g., Garrison, Jackson, Marsteller, McKeown, & Addy, 1990; Roberts, Lewinsohn, & Seeley, 1991). Rather than mere "adolescent turmoil," elevated self-report scores indicate impaired functioning, and may portend the later development of diagnosable disorders.

High rates of depression in youths appear to reflect increasing prevalence over previous decades. Earlier reports of birth cohort effects showing increased rates of major depression in those born more recently (e.g., Klerman et al., 1985) have been replicated in the United States and internationally by the Cross-National Collaborative Group (1992), indicating growing rates of childhood or adolescent onset of depression among those born in more recent decades. Recent results from the NCS also show clear evidence of increasing prevalence of major depressive episode in those born since 1960 (Kessler et al., 2001). These findings confirm the view that depression is a disorder of young onset.

Various analyses of the sources of such increased rates have generally ruled out methodological artifacts, such as memory or increasing willingness to admit to depressive experiences (e.g., Murphy, Laird, Monson, Sobol, & Leighton, 2000). The cause of the increases is not known, but it is often suggested that at least some of the increase may be due to social changes that contribute to vulnerability to depression (such as family disruption and exposure to greater stressors, along with reduced access to resources and supports). The role of such social and psychological factors is discussed more fully in later sections.

Gender Differences

The basic finding of higher rates of depressive diagnoses and symptoms in girls during adolescence is well established (e.g., Cohen et al., 1993; Fergusson, Horwood, & Lynskey, 1993; Lewinsohn et al., 1993; McGee et al., 1990; Reinherz, Giaconia, Lefkowitz, Pakiz, & Frost, 1993; see also Nolen-Hoeksema & Girgus, 1994). Studies of preadolescent children vary in their reports of whether boys' and girls' rates are equal or whether boys' rates exceed girls' rates (e.g., Angold & Rutter, 1992) prior to adolescence. There are also slightly divergent findings about the age at which adolescent girls' rates increase and differences appear, but most studies concur that it is about 13–15 years (e.g., Angold & Rutter, 1992; Cohen et al., 1993; Cooper & Goodyer, 1993; Petersen et al., 1991). Hankin et al. (1998) noted that the greatest increases in diagnosed depression in young women occurred between ages 15 and 18 in a New Zealand sample.

The issues of why sex differences occur and why they emerge in adolescence have been explored from numerous perspectives, which variously focus on hormonal changes, stress and coping processes, changing social roles, and interactions among these variables. A complete discussion is beyond the scope of this chapter (for reviews, see Cyranowski, Frank, Young, & Shear, 2000; Nolen-Hoeksema & Girgus, 1994; Nolen-Hoeksema, 2002). Initial studies suggested that hormonal levels and pubertal status as such did not appear to coincide precisely with depression level (e.g., Angold & Rutter, 1992). However, a more recent report in an epidemiological sample of girls did find an association between depressive symptoms and levels of female estradiol and testosterone in adolescence (Angold, Costello, Erkanli, & Worthman, 1999). Nolen-Hoeksema (2002) and Cyranowski et al. (2000) observe that complex associations among gonadal hormones and brain neurotransmitters may affect mood and biological processes in response to stressful circumstances in adolescence in vulnerable individuals. These investigators also note the likely importance to females of social relationships, mediated by both biological sex differences in affiliative needs and socialization experiences. Such gender differences may result in females' greater exposure and sensitivity to interpersonal stressful life events (Rudolph, 2002; Rudolph & Hammen, 1999). Girls may also be exposed more often to traumatic sexual abuse experiences, which may further affect their biological and psychological reactivity to social stressors. In addition, there are differences between the genders in the ways they cope with depressed mood and stressful life events, with women tending to adopt a more passive, internalized, ruminative style, compared with males' more active and instrumental coping (Nolen-Hoeksema, 2000). It appears that complex integrative models are necessary to account for the emergence of marked sex differences in rates of depression in dolescence.

Socioeconomic, Ethnic, and Cultural Differences

Effects of socioeconomic status (SES) on depression have been well documented in adults. Findings in children and adolescents are generally consistent with those in adults (see Bird et al., 1988; Reinherz et al., 1993). Studies of symptom levels rather than diagnoses also have linked depression to lower SES (e.g., Gore, Aseltine, & Colton, 1993; Offord et al., 1992, using a broad category of "emotional disorder"). Costello et al. (1996) found that low income was associated with significantly more depressive and other disorders in children; overall, the poorest children had 3.2 higher rates for any disorder.

SES is measured in various ways and probably is not a very useful variable in understanding mechanisms of depression. Social disadvantage conferred by low SES not only may consist of low income and restricted parental education; it also may include chronic stress, family disruption, racial discrimination, blocked access to opportunities, and greater exposure to environmental adversities. As we explore later in greater detail, there is fairly consistent evidence of links between childhood depression and various indicators of adversity.

Few studies have included sufficient ethnically diverse samples to examine differences in depression rates. One of the largest studies to date (5,423 students in grades 6–8) examined rates of major depression in nine ethnic groupings, and found comparable rates for all groups, except for higher rates among those of Mexican descent (Roberts, Roberts, & Chen, 1997). Most studies generally have found few differences in depression between European American and African American youths (e.g., Costello et al., 1996). One study found that African American girls did not show the same increases in depression rates from pre- to postpuberty that are commonly found in European Americans (Hayward, Gotlib, Schraedley, & Litt, 1999). Further studies are needed to explore other race/ethnicity effects, and to separate out (1) effects that might be caused by different cultural expressions of depressive symptoms and (2) adverse conditions that might be associated with ethnic status.

DEVELOPMENTAL COURSE AND PROGNOSIS OF DEPRESSION

Age of Onset

Adult depression is currently viewed largely as a disorder of adolescent onset. Retrospective assessment among community adults typically indicates that middle to late adolescence is the most common age at onset of first major depression or significant symptoms (e.g., Burke, Burke, Regier, & Rae, 1990). As indicated previously, depression in young children is relatively rare, but becomes more frequent in school-age groups. Among clinic samples of depressed children, the longitudinal studies of Kovacs, Feinberg, Crouse-Novak, Paulauskas, & Finkelstein (1984) found onset of major depression at about 11 years of age, significantly older than onset of dysthymic disorder. In their community sample of adolescents, Lewinsohn et al. (1993) reported mean onset of major depression at about 14 years and mean onset of dysthymic disorder at about 11 years for both boys and girls. As discussed in the section on gender and depression, early adolescence is the most common age of onset for girls in particular.

Age-of-onset information not only suggests that depression is commonly a disorder of relatively young onset, but also has implications for prognosis. Earlier onset of depression, as with most disorders, appears to predict a more protracted or more severe course of disorder in both children (e.g., Kovacs, Feinberg, Crouse-Novak, Paulauskas, & Finkelstein, 1984) and adults (e.g., Bland, Newman, & Orn, 1986; Hammen, Davila, Brown, Gitlin, & Ellicott, 1992). However, as indicated below, whereas prepubertal onset of major depressive disorder bodes ill for later adjustment, it may not specifically portend continuing depressive disorders.

Duration and Course of Depressive Episodes

Several aspects of course have implications for understanding children's depression and outcomes: duration of episodes, "double depression," recurrence, and continuity of episodes and of impairment from childhood or adolescence into adulthood.

Duration

Reviews of research on clinical features of depression have been based on a small number of samples, many of which are clinical populations that often combine children and adolescents. The reviews report that major depressive episodes have a mean duration (time to recovery) of 7–9 months (Birmaher et al., 1996; Kovacs, 1996), which is similar to that of adults. This estimate includes both clinical (inpatient and outpatient) and community samples (e.g., Lewinsohn, Clarke, Seeley, & Rohde, 1994). The vast majority of major depressive episodes remit within a few months, but a small group (approximately 6–10%) may have prolonged episodes. Thus the median time to recovery is shorter than the mean number of months' duration. As an example of a nonclinical and prospective assessment, Rao, Hammen, and Daley (1999) found a median of 8 weeks' duration of major depressive episode over the course of a 5-year study in a community sample of adolescent women. Similar median durations were reported by Lewinsohn, Clarke, et al. (1994) in their community sample.

Dysthymia and Double Depression

Dysthymic disorder by definition is lengthy (at least 1 year's duration), although presumably with less severe symptoms than a major depressive episode. As noted previously, there is controversy over whether dysthymia is a valid diagnosis (Goodman et al., 2000). However, there is agreement that many affected children go on to develop "double depression." Birmaher et al. (1996) summarized studies suggesting a mean episode length of 4 years for dysthymic disorder. They reviewed studies suggesting that approximately 70% or more of children with dysthymic disorder go on to develop episodes of major depression. Kovacs et al. (1994) observed that dysthymic children typically experienced their first major depressive episode 2–3 years after the onset of dysthymia. She and her colleagues argued that early-onset dysthymia is a risk factor for recurrent or chronic mood disorder. Moreover, the combination of dysthymia and major depression appears to be associated with considerable impairment—more than that caused by either disorder alone, according to the MECA study (Goodman et al., 2000).

Recurrence

Depression is increasingly recognized as a chronic or recurrent disorder in adults (e.g., Judd et al., 1998), and this view has been extended to children in recent years. Research on adults has shown that about 40% experience a recurrence of major depression within 2 years, and over 80% within 5–7 years (e.g., Coryell et al., 1994; Solomon et al., 2000). Patterns of recurrence in depressed youngsters are remarkably similar, based on both clinical and community samples of children and adolescents (e.g., Asarnow et al., 1988; Emslie et al., 1997; Kovacs, Feinberg, Crouse-Novak, Paulauskas, Pollock, & Finkelstein, 1984).

Studies of community samples of diagnosed adolescents also have indicated high rates of recurrence—approximately 40% over 3–5 years (Lewinsohn, Clarke, et al., 1994; Rao et al., 1999). Rates of recurrence in community samples of children followed over time have been based on self-reported depressive symptoms, rather than diagnoses. Such studies suggest considerable stability of depressive symptoms over 3–6 years (e.g., Garrison et al., 1990; Verhulst & van der Ende, 1992). For instance, Verhulst and van der Ende (1992) observed that the majority of those scoring high at the first testing remained higher scorers over 6 years, and that 16% of the youngsters had high scores at all four testings.

Continuity of Depressive Episodes into Different Developmental Periods

There is also growing evidence that early onsets of depression portend a potentially lifelong course, with continuity between childhood or adolescent depression and adult depression. Long-term follow-ups of children are rare, but two are noteworthy. Reinherz, Giaconia, Hauf, Wasserman, and Paradis (2000) followed 360 community children from age 5 to age 21; they found that presence of major depressive episodes by age 21 was predicted by reports of depressive/anxious symptoms by teachers at age 6, and by self and parents at age 9. In the largest follow-up study of the continuity of clinically ascertained childhood depression into adulthood, Weissman et al. (1999) found that a subgroup of 108 prepubertally depressed youngsters in treatment who were followed for 10–15 years had major depressive episodes in adulthood. About one-third of the subgroup of youngsters whose families had histories of major depression or who had recurrent depression in childhood went on to have continuing major depressive episodes in adulthood. However, it is important to note that the majority of prepubertally depressed children did *not* go on to have adult depressive experiences. These youngsters had high rates of psychological disorders and significant maladjustment, but there was poor specificity for depressive disorders. Similar results were reported by Harrington,

Fudge, Rutter, Pickles, and Hill (1990) in a follow-back study of the adult functioning of individuals who had been treated for depression as children or adolescents. In further analyses, Harrington, Fudge, Rutter, Pickles, and Hill (1991) found continuity of depression into adulthood—but less for those with comorbid conduct disorder than for those with only depressive disorder as youngsters. Those with conduct disorder had considerable impairment as adults, but were less likely to have continued depression. Thus, across these studies, *childhood* onset of depression may predict significant disorder but not specifically recurring depression, except in subsamples characterizd by less comorbidity, recurrent depressive episodes, and family history of depression. Many children presenting with depression plus externalizing disorders may have an etiologically different depression, or actually may not have depressive disorder as such; rather, they may suffer from marked emotional and behavioral dysregulation that eventually coalescences into nondepressive psychopathology.

In contrast, data on continuity of *adolescent* depression into adulthood are strongly consistent. Several large-scale community samples reported on the outcomes in adulthood of those who had been found to have a diagnosis of major depressive disorder during adolescence. The Dunedin (New Zealand) Multidisciplinary Health and Development (Bardone, Moffitt, Caspi, Dickson, & Silva, 1996), the Ontario Child Health Study (Fleming, Boyle, & Offord, 1993), the Oregon Adolescent Depression Project (Lewinsohn, Rohde, Klein, & Seeley, 1999), and the Upstate New York study (Pine et al., 1998) all reported high rates of recurrence of major depression in young adulthood. Finally, one large-scale 10-year study of clinic-referred adolescents followed up to a mean age of 26 found that only 37% survived without an episode of major depression in adulthood (Weissman et al., 1999).

Continuity of Impairment

It is perhaps unsurprising that youthful depression not only is predictive of recurrent episodes, but also predicts more general maladjustment. The development of new comorbid nondepressive disorders, such as substance abuse, anxiety disorders, and personality disorders, is commonly observed; suicide and attempted suicide are also evident among those with juvenile onset of depression (e.g., Lewinsohn et al., 1999; Weissman et al., 1999). Studies that have included indicators of psychosocial functioning have reported significant social problems in early adulthood, such as marital/relationship discord, unwanted pregnancies, and occupational and economic impairment (Bardone et al., 1996; Gotlib, Lewinsohn, & Seeley, 1998; Rao et al., 1999; Weissman et al., 1999). Such disruptions occurring in highly formative periods of establishing family and work roles may signal high risk for recurrent depression and problematic environments.

THEORETICAL MODELS OF CHILDHOOD DEPRESSION

Theoretical conceptualizations of the etiology, concomitants, and consequences of childhood depression largely originated as adaptations of adult models. However, developmental psychopathologists have underscored the potential problems of uniformly applying adult models to children. This concern has provided an impetus for the introduction of developmentally sensitive models that account for the complex ontogenic processes involved in the evolution and persistence of vulnerability (see Cicchetti & Toth, 1998). We first present the major theoretical approaches, emphasizing developmental issues that arise when these models are applied to the child depression literature, and summarizing relevant empirical findings. Then we describe a multidimensional developmental model that integrates these separate theories. We present some representative examples of early studies, but highlight contemporary trends in theory and research during the past decade, including several recurring themes: (1) an emphasis on developmental perspectives; (2) an interest in understanding the origins of vulnerability factors and the mechanisms underlying their effects; (3) the use of prospective designs to distinguish among the causes, correlates, and consequences of depression; (4) a consideration of the specificity of theories and empirical findings to depression; and (5) an acknowledgment of depression comorbidity. The issue of comorbidity is particularly important to consider when one is interpreting the often inconsistent findings that emerge across studies, which may result in part from a failure to account for comorbid disorders.

Biological Models

Genetic Influences

The predominance of evidence concerning genetic influences on depression comes from studies of adult probands, which indicate clearly that show clear evidence that depression runs in families (for a review, see Sullivan, Neale, & Kendler, 2000). The results of family aggregation studies and biometric modeling based on twin populations suggest that a combination of genetic and environmental factors explain variance in depression. Recently, research has focused on genetic factors in child and adolescent depression.

There have been numerous "top-down" studies of children of depressed parents, with clear evidence of considerable risk to children for development of depressive, anxiety, and behavioral disorders and impaired functioning. Indeed, having a parent with major depression is one of the strongest predictive factors in childhood or adolescent depression (for a review, see Beardslee, Versage, & Gladstone, 1998). Over time, children of depressed parents may display considerable maladjustment, as well as recurrent depression (e.g., Hammen, Burge, Burney, & Adrian, 1990; Weissman, Warner, Wickramaratne, Moreau, & Olfson, 1997). Although genetic transmission of depression may be one explanation for such risk, these designs cannot rule out the influence of adverse psychosocial factors—such as disordered parent–child relationships, stressful life events and conditions, and parental marital/couple discord—which are common in families with depressed parents (for a review, see Goodman & Gotlib, 1999). The association of several of these factors with children's depression is reviewed in later sections of this chapter.

Several genetically informative studies with child probands have been conducted. Using different designs and samples, earlier studies reported heritability rates of about 35% (e.g., Rende, Plomin, Reiss, & Hetherington, 1993; Wierzbicki, 1987). More recently, a study of depressive symptoms in 411 British child and adolescent twin pairs by Thapar and McGuffin (1994) found much stronger evidence of heritability in adolescents, whereas children's depressive symptoms were strongly associated with environmental factors. Eaves et al. (1997) reported on a sample of 1,412 twin pairs aged 8–16 in the Virginia Twin Study of Adolescent Behavioral Development. They found a moderate genetic effect, and also significant individual environmental effects; however, the results differed by informant, and no age effects were reported. In a later analysis of the Virginia Twin Study data, Silberg et al. (1999) found increased heritability effects only for adolescent girls. About 30% of the variance in adolescent girls' depression was attributed to genetic effects, with the rest due to individual environmental effects. Interestingly, part of the genetic risk for depression appeared to be attributable to genetic effects on the occurrence of stressful life events.

Overall, results from genetic studies appear to vary by age, gender, and informant, as well as by whether symptoms or diagnoses (as well as mild or more severe depression) are the focus of attention. Replication and further elaboration of results are needed. Moreover, as with adult studies, it remains unclear what is inherited, with possibilities including traits of temperament and emotionality, stress generation and reactivity, and disordered neurobiological processes. Finally, in view of the evidently large impact of individual environmental factors, further studies that integrate genetic and psychosocial processes are needed.

Brain and Neurochemistry

Neuroendocrine Regulation and Neurotransmitters. There has been considerable interest in abnormalities of the hypothalamic–pituitary–adrenal (HPA) axis in adult depression, consistent with the possibility that depression is linked to dysregulation of the processes associated with responses to stress. Adult depressives commonly demonstrate three related abnormalities: higher basal cortisol, abnormal cortisol regulation indicated by the dexa-methasone suppression test (DST), and abnormalities of corticotropin-releasing factor (CRF). As reviewed by Birmaher et al. (1996) and Kaufman, Martin, King, and Charney (2001), however, similar patterns have not been observed consistently in child and adolescent samples. Basal cortisol secretion generally has not been shown to differ between depressed and normal children or adolescents; when group differences have been found, they tend to be subtle alternations in normal diurnal patterns (Kaufman et al., 2001). On the other hand, there is clear evidence of nonsuppression on the DST in child and adolescent samples, with rates generally similar to those of depressed adults. Somewhat higher rates of nonsuppression have been found in child than adolescent samples, and in inpatients than outpatients. Yet studies of CRF infusion generally have failed to show the same cortisol or corticotropin responses as those found in depressed adults (Kaufman et al., 2001).

Despite inconsistent evidence of disturbed HPA functioning in depressed youngsters, increasingly sophisticated models and methods suggest the desirability of continued study of neurohormonal stress processes. For instance, one important new line of research concerns the influence of exposure to severe stress on the developing brains of infants and children. There is considerable preclinical research suggesting that early exposure to adverse conditions promotes alterations in CRF circuits and behavioral changes consistent with depression and anxiety in animals (for a review, see Heim & Nemeroff, 2001). Moreover, these authors speculate—and present some support based on preclinical and some human data—that early adversity may be associated with abnormalities of HPA functioning, which sensitize the organism to subsequent stress. Consistent with this model, for example, Goodyer, Herbert, Tamplin, and Altham (2000b) found that among a group of 180 adolescents at risk for depression, those with high levels of either baseline cortisol or the adrenal steroid hormone dehydroepiandrosterone, as well as recent stressful life events, experienced major depressive episodes over a 1-year follow-up. It is possible that markers of HPA axis dysregulation—possibly acquired via early exposure to adversity or even genetically—may provide a susceptibility to depression or certain anxiety disorders when stressors are encountered. The various issues requiring further exploration include identifying (1) particular alterations in the brain and neuroregulatory systems of the developing organism exposed to stress, (2) developmental processes involved in stress responses, (3) effects of depressive experiences on subsequent neuroregulatory processes, and (4) specificity of such mechanisms to depressive disorders.

A further biological marker examined in relation to adult depression is growth hormone (GH). Adults with depression have been found to hyposecrete GH after various pharmacological challenges. Blunted GH response has also been observed during remission from depressive episodes, suggesting that it may be a stable marker or "scar" of depression (Dinan, 1998). Studies of responses of children and adolescents to growth hormone challenge paradigms have indicated similar patterns. For instance, Dahl et al. (2000) observed blunted responses to growth-hormone-releasing hormone (GHRH) in children diagnosed with major depressive disorder compared to normal controls. Moreover, the depressed children continued to display low GH response when retested during remission of their depression. Using the GHRH challenge procedure, Birmaher et al. (2000) compared youngsters who were at risk for depression (due to parental depression), but who had never been depressed, to low-risk children. As predicted, the high-risk youths secreted significantly less GH than the low-risk youths. These studies suggest that GH response may be a trait marker of predisposition to depression in children. Because most of the participants in these studies were children, the question of whether the results are generalizable to adolescents remains (e.g., Kaufman et al., 2001). In contrast to the GH probe studies, most research has failed to find robust evidence of *basal* GH differences, suggesting that an overall dysregulation of the GH process (rather than abnormal levels as such) is associated with risk for depression (e.g., Birmaher et al., 2000). To date, the precise role of GH secretion is unknown, but it appears to be a marker of central noradrenergic and serotonergic processes (Birmaher et al., 2000).

Serotonergic neurotransmitter processes, along with other catecholeamine neurotransmitters, have been strongly implicated in adult depression; this implication is based not only on pharmacological challenges (e.g., tryptophan depletion; Bremner et al., 1997), but also on the successful treatment of depressive disorders with selective serotonin reuptake inhibitors (SSRI). However, responses of children and adolescents to serotonergic probes have been varied and inconsistent with patterns observed in depressed adults (e.g., Kaufman et al., 2001). Moreover, it is well known that traditional tricyclic antidepressant medications have little therapeutic effect on children and adolescents, although studies have increasingly suggested positive effects of SSRIs (e.g., Emslie et al., 1997). In their review, Kaufman et al. (2001) suggest that there appear to be developmental differences in serotonergic and other neurotransmitter mechanisms, which require further exploration.

Sleep–Wake Cycle. Studies of dysfunctions in sleep behaviors and electroencephalographic patterns have been well established in depressed adults. Reviews of sleep studies in depressed children and adolescents, however, have shown that adolescent patterns are more similar to those of adults than are those of children (Birmaher et al., 1996; Kaufman et al., 2001). Reduced rapid-eye-movement (REM) latency is an especially consistent finding in adolescents, and increased REM density also is observed. Unlike studies of adults, however, no studies of youngsters have detected stage 3 and 4 (delta) sleep pattern differences. Clearly, developmental differences across the life cycle in the nature and function of sleep need to be taken into account in studies of sleep patterns as markers of mechanisms underlying depression.

Structural and Functional Brain Findings. Studies of the anatomy and neural circuitry of the adult brain have been the focus of considerable research in psychopathology generally, with much of the work based on samples of depressed adult patients. The vast scope of this work has included imaging studies of prefrontal cortex anatomy and function, and studies of the amygdala and hippocampus in particular (for a review, see Kaufman et al., 2001). To date, however, relatively little work has been conducted with depressed children using noninvasive imaging; such studies could help to detail developmental differences in both normal and depressed samples.

Electrophysiological research on frontal brain activity by Davidson and colleagues has resulted in a model of emotional reactivity in adults, which may have considerable promise as a vulnerability factor for negative emotional states such as depression (e.g., Davidson, 1993, 2000). He observed that depressed patients, and even previously depressed but remitted patients, showed relative left frontal hypoactivation. Davidson has proposed that decreased left prefrontal activation represents an underactivation of an approach system, thus reducing the person's experiencing of pleasure and motivation to interact positively with the environment, while increasing the likelihood of developing depressive symptoms. Interestingly, several studies have found that infants and toddlers of depressed mothers display relative left frontal hypoactivation (e.g., Dawson, Frey, Panagiotides, Osterling, & Hessl, 1997; Jones, Field, Fox, Lundy, & Davalos, 1997). Investigators have speculated that the patterns may be genetically transmitted—or acquired prenatally or in early stressful interactions with a depressed mother—and may represent a mechanism of risk for development of depression.

Cognitive Models

Cognitive theories emphasize the role of negative or maladaptive belief systems in the onset and course of disorder. Several significant advances in depression research have involved reformulations of cognitive theories. Most importantly, although original cognitive theories included an implicit or explicit emphasis on cognitive appraisals in the context of particular life experiences, early empirical studies most commonly assessed cognitions in isolation. In contrast, more recent work has embedded cognitive vulnerability within integrative models that more accurately reflect diathesis–stress perspectives on depression. Another recent trend has expanded on cognitive vulnerability by considering the intersection of cognitive and interpersonal models of depression. Finally, research has focused on investigating the developmental origins of cognitive vulnerability to depression. Progress in each of these areas is discussed in later sections.

Information-Processing/Cognitive Schemas

Cognitive theories were pioneered by Beck (e.g., Beck, Rush, Shaw, & Emery, 1979). Beck's information-processing model implicates three aspects of cognitive functioning in depression. First, depressed individuals are believed to engage in systematic biases or errors in thinking, which lead to idiosyncratic interpretations of situations and events—that is, negative "automatic thoughts." Second, depressed individuals are believed to exhibit negative cognitive "schemas," which are viewed as internal structures that guide information processing and stimulate the self-critical beliefs characteristic of depression. Finally, depression is associated with the "negative cognitive triad," or a tendency to possess negative perceptions of the self, world, and future (i.e., views of the self as worthless or inadequate, of the world as mean or unfair, and of the future as hopeless). The theory maintains that these cognitive styles heighten one's susceptibility to depression, especially when activated by external stressors. Because the rigid nature of cognitive schemas renders them highly resistant to change, depressed individuals may be vulnerable to persistent difficulties.

Early studies mainly gathered indirect support for the operation of depressogenic schemas by examining the end products of impaired information processing, such as self-critical beliefs or negative thoughts about the world (for reviews, see Garber & Hilsman, 1992; Kaslow, Adamson, & Collins, 2000; Weisz, Rudolph, Granger, & Sweeney, 1992). Studies have consistently linked depression to diminished self-worth, irrational beliefs, dysfunctional attitudes, negative automatic thoughts, and pessimism (Garber, Weiss, & Shanley, 1993; Gotlib, Lewinsohn, Seeley, Rohde, & Redner, 1993; Hops, Lewinsohn, Andrews, & Roberts, 1990; Kaslow, Rehm, & Siegel, 1984; Laurent & Stark, 1993). Other early studies demonstrated that depressed youths have biased information processing in the form of cognitive errors and maladaptive patterns of stimulus appraisal (e.g., Leitenberg, Yost, & Carroll-Wilson, 1986).

More direct investigations of information-processing theories have yielded mixed evidence for depressive biases. These studies typically have investigated two stages of information processing—attention and memory—through the use of laboratory paradigms. Studies of attentional processes usually have not revealed a significant bias toward depression-related words in depressed children (for a review, see Garber & Kaminski, 2000). In contrast, studies of memory biases have revealed idiosyncratic processing of self-referent adjectives (Hammen & Zupan, 1984; Neshat Doost, Taghavi, Moradi, Yule, & Dalgleish, 1998; Prieto, Cole, & Tageson, 1992); these negative self-schemas may emerge with increasing age (Cole & Jordan, 1995). Consistent with an information-processing perspective, depressed youths also engage in higher levels of self-verification (i.e., seeking out negative feedback) of negative self-views than nondepressed youths do (Joiner, Katz, & Lew, 1997).

Attributional Style/Control-Related Beliefs

A second set of cognitive theories involves reformulations of Seligman's (1975) learned helplessness model. The original version posited that depression stems from the experience of uncontrollable, noncontingent events. A revision of this model (Abramson, Seligman, & Teasdale, 1978) relies more heavily on cognitions by introducing the notion of a "depressive attributional style," or a predisposition to attribute negative outcomes to internal, global, and stable factors, and positive outcomes to external, specific, and unstable factors. In the most recent version of this model, Abramson, Metalsky, and Alloy (1989) have described a subtype of "hopelessness" depression, which evolves from the interaction between exposure to negative events and a depressogenic attributional style involving pessimistic expectations about the future. Related cognitive perspectives (e.g., Rehm, 1977; Weisz, Sweeney, Proffitt, & Carr, 1994) draw from theories of self-regulation, which emphasize the joint contribution of one's expectations regarding outcomes (e.g., perceptions of control and competence, outcome contingencies) and one's personal investment in outcomes (e.g., goals, standards, values) to the determination of behavior and emotion. For example, depressed individuals may engage in setting unrealistic and perfectionistic standards for themselves, or may believe that their efforts to achieve their goals will be futile. Competence-based models of depression focus in particular on the perceived-competence aspect of self-regulation (Cole, 1991; Cole, Martin, & Powers, 1997; Harter & Whitesell, 1996).

Cross-sectional studies have consistently linked depression with negative attributional style and hopelessness about the future (for reviews, see Garber & Hilsman, 1992; Gladstone & Kaslow, 1995). Both self-report questionnaires and laboratory tasks have also documented associations between depression and maladaptive control-related beliefs and self-regulatory processes (e.g., negative self-evaluation, standard setting, perfectionism) (Cole & Rehm, 1986; Kaslow et al., 1984; Kendall, Stark, & Adam, 1990; Weisz et al., 1994), although these findings have not always been consistent.

Recent Research and Commentary

Although ample evidence links child depression to dysfunctional attitudes about the self and biased cognitive appraisal processes, until recently many investigations of cognitive theories of depression suffered from relatively simple empirical designs that did not map onto the complexity of the conceptual models. Significant progress has been made to address some of the ongoing controversies and questions about the position of cognitive theories as useful conceptual frameworks. As a result of these efforts, cognitive theories remain central to understanding the etiology and persistence of depression.

Cognitive theories of depression have historically been presented as vulnerability models that emphasize the etiological significance of dysfunctional cognitions. Yet many studies have not included prospective designs suitable for testing causal mechanisms, leading investigators to question whether depressive cognitions represent antecedents, correlates, or consequences of depression (Haaga, Dyck, & Ernst, 1991). A related controversy concerns the status of depressive cognitions: Are they stable traits that operate regardless of mood state, or latent characteristics that are reactive to particular triggers or are accessible only in the context of a depressive state? Questions about the trait-like nature of depressive cognitions were heightened by early studies demonstrating instability during symptom remission, or a failure of cognitions to predict future depression (Gotlib et al., 1993; Hammen, Adrian, & Hiroto, 1988), although some studies have supported the predictive validity of dysfunctional cognitions in children (Lewinsohn, Roberts, et al., 1994; Nolen-Hoeksema, Girgus, & Seligman, 1992; Rudolph, Kurlakowsky, & Conley, 2001).

Others have argued that conclusions about the predictive validity and stability of depressive cognitions cannot be drawn from studies that overlook the contextual component of cognitive theories—namely, the fact that depressive cognitions may remain latent until activated by particular mood states or events (Abramson et al., 1989; Persons & Miranda, 1992). Two approaches have been used to test this idea. First, priming studies assess vulnerability under conditions of cognitive activation; such activation is achieved by using negative mood induction techniques that are presumed to prime depressogenic schemas. One study of at-risk children (the children of depressed mothers) supports this idea. Specifically, this at-risk group demonstrated less positive self-concepts and greater information-processing biases when primed with a negative mood induction than did low-risk children (Taylor & Ingram, 1999). Second, investigations of diathesis–stress models provide more direct tests of the assumption that depressogenic cognitions are triggered by negative life events. These models are discussed in more detail in our section on life stress models. In brief, recent research using a diathesis–stress approach supports many of the more specific claims of cognitive theories.

Contemporary research on cognitive models of depression has also benefited from the application of more developmentally sensitive frameworks. Developmental issues that have been addressed include the bidirectional influence of cognitions and depression, changes in the association between cognitions and depression across age, and the origins of cognitive vulnerability to depression.

Although dysfunctional cognitions have been found to predict future depressive symptoms, several studies have revealed reciprocal influences of depression on subsequent cognitions. For example, Nolen-Hoeksema et al. (1992) noted a *deterioration* in attributional style following depression onset, and stability of pessimistic attributions even after a significant decline in symptoms. The authors interpreted these results as evidence that depression may leave a cognitive "scar," by leading children to develop a negative explanatory style. Similarly, Cole, Martin, Peeke, Seroczynski, and Hoffman (1998) have shown that depressive symptoms predict future underestimation of competence (see also McGrath & Repetti, 2002). Expanding on this model, Pomerantz and Rudolph (2002) found that negative views of self and the world mediated the association between negative affect and subsequent underestimation of competence. Together, these studies demonstrate the need to consider the interplay between cognitions and depression across development.

Recent cognitive perspectives also have emphasized possible developmental differences in the cognition–depression association. Several studies have revealed that the link between attributional style and depression becomes stronger across age (Abela, 2001; Nolen-Hoeksema et al., 1992; Turner & Cole, 1994). It has therefore been suggested that stable cognitive vulnerability may emerge over time as children develop the capacity for more abstract reasoning and generalization about the future (Turner & Cole, 1994).

Progress in elaborating on developmental aspects of cognitive models has also been made through the generation of theory and empirical research regarding the antecedents of cognitive vulnerability. Until recently, relatively little was known about how depression-related cognitions develop over time. However, several models have now been proposed to account for the emergence of negative cognitions. These models focus on the role of social learning, socialization by parents, exposure to early disruptions, current stressful contexts, and negative environmental feedback in precipitating depressogenic views of self and the world. Several studies have provided support for these models. For example, maternal negative attributional style, family disruptions (e.g., parent–child separations), parent socialization styles, external appraisals of competence, and stressful life circumstances have been found to predict several types of depression-related cognitions over time (Alloy et al., 2001; Cole, Jacquez, & Maschman, 2001; Garber & Flynn, 2001; Rudolph, Kurlakowsky, & Conley, 2001). These studies suggest that children not only learn to imitate maternal cognitive styles through observation, but also internalize aversive interactions and stressful events in the form of self-blaming cognitive styles, negative beliefs about their own self-worth and adequacy, and a sense of uncertainty or hopelessness about future outcomes in their lives.

Another advance involves the extension of traditional cognitive theories to the interpersonal domain by considering not only self-representations, but also representations of relationships (Blatt & Homann, 1992; Cummings & Cicchetti, 1990; Hammen, 1992a; Rudolph, Hammen, & Burge, 1997). Indeed, research has shown that depressive symptoms are associated with negative interpersonal expectancies and perceptions, biased processing of interpersonal information, and maladaptive relationship-oriented beliefs (Hammen et al., 1995; Rudolph & Clark, 2001; Rudolph et al., 1997; Shirk, Van Horn, & Leber, 1997). This research forms an important basis for building cognitive–interpersonal models of depression (see Gotlib & Hammen, 1992), which are discussed in more detail in the section on integrative models.

Behavioral/Interpersonal Models

Traditional behavioral models conceptualized depression as a consequence of skill deficits and an ensuing inability to elicit positive feedback. For example, Lewinsohn (1974) viewed depression as a reaction to low rates of response-contingent positive reinforcement. This lack of positive feedback may result from competence deficits that interfere with the achievement of success or the formation of satisfactory relationships, from the unavailability of reinforcers in the environment, or from a decreased ability to appreciate positive experiences. Any one of these sources of reduced reinforcement may lead to withdrawal, further functional impairment, and intensified feelings of depression. Similarly, in their competence-based model of depression, Cole and colleagues (Cole, Martin, Powers, & Truglio, 1996; Cole, Martin, & Powers, 1997) suggest that negative competence-related feedback is internalized by the child in the form of negative self-perceptions, which increase risk for depression. Building on these models, interpersonal theories of depression have emphasized the transactional nature of social experience. In this vein, researchers have argued that depressive symptoms and qualities of depression-prone individuals may foster problematic relationships (Coyne, 1976; Gotlib & Hammen, 1992; Hammen, 1992a; Joiner, Coyne, & Blalock, 1999). These interactional perspectives regard the link between depression and social impairment as a bidirectional partnership, in that depressed individuals both *react* and *contribute* to interpersonal difficulties. Thus depressive behaviors may provoke aversive interpersonal encounters and rejection, which maintain or heighten depressed affect. A growing data base confirms the presence of social impairment and other competence deficits in depressed youngsters, including difficulties in relationships; maladaptive problem solving, coping, and emotion regulation; and school-related dysfunction.

Interpersonal Relationships

Much of the early research on interpersonal relationships in depressed children relied on self-reports of social competence and quality of peer relations. This work has consistently linked depressive symptoms with decreased perceptions of competence and poor peer relationships and friendships (for reviews, see Gotlib & Hammen, 1992; Weisz et al., 1992). Reports of problematic interpersonal styles range from increased impulsivity and aggression to decreased social activity, passivity, and withdrawal. Consistent with self-perceptions, teachers report deficits in prosocial behavior and higher levels of aggression and withdrawal in depressed children (Rudolph & Clark, 2001). Interviews of depressed children and their parents also reveal impairments in the ability to form high-quality friendships (Goodyer, Wright, & Altham, 1990; Puig-Antich et al., 1993). Not surprisingly, given these deficits, depressed children tend to be described by peers and teachers as less popular and more socially rejected or isolated than their nondepressed counterparts (Cole, 1990; Patterson & Stoolmiller, 1991; Rudolph & Clark, 2001; Rudolph, Hammen, & Burge, 1994).

Only a few studies have used observational methods to examine the peer interactions of depressed children. In one inpatient sample, depressed youths were found to engage in less social activity and to exhibit less affect-related expression than nondepressed psychiatric controls (Kazdin, Esveldt-Dawson, Sherick, & Colbus, 1985). Altmann and Gotlib (1988) discovered that depressive symptoms in school children were associated with a greater amount of time spent alone on the playground and with more aversive and aggressive behavior. Assessing more specific interpersonal behaviors, Rudolph et al. (1994) found that children with depressive symptoms showed more difficulty negotiating peer conflict and more emotional dysregulation during stressful peer encounters. Moreover, several observational studies have revealed that depressed children elicit negative reactions from peers during dyadic transactions (Baker, Milich, & Manolis, 1996; Connolly, Geller, Marton, & Kutcher, 1992; Rudolph et al., 1994). Interestingly, recent research has confirmed early predictions of interpersonal theories that a tendency to engage in excessive reassurance seeking may in part explain this interpersonal disruption in the peer relationships of depressed youths (for a review, see Joiner, Metalsky, Katz, & Beach, 1999).

Social Problem Solving, Coping, and Emotion Regulation

Another line of research has been directed toward identifying specific competence deficits in the form of dysfunctional problem solving, coping, and emotion regulation. In general, studies have revealed that depressed children endorse fewer sociable and assertive and more hostile problem-solving strategies (Quiggle, Garber, Panak, & Dodge, 1992; Rudolph, Kurlakowsky, & Conley, et al., 1994). Moreover, depression is linked to lower levels of active or problem-focused coping, and elevated levels of passive or ruminative coping and helpless responses to challenge (Ebata & Moos, 1991; Herman-Stahl & Petersen, 1999; Nolen-Hoeksema et al., 1992; Rudolph, Kurlakowsky, & Conley, 2001). Depressed youngsters may experience particular difficulty regulating their emotions in arousing situations (Zahn-Waxler, Klimes-Dougan, & Slattery, 2000). For example, depressed children and adolescents are more likely to show increased avoidance and descreased assertiveness in the face of negative affect or conflict (Garber, Braafladt, & Zeman, 1991; Kobak & Ferenz-Gillies, 1995). These coping and emotion-regulating responses are similar to those observed in depressed adults, who display a passive/ruminative response style that entails excessive attention to depressive symptoms and their potential causes and consequences, and that interferes with active and effective problem solving (Nolen-Hoeksema, 1991). In recent years, increasingly complex, multidimensional models of coping have been generated that will allow for more fine-grained analyses of particular types of responses to stress and challenge in depressed children (e.g., Compas, Connor-Smith, Saltzman, Thomsen, & Wadsworth, 2001).

Achievement and School-Related Functioning

Contradictory evidence exists as to whether depression is associated with academic and cognitive difficulties. Studies have linked depression to lower *perceived* cognitive competence and negative academic self-concept (Asarnow, Carlson, & Guthrie, 1987). Some investigators have found an association between depressive symptoms and impaired cognitive performance on laboratory tasks (Ward, Friedlander, & Silverman, 1987), whereas others have reported no differences between depressed and nondepressed children in actual performance, despite discrepancies in self-evaluation (Kendall et al., 1990). Studies using academic grades as the criterion have generally shown significant negative associations between depressive symptoms and grades (Forehand, Brody, Long, & Fauber, 1988). As early as first grade, depression is associated with compromised academic achievement and concentration problems (Ialongo, Edelsohn, Werthamer-Larson, Crockett, & Kellam, 1996). Finally, interviews with depressed adolescents and their mothers reveal more behavior problems at school, less positive relationships with teachers, and lower academic achievement in comparison to nonpsychiatric controls (Puig-Antich et al., 1993).

Multidimensional Competence-Based Models

In an effort to examine the joint contribution of multiple competence domains to depression, several investigators have evaluated multidimensional competence-based models (Blechman, McEnroe, Carella, & Audette, 1986; Cole et al., 1996; Patterson & Stoolmiller, 1991; Seroczynski, Cole, & Maxwell, 1997). Findings from these studies confirm that deficits in different competence domains (e.g., academic, social, behavioral) exert cumulative effects on depression, although social incompetence often emerges as a stronger predictor than other competence difficulties.

Recent Research and Commentary

Considerable evidence indicates that depressed children demonstrate behavioral and interpersonal deficits and encounter negative feedback and aversive interpersonal environments in their everyday lives. Yet controversy has arisen regarding several aspects of behavioral and interpersonal models of child depression. Advances in both theory and empirical research have addressed some of these issues and have provided a more sophisticated perspective on these models.

Progress on the theoretical front is reflected in the elucidation of the likely cyclical processes linking interpersonal disruption and depression (Gotlib & Hammen, 1992; Joiner, Coyne, & Blalock, 1999). That is, competence difficulties are presumed to evoke negative interpersonal consequences that lead to depressive symptoms, which then create further dysfunctional behaviors and negative feedback that perpetuate or exacerbate symptoms. Consistent with this feedback loop, longitudinal research has provided support for both directions of influence—skill deficits and interpersonal problems leading to depression, and depression leading to incompetence and troubled relationships. In support of the etiological role of interpersonal difficulties, investigators have demonstrated that social difficulties and poor-quality friendships predict increases in depression over time (Boivin, Hymel, & Bukowski, 1995; Cole et al., 1996; Goodyer et al., 1990; Panak & Garber, 1992). Furthermore, longitudinal studies have revealed that the interpersonal difficulties displayed by depressed children are enduring characteristics that remain even when symptoms have remitted (Lewinsohn, Roberts, et al., 1994; Puig-Antich et al., 1985b). Together, these findings suggest that impaired social functioning and low rates of environmental reinforcement constitute a risk factor for depression onset or relapse.

Nevertheless, other research demonstrates that depression impairs competence. For example, depressive symptoms have been found to predict helpless behavior (Nolen-Hoeksema et al., 1992) and academic problems (Ialongo, Edelsohn, & Kellam, 2001) over time. Observational research also reveals that depressed children induce negative affect and elicit aversive responses from unfamiliar peers (Baker et al., 1996; Connolly et al. 1992; Rudolph et al., 1994), suggesting that characteristics of the depressed children undermine the quality of their interactions. In sum, research supports the continued examination of transactional models that consider the interplay between interpersonal impairment and depression.

Theoretical advances also have been made in reconciling cognitive and interpersonal models of depression. Although cognitive models traditionally view the negative belief systems of depressed youngsters as biased, the presence of significant competence deficits in depressed individuals suggests that negative cognitions actually may represent accurate appraisals of personal deficits and environmental realities. Recent efforts to elucidate this issue provide support for both the cognitive distortion and the skill deficit models. In one study, perceptions of self and peers were compared in depressed and nondepressed children with different levels of social status. Consistent with a skill deficit model, depressed children were sensitive to actual differences in their social status; that is, depressed/unpopular children endorsed more negative conceptions of relationships than did depressed/accepted children. However, consistent with a cognitive distortion model, comparisons of depressed and nondepressed children within the same social status categories revealed that the conceptions of depressed children were more negative than was warranted by their social status (Rudolph & Clark, 2001). In another systematic effort to address this issue, Cole, Martin, et al. (1998) have shown that depression is associated with the underestimation of competence relative to others' evaluations, but this cognitive tendency seems to be more a consequence than a predictor of depression. This work clearly points to the importance of supplementing self-reports of interpersonal functioning with other types of measures.

Family Models

A major emphasis in contemporary developmental psychopathology models of depression is placed on the contribution of family influences to the etiology of depression. In earlier sections, we have discussed genetic contributions; here we focus on psychosocial factors within the family.

Psychodynamic Theories

Disruptions of caregiving relationships figured prominently in early etiological formulations of depression. Psychoanalytic and object relations theories both proposed the experience of loss as a primary vulnerability factor for depression —either actual physical loss through death or separation, or symbolic loss through emotional deprivation, rejection, or inadequate parenting (Fairbairn, 1952; Freud, 1917/1957). These theories held in common the notion that depression arises from anger or hostility that initially is felt toward the lost object, but then is directed inward in the form of self-criticism. Because children historically were believed to lack introjective abilities, early theories failed to recognize the occurrence of childhood depression. Rather, their emphasis lay in explaining how problematic childhood relationships may contribute to risk for depression in adults.

Attachment Theory

Contemporary conceptualizations have expanded on these approaches to account for early onset of depression. Most notably, attachment theory focuses on the adverse impact of dysfunctional parent–child relationships on children's subsequent functioning (Bowlby, 1969, 1980). Bowlby contended that establishment of a secure attachment relationship is dependent upon the ability of the caregiver to impart a sense of security and trust to the infant and to comfort the infant when distressed. In the absence of conditions that would cultivate a healthy bond (e.g., accessibility, contingent responsivity, emotional supportiveness), the infant presumably becomes vulnerable to later adjustment problems. Based on Bowlby's original work that hypothesized depressive (and other psychopathological) reactions to disruptions in the attachment bond, theorists have implicated insecure attachment and ensuing "internal working models" of relationships (Bowlby, 1969, 1980; Main, Kaplan, & Cassidy, 1985) as specific risk factors for depression (e.g., Blatt & Homann, 1992; Cummings & Cicchetti, 1990; Hammen, 1992a).

Complementing these conceptual advances, a considerable body of evidence has been gathered documenting an association between family experiences and childhood depression. Two separate areas of research have yielded important information about family functioning: studies of interactions between depressed parents and their offspring (high-risk studies), and studies of the families of depressed youngsters (for reviews, see Goodman & Gotlib, 1999; Gotlib & Hammen, 1992; Kaslow, Deering, & Racusin, 1994).

Parent–Child Relationships: High-Risk Studies

As discussed earlier, the observed aggregation of depression in families may be due in part to genetic factors, but evidence indicates the additional influence of psychosocial factors in maintaining this generational cycle (Goodman & Gotlib, 1999; Hammen, 1991a). Specifically, a burgeoning body of research attests to ongoing and pervasive patterns of dysfunctional interactions in families with affectively disordered parents (for reviews, see Cummings & Davies, 1999; Gelfand & Teti, 1990; Goodman & Gotlib, 1999; Hammen, 1991a). Because of the high risk for depression in offspring, these studies may advance our understanding of family processes relevant to child depression.

In the period since Weissman, Paykel, and Klerman (1972) reported a variety of persisting interactional difficulties among clinically depressed women with their children and families, there have been many studies of mother–child interactions as a possible mediator of the maladaptive impact of parental depression. Observations of mother–infant interactions (based largely on nonclinical samples) often revealed two common patterns: one of withdrawal and disengagement, flat affect, and lack of contingent responding (e.g., Field, Healy, Goldstein, & Guthertz, 1990), and one of hostility and intrusiveness (e.g., Cohn, Matias, Tronick, Connell, & Lyons-Ruth, 1986). Similar patterns of decreased responsiveness and involvement or increased negativity were seen in observations of depressed mothers with their toddler and preschool children (e.g., Breznitz & Sherman, 1987; Goodman & Brumley, 1990; Radke-Yarrow, 1998) and their school-age children and adolescents (e.g., Gordon et al., 1989; Hops et al., 1987; Radke-Yarrow, 1998).

Recent research has attempted to clarify the parenting characteristics that are most likely to be associated with children's depression and other adverse outcomes. Lovejoy, Graczyk, O'Hare, and Neuman (2000) identified three variables representing the foci of most studies of depressed mothers and their children: negative/hostile interactions (negative affect, criticism, negative facial expression); positive behaviors (pleasant affect, praise, affectionate contact); and disengagement (ignoring, withdrawal, silence, gaze aversion). A meta-analysis of 46 somewhat overlapping studies revealed several significant patterns (Lovejoy et al., 2000). Overall, depressed mothers differed significantly from nondepressed mothers, displaying more negative and disengaged behaviors (associated with moderate effect sizes) and fewer positive behaviors (characterized by small effect sizes). The effects of possible moderating variables were also explored, including timing of depression (current or lifetime), SES, nature of depression, child age, and type of observation. The most noteworthy effect was that negative interactions were more pronounced among currently depressed women than among those with lifetime diagnoses; no other moderators were significant (Lovejoy et al., 2000).

The Lovejoy et al. (2000) meta-analysis confirms prior observations that depression is associated with maladaptive parenting. However, the meaning and mechanisms of the effects remain unclear. As noted in a detailed review by Goodman and Gotlib (1999), there are many possible contributors to offspring risk, and parenting behaviors are embedded in complex and maladaptive environmental conditions, so that it may be difficult to determine the extent to which parenting behaviors as such affect children's outcomes. Several studies have suggested that quality of parenting behaviors does indeed predict children's adjustment (e.g., Hammen, Burge, & Stansbury, 1990; Johnson, Cohen, Kasen, Smailes, & Brook, 2001; National Institute of Child Health and Human Development [NICHD] Early Child Care Research Network, 1999). Considerable work is needed to clarify the mechanisms of the effects, however, as will be discussed at the end of this section.

Parent–Child Relationships: Parents of Depressed Children

Until recently, much of the research examining the family functioning of depressed children relied on self-report measures. Investigators have assessed various parenting dimensions (including warmth/acceptance vs. rejection, and autonomy vs. control/overprotection), as well as more general aspects of parent–child relationships (such as attachment, trust, support, and availability). This research has consistently revealed more negative perceptions of family interactions in depressed than in nondepressed children. Collectively, these studies have linked depression to many types of perceived family dysfunction, including decreased parental psychological availability (Kaslow et al., 1984) and acceptance (Rudolph et al., 1997), decreased family support (Hops et al., 1990), and insecure parent–child attachment (Pappini, Roggman, & Anderson, 1991; Pavlidis & McCauley, 2001). Similarly, studies of young adults reveal a link between depression and recall of early parent–child relationships characterized by low maternal care, nurturance, and affection, and high punitiveness, rejection, and overprotection (Lamont, Fischoff, & Gottlieb, 1976; Parker, 1981; for a review, see Blatt & Homann, 1992).

Although self-reports of family relationships are subject to reporting biases that may be influenced by depressed mood, these patterns typically have been corroborated by other methods. For example, interviews with the parents of depressed children revealed that mother–child relationships were marked by poorer communication, decreased warmth, and increased hostility compared to those of nondepressed groups (Puig-Antich et al., 1993). Examination of family variables during and after children's depressive episodes revealed only partial improvement after recovery (Puig-Antich et al., 1985a, 1985b). Moreover, research in the area of expressed emotion has revealed higher levels of criticism and emotional overinvolvement in the descriptions made by parents about their depressed children than about nondepressed children (Asarnow, Tompson, Hamilton, Goldstein, & Guthrie, 1994).

Disruption in family relationships has been confirmed in a few observational studies. Such observations reveal that the mothers of depressed children set higher standards for their children's success (Cole & Rehm, 1986); are more dominant in parent–child interactions (Kobak, Sudler, & Gamble, 1991); and show less support, validation, and positive behavior (e.g., smiling, approving) toward their children (Messer & Gross, 1995; Sheeber & Sorenson, 1998). Depressed youths in turn demonstrate less effective problem solving, fewer supportive and positive behaviors, less positive communication (Forehand et al., 1988; Messer & Gross, 1995; Sheeber & Sorenson, 1998), and less autonomous assertion (Kobak & Ferenz-Gillies, 1995) during parent–child interactions than nondepressed youths do. Less consistent evidence is available to support overtly hostile or conflictual behavior in depressed children or their parents, despite higher self-reported levels of family conflict (e.g., Sheeber & Sorenson, 1998).

Contextual Family Variables

In addition to specific aversive qualities of parent–child interactions, other negative family circumstances have been linked to depression. Substantial data indicate differences in the family atmosphere and home environment of depressed youngsters and offspring of depressed parents, including increased family, marital/couple, and sibling discord (Cole & McPherson, 1993; Kashani, Burbach, & Rosenberg, 1988; Kaslow et al., 1994). Families with depressed members are perceived as less cohesive and adaptable, less open to emotional expressiveness, less democratic, more hostile and rejecting, more conflictual and disorganized, and less likely to engage in pleasant activities (e.g., Hops et al., 1990; McKeown et al., 1997; Oliver, Handal, Finn, & Herdy, 1987; Sheeber & Sorenson, 1998). Moreover, an aversive family environment predicts future depressive symptoms in children (Garrison et al., 1990; Sheeber, Hops, Alpert, Davis, & Andrews, 1997).

Parental and child depression also occur in the context of increased family stressors, including negative life events and chronic strain—for example, marital/couple discord, maternal adversity, decreased family support, and abuse and neglect (Goodyer, Wright, & Altham, 1988; Hammen et al., 1987; Kashani & Carlson, 1987). Moreover, using microanalytic behavioral observation techniques, research has demonstrated that children's responses to aversive interparental behavior predicted increases in subsequent depression (Davis, Sheeber, Hops, & Tildesley, 2000), confirming that general family discord creates risk for depression in children.

Recent Research and Commentary

Research examining depression within the family context has reflected several critical trends over the past decade. Much of the earlier evidence about family dysfunction came from offspring studies, whereas recent studies have placed an increasing focus on the families of depressed children. These two distinct areas of investigation are important for determining whether similar processes apply to these two groups. Also, the growing use of multiple assessment methods (e.g., Sheeber et al., 1997) has added much to our knowledge in this area by addressing the possible biases of self-report data.

Another important empirical advance, which has substantial implications for emerging theories of family relations and depression, is the use of prospective designs. Because much of the early research on family adjustment was cross-sectional in nature, questions concerning the direction of influence between family dysfunction and child depression could not be answered. Although one feasible hypothesis would assign problematic parent–child relationships and stressful family environments an etiological role in depression, other processes must be considered. First, the observed associations may reflect the operation of a third variable (such as a common genetic vulnerability) that underlies parental psychopathology and parenting difficulties, and at the same time increases children's susceptibility to depression.

Second, we must consider an alternate pathway whereby children's symptoms or dysfunctional behavior evoke negative responses from their parents and impede adaptive family functioning. Indeed, evidence supports this type of transactional framework. Hammen and colleagues tested a bidirectional model and found that depressed mothers and their offspring exerted mutual negative influences on each other (Hammen, Burge, & Stansbury, 1990; Radke-Yarrow, 1998). Likewise, Messer and Gross (1995) observed more negative interchanges and less positive reciprocity between depressed children and their parents than in nondepressed families. Thus impaired parental behavior may result partly from the unrewarding nature of interactions with a depressed child. Researchers therefore may do well to include a stronger emphasis on the reciprocal nature of parent–child relationships, the behavior of depressed children during family interactions, and the more global impact of child depression on the family.

A third explanation for family–depression linkages may be that maladaptive family patterns represent state-dependent concomitants of the acute episode of illness. On balance, however, relevant research tends to find that family interaction problems are relatively stable even when symptoms remit (e.g., Billings & Moos, 1985; Puig-Antich et al., 1985b). Moreover, a growing body of research assessing temporal associations between family relationships and depression has yielded support for causal hypotheses by showing that the quality of parent–child interactions and the quality of the family environment predict changes in children's depression over time (Asarnow, Goldstein, Tompson, & Guthrie, 1993; Hops et al., 1990; McKeown et al., 1997; Sheeber et al., 1997).

Finally, recent research has only just begun to move beyond the documentation of dysfunction in the families of depressed individuals to specify the mechanisms by which parental depression and family disturbances confer risk for depression in youngsters. Understanding these processes no doubt will require adopting a developmental perspective that considers stage-specific consequences of parental depression and dysfunctional parenting. Maladaptive parent–child interactions associated with depression may interfere with the mastery of different developmental tasks throughout childhood, leading to insecure attachment and poor emotion regulation, as well as to a failure to acquire skills necessary for effective interpersonal behavior, problem solving, and conflict resolution. Decreased stimulation and contingent responding also may result in suboptimal cognitive development. These deficits may leave children with poor coping skills and dysfunctional cognitions about themselves and others, eventually leading to impaired social functioning and depressive reactions (see Goodman & Gotlib, 1999). Thus ineffective parenting may influence children's risk for depression through different channels across development, and the specific influence of parental depression may depend on the age at which a child is exposed.

Preliminary research supports the role of several mechanisms of vulnerability in the children of depressed parents. For example, there is some evidence from observational studies that dysfunctional styles of parent–child interaction are indeed associated with maladaptive social skills and problem-solving deficits, attachment difficulties, and other indicators of impairment that might eventuate in depression (e.g., Goodman, Brogan, Lynch, & Fielding, 1993; Jaenicke et al., 1987; NICHD Early Child Care Research Network, 1999; Teti, Gelfand, Messinger, & Isabella, 1995). The NICHD Early Child Care Research Network (1999) study is an elegant example of attempts to clarify processes linking maternal depression and children's outcomes over a longitudinal course, evaluating quality of mother–child interaction as a moderator. This study found that observed maternal sensitivity among depressed women toward their infants moderated the effects of the depression, in that relatively more sensitive and responsive women had children with better language development and fewer behavioral problems at 36 months (NICHD Early Child Care Research Network, 1999).

Depression in parents has also been linked to cognitive vulnerability in children. The offspring of depressed parents manifest low self-worth, negative attributional styles, and hopelessness (Garber & Flynn, 2001). Moreover, this group displays more negatively biased processing of self-referent information when in a negative mood state than a low-risk group does (Taylor & Ingram, 1999). These negative views of self and the world may arise through modeling of parental cognitive styles, internalization of negative parental feedback, and reactions to maladaptive parenting styles (Garber & Flynn, 2001; Garber, Robinson, & Valentiner, 1997; Goodman, Adamson, Riniti, & Cole, 1994; Randolph & Dykman, 1998).

Elaborating on possible interpersonal mechanisms of transmission, Hammen and Brennan (2001) have suggested that one of the pathways to depression among offspring of depressed mothers is through persisting interpersonal difficulties. They found that depressed adolescents of depressed mothers were significantly more impaired interpersonally than were depressed adolescents of nondepressed mothers, despite lack of differences in the severity of current depression. These results may imply risk for more recurrent depression in the offspring of depressed mothers, to the extent that their interpersonal difficulties create stressors that trigger depressive experiences.

Finally, mother–infant interactions associated with maternal depression may influence the development of neural circuits for emotion expression and regulation (e.g., Dawson et al., 1997; Goodman & Gotlib, 1999). These changes in brain structure or function may then leave children at risk for emotion dysregulation and consequent sensitivity to depression.

Additional work of this sort is needed to examine other pathways through which depression vulnerability is transmitted across generations. This process is most likely to involve multiple pathways—including genetic and biological risk factors, deficits in children's behavioral competence, increases in exposure to stress in the family context, decreases in family support, and changes in the ways in which children view themselves and the world.

Life Stress Models

Life stress theories of depression have progressed in complexity in the past two decades. This evolution has been described in depth elsewhere (Garber & Hilsman, 1992; Gotlib & Hammen, 1992; Hammen, 1992b); below we briefly summarize several variants of the life stress approach. Advances in life stress theory and research are discussed, including focused efforts to examine diathesis–stress models of depression, attempts to understand the pathways linking stress and depression, the identification of specific types of stress that constitute risk for depression, and elaboration of transactional approaches to life stress research.

Stress Exposure Models

The original life stress theories viewed depression as a response to the experience of negative life events (Brown & Harris, 1978; Paykel, 1979). From this perspective, stress is viewed as a precursor and contributor to depression onset, persistence, or recurrence. To avoid the confounds associated with symptom-related stress, researchers initially concentrated on "fateful" life events, or events whose occurrence is independent of an individual. Furthermore, to avoid the confounds associated with idiosyncratic *perceptions* of events, researchers used the "contextual threat" method (Brown & Harris, 1978) to determine the *objective* impact of stress, independent of individuals' subjective reactions.

A great deal of attention has been paid to testing life stress models of depression in children. Early studies supported concurrent links between stress and depression across development (e.g., Kashani et al., 1986, with preschoolers; Mullins et al., 1985, with school-age children; Goodyer et al., 1990, with children and adolescents; Burt, Cohen, & Bjorck, 1988, and Hops et al., 1990, with adolescents). Longitudinal studies also have supported stress exposure models by demonstrating that the experience of stress precedes the onset, recurrence, and exacerbation of depressive symptoms (e.g., Ge, Lorenz, Conger, Elder, & Simons, 1994; Goodyer, Herbert, Tamplin, & Altham, 2000a).

Diathesis–Stress Models

Diathesis–stress models view depression as a function of the interaction between personal vulnerability and external stress. Most commonly, as discussed earlier, vulnerability has been construed as a stable cognitive propensity toward depression-inducing interpretations of events. Exposure to events is presumed to serve as a trigger that activates this underlying cognitive predisposition. Even more specifically, several theorists have speculated that a key determinant of depression may be the *match* between a particular cognitive vulnerability and the nature of the stressful event. In this respect, psychodynamic, cognitive, and life stress models converge in the notion that individual vulnerability may be understood in terms of a tendency to base one's self-worth either on success in interpersonal relationships (called "dependency" or "sociotropy") or on individual achievement/mastery (called "autonomy") (Beck, 1983; Blatt & Homann, 1992). Negative events would therefore induce depression to the extent that they precipitate a loss of self-worth in an individual's specific area of vulnerability.

A growing number of researchers have examined cognition–stress interactions, allowing for more comprehensive tests of both cognitive and life stress theories of depression. Several studies have discovered significant interactions (Lewinsohn, Joiner, & Rohde, 2001; Robinson, Garber, & Hilsman, 1995), with results often stronger for older than for younger children (Abela, 2001; Turner & Cole, 1994). Support for diathesis–stress models has also been obtained in studies using broader conceptualizations of stress beyond life events. For example, conceptualizing stress as an increase in peer rejection, Panak and Garber (1992) found that attributional style moderated the impact of stress on depressive symptoms 1 year later. Conceptualizing stress in terms of the experience of a stressful developmental transition—namely entrance into middle school—Rudolph, Lambert, Clark, and Kurlakowsky (2001) found that maladaptive self-regulatory beliefs predicted increases in depressive symptoms over a 6-month period in adolescents who experienced a stressful transition but not in adolescents who did not.

Only a few studies have tested cognition–stress "match" models in depressed children. Turner and Cole (1994) found that cognitions about the social and academic domains moderated the effects of negative daily events and activities in the same domain in older children. Hammen and Goodman-Brown (1990) assessed the relative value placed by each *individual* child on particular competence domains (interpersonal vs. achievement). As predicted, the authors found an increased risk for the development of depression only in those children who experienced a preponderance of negative life events congruent with their specific vulnerabilities, particularly for the interpersonal schema types. Similarly, negative interpersonal beliefs and schemas have been found to confer risk for depression in the face of interpersonal stress (Hammen et al., 1995; Shirk, Boergers, Eason, & Van Horn, 1998). Such studies confirm the need for a focus on domain-specific negative cognitions.

Mediation Models

An aspect of life stress models that has not been well elaborated concerns the *process* by which stress increases risk for depression. In an effort to understand possible developmental differences in cognition–stress interactions, Cole and colleagues (Cole & Turner, 1993; Tram & Cole, 2000) have argued that the absence of stable cognitive styles in early childhood diminishes the likelihood that negative cognitions moderate the impact of stress on depression. Instead, they have suggested that adverse environmental events or other forms of pathogenic feedback are internalized in the form of negative cognitions, which then predispose the child to depression. In this case, depressogenic cognitions would *arise from* rather than *interact with* life stress. Other similar models have been proposed, wherein stressful life circumstances contribute to the development of maladaptive cognitions that increase risk for depression (Alloy et al., 2001; Garber & Flynn, 2001; Rudolph, Kurlakowsky, & Conley, 2001). Preliminary tests of these models have provided support for the proposed pathways. Continued research is needed to identify other mechanisms linking life stress with depression.

Stress Generation Models

Whereas traditional life stress research focused on "fateful" life events, Hammen (1991b, 1992b) has proposed an alternative stress generation model of depression. This model suggests that depression and associated characteristics may promote dysfunction, such that depressed individuals actually *generate* stressful circumstances, which in turn trigger depressive reactions. To apply this model to children, early onset of depression may interrupt normal development and the acquisition of skills, leading to stress and risk for future maladjustment.

Several studies have provided support for a stress generation model in children. Depressive symptoms have been linked to self-generated stress, particularly within interpersonal relationships (Rudolph & Hammen, 1999; Rudolph et al., 2000; Williamson, Birmaher, Anderson, Al-Shabbout, & Ryan, 1995). Moreover, the offspring of depressed mothers have been found to display significantly higher rates of life events that they at least partially caused (Adrian & Hammen, 1993). These results are compatible with the hypothesis that life stress may be not only a *cause* of subsequent symptoms, but also a *consequence* of disorder-related impairment; yet they leave open the question of whether depression precedes event occurrence. In a prospective study of stress generation, Cohen, Burt, and Bjorck (1987) demonstrated that depressive symptoms in adolescents predicted the occurrence of subsequent controllable negative events, whereas controllable stress failed to predict subsequent symptoms.

Miscellaneous Environmental Influences

Investigators have also assessed the impact of other environmental and demographic risk factors and adverse conditions on child depression. For example, depression has been linked to social disadvantage, parental unemployment, remarriage of a parent, living in a single-parent household, and coming from a larger family (for a review, see Kaslow et al., 1994). Gore, Aseltine, and Colton (1992) hypothesized that stress and poor-quality social support act as proximal risk factors that mediate the impact of background variables (i.e., family structure, gender, SES, parent health) on depression. Findings from this study confirmed that depression was directly associated with being a girl, living in a family with a lower standard of living and a lower level of parental education (in girls only), and having parents with higher levels of physical and mental illness. Depression was unrelated to family structure (i.e., single-parent or stepparent household) when economic conditions were controlled. Finally, stress and social support accounted for the effects on depression of some background variables (i.e., parental mental illness and standard of living), but not others (i.e., gender, parental education).

Recent Research and Commentary

Theory and empirical research examining life stress conceptualizations of depression in children have advanced in sophistication in many ways. Importantly, conceptual models have begun to take into account the transactional relations between children and their social contexts across development, allowing for more dynamic and interactive perspectives. To date, however, research has remained somewhat limited in terms of delineating which environmental stresses are most influential in creating risk for depression, and which personal characteristics and external resources of children determine how they react and contribute to these stresses. Some preliminary ideas have been generated that will undoubtedly set the course for upcoming research on child depression.

Whereas early life stress research focused primarily on the impact of cumulative events across multiple life domains, investigators have begun to question whether particular types of stress may play a particularly salient role in depression. Although specific-vulnerability models have focused on both interpersonal and achievement stress, some researchers have suggested that interpersonal stress and disruption may be most strongly associated with depression. In particular, developmental perspectives on depression highlight the critical role of relationships in the formation of self-perceptions, affect regulation, competence, and other processes integral to depression (Cicchetti & Toth, 1998; Hammen, 1992a; Rudolph, 2002). Research has supported the link between interpersonal stress (e.g., separation, conflict) and depression. For example, "exit" or "loss" events have been found to be significantly associated with risk for depression (Eley & Stevenson, 2000; Goodyer & Altham, 1991). Others have demonstrated that particular forms of interpersonal stress, such as romantic relationship breakups (Monroe, Rohde, Seeley, & Lewinsohn, 1999), peer rejection (Panak & Garber, 1992), and friendship disruption (Eley & Stevenson, 2000; Rudolph, 2002), are strongly associated with depression. Moreover, direct comparisons of the association between interpersonal and noninterpersonal stress and depression have confirmed a particularly strong role of interpersonal stress, especially with regard to the generation of dependent stress (Rudolph & Hammen, 1999; Rudolph et al., 2000).

Life stress research is also marked by limited information regarding the predictors of stress reactions and stress generation. Despite widespread acknowledgment of the importance of diathesis–stress models, life stress researchers have considered a relatively restricted domain of individual vulnerabilities—cognitive or otherwise—as potential moderators of stress in children. Several likely candidates should be on the agenda for future research. For instance, other potential risk or protective factors include genetic and biological influences, coping repertoires and problem-solving skills, beliefs about control and self-efficacy, and sociodemographic variables. In this vein, several investigators have examined whether boys and girls show different reactions to stress. Although evidence is mixed, some studies have suggested that girls are more vulnerable to depressive reactions to stress than boys (Ge et al., 1994; Schraedley, Gotlib, & Hayward, 1999), particularly in the context of interpersonal stress (Goodyer & Altham, 1991; Rudolph, 2002; Rudolph & Hammen, 1999). External resources also may intervene in the stress–depression link. For example, many researchers have pointed out the potential buffering effects of social support, but minimal empirical research has examined this prediction in depressed children. Conversely, increased parental strain or psychopathology may exacerbate children's sensitivity to life stress. The determinants of children's vulnerability and resilience to depression in the face of stress deserve further exploration, as we are still far from tapping the many possibilities offered by this line of research.

Another critical elaboration of life stress models involves identification of the mechanisms underlying stress generation. Although stress generation models focus in part on depressive symptoms themselves as predictors of stress, personal characteristics of individuals, perhaps associated with depression, also may lead to the creation of stressful circumstances. Indeed, several factors have been implicated as determinants of stress generation, including demographic variables such as age and sex (Rudolph & Hammen, 1999; Rudolph et al., 2000), personality styles (Nelson, Hammen, Daley, Burge, & Davila, 2001), conceptions of relationships (Caldwell & Rudolph, 2002), social competence (Herzberg et al., 1998), and interpersonal problem solving (Davila, Hammen, Burge, Paley, & Daley, 1995).

General Commentary on Theoretical Models of Childhood Depression

Research on childhood depression has clearly advanced in many ways. Throughout the chapter, we have identified areas of progress, as well as theoretical, empirical, and methodological gaps that still remain. A few general issues are worth noting that apply across different etiological models and empirical studies.

Distinguishing Levels of Depression

As discussed earlier, a controversial issue in depression theory and research concerns the continuity among depressive mood, syndromes, and disorders. Much of the research on childhood depression continues to focus on groups of children who show elevated symptom scores on self-report measures (although there are certainly some notable exceptions). Although research suggests that at least a certain subgroup of these children—particularly those with prolonged distress and significant impairment—are likely to meet criteria for a depressive disorder either concurrently or in the future, studies of clinically diagnosed children are essential for validation of current theories. Moreover, tests of etiological models need to be informed by descriptive work on the characteristics of depression, developmental changes in the phenomenology of depression, and the continuity of depression across the life span, with a focus on determining whether the same models apply across different levels and manifestations of depression.

Constructing and Testing Disorder-Specific Models

One challenging task for child depression researchers is the development of disorder-specific theories that explain the emergence, progression, and consequences of depression versus other forms of disorder. Evidence for the specificity of existing models is mixed. Regarding cognitive models, some studies have demonstrated syndrome-specific beliefs and information-processing patterns (Epkins, 2000; Joiner et al., 1997; Kaslow et al., 1984; Rudolph & Clark, 2001), whereas others have found only partial or no evidence for specificity (Garber et al., 1993; Gotlib et al., 1993; Laurent & Stark, 1993). Life stress is a general predictor of psychopathology (Compas, Howell, Phares, Williams, & Giunta, 1989; Goodyer & Altham, 1991), although studies suggest that more specific life stress models may be developed, based on the analysis of particular types of stress (Eley & Stevenson, 2000; Rudolph & Hammen, 1999; Rudolph et al., 2000) or the interaction of stress with cognitive vulnerability (Lewinsohn et al., 2001; Robinson et al., 1995). Likewise, competence deficits and disruption in the peer and family relationships of depressed youths seem to mirror many of those difficulties seen in children with other forms of psychopathology (Armsden, McCauley, Greenberg, Burke, & Mitchell, 1990; Goodyer et al., 1990). However, some investigations have identified certain types of peer difficulties (Rudolph & Clark, 2001; Rudolph et al., 1994) and family dysfunction (Armsden et al., 1990; Sheeber et al., 1997) that specifically characterize children with depression; these findings suggest that the delineation of more specific models of risk will require linking particular dimensions or constellations of interpersonal styles and family characteristics to particular disorders. Integrative models of depression also hold promise in efforts to construct disorder-specific models, because specificity may depend on combinations of risk factors rather than the impact of any one risk factor in isolation.

Understanding Diagnostic Comorbidity

Efforts to develop disorder-specific models are complicated by the high rates of comorbidity between depression and other forms of psychopathology, which make it difficult to determine whether particular processes are linked to depressive symptoms themselves or to co-occurring problems. Investigations of comorbidity have begun to shed light on how co-occurring problems may influence depression-related processes. For example, research on interpersonal competence in depressed children has revealed quite heterogeneous interpersonal profiles, ranging from passivity, withdrawal, and peer isolation to aggressiveness, impulsivity, and peer rejection. Preliminary evidence suggests that comorbidity may contribute to these intragroup differences. Specifically, children with depressive and externalizing symptoms account for the high levels of aggression and peer rejection in depressed children (Cole & Carpentieri, 1990; Rudolph et al., 1994; Rudolph & Clark, 2001). Comorbid depression has also been linked to particularly high levels of parental criticism (Asarnow et al., 1994) and stress generation (Daley et al., 1997; Rudolph et al., 2000). Patterns of maladaptive cognitive and family processes in groups with comorbidity have been less consistent (Dadds, Sanders, Morrison, & Rubgetz, 1992; Gotlib et al., 1993; Laurent & Stark, 1993).

These complex patterns of findings associated with depression comorbidity illustrate the need to consider subtypes of depressed children with and without co-occuring symptoms when researchers are developing and testing models of depression. In terms of model development, conceptual models should be able to explain the phenomenon of comorbidity. In terms of model validation, the presence of unidentified comorbid subgroups may create contradictory findings across studies.

TOWARD AN INTEGRATIVE, DEVELOPMENTAL THEORY OF YOUTH DEPRESSION

Throughout the chapter to this point, we have identified methodological and empirical gaps in the study of child and adolescent depression. In addition, conceptual issues remain that highlight the differences between the child and adult depression fields. The abundance of well-validated theories of adult depression has represented both an asset and a liability for child depression researchers. On the one hand, adult models have been indispensable as guides to research in youngsters. Yet, as a consequence, early research on child depression suffered from a relative dearth of developmentally grounded theories. Thus these early models often neglected to take into account two critical and distinct components of child depression: the impact of development on depression, and the impact of depression, on development.

Prompted by the emergence of the field of developmental psychopathology, however, theories of childhood depression have begun to adopt multidimensional, developmental, transactional perspectives (e.g., Cicchetti & Toth, 1998; Cummings & Cicchetti, 1990; Gotlib & Hammen, 1992; Hammen, 1992a). Contemporary integrative models, which reflect the convergence of biological, cognitive, interpersonal, family, and life stress approaches, share many common features: the contribution of early family socialization to subsequent functioning; the emergence of internal representations or working models of relationships; the interplay between individual vulnerabilities—both psychological and biological—and external experience; and the role of depression both as a consequence of prior disturbance and as a risk factor for future difficulties.

Figure 5.1 depicts one multidimensional developmental model of depression. The model is intended to highlight the complex and reciprocal interplay among personal characteristics, interpersonal experiences, and depressive symptoms. However, there are clearly many other variables and pathways that may be involved in shaping children's adjustment over time.

In brief, the model proposes that experiences within the family are encoded in memory as a set

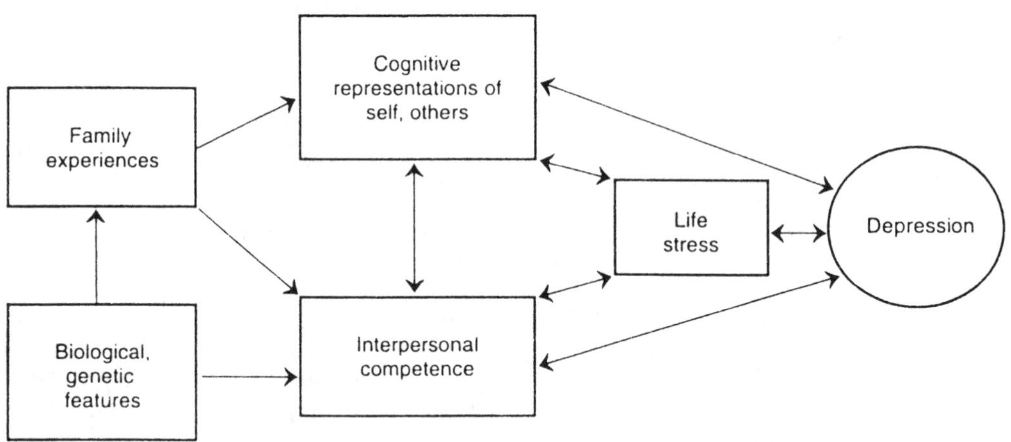

FIGURE 5.1. Multifactorial, transactional model of child and adolescent depression.

of beliefs about the self and others and expectations about future interpersonal encounters. Children who are exposed to caregiving styles characterized by insensitivity or rejection presumably develop generalized internal representations of the self as incompetent or unworthy, of others as hostile or unresponsive, and of relationships as aversive or unpredictable. Dysfunctional relationships and negative cognitive styles in turn are believed to interfere with the maturation of skills for emotion and behavior regulation. This backdrop of cognitive, affective, and social impairment may precipitate depression directly or may drive maladaptive interpersonal behavior that is met with conflict, rejection, or isolation, leading to depression. Alternatively, negative cognitive representations and poor relationships may augment children's vulnerability to depression when they are faced with high levels of stress. Depression then may compromise future development by disrupting important social bonds, undermining existing competencies, inducing stress, and reaffirming children's negative views of themselves and the world.

Genetic and biological vulnerability may enter into the picture at several points. Individual differences in temperament are likely to shape the nature of parent–child relationships and children's selection of and experiences within various interpersonal contexts. Biological vulnerability, such as a tendency toward neuroendocrine hyperarousal, will inevitably interact with psychosocial resources in determining children's ability to cope with external stress and their ensuing sensitivity to depression (Post, 1992); genetic factors may even account for heightened exposure to stress (Kendler, 1995).

According to a developmental perspective, depression onset early in childhood may be particularly deleterious. First, impairment during critical periods may redirect typical developmental trajectories, such that children are unable to compensate for skills that they have failed to learn. Second, early formation of negative and inflexible cognitive schemas may reduce the likelihood that children will attend to or incorporate future disconfirmatory feedback. Third, the connections among cognitive appraisal mechanisms, affective tendencies, behavioral patterns, and external stress may strengthen over time, resulting in a decreased threshold for activation of these networks as children enter adolescence and adulthood (see Teasdale, 1983). Finally, the cumulative impact of chronic psychological and social stress over time may alter biological processes presumed to underlie depression vulnerability, particularly in young children, whose systems are not fully matured (Gold, Goodwin, & Chrousos, 1988).

Reflecting the conceptual sophistication of contemporary models of child depression, empirical investigations have emphasized the interplay among biological, psychological, and social processes. For example, data support cognitive–interpersonal models that consider the joint contributions of parent–child and family dysfunction, attachment, interpersonal schemas, interpersonal stress, and relationship processes to depression vulnerability (Hammen et al., 1995; Kobak et al., 1991; Rudolph et al., 1997; Stark, Humphrey, Laurent, Livingston, & Christopher, 1993), although further research using prospective designs is needed to confirm the temporal associations among these variables. A growing body of research also confirms the dynamic interactions among genetic and biological characteristics and psychosocial processes in the emergence of depression vulnerability. For instance, evidence points to a genetic liability to stress exposure and reactivity (Kendler, 1995; Kendler, Neale, Kessler, Heath, & Eaves, 1993). Studies also support the interface of psychosocial factors and biological reactivity to stress in the prediction of depression (e.g., Goodyer, Herbert, & Altham, 1998; Goodyer et al., 2000b). Understanding how genetic or biological predispositions to depression are translated into psychological manifestations of vulnerability represents a fascinating area for future research.

Contemporary theory and research clearly point to the need for comprehensive and developmental models that incorporate multiple domains of functioning and account for the reciprocal interplay among these domains across development. Many exciting directions have emerged in recent years. These novel ideas need to be pursued using state-of-the-art methodologies that carefully track the emergence and progression of risk factors and depression across development.

BIPOLAR DISORDERS IN ADOLESCENTS AND CHILDREN

Just as depression was "discovered" to occur in children some 20 years ago, there has been a similar recent interest in bipolar disorders in children. Spurred in part by increased awareness and effective treatments of bipolar disorders in adults, the relatively recent focus on youth bipolarity has also been stimulated by the hypothesis that early diagnosis and treatment of bipolar youngsters may actually make the course more benign (and, conversely, that misidentification may lead to treatments that make the disorder worse). A certain fervor has accompanied the "discovery" of bipolar disorders in children, and controversy has arisen mainly around the problems of accurate diagnosis.

To provide a context for discussion of childhood bipolarity, key diagnostic features of bipolar disorders as applied to adults should be noted. Bipolar disorders are recurrent and cycling by definition, but cycles of depression and mania/hypomania may be quite variable from person to person in polarity, cyclicity, frequency, and status between episodes. Bipolar I disorder as defined by DSM-IV (American Psychiatric Association, 1994) involves a history of major depression and mania, whereas bipolar II disorder refers to a history of major depression and hypomania. Mania is defined by a period of abnormally elevated (or irritable) mood of at least 1 week's duration, accompanied by such features as grandiosity, decreased need for sleep, increased talkativeness, racing thoughts or flight of ideas, distractibility, increased goal-directed activity or agitation, and excessive involvement in pleasurable but potentially harmful activities (such as excessive spending, extreme levels of sexual activity, or obviously foolish business investments). Hypomania is marked by less severe symptoms of mania, and may be of briefer duration. Cyclothymia is a disorder in the bipolar spectrum that includes chronic, mild fluctuations of mood in which depressions and hypomanias do not meet criteria for major depression or mania, and symptom-free intervals are brief.

Diagnostic Issues and Course Features for Bipolar Disorders in Adolescents

Bipolar disorders often emerge in adolescence. Faedda et al. (1995) summarized 28 studies that reported onset by age; overall, 25% of bipolar patients had onset before the age of 20 (a likely underestimate, due to prior diagnostic practices that might have reflected biases of the day, such as exclusion of child samples). Dating age of onset is difficult, due to different definitions of onset (first symptoms, first diagnosable disorder, first official diagnosis?). In recent years, however, greater knowledge of bipolar disorders among clinicians as well as patients, combined with acceptance of their appearance in adolescents, has led to greater recognition of bipolar I and bipolar II disorders (as defined by adult DSM-IV criteria) in teenagers. A retrospective self-report survey of 500 members of the National Depressive and Manic–Depressive Association found that 60% of respondents with bipolar disorders reported symptom onset in childhood or adolescence (Lish, Dime-Meehan, Whybrow, Price, & Hirschfeld, 1994).

Diagnostic Obstacles in Adolescence

Despite acceptance of adult criteria for adolescent-onset bipolar disorders, accurate diagnosis may be difficult. There are several major obstacles. One is misperception of the symptoms, especially when they are compounded by comorbid conditions; they are often viewed as behavior disturbances or excessive teenage emotional and behavioral dysregulation. For many years, bipolar I disorder in youths was often misdiagnosed as schizophrenia, or recognition was obscured by co-occurring drug or alcohol abuse, conduct problems, ADHD, or mixed symptoms. Bizarre preoccupations, irritability and defiance, mood swings, and deviant behaviors may be easily misconstrued, especially in the absence of a history of specific episodes.

A second diagnostic obstacle is that many bipolar disorders initially present as depression, so that bipolarity may be diagnosed only by following the person over time and observing the presence of hypomania or mania. A significant number of initial diagnoses of unipolar depression "switch" over time. A review of seven studies of over 250 severely depressed children and adolescents followed 2–4 years reported a mean switch rate from depression to mania of about 25% (Faedda et al., 1995; see also Kovacs, 1996). Weissman et al. (1999) recontacted 10–15 years later a mostly outpatient sample initially diagnosed with major depression during adolescence. Participants had a substantial risk for recurrence of major depression, but notably, 4.1% had developed bipolar I disorder, and 1.4% bipolar II disorder.

A third diagnostic obstacle is even more problematic: Some adolescents who have displayed severe childhood symptomatology of varying sorts, but may have eluded accurate diagnosis, may have childhood-onset bipolar disorders. This is a controversial topic, discussed below.

Course Features in Adolescence

It appears that some adolescents present with an initial, rapid-onset mania that must be distinguished from schizophrenia if psychotic symptoms are present, or from attention-deficit and disruptive behavior disorders that are either comorbid conditions or behavioral manifestations of the underlying bipolarity. Several studies have reported that between one-third and one-half of adolescent bipolar patients have prominent psychotic symptoms (e.g., Faraone, Biederman, Wozniak, et al., 1997; Kafantaris, Coletti, Dicker, Padula, & Pollack, 1998). Kafantaris et al. (1998) found that half of the bipolar youths in their study who presented with psychotic mania had no prior psychiatric history, and seemed to have an acute onset after functioning well. They suggested that this subgroup might have "classic" bipolar I disorder, with discrete episodes of depression and mania, and well intervals (a subtype often responsive to lithium).

Other youngsters initially may present with depressive disorders, and a bipolar diagnosis must await onset of manic or hypomanic episodes. Adolescents—and children—who present with severe depression, especially with psychotic features; who have a family history of bipolar disorders; and who develop hypomania in response to antidepressant treatment are thought to be especially at risk for the development of bipolar disorders. The prognostic significance of first presentation of bipolar disorders as depression is not clear, but Strober et al. (1995) found that although the great majority of adolescent bipolar inpatients recovered relatively rapidly, patients with index episodes of depression took longer to recover than those who had manic or mixed states.

Diagnostic Issues and Course Features for Bipolar Disorders in Children

There is wide consensus that bipolar disorders do exist in children, but they are considered to be rare, at least in their classic forms. Some have begun to argue that "atypical" bipolar disorders, or DSM-IV bipolar disorder not otherwise specified, may be relatively more common but often undiagnosed in children. There is considerable interest in—and, indeed, controversy over—the appropriate diagnostic criteria.

Clinical Features in Childhood

One of the major obstacles to diagnosis of bipolarity in prepubertal children is that it does not resemble adult bipolar disorders in certain key ways. For instance, it typically is not characterized by an acute onset of episodes, periods of relatively good functioning between episodes, or distinct episodes of elevated mood or irritability (Geller & Luby, 1997). Moreover, some adult symptoms (such as euphoria and grandiosity) are relatively rare (e.g., Carlson, 1999).

Bipolar children may present clinically with chronic symptoms that include exacerbations of mood states or ultrarapid mood shifts. Geller et al. (1998), for example, studied a carefully defined sample with a mean age at onset of 8.1 years. These investigators found that 75% had ultradian cycles (variation within a 24-hour period). Moreover, these children were chronically ill, and had been manic for a mean of 3 years before entering the study. The presentation of "mixed" episodes is also common (e.g., Biederman, 1998), with dysphoric and especially intensely irritable mood. Irritability, rage, and aggressiveness are noted as prominent features for many bipolar children (e.g., Carlson & Kelley, 1998; Faraone, Biederman, Wozniak, et al., 1997). Many are seen as out of control and destructive, with severe impairment in social and academic functioning. Psychotic features may be present; Geller et al. (1998) reported that 60% of their child bipolar sample had delusions. Suicidal thoughts and behaviors may also be prominent.

The picture of severely impaired, chronic, disorganized, and dysregulated children is compounded by the frequent if not typical comorbidity with various other disorders. Mania presenting alone is quite rare. As discussed below, ADHD may be a frequent co-occurring disorder, but conduct disorder (e.g., Biederman, Faraone, Chu, & Wozniak, 1999; Kovacs & Pollack, 1995), oppositional defiant disorder, substance use disorders, depression, and anxiety disorders are also common. As we note, symptoms of hyperactivity, heightened energy and restlessness, distractibility, racing thoughts and pressure to talk, and impulsivity may make it difficult to distinguish between severe ADHD and mania.

Diagnostic Controversies in Childhood

There are several types of diagnostic concerns. One is a relative lack of developmental data on the expression of symptomatology. It is hypothesized that if we knew more about the ability of children of different levels of maturity to experience and express different symptoms of bipolar disorders, we would have greater guidance in adjusting the diagnostic criteria accordingly. It is possible, for example, that studies of children at risk due to parental bipolarity might help to shed light on childhood manifestations of symptoms and prodromal expressions of bipolar disorders.

Another diagnostic concern is the apparent overlap or similarity of ADHD and prepubertal bipolar disorders. Biederman and colleagues (Biederman, 1998; Faraone, Biederman, Wozniak, et al., 1997; Wozniak et al., 1995) have shown extremely high rates of ADHD among children diagnosed with mania, as well as elevated rates of mania in children diagnosed with ADHD (e.g., 21% over a 4-year follow-up; Biederman et al., 1996). Similar high rates of ADHD in bipolar youngsters also have been reported by Geller et al. (1998).

Some might argue that there is a true comorbidity of these conditions, and that ADHD may even mask true bipolar disorders (Biederman, 1998). Biederman and colleagues have also suggested that there might even be a genetic subtype of co-occurring ADHD and bipolarity (e.g., Faraone, Biederman, Mennin, Wozniak, & Spencer, 1997). Geller et al. (1998), however, have suggested that ADHD in young bipolar samples may be a "phenocopy" ADHD, driven by developmentally prevalent high energy in children. With age, Geller et al. predict that the ADHD will "decrease" to population levels by adulthood. Thus ADHD may be a prodrome or developmentally expressed version of bipolarity in children, rather than a separate disorder. Obviously, longitudinal follow-up of young bipolar samples may help to resolve the various diagnostic issues through clarification of clinical course and outcome.

Yet another diagnostic concern is that clinicians have started to label unknown conditions as "bipolar disorders," lumping confusing but diverse disorders under the umbrella term of "bipolar disorders." According to this perspective, a "bipolar disorder"—especially manic-like symptoms—may be a condition of extreme labile and aggressive temperament, a severe disorder of chronic hyperarousal and emotional and behavioral dysregulation, or even a condition secondary to brain injury or organic disorder (e.g., Carlson & Kelley, 1998). Carlson (1998) notes that there are several nonspecific terms used in the child psychiatry literature to describe children with multiple, severe, disruptive behaviors that do not fit any typical diagnostic picture ("multidimensionally impaired," "multiple complex developmental disorder"), as well as children suffering from some forms of head injury, pervasive developmental disorder, or other medical conditions. According to this perspective, clinicians need to be cautious not to overdiagnose conditions as bipolar disorders that are simply not yet classifiable or understood.

Epidemiology of Juvenile Bipolar Disorders

Epidemiological surveys that include children and adolescents are rare, and few have included bipolar disorders as an option for juvenile populations. One important exception, the Oregon Adolescent Depression Project, was a school-based survey of 14- to 18-year-olds. Lewinsohn, Klein, and Seeley (1995) interviewed 1,700 youths, and reported a lifetime prevalence of about 1% for bipolar disorders, chiefly bipolar II disorder and cyclothymia. An additional 5.7% of the youths had significant subsyndromal bipolar symptoms with functional impairment. Furthermore, according to Klein, Lewinsohn, and Seeley (1996), hypomanic personality traits in the Oregon sample were also associated with various indices of impaired functioning. Among those adolescents with a past history of depression, hypomanic traits predicted more symptomatology, history of recurrent depression, comorbid conditions, and higher rates of attempted suicide. It is unclear whether hypomanic traits predict eventual Axis I bipolar disorders, or whether they may reflect stable personality traits. Other community and treatment samples of adolescents in the United States and Europe have yielded rates of mania and hypomania that approximate the adult norms of about 1% (e.g., Thomsen, Moller, Dehlholm, & Brask, 1992; Verhulst, van der Ende, Ferdinand, & Kasius, 1997). Costello et al. (1996) found no cases of mania in their epidemiological survey of children, but reported hypomania at about 0.1%.

Taken together, these sparse findings in representative community and psychiatric samples illustrate several patterns generally accepted and confirmed by clinical studies. First, childhood bipolar I disorder appears to be quite rare—although this view is often challenged by some clinicians, advocacy groups, and investigators. As noted above, developmentally appropriate criteria and longitudinal studies will help to resolve this issue by improving diagnostic validity. Second, adolescent bipolar disorders occur at about the same rate as in the general adult population. Third, subsyndromal forms of bipolar disorder may be identified in juvenile samples, and can reflect prodromal or stable dimensional traits of the bipolar spectrum that may be associated with impairment of functioning. Longitudinal studies of behavioral and offspring high-risk groups are needed to help clarify the outcomes of early subclinical forms of bipolar disorders.

Etiological Hypotheses and Implications of Early Identification of Bipolar Disorders

Bipolar disorders are considered to be among the most genetically controlled forms of major mental illness, and increasingly sophisticated genetic analyses are underway to identify potential gene loci. The mechanisms of the disorders are as yet unknown, although various neural circuits are under investigation (e.g., Blumberg et al., 1999, 2000). Imperfect concordance between monozygotic twins, however, makes it clear that interactions among vulnerability and environmental factors play a role in expression of these disorders. Identification of endophenotypes thought to reflect risk for bipolar disorders is viewed as a high priority in the field, and would be especially important if coupled with efforts to identify developmentally related expression of mood and behavioral regulation.

The high-risk methodology (i.e., the study of children of bipolar parents) has been employed relatively less in bipolar than in unipolar families. Nevertheless, a meta-analysis by Lapalme, Hodgins, and LaRoche (1997) concluded that 52% of the offspring of bipolar parents met criteria for some diagnosis, compared with 29% of the offspring of parents with no disorders. In total, 26.5% of the offspring of bipolar parents had an *affective* disorder (including major, minor, and intermittent depression and dysthymia, as well as mania, hypomania, cyclothymia, and hyperthymic states), compared with 8.3% of children of parents wth no disorders. *Bipolar* disorders occurred in 5.4% of the offspring of bipolar parents, whereas none of the children of parents with no disorders were bipolar. Several high-risk investigators have included subsyndromal and temperament measures thought to reflect the bipolar spectrum (e.g., Grigoroiu-Serbanescu et al., 1989; Grigoroiu-Serbanescu, Christodorescu, Totoescu, & Jipescu, 1991; Klein, Depue, & Slater, 1985). It is an intriguing question whether such traits reflect prodromal signs of later bipolarity, or indicate stable subclinical states with heritable components. Also, because many of the offspring studies included only older children and adolescents, it would be of interest to carefully evaluate the characteristics of younger children as well.

It is further hypothesized that the episodes of a bipolar disorder themselves, and an affected individual's experiences of stressors, may alter the brain and "sensitize" the organism to react with episodes to increasingly milder triggering events; this hypothesis is similar to models of kindling and behavioral sensitization observed in experimental studies of animals (e.g., Post, 1992). Therefore, one important implication is that fewer (early) episodes may predict a more benign course of disorder. Some investigators and clinicians have urged rapid institution of mood stabilizer treatment of presumed bipolar disorders, in the hope of improving the eventual course.

The opposite problem is that some pharmacological interventions for children's disorders may actually worsen the course. It is known, for instance, that treatment of apparent depression with antidepressants may precipitate hypomania—and even rapid cycling—in individuals who are believed to have underlying bipolar disorders. Rapid cycling is especially disruptive and difficult to treat. Also, psychostimulant treatment due to misdiagnosis of a bipolar disorder as ADHD may worsen the underlying mood disorder and exacerbate symptoms of mania. Considerable research is needed to clarify the effects of various pharmacological interventions and preventive treatments.

Conclusions about Bipolar Disorder in Youngsters

A rapidly moving "bandwagon" effect leading to the diagnosis of bipolar disorders in children should be viewed with great caution. Nevertheless, bipolar disorders and their subclinical forms represent much unmapped territory that may provide important clinical discoveries with significant implications. This is a topic that strongly reminds us of the need for developmental understanding of symptom expression, and for the study of prodromes and endophenotypes potentially arising in young populations before a full clinical disorder emerges. Such studies have proven to be highly productive in the schizophrenia field, yielding not only clinical but also neurobiological understanding of the disorder. This topic has not been of major interest to psychologists to date, but increased focus by developmental psychopathologists and researchers with the assessment, diagnostic, and conceptual tools that have added such substance to the childhood and adolescent (unipolar) depression field in recent years have much to contribute.

ACKNOWLEDGMENTS

Preparaton of this chapter was supported in part by National Institute of Mental Health (NIMH) Grant No. 2R01MH52239 awarded to Constance Hammen, and by a William T. Grant Foundation Faculty Scholars Award and NIMH Grant No. MH59711-01 awarded to Karen D. Rudolph. We would like to express our thanks to Alison J. Dupre and Megan Flynn for their assistance in preparation of this chapter.

REFERENCES

Abela, J. R. Z. (2001). The hopelessness theory of depression: A test of the diathesis–stress and causal mediation components in third and seventh grade children. *Journal of Abnormal Child Psychology*, *29*, 241–254.

Abramson, L. Y., Metalsky, G. I., & Alloy, L. B. (1989). Hopelessness depression: A theory-based subtype of depression. *Psychological Review*, *96*, 358–372.

Abramson, L. Y., Seligman, M. E. P., & Teasdale, J. D. (1978). Learned helplessness in humans: Critique and reformulation. *Journal of Abnormal Psychology*, *37*, 49–74.

Achenbach, T. M. (1991). The derivation of taxonomic constructs: A necessary stage in the development of developmental psychopathology. In D. Cicchetti & S. Toth (Eds.), *Rochester Symposium on Developmental Psychopathology: Vol. 3. Models and integrations* (pp. 43–74). Hillsdale, NJ: Erlbaum.

Achenbach, T. M., & Edelbrock, C. (1978). The classification of child psychopathology: A review and analysis of empirical efforts. *Psychological Bulletin*, *85*, 1275–1301.

Achenbach, T. M., McConaughy, S. H., & Howell, C. T. (1987). Child/adolescent behavioral and emotional problems: Implications of cross-informant for situational stability. *Psychological Bulletin*, *101*, 213–232.

Adrian, C., & Hammen, C. (1993). Stress exposure and stress generation in children of depressed mothers. *Journal of Consulting and Clinical Psychology*, *61*, 354–359.

Allgood-Merten, B., Lewinsohn, P., & Hops, H. (1990). Sex differences and adolescent depression. *Journal of Abnormal Psychology*, *99*, 55–63.

Alloy, L. B., Abramson, L. Y., Tashman, N. A., Berrebbi, D. S., Hogan, M. E., Whitehouse, W. G., Crossfield, A. G., & Morocco, A. (2001). Developmental origins of cognitive vulnerability to depression: Parenting, cognitive, and inferential feedback styles of the parents of individuals at high and low cognitive risk for depression. *Cognitive Therapy and Research*, *25*, 397–423.

Altmann, E. O., & Gotlib, I. H. (1988). The social behavior of depressed children: An observational study. *Journal of Abnormal Child Psychology*, *16*, 29–44.

Ambrosini, P. J. (2000). Historical development and present status of the Schedule for Affective Disorders and Schizophrenia for School-Age Children (K-SADS). *Journal of the American Academy of Child and Adolescent Psychiatry*, *39*, 49–58.

American Psychiatric Association. (1994). *Diagnostic and statistical manual of mental disorders* (4th ed.). Washington, DC: Author.

Angold, A., Costello, E. J., & Erkanli, A. (1999). Comorbidity. *Journal of Child Psychology and Psychiatry*, *40*, 57–87.

Angold, A., Costello, E. J., Erkanli, A., & Worthman, C. M. (1999). Pubertal changes in hormones of adolescent girls. *Psychological Medicine*, *29*, 1043–1053.

Angold, A., & Rutter, M. (1992). Effects of age and pubertal status on depression in a large clinical sample. *Development and Psychopathology*, *4*, 5–28.

Armsden, G. C., McCauley, E., Greenberg, M. T., Burke, P. M., & Mitchell, J. R. (1990). Parent and peer attachment in early adolescent depression. *Journal of Abnormal Child Psychology*, *18*, 683–697.

Asarnow, J. R., Carlson, G. A., & Guthrie, D. (1987). Coping strategies, self-perceptions, hopelessness, and perceived family environments in depressed and suicidal children. *Journal of Consulting and Clinical Psychology*, *55*, 361–366.

Asarnow, J., Goldstein, M., Carlson, G., Perdue, S., Bates, S., & Keller, J. (1988). Childhood-onset depressive disorders: A follow-up study of rates of rehospitalization and out-of-home placement among child psychiatric inpatients. *Journal of Affective Disorders*, *15*, 245–253.

Asarnow, J. R., Goldstein, M. J., Tompson, M., & Guthrie, D. (1993). One-year outcomes of depressive disorders in child psychiatric inpatients: Evaluation of the prognostic power of a brief measure of expressed emotion. *Journal of Child Psychology and Psychiatry*, *34*, 129–137.

Asarnow, J. R., Tompson, M., Hamilton, E. B., Goldstein, M. J., & Guthrie, D. (1994). Family-expressed emotion, childhood-onset depression, and childhood-onset schizophrenia spectrum disorders: Is expressed emotion a nonspecific correlate of child psychopathology or a specific risk factor for depression? *Journal of Abnormal Child Psychology*, *22*, 129–146.

Avenevoli, S., Stolar, M., Li, J., Dierker, L., & Merikangas, K. R. (2001). Comorbidity of depression in children and adolescents: Models and evidence from a prospective high-risk family study. *Biological Psychiatry*, *49*, 1071–1081.

Baker, M., Milich, R., & Manolis, M. (1996). Peer interactions of dysphoric adolescents. *Journal of Abnormal Child Psychology*, *24*, 241–255.

Bardone, A., Moffitt, T., Caspi, A., Dickson, N., & Silva, P. (1996). Adult mental health and social outcomes of adolescent girls with depression and conduct disorder. *Development and Psychopathology*, *8*, 811–829.

Beardslee, W. R., Versage, E. M., & Gladstone, T. R. (1998). Children of affectively ill parents: A review of the past 10 years. *Journal of the American Academy of Child and Adolescent Psychiatry*, *37*, 1134–1141.

Beck, A. T. (1983). Cognitive therapy of depression: New perspectives. In P. J. Clayton & J. E. Barrett (Eds.), *Treatment of depression: Old controversies and new approaches* (pp. 265–290). New York: Raven Press.

Beck, A. T., Rush, A. J., Shaw, B. F., & Emery, G. (1979). *Cognitive therapy of depression.* New York: Guilford Press.

Berman, A., & Jobes, D. (1991). *Adolescent suicide: Assessment and intervention.* Washington, DC: American Psychological Association.

Biederman, J. (1998). Resolved: Mania is mistaken for ADHD in prepubertal children. *Journal of the American Academy of Child and Adolescent Psychiatry, 37,* 1091–1093.

Biederman, J., Faraone, S. V., Chu, M. P., & Wozniak, J. (1999). Further evidence of a bidirectional overlap between juvenile mania and conduct disorder in children. *Journal of the American Academy of Child and Adolescent Psychiatry, 38,* 468–476.

Biederman, J., Faraone, S., Mick, E., Wozniak, J., Chen, L., Ouellette, C., Marrs, A., Moore, P., Garcia, J., Mennin, D., & Lelon, E. (1996). Attention-deficit hyperactivity disorder and juvenile mania: An overlooked comorbidity? *Journal of the American Academy of Child and Adolescent Psychiatry, 35,* 997–1008.

Billings, A. G., & Moos, R. H. (1985). Children of parents with unipolar depression: A controlled 1-year follow-up. *Journal of Abnormal Child Psychology, 14,* 149–166.

Bird, H. R., Canino, G., Rubio-Stipec, M., Gould, M. S., Ribera, J., Sesman, M., Woodbury, M., Huertas-Goldman, S., Pagan, A., Sanchez-Lacay, A., & Moscoso, M. (1988). Estimates of the prevalence of childhood maladjustment in a community survey in Puerto Rico. *Archives of General Psychiatry, 45,* 1120–1126.

Birmaher, B., Dahl, R. E., Williamson, D. E., Perel, J. M., Brent, D. A., Axelson, D. A., Kaufman, J., Dorn, L. D., Stull, S., Rao, U., & Ryan, N. D. (2000). Growth hormone secretion in children and adolescents at high risk for major depressive disorder. *Archives of General Psychiatry, 57,* 867–872.

Birmaher, B., Ryan, N. D., Williamson, D. E., Brent, D. A., Kaufman, J., Dahl, R. E., Perel, J., & Nelson, B. (1996). Childhood and adolescent depression: A review of the past 10 years. Part I. *Journal of the American Academy of Child and Adolescent Psychiatry, 35,* 1427–1439.

Bland, R. C., Newman, S. C., & Orn, H. (1986). Recurrent and nonrecurrent depression: A family study. *Archives of General Psychiatry, 43,* 1085–1089.

Blatt, S. J., & Homann, E. (1992). Parent–child interaction in the etiology of dependent and self-critical depression. *Clinical Psychology Review, 12,* 47–91.

Blechman, E. A., McEnroe, M. J., Carella, E. T., & Audette, D. P. (1986). Childhood competence and depression. *Journal of Abnormal Psychology, 95,* 223–227.

Blumberg, H. P., Stern, E., Martinez, D., Ricketts, S., de Asis, J., White, T., Epstein, J., McBride, P. A., Eidelberg, D., Kocsis, J. H., & Silbersweig, D. A. (2000). Increased anterior cingulate and caudate activity in bipolar mania. *Biological Psychiatry, 48,* 1045–1052.

Blumberg, H. P., Stern, E., Ricketts, S., Martinez, D., de Asis, J., White, T., Epstein, J., Isenberg, N., McBride, P. A., Kemperman, I., Emmerich, S., Dhawan, V., Eidelberg, D., Kocsis, J. H., & Silbersweig, D. A. (1999). Rostral and orbital prefrontal cortex dysfunction in the manic state of bipolar disorder. *American Journal of Psychiatry, 156,* 1986–1988.

Boivin, M., Hymel, S., & Bukowski, W. M. (1995). The roles of social withdrawal, peer rejection, and victimization by peers in predicting loneliness and depressed mood in childhood. *Development and Psychopathology, 7,* 765–785.

Bowlby, J. (1969). *Attachment and loss: Vol. 1. Attachment.* New York: Basic Books.

Bowlby, J. (1980). *Attachment and loss: Vol. 3. Loss: Sadness and depression.* New York: Basic Books.

Boyle, M., & Pickles, A. (1997). Influence of maternal depressive symptoms on ratings of childhood behavior. *Journal of Abnormal Child Psychology, 25,* 399–412.

Bremner, J. D., Innis, R. B., Salomon, R. M., Staib, L. H., Ng, C. K., Miller, H. L., Bronen, R. A., Krystal, J. H., Duncan, J., Rich, D., Price, L. H., Malison, R., Dey, H., Soufer, R., & Charney, D. S. (1997). Positron emission tomography measurement of cerebral metabolic correlates of tryptophan depletion-induced depressive relapse. *Archives of General Psychiatry, 54,* 364–374.

Breznitz, Z., & Sherman, T. (1987). Speech patterning of natural discourse of well and depressed mothers and their young children. *Child Development, 58,* 395–400.

Brown, G. W., & Harris, T. (1978). *Social origins of depression: A study of psychiatric disorders in women.* New York: Free Press.

Burke, K. C., Burke, J. D., Regier, D. A., & Rae, D. S. (1990). Age at onset of selected mental disorders in five community populations. *Archives of General Psychiatry, 47,* 511–518.

Burt, C. E., Cohen, L. H., & Bjorck, J. P. (1988). Perceived family environment as a moderator of young adolescents' life stress adjustment. *American Journal of Community Psychology, 16,* 101–122.

Caldwell, M., & Rudolph, K. D. (2002). *Mechanisms of stress-generation among early adolescents.* Manuscript in preparation.

Carlson, G. A. (1998). Mania and ADHD: Comorbidity or confusion? *Journal of Affective Disorders, 51,* 177–187.

Carlson, G. A. (1999). Juvenile mania vs. ADHD [Letter to the editor]. *Journal of the American Academy of Child and Adolescent Psychiatry, 50,* 353–354.

Carlson, G. A., & Cantwell, D. (1980). Unmasking masked depression in children and adolescents. *American Journal of Psychiatry, 137,* 445–449.

Carlson, G. A., & Kashani, J. (1988). Phenomenology of major depression from childhood through adulthood: Analysis of three studies. *American Journal of Psychiatry, 145,* 1222–1225.

Carlson, G. A., & Kelley, K. L. (1998). Manic symptoms in psychiatrically hospitalized children: What do they mean? *Journal of Affective Disorders, 51,* 123–135.

Chambers, W., Puig-Antich, J., Tabrizi, M., & Davies, M. (1982). Psychotic symptoms in prepubertal major depressive disorder. *Archives of General Psychiatry, 39,* 921–927.

Cicchetti, D., & Toth, S. L. (1998). The development of depression in children and adolescents. *American Psychologist, 53,* 221–241.

Clark, L. A., & Watson, D. (1991). Tripartite model of anxiety and depression: Psychometric evidence and taxonomic implications. *Journal of Abnormal Psychology, 100,* 316–336.

Cohen, L. H., Burt, C. E., & Bjorck, J. P. (1987). Life stress and adjustment: Effects of life events experienced by young adolescents and their parents. *Developmental Psychology, 23,* 583–592.

Cohen, P., Cohen, J., Kasen, S., Velez, C. N., Hartmark, C., Johnson, J., Rojas, M., Brook J., & Streuning, E. L. (1993). An epidemiological study of disorders in late childhood and adolescence: I. Age- and gender-specific prevalence. *Journal of Child Psychology and Psychiatry, 34*, 851–867.

Cohn, J. F., Matias, R., Tronick, E., Connell, D., & Lyons-Ruth, K. (1986). Face-to-face interactions of depressed mothers and their infants. In E. Tronick & T. Field (Eds.), *New directons for child development: No. 34. Maternal depression and infant disturbance* (pp. 31–46). San Francisco: Jossey-Bass.

Cole, D. A. (1990). The relation of social and academic competence to depressive symptoms in childhood. *Journal of Abnormal Psychology, 99*, 422–429.

Cole, D. A. (1991). Preliminary support for a competency-based model of depression in children. *Journal of Abnormal Psychology, 100*, 181–190.

Cole, D. A., & Carpentieri, S. (1990). Social status and the comorbidity of child depression and conduct disorder. *Journal of Consulting and Clinical Psychology, 58*, 748–757.

Cole, D. A., Jacquez, F. M., & Maschman, T. L. (2001). Social origins of depressive cognitions: A longitudinal study of self-perceived competence in children. *Cognitive Therapy and Research, 25*, 377–395.

Cole, D. A., & Jordan, A. E. (1995). Competence and memory: Integrating psychosocial and cognitive correlates of child depression. *Child Development, 66*, 459–473.

Cole, D. A., Martin, J. M., Peeke, L. G., Seroczynski, A. D., & Hoffman, K. (1998). Are cognitive errors of underestimation predictive or reflective of depressive symptoms in children?: A longitudinal study. *Journal of Abnormal Psychology, 107*, 481–496.

Cole, D. A., Martin, J. M., & Powers, B. (1997). A competency-based model of child depression: A longitudinal study of peer, parent, teacher, and self-evaluations. *Journal of Child Psychology and Psychiatry, 38*, 505–514.

Cole, D. A., Martin, J. M., Powers, B., & Truglio, R. (1996). Modeling causal relations between academic and social competence and depression: A multitrait–multimethod longitudinal study of children. *Journal of Abnormal Psychology, 105*, 258–270.

Cole, D. A., & McPherson, A. E. (1993). Relation of family subsystems to adolescent depression: Implementing a new family assessment strategy. *Journal of Family Psychology, 7*, 119–133.

Cole, D. A., Peeke, L. G., Martin, J. M., Truglio, R., & Seroczynski, A. D. (1998). A longitudinal look at the relation between depression and anxiety in children and adolescents. *Journal of Consulting and Clinical Psychology, 66*, 451–460.

Cole, D. A., & Rehm, L. P. (1986). Family interaction patterns and childhood depression. *Journal of Abnormal Child Psychology, 14*, 297–314.

Cole, D. A., Truglio, R., & Peeke, L. (1997). Relation between symptoms of anxiety and depression in children: A multitrait–multimethod–multigroup assessment. *Journal of Consulting and Clinical Psychology, 65*, 110–119.

Cole, D. A., & Turner, J. E. (1993). Models of cognitive mediation and moderation in child depression. *Journal of Abnormal Psychology, 102*, 271–281.

Compas, B. E., Connor-Smith, J. K., Saltzman, H., Thomsen, A. H., & Wadsworth, M. E. (2001). Coping with stress during childhood and adolescence: Problems, progress, and potential in theory and research. *Psychological Bulletin, 127*, 87–127.

Compas, B. E., Ey, S., & Grant, K. E. (1993). Taxonomy, assessment, and diagnosis of depression during adolescence. *Psychological Bulletin, 114*, 323–344.

Compas, B. E., Howell, D. C., Phares, V., Williams, R. A., & Giunta, C. T. (1989). Risk factors for emotional/behavioral problems in young adolescents: A prospective analysis of adolescent and parental stress and symptoms. *Journal of Consulting and Clinical Psychology, 57*, 732–740.

Connolly, J., Geller, S., Marton, P., & Kutcher, S. (1992). Peer responses to social interaction with depressed adolescents. *Journal of Clinical Child Psychology, 21*, 365–370.

Conrad, M., & Hammen, C. (1989). Role of maternal depression in perceptions of child maladjustment. *Journal of Consulting and Clinical Psychology, 57*, 663–667.

Cooper, P. J., & Goodyer, I. (1993). A community study of depression in adolescent girls: I. Estimates of symptom and syndrome prevalence. *British Journal of Psychiatry, 163*, 369–374.

Coryell, W., Akiskal, H., Leon, A., Winokur, G., Maser, J., Mueller, T., & Keller, M. (1994). The time course of nonchronic major depressive disorder: Uniformity across episodes and samples. *Archives of General Psychiatry, 51*, 405–410.

Costello, E. J., Angold, A., Burns, B. J., Stangl, D. K., Tweed, D. L., Erkanli, A., & Worthman, C. M. (1996). The Great Smoky Mountains Study of Youth: Goals, design, methods, and the prevalence of DSM-III-R disorders. *Archives of General Psychiatry, 53*, 1129–1136.

Coyne, J. C. (1976). Depression and the response of others. *Journal of Abnormal Psychology, 85*, 186–193.

Cross-National Collaborative Group. (1992). The changing rate of major depression: Cross-national comparisons. *Journal of the American Medical Association, 268*, 3098–3105.

Cummings, E. M., & Cicchetti, D. (1990). Toward a transactional model of relations between attachment and depression. In M. T. Greenberg, D. Cicchetti, & E. M. Cummings (Eds.), *Attachment in the preschool years: Theory, research, and intervention* (pp. 339–372). Chicago: University of Chicago Press.

Cummings, E. M., & Davies, P. T. (1999). Depressed parents and family functioning: Interpersonal effects and children's functioning and development. In T. E. Joiner & J. C. Coyne (Eds.), *The interactional nature of depression: Advances in interpersonal approaches* (pp. 299–327). Washington, DC: American Psychological Association.

Cyranowski, J. M., Frank, E., Young, E., & Shear, M. K. (2000). Adolescent onset of the gender difference in lifetime rates of major depression. *Archives of General Psychiatry, 57*, 21–27.

Dadds, M. R., Sanders, M. R., Morrison, M., & Rebgetz, M. (1992). Childhood depression and conduct disorder: II. An analysis of family interaction patterns in the home. *Journal of Abnormal Psychology, 101*, 505–513.

Dahl, R. E., Birmaher, B., Williamson, L. D., Perel, J., Kaufman, J., Brent, D. A., Axelson, D. A., & Ryan, N. D. (2000). Low growth hormone response to growth hormone-releasing hormone in child depression. *Biological Psychiatry, 48*, 981–988.

Daley, S. E., Hammen, C., Burge, D., Davila, J., Paley, B., Lindberg, N., & Herzberg, D. S. (1997). Predictors of the generation of episodic stress: A longitudinal study of late adolescent women. *Journal of Abnormal Psychology, 106*, 251–259.

Davidson, R. J. (1993). Cerebral asymmetry and emotion: Conceptual and methodological conundrums. *Cognition and Emotion, 7*, 115–138.

Davidson, R. J. (2000). Affective style, psychopathology, and resilience: Brain mechanisms and plasticity. *American Psychologist*, *55*, 1196–1214.

Davila, J., Hammen, C., Burge, D., Paley, B., & Daley, S. E. (1995). Poor interpersonal problem solving as a mechanism of stress generation in depression among adolescent women. *Journal of Abnormal Psychology*, *104*, 592–600.

Davis, B., Sheeber, L., Hops, H., & Tildesley, E. (2000). Adolescent responses to depressive parental behaviors in problem-solving interactions: Implications for depressive symptoms. *Journal of Abnormal Child Psychology*, *28*, 451–465.

Dawson, G., Frey, K., Panagiotides, H., Osterling, J., & Hessl, D. (1997). Infants of depressed mothers exhibit atypical frontal brain activity: A replication and extension of previous findings. *Journal of Child Psychology and Psychiatry*, *38*, 179–186.

Dinan, T. G. (1998). Psychoneuroendocrinology of depression: growth hormone. *Psychoneuroendocrinology*, *21*, 325–339.

Eaves, L. J., Silberg, J. L., Maes, H. H., Simonoff, E., Pickles, A., Rutter, M., Neale, M. C., Reynolds, C. A., Erikson, M. T., Heath, A. C., Loeber, R., Truett, K. R., & Hewitt, J. K. (1997). Genetics and devolopmental psychopathology: 2. The main effects of genes and environment on behavioral problems in the Virginia Twin Study of Adolescent Behavioral Development. *Journal of Child Psychology and Psychiatry*, *38*, 965–980.

Ebata, A. T., & Moos, R. H. (1991). Coping and adjustment in distressed and healthy adolescents. *Journal of Applied Developmental Psychology*, *12*, 33–54.

Eley, T. C., & Stevenson, J. (2000). Specific live events and chronic experiences differentially associated with depression and anxiety in young twins. *Journal of Abnormal Child Psychology*, *28*, 383–394.

Emslie, G. J., Rush, A. J., Weinberg, W. A., Kowatch, R. A., Hughes, C. W., Carmody, T., & Rintelmann, J. (1997). A double-blind, randomized, placebo-controlled trial of fluoxetine in children and adolescents with depression. *Archives of General Psychiatry*, *54*, 1031–1037.

Epkins, C. C. (2000). Cognitive specificity in internalizing and externalizing problems in community and clinic-referred children. *Journal of Clinical Child Psychology*, *29*, 199–208.

Faedda, G., Baldessarini, R., Suppes, T., Tondo, L., Becker, I., & Lipschitz, D. (1995). Pediatric-onset bipolar disorder: A neglected clinical and public health problem. *Harvard Review of Psychiatry*, *3*, 171–195.

Fairbairn, W. (1952). *An object relations theory of the personality*. New York: Basic Books.

Faraone, S. V., & Biederman, J. (1997). Do attention deficit hyperactivity disorder and major depression share familial risk factors? *Journal of Nervous and Mental Disease*, *185*, 533–541.

Faraone, S. V., Biederman, J., Mennin, D., Wozniak, J., & Spencer, T. (1997). Attention-deficit hyperactivity disorder with bipolar disorder: A familial subtype? *Journal of the American Academy of Child and Adolescent Psychiatry*, *36*, 1378–1387.

Faraone, S. V., Biederman, J., Wozniak, J., Mundy, E., Mennin, D., & O'Donnell, D. (1997). Is comorbidity with ADHD a marker for juvenile-onset mania? *Journal of the American Academy of Child and Adolescent Psychiatry*, *36*, 1046–1055.

Fergusson, D. M., Horwood, J., & Lynskey, M. T. (1993). Prevalence and comorbidity of DSM-III-R diagnoses in a birth cohort of 15 year olds. *Journal of the American Academy of Child and Adolescent Psychiatry*, *32*, 1127–1134.

Fergusson, D. M., Lynskey, M., & Horwood, L. J. (1993). The effect of maternal depression on maternal ratings of child behavior. *Journal of Abnormal Child Psychology*, *21*, 245–269.

Field, T., Healy, B., Goldstein, S., & Guthertz, M. (1990). Behavior-state matching and synchrony in mother–infant interactions of nondepressed versus depressed dyads. *Developmental Psychology*, *26*, 7–14.

Fleming, J. E., Boyle, M. H., & Offord, D. R. (1993). The outcome of adolescent depression in the Ontario Child Health Study follow-up. *Journal of the American Academy of Child and Adolescent Psychiatry*, *32*, 28–33.

Fleming, J. E., & Offord, D. R. (1990). Epidemiology of childhood depressive disorders: A critical review. *Journal of the American Academy of Child and Adolescent Psychiatry*, *29*, 571–580.

Fombonne, E. (1994). The Chartres study: I. Prevalence of psychiatric disorders among French school-aged children. *British Journal of Psychiatry*, *164*, 69–79.

Forehand, R., Brody, G. H., Long, N., & Fauber, R. (1988). The interactive influence of adolescent and maternal depression on adolescent social and cognitive functioning. *Cognitive Therapy and Research*, *12*, 341–350.

Freud, S. (1957). Mourning and melancholia. In J. Strachey (Ed. and Trans.), *The standard edition of the complete psychological works of Sigmund Freud* (Vol. 14, pp. 237–260). London: Hogarth Press. (Original work published 1917)

Garber, J., Braafladt, N., & Zeman, J. (1991). The regulation of sad affect: An information-processing perspective. In J. Garber & K. A. Dodge (Eds.), *The development of emotion regulation and dysregulation* (pp. 208–240). New York: Cambridge University Press.

Garber, J., & Flynn, C. A. (2001). Predictors of depressive cognitions in young adolescents. *Cognitive Therapy and Research*, *25*, 353–376.

Garber, J., & Hilsman, R. (1992). Cognitions, stress, and depression in children and adolescents. *Child and Adolescent Psychiatric Clinics of North America*, *1*, 129–167.

Garber, J., & Kaminski, K. M. (2000). Laboratory and performance-based measures of depression in children and adolescents. *Journal of Clinical Child Psychology*, *29*, 509–525.

Garber, J., Robinson, N. S., & Valentiner, D. (1997). The relation between parenting and adolescent depression: Self-worth as a mediator. *Journal of Adolescent Research*, *12*, 12–33.

Garber, J., Weiss, B., & Shanley, N. (1993). Cognitions, depressive symptoms, and development in adolescents. *Journal of Abnormal Psychology*, *102*, 47–57.

Garrison, C. Z., Jackson, K. L., Marsteller, F., McKeown, R., & Addy, C. (1990). A longitudinal study of depressive symptomatology in young adolescents. *Journal of the American Academy of Child and Adolescent Psychiatry*, *29*, 581–585.

Ge, X., Lorenz, F. O., Conger, R. D., Elder, G. G., & Simons, R. L. (1994). Trajectories of stressful life events and depressive symptoms during adolescence. *Developmental Psychology*, *30*, 467–483.

Gelfand, D. M., & Teti, D. M. (1990). The effects of maternal depression on children. *Clinical Psychology Review*, *10*, 320–354.

Geller, B., & Luby, J. (1997). Child and adolescent bipolar disorder: Review of the past 10 years. *Journal of the American Academy of Child and Adolescent Psychiatry, 36*, 1168–1176.

Geller, B., Williams, M., Zimerman, B., Frazier, J., Beringer, L., & Warner, K. (1998). Prepubertal and early adolescent bipolarity differentiate from ADHD by manic symptoms, grandiose delusions, ultra-rapid or ultradian cycling. *Journal of Affective Disorders, 51*, 81–91.

Gladstone, T. R. G., & Kaslow, N. J. (1995). Depression and attributions in children and adolescents: A meta-analytic review. *Journal of Abnormal Child Psychology, 23*, 597–606.

Gold, P. W., Goodwin, F. K., & Chrousos, G. P. (1988). Clinical and biochemical manifestations of depression: Relation to the neurobiology of stress. *New England Journal of Medicine, 319*, 348–353.

Goodman, S. H., Adamson, L. B., Riniti, J., & Cole, S. (1994). Mothers' expressed attitudes: Associations with maternal depression and children's self-esteem and psychopathology. *Journal of the American Academy of Child and Adolescent Psychiatry, 33*, 1265–1274.

Goodman, S. H., Brogan, D., Lynch, M. E., & Fielding, B. (1993). Social and emotional competence in children of depressed mothers. *Child Development, 64*, 516–531.

Goodman, S. H., & Brumley, H. E. (1990). Schizophrenic and depressed mothers: Relational deficits in parenting. *Developmental Psychology, 26*, 31–39.

Goodman, S. H., & Gotlib, I. H. (1999). Risk for psychopathology in the children of depressed mothers: A developmental model for understanding mechanisms of transmission. *Psychological Review, 106*, 458–490.

Goodman, S. H., Schwab-Stone, M., Lahey, B., Shaffer, D., & Jensen, P. (2000). Major depression and dysthymia in children and adolescents: Discriminant validity and differential consequences in a community sample. *Journal of the American Academy of Child and Adolescent Psychiatry, 39*, 761–770.

Goodyer, I. M., & Altham, P. M. E. (1991). Lifetime exit events and recent social and family adversities in anxious and depressed school-age children and adolescents: I. *Journal of Affective Disorders, 21*, 219–228.

Goodyer, I. M., & Cooper, P. (1993). A community study of depression in adolescent girls: II. The clinical features of identified disorder. *British Journal of Psychiatry, 163*, 374–380.

Goodyer, I. M., Herbert, J., & Altham, P. M. E. (1998). Adrenal steroid secretion and major depression in 8- to 16-yr-olds: III. Influences of cortisol/DHEA ratio at presentation on subsequent rates of disappointing life events and persistent major depression. *Psychological Medicine, 28*, 265–273.

Goodyer, I. M., Herbert, J., Tamplin, A., & Altham, P. M. E. (2000a). First-episode major depression in adolescents: Affective, cognitive and endocrine characteristics of risk status and predictors of onset. *British Journal of Psychiatry, 176*, 142–149.

Goodyer, I. M., Herbert, J., Tamplin, A., & Altham, P. M. E. (2000b). Recent life events, cortisol, dehydroepiandrosterone and the onset of major depression in high-risk adolescents. *British Journal of Psychiatry, 177*, 499–504.

Goodyer, I. M., Wright, C., & Altham, P. M. E. (1988). Maternal adversity and recent life events in anxious and depressed school-age children. *Journal of Child Psychology and Psychiatry, 29*, 651–667.

Goodyer, I. M., Wright, C., & Altham, P. M. E. (1990). The friendships and recent life events of anxious and depressed school-age children. *British Journal of Psychiatry, 156*, 689–698.

Gordon, D., Burge, D., Hammen, C., Adrian, C., Jaenicke, C., & Hiroto, D. (1989). Observations of interactions of depressed women with their children. *American Journal of Psychiatry, 146*, 50–55.

Gore, S., Aseltine, R. H., & Colton, M. E. (1992). Social structure, life stress and depressive symptoms in a high school-aged population. *Journal of Health and Social Behavior, 33*, 97–113.

Gore, S., Aseltine, R. H., & Colton, M. E. (1993). Gender, social-relational involvement, and depression. *Journal of Research on Adolescence, 3*, 101–125.

Gotlib, I. H., & Hammen, C. (1992). *Psychological aspects of depression: Toward a cognitive–interpersonal integration*. Chichester, England: Wiley.

Gotlib, I. H., Lewinsohn, P. M., & Seeley, J. R. (1995). Symptoms versus a diagnosis of depression: Differences in psychosocial functioning. *Journal of Consulting and Clinical Psychology, 63*, 90–100.

Gotlib, I. H., Lewinsohn, P. M., & Seeley, J. R. (1998). Consequences of depression during adolescence: Marital status and marital functioning in early adulthood. *Journal of Abnormal Psychology, 107*, 686–690.

Gotlib, I. H., Lewinsohn, P. M., Seeley, J. R., Rohde, P., & Redner, J. E. (1993). Negative cognitions and attributional style in depressed adolescents: An examination of stability and specificity. *Journal of Abnormal Psychology, 102*, 607–615.

Grigoroiu-Serbanescu, M., Christodorescu, D., Jipescu, I., Totoescu, A., Marinescu, E., & Ardelean, V. (1989). Psychopathology in children aged 10–17 of bipolar parents: Psychopathology rate and correlates of the severity of the psychopathology. *Journal of Affective Disorders, 16*, 167–179.

Grigoroiu-Serbanescu, M., Christodorescu, D., Totoescu, A., & Jipescu, I. (1991). Depressive disorders and depressive personality traits in offspring aged 10–17 of bipolar and of normal parents. *Journal of Youth and Adolescence, 20*, 135–148.

Haaga, D. A., Dyck, M. J., & Ernst, D. (1991). Empirical status of cognitive theory of depression. *Psychological Bulletin, 110*, 215–236.

Hammen, C. (1991a). *Depression runs in families: The social context of risk and resilience in children of depressed mothers*. New York: Springer-Verlag.

Hammen, C. (1991b). The generation of stress in the course of unipolar depression. *Journal of Abnormal Psychology, 100*, 555–561.

Hammen, C. (1992a). Cognitive, life stress, and interpersonal approaches to a developmental psychopathology model of depression. *Development and Psychopathology, 4*, 191–208.

Hammen, C. (1992b). Life events and depression: The plot thickens. *American Journal of Community Psychology, 20*, 179–193.

Hammen, C., Adrian, C., Gordon, D., Burge, D., Jaenicke, C., & Hiroto, D. (1987). Children of depressed mothers: Maternal strain and symptom predictors of dysfunction. *Journal. of Abnormal Psychology, 96*, 190–198.

Hammen, C., Adrian, C., & Hiroto, D. (1988). A longitudinal test of the attributional vulnerability model in children at risk for depression. *British Journal of Clinical Psychology, 27*, 37–46.

Hammen, C., & Brennan, P. A. (2001). Depressed adolescents of depressed and nondepressed mothers: Tests of an interpersonal impairment hypothesis. *Journal of Consulting and Clinical Psychology, 69*, 284–294.

Hammen, C., Burge, D., & Stansbury, K. (1990). Relationship of mother and child variables to child outcomes in a high risk sample: A causal modeling analysis. *Developmental Psychology, 26*, 24–30.

Hammen, C., Burge, D., Burney, E., & Adrian, C. (1990). Longitudinal study of diagnoses in children of women with unipolar and bipolar affective disorder. *Archives of General Psychiatry, 47*, 1112–1117.

Hammen, C., Burge, D., Daley, S. E., Davila, J., Paley, B., & Rudolph, K. D. (1995). Interpersonal attachment cognitions and prediction of symptomatic responses to interpersonal stress. *Journal of Abnormal Psychology, 104*, 436–443.

Hammen, C., Davila, J., Brown, G., Gitlin, M., & Ellicott, A. (1992). Stress as a mediator of the effects of psychiatric history on severity of unipolar depression. *Journal of Abnormal Psychology, 101*, 45–52.

Hammen, C., & Goodman-Brown, T. (1990). Self-schemas and vulnerability to specific life stress in children at risk for depression. *Cognitive Therapy and Research, 14*, 215–227.

Hammen, C., & Zupan, B. A. (1984). Self-schemas, depression, and the processing of personal information in children. *Journal of Experimental Child Psychology, 37*, 598–608.

Hankin, B. L., Abramson, L. Y., Moffitt, T. E., Silva, P. A., McGee, R., & Angell, K. E. (1998). Development of depression from preadolescence to young adulthood: Emerging gender differences in a 10-year longitudinal study. *Journal of Abnormal Psychology, 107*, 128–140.

Harrington, R., Fudge, H., Rutter, M., Pickles, A., & Hill, J. (1990). Adult outcomes of childhood and adolescent depression: Psychiatric status. *Archives of General Psychiatry, 47*, 465–473.

Harrington, R., Fudge, H., Rutter, M., Pickles, A., & Hill, J. (1991). Adult outcomes of childhood and adolescent depression: II. Links with antisocial disorders. *Journal of the American Academy of Child and Adolescent Psychiatry, 30*, 434–439.

Harter, S., & Whitesell, N. R. (1996). Multiple pathways to self-reported depression and psychological adjustment among adolescents. *Development and Psychopathology, 8*, 761–777.

Hays, R. D., Wells, K. B., Sherbourne, C. D., Rogers, W., & Spritzer, K. (1995). Functioning and well-being outcomes of patients with depression compared with chronic general medical illness. *Archives of General Psychiatry, 52*, 11–19.

Hayward, C., Gotlib, I. H., Schraedley, P. K., & Litt, I. F. (1999). Ethnic differences in the association between pubertal status and symptoms of depression in adolescent girls. *Journal of Adolescent Health, 25*, 143–149.

Heim, C., & Nemeroff, C. B. (2001). The role of childhood trauma in the neurobiology of mood and anxiety disorders: Preclinical and clinical studies. *Biological Psychiatry, 49*, 1023–1039.

Herman-Stahl, M., & Petersen, A. C (1999). Depressive symptoms during adolescence: Direct and stress-buffering effects of coping, control beliefs, and family relationships. *Journal of Applied Developmental Psychology, 20*, 45–62.

Herzberg, D. S., Hammen, C., Burge, D., Daley, S. E., Davila, J., & Lindberg, N. (1998). Social competence as a predictor of chronic interpersonal stress. *Personal Relationships, 5*, 207–218.

Hops, H., Biglan, A., Sherman, L., Arthur, J., Friedman, L., & Osteen, V. (1987). Home observations of family interactions of depressed women. *Journal of Consulting and Clinical Psychology, 55*, 341–346.

Hops, H., Lewinsohn, P. M., Andrews, J. A., & Roberts, R. E. (1990). Psychosocial correlates of depressive symptomatology among high school students. *Journal of Clinical Child Psychology, 3*, 211–220.

Ialongo, N., Edelsohn, G., & Kellam, S. G. (2001). A further look at the prognostic power of young children's reports of depressed mood and feelings. *Child Development, 72*, 736–747.

Ialongo, N., Edelsohn, G., Werthamer-Larsson, L., Crockett, L., & Kellam, S. G. (1996). Social and cognitive impairment in first-grade children with anxious and depressive symptoms. *Journal of Clinical Child Psychology, 25*, 15–24.

Jacobsen, R. H., Lahey, B. B., & Strauss, C. C. (1983). Correlates of depressed mood in normal children. *Journal of Abnormal Child Psychology, 11*, 29–40.

Jaenicke, C., Hammen, C., Zupan, B., Hiroto, D., Gordon, D., Adrian, C., et al. (1987). Cognitive vulnerability in children at risk for depression. *Journal of Abnormal Child Psychology, 15*, 559–572.

Johnson, J. G., Cohen, P., Kasen, S., Smailes, E., & Brook, J. S. (2001). Association of maladaptive parental behavior with psychiatric disorder among parents and their offspring. *Archives of General Psychiatry, 58*, 453–460.

Joiner, T. E., Coyne, J. C., & Blalock, J. (1999). On the interpersonal nature of depression: Overview and synthesis. In T. E. Joiner & J. C. Coyne (Eds.), *The interactional nature of depression* (pp. 3–19). Washington, DC: American Psychological Association.

Joiner, T. E., Katz, J., & Lew, A. S. (1997). Self-verification and depression among youth psychiatric inpatients. *Journal of Abnormal Psychology, 106*, 608–618.

Joiner, T. E., Metalsky, G. I., Katz, J., & Beach, S. R. H. (1999). Depression and excessive reassurance-seeking. *Psychological Inquiry, 10*, 269–278.

Jones, N. A., Field, T., Fox, N. A., Lundy, B., & Davalos, M. (1997). EEG activation in 1-month-old infants of depressed mothers. *Development and Psychopathology, 9*, 491–505.

Judd, L., Akiskal, A., Maser, J. D., Zeller, P. J., Endicott, J., Coryell, W., Paulus, M. P., Kunovac, J. L., Leon, A. C., Mueller, T. I., Rice, J. A. & Keller, M. B. (1998). A prospective 12-year study of subsyndromal and syndromal depressive symptoms in unipolar major depressive disorders. *Archives of General Psychiatry, 55*, 694–700.

Kafantaris, V., Coletti, D. J., Dicker, R., Padula, G., & Pollack, S. (1998). Are childhood psychiatric histories of bipolar adolescents associated with family history, psychosis, and response to lithium treatment? *Journal of Affective Disorders, 51*, 153–164.

Kashani, J. H., Burbach, D. J., & Rosenberg, T. K. (1988). Perception of family conflict resolution and depressive symptomatology in adolescents. *Journal of the American Academy of Child and Adolescent Psychiatry, 27*, 42–48.

Kashani, J. H., & Carlson, G. A. (1987). Seriously depressed preschoolers. *American Journal of Psychiatry, 144*, 348–350.

Kashani, J. H., Holcomb, W. R., & Orvaschel, H. (1986). Depression and depressive symptoms in preschool children from the general population. *American Journal of Psychiatry, 143*, 1138–1143.

Kashani, J., Rosenberg, T., & Reid, J. (1989). Developmental perspectives in child and adolescent depressive symptoms in a community sample. *American Journal of Psychiatry, 146*, 871–875.

Kaslow, N. J., Adamson, L. B., & Collins, M. H. (2000). A developmental psychopathology perspective on the cognitive components of child and adolescent depression. In A. J. Sameroff, M. Lewis, & S. M. Miller (Eds.), *Handbook of developmental psychopathology* (2nd ed., pp. 491–510). New York: Kluwer Academic/Plenum.

Kaslow, N. J., Deering, C. G., & Racusin, G. R. (1994). Depressed children and their families. *Clinical Psychology Review, 14*, 39–59.

Kaslow, N. J., Rehm, L. P., & Siegel, A. W. (1984). Social-cognitive and cognitive correlates of depression in children. *Journal of Abnormal Child Psychology, 12*, 605–620.

Kaufman, J., Martin, A., King, R. A., & Charney, D. (2001). Are child-, adolescent-, and adult-onset depression one and the same disorder? *Biological Psychiatry, 49*, 980–1001.

Kazdin, A. E., Esveldt-Dawson, K., Sherick, R. B., & Colbus, D. (1985). Assessment of overt behavior and childhood depression among psychiatrically disturbed children. *Journal of Consulting and Clinical Psychology, 53*, 201–210.

Kendall, P. C., Stark, K. D., & Adam, T. (1990). Cognitive deficit or cognitive distortion in childhood depression. *Journal of Abnormal Child Psychology, 18*, 255–270.

Kendler, K. S. (1995). Adversity, stress and psychopathology: A psychiatric genetic perspective. *International Journal of Methods in Psychiatric Research, 5*, 163–170.

Kendler, K. S., Neale, M. C., Kessler, R. C., Heath, A. C., & Eaves, L. J. (1992). Major depression and generalized anxiety disorder: Same genes, (partly) different environments? *Archives of General Psychiatry, 49*, 716–722.

Kendler, K. S., Neale, M. C., Kessler, R. C., Heath, A. C., & Eaves, L. J. (1993). A twin study of recent life events and difficulties. *Archives of General Psychiatry, 50*, 789–796.

Kessler, R. C., Avenevoli, S., & Merikangas, K. R. (2001). Mood disorders in children and adolescents: An epidemiologic perspective. *Biological Psychiatry, 49*, 1002–1014.

Kessler, R. C., & Walters, E. E. (1998). Epidemiology of DSM-III-R major depression and minor depression among adolescents and young adults in the National Comorbidity Survey. *Depression and Anxiety, 7*, 3–14.

Klein, D. N., Depue, R. A., & Slater, J. F. (1985). Cyclothymia in the adolescent offspring of parents with bipolar affective disorder. *Journal of Abnormal Psychology, 94*, 115–127.

Klein, D. N., Lewinsohn, P. M., & Seeley, J. R. (1996). Hypomanic personality traits in a community sample of adolescents. *Journal of Affective Disorders, 38*, 135–143.

Klerman, G. L., Lavori, P. W., Rice, J., Reich, T., Endicott, J., Andreasen, N. C., Keller, M. B., & Hirschfeld, R. M. A. (1985). Birth cohort trends in rates of major depressive disorder among relatives of patients with affective disorder. *Archives of General Psychiatry, 42*, 689–693.

Kobak, R. R., & Ferenz-Gillies, R. (1995). Emotion regulation and depressive symptoms during adolescence: A functionalist perspective. *Development and Psychopathology, 7*, 183–192.

Kobak, R. R., Sudler, N., & Gamble, W. (1991). Attachment and depressive symptoms during adolescence: A developmental pathways analysis. *Development and Psychopathology, 3*, 461–474.

Kovacs, M. (1980). Rating scales to assess depression in school-aged children. *Acta Paedopsychiatrica, 46*, 305–315.

Kovacs, M. (1990). Comorbid anxiety disorders in childhood-onset depressions. In J. D. Maser & C. R. Cloninger (Eds.), *Comorbidity of mood and anxiety disorders* (pp. 272–281). Washington, DC: American Psychiatric Press.

Kovacs, M. (1996). Presentation and course of major depressive disorder during childhood and later years of the life span. *Journal of the American Academy of Child and Adolescent Psychiatry, 35*, 705–715.

Kovacs, M., Akiskal, H. S., Gatsonis, C., & Parrone, P. L. (1994). Childhood-onset dysthymic disorder: Clinical features and prospective naturalistic outcome. *Archives of General Psychiatry, 51*, 365–374.

Kovacs, M., Feinberg, T. L., Crouse-Novak, M. A., Paulauskas, S. L., & Finkelstein, R. (1984). Depressive disorders in childhood: I. A longitudinal prospective study of characteristics and recovery. *Archives of General Psychiatry, 41*, 229–237.

Kovacs, M., Feinberg, T. L., Crouse-Novak, M. A., Paulauskas, S. L., Pollock, M., & Finkelstein, R. (1984). Depressive disorders in childhood: II. A longitudinal study of the risk for a subsequent major depression. *Archives of General Psychiatry, 41*, 643–649.

Kovacs, M., Gatsonis, C., Paulauskas, S. L., & Richards, C. (1989). Depressive disorders in childhood: IV. A longitudinal study of comorbidity with and without risk for anxiety disorders. *Archives of General Psychiatry, 46*, 776–782.

Kovacs, M., Paulauskas, S., Gatsonis, C., & Richards, C. (1988). Depressive disorders in childhood: III. Longitudinal study of comorbidity with and risk for conduct disorders. *Journal of Affective Disorders, 15*, 205–217.

Kovacs, M., & Pollock, M. (1995). Bipolar disorder and comorbid conduct disorder in childhood and adolescent. *Journal of the American Academy of Child and Adolescent Psychiatry, 34*, 715–723.

Lamont, J., Fischoff, S., & Gottlieb, H. (1976). Recall of parental behaviors in female neurotic depressives. *Journal of Clinical Psychology, 32*, 762–765.

Lapalme, M., Hodgins, S., & LaRoche, C. (1997). Children of parents with bipolar disorder: A meta-analysis of risk for mental disorders. *Canadian Journal of Psychiatry, 42*, 623–631.

Laurent, J., & Ettelson, R. (2001). An examination of the tripartite model of anxiety and depression and its application to youth. *Clinical Child and Family Psychology Review, 4*, 209–230.

Laurent, J., & Stark, K. D. (1993). Testing the cognitive content-specificity hypothesis with anxious and depressed youngsters. *Journal of Abnormal Psychology, 102*, 226–237.

Leitenberg, H., Yost, L. W., & Carroll-Wilson, M. (1986). Negative cognitive errors in children: Questionnaire development, normative data, and comparisons between children with and without self-reported symptoms of depression, low self-esteem, and evaluation anxiety. *Journal of Consulting and Clinical Psychology, 54*, 528–536.

Lewinsohn, P. M. (1974). A behavioral approach to depression. In R. Friedman & M. Katz (Eds.), *The psychology of depression: Contemporary theory and research* (pp. 157–185). Washington, DC: Winston-Wiley.

Lewinsohn, P. M., Clarke, G., Seeley, J., & Rohde, P. (1994). Major depression in community adolescents: Age at onset, episode duration, and time to recurrence. *Journal of the American Academy of Child and Adolescent Psychiatry, 33*, 809–818.

Lewinsohn, P. M., Hops, H., Roberts, R. E., Seeley, J. R., & Andrews, J. A. (1993). Adolescent psychopathology: I. Prevalence and incidence of depression and other DSM-III-R disorders in high school students. *Journal of Abnormal Psychology, 102*, 133–144.

Lewinsohn, P. M., Joiner, T. E., & Rohde, P. (2001). Evaluation of cognitive diathesis–stress models in predicting major depressive disorder in adolescents. *Journal of Abnormal Psychology, 110*, 203–215.

Lewinsohn, P. M., Klein, D. N., & Seeley, J. R. (1995). Bipolar disorders in a community sample of older adolescents: Prevalence, phenomenology, comorbidity, and course. *Journal of the American Academy of Child and Adolescent Psychiatry, 34*, 454–463.

Lewinsohn, P. M., Roberts, R. E., Seeley, J. R., Rohde, P., Gotlib, I. H., & Hops, H. (1994). Adolescent psychopathology: II. Psychosocial risk factors for depression. *Journal of Abnormal Psychology, 103*, 302–315.

Lewinsohn, P. M., Rohde, P., Klein, D. M., & Seeley, J. R. (1999). Natural course of adolescent major depressive disorder: I. Continuity into young adulthood. *Journal of the American Academy of Child and Adolescent Psychiatry, 38*, 56–63.

Lewinsohn, P. M., Rohde, P., & Seeley, J. R. (1994). Psychosocial risk factors for future adolescent suicide attempts. *Journal of Consulting and Clinical Psychology, 62*, 297–305.

Lewinsohn, P. M., Zinbarg, R., Seeley, J. R., Lewinsohn, M., & Sack, W. H. (1997). Lifetime comorbidity among anxiety disorders and between anxiety disorders and other mental disorders in adolescents. *Journal of Anxiety Disorders, 11*, 377–394.

Lish, J. D., Dime-Meenan, S., Whybrow, P. C., Price, R. A., & Hirschfeld, R. M. A. (1994). The National Depressive and Manic–Depressive Association (DMDA) survey of bipolar members. *Journal of Affective Disorders, 31*, 281–294.

Lovejoy, C. M., Graczyk, P. A., O'Hare, E., & Neuman, G. (2000). Maternal depression and parenting behavior: A meta-analytic review. *Clinical Psychology Review, 20*, 561–592.

Main, M., Kaplan, N., & Cassidy, J. (1985). Security in infancy, childhood, and adulthood: A move to the level of representation. In I. Bretherton & E. Waters (Eds.), Growing points in attachment theory and research. *Monographs of the Society for Research in Child Development, 50* (1–2, Serial No. 209), 66–104.

McCauley, E., Myers, K., Mitchell, J., Calderon, R., Schloredt, K., & Treder, R. (1993). Depression young people: Initial presentation and clinical course. *Journal of the American Academy of Child and Adolescent Psychiatry, 32*, 714–722.

McGee, R., Feehan, M., Williams, S., Partridge, F., Silva, P. A., & Kelly, J. (1990). DSM-III disorders in a large sample of adolescents. *Journal of the American Academy of Child and Adolescent Psychiatry, 29*, 611–619.

McGrath, E. P., & Repetti, R. L. (2002). A longitudinal study of children's depressive symptoms, self-perceptions, and cognitive distortions about the self. *Journal of Abnormal Psychology, 111*, 77–87.

McKeown, R. E., Garrison, C. Z., Jackson, K. L., Cuffe, S. P., Addy, C. L., & Waller, J. L. (1997). Family structure and cohesion, and depressive symptoms in adolescents. *Journal of Research on Adolescence, 7*, 267–281.

Messer, S. C., & Gross, A. M. (1995). Childhood depression and family interaction: A naturalistic observation study. *Journal of Clinical Child Psychology, 24*, 77–88.

Mitchell, J., McCauley, E., Burke, P. M., & Moss, S. J. (1988). Phenomenology of depression in children and adolescents. *Journal of the American Academy of Child and Adolescent Psychiatry, 27*, 12–20.

Monroe, S. M., Rohde, P., Seeley, J. R., & Lewinsohn, P. M. (1999). Life events and depression in adolescence: Relationship loss as a prospective risk factor for first onset of major depressive disorder. *Journal of Abnormal Psychology, 108*, 606–614.

Murphy, J. M., Laird, N. M., Monson, R. R., Sobol, A. M., & Leighton, A. H. (2000). A 40–year perspective on the prevalence of depression: The Stirling County Study. *Archives of General Psychiatry, 57*, 209–215.

National Institute of Child Health and Human Development (NICHD) Early Child Care Research Network. (1999). Chronicity of maternal depressive symptoms, maternal sensitivity, and child functioning at 36 months. *Developmental Psychology, 35*, 1297–1310.

Nelson, D. R., Hammen, C., Daley, S. E., Burge, D., & Davila, J. (2001). Sociotropic and autonomous personality styles: Contributions to chronic life stress. *Cognitive Therapy and Research, 25*, 61–76.

Neshat Doost, H. T., Taghavi, M. R., Moradi, A. R., Yule, W., & Dalgleish, T. (1998). Memory for emotional trait adjectives in clinically depressed youth. *Journal of Abnormal Psychology, 107*, 642–650.

Nolen-Hoeksema, S. (1991). Responses to depression and their effects on the duration of depressive episodes. *Journal of Abnormal Psychology, 100*, 569–582.

Nolen-Hoeksema, S. (2000). The role of rumination in depressive disorders and mixed anxiety/depressive symptoms. *Journal of Abnormal Psychology, 109*, 504–511.

Nolen-Hoeksema, S. (2002). Gender differences in depression. In I. Gotlib & C. Hammen (Eds.), *Handbook of depression* (pp. 492–509). New York: Guilford Press.

Nolen-Hoeksema, S., & Girgus, J. S. (1994). The emergence of gender differences in depression during adolescence. *Psychological Bulletin, 115*, 424–443.

Nolen-Hoeksema, S., Girgus, J. S., & Seligman, M. E. P. (1992). Predictors and consequences of childhood depressive symptoms: A 5–year longitudinal study. *Journal of Abnormal Psychology, 101*, 405–422.

Offord, D. R., Boyle, M. H., Racine, Y. A., Fleming, J. E., Cadman, D. T., Blum, H, M., Byrne, C., Links, P. S., Lipman, E. L., MacMillan, H. L., Grant, N. I. R., Sanford, M. N., Szatmari, P., Thomas, H., & Woodward, C. A. (1992). Outcome, prognosis, and risk in a longitudinal follow-up study. *Journal of the American Academy of Child and Adolescent Psychiatry, 31*, 916–923.

Oliver, J. M., Handal, P. J., Finn, T., & Herdy, S. (1987). Depressed and nondepressed students and their siblings in frequent contact with their families. *Cognitive Therapy and Research, 11*, 501–515.

Panak, W. F., & Garber, J. (1992). Role of aggression, rejection, and attributions in the prediction of depression in children. *Development and Psychopathology, 4*, 145–165.

Pappini, D., Roggman, L., & Anderson, J. (1991). Early-adolescent perceptions of attachment to mother and father: A test of the emotional-distancing and buffering hypothesis. *Journal of Early Adolescence, 11*, 258–275.

Parker, G. (1981). Parental reports of depressives: An investigation of several explanations. *Journal of Affective Disorders, 3*, 131–140.

Patterson, G. R., & Stoolmiller, M. (1991). Replications of a dual failure model for boys' depressed mood. *Journal of Consulting and Clinical Psychology, 59*, 491–498.

Pavlidis, K., & McCauley, E. (2001). Autonomy and relatedness in family interactions with depressed adolescents. *Journal of Abnormal Child Psychology, 29*, 11–21.

Paykel, E. S. (1979). Recent life events in the development of the depressive disorders: Implications for the effects of stress. In R. A. Depue (Ed.), *The psychobiology of the depressive disorders* (pp. 245–262). New York: Academic Press.

Persons, J. B., & Miranda, J. (1992). Cognitive theories of vulnerability to depression: Reconciling negative evidence. *Cognitive Therapy and Research, 16*, 485–502.

Petersen, A. C., Sarigiani, P. A., & Kennedy, R. E. (1991). Adolescent depression: Why more girls? *Journal of Youth and Adolescence, 20*, 247–271.

Pfeffer, C. R. (2001). Diagnosis of childhood and adolescent suicidal behavior: Unmet needs for suicide prevention. *Biological Psychiatry, 49*, 1055–1061.

Pine, D. S., Cohen, P., Gurley, D., Brook, J. S., & Ma, Y. (1998). The risk for early-adulthood anxiety and depressive disorders in adolescents with anxiety and depressive disorders. *Archives of General Psychiatry, 55*, 56–64.

Polaino-Lorente, A., & Domenech, E. (1993). Prevalence of childhood depression: Results of the first study in Spain. *Journal of Child Psychology and Psychiatry, 34*, 1007–1017.

Pomerantz, E. M., & Rudolph, K. D. (in press). What ensues from emotional distress?: Implications for the development of competence estimation. *Child Development.*

Post, R. M. (1992). Transduction of psychosocial stress into the neurobiology of recurrent affective disorder. *American Journal of Psychiatry, 149*, 999–1010.

Prieto, S. L., Cole, D. A., & Tageson, C. W. (1992). Depressive self-schemas in clinic and nonclinic children. *Cognitive Therapy and Research, 16*, 521–534.

Puig-Antich, J. (1982). Major depression and conduct disorder in prepuberty. *Journal of the American Academy of Child and Adolescent Psychiatry, 21*, 118–128.

Puig-Antich, J., Chambers, W. J., & Tabrizi, M. A. (1983). The clinical assessment of current depressive episodes in children and adolescents: Interviews with parents and children. In D. P. Cantwell & G. A. Carlson (Eds.), *Affective disorders in childhood and adolescence* (pp.157–179). New York: Spectrum.

Puig-Antich, J., Kaufman, J., Ryan, N. D., Williamson, D. E., Dahl, R. E., Lukens, E., et al. (1993). The psychosocial functioning and family environment of depressed adolescents. *Journal of the American Academy of Child and Adolescent Psychiatry, 32*, 244–253.

Puig-Antich, J., Lukens, E., Davies, M., Goetz, D., Brennan-Quattrock, J., & Todak, G. (1985a). Psychosocial functioning in prepubertal major depressive disorders: I. Interpersonal relationships during the depressive episode. *Archives of General Psychiatry, 42*, 500–507.

Puig-Antich, J., Lukens, E., Davies, M., Goetz, D., Brennan-Quattrock, J., & Todak, G. (1985b). Psychosocial functioning in prepubertal major depressive disorders: II. Interpersonal relationships after sustained recovery from affective episode. *Archives of General Psychiatry, 42*, 511–517.

Quiggle, N. L., Garber, J., Panak, W. F., & Dodge, K. A. (1992). Social information processing in aggressive and depressed children. *Child Development, 63*, 1305–1320.

Radke-Yarrow, M. (1998). *Children of depressed mothers: From early childhood to maturity*. Cambridge, England: Cambridge University Press.

Radloff, L. (1977). The CES-D Scale: A new self-report depression scale for research in the general population. *Applied Psychological Measurement, 1*, 385–401.

Randolph, J. J., & Dykman, B. M. (1998). Perceptions of parenting and depression-proneness in the offspring: Dysfunctional attitudes as a mediating mechanism. *Cognitive Therapy and Research, 22*, 377–400.

Rao, U., Hammen, C., & Daley, S. (1999). Continuity of depression during the transition to adulthood: A 5-year longitudinal study of young women. *Journal of the American Academy of Child and Adolescent Psychiatry, 38*, 908–915.

Rehm, L. P. (1977). A self-control model of depression. *Behavior Therapy, 8*, 787–804.

Reinherz, H. Z., Giaconia, R. M., Hauf, A. M. C., Wasserman, M. S., & Paradis, A. D. (2000). General and specific childhood risk factors for depression and drug disorders by early adulthood. *Journal of the American Academy of Child and Adolescent Psychiatry, 39*, 223–231.

Reinherz, H. Z., Giaconia, R. M., Lefkowitz, E. S., Pakiz, B., & Frost, A. K. (1993). Prevalence of psychiatric disorders in a community population of older adolescents. *Journal of the American Academy of Child and Adolescent Psychiatry, 32*, 369–377.

Rende, R. D., Plomin, R., Reiss, D., & Hetherington, E. M. (1993). Genetic and environmental influences on depressive symptomatology in adolescence: Individual differences and extreme scores. *Journal of Child Psychology and Psychiatry, 8*, 1387–1398.

Renouf, A., & Kovacs, M. (1994). Concordance between mothers' reports and children's self-reports of depressive symptoms: A longitudinal study. *Journal of the American Academy of Child and Adolescent Psychiatry, 33*, 208–216.

Richters, J. E. (1992). Depressed mothers as informants about their children: A critical review of the evidence for distortion. *Psychological Bulletin, 112*, 485–499.

Roberts, R. E., Attkisson, C. C., & Rosenblatt, A. (1998). Prevalence of psychopathology among children and adolescents. *American Journal of Psychiatry, 155*, 715–725.

Roberts, R. E., Lewinsohn, P. M., & Seeley, J. R. (1991). Screening for adolescent depression: A comparison of depression scales. *Journal of the American Academy of Child and Adolescent Psychiatry, 30*, 58–66.

Roberts, R. E., Roberts, C. R., & Chen, Y. R. (1997). Ethonocultural differences in prevalence of adolescent depression. *American Journal of Community Psychology, 25*, 95–110.

Robinson, N. S., Garber, J., & Hilsman, R. (1995). Cognitions and stress: Direct and moderating effects on depressive versus externalizing symptoms during the junior high school transition. *Journal of Abnormal Psychology, 104*, 453–463.

Rohde, P., Lewinsohn, P., & Seeley, J. (1991). Comorbidity of unipolar depression: II. Comorbidity with other mental disorders in adolescents and adults. *Journal of Abnormal Psychology, 100*, 214–222.

Rudolph, K. D. (2002). Gender differences in emotional responses to interpersonal stress during adolescence. *Journal of Adolescent Health, 30*, 3–13.

Rudolph, K. D., & Clark, A. G. (2001). Conceptions of relationships in children with depressive and aggressive symptoms: Social-cognitive distortion or reality? *Journal of Abnormal Child Psychology*, *29*, 41–56.

Rudolph, K. D., & Hammen, C. (1999). Age and gender as determinants of stress exposure, generation, and reactions in youngsters: A transactional perspective. *Child Development*, *70*, 660–677.

Rudolph, K. D., Hammen, C., & Burge, D. (1994). Interpersonal functioning and depressive symptoms in childhood: Addressing the issues of specificity and comorbidity. *Journal of Abnormal Child Psychology*, *22*, 355–371.

Rudolph, K. D., Hammen, C., & Burge, D. (1997). A cognitive–interpersonal approach to depressive symptoms in preadolescent children. *Journal of Abnormal Child Psychology*, *25*, 33–45.

Rudolph, K. D., Hammen, C., Burge, D., Lindberg, N., Herzberg, D. S., & Daley, S. E. (2000). Toward an interpersonal life-stress model of depression: The developmental context of stress generation. *Development and Psychopathology*, *12*, 215–234.

Rudolph, K. D., Kurlakowsky, K. D., & Conley, C. S. (2001). Developmental and social-contextual origins of depressive control-related beliefs and behavior. *Cognitive Therapy and Research*, *25*, 447–475.

Rudolph, K. D., Lambert, S. F., Clark, A. G., & Kurlakowsky, K. D. (2001). Negotiating the transition to middle school: The role of self-regulatory processes. *Child Development*, *72*, 929–946.

Rudolph, K. D., Lambert, S. M., Osborne, L., Gathright, T., & Kumar, S. (2002). *Developmental considerations in anxiety and depression: The emergence of sex differences across early adolescence*. Manuscript submitted for publication.

Rutter, M. (1986). The developmental psychopathology of depression: Issues and perspectives. In M. Rutter, C. E. Izard, & P. B. Read (Eds.), *Depression in young people: Clinical and developmental perspectives* (pp. 3–30). New York: Guilford Press.

Ryan, N. D., Puig-Antich, J., Ambrosini, P., Rabinovich, H., Robinson, D., Nelson, B., Iyengar, S., & Twomey, J. (1987). The clinical picture of major depression in children and adolescents. *Archives of General Psychiatry*, *44*, 854–861.

Schraedley, P. K., Gotlib, I. H., & Hayward, C. (1999). Gender differences in correlates of depressive symptoms in adolescents. *Journal of Adolescent Health*, *25*, 98–108.

Seligman, M. E. P. (1975). *Helplessness: On depression, development, and death*. San Francisco: Freeman.

Seroczynski, A. D., Cole, D. A., & Maxwell, S. E. (1997). Cumulative and compensatory effects of competence and incompetence on depressive symptoms in children. *Journal of Abnormal Psychology*, *106*, 586–597.

Shaffer, D., Fisher, P., Lucas, C.P., Dulcan, M.K., & Schwab-Stone, M.E. (2000). NIMH Diagnostic Interview Schedule for Children Version IV (NIMH DISC-IV): Description, differences from previous versions, and reliability of some common diagnoses. *Journal of the American Academy of Child and Adolescent Psychiatry*, *39*, 28–38.

Sheeber, L., Hops, H., Alpert, A., Davis, B., & Andrews, J. A. (1997). Family support and conflict: Prospective relations to adolescent depression. *Journal of Abnormal Child Psychology*, *25*, 333–344.

Sheeber, L., & Sorenson, E. (1998). Family relationships of depressed adolescents: A multimethod assessment. *Journal of Clinical Child Psychology*, *27*, 268–277.

Shirk, S. R., Boergers, J., Eason, A., & Van Horn, M. (1998). Dysphoric interpersonal schemata and preadolescents' sensitization to negative events. *Journal of Clinical Child Psychology*, *27*, 54–68.

Shirk, S. R., Van Horn, M., & Leber, D. (1997). Dysphoria and children's processing of supportive interactions. *Journal of Abnormal Child Psychology*, *25*, 239–249.

Silberg, J., Pickles, A., Rutter, M., Hewitt, J., Simonoff, E., Maes, H., Carbonneau, R., Murrelle, L., Foley, D., & Eaves, L. (1999). The influence of genetic factors and life stress on depression among adolescent girls. *Archives of General Psychiatry*, *56*, 225–232.

Silberg, J. L., Rutter, M., & Eaves, L. (2001). Genetic and environmental influences on the temporal association between earlier anxiety and later depression in girls. *Biological Psychiatry*, *49*, 1040–1049.

Solomon, D. A., Keller, M. B., Leon, A. C., Mueller, T. I., Lavori, P. W., Shea, T., Coryell, W., Warshaw, M., Turvey, C., Maser, J. D., & Endicott, J. (2000). Multiple recurrences of major depressive disorder. *American Journal of Psychiatry*, *157*, 229–233.

Stark, K. D., Humphrey, L. L., Laurent, J., Livingston, R., & Christopher, J. (1993). Cognitive, behavioral, and family factors in the differentiation of depressive and anxiety disorders during childhood. *Journal of Consulting and Clinical Psychology*, *5*, 878–886.

Strober, M., Lampert, C., Schmidt, S., & Morrell, W. (1993). The course of major depressive disorder in adolescents: Recovery and risk of manic switching in a 24-month prospective, naturalistic follow-up of psychotic and non-psychotic subtypes. *Journal of the American Academy of Child and Adolescent Psychiatry*, *32*, 34–42.

Strober, M., Schmidt-Lackner, S., Freeman, R., Bower, S., Lampert, C. & DeAntonio, M. (1995). Recovery and relapse in adolescents with bipolar affective illness: A five-year naturalistic, prospective follow-up. *Journal of the American Academy of Child and Adolescent Psychiatry*, *34*, 724–731.

Sullivan, P. F., Neale, M. C., & Kendler, K. S. (2000). Genetic epidemiology of major depression: Review and meta-analysis. *American Journal of Psychiatry*, *157*, 1552–1562.

Taylor, L., & Ingram, R. E. (1999). Cognitive reactivity and depressotypic information processing in children of depressed mothers. *Journal of Abnormal Psychology*, *108*, 202–210.

Teasdale, J. D. (1983). Negative thinking in depression: Cause, effect, or reciprocal relationship? *Advances in Behaviour Research and Therapy*, *5*, 3–25.

Teti, D. M., Gelfand, D. M., Messinger, D. S., & Isabella, R. (1995). Maternal depression and the quality of early attachment: An examination of infants, preschoolers, and their mothers. *Developmental Psychology*, *31*, 364–376.

Thapar, A., & McGuffin, P. (1994). A twin study of depressive symptoms in childhood. *British Journal of Psychiatry*, *165*, 259–265.

Thapar, A., & McGuffin, P. (1997). Anxiety and depressive symptoms in childhood: A genetic study of comorbidity. *Journal of Child Psychology and Psychiatry*, *38*, 651–656.

Thomsen, P. H., Moller, L. L., Dehlholm, B., & Brask, B. H. (1992). Manic-depressive psychosis in children younger than 15 years: A register-based investigation of 39 cases in Denmark. *Acta Psychiatrica Scandinavica*, *85*, 401–406.

Tram, J. M., & Cole, D. A. (2000). Self-perceived competence and the relation between life events and depressive symptoms in adolescence: Mediator or moderator? *Journal of Abnormal Psychology*, *109*, 753–760.

Turner, J. E., & Cole, D. A. (1994). Developmental differences in cognitive diatheses for child depression. *Journal of Abnormal Child Psychology*, *22*, 15–32.

Verhulst, F. C., & van der Ende, J. (1992). Six-year developmental course of internalizing and externalizing problem behaviors. *Journal of the American Academy of Child and Adolescent Psychiatry*, *31*, 924–931.

Verhulst, F. C., van der Ende, J., Ferdinand, R. F., & Kasius, M. C. (1997). The prevalence of DSM-III-R diagnoses in a national sample of Dutch adolescents. *Archives of General Psychiatry*, *54*, 329–336.

Ward, L. G., Friedlander, M. L., & Silverman, W. K. (1987). Children's depressive symptoms, negative self-statements, and causal attributions for success and failure. *Cognitive Therapy and Research*, *11*, 215–227.

Weiss, B., Weisz, J. R., Politano, M., Carey, M., Nelson, W. M., & Finch, A. J. (1991a). Developmental differences in the factor structure of the Children's Depression Inventory. *Psychological Assessment: A Journal of Consulting and Clinical Psychology*, *3*, 38–45.

Weiss, B., Weisz, J. R., Politano, M., Carey, M., Nelson, W. M., & Finch, A. J. (1991b). Relations among self-reported depressive symptoms in clinic-referred children versus adolescents. *Journal of Abnormal Psychology*, *101*, 391–397.

Weissman, M. M., Paykel, E. S., & Klerman, G. L. (1972). The depressed woman as a mother. *Social Psychiatry*, *7*, 98–108.

Weissman, M. M., Warner, V., Wickramaratne, P., Moreau, D., & Olfson, M. (1997). Offspring of depressed parents: 10 years later. *Archives of General Psychiatry*, *54*, 932–940.

Weissman, M. M., Wickramarante, P., Warner, V., John, K., Prusoff, B. A., Merikangas, K. R., & Gammon, D. (1987). Assessing psychiatric disorders in children: Discrepancies between mothers' and children's reports. *Archives of General Psychiatry*, *44*, 747–753.

Weissman, M. M., Wolk, S., Goldstein, R. B., Moreau, D., Adams, P., Greenwald, S., Klier, C. M., Ryan, N. D., Dahl, R. E., & Wickramaratne, P. (1999). Depressed adolescents grown up. *Journal of the American Medical Association*, *281*, 1707–1713.

Weisz, J. R., Rudolph, K. D., Granger, D. A., & Sweeney, L. (1992). Cognition, competence, and coping in child and adolescent depression: Research findings, developmental concerns, therapeutic implications. *Development and Psychopathology*, *4*, 627–653.

Weisz, J. R., Sweeney, L., Proffitt, V., & Carr, T. (1994). Control-related beliefs and self-reported depressive symptoms in late childhood. *Journal of Abnormal Psychology*, *102*, 411–418.

Wickramaratne, P. J., & Weissman, M. M. (1998). Onset of psychopathology in offspring by developmental phase and parental depression. *Journal of the American Academy of Child and Adolescent Psychiatry*, *37*, 933–941.

Wierzbicki, M. (1987). Similarity of monozygotic and dizygotic child twins in level and lability of subclinically depressed mood. *American Journal of Orthopsychiatry*, *57*, 33–40.

Williamson, D. E., Birmaher, B., Anderson, B. P., Al-Shabbout, M., & Ryan, N. D. (1995). Stressful life events in depressed adolescents: The role of dependent events during the depressive episode. *Journal of the American Academy of Child and Adolescent Psychiatry*, *34*, 591–598.

World Health Organization. (1993). *The ICD-10 classification of mental and behavioural disorders: Diagnostic criteria for research*. Geneva: Author.

Wozniak, J., Biederman, J., Kiely, K., Ablon, J. S., Faraone, S. V., Mundy, E., & Mennin, D. (1995). Mania-like symptoms suggestive of childhood-onset bipolar disorder in clinically referred children. *Journal of the American Academy of Child and Adolescent Psychiatry*, *34*, 867–876.

Zahn-Waxler, C., Klimes-Dougan, B., & Slattery, M. (2000). Internalizing problems of childhood and adolescence: Prospects, pitfalls, and progress in understanding the development of anxiety and depression. *Development and Psychopathology*, *12*, 443–466.

CHAPTER SIX

Childhood Anxiety Disorders

Anne Marie Albano
Bruce F. Chorpita
David H. Barlow

Anxiety disorders are widely recognized as among the most common psychiatric disorders affecting children and adolescents (Anderson, Williams, McGee, & Silva, 1987; Bell-Dolan & Brazeal, 1993; Costello & Angold, 1995; Gurley, Cohen, Pine, & Brook, 1996; Kashani & Orvaschel, 1988; Orvaschel & Weissman, 1986), and yet these disorders are not well understood with regard to youths (Zahn-Waxler, Klimes-Dougan, & Slattery, 2000). Transient fears and anxieties are considered part of normal development; however, for some children, this developmental expectation may serve to mask the presence of an emerging or existing anxiety disorder (Muris, Merckelbach, Mayer, & Prins, 2001). High and stable levels of anxiety are associated with severe impairment in functioning, expressed in its most disabling form through a child's avoidance of such activities as school, peer involvement, and the attainment of stage-related developmental tasks (Albano & Detweiler, 2001; Bell-Dolan & Brazeal, 1993). Long-term outcomes of anxiety disorders in childhood and adolescence are still not well understood, and conflicting evidence exists suggesting a more optimistic prognosis in some studies (e.g., Last, Perrin, Hersen & Kazdin, 1996; Last, Hansen, & Franco, 1997), while others show an increased risk for additional anxiety disorders, depression, and other negative mental health outcomes over time (Berg et al., 1989; Feehan, McGee, & Williams, 1993; Ferdinand & Verhulst, 1995; Flament et al., 1990; Keller et al., 1992; Pine, Cohen, Gurley, Brook, & Ma, 1998). The third edition of the *Diagnostic and Statistical Manual of Mental Disorders* (DSM-III; American Psychiatric Association, 1980) introduced a separate section delineating three anxiety disorders unique to childhood and adolescence: separation anxiety disorder (SAD), avoidant disorder of childhood or adolescence, and overanxious disorder (OAD). Consequently, a multitude of studies emerged documenting the incidence and prevalence of these three disorders along with the "adult" anxiety disorders in youths. Advances in child psychopathology research focused on the anxiety disorders resulted in further nosological changes to DSM's fourth edition (DSM-IV; American Psychiatric Association, 1994). Although SAD is the only remaining childhood anxiety disorder per se, several criteria for the "adult" anxiety disorders include descriptors for their application to children. However, developmental epidemiologists and clinical scientists caution that the DSM-IV categories, while guiding clinicians toward modifying certain criteria for youths, do not actually reflect a developmental psychopathology perspective (Angold & Costello, 1995; Cantwell & Baker, 1988). As noted by March and Albano (2002), a clinician is left to his or her own devices in translating these criteria for each child by taking into account demographic and developmental variables, such as age, gender, race, cultural background, socioeconomic status (SES), and cognitive level. This leaves much room for wide variation among clinicians, due to differences in training, experience, theoretical orientation, familiarity with normal development, and understanding of the processes involved in the development and expression of psychopathology.

The present chapter examines the prevalence, expression, and developmental patterns of specific anxiety disorders in children and adolescents. Attention is directed toward clinical variables (e.g., age at onset, severity, comorbidity) and sociodemographic variables (e.g., gender, race, SES) relative to each disorder. Clinical impairment in functioning is specified within a developmental context. These issues are discussed in terms of the course of childhood anxiety disorders. Moreover, we review the research literature pertaining to proposed mechanisms involved in the etiology of these disorders, which involve exciting and provocative areas of inquiry and investigation. We then highlight recent studies suggesting serious long-term negative outcomes for youths with anxiety disorders. The chapter concludes with a review of current issues in the study of childhood anxiety and future directions.

BRIEF HISTORICAL CONTEXT

The study of children's anxieties and fears has been described in the literature for decades (for reviews, see Albano, Causey, & Carter, 2001; Barrios & Hartmann, 1997). Case studies of childhood fears formed the foundation for the development of both psychoanalytic and behavioral theory. In the classic case study of "Little Hans," Freud (1909/1955) defined and described several key unconscious processes operating in the development of phobia, such as the ego defense mechanisms of repression and displacement. Furthermore, this case provided Freud with rich clinical data for the explication of the "Oedipal stage," perhaps the most controversial and critical stage of psychosexual development. Although the study of Little Hans has since been reformulated beyond Freud's initial conceptualization (e.g., A. Freud, 1965), its value and place in psychoanalytic theory remain firmly ingrained. Similarly, the conditioned fear of a white laboratory rat in young Albert provided early support for the classical conditioning of anxiety and the foundations of behavioral theory (Harris, 1979; Watson & Rayner, 1920). As students of psychology are well aware, prior to the classic experiment, little Albert was fearless of white rats and similar white furry stimuli. Repeated pairings of a neutral stimulus (a white rat) and an aversive stimulus (loud noise) resulted in the development of a conditioned reaction of fear of the rat in 1-year-old Albert. In addition, Albert's fear generalized to a range of white stimuli (including cotton), providing Watson and Rayner with an experimental paradigm upon which to base the core principles of behavioral theory. Additional support for the theory was soon to follow in yet another case study of a child, as Mary Cover Jones (1924a, 1924b) validated the behavioral tenet that all behavior is learned and hence can also be unlearned. Utilizing techniques incorporating modeling and desensitization, Jones described the treatment of 3-year-old Peter's fear of rabbits, which was successfully resolved.

Although these and similar case studies of children served to further the interest in and support for specific theoretical models and related therapeutic interventions, the study of pathological anxiety conditions in children was essentially ignored until only the latter part of the 20th century. This fact is both surprising and humbling, when one considers that there existed a wealth of information and research spanning most of the last 60 years of the 1900s focused on the developmental progression of children's fears and phobias. Several comprehensive reviews describe the historical progression of this research (Barrios & Hartmann, 1997; Barrios & O'Dell, 1998; King, Hamilton, & Ollendick, 1988; Ollendick & King, 1991). To summarize, prior to the publication of DSM-III (American Psychiatric Association, 1980), fears and anxiety reactions in children were largely ignored in psychiatric nosological systems; rather, they were studied as part of research investigating normative developmental reactions and classified according to etiology (Hebb, 1946) or empirically based factor groupings (Miller, Barrett, Hampe, & Noble, 1972; Ollendick, 1983a; Scherer & Nakamura, 1968). Such research demonstrated that subclinical fears are common in children (e.g., Miller, 1983; Ollendick, 1983a), that the number of fears reported by children declines with age (MacFarlane, Allen, & Honzik, 1954), and that the focus of the fear changes over time (e.g., Bauer, 1976). In addition, across studies, girls have consistently endorsed a greater number of fears and anxieties than boys (Abe & Masui, 1981; Essau, Conradt, & Petermann, 1999; La Greca, 2001; Lapouse & Monk, 1958, 1959; Lewinsohn, Gotlib,

Lewinsohn, Seeley, & Allen, 1998; Mackinaw-Koons & Vasey, 2000).

In contrast to the wealth of studies examining subclinical fears in children, formal psychiatric classification systems have acknowledged the presence of pathological phobic reactions only since the early 1950s. The publication of DSM's first edition (American Psychiatric Association, 1952) first identified phobias as psychoneurotic reactions, and subsequently in DSM-II (American Psychiatric Association, 1968), the diagnostic category changed to phobic neuroses. DSM-II introduced overanxious reaction as a distinct diagnostic category for children and adolescents. These early DSM systems were heavily tied to psychoanalytic theory, purporting an unconscious process or conflict as the etiological mechanism for phobic or overanxious reactions (Barlow, 2002). The inclusion of overanxious reaction in the psychiatric nomenclature marked the beginning, albeit meager, of attention to pathological anxiety states in children and adolescents. Although this category provided clinicians with a framework for understanding anxiety in youths, research attention to the study of anxiety in children was not to occur in earnest until the 1980s. This lag in attention to childhood anxiety conditions may have been due in part to long-standing disagreements within the field as to what constituted a clinical anxiety state, distinct from transient developmental fears and anxieties (Barrios & Hartmann, 1997; Strauss & Last, 1993). DSM-III (American Psychiatric Association, 1980) and DSM-III-R (American Psychiatric Association, 1987) represent the first attempts in the history of modern classification systems of psychopathology to delineate developmentally appropriate diagnostic criteria for phobias and other anxiety disorders in children and adolescents. SAD, avoidant disorder of childhood or adolescence, and OAD earned notoriety as the three distinct anxiety disorders of childhood. In total, children could be diagnosed with these three anxiety disorders in addition to such adult anxiety disorders as phobic disorders, obsessive–compulsive disorder (OCD), and posttraumatic stress disorder. Thus the DSM-III and subsequent DSM-III-R sparked a legion of studies examining the epidemiology and clinical characteristics of anxiety disorders in childhood (e.g., Flament et al., 1988; Francis, Last, & Strauss, 1987; Last, Francis, Hersen, Kazdin, & Strauss, 1987; Last, Hersen, Kazdin, Finkelstein, & Strauss, 1987; Last & Strauss, 1989a). Consequently, such studies have culminated in changes and revisions in criteria for diagnosing anxiety disorders, evidenced in DSM-IV (American Psychiatric Association, 1994). As noted above and discussed throughout this chapter, studies must continue to examine these disorders from a developmental psychopathology perspective; as such, it can be expected that further refinement of the diagnostic categories will occur in future editions of the DSM.

Researchers have witnessed a plethora of studies in the broad area of anxiety disorders, attending to the clinical course and expression of these conditions in children, along with the continuity of anxiety from childhood throughout the life span (e.g., Ferdinand & Verhulst, 1995; Pine et al., 1998). Still, the systematic examination of anxiety disorders in children continues to lag far behind adult psychopathology research, and several pressing issues underscore the crucial necessity for ongoing study in this area. First, anxiety disorders are among the most common and most prevalent psychiatric disorders in youths (Achenbach, Howell, McConaughy, & Stanger, 1995; Costello & Angold, 1995; Gurley et al., 1996; Shaffer et al., 1996), and they constitute the primary reason for the referral of children and adolescents for mental health services (Beidel, 1991). Yet fewer than 20% of all children requiring mental health services for any disorder actually receive the necessary intervention (Kendall, 1994; Tuma, 1989). This underutilization of mental health services may partially result from inadequate identification of psychiatric disorders in children, particularly internalizing problems such as anxiety disorders. Children presenting with externalizing conditions, such as conduct disorder and attention-deficit/hyperactivity disorder (ADHD), are more easily recognized by adult caretakers, particularly when the symptoms of these disorders begin to interfere with daily functioning and cause disruption in school and familial activities. In fact, research indicates that children with anxiety disorders are rated on some measures (e.g., teachers' perception of global competence) as just as impaired as children with externalizing disorders (Benjamin, Costello, & Warren, 1990). Still, children with internalizing disorders suffer for the most part in silence and are not easily identified as problematic. The limited utilization of mental health services in response to anxiety disorders in children and adolescents may well reflect the limited knowledge of what constitutes this type of mental health problem in children. Consequently, the result is a failure to recognize and intervene early in the development of these disorders.

Contributing to the problem of identifying pathological anxiety conditions in children is our inadequate understanding of what constitutes normal, developmentally appropriate anxiety reactions. Because all children are expected to display separation anxiety or specific fears at various times in their young lives, the intensity and duration of these developmentally appropriate episodes have not been adequately studied in comparison to pathological anxiety states. Early studies on the prevalence of fears, worries, and anxieties in children and adolescents reported estimates ranging from 3% to 18% (e.g., Abe & Masui, 1981; Orvaschel & Weissman, 1986; Werry & Quay, 1971). However, Bell-Dolan, Last, and Strauss (1990) examined the prevalence of anxiety symptoms in a sample on 62 never-psychiatrically-ill children and adolescents. A variety of anxiety symptoms—particularly fears of heights, public speaking, and somatic complaints—were endorsed by approximately 20% of the subjects. These findings were higher than previous estimates reported in the literature, suggesting that anxiety symptoms at subclinical or clinical levels may occur with greater frequency in youths than previously expected. Overall, Bell-Dolan et al. (1990) called for greater attention toward examining the patterns of expression of anxiety symptoms in children, and for investigations into developmental and situational factors influencing these symptoms.

Second, research has demonstrated the negative impact of childhood anxiety on a broad range of psychosocial factors, including academic performance, family functioning, and social functioning (Dweck & Wortman, 1982; Ialongo, Edelsohn, Werthamer-Larsson, Crockett, & Kellam, 1994, 1995; Strauss, Frame, & Forehand, 1987; Turner, Beidel, & Costello, 1987). Impairment in functioning may be adversely affected by the consistent findings of high comorbidity among the anxiety disorders and comorbidity of anxiety with such disorders as depression and ADHD (Brady & Kendall, 1992; Essau, Conradt, & Petermann, 2000; Keller et al., 1992; Lewinsohn, Zinbarg, Seeley, Lewinsohn, & Sack, 1997; Pawlak, Pascual-Sanchez, Rae, Fischer, & Ladame, 1999). In cases where anxiety is comorbid with an externalizing disorder or depression of sufficient intensity, it is likely that the latter disorder will become the focus of treatment and overshadow the anxiety disorder. Given that the impairment experienced by anxious children and adolescents cuts across a wide range of activities and situations, and that the diagnostic picture may be complicated by anxiety comorbidity, ongoing studies are sorely needed to evaluate fully the impact and course of anxiety disorders in youths.

Finally, empirical data consistently support the findings that anxiety disorders have an early onset in childhood and adolescence and run a chronic course well into adulthood (Achenbach et al., 1995; Ferdinand & Verhulst, 1995; Klein, 1995; Pine et al., 1998). Thus the impairments associated with anxiety in youths hold long-term implications for adult functioning (Kendall, 1992). Research suggests that anxiety symptoms may actually worsen over time (cf. Kendall, 1994) and lead to serious adult outcomes, such as continuing anxiety disorders, major depression, suicide attempts, and psychiatric hospitalization (Achenbach et al., 1995; Alloy, Kelly, Mineka, & Clements, 1990; Ferdinand & Verhulst, 1995; Woodward & Ferguson, 2001). Attention to basic psychopathology research serves to advance our understanding of the nature and course of such disorders; more importantly, it holds implications for the development of empirically based and efficacious prescriptive treatment protocols for the range of anxiety disorders in youths.

DESCRIPTION OF THE DISORDERS

In DSM-IV (American Psychiatric Association, 1994), children can be diagnosed with any of nine anxiety disorders: SAD, panic disorder, agoraphobia, generalized anxiety disorder (GAD, which includes the former diagnosis of OAD), social phobia, specific (formerly simple) phobia, OCD, posttraumatic stress disorder, and acute stress disorder. These disorders share anxiety as the predominant feature, expressed through specific and discrete cognitive, physiological, and behavioral reactions. What distinguishes one anxiety disorder from the next is the focus of a child's anxiety. In this section, we define the core and related symptoms of specific anxiety disorders affecting children and adolescents. A listing of DSM-IV criteria is provided in tabular form for each disorder. The reader interested in posttraumatic stress disorder and related reactions is referred to Fletcher (Chapter 7, this volume) for a comprehensive review.

Separation Anxiety Disorder

Core Symptoms

SAD is the only childhood anxiety disorder to have survived the latest revision of American psychiatric nomenclature. First described in DSM-III, SAD was retained in the childhood disorders section of DSM-IV (American Psychiatric Association, 1994). The essential feature of SAD is excessive anxiety and fear concerning separation from home or from those to whom the child is attached. Such anxiety must be inappropriate for the child's age and expected developmental level, given that separation anxiety is a normal developmental phenomenon from approximately 7 months to 6 years of age (Bernstein & Borchardt, 1991). The core fear of this disorder is evidenced through recurrent distress when separation is anticipated or occurs, avoidance of separation situations, and impairment in important areas of functioning. The primary cognitive distortion displayed by children with SAD is an overwhelming fear of losing or becoming separated from major attachment figures through catastrophic means. For example, children with SAD often fear that harm may befall a parent through accident, assault, or other catastrophe, or that they themselves may become lost or get kidnapped and thus never see their parents again. It is common for younger children with SAD to report recurrent nightmares characterized by separation themes (Bell-Dolan & Brazeal, 1993); however, nightmares are also associated with SAD symptoms in adolescents (Nielsen et al., 2000).

Children with SAD display a wide range of concomitant avoidance behaviors. Avoidance behaviors can be described along a continuum of severity, although no formal classification of such avoidance exists. Mild avoidance behavior may be characterized by a child's wanting the parents to be available by phone during school hours or to be easily accessible when he or she is attending parties or other outings. Parents may notice the child's hesitation to leave home, procrastination during the morning routine, and incessant questioning about schedules. Moderate degrees of avoidance are often characterized by refusal to attend sleepovers or outings requiring a separation of several hours from the parents. Younger children become very "clingy" with parents, often following their parents from room to room, whereas older children become reluctant to leave home or engage in peer activities in the absence of their parents (Bell-Dolan & Brazeal, 1993). Children who evidence severe avoidance behavior may refuse to attend school or to sleep in their own rooms, and tend to shadow or cling to their parents at all times. These children can become desperate in their attempts to contact parents, feigning illness and concocting fantastic excuses in their effort to escape or avoid the separation situation. It is not uncommon for children with SAD to leave schools or camps and attempt to reach home by walking or running away, despite the structure and supervision of responsible adults.

The progression from mild to severe avoidance occurs through an insidious process, beginning with deceivingly innocuous requests or complaints on the part of the child. For example, complaints of nightmares may first allow the child intermittent access to sleeping with the parents. Within a relatively short period of time, the child will be sleeping with one or both parents on a consistent basis. We have observed this pattern in children up to 13 years of age. Similarly, morning routines become disrupted by somatic complaints, resulting in delaying attendance or sporadic absence from school. This pattern of avoidance reaches its peak when the child clings and cries in anticipation of a separation situation, and refuses to attend required activities such as school or to allow the parents to leave for work. Likewise, physical symptoms progress from nonspecific complaints of stomachaches or headaches (Livingston, Taylor, & Crawford, 1988) to more serious concerns evidenced by children who vomit and experience panic attacks at separation. Observation of children with SAD invariably reveals a pattern to these complaints, as the symptoms occur on a fairly regular basis on weekdays but not on weekends or school holidays (Kearney, 2001). According to DSM-IV, children must evidence at least three of eight symptoms for at least 4 weeks to qualify for a diagnosis of SAD. Moreover, the disturbance must be accompanied by clinically significant distress or impairment in social, academic, or other important areas of functioning. Table 6.1 presents DSM-IV criteria for SAD.

SAD is most often diagnosed in prepubertal children (Bowen, Offord, & Boyle, 1990; Kashani & Orvaschel, 1988), although it can occur at any age (Bell-Dolan & Brazeal, 1993; Nielsen et al., 2000). In one study examining the developmental differences in the expression of separation anxiety symptoms, Francis et al. (1987) found age differences but not gender differences with re-

TABLE 6.1. DSM-IV Diagnostic Criteria for Separation Anxiety Disorder (SAD)

A. Developmentally inappropriate and excessive anxiety concerning separation from home or from those to whom the individual is attached, as evidenced by three (or more) of the following:

(1) recurrent excessive distress when separation from home or major attachment figures occurs or is anticipated
(2) persistent and excessive worry about losing, or about possible harm befalling, major attachment figures
(3) persistent and excessive worry that an untoward event will lead to separation from a major attachment figure (e.g., getting lost or being kidnapped)
(4) persistent reluctance or refusal to go to school or elsewhere because of fear of separation
(5) persistently and excessively fearful or reluctant to be alone or without major attachment figures at home or without significant adults in other settings
(6) persistent reluctance or refusal to go to sleep without being near a major attachment figure or to sleep away from home
(7) repeated nightmares involving the theme of separation
(8) repeated complaints of physical symptoms (such as headaches, stomachaches, nausea, or vomiting) when separation from major attachment figures occurs or is anticipated

B. The duration of the disturbance is at least 4 weeks.

C. The onset is before age 18 years.

D. The disturbance causes clinically significant distress or impairment in social, academic (occupational), or other important areas of functioning.

E. The disturbance does not occur exclusively during the course of a Pervasive Developmental Disorder, Schizophrenia, or other Psychotic Disorder and, in adolescents and adults, is not better accounted for by Panic Disorder With Agoraphobia.

Specify if:
Early Onset: if onset occurs before age 6 years

Note. From American Psychiatric Association (1994, p. 113).

gard to which DSM-III criteria were most frequently endorsed. Young prepubertal children (ages 5–8) were most likely to report fears of harm befalling attachment figures, nightmares, or school refusal; children ages 9–12 endorsed excessive distress at the time of separation; and adolescents (ages 13–16) most often endorsed somatic complaints and school refusal. Moreover, younger children endorsed a greater number of symptoms than the adolescents did.

Related Symptoms

Children diagnosed with SAD are more likely to report somatic complaints than children diagnosed with phobic disorders (Last, 1991). Children with SAD may also drop out of activities such as clubs or sports if their parents are not actively involved, but not for lack of interest in the activity. Friendships may wane due to a child's repeated refusal to attend activities away from home, although children with SAD in general are socially skilled and well liked by peers (Last, 1989). Academic performance can be compromised by repeated requests to leave class and by a child's distress and preoccupation with separation concerns. In extreme form, children with SAD who refuse to attend school miss important social and academic experiences available only in the school setting (Kearney, 2001). At times, efforts are made to provide these children with tutoring and assignments to complete at home; however, repeated absences place a child at risk for failure to meet the standards for attendance set forth in state regulations. Consequently, some children are then required to repeat the academic year and, in extreme cases, are remanded to the legal system for compliance with school attendance.

Children who present with SAD often report a variety of specific fears in addition to their separation anxiety, such as fears of monsters, animals, insects, and the dark (Last, 1989; Ollendick & Huntzinger, 1990); such fears may or may not be of phobic proportions (Last, 1989). The most common fear expressed by children with SAD is of getting lost (Last, Francis, & Strauss, 1989). This fear differentiated children with SAD from children diagnosed with OAD and those with a "phobia of school" (Last et al., 1989). Moreover, the fears endorsed by children with SAD were different from those reported by children in the general population (cf. Last et al., 1989; Ollendick, Matson, & Helsel, 1985). Approximately one-third of children with SAD present with concurrent GAD that is usually secondary to the separation anxiety; one-third of children with SAD present with a comorbid depressive disorder that develops several months following the onset of SAD (Last, Strauss, & Francis, 1987). Children with SAD may threaten to harm themselves in attempts to escape or avoid separations; however, serious suicidal symptomatology is rarely associated with SAD (Last, 1989).

Social Phobia

Core Symptoms

In DSM-IV, the essential feature of social phobia is a marked and persistent fear of one or more social or performance situations in which the person fears that embarrassment may occur. Upon exposure to the social or performance situation, the person almost invariably experiences an immediate anxiety response that may take the form of a panic attack. Individuals with social phobia may either avoid these situations or endure them with extreme distress. Due to cognitive-developmental limitations, children and adolescents may fail to recognize that this fear is unreasonable and excessive, although such insight is required to make the diagnosis in adults. In children and adolescents, the symptoms must be present for a minimum of 6 months and cause significant interference in functioning or marked distress in order to warrant the diagnosis.

The DSM-III-R diagnosis of avoidant disorder of childhood or adolescence has been subsumed within social phobia in DSM-IV. The essential feature of avoidant disorder was defined as an excessive shrinking from contact with unfamiliar people, for a minimum of 6 months and of sufficient intensity to interfere with the child's ability to foster and perform in peer relationships. Although social phobia and avoidant disorder shared many characteristics in DSM-III-R, the latter did not require that the fear focus on social evaluation, but solely on contact with unfamiliar people (Vasey, 1995). Thus social phobia in DSM-IV was expanded to include a fear of situations where the person is exposed to unfamiliar people. DSM-IV requires the qualifier "generalized" if the fear includes most social situations; however, subtype distinctions in youths are only just beginning to receive research attention (e.g., Hofmann et al., 1999; Wittchen, Stein, & Kessler, 1999). Preliminary data suggest that the generalized subtype is the most common form of social phobia in children and adolescents (Beidel & Morris, 1993; Hofmann et al., 1999). Moreover, adolescents with generalized social phobia may be distinguished from those with the nongeneralized form by an earlier age of onset, greater impairment in functioning, higher risk for the development of comorbid conditions, and a greater likelihood of earlier inhibited temperament or familial adversities (see Velting & Albano, 2001, for a review). DSM-IV diagnostic criteria for social phobia are provided in Table 6.2.

Children and adolescents with social phobia often have few friends, are reluctant to join group activities, endorse feelings of loneliness on self-report measures (Beidel, Turner, & Morris, 1999; La Greca, 2001) and are considered shy and quiet by their parents and peers. In school situations, these children are extremely fearful of a wide range of situations, including reading aloud or speaking in class, asking the teacher for help, unstructured peer encounters, gym activities, working on group projects, taking tests, and eating in the cafeteria (Beidel et al., 1999; Hofmann et al., 1999). Children with social phobia may be described by teachers as "loners." During unstructured class time, these children are typically off by themselves or in the company of one specific friend. Children and adolescents with social phobia are reluctant to attend extracurricular events such as club meetings or school dances, and need much encouragement to attend parties or similar social activities. Similar avoidance behavior may be observed in family situations. Younger children shrink away from extended family gatherings, avoid answering the telephone or doorbell, and are reticent when meeting friends of family members. Older children may refuse to order for themselves in restaurants. Adolescents with social phobia lag behind peers in meeting age-specific developmental challenges such as dating and seeking employment. It is not uncommon for the parents of these adolescents to lament over *not* having to deal with typical

TABLE 6.2. DSM-IV Diagnostic Criteria for Social Phobia

A. A marked and persistent fear of one or more social or performance situations in which the person is exposed to unfamiliar people or to possible scrutiny by others. The individual fears that he or she will act in a way (or show anxiety symptoms) that will be humiliating or embarrassing. **Note**: In children, there must be evidence of the capacity for age-appropriate social relationships with familiar people and the anxiety must occur in peer settings, not just in interactions with adults.

B. Exposure to the feared social situation almost invariably provokes anxiety, which may take the form of a situationally bound or situationally predisposed Panic Attack. **Note**: In children, the anxiety may be expressed by crying, tantrums, freezing, or shrinking from social situations with unfamiliar people.

C. The person recognizes that the fear is excessive or unreasonable. **Note**: In children, this feature may be absent.

D. The feared social or performance situations are avoided or else are endured with intense anxiety or distress.

E. The avoidance, anxious anticipation, or distress in the feared social or performance situation(s) interferes significantly with the person's normal routine, occupational (academic) functioning, or social activities or relationships, or there is marked distress about having the phobia.

F. In individuals under age 18 years, the duration is at least 6 months.

G. The fear or avoidance is not due to the direct physiological effects of a substance (e.g., a drug of abuse, a medication) or a general medical condition and is not better accounted for by another mental disorder (e.g., Panic Disorder With or Without Agoraphobia, Separation Anxiety Disorder, Body Dysmorphic Disorder, a Pervasive Developmental Disorder, or Schizoid Personality Disorder).

H. If a general medical condition or another mental disorder is present, the fear in Criterion A is unrelated to it, e.g., the fear is not of Stuttering, trembling in Parkinson's disease, or exhibiting abnormal eating behavior in Anorexia Nervosa or Bulimia Nervosa.

Specify if:

Generalized: if the fears include most social situations (also consider the additional diagnosis of Avoidant Personality Disorder)

Note. From American Psychiatric Association (1994, pp. 416–417). Copyright 1994 by the American Psychiatric Association. Reprinted by permission.

teenage behavior, such as tying up the telephone lines or always being on the go.

In feared situations, a child with social phobia will experience excessive concerns about embarrassment, negative evaluation, and rejection. Observations and responses of such children reveal their thoughts to be characterized by negative self-focus and self-deprecation, and to be accompanied by a range of autonomic symptoms and sensations (Albano, 1995; Albano, DiBartolo, Heimberg, & Barlow, 1995; Albano, Marten, Holt, Heimberg, & Barlow, 1995; Beidel et al., 1999; Spence, Donovan, & Brechman-Toussaint, 1999). Complaints of stomachaches and illness are common, especially among younger children. Older children and adolescents become overly concerned with the physical manifestations of anxiety, much like adults with social phobia. Fears of blushing or shaking during an oral report, of an unsteady voice while speaking to peers, or of sweating that others may notice serve to magnify the child's social phobia. Research has demonstrated that the aforementioned physical responses of children with social phobia are consistent with those of adults with the disorder (see Beidel & Morris, 1993, 1995). Behaviorally, younger children may manifest excessive clinging and crying, while older children are likely to shrink from social contact and avoid being the focus of attention.

Social phobia is most often diagnosed in adolescents but does occur earlier in childhood (Beidel et al., 1999; Vasey, 1995). Strauss and Last (1993) examined the sociodemographic differences between children with DSM-III-R simple (specific) phobias (n = 38) and children with social phobia (n = 29) aged 4 through 17 years. Results indicated that both groups of children were referred for treatment approximately 3 years following the onset of their phobias, and that equal proportions of male and female children were referred for both types of disorders (Strauss & Last, 1993). Children with simple phobias were found to be younger and to have an earlier age at onset. Consistent with this pattern, a significantly higher proportion of children with social phobia were found to be postpubertal. These results corroborate epidemiological studies of adolescents (Essau et al., 2000; Wittchen et al., 1999), along with retrospective reports of adults with social phobia who placed the age of onset of their disorder in adolescence (Thyer, Parrish, Curtis, Nesse, & Cameron, 1985).

Related Symptoms

In the large National Comorbidity Survey, social phobia was identified as the most common anxiety disorder affecting adults and the third most common adult psychiatric disorder overall (Kessler et al., 1994). Still, information regarding this anxiety disorder in children and adolescents has been slow to emerge. Children with social phobia present with significantly higher levels of depressed mood than normal children (Beidel et al., 1999; Francis, Last, & Strauss, 1992; La Greca & Lopez, 1998). Moreover, as compared to their nonanxious peers, these children generally endorse significantly lower perceptions of cognitive competence and higher trait anxiety (Beidel, 1991; Beidel et al., 1999), with higher self-reported state anxiety observed during an evaluative task (Beidel, 1991). Youths with social phobia typically present with higher levels of overall fearfulness and general emotional overresponsiveness (Beidel et al., 1999). Several investigators have observed impaired social skills in children with social phobia aged 7–14 years (Beidel et al., 1999; Spence et al., 1999).

Children and adolescents who fear being the focus of attention during meals may refuse to eat during school hours. These children may spend their lunch time in study hall or the library, avoiding the social activity of the school cafeteria. One teenage girl seen at our clinic spent every lunch period during her freshman year of high school sitting in a bathroom stall. Ironically, the attention that these children attempt to avoid often comes back on them in the form of "growling" stomachs caused by hunger. Children and adolescents with social phobia may avoid school for a variety of reasons (Kearney, 2001). Younger children may refuse to attend school because of fears of being teased or rejected by peers or fears of being called on by the teacher to read before the class. School refusal in an adolescent may be prompted by concerns about appearance, especially if the adolescent is required to change clothes in a locker room for gym class. Youths with social phobia go to great lengths to appear calm before their peers and to avoid any sort of attention at all costs. Therefore, children entering the middle school years who are sensitive to negative evaluation may be particularly vulnerable to social phobia. Changing classes, using lockers, larger classrooms, and working in groups will increase the number and types of social-evaluative situations to which a child may be exposed. Hence, middle school children who are school refusing constitute a significant proportion of the children referred to our anxiety clinics with social phobia. For children with significant school refusal behavior, the complications of nonattendance described for children with SAD will also apply.

Obsessive–Compulsive Disorder

Core Symptoms

The essential features of OCD are recurrent and intrusive obsessions and compulsions that are time-consuming (greater than 1 hour per day) and cause either marked distress for an individual or significant impairment in functioning (American Psychiatric Association, 1994). The symptoms of OCD in children and adolescents are consistent with those found in adults (see Table 6.3 for the DSM-IV criteria list). Children will report obsessions involving contamination fears, sexual themes, religiosity, or aggressive/violent images. Some children complain of an inability to stop "hearing" intrusive and recurrent songs or rhymes. Fears of catching a life-threatening illness (e.g., cancer or AIDS), and excessive concern with morality and religion, have also been reported. Compulsions involving repetition, washing, checking, ordering, and arranging are also common in child cases (Flament et al., 1988; Last & Strauss, 1989b; Riddle et al., 1990). Washing rituals have been identified as the most common symptom of OCD, affecting more than 85% of children in the National Institute of Mental Health (NIMH) cohort (Swedo, Rapoport, Leonard, Lenane, & Cheslow, 1989). Excessive washing may be expressed in repeated handwashing and elaborate bathing or shower rituals. Children with OCD often report that a specific washing and grooming pattern must be followed daily; if it

TABLE 6.3. DSM-IV Diagnostic Criteria for Obsessive–Compulsive Disorder (OCD)

A. Either obsessions or compulsions:

Obsessions as defined by (1), (2), (3), and (4):

(1) recurrent and persistent thoughts, impulses, or images that are experienced, at some time during the disturbance, as intrusive and inappropriate and that cause marked anxiety or distress

(2) the thoughts, impulses, or images are not simply excessive worries about real-life problems

(3) the person attempts to ignore or suppress such thoughts, impulses, or images, or to neutralize them with some other thought or action

(4) the person recognizes that the obsessional thoughts, impulses, or images are a product of his or her own mind (not imposed from without as in thought insertion)

Compulsions as defined by (1) and (2):

(1) repetitive behaviors (e.g., hand washing, ordering, checking) or mental acts (e.g., praying, counting, repeating words silently) that the person feels driven to perform in response to an obsession, or according to rules that must be applied rigidly

(2) the behaviors or mental acts are aimed at preventing or reducing distress or preventing some dreaded event or situation; however, these behaviors or mental acts either are not connected in a realistic way with what they are designed to neutralize or prevent or are clearly excessive

B. At some point during the course of the disorder, the person has realized that the obsessions or compulsions are excessive or unreasonable. **Note**: This does not apply to children.

C. The obsessions or compulsions cause marked distress, are time consuming (take more than 1 hour a day), or significantly interfere with the person's normal routine, occupational (or academic) functioning, or usual social activities or relationships.

D. If another Axis I disorder is present, the content of the obsessions or compulsions is not restricted to it (e.g., preoccupation with food in the presence of an Eating Disorder; hair pulling in the presence of Trichotillomania; concern with appearance in the presence in the presence of Body Dysmorphic Disorder; preoccupation with drugs in the presence of a Substance Use Disorder; preoccupation with having a serious illness in the presence of Hypochondriasis; preoccupation with sexual urges or fantasies in the presence of a Paraphilia; or guilty ruminations in the presence of Major Depressive Disorder).

E. The disturbance is not due to the direct physiological effects of a substance (e.g., a drug of abuse, a medication) or a general medical condition.

Specify if:

With Poor Insight: if, for most of the time during the current episode, the person does not recognize that the obsessions and compulsions are excessive or unreasonable

Note. From American Psychiatric Association (1994, pp. 422–423).

is interrupted, then it must be repeated until "perfect."

Compulsions associated with OCD must be distinguished from normal developmental rituals found in childhood. Nonanxious children will at times display preferences or ritual-like behaviors that are relatively innocuous. For example, arranging dolls or toys in a specified order, and nighttime rituals with parents and siblings, are common in children. What distinguishes OCD from transient rituals or behavioral preferences is a child's distress if the ritual is prevented or the sequence interrupted. Normal developmental rituals are not excessive, differ in content from typical OCD rituals (e.g., washing), and typically dissipate by age 9 years (Leonard, Goldberger, Rapoport, Cheslow, & Swedo, 1990; Leonard et al., 1993). DSM-IV does not require children to recognize the excessive and unreasonable nature of OCD symptoms. Parents may become alert to OCD when the disorder begins to interfere with the child's or the family's functioning. For example, excessive slowness in grooming, touching, and arranging all personal belongings and repeated checking of locks will intrude upon family plans and could interfere with school attendance. Parents may observe their child repeating nonsensical behavioral patterns, such as tapping and touching food before eating, or going back and forth through doorways for a certain number of times. One 12-year-old boy at our clinic had to repeat a series of dance-like footsteps prior to entering any room. This behavior caused him considerable embarrassment in peer situations, especially in middle school when he was required to change classes. In children, obsessions without compulsions are relatively rare, as is also true for adults. Conversely, in very young children (ages 6–8), rituals typically occur without cognitive obsessions (Swedo et al., 1989). These children may describe an irresistible urge or ritual without an identifiable cognitive precipitant. Interestingly, the literature reveals that in 90% of children with OCD, the symptom patterns change over time (Swedo et al., 1989). For example, parents will report early symptoms involving checking locks and cupboards, with such behaviors later being replaced by counting or arranging rituals.

Investigators have noted that as many as 50–60% of children diagnosed with OCD experience severe impairment in global functioning (Berg et al., 1989; Last & Strauss, 1989b; Whitaker et al., 1990). Such impairment reflects the interference of the disorder in a child's personal, social, and academic life. Children and adolescents with elaborate nighttime rituals are unable to invite friends to sleepovers and, likewise, must refuse to accept similar invitations. With increasing complexity, ordering and arranging rituals become difficult to hide from schoolmates. These rituals become more elaborate and time-consuming as they evolve topographically, reflecting ever-increasing anxiety in the child. Homework may become an overwhelming struggle, as a child may spend hours with repeated checking and erasing. A straightforward multiple-choice test can trigger continuous checking rituals due to obsessional doubting, with the child failing to complete the test within the allotted time. Adolescents are particularly challenged by OCD. Instead of gaining independence from the family and testing skills in autonomous activities, adolescents with OCD will find their increased independence extremely anxiety-provoking and difficult to master. Rituals may keep the adolescent from engaging in usual teenage activities, such as dating, working, or driving. Moreover, leaving home for college can be particularly challenging, due to the impact of leaving a family system that has evolved around the OCD. The potential for being "discovered" by college peers may increase the adolescent's anxiety, and reinforce feelings of uncontrollability and helplessness.

Studies of OCD in children and adolescents place the mean age of onset between 10 years and 12.5 years (Leonard & Rapoport, 1991; Wewetzer et al., 2001), although onset has been reported in cases younger than 7 years (Swedo et al., 1989). Onset appears earlier in male than in female children, resulting in a predominance of boys in younger samples. However, gender differences disappear by middle childhood, with equal male-to-female ratios reported in older samples of children with OCD. Interestingly, one study found female adolescents reporting more symptoms of compulsions and male adolescents reporting more obsessions (Valleni-Basile et al., 1994). Moreover, epidemiological surveys of adolescents find females typically reporting more symptoms and greater impairment than boys (e.g., Berg et al., 1989; Maggini et al., 2001).

Related Symptoms

Other anxiety disorders and depression are the most common associated features of OCD (Swedo et al., 1989; Wewetzer et al., 2001). Although higher severity of depressive symptoms has been associated with an earlier onset of OCD (Rapoport et al., 1981), concurrent mood disorders are typically more prevalent in older children (Geller et al., 2001). Earlier age of onset has been associated with increased risk of ADHD and other anxiety disorders, including specific phobia, GAD, and SAD (Geller et al., 2001; Last & Strauss, 1989b; March, Leonard, & Swedo, 1995). Although obsessions may involve seemingly bizarre content, thought disorder is not usually an associated feature of OCD (Wolff, 1989). There is a high incidence of OCD in children and adults with Tourette's disorder (35–50%); the incidence of Tourette's disorder in children and adults with OCD is lower, with estimates ranging between 5% and 7% (American Psychiatric Association, 1994; Geller et al., 2001).

Specific Phobias

Core Symptoms

Specific phobia (called simple phobia prior to DSM-IV) refers to a marked and persistent fear of circumscribed objects or situations; this fear is unrelated to fears of embarrassment in public or performance situations (social phobia) or fears of having a panic attack (panic disorder). Exposure to the phobic stimulus almost immediately provokes an anxiety response that may take the form of a panic attack. The phobic stimulus is avoided or may be endured with distress. Children may not recognize that the fear is excessive or unreasonable. Moreover, for children and adolescents, the fear must have persisted for 6 months and cause marked interference in functioning or distress to warrant the diagnosis (see Table 6.4). Silverman and Rabian (1993) differentiate specific phobias from normal developmental fears as follows: A phobic reaction is excessive and out of proportion to the demands of the situation, occurs without volition, leads to avoidance, persists over time, and is maladaptive. Moreover, the convictions associated with a phobic reaction persist despite disconfirmatory evidence or attempts to reason with the child or adolescent. Table 6.5 lists the DSM-IV subtypes that have been delineated to indicate the focus of the fear or avoidance in specific phobias.

Common specific phobias of childhood include phobias of heights, darkness, loud noises (including thunder), injections, insects, dogs, and other small animals (Essau et al., 2000; King, 1993; Silverman & Rabian, 1993; Strauss & Last, 1993). School phobia is also common in children, but the principal motivating condition for the school refusal behavior must be delineated for accurate differential diagnosis and prescriptive treatment planning (Kearney, 2001). A child would be diagnosed with a specific phobia of school if the fear were circumscribed to a particular school-related situation (e.g., fire drills) as opposed to embarrassment or humiliation, in which case social phobia would be the appropriate diagnosis. Responses of phobic children are manifested across the three components of anxiety (cognitive, behavioral, and physiological). Cognitions of phobic children are characterized by catastrophic predictions of some dreadful event's occurring upon

TABLE 6.4. DSM-IV Diagnostic Criteria for Specific Phobia

A. Marked and persistent fear that is excessive or unreasonable, cued by the presence or anticipation of a specific object or situation (e.g., flying, heights, animals, receiving an injection, seeing blood).

B. Exposure to the phobic stimulus almost invariably provokes an immediate anxiety response, which may take the form of a situationally bound or situationally predisposed Panic Attack. **Note**: In children, the anxiety may be expressed by crying, tantrums, freezing, or clinging.

C. The person recognizes that the fear is excessive or unreasonable. **Note**: In children, this feature may be absent.

D. The phobic situation(s) is avoided or else is endured with intense anxiety or distress.

E. The avoidance, anxious anticipation, or distress in the feared situation(s) interferes significantly with the person's normal routine, occupational (or academic) functioning, or social activities or relationships, or there is marked distress about having the phobia.

F. In individuals under age 18 years, the duration is at least 6 months.

G. The anxiety, Panic Attacks, or phobic avoidance associated with the specific object or situation are not better accounted for by another mental disorder, such as Obsessive–Compulsive Disorder (e.g., fear of dirt in someone with an obsession about contamination), Posttraumatic Stress Disorder (avoidance of stimuli associated with a severe stressor), Separation Anxiety Disorder (e.g., avoidance of school), Social Phobia (e.g., avoidance of social situations because of fear of embarrassment), Panic Disorder With Agoraphobia, or Agoraphobia Without History of Panic Disorder.

Specify type:

Animal Type
Natural Environment Type (e.g., heights, storms, water)
Blood–Injection–Injury Type
Situational Type (e.g., airplanes, elevators, enclosed places)
Other Type (e.g., phobic avoidance of situations that may lead to choking, vomiting, or contracting an illness; in children, avoidance of loud sounds or costumed characters)

Note. From American Psychiatric Association (1994, pp. 410–411).

TABLE 6.5. Specific Phobia Subtypes

Subtype	Description
Animal	Fear cued by animals or insects.
Natural	Fear cued by objects in the natural environment, such as storms, heights, darkness, or water.
Blood–injection–injury	Fear cued by seeing blood or an injury, or receiving an injection or other invasive medical procedure.
Situational	Fear cued by a specific situation, such as public transportation, tunnels, bridges, elevators, flying, driving, or enclosed places.
Other	Fear cued by such stimuli as loud noise or costumed characters; fear and avoidance of such situations as vomiting, choking, or contracting an illness.

exposure to the feared stimulus. Most common are fears of threats to personal safety, such as fearing being bitten by a dog, struck by lightning, or stung by an insect. Children with specific phobias also report anticipatory anxiety in the form of "What if . . ." statements (Silverman & Rabian, 1993). For example, a child with a phobia of thunderstorms may lament, "What if it storms on my way to school, and I get struck by lightning?" These catastrophic and worrisome thoughts preoccupy the child and result in extreme distress and interference in functioning. Behaviorally, avoidance is the predominant response of children with specific phobias. Avoidance may take the form of screaming, crying, having tantrums, or hiding in anticipation of confronting the feared stimulus. When contact with the phobic stimulus is unavoidable, clinging and begging the parents for help to escape the confrontation is not uncommon. Moreover, these children are apprehensive and hypervigilant for the feared stimulus. For example, children fearful of thunderstorms may scan the weather channels and watch the sky prior to leaving home. Children with dog phobias may go to great lengths to avoid walking down a street where a dog may be penned behind a fence. Significant avoidance behavior is associated with the intensity of the fear and degree of interference in functioning (Silverman & Rabian, 1993). Children with specific phobias report physiological symptoms consistent with panic sensations, including rapid heart rate, sweating, hyperventilation, shakiness, and stomach upset.

Phobias of animals, darkness, insects, blood, and injury usually begin before age 7 years and are not typically linked to any traumatic event at onset (Marks & Gelder, 1966). These phobias parallel the onset of normal subclinical fears in children, although the phobic diagnosis suggests stability of the fear over time. Our understanding of the patterns of onset for childhood phobias is largely based on the retrospective report of adult patients with phobias. For example, adult patients place the onset of animal phobia at 7 years, blood phobia at 9 years, and dental phobia at 12 years (Öst, 1987). Similarly, Liddell and Lyons (1978) reported the age of onset to be 8.8 years for blood phobia, 10.8 years for dental phobia, and 11.9 years for thunderstorm phobia. Evidence suggests that specific phobias occur across the life span, with elevations between the ages of 10 and 13 years (Strauss & Last, 1993).

Related Symptoms

Typically, a child with a specific phobia is brought to treatment when the intensity of the phobia causes significant interference with normal routines and functioning within the family. Some specific phobia stimuli can be avoided with little disruption in routine; for example, small animals can be kept out of sight of a child visiting a relative's home. However, when a particular situation cannot be altered or avoided, a child can become oppositional and aggressive in his or her struggle for escape. It is not uncommon for a child with a needle phobia to have to be held down by several adults for required injections. Children attempting to avoid specific situations may hide from parents, shout in rage, and attempt to punch or kick to avoid the stimulus. The intensity of such behavior represents the degree of distress experienced by a child and serves to reinforce frustration and helplessness on the part of the parents. Essau et al. (2000) report depression and somatic symptoms as the most common associated features of specific phobias in adolescents.

A vasovagal fainting response occurs in approximately 70–75% of blood–injection–injury phobias (American Psychiatric Association, 1994; Antony, 1994). Estimates specific to children and adolescents are lacking at present. This physiological response is characterized by an initial brief acceleration of heart rate, followed by an immediate deceleration of heart rate and drop in blood pressure. This deceleration is unique to this subtype of specific phobia and is in contrast to the usual sustained acceleration of heart rate found in other specific phobia subtypes. In severe cases, children and adolescents who display this response may faint on exposure to stimuli that evoke images of blood or injury. Reading about bloody scenes in stories, viewing blood or injuries on television, or hearing about accidents and trauma in news reports may all evoke this fainting response. In a severe case of a 16-year-old girl, fainting occurred on average of four to eight times per week (Albano, Mitchell, Zarate, & Barlow, 1992). Even common everyday sayings, such as "Cut it out!", would evoke a sufficiently strong visual image of blood resulting in the fainting response for this particular adolescent. In this case, in addition to the potential detrimental effects of avoiding medical and dental care, this child was exposed to excessive teasing and ridicule from peers.

Generalized Anxiety Disorder

Core Symptoms

The essential feature of GAD is excessive and uncontrollable anxiety and worry about a number of events and activities, occurring more days than not, for at least 6 months. In addition, diagnosis of GAD in children requires the presence of at least one accompanying physiological symptom. Table 6.6 outlines the diagnostic criteria for GAD. In DSM-IV, the former diagnosis of OAD has been subsumed under the revised GAD; hence our understanding of the symptoms and clinical presentation of GAD in youths is based largely on studies of children with OAD. Research suggests minimal and nonsignificant differences between the DSM-III-R and DSM-IV criteria, suggesting that past research on OAD can be applied to understanding GAD in youths (e.g., Kendall & Warman, 1996; Tracey, Chorpita, Douban, & Barlow, 1997). The uncontrollable worry characteristic of GAD may be focused on a number of general life concerns, including the future, past behavior, and competence in such areas as sports, academics, and peer relationships. Children with GAD are typically described as "little worriers" by adult caretakers.

Unrealistic and excessive worrying about future events was present in over 95% of a clinic sample of children with GAD (Strauss, Lease, Last, & Francis, 1988). The most frequently reported worries of a clinical sample of youths with GAD included tests/grades, natural disasters, being physically attacked, future school performance, and being bullied or scapegoated by peers (Weems, Silverman, & La Greca, 2000). It is not uncommon for children with GAD to worry about a number of adult concerns as well, such as family finances (Bell-Dolan & Brazeal, 1993). Children with GAD may experience worry concerning performance in school, athletics, social relationships, and so on, to the point of being perfectionistic (Bell-Dolan & Brazeal, 1993; Strauss, 1990). Consequently, these children place exceedingly high standards for achievement on themselves and are brutal in their self-reproach if they fail to meet these standards. In fact, worry associated with GAD persists in the absence of objective cause for concern. For example, children and adolescents with GAD who receive A's on homework and tests will continue to worry about failure or falling below some self-generated standard.

Children with GAD are described as markedly self-conscious and require frequent reassurance from others (Eisen & Kearney, 1995; Silverman & Ginsburg, 1995; Strauss, 1990). As in children with specific phobias, "What if . . ." statements also pervade these children's thinking. Unlike those in specific phobias, however, cognitive distortions in GAD are fairly continuous and not circumscribed to a particular stimulus or situation. Children with GAD overestimate the likelihood of negative consequences, exaggerate the predicted outcomes to a catastrophic degree, and underestimate their ability to cope with less than ideal circumstances. Research has demonstrated that although nonreferred children also worry about low-frequency events (Silverman, La Greca, & Wasserstein, 1995), children with GAD may not recognize that such events have a low probability of occurrence. As opposed to the *number* of worries, it has been found that the *intensity* of children's worries differentiated clinic-referred children from nonreferred controls (Muris, Meesters, Merckelbach, Sermon, & Zwakhalen, 1998; Perrin & Last, 1997; Weems et al., 2000). In fact, these studies demonstrated that nonreferred children report just as many worries as clinical samples, suggesting that the

TABLE 6.6. DSM-IV Diagnostic Criteria for Generalized Anxiety Disorder (GAD)

A. Excessive anxiety and worry (apprehensive expectation), occurring more days than not for at least 6 months, about a number of events or activities (such as work or school performance).

B. The person finds it difficult to control the worry.

C. The anxiety and worry are associated with three (or more) of the following six symptoms (with at least some symptoms present for more days than not for the past 6 months). **Note**: Only one item is required in children.

(1) restlessness or feeling keyed up or on edge
(2) being easily fatigued
(3) difficulty concentrating or mind going blank
(4) irritability
(5) muscle tension
(6) sleep disturbance (difficulty falling or staying asleep, or restless unsatisfying sleep)

D. The focus of the anxiety and worry is not confined to features of an Axis I disorder, e.g., the anxiety or worry is not about having a Panic Attack (as in Panic Disorder), being embarrassed in public (as in Social Phobia), being contaminated (as in Obsessive–Compulsive Disorder), being away from home or close relatives (as in Separation Anxiety Disorder), gaining weight (as in Anorexia Nervosa), having multiple physical complaints (as in Somatization Disorder), or having a serious illness (as in Hypochondriasis), and the anxiety and worry do not occur exclusively during Posttraumatic Stress Disorder.

E. The anxiety, worry, or physical symptoms cause clinically significant distress or impairment in social, occupational, or other important areas of functioning.

F. The disturbance is not due to the direct physiological effects of a substance (e.g., a drug of abuse, a medication) or a general medical condition (e.g., hyperthyroidism) and does not occur exclusively during a Mood Disorder, a Psychotic Disorder, or a Pervasive Developmental Disorder.

Note. From American Psychiatric Association (1994, pp. 435–436). Copyright 1994 by the American Psychiatric Association. Reprinted by permission.

intensity of worry may be the mechanism leading to a sense of uncontrollability over the worry process (Weems et al., 2000).

Studies examining DSM-III and DSM-III-R diagnoses suggested that OAD/GAD may begin at any age in childhood, with one study reporting OAD present as early as age 4 years (Beitchman, Wekerle, & Hood, 1987). The reported mean age of onset of OAD/GAD ranges from 10.8 years (Last, Strauss, & Francis, 1987) to 13.4 years (Last, Hersen, et al., 1987). OAD/GAD occurs in approximately 3% of children, whereas estimates in adolescents can be as high as 10.8% (Costello, Stouthamer-Loeber, & DeRosier, 1993). In clinic-referred samples, children with OAD/GAD are older than children with SAD or specific phobias (e.g., Albano, Chorpita, DiBartolo, & Barlow, 1995). Strauss, Lease, et al. (1988) examined the developmental characteristics of children with OAD and found that older children presented with a higher total number of overanxious symptoms and self-reported significantly higher levels of anxiety and depression than younger children.

Related Symptoms

In a study examining the developmental characteristics of DSM-III-defined OAD, Strauss, Last, Hersen, and Kazdin (1988) found a sample of 55 children to present with a high rate of concurrent anxiety and affective disorders. Younger children (ages 5–11) tended to present with comorbid separation anxiety concerns and attention deficit disorder, whereas major depression and simple (specific) phobia were more common to the older children with OAD (ages 12–19; Strauss, Lease, et al., 1988). Masi, Favilla, Mucci, and Millipiedi (2000a) examined 108 children and adolescents with GAD, and found those with comorbid depression (n = 55) to report significantly more anxiety symptoms and more severe functional impairment than youths with pure GAD and no depressive comorbidity. Age, gender, and SES did not differentiate these two groups. Eisen and Engler (1995) identified headaches, stomachaches, muscle tension, sweating, and trembling as the most commonly reported physical complaints of children with OAD/GAD. Accordingly, many children with OAD/GAD are referred for treatment by their pediatricians or by gastrointestinal specialists (Bell-Dolan & Brazeal, 1993). The criteria for OAD in DSM-III-R were rather vague with regard to somatic complaints. A child could endorse some physical complaint for which no physical basis could be established (e.g., headaches or stomachaches), or endorse marked feelings of tension or inability to relax. However, the child could meet full criteria for OAD in the absence of any somatic symptom, because DSM-III-R required four of seven symptoms for diagnosis (only two were somatic in nature). DSM-IV outlines six specific somatic symptoms, of which one is required to make the diagnosis in children and adolescents. Tracey et al. (1997) found only the muscle tension symptom to be infrequently endorsed by both children and their parents in a clinical sample using DSM-IV criteria. In addition to the aforementioned symptoms, disturbing dreams has been associated with GAD in adolescents, especially girls (Nielsen et al., 2000).

Panic Disorder

Core Symptoms

At one time, panic disorder was considered an anxiety disorder of adulthood that did not occur in children and only rarely occurred in adolescents (see Kearney & Silverman, 1992; Moreau & Weissman, 1992; Nelles & Barlow, 1988). Because of the cognitive nature of this disorder, children were thought to be incapable of forming catastrophic misinterpretations of bodily sensations. However, literature is accumulating supporting the existence of panic attacks and panic disorder in youths (e.g., Essau et al., 1999; Hayward et al., 1992; Kearney, Albano, Eisen, Allan, & Barlow, 1997; Moreau & Follett, 1993; Ollendick, 1995; Ollendick, Mattis, & King, 1994; Vitiello, Behar, Wolfson, & Delaney, 1987; Vitiello, Behar, Wolfson, & McLeer, 1990). Panic disorder is defined by the occurrence of at least one unexpected panic attack, followed by a minimum of 1 month of any one (or more) of the following: persistent fear of experiencing future attacks, worry about the implications of the attack or its consequences, or a significant change in behavior related to the attacks (American Psychiatric Association, 1994). In addition, the panic attacks cannot result from the direct physiological effects of a substance (e.g., medications or caffeine), or from a general medical condition (e.g., hyperthyroidism).

Table 6.7 outlines the DSM-IV criteria for a panic attack (which is not a codable disorder, and which can in fact occur in other disorders besides panic disorder—e.g., in severe specific phobia or social phobia). Table 6.8 gives the DSM-IV diagnostic criteria for panic disorer without and with agoraphobia. The diagnosis of panic disorder in children may be difficult to establish because of their cognitive-developmental limitations. Young children report a fear of becoming sick, without specific reference to autonomic symptoms and misinterpretation of such symptoms. In our clinical practice, prepubescent children almost never verbalize specific fears of dying, going crazy, or losing control because of the presence of physiological symptoms. More often, these children report nonspecific anxiety about suddenly becoming ill, or express a fear of vomiting that the children find difficult to predict or control. In early adolescence, fears of specific autonomic symptoms begin to occur, including fears of breathlessness, tachycardia, depersonalization, and dizziness.

Kearney et al. (1997) compared a clinical sample of youths diagnosed with panic disorder (n = 20; 12 females; aged 8–17 years; 18 with agoraphobia, 2 without agoraphobia) to a clini-

TABLE 6.7. DSM-IV Criteria for Panic Attack

Note: A Panic Attack is not a codable disorder. Code the specific diagnosis in which the Panic Attack occurs (e.g., . . . Panic Disorder With Agoraphobia . . .)

A discrete period of intense fear or discomfort, in which four (or more) of the following symptoms developed abruptly and reached a peak within 10 minutes:

(1) palpitations, pounding heart, or accelerated heart rate
(2) sweating
(3) trembling or shaking
(4) sensations of shortness of breath or smothering
(5) feeling of choking
(6) chest pain or discomfort
(7) nausea or abdominal distress
(8) feeling dizzy, unsteady, lightheaded, or faint
(9) derealization (feelings of unreality) or depersonalization (being detached from oneself)
(10) fear of losing control or going crazy
(11) fear of dying
(12) chills or hot flushes

Note. From American Psychiatric Association (1994, p. 395).

TABLE 6.8. DSM-IV Diagnostic Criteria for Panic Disorder Without and With Agoraphobia

Panic Disorder Without Agoraphobia

A. Both (1) and (2):

(1) recurrent unexpected Panic Attacks (see [Table 6.7])
(2) at least one of the attacks has been followed by 1 month (or more) of one (or more) of the following:

(a) persistent concern about having additional attacks
(b) worry about the implications of the attack or its consequences (e.g., losing control, having a heart attack, "going crazy")
(c) a significant change in behavior related to the attacks

B. Absence of Agoraphobia . . .

C. The Panic Attacks are not due to the direct physiological effects of a substance (e.g., a drug of abuse, a medication) or a general medical condition (e.g., hyperthyroidism).

D. The Panic Attacks are not better accounted for by another mental disorder, such as Social Phobia (e.g., occurring on exposure to feared social situations), Specific Phobia (e.g., on exposure to a specific phobic situation), Obsessive–Compulsive Disorder (e.g., on exposure to dirt in someone with an obsession about contamination), Posttraumatic Stress Disorder (e.g., in response to stimuli associated with a severe stressor), or Separation Anxiety Disorder (e.g., in response to being away from home or close relatives).

Panic Disorder With Agoraphobia

A. Both (1) and (2):

(1) recurrent unexpected Panic Attacks (see [Table 6.7])
(2) at least one of the attacks has been followed by 1 month (or more) of one (or more) of the following:

(a) persistent concern about having additional attacks
(b) worry about the implications of the attack or its consequences (e.g., losing control, having a heart attack, "going crazy")
(c) a significant change in behavior related to the attacks

B. The presence of Agoraphobia . . .

C. The Panic Attacks are not due to the direct physiological effects of a substance (e.g., a drug of abuse, a medication) or a general medical condition (e.g., hyperthyroidism).

D. The Panic Attacks are not better accounted for by another mental disorder, such as Social Phobia (e.g., occurring on exposure to feared social situations), Specific Phobia (e.g., on exposure to a specific phobic situation), Obsessive–Compulsive Disorder (e.g., on exposure to dirt in someone with an obsession about contamination), Posttraumatic Stress Disorder (e.g., in response to stimuli associated with a severe stressor), or Separation Anxiety Disorder (e.g., in response to being away from home or close relatives).

Note. From American Psychiatric Association (1994, pp. 402–403).

cal group matched for age and gender and meeting criteria for one or more anxiety disorder other than panic disorder. The symptoms most frequently reported by the group with panic disorder were tachycardia, nausea, hot or cold flashes, shaking or jitteriness, dizziness, sweating, dyspnea, depersonalization, derealization, and headaches. There were no differences in symptom report due to age. The symptoms reported by Kearney et al.'s sample are similar to those found in a large epidemiological study of adolescents conducted in Germany (Essau et al., 1999), where palpitations, trembling/shaking, nausea, chills or hot flashes, and abdominal distress were most frequently endorsed. Moreau and Follett (1993) found only depersonalization (feeling "out of one's body") to be rarely reported by prepubescent children in a clinical sample. In addition to the above–described symptoms, several investigators have noted the co-occurrence of panic attacks and refusal to eat due to fear of vomiting in children and adolescents (Ballenger,

Carek, Steele, & Cornish-McTighe, 1989; Bradley & Hood, 1993; Manassis & Kalman, 1990).

There is a serious paucity of literature examining age and gender patterns in childhood panic disorder. The extant literature is comprised largely of case reports and uncontrolled studies (e.g., Alessi & Magen, 1988; Alessi, Robbins, & Dilsaver, 1987; Ballenger et al., 1989; Moreau, Weissman, & Warner, 1989; Vitiello et al., 1990). In a review of this literature, Ollendick et al. (1994) suggested that panic attacks are common among adolescents, with 40–60% of adolescents surveyed reporting having experienced a panic attack. Panic attacks and panic disorder occur in children, but with less frequency than in adolescents (Ollendick et al., 1994). Results of an investigation of panic attacks in younger children revealed an interesting developmental trend (Hayward et al., 1992). Of 754 children aged 10.3 to 15.6 years, the increased occurrence of panic attacks was associated with pubertal progression as assessed through the Tanner self-staging method. Overall, panic attacks were more commonly reported by female subjects evidencing advanced pubertal development, regardless of age (Hayward et al., 1992). This apparent association of pubertal development and panic attacks warrants further study. Consistent with the gender pattern for adults with the disorder, panic disorder appears to be more common among female than male adolescents (Kearney & Allan, 1995; Ollendick et al., 1994).

Related Symptoms

In addition to panic symptoms, children and adolescents with panic disorder may display concomitant agoraphobia, defined as the fear of being in situations from which escape may be difficult or embarrassing, or in which help is not readily available in the event of a panic attack (Essau et al., 1999; Kearney et al., 1997; Masi, Favilla, Mucci, & Millepiedi, 2000b). In the Kearney et al. 1997) sample, the situations reported as most often avoided by youths with panic disorder were restaurants/school cafeterias, crowds, small rooms, auditoriums, elevators, parks, grocery stores, shopping malls, being home alone, and movie theaters. A child with panic disorder may also avoid such school situations as riding the bus or going to gym class, or may present with an outright refusal to attend school. Typically a parent or close friend becomes the child's "safety person," in whose presence activities are endured. To ensure attendance, a parent may attempt to accompany the child during the school day. Although this behavior resembles SAD, the differential diagnosis must be made according to the focus of the child's fear. In panic disorder, the fear is of the physical sensations accompanying the panic attack or of having the attack itself, and is not triggered by the fear of becoming lost or separated from a parent or loved one. Youths with panic disorder may also present with comorbid GAD, specific phobias, SAD, and depression (Essau et al., 1999; Kearney et al., 1997; Masi et al., 2000b).

DEFINITIONAL AND DIAGNOSTIC ISSUES

When one is evaluating a child or adolescent patient with anxiety, care must be taken in differentiating normal from pathological anxiety conditions. Anxiety is a basic human emotion, characterized by a diffuse, uncomfortable sense of apprehension, and often accompanied by autonomic symptoms (Barlow, 2002). At its basic level, anxiety serves an adaptive function to alert an individual to novel or threatening situations, and thus to allow the person to confront or flee such situations. Thus anxiety is also an integral part of the normal developmental progression from dependency to autonomy. Through repeated exposure to new and untried situations, individuals become "experienced" in the cycle of anxious arousal and the resultant habituation and abatement of sensations. For example, anxiety is considered normal for young children who confront such situations as the dark, separation from caretakers, or the first day of school. Similarly, adolescents will experience anxiety when learning to drive, or on their first date or job interview. Pathological anxiety, however, may be distinguished from normal, expected levels of anxiety on the basis of the intractability of the anxiety, the pervasiveness of the fear and avoidance, and the degree of interference in the child's daily functioning (Albano et al., 2001; Barrios & Hartmann, 1997). DSM-IV attempts to account for each of these variables in the criteria for the individual anxiety disorders. Specific time intervals for the presence of significant symptomatology are specified within each diagnostic category. In addition, evidence of distress and significant interference in the child's normal routines (academic, social, occupational) are also required. These criteria alert the clinician to examine the presenting complaint in terms of normal, transient anxiety and fear experiences that are an expected and necessary part of development. Research demonstrates that when structured diagnostic interviews and standardized self-report measures are utilized, children with anxiety disorders can be differentiated from nonclinical controls (Dierker et al., 2001; Schniering, Hudson, & Rapee, 2000).

The DSM system represents the categorical classification approach, attempting to separate disorders into clinically derived and mutually exclusive diagnostic classes based upon a hierarchical model. The DSM system has been widely used by clinicians and researchers, fostering efficient means of communication among health care professionals. However, there exists considerable debate as to the usefulness of categorical systems such as DSM, largely due to the dissatisfaction with the categorical approach to psychopathology in general (e.g., Achenbach, 1980, 1988; Rutter & Tuma, 1988). Brown and Barlow (2002) present a thorough review of the problems inherent in the DSM system, which include (1) diagnostic unreliability caused by disagreements among diagnosticians; (2) a frequent assignment of, and high diagnostic unreliability for, categories capturing symptoms but not full criteria, by way of the "not otherwise specified" category; (3) false comorbidity rates due to certain hierarchy rules for rendering a differential diagnosis; and (4) failure to include specifiers for many disorders to assess information regarding levels of severity and intensity of disorders. Thus categorical systems such as the DSM rely primarily on the dichotomous nature of diagnosis, resulting in problems with discriminative validity because of symptom overlap among the anxiety disorders, as well as between the anxiety disorders and other DSM categories. For example, Brown and Barlow (2002) call attention to the fact that the important definitional features of the anxiety disorders (such as worry, panic attacks, social anxiety, and negative affect) are shared to some degree among the different anxiety disorder categories, in addition to being present in varying degrees in all emotional disorders and in persons not meeting the threshold for particular diagnoses. Categorical systems explicitly require that a certain number of symptoms must be present to assign a diagnosis. If symptoms of several different diagnoses are present in a child, but the child does not display the minimum number of required symptoms for any one diagnosis, then no diagnosis is assigned. Consequently, the child fails to meet the "threshold" for any disorder (Frances, Widiger, & Fyer, 1990). Among the problems with this threshold approach is that appropriate treatment planning can be seriously compromised (Eisen & Kearney, 1995) because of the failure to identify subclinical and prodromal syndromes.

One alternative to categorical classification is an empirically derived dimensional system of classification. Dimensional systems are based on a quantitative analysis of those behaviors or symptoms that are correlated and cluster together most often (Eisen & Kearney, 1995). The best-known dimensional approach is Achenbach's "internalizing–externalizing" system (Achenbach, 1991, 1993; Achenbach & Edelbrock, 1983). Based on extensive empirical studies using the Child Behavior Checklist (CBCL; Achenbach, 1993), two broad-band factors, Internalizing/Overcontrolled and Externalizing/Undercontrolled, have been delineated. An anxious child may score highest on the Anxious/Depressed and Somatic Complaints narrow-band factors, with lesser loadings on conceptually unrelated factors, such as Delinquent Behavior and Aggressive Behavior. Developmental variables are accounted for in this system, which also provides clinical profiles for specific populations of children and adolescents. Although this system is grounded in empirical research, it has the disadvantage of not being widely adopted by clinicians and researchers. An additional disadvantage of the system is the high correlation between the two broad-band factors when psychopathology is extensive (Hinshaw, 1992).

Clinical researchers are moving toward a combined approach to understanding psychopathology. For example, the current approach toward defining school refusal behavior represents a combination of an empirically derived categorical and dimensional system (Kearney, 2001; Kearney & Silverman, 1993). Briefly, school refusal behavior is hypothesized to occur along four functional dimensions: (1) avoidance of negative affect (e.g., anxiety and depression); (2) escape from aversive social and/or evaluative situations (e.g., peer interactions, tests); (3) attention seeking (e.g., disruptive behavior); and (4) positive tangible reinforcement (e.g., watching television and sleeping late rather than attending class).

Conditions 1 and 2 describe children who refuse school for negative reinforcement, whereas conditions 3 and 4 describe children who refuse school for positive reinforcement (Kearney, 1995, 2001). This functional approach toward defining school refusal behavior (Kearney & Silverman, 1990) is grounded in sound psychometric properties and allows for individual and developmental differences. Moreover, the system bridges the gap between assessment and treatment planning. The development of treatment goals and focus of treatment interventions can be derived from knowledge about the function of the school refusal behavior. Specifically, treatment success is enhanced by adapting specific therapeutic procedures and foci to specific functional components of a child's problem (e.g., Kearney & Albano, 2000).

Research on the classification of psychological disorders has contributed to the delineations represented in the fourth edition of DSM. DSM-IV is based on the prototypical approach to classification (Barlow, 2002). Similar to the functional model of school refusal behavior, the prototypical approach also combines some features of both the categorical and dimensional approaches. Briefly, this approach identifies essential symptoms of a disorder and concurrently allows for nonessential variations of symptoms to occur. Although this represents an improvement over previous editions of DSM, problems continue to accompany diagnosis with DSM-IV. First, the problem of diagnostic comorbidity as described above continues to blur diagnostic decisions (Brown & Barlow, 2002; Barlow & Durand, 1995). Second, DSM-IV fails to provide operational definitions for the individual diagnostic criteria. For example, the term "persistent" is used throughout the criteria for SAD (see Table 6.1), but as noted by Kearney, Eisen, and Schaefer (1995), specific guidelines for defining the term "persistent" are not provided in DSM-IV, leaving the criteria open to interpretation and variability across clinicians. Third, DSM-IV also fails to consider the variability of each diagnostic category across different developmental periods. Except for the disorders of infancy, childhood, or adolescence, diagnostic criteria are based on the clinical presentation of each disorder in adults. The various versions of the DSM system have repeatedly been criticized as being highly "adultomorphistic" (e.g., Phillips, Draguns, & Bartlett, 1975); that is, adult parameters of a disorder are automatically applied to children and adolescents. Thus the reliability and validity of diagnoses as applied to clinically referred children become questionable, especially when developmental fluctuations are left up to individual clinicians' judgment.

Clinical scientists interested in the anxiety disorders have turned toward the development of sensitive and specific self-report measures incorporating both dimensional and categorical elements, in order to provide reliable and feasible means of capturing both these qualities of anxiety states, along with accessing information to guide the clinician toward the appropriate DSM-IV anxiety diagnosis of the child or adolescent. Although not meant to replace more detailed diagnostic interview schedules, two specific measures have been developed that serve as screening tools for dimensional symptoms and yet also match specific DSM categories. The Multidimensional Anxiety Scale for Children (MASC; March, Parker, Sullivan, Stallings, & Conners, 1997) is a 39-item self-report rating scale that has shown robust psychometric properties in clinical, epidemiological, and treatment studies. The MASC includes four factors: Physical Symptoms (Tense/Restless and Somatic/Autonomic subfactors), Social Anxiety (Humiliation/Rejection and Public Performance subfactors), Harm Avoidance (Anxious Coping and Perfectionism subfactors), and Separation/Panic Anxiety. Each factor maps to a specific DSM-IV category, in addition to providing dimensional information about symptom expression and severity. Three-week test–retest reliability for the MASC is .79 in clinical samples (March et al., 1997) and .88 in school-based samples (March & Sullivan, 1999). The MASC was shown to be sensitive and specific in identifying anxiety disorders in a nonreferred school sample of adolescents, and in discriminating youths with anxiety disorders from nonclinical and depressed youths (Dierker et al., 2001). The Screen for Child Anxiety Related Emotional Disorders (SCARED; Birmaher et al., 1997, 1999) is a 41-item child and parent self-report instrument that assesses DSM-IV symptoms of panic disorder, SAD, social phobia, and GAD, as well as symptoms of school refusal. Again, the SCARED provides dimensional information and is useful as a screening tool in various clinical and research contexts. The SCARED has shown very good psychometric properties in two different large clinical samples (Birmaher et al., 1997, 1999) and in a community sample (Muris, Merckelbach, et al., 1998).

Both the MASC and the SCARED represent moves toward integrating the categorical and dimensional approaches of classification and explication of psychopathology. Although these measures (much like the CBCL) are not meant to replace diagnostic interviews or other formal psychiatric assessment paradigms, they possess high utility in clinical and research applications, and in furthering our understanding of the specific age- and stage-related expression of anxiety symptoms and disorders in youths. Sophisticated statistical methods may allow comparisons of these self-report methods with more structured diagnostic assessments in large samples (e.g., Dierker et al., 2001); the resulting data will allow investigators to examine the sensitivity of these measures, while also evaluating the validity of DSM diagnoses within a developmental context.

Clearly, the classification of psychopathology in children and adolescents remains controversial and represents a fast-growing and exciting field (Kearney, Eisen, & Schaefer, 1995). The process of refining the aforementioned systems of classification will continue as our science advances. Of critical importance for improving the reliability and validity of diagnosis in children will be greater attention to the explication of developmental factors and variations in the etiology and maintenance of symptoms, along with studies focused on the expression of such symptoms in nonreferred children (see Vasey & Dadds, 2001).

DEVELOPMENTAL COURSE AND PROGNOSIS

A question haunting most parents of anxious youths and causing an uncomfortable pause when posed to clinical scientists is "Will my child always have this problem?" Anxiety symptoms are common in children and adolescents, and information on the natural history of anxiety disorders in youths is slowly emerging. The extant literature is limited by a variety of methodological constraints, including small sample size, failure to conduct "blind" diagnostic assessments, lack of adequate follow-up assessments, and absence of appropriate psychiatric and nonreferred control groups. Nevertheless, evidence is accumulating to suggest that certain anxiety disorders in childhood begin relatively early (Spence, Rapee, McDonald, & Ingram, 2001); render a child prone to the development of comorbid conditions; and, if left untreated, may span a chronic course into adulthood. Moreover, pathways from anxiety disorders to significant psychiatric and psychosocial consequences in adulthood have been documented in recent studies (e.g., Achenbach et al., 1995; Ferdinand & Verhulst, 1995; Pine et al., 1998).

SAD has an acute and early onset (Last, Hersen, et al., 1987) often occurring after a major stressor (e.g., the start of school, a prolonged illness, the death of a parent, or a move to a new school or neighborhood) or at a period of developmental change (Last, 1989). Several studies have tracked the long-term course of SAD in children (Cantwell & Baker, 1989; Keller et al., 1992), suggesting a variable course with recurrence tied to school holidays, prolonged illness, or a change in residence and/or school. Complete remission of all signs and symptoms may extend for years, with a relapse seeming to occur from "out of the blue" (see Black, 1995). However, clinical observation suggests that relapse occurs during times of significant developmental changes and demands or periods of increased stress. Children who do not recover completely from SAD may be at greater risk for developing anxiety or depressive disorders during adolescence and adulthood (Pine et al., 1998). Interestingly, children with early symptoms of SAD were found to have a decreased risk for the initiation of alcohol abuse in adolescence (Kaplow, Curran, Angold, & Costello, 2001), although this research must be replicated. Several studies suggest that children with SAD are at increased risk of developing depression and social phobia, and that girls with SAD are especially at risk for panic disorder and agoraphobia (Biederman et al., 1993b; Black & Robbins, 1990; Gittelman & Klein, 1985; Moreau & Follett, 1993).

In contrast to the wealth of literature documenting the natural course of fears in children, very little empirical research has been conducted on the course of phobic disorders in childhood. In a classic and widely cited study, Agras, Chapin, and Oliveau (1972) followed a community sample of individuals with phobias, consisting of 10 children (under the age of 20 years) and 20 adults. Subjects were followed over a 5-year period, during which none received treatment for his or her phobia. Results suggested that many phobic conditions resolve without active intervention, and that children improve more rapidly than adults. Ollendick (1979) subsequently criticized the Agras et al. (1972) data, noting that the children were not completely asymptomatic over the course of the follow-up assessment. Similarly, in a study of 62 children (aged 6–15 years) treated for phobias, Hampe, Noble, Miller, and Barrett (1973) found 7% of the sample to exhibit phobias at 2-year follow-up. Using DSM-IV criteria, Essau et al. (2000) examined the prevalence and comorbidity associated with fears and specific phobias in 1,035 German adolescents aged 12–17 years, and found significant psychosocial impairment associated with phobias. Overall, these studies suggest that symptoms of phobias persist over time for a proportion of youths and are consistent with the retrospective reports of adults with phobias (e.g., Öst, 1987; Thyer, Parrish, et al., 1985). These data must be interpreted with caution, however, as each investigation was limited by methodological constraints.

The literature on the course of childhood OCD documents consistent findings supporting the chronicity and intractability of this anxiety disorder in youths. As in adults, OCD appears to follow a chronic but fluctuating course (Swedo et al., 1989). In a 2-year epidemiological follow-up study of adolescents, 31% of those who had received an initial current or lifetime diagnosis of OCD received a current diagnosis at follow-up, and an additional 25% received a residual diagnosis of subclinical OCD symptoms. Of those who had received an initial current or lifetime subclinical OCD diagnosis, 10% received a current diagnosis of OCD, and an additional 40% received a residual diagnosis of subclinical OCD symptoms (Berg et al., 1989). Similarly, Leonard et al. (1993) reported the results of a prospective 2- to 7-year follow-up study of 54 pediatric patients with OCD. Subjects in this study participated in controlled pharmacological treatment followed by a variety of uncontrolled treatments, including behavior therapy. At follow-up, 43% of the subjects continued to meet diagnostic criteria for OCD, and only 11% were considered totally asymptomatic. Seventy percent of subjects were still taking psychoactive medication at follow-up. Overall, the authors considered that the group improved from baseline despite continued OCD symptomatology, and they reported only 10 subjects (19%) as unchanged or worse.

Recently, Wewetzer et al. (2001) published a follow-up study of 55 patients treated for OCD as youths in the years between 1980 and 1991. The mean age of onset for their sample was 12.5 years, with follow-up occurring 11.2 years after treatment. At follow-up, 36% of patients were still suffering with OCD, while 71% met criteria for some form of psychiatric disorder. Of the patients with OCD, 70% had at least one additional clinical disorder (mainly anxiety or depression). Axis II disorders were present in 12.7% (paranoid personality disorder) to 25.5% (obsessive–compulsive personality disorder) of patients. Factors predictive of more severe OCD symptoms in adulthood included inpatient treatment, early termination of treatment, and tics in childhood or adolescence. These studies well illustrate the chronicity of OCD and support the published expert consensus statement, which concludes that young patients with OCD who receive a combination of pharmacological and cognitive-behavioral therapy "can expect substantial improvement but not complete remission of symptoms over time" (March et al., 1995, p. 257).

The limited data on GAD, interpreted from studies of children with OAD, suggest that the disorder is unstable over time (e.g., Cantwell & Baker, 1989; Last, Hersen, et al., 1987; Last et al., 1992). For example, in a 5-year follow-up study of eight children diagnosed with OAD, Cantwell and Baker (1989) found that an equal percentage of children either maintained or did not meet the diagnosis (25% each). However, the majority of the sample (50%) received an alternative diagnosis at follow-up. In a community study, Kaplow et al. (2001) found that children with elevated levels of GAD symptoms early in childhood were at an increased risk for the initiation of alcohol use in adolescence, even after depressive symptoms were controlled for. The authors suggest that alcohol may be used as a self-medication strategy to control excessive worry.

The natural course of panic disorder in children and adolescents has not been studied. Investigations with adult patients suggest that panic disorder tends to be a chronic and recurrent illness (see Barlow, 2002; Breier, Charney, & Heninger, 1986; Keller & Baker, 1992). The field remains split on whether SAD is a precursor to, or early manifestation of, panic disorder in adults. Some studies suggest that a common biological mechanism, related to respiratory functions, places a child at risk for SAD and eventually panic disorder (e.g., Pine et al., 2000); others argue that equal rates of childhood SAD can be found in patients with social phobia and those with panic disorder (Otto et al., 2001), and thus that a continuity hypothesis is not supported. A history of any childhood anxiety disorder (in addition to comorbid depression and personality disorder) has been associated with the chronicity and stability of panic disorder in adults (Pollack, Otto, Rosenbaum, & Sachs, 1992).

Social phobia has received increased attention with regard to its natural history and long-term course. Youths with social phobia are at a high risk for developing major depression (Last et al., 1992), with the likelihood increasing over time. Epidemiological studies indicate that social phobia in early adolescence is a direct pathway to the development of substance use disorders by middle to late adolescence (Kessler et al., 1994). It is likely that adolescents stumble into the vicious cycle of drinking to ease their social anxiety about entering challenging situations, and then coming to rely on use of alcohol to continue their social behavior. Social phobia (in addition to other anxiety disorders) is also associated with significant impairment in role functioning, delayed or unstable marriage, and an overall poor quality of life (Forthofer, Kessler, Story, & Gotlib, 1996; Kessler, Foster, Saunders, & Stang, 1995; Kessler & Frank, 1997). As compared to peers without the disorder, females with social phobia are more likely to fail to complete high school and enter college, while both males and females with the disorder who enter college fail to matriculate (Kessler et al., 1995). Such truncated educational attainment is associated with a number of adverse life course and societal consequences (see Kessler et al., 1995), including longer dependency on the family of origin, less training for and entering into the work force, and greater demands on the social welfare and health care system.

Thus evidence is amassing indicating that anxiety disorders in childhood lead to severe emotional, social, health, and economic consequences over the long term, especially when left untreated. In addition to the studies cited above, a follow-up study of a New Zealand adolescent cohort (Woodward & Ferguson, 2001) found associations between presence of an anxiety disorder at ages 14–16, and later risks for mental health problems, educational problems, and social role outcomes in 964 respondents available at ages 18–21 years. Significant linear associations were identified linking the number of anxiety disorders in early adolescence to later risks for anxiety disorders; major depression; nicotine, alcohol, and illicit drug dependence; suicidal behavior; educational underachievement; and early parenthood. After controls for personal disadvantages and social/familial factors, the relationships between the number of anxiety disorders in adolescence and later risks of suicidal behavior, nicotine and alcohol dependence, and early parenthood were reduced to nonsignificant levels. These results suggested that these outcomes were sequelae of the risk factors and life consequences associated with anxiety, rather than direct effects of anxiety disorders on later life course development. However, despite controls for a wide range of confounding factors, significant associations remained between the number of anxiety disorders in adolescence and later risks for anxiety disorders, major depression, illicit drug dependence, and failure to attend college.

Two specific outcomes of childhood anxiety are beginning to receive increased attention by investigators. The first pertains to anxiety in youths as a pathway to the onset of cigarette smoking, regular use of cigarettes, and eventual nicotine dependence. In a community sample of 688 adolescents (51% female; mean age 16 years at baseline, 22 years at follow-up), heavy cigarette smoking during adolescence was associated with a higher risk of agoraphobia, GAD, and panic disorder in adulthood, but not OCD or social phobia (Johnson et al., 2000). These results remained significant after controls for a number of factors, including age, sex, temperament, alcohol and drug use, anxiety, depression, parental smoking, and educational level. In contrast to the negative finding for social phobia, the Early Developmental Stages of Psychopathology Study utilized a prospective, longitudinal design to follow a community sample of 3,021 adolescents and young adults over a 4-year period (Sonntag, Wittchen, Hofler, Kessler, & Stein, 2001). At baseline, 35.7% of the total sample smoked on a regular basis, and 18.7% met DSM-IV criteria for nicotine dependence. Of the 7.2% who met criteria for social phobia, most reported that the first onset of their social fears predated the use of tobacco. Both subclinical social fears and social phobia were significantly associated with higher rates of nicotine dependence. In fact, even when comorbid depression was controlled for, baseline nonusers with social fears and baseline nondependent users with social fears had an increased risk of onset of nicotine dependence during the follow-up period. These studies—in addition to those previously discussed with regard to alcohol use among adolescents with GAD and social phobia—indicate that investigators and mental health professionals must attend to the risk for, and use of, various substances by youths with anxiety disorders. Their impact on general physical health, in addition to serious mental health outcomes, warrants further attention and investigation.

A second and more troubling outcome of early anxiety may well be the attempt and/or completion of suicide. Research is mounting suggesting that adolescents with anxiety disorders who develop major depression are at a high risk for attempting suicide (Pawlak et al., 1999). In comparing a sample of 80 female adolescents (aged 15–20 years), half of whom attempted suicide and half of whom did not, Pawlak and colleagues found that comorbid major depression significantly distinguished those with anxiety disorders who attempted suicide from those with anxiety disorders who did not. Similarly, Nelson and colleagues (2000) found an elevated risk for suicide-related symptoms (ideation, attempts) and alcohol dependence in adolescents with social phobia and comorbid major depressive disorder. Although this study was limited to a population-based adolescent female twin sample, earlier studies of shy (not diagnosed) adolescents revealed a higher risk for suicidal attempts (see Zimbardo & Radl, 1981). Finally, a study of a clinical sample of 1,979 youths aged 5–19 years revealed two specific findings relevant to anxiety disorders and suicidal symptoms (Strauss et al., 2000). Younger subjects (<15 years) who attempted suicide had a significantly lower prevalence of SAD than youths with suicidal ideation and nonsuicidal youths. However, in older youths (>15 years), GAD was more prevalent in those with ideation than in nonsuicidal patients. Although the results of this study are not straightforward with regards to the relation between anxiety and suicide in youths, clinicians must take heed. Suicidality has been largely understudied in anxious youths, probably because of the idea that anxiety is not like depression and hence there is no risk. However (as we will see below), anxiety and depression are highly comorbid conditions, and the aforementioned studies point to this combination of psychiatric disorders—with or without the addition of alcohol use—as potentially fatal for many youths. It is time to take our heads out of the sand and give careful attention to suicidal symptoms in youths with anxiety disorders, in order to effect preventive intervention strategies to save lives.

EPIDEMIOLOGY

Population Studies

The incidence and course of anxiety disorders in children and adolescents have been explored in a number of studies using community and clinical samples. Typically, epidemiological samples show lower rates of anxiety disorders than clinical studies do; however, this is to be expected, as youths who are suffering with these conditions will be brought to treatment (especially as impairment and distress escalate). The extant literature on community rates of anxiety disorders consists mainly of studies using DSM-III or DSM-III-R criteria, as studies using DSM-IV criteria are still in progress. Of 15 epidemiological studies, 11 estimate the prevalence of childhood anxiety disorders at greater than 10% (Pine, 1994). In the United States, four of five large surveys estimated prevalence to be 12–20% (Achenbach et al., 1995; Gurley et al., 1996; Shaffer et al., 1996). For example, in two cross-sectional epidemiological studies (Kashani, Orvaschel, Rosenberg, & Reid, 1989; Kashani & Orvaschel, 1988), 21% of children sampled (aged 8, 12, or 17 years) reported symptoms consistent with the diagnosis of an anxiety disorder. Prevalence rates reported for these samples were 12.9% and 12.4% for SAD and OAD, respectively; 3.3% for simple (specific) phobia; and 1.1% for social phobia. Similar findings were obtained in a longitudinal study conducted in New Zealand (Anderson et al., 1987; McGee et al., 1990). In a sample of 792 children evaluated at age 11 years, the prevalence rates were 3.5% for SAD, 2.9% for OAD, 2.4% for simple phobia, and 1.0% for social phobia. When the children were reassessed at age 15 years (McGee et al., 1990), the overall prevalence rates were 5.9% for OAD/GAD, 2.0% for SAD, 3.6% for simple phobia, and 1.1% for social phobia. The rates reported for simple and social phobia are misleading, however, because the most common simple fear was the fear of public speaking. According to the criteria and descriptions outlined in DSM-III-R (American Psychiatric Association, 1987), phobia of public speaking should be considered a social phobia. In contrast to the New Zealand study, rates as high as 6.3% for social phobia were reported in a 6-month prevalence study of Dutch adolescents, with 9.2% of youths meeting criteria for specific phobia (Verhulst, van der Ende, Ferdinand, & Kasius, 1997). Essau et al. (2000) found a lifetime rate of 3.5% for specific phobia in a community sample of adolescents in Germany. Animal phobia and natural environment phobia were the most common subtypes in this sample, with high levels of psychosocial impairment reported during the worst episode of the disorder. Despite this impairment, few adolescents had received any help for their disorder.

The first epidemiological study of OCD in children was conducted on the Isle of Wight (Rutter, Tizard, & Whitmore, 1970). Of the 2,199 children studied (aged 10 and 11), 0.3% were identified as having "mixed obsessional/anxiety disorders." Results of the NIMH adolescent OCD study revealed a weighted point prevalence rate of 0.8% and a lifetime prevalence of 1.9% for the general adolescent population (Flament et al., 1988). These findings are more consistent with the estimated 2% prevalence in the general adult population (Karno, Golding, Sorenson, & Burnam, 1988). However, Valleni-Basile et al. (1994) reported a 3% prevalence rate for clinical OCD and 19% for subclinical OCD in their community sample of adolescents. A prevalence of 4% was found in a study of older Israeli adolescents (Zohar et al., 1992), and also in a community sample of Italian adolescents (Maggini et al., 2001). Overall, these studies suggest that OCD is a relatively common disorder in adolescents.

Controversy regarding the occurrence of panic disorder in youths has probably contributed to the paucity of studies investigating the epidemiology of this disorder in children and adolescents. Panic disorder was not mentioned in the most widely cited epidemiological studies of anxiety disorders in youth (e.g., Anderson et al., 1987; Kashani & Orvaschel, 1988; Rutter et al., 1970). However, several investigators have reported on the prevalence of this disorder in children and adolescents. In a sample of 388 adolescents aged 12–19 years, Warren and Zgourides (1988) reported that 4.7% of the sample met DSM-III diagnostic criteria for panic disorder. In addition, 60% of the sample reported having experienced at least one panic attack, and 31.9% reported having at least one attack meeting DSM-III criteria. Macaulay and Kleinknecht (1989) assessed 660 adolescents (aged 13–18) with a battery of panic-related questionnaires. In this sample, the authors found that 35.7% reported no panic attacks, 47.5% reported mild panic, 10.4% reported moderate panic, and 5.4% reported severe panic. The frequency of panic reported by the subgroup with severe panic averaged slightly less than DSM-III-R criteria (3.8 attacks as opposed to 4 attacks in 4 weeks). Moreover, 73.3% of the adolescents in this group were females. Other epidemiological studies suggest a lifetime prevalence for panic disorder ranging from about 0.3% to 1% for adolescents (Lewinsohn, Hops, Roberts, Seeley, & Andrews, 1993; Verhulst et al., 1997; Whitaker et al., 1990). These data are fairly consistent with the adult lifetime prevalence rates, estimated to be about 1.5% (see Ollendick et al., 1994).

Clinical Samples

Among clinic-referred samples of anxious children, Last, Francis, et al. (1987) reported that 33% of their sample received a primary DSM-III diagnosis of SAD, 15% had primary school phobia (described as social in origin), 15% had OAD, and 15% presented with a major affective disorder. High comorbidity rates were evidenced among childhood anxiety disorders, with one or more concurrent anxiety disorder diagnosed in 41% of the children with primary SAD, 63% of the sample with school (social) phobia, and 56% of the children with primary OAD (Last, Hersen, et al., 1987). Prior research has consistently reported a higher prevalence of OCD in community than in clinic samples (see March et al., 1995). It has been suggested that a bias toward considering OCD as rare may have led clinicians to consider alternative diagnoses, such as schizophrenia (Valleni-Basile et al., 1994).

Last, Perrin, Hersen, and Kazdin (1996) examined prospectively the course and outcome of DSM-III-R anxiety disorders in a clinical sample of 84 children over a 3- to 4-year period. The authors found that 82% of children were recovered from their initial anxiety disorders at the end of the follow-up period, and that 68% of these children had recovered during the first year. Only 8% of children evidenced a relapse of anxiety disorders after a period of remission. SAD had the highest rate of recovery (96%) and specific phobia the poorest (69%). The majority of children with OAD recovered during follow-up (80%); however, this disorder showed the slowest time to recovery and the highest rate of new disorders during follow-up (35%).

The systematic study of anxious youths in community and clinical samples provides invaluable information concerning the incidence and prevalence of these disorders, patterns of comorbidity, demographic factors, and examination of factors related to course and clinical outcome. However, much more research is needed to increase our understanding of the nature of these disorders and to develop effective interventions for youths.

SOCIODEMOGRAPHIC VARIABLES

Racial and Socioeconomic Factors

Lower SES and lower parental education level have been associated with a greater prevalence and risk of SAD (Bird, Gould, Yager, Staghezza, & Canino, 1989; Last, Hersen, et al., 1987; Valez, Johnson, & Cohen, 1989). In addition, reported samples of children with SAD have been predominantly European American. Samples of children with phobic disorders (simple [specific] and social combined) are predominantly European American and of and middle to low middle SES (Strauss & Last, 1993). In a study examining a community (n = 2,384) and clinical (n = 217) sample of youths, Compton, Nelson, and March (2000) found in the community sample that European American children endorsed more symptoms of social phobia and fewer symptoms of SAD than African American children, regardless of age. The opposite held true for African American youths, who reported low social anxiety but higher separation anxiety. Results were similar for the clinical sample. No information is available on the demographic composition of GAD in children and adolescents; however, children with OAD are predominantly from middle- to upper-income families in clinical samples (e.g., Last, Hersen, et al., 1987; Last et al., 1992) and predominantly European American (e.g., Last, Hersen, et al., 1987). No particular pattern has emerged for socioeconomic or racial data in children and adolescents with OCD (e.g., Last & Strauss, 1989b; Valleni-Basile et al., 1994).

In a study designed to evaluate racial similarities and differences in youths with anxiety disorders, Last and Perrin (1993) compared a clinical sample of African American children (n = 30) to one of European American children (n = 139) on sociodemographic variables, clinical characteristics, and lifetime rates of DSM-III-R anxiety disorders. The results suggest that African American and European American children seeking treatment for anxiety disorders are more similar than different, as no significant differences were found with regard to age, sex, duration of disorder, or lifetime history of a mood disorder. There was a trend toward significance in two findings: European American children were more likely to present with school refusal and higher diagnostic severity ratings, and African American children were more likely to have a history of posttraumatic stress disorder. Moreover, African American children tended to score higher on the Fear Survey Schedule for Children—Revised (FSSC-R; Ollendick, 1983b; cf. Neal, Lilly, & Zakis, 1993).

Costello, Keeler, and Angold (2001) examined the effects of poverty on the prevalence of psychiatric disorders in a community sample of rural black and white children aged 9–17. In this sample, black children (n = 541) were three times as likely as white children (n = 379) to be living in poverty; yet the association between poverty and a list of risk factors (e.g., unemployment, parent arrest, family size, parental psychopathology, dangerous environment, welfare status, multiple moves, abuse) for psychiatric disorders was not different between the groups. The prevalence of psychiatric disorder increased for all children with the number of risk factors, but most markedly for white children. When relative poverty level (defined as being in the bottom two-thirds for income of the comparison nonpoor racial/ethnic group) was examined, an excess of psychiatric disorders was found for poor white children overall, especially anxiety.

Sex Differences

Several studies have reported a greater prevalence of SAD in female than in male children (Anderson et al., 1987; Compton et al., 2000; Costello, 1989; Last, Hersen, et al., 1987), although others have reported no differences (Last et al., 1992; Bird et al., 1989). Last et al. (1992) reported that 44.3% of their sample with social phobia were female children; however, Beidel and Turner (as cited in Beidel & Morris, 1995) reported that 70% of their sample were female children. In contrast, the clinical sample in Compton et al. (2000) had higher rates for social anxiety in males than in females. In a community study examining the relative prevalence of DSM-III phobic disorders, Anderson et al. (1987) found a male-to-female ratio of 6:1 for such disorders (excluding social phobia) in children and adolescents. Strauss and Last (1993) reported equal proportions of males and females in their clinic-referred sample of children with simple phobias. This apparent discrepancy between these studies may reflect either methodological differences or the possibility that male and female children are referred for treatment of these disorders at a similar rate (Strauss & Last, 1993). Using DSM-IV criteria, Essau et al. (2000) found more girls than boys meeting criteria for specific phobia in a community sample of German adolescents. A clear and stable gender difference for the blood phobia subtype has emerged, with the majority of cases being female ones (Marks, 1988).

Male cases predominate in samples of children with OCD (Swedo et al., 1989; Last & Strauss, 1989b); however, this finding may be a function of age (see "Obsessive–Compulsive Disorder," above). Male and female rates of OCD in adolescence are equivalent (Flament et al., 1988; Valleni-Basile et al., 1994). Several studies examining gender differences in OAD have suggested a preponderance of male cases (Cantwell & Baker, 1989; Verhulst, Akkerhuis, & Althaus, 1985; Verhulst & Akkerhuis, 1988), but referral biases may have contributed to these results. The gender ratio generally reported in both community and clinical samples is nearly 1:1, although it has been suggested that the disorder may be more common in females (Eisen & Kearney, 1995). GAD has been diagnosed more frequently in female adolescents than in males (Bowen et al., 1990; McGee et al., 1990).

In a study of gender differences in anxiety disorders and anxiety symptoms in adolescents, Lewinsohn et al. (1998) found a preponderance of female cases of anxiety disorders in their longitudinal cohort from the Oregon Adolescent Depression Project. Incidence data revealed that by the age of 6 years, twice as many girls as boys had experienced an anxiety disorder. Boys and girls were not found to differ with respect to age of onset or duration of their first anxiety episode. A number of psychosocial variables were significantly associated with gender, with girls reporting significantly more major life events, higher self-consciousness, lower self-esteem, more physical illness, poorer self-rated physical health, less exercise, a greater number of physical symptoms, greater emotional reliance, and more social support from friends. When examining their findings with relation to these and other psychosocial variables, the authors suggested that some sort of genetic factor, rather than purely environmental factor, may lead to girls' having an increased vulnerability to anxiety. However, these results must be interpreted with caution, as the authors also noted that differential reporting of symptoms by boys and girls may have affected these results.

Interestingly, Ginsburg and Silverman (2000) found that children reporting higher levels of masculinity, based on self-report responses to a sex role inventory, experienced less overall fearfulness than peers reporting lower levels of masculinity. Masculinity is associated with instrumental traits including approaching novel or challenging situations, self-reliance, determinism, and persistence. A clinic sample of 66 youths (aged 6–11; 41 boys, 25 girls) completed the sex role inventory in addition to the FSSC-R (Ollendick, 1983b). Children who rated themselves as high in masculine traits reported a lower number and intensity of fears related to social anxiety (failure and criticism, oral reports, looking foolish), fears of the unknown, and medical fears. Although this finding is consistent with theories of gender development and prior research in childhood fears, levels of femininity were unrelated to fearfulness in this sample, contrary to prior research. The authors hypothesized that traditional feminine traits associated with fearfulness in adults may be underdeveloped in younger children, and hence may exert less influence on fearfulness. Based on the results of this study, it was suggested that interventions designed to address fearfulness in youths should focus on teaching or refining masculine/instrumental traits to reduce fear and avoidance behavior.

In summary, little research has focused directly on the demographic composition of anxiety disorders in children and adolescents; consequently, the available data are limited by referral and methodological constraints. It is extremely difficult to draw any firm conclusions regarding racial, socioeconomic, or gender patterns in youthful anxiety disorders. Studies vary on selection and recruitment procedures, geographical boundaries, incentives for participation, and opportunities for treatment. Cultural or racial biases may influence whether or not children from specific minority groups are referred for treatment of internalizing disorders such as anxiety. Moreover, in research on clinic-referred samples, the majority of studies in the literature were carried out at specialty clinics for anxiety disorders in youth. Thus, within clinic-referred samples, there is the potential for ascertainment bias in the patient population. Families who seek mental health services may have been in a better position to be referred for or to afford such services. The literature is best interpreted with these caveats in mind.

CULTURAL VARIATIONS

Investigations of the cultural aspects of childhood anxiety play an important role in determining which patterns of behavior are universal and which might be specific to particular groups or settings. By highlighting determinants of anxiety not accounted for by existing biological and psychosocial theory, cross-cultural perspectives help to clarify the underlying validity of our present conceptualization of childhood anxiety. Although cultural influences have received some attention in the adult anxiety literature (e.g., Barlow, 2002; Brown, Eaton, & Sussman, 1990; Friedman & Paradis, 1991; Neal & Turner, 1991), there are still very few studies of child populations. The majority of the research has involved cross-cultural assessment using self-report measures developed in the United States. Only a few studies have examined differences in diagnostic patterns across cultural groups (Neal & Turner, 1991). The FSSC-R (Ollendick, 1983b), an 80-item inventory of different fear stimuli and situations, has been used to assess differences in patterns of childhood fears across numerous cultural groups. The FSSC-R has been translated into a variety of languages and administered to children and adolescents in the United States, Portugal, Italy, Turkey, Australia, the Netherlands, Northern Ireland, China, and the United Kingdom (see Fonesca, Yule, & Erol, 1994, for a review). Examination of the main differences across groups is limited to those countries that have received the same 80-item adaptation—that is, Australia, the United States, the United Kingdom, Portugal, China, and the Netherlands. Results showed relatively similar scores for most of these countries; however, the Dutch sample scored lower and the Portuguese sample scored higher than the other countries on total fear (Fonesca et al., 1994). One possible explanation for this difference is that the tendency for Latin cultures is to express fears more spontaneously, whereas Nordic cultures tend to control or conceal emotions (Fonesca et al., 1994). Across all groups, girls were found to score higher than boys. This does not necessarily imply a universal, "culture-free" gender pattern for fears, however, because the role of women in these cultures is fairly homogeneous and may involve a higher risk for the development of anxiety (cf. Nolen-Hoeksema, 1987).

Examination of the most common fears across cultures shows striking commonalities. For children in the United Kingdom, the United States, Turkey, Portugal, and Australia, the fear of being hit by a car was the most frequently endorsed childhood fear. Fears of not being able to breathe, a bomb attack or war, fire, a burglar, falling from a height, and death ranked in the top 10 fears of children from at least four of these countries. In addition, items appended to the original 80-item measure revealed that fear of a parent's death was considerable in all countries tested (United Kingdom, Turkey, Portugal), with endorsement ranging from 73% to 84% (Fonesca et al., 1994).

In a manner similar to the work of Ollendick and colleagues, Spielberger and colleagues (Spielberger & Diaz-Guerrero, 1986; Spielberger, Diaz-Guerrero, & Strelau, 1990) have fostered research examining self-reported trait anxiety across different cultures. The State–Trait Anxiety Inventory for Children (STAIC; Spielberger, 1973) is a measure of general anxiety or negative affect in school-age children. At present, the majority of the cross-cultural research with the STAIC has involved validation of the instrument in a variety of countries. Currently, adaptations have been developed for Polish, Hungarian, Russian, Jordanian, Lebanese, and Bengali populations, most of which consisted of students in middle to late adolescence. In one comparative study, Ahlawat (1986) found similar factor structures between the Arabic STAIC and the American version. In addition, sex differences were similar to those found in the United States, with girls scoring higher in trait anxiety than boys. In general, support for the use of the STAIC across different cultures is growing. These developments are particularly noteworthy, given that not all attempts to validate self-report measures of childhood anxiety across cultures have been successful (e.g., Wilson, Chibaiwa, Majoni, Masakume, & Nkoma, 1990).

Guida and Ludlow (1989) examined the phenomenon of test anxiety in children from different cultural groups and evaluated the effects of SES, subject sex, and cultural background on self-reported test anxiety. Using the Test Anxiety Scale for Children (TASC; Sarason, Davidson, Lightfall, Waite, & Ruebush, 1960), the investigators compared samples of urban African American children, middle-class American children, upper-class American children, and a large sample of Chilean students. In the comparative analyses, the Chilean students scored higher on test anxiety than the American samples. Across groups, children with high SES scored lower on the TASC than children with low SES. Within low-SES subjects, there was also a tendency for girls to score higher than boys on the test anxiety measure.

In an investigation of cultural influences on general child pathology, Weisz et al. (1987) used parent self-report measures to compare American children with children living in Thailand. The general pattern suggested that Thai children manifested more internalizing behavior (e.g., being withdrawn, anxious, or depressed) than American children did. The authors interpreted these findings as consistent with their hypothesis that the more emotionally controlled Thai culture would contribute to higher internalizing behavior in Thai children. Such findings are particularly interesting in light of the extant findings concerning the influence of a controlled environment on the development of anxiety and negative affect (e.g., Parker, 1983; Mineka, 1985).

In the literature examining cultural issues in childhood anxiety, diagnostic studies are certainly the fewest in number (see Neal & Turner, 1991). In one study using DSM-III nosology, Anderson et al. (1987) found SAD to be the most frequent childhood anxiety diagnosis in a New Zealand population. In another investigation, Orvaschel (1988) found a significantly lower prevalence of anxiety disorders among European American children than among children from other ethnic groups. However, the size of the latter group ($n = 8$) was too small to be representative of the population in general. Costello, Farmer, Angold, Burns, and Erkanli (1997) found that American Indian children had a slightly lower overall prevalence of psychiatric disorders than a comparison European American sample (16.7% vs 19.2%), although substance abuse or dependence was significantly more common in the American Indian youths (1.2% vs 0.1%). Moreover, comorbidity of substance use disorders and other psychiatric disorders was more common among the American Indian youths. This study did not find significant differences in prevalence rates for the anxiety disorders between the two groups. However, in an examination of depression, anxiety, and substance misuse among American Indian and Alaskan Native adolescents, Dinges and Duong-Tran (1993) found that in adolescents diagnosed with depression (via the Diagnostic Interview Schedule for Children), stressful life events had a significant relationship to comorbidity in both groups.

In general, the diversity of findings obscures any unified theory of cultural influence at present. There is undoubtedly a need for more comparative cultural studies using diagnostic criteria, and for lines of research to continue to follow up the investigations of existing assessment studies. Cultural differences in the expression and conceptualization of anxiety disorders in adults have been well documented (see Barlow, 2002). Of interest to the cross-cultural study of children with anxiety disorders is the examination of cultural differences in the interpretation of the course of these disorders, symptom presentation, and intervention approaches. Culture-specific symptoms and syndromes of anxiety have not been explored in children. For example, isolated sleep paralysis has been found to be more prevalent in African Americans than in European Americans, and is conceptualized as a form of nocturnal panic (Barlow & Durand, 1995). Whether this phenomenon occurs in African American children has yet to be evaluated. The efforts to understand the role of culture in childhood anxiety are only in their earliest stages.

ETIOLOGICAL MODELS OF ANXIETY DISORDERS IN CHILDREN

We have suggested that the development of anxiety and its disorders is a function of an interacting set of three dispositions. The first disposition consists of a heritable biological diathesis. The second is best described as a generalized psychological vulnerability, characterized by a sense of impending uncontrollable and unpredictable threat or danger. And the third is a specific psychological vulnerability, growing out of early learning experiences that focus anxiety on certain circumstances. This model has come to be called the "triple-vulnerability" model of anxiety development (Barlow, 2000, 2002). We review each of these dispositions in turn.

Genetics

Over the past 15 years, important gains have been made in understanding the role of genetics in the development of anxiety disorders in children (Eley, 2001). Although many of the details have yet to be clearly articulated, the collective findings to date suggest that genes play a significant role in transmission of a general risk factor for anxiety (Barlow, 2002), accounting on average for about one-third of the variance in anxiety measures. The earliest twin studies on anxiety disorders were conducted prior to the acceptance of DSM-III or DSM-III-R terminology. In the first large-scale twin study using DSM criteria, Torgersen (1983) studied a sample of 85 same-sex twin pairs (aged 18–66) to investigate the possibility of genetic transmission of anxiety disorders. Results demonstrated considerably high monozygotic concordance for the anxiety disorders other than GAD. Concordance rates were highest for panic disorder with and without agoraphobia. These data were interpreted to suggest that there is high heritability for most of the anxiety disorders, but not for GAD; however, it has since been shown that the heritability at the level of disorders is unlikely (Eley, 2001). That is, investigators have recently argued that genes play their greatest role in contributing to a general risk factor for most of the anxiety disorders as well as depression (e.g., Kendler, Neale, Kessler, Heath, & Eaves, 1992; Turner et al., 1987). Viewed in this manner, nonspecific anxiety disorder concordance rates have received increasing conceptual and empirical attention.

Some of the earliest data to support the notion of a general vulnerability emerged from the work of Turner et al. (1987). Using a structured diagnostic interview (the Anxiety Disorders Interview Schedule; DiNardo, O'Brien, Barlow, Waddell, & Blanchard, 1983) these investigators classified adults into a group with anxiety disorders, a group with dysthymia, and a normal control group. Fifty-nine children of clinically anxious adults were found to have more worries, more somatic complaints, more intense fears, and were more withdrawn than children of controls, when assessed with the FSSC-R (Ollendick, 1983b), the STAIC (Spielberger, 1973), and a semistructured interview schedule (the Child Assessment Schedule, or CAS; Hodges, McKnew, Cytryn, Stern, & Kline, 1982). In addition, information from the CAS suggested that the children studied were seven times as likely to meet criteria for an anxiety disorder as offspring of the normal controls were, and two times as likely as offspring of the dysthymic controls were. These findings were consistent with the idea of a general familial risk factor for anxiety disorders; the child self-report data suggest that symptoms in these children may be better understood as dimensional than as categorical (i.e., frequency of symptoms vs. disorder presence or absence).

In a similar investigation, Last, Hersen, Kazdin, Orvaschel, and Perrin (1991) assessed psychopathology in the first- and second-degree relatives of children with anxiety disorders. Results indicated that relatives of clinically anxious children showed a higher prevalence of anxiety than relatives of normal controls, as well as relatives of controls with ADHD. Consistent with previous familial studies, there were no significant findings to indicate that specific anxiety diagnoses in children also exist in their relatives. The pattern once again suggested a family influence for general anxiety proneness.

Emerging twin data have increasingly supported this same position. For example, Stevenson, Batten, and Cherner (1992), in a study of 319 same-sex twin pairs aged 8–18, examined the heritability of fears or phobic symptoms as assessed by the FSSC-R (Ollendick, 1983b). Their results showed that heritability accounted for 29% of the variance, with shared and unshared environment each accounting for about a third of the variance as well. Shortly thereafter, Thapar and McGuffin (1994) studied anxiety symptoms in 376 same-sex twin pairs aged 8–16 years and found more somewhat more complicated results. These investigators used both parent and adolescent reports (only twins aged 12–16 completed the self-report measure), and found that heritability accounted for over half of the variance in parent reports, but was not significant for adolescent reports. Subsequent research has, however, found significant effects of genes on self-reported anxiety (Topolski et al., 1997) and parent-reported anxiety as well (Eaves et al., 1997).

Some more recent evidence from child research supports the idea that this general risk factor is also related to depression. In a study of 395 same-sex twin pairs aged 8–16 years, Eley and Stevenson (1999a) examined the effects of genes on an anxiety factor from which depression variance had been partialed out. Using this method, the investigators found that heritability accounted for only 10% of the variance, suggesting that those aspects of anxiety that are most closely related to depression are more involved in genetic transmission. In a more direct look at the relation of genes to anxiety and depression in children, Thapar and McGuffin (1997) did indeed find that most of the covariance between anxiety and depression was accounted for by a common, heritable factor. Eley and Stevenson (1999b) also found that genetic variance accounted for nearly all of the correlation of anxiety and depression measures, whereas environmental factors were specific to either anxiety or depression.

Such findings are consisted with earlier findings from the adult literature. For example, Kendler et al. (1992) found in 1,033 female twin pairs that genetic variance represented a common influence on the presence of both GAD and major depressive disorder. In addition, Kendler and colleagues demonstrated that family environment played no significant role in the etiology of either major depression or GAD. The implications, then, are that a shared genetic risk factor may be responsible for a general vulnerability for anxiety or depression, and that unique experience modifies the specific expression of this vulnerability.

Temperament

An accumulation of findings over the past several years suggests that this general vulnerability may be linked to child "temperament," which refers to the possibly heritable, early manifestations of personality, including emotionality and behavioral style (see Lonigan & Philips, 2001, for a review). One of the more important models of temperament and its relation to anxiety has come from the work of Kagan and colleagues on behavioral inhibition (e.g., Biederman et al., 1990, 1993a, 1993b; Hirshfeld et al., 1992; Kagan, 1994, 1997; Rosenbaum et al., 1988, 1992; Rosenbaum, Biederman, Hirshfeld, Bolduc, & Chaloff, 1991). The term "behavioral inhibition" (Kagan, 1997) refers to a particular temperamental style, evidenced by a child's degree of sociability as displayed by observable behaviors manifested along the approach–withdrawal dimension. The criteria by which behavioral inhibition is measured include both behavior (speech latency and frequency to peers and adults, proximity to caretaker, physical inactivity, verbalization of distress) and physiology (heart rate, heart rate variability, blood pressure, pupil dilation, muscle tension, cortisol level, urinary norepinephrine levels, and vocal pitch). Behavioral inhibition is distinct from most other models of temperament in that it is a categorical model, asserting that the emotional and behavioral profiles of children at the extremes are qualitatively different from those of average children.

As a result of years of longitudinal research, Kagan, Reznick, and Snidman (1988) reported on the distinction and course of inhibited and uninhibited children. According to their findings, approximately 15% of European American children are born predisposed to be inhibited as infants. These children then become shy and fearful as toddlers, and quiet, cautious, and introverted by the start of their primary school years. In standardized behavioral test situations, these children consistently refrain from spontaneous vocalizations when in the presence of a stranger, and cry and cling to their mothers instead of exploring play settings and approaching other children. At the other end of the scale, about 15% of European American children demonstrate an opposing temperament of being sociable, bold, and gregarious. Moreover, unlike the inhibited children, these children are untroubled by novel stimuli. Kagan and his colleagues have followed two independent cohorts of children over an extended (7-year) period. Children were originally identified as inhibited or uninhibited at either 21 or 31 months of age during standardized behavioral tests when exposed to unfamiliar settings, people, and objects. These differences in behavior were largely maintained through repeated assessments at 4, 5, and 7 years of age, suggesting that such differences represent an enduring temperamental trait (see Kagan, Reznick, & Gibbons, 1989; Kagan, Reznick, & Snidman, 1987; Kagan et al., 1988).

Kagan's original work on behavioral inhibition was designed to examine temperamental styles of infants, and as such no specific hypotheses regarding psychopathology were postulated. However, as attention turned toward the serious study of childhood anxiety disorders, the similarities between inhibited and anxious children became more apparent. In a series of studies, Biederman and colleagues (e.g., Biederman et al., 1993b; Rosenbaum, Biederman, Hirshfeld, Bolduc, & Chaloff, 1991) assessed behavioral inhibition in high-risk children of parents with panic disorder with agoraphobia. These children were compared with children of parents with other psychiatric diagnoses, including major depression; with the inhibited and uninhibited children in Kagan's original longitudinal studies of behavioral inhibition; and with a pediatric outpatient control group who had no history of anxiety or depression.

Parental panic disorder with agoraphobia, either alone or with comorbid major depressive disorder, was associated with behavioral inhibition in 85% and 70% of the children, respectively. Parental major depression alone was associated with a 50% rate of inhibition in offspring, whereas for parents with a psychiatric disorder other than major depression or panic disorder with agoraphobia, the rate of behavioral inhibition was 15.4%. Furthermore, evaluation of the children revealed a greater prevalence of anxiety disorders in the inhibited children than in the not-inhibited and pediatric controls. These results were taken as evidence that behavioral inhibition is an expression of familial vulnerability to anxiety disorders (Biederman, Rosenbaum, Bolduc, Faraone, & Hirshfeld, 1991; Biederman et al., 1993a). Finally, assessments conducted on the parents and siblings of the children from the Kagan et al. (1988) longitudinal cohort and compared with evaluations of first-degree relatives of normal control children (Rosenbaum, Biederman, Hirshfeld, Bolduc, Faraone, et al., 1991) revealed that parents of inhibited children had higher rates of social phobia, history of childhood anxiety disorders (i.e., avoidant disorder and OAD), and continuity of anxiety from childhood through adulthood. Moreover, siblings of inhibited children had higher rates of phobias than siblings of control children.

Other models of temperament and anxiety have focused more directly on the organization of biological systems that underlie motivation and emotion (e.g., Gray & McNaughton, 1996). Gray (1982) detailed the operations of a functional brain system termed the "behavioral inhibition system" (BIS), involving the septal area, the hippocampus, and the Papez circuit, as well as the neocortical inputs to the septo-hippocampal system, dopaminergic ascending input to the prefrontal cortex, cholinergic ascending input to the septo-hippocampal system, noradrenergic input to the hypothalamus, and the descending noradrenergic fibers of the locus coeruleus. According to Gray, this system is the substrate of a reactive motivational system and is activated by signals for punishment, signals for nonreward, and novelty. The primary short-term outputs of the BIS involve narrowing of attention, inhibition of gross motor behavior, increased stimulus analysis (e.g., vigilance or scanning), increased central nervous system arousal (e.g., alertness), and priming of hypothalamic motor systems for possible rapid action that may be required (i.e., possible activation of the fight–flight system). Its phenomenology is characterized by increased caution, vigilance, and processing of threat-relevant information. Gray's model of inhibition, independent of Kagan's work, has inspired rich theorizing regarding the relation of biological and temperamental factors to anxiety and anxiety disorders (e.g., Barlow, Chorpita, & Turovsky, 1996; Chorpita, 2001; Derryberry & Reed, 1996; Fowles, 1995; Lonigan & Philips, 2001).

In yet another line of temperament research, efforts have focused on the relation of anxiety disorders and depression to broader personality and affective variables, such as those represented in the "Big Five" model (i.e., Surgency/Extraversion, Agreeableness, Conscientiousness, Emotional Stability/Neuroticism, and Openness). Perhaps the greatest accumulation recent research in this area involves study of Clark and Watson's (1991) tripartite model of emotion and its relation to anxiety and depression in children (see also Mineka, Watson, & Clark, 1998). The original tripartite model posited factors of Positive Affect (PA), Negative Affect (NA), and Physiological Hyperarousal (PH), to account for the relation of anxiety and depression (the former two of which have been likened to Surgency/Extraversion and Emotional Stability/Neuroticism, respectively; e.g., Ahadi, Rothbart, & Ye, 1993; Lonigan & Philips, 2001). Clark and Watson (1991) articulated these relations as follows: NA represents a factor common to anxiety and depression; (low) PA represents a factor specific to depression; and PH represents a factor specific to anxiety. Considerable evidence has shown that both NA and PA appear to be temperamental constructs, acting as risk factors for anxiety and mood disorders (e.g., Mineka et al., 1998; Lonigan & Phillips, 2001; Watson, Clark, & Harkness, 1994).

Given the implications of this model for understanding both the etiology and comorbidity of anxiety and depression (Brady & Kendall, 1992), there have been growing efforts to investigate the validity of the tripartite model of emotion in child and adolescent samples (e.g., Chorpita, Albano, & Barlow, 1998; Joiner, Catanzaro, & Laurent, 1996; Lonigan, Carey, & Finch, 1994; Lonigan, Hooe, David, & Kistner, 1999). Thus far, the collective findings support a model in children and adolescents roughly consistent with the tripartite model in adults (e.g., Chorpita, Albano, & Barlow, 1998; Joiner et al., 1996). For example, Lonigan et al. (1994) found that measures related to low PA best discriminated children with depressive disorders from those with anxiety disorders. More recently, Lonigan et al. (1999) examined the relations of PA and NA measures with anxiety and depression measures in a school sample of 365 children and adolescents; they found that NA and PA measures performed in a manner consistent with findings from adult samples, and that such findings were uniform across children and adolescents.

Amidst a gathering of empirical support for the tripartite model, some recent revisions to the model (Brown, Chorpita, & Barlow, 1998; Mineka et al., 1998) have suggested that PH is not uniformly related to all anxiety disorders. For example, in a sample of 350 adults with anxiety disorders, Brown et al. (1998) found that PH was related positively to measures of panic disorder, but not to the other anxiety disorders measured. These results were first partially replicated in a sample of 100 children with anxiety and mood disorders (Chorpita, Plummer, & Moffitt, 2000). As had been done in previous studies in the child literature, tripartite scales were constructed by summing items from anxiety and depression measures that were selected to represent the tripartite constructs of NA, PA, and PH. Although consistencies with findings in the adult literature were enough to encourage continued research, the number of inconsistencies raised some questions about the utility of these early measurement strategies (Lonigan et al., 1999). The model outlined by Brown et al. (1998) in adults has thus been evaluated once more in a nonclinical sample of 1,578 children in grades 3 through 12, using a measure empirically designed to tap the tripartite factors in children (Chorpita, 2002). The results of that investigation were consistent with previous observations in adult samples (e.g., PH was positively related with panic only, and was not significantly positively correlated with other anxiety dimensions). The model also appeared robust across different grade levels and both genders (Chorpita, 2002).

One particularly interesting feature in this line of investigation is that the relation between the general vulnerabilities in the model (i.e., NA) and generalized anxiety measures tend to be among the strongest links. Indeed, the initial research in this area actually used measures of anxiety as the measures for NA, and a diversity of findings suggests that many of the early anxiety measures are indeed better measures of a broad negative emotionality (Stark & Laurent, 2001). The similarity between NA and the general experience of anxious emotion has been raised elsewhere (Chorpita & Barlow, 1998); in the context of anxiety and depressive disorders, it speaks to the idea that anxiety itself (e.g., heightened activity of Gray's BIS) may represent the risk factor for anxiety disorders as well as depression. This notion is consistent with much of the patterns found in adult research, such as the tendency for anxiety disorders to precede depression but not the reverse, as well as the asymmetric comorbidity whereby depression is often comorbid with anxiety disorders but anxiety disorders more often occur in the absence of depression. Recent findings in the child literature lend further support to this idea. Cole, Peeke, Martin, Truglio, and Ceroczynski (1998) followed 330 children over a 3-year period and found that even when past depression scores were controlled for, heightened anxiety symptoms predicted future high depression, but not the reverse.

Overall, the collective work in the area of temperament, affect, and anxiety continues to speak to the idea that negative emotions are characterized by a single temperamental risk factor, with some additional evidence that other factors may play an important role (e.g., "effortful control"; Lonigan & Philips, 2001). Problems remain with respect to strategies by which to better measure these important dimensions of temperament, as well as anxiety and depression—particularly given the recent demonstrations that the most widely used measures of anxiety and depression appear to be nonspecific and are not well validated as measures of anxiety or depressive disorders (Chorpita et al., 2000; Chorpita & Daleiden, in press; Stark & Laurent, 2001). Furthermore, difficult work lies ahead with respect to integration of the different models and constructs proposed to underlie anxiety and depressive disorders (Chorpita, 2001; Rapee, 2001).

Psychosocial Factors

In light of the review above, it is clear that any psychosocial influences might better be considered biopsychosocial in nature, given their important dynamic interaction with aspects of biology and temperament. In addition, more recent theorizing suggests that just as the general biological influences for anxiety overlap heavily with those for depression, so too do the general psychological influences for anxiety. Within this context, recent work has focused on detailing possible mechanisms or processes that may establish or intensify risk for negative emotions, including coping strategies (Kendall, 1992), social/familial transmission (Barrett, Rapee, Dadds, & Ryan, 1996; Chorpita, Albano, & Barlow, 1998), information processing (Vasey, Daleiden, Williams, & Brown, 1995; McNally, 1996), and complex forms of conditioning (Bouton, Mineka, & Barlow, 2001).

One recurrent and possibly organizing theme throughout much of this growing literature involves the role of perceptions of control in both the expression and the development of negative emotions (Barlow, 2000, 2002; Barlow et al., 1996; Chorpita & Barlow, 1998; Chorpita, 2001). Issues concerning control and experience with control are ubiquitous among the major theories of anxiety and depression (Alloy et al., 1990; Barlow, 2002), and recent theorizing suggests that a history of lack of control may put individuals at eventual risk for experiencing chronic negative emotional states through the development of a generalized psychological vulnerability (Barlow, 2000; Chorpita, 2001; Chorpita & Barlow, 1998).

Chorpita and Barlow (Chorpita, 2001; Chorpita & Barlow, 1998) have proposed a model outlining the development of anxiety with respect to psychological variables related to control (see Figure 6.1). This model suggests that a sense of diminished control acts as a mediator between stressful events and NA early in development, and that over time this sense of diminished control becomes a moderator of the expression of NA. The model speculates further that the establishment of a sense of high or low control occurs in a sequence of domains, depicted in Figure 6.1 as minimally including aspects of the caregiver, the environment, and the self. If such a sequence exists, it is likely that the establishment of a sense of diminished control within an earlier domain influences the likelihood of developing that same cognitive pattern within the subsequent domain. Thus, within the first column, the relation between events and emotion is purely mediational, with experience acting on the establishment of a general sense of limited control, which has immediate effects on anxious emotion. If a low sense of control is firmly established within this first domain, this sense may then moderate or color the nature of events encountered in the second domain (diagonal arrow). In the second domain, this sequence is played out again, and so on until early adulthood. By this time it is possible that the cumulative developmental effects have established a fixed psychological vulnerability that amplifies the emotional responses to events. It is clear from the figure that if the child begins in the first column with high BIS activity, anxiety, or NA, and life events are frequently uncontrollable, the child is likely to enter the next domain processing events as uncontrollable, even when they are not. Thus, over the course of development, the actual nature of the events for the child become less influential as cognitive factors begin to color experience to a greater and greater degree.

Clearly, the evidence for such a detailed network is far from complete. Nevertheless, a diversity of research supports one section or another of the model. For example, it is well known that the moderational structure in the rightmost part of Figure 6.1 is operative with anxiety and mood disorders (e.g., Sanderson et al., 1989). A number of studies support the idea of temperamental stability (Hirshfeld et al., 1992) and of memory as a mechanism for the stability of cognitive vulnerabilities (e.g., Daleiden, 1998). Finally, new evidence supports the mediational structure in the second column of the figure as well (see Figure 6.1; Chorpita, Brown, & Barlow, 1998). As mentioned earlier, the main task facing researchers may be largely one of integrating the diversity of constructs.

Parenting

Research involving the establishment of maintenance of a general vulnerability points to the role of the early environment, particularly the influence of parents (McClure, Brennan, Hammen, & Le Brocque, 2001; Rapee, 1997). Research over the past several years has identified relevant modeling or conditioning processes in family interactions that may serve to increase anxious cognition (Barrett, Rapee, & Dadds, 1993; Dadds, Heard, & Rapee, 1992). In a group of studies, children were asked to generate interpretations and plans of action in response to an ambiguous description of a hypothetical scene, similar to the ambiguous-situation paradigm developed for adults by Butler and Mathews (1983). The parents completed the same procedure, after which the family members discussed their answers together to arrive at a mutual solution. The degree to which parents modeled, prompted, and re-

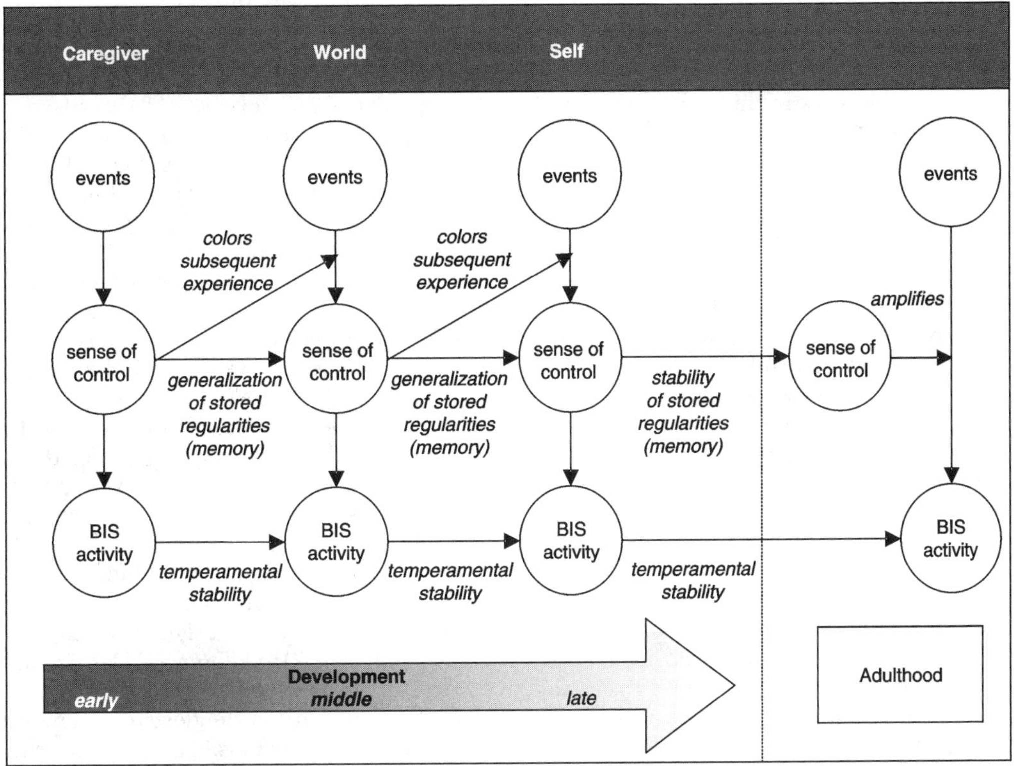

FIGURE 6.1. A model of the development of anxiety with respect to psychological variables related to control. From Chorpita (2001). Copyright 2001 by Oxford University Press. Reprinted by permission

warded anxiety in their children was assessed during the discussion. Results indicated not only that children with anxiety disorders interpreted more threat than controls, but that they were also more sensitive to adopting a more anxious interpretation following the discussion with their parents (Barrett et al., 1993). We reported similar findings (Chorpita, Albano, & Barlow, 1996), but a similar study of parental influence on children's anxious expectations failed to find any effect of parent anxiety (Cobham, Dadds, & Spence, 1998).

Lending more support to the idea that parental behavior may influence the expression of anxiety phenomena, subsequent findings demonstrated that children and their parents who received a family intervention targeting these same communication variables responded better to treatment than those children who received traditional cognitive-behavioral treatment alone (Barrett, Dadds, Rapee, & Ryan, 1994). The notion that anxious behavior among parents is further supported by another treatment outcome study in which children with anxiety disorders and their parents were randomly assigned either to child-focused cognitive-behavioral therapy or to such therapy plus parent anxiety management. Among the children whose parents had the elevated anxiety, cognitive-behavioral therapy was successful for only 39% of cases, compared with 77% of cases when parent anxiety management was added. The results clearly suggest that child anxiety and anxiety disorders are clearly influenced by parents' anxiety in some way.

Recent evidence suggests that parenting also exerts a significant impact on symptoms in youths exposed to trauma. In a study of 339 war-exposed Bosnian children aged 9–14, it was found that children's reports of posttraumatic stress symptoms were significantly associated not only with exposure, but also with maternal distress (Smith, Perrin, Yule, & Rabe-Hesketh, 2001). Other lines of research examining psychosocial mechanisms of transmission have suggested that broader dimensions of parenting style, such as control and warmth, are related to anxiety in offspring (e.g., Parker, 1983; Solyom, Silberfeld, & Solyom, 1976).

Gerlsma, Emmelkamp, and Arrindell (1990) have summarized the extensive literature on the effects of parenting rearing style on depression and anxiety. Much of the work in this area stems from attachment theory (Bowlby, 1973), which posits the relevance of unsuitable or disrupted parenting style as a determinant of anxiety. Research progressing along several different lines has demonstrated the importance of inadequate affection and excessive parental control as part of the early experiences of adults with anxiety disorders (e.g., Ehiobuche, 1988; Parker, 1981). Most findings implicate "affectionless control" (Parker, 1983) as a key variable in predicting general predisposition to anxiety or phobias (Gerlsma et al., 1990), with effect sizes generally larger for maternal rearing style. Alnæs and Torgersen (1990), however, have emphasized that lack of paternal care may play an important role as well, particularly in the discrimination of anxiety and depression.

Attempting to identify how parental rearing style might discriminate among different anxiety disorders, Silove, Parker, Hadzi-Pavlovic, Manicavasagar, and Blaszczynski (1991) investigated parental rearing style in patients with DSM-III-R diagnoses of panic disorder and GAD. Results tentatively suggest that insufficient affection played a role for both disorders; however, control or overprotection seemed to be the more important variable associated with panic disorder. In general, the findings in the area of parental rearing style are limited by the fact that most assessment of this construct has been conducted retrospectively, requiring individuals with anxiety to describe their perceptions of early parenting experiences. Although some evidence exists that these retrospective accounts may not be state-dependent or otherwise biased (e.g., Parker, 1979), there is clearly a need to validate this line of work with an emphasis on cross-sectional or prospective designs (cf. Messer & Beidel, 1994).

In a partial test of the model outlined in Figure 6.2, Chorpita, Brown, and Barlow (1998) examined whether a family environment characterized by a high degree of parental control predicted an increase in cognitive perception of uncontrollability, and whether that in turn predicted anxiety and elevations in the severity of anxiety. In a mixed sample of 62 children with anxiety disorders and 31 without, measures of control mediated between family environment and children's anxious emotion—a finding consistent with the model.

In an observational study of parents of children with anxiety disorders ($n = 43$), parents of children with oppositional defiant disorder ($n = 20$), and parents of controls ($n = 32$), Hudson and Rapee (2001) found similar evidence of an association between intrusive parenting and anxiety. Rapee (2001) has proposed that temperamentally anxious children tend to elicit more intrusive behavior from parents and are more likely to be encouraged to avoid challenges by their parents. Consistent with this idea, Hudson and Rapee (2001) found that mothers of anxious children were more intrusive and more critical when working with their children on two challenging puzzle tasks. The results were similar for mothers of oppositional children, however, suggesting that the interaction between parenting style and child psychopathology was not specific to anxiety on the dimensions measured.

In a subsequent test of Rapee's model, Gerull and Rapee (2002) examined whether parental modeling of anxiety had a significant impact on child behavior in 30 toddlers aged 15–20 months. Children were presented with a rubber snake and a rubber spider in independent trials, and their degree of approach or avoidance was measured. Children whose mothers' expressions were negative toward a toy in an earlier trial were less likely to approach that toy in subsequent tests and were more likely to show a negative emotional reaction to that toy. These observations are consistent with earlier developmental work showing that children at this age use the emotional reactions of others to determine the meaning of a novel stimulus.

Finally, we posit a third set of psychological vulnerabilities, which predisposes an individual to focus anxiety on some specific object or event. Bouton et al. (2001) have reviewed evidence for the acquisition for this specific vulnerability in early learning experiences in some detail. Thus individuals with panic disorder have evidence in their backgrounds for early learning experiences encouraging sick role behavior and/or negative evaluations of somatic symptoms (Ehlers, 1993). To take one example, Craske, Poulton, Tsao, and Plotkin (2001) noticed a marked sensitivity to respiratory symptoms among individuals who had witnessed chronic obstructive pulmonary disease among their relatives while growing up. Other investigators have noted that parents of anxious children spend a great deal of time discussing the potentially threatening nature of ambiguous

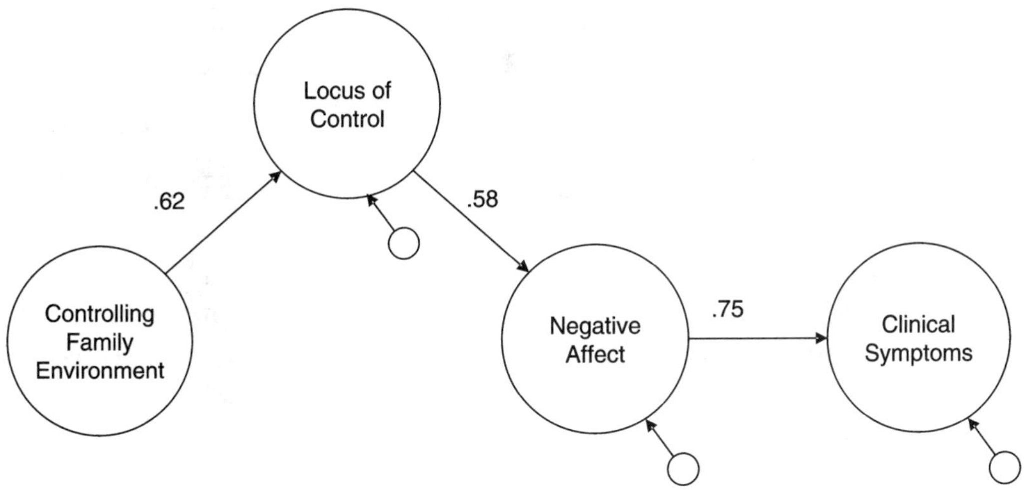

FIGURE 6.2. A partial test of a model linking a controlling family environment with child locus of control, negative emotion, and clinical symptoms of anxiety. From Chorpita (2001). Copyright 2001 by Oxford University Press. Reprinted by permission.

situations with their children by misinterpreting ambiguous cues as threatening, and hence reinforce escape or avoidant tendencies in ambiguous situations (Barrett et al., 1996). This is particularly true when the parents themselves report or display high levels of anxiety (Albano, Logsdon-Conradsen, & Barlow, 1999). Thus vicarious learning of anxiety focused on a variety of key features or situations seems to serve as a specific type of psychological vulnerability for the development of individual anxiety disorders (Barlow, 2002). Figure 6.3 displays the synergistic interaction of generalized biological and psychological vulnerabilities with the specific psychological vulnerability, which, when precipitated by a stressful life event, may lead to the occurrence of panic attacks and/or individual anxiety disorders.

COMMON COMORBIDITIES

The issue of comorbidity in the childhood anxiety disorders plays a critical role in the understanding of childhood anxiety more generally (e.g., Caron & Rutter, 1991). Certainly, the study of comorbid anxiety syndromes is essential to understanding the underlying risk factors, the relationships among anxiety symptoms, the developmental continuities and discontinuities, and the validity of the major anxiety syndromes themselves. Comorbid disorders in childhood tend to occur more often than "pure" diagnostic profiles (e.g., Anderson et al., 1987). As such, it is difficult to draw meaningful conclusions about the characteristics of any particular childhood anxiety syndrome without consideration of the comorbid disorders, their potential influences, and their underlying latent constructs (cf. Lillienfeld, Waldman, & Israel, 1994).

Disagreements about how comorbidity itself should best be defined continue. For example, the categorical nosology of the DSM classification system for anxiety disorders allows examination of comorbidity at the syndrome level only; meanwhile, others have argued that symptom comorbidity, or covariability within dimensional classification systems (cf. Achenbach & Edelbrock, 1983), might have greater utility (e.g., Brown & Barlow, 1992, 2002; Frances et al., 1990). In addition, Caron and Rutter (1991) have proposed that syndromal comorbidity might arise for numerous reasons, many of which can be artifactual. These reasons include referral effects (e.g., Berkson, 1946), symptom criterion overlap, artificial dichotomizing of dimensional syndromes, and developmental progression (e.g., social phobia leading to depression or GAD in adolescence). Such conceptual disagreements about comorbidity more generally may in part be responsible for the relative lack of research ex-

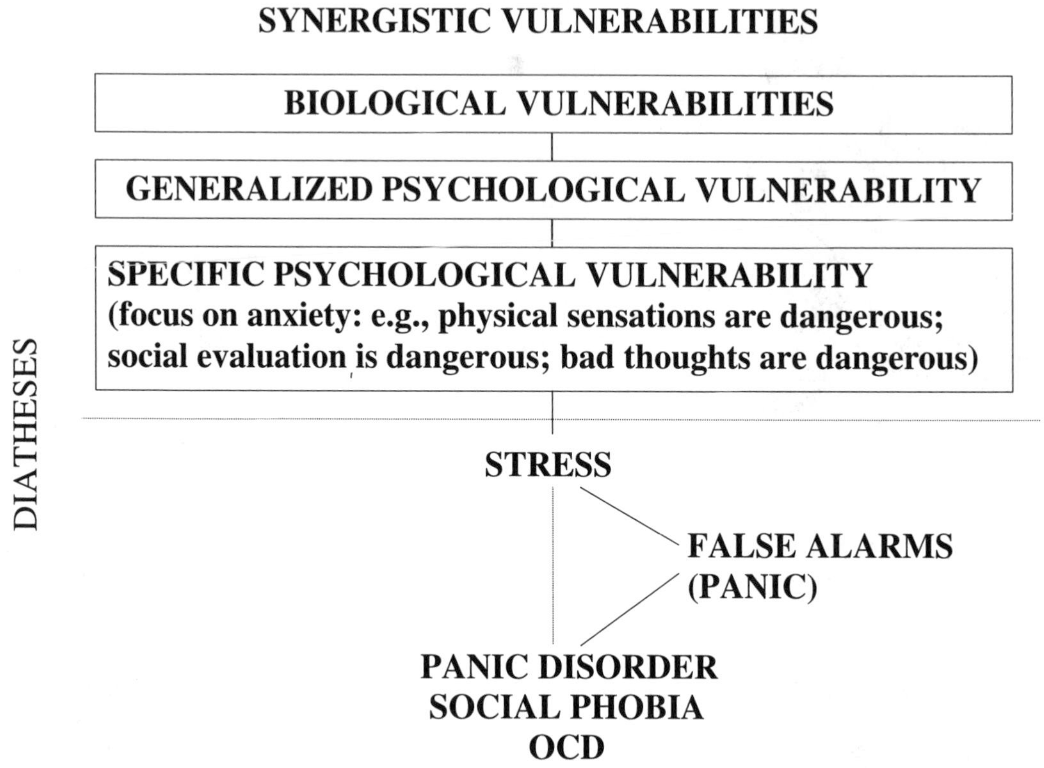

FIGURE 6.3. Triple vulnerabilities in the development of certain anxiety and related disorders. From Barlow (2002). Copyright 2002 by The Guilford Press. Reprinted by permission.

amining comorbidity among childhood anxiety disorders.

Early research attention given to the comorbidity of childhood anxiety disorders involved an investigation by Last, Strauss, and Francis (1987). Using DSM-III diagnostic criteria, the investigators examined the co-occurrence of diagnoses in an outpatient population of 73 children. The results demonstrated that children with OAD demonstrated the highest rate of comorbidity, with 9% having three or more additional clinical diagnoses. In addition, children assigned principal diagnoses of OAD most frequently received social phobia or avoidant disorder as additional diagnoses. Overall, the patterns demonstrated high diagnostic comorbidity for all of the anxiety disorders studied, with additional diagnoses assigned to as many as 80% of cases for selected anxiety diagnoses (SAD, OAD, school phobia), and with additional anxiety diagnoses assigned to 100% of the children with a principal diagnosis of major depression. Studies using DSM-IV criteria, although fewer in number, find patterns of comorbidity similar to those in studies of the DSM-III anxiety disorders. For example, in a large community sample of German adolescents, one-third of the youths with specific phobias also met criteria for depressive and somatoform disorders (Essau et al., 2000).

Existing studies on OCD have found many disorders to be comorbid with this diagnosis. For example, the NIMH study of 70 children and adolescents found that only 26% of the sample presented with OCD alone (Swedo et al., 1989). For this sample, the most common comorbid DSM-III disorders were tic disorders (30%, excluding Tourette's disorder), major depression (26%), specific developmental disorder (24%), simple phobia (17%), OAD (16%), adjustment disorder with depressed mood (13%), oppositional disorder (11%), and attention deficit disorder (10%). Similar rates of comorbidity have been reported in both community and clinical samples (e.g., Albano, Chorpita, et al., 1995; Flament et al., 1988; Last & Strauss, 1989b; Riddle et al., 1990; Valleni-Basile et al., 1994). It has been suggested that high rates of comorbidity among OCD and other anxiety and mood disorders are reflective of these disorders' being associated features of OCD and/or of OCD symptoms' being features of other disorders (Valleni-Basile et al., 1994). Further research is necessary to explore fully the hypothesis that anxiety and depression exist on a continuum representing the same underlying construct.

Often the study of comorbidity involves attempts to clarify difficult diagnostic boundary issues. Because closely related diagnostic categories that often co-occur may actually represent one underlying syndrome, it is important to examine the validity of such disorders. For example, children diagnosed with DSM-III-R avoidant disorder of childhood or adolescence were found to be indistinguishable from children with DSM-III-R social phobia on measures of fear and depression, SES, and gender and ethnicity ratios (Francis et al., 1992). In fact, these two disorders appeared to be best differentiated by age at intake, suggesting that avoidant disorder may be a temporal precursor to social phobia (i.e., developmental progression; cf. Caron & Rutter, 1991). Consistent with these findings, avoidant disorder of childhood or adolescence was not included in DSM-IV; however, the social phobia criteria were modified to account for developmental variation (see "Description of the Disorders," above).

The issue of whether high comorbidity indicates invalid division of latent constructs becomes more complex when one considers the more heterogeneous and yet common syndromes of childhood, such as school refusal or test anxiety. Indeed, because these syndromes are unique to childhood, their nosology has received relatively less empirical attention than the disorders common to both children and adults. Consequently, their relationship to DSM diagnostic nosology has been the subject of debate (e.g., Beidel & Turner, 1988; Kearney & Silverman, 1996). In a study of test anxiety, for example, Beidel and Turner found it to be comorbid with DSM-III diagnoses of social phobia (24%), simple phobia (4%), SAD (4%), and OAD (24%). Although it might be argued that test anxiety is perhaps best conceptualized along the dimension of DSM nosology, it is interesting to note that 40% of the test-anxious sample did not meet criteria for any DSM-III diagnosis.

Similar quandaries have arisen in the area of school refusal (Kearney & Silverman, 1996). Several attempts have been made to understand school refusal as a symptom of anxiety or mood disorders (Bernstein & Garfinkel, 1986; Last & Francis, 1988; Last, Francis, et al., 1987; Last & Strauss, 1990; Ollendick & Mayer, 1984), and there has been considerable debate as to how the phenomenon is principally related to the most frequently comorbid diagnostic categories, specific (simple) phobia and SAD (Last & Strauss, 1990). Complicating the issue still further, many researchers continue to use the terms "school phobia" and "school refusal" interchangeably, considering the school refusal syndrome to be more or less conceptually equivalent to simple phobia of school (Burke & Silverman, 1987). Evidence does not support this contention, however (Kearney & Silverman, 1996). In fact, the comorbidity of school refusal and DSM anxiety disorders suggests no clear overlap at all (e.g., Kearney, Eisen, & Silverman, 1995; Last & Francis, 1988; Last & Strauss, 1990). Rather, as noted earlier in this chapter, it appears that the school refusal syndrome may best be conceptualized along dimensions other than those included in DSM nosology (e.g., function of symptomatic behaviors).

The comorbidity of SAD and panic disorder with agoraphobia continues to spur debate among clinical scientists as to whether one is a precursor to the other. Although these disorders can share features of restricted range of activity, necessity of a "safe" person, and the experience of fear without an external stressor, the data supporting their relationship are indeterminate (Ollendick et al., 1994; Otto et al., 2001). Data from the retrospective studies attempting to assess longitudinal comorbidity suggest that the link between SAD and panic disorder with agoraphobia is not a strong one (Thyer, Neese, Cameron, & Curtis, 1985; Thyer, Neese, Curtis, & Cameron, 1986; van der Molen, van den Hout, van Dieren, & Greiz, 1989); however, contrary evidence has also been noted (e.g., Alessi & Magen, 1988). Evaluating children for lifetime history of anxiety disorders, Last et al. (1992) found no significant relationship between SAD and the subsequent diagnosis of panic disorder. In fact, their data supported the notion that OAD/GAD may be the most frequent diagnosis to precede panic disorder, having emerged prior to panic disorder in 90% of their subjects. Although not consistent with existing speculation about the relationship of panic disorder and SAD, such findings compare favorably with existing theories about the relationship of chronic arousal and panic attacks (Barlow, 2002).

Research on comorbidity of the anxiety disorders has often extended into the realm of depressive disorders as well, notably major depression and dysthymia. For example, Strauss, Last, et al. (1988) examined anxiety and depression in 106 outpatient children and adolescents, using DSM-III criteria. For children diagnosed with an anxiety disorder, comorbidity with depression was extensive (28%), and those children with comorbid anxiety and depression showed more severe anxiety symptomatology than those children with anxiety disorders alone. In a similar manner, Strauss, Lease, et al. (1988), examined a broad age range of 55 children and adolescents diagnosed with DSM-III OAD. In a median-split analysis of the sample, comorbid depression was found in 50% of the older children (aged 12–19 years) and in 20% of the younger children (aged 5–11 years). In a review of the extant literature, Brady and Kendall (1992) found that 15.9% to 61.9% of youths identified as anxious or depressed have comoribid anxiety and depressive disorders, and that measures of anxiety and depression are highly correlated. Moreover, younger children tend to present with anxiety only, whereas older child and adolescents tend to show the comorbidity and also present as more impaired and symptomatic. This not only suggests the overlap between the latent constructs of anxiety and depression; it also supports the possibility of a developmental progression, whereby anxiety precedes depression and leads to the more detrimental outcomes discussed earlier in this chapter. In the prospective, longitudinal Oregon Adolescent Depression Study, youths with a lifetime anxiety disorder (n = 134) demonstrated an intra-anxiety comorbidity rate of 18.7% and were predominantly female, whereas the lifetime comorbidity rate between anxiety and other mental disorders (primarily major depressive disorder) was 73.1% and was not associated with being female (Lewinsohn et al., 1997). Further research using prospective longitudinal designs are needed to examine patterns of anxiety expression and the development of comorbid conditions as they relate to demographic and developmental factors.

CURRENT ISSUES AND FUTURE DIRECTIONS

The inclusion of the childhood anxiety disorders section within DSM-III sparked a legion of studies on the classification and diagnosis of these disorders in youth. Clearly, the increased attention to understanding the phenomenology and classification of these disorders has illuminated the high prevalence of these conditions in the general child and adolescent population. Investigators are turning toward explicating cognitive-developmental variations in the expression of various disorders in youths (e.g., Ollendick et al., 1994; Vasey, Crnic, & Carter, 1994; Vasey & Dadds, 2001). However, clinical scientists have been cautioned to approach the study of these conditions from a developmental psychopathology perspective, to understand the multiple pathways involved in the etiology and maintenance of these disorders (Angold & Costello, 1995; Vasey & Dadds, 2001). Moreover, the structure and process of classification in children and adolescents remain areas of considerable study and debate. The utility of the categorical, dimensional, and integrated systems of classification must be explored further, with attention to developmental and age-related issues impacting upon the presence and expression of symptoms and syndromes.

Studies of both epidemiological and clinic-referred samples have furthered our understanding of the devastating impact of anxiety disorders on all areas of a child's functioning. Although the existing literature is growing, many questions remain regarding the expression, diagnosis, and treatment of these disorders in youths. Specifically, longitudinal studies are needed to explore fully the natural history of these disorders and the patterns of symptom expression in nonreferred youths. Only with the systematic study of nonreferred children will investigators begin to appreciate and understand those factors involved in the etiology and maintenance of these disorders. Disturbing data is emerging suggesting that anxiety disorders in youths lead to secondary disorders, such as substance abuse and dependence, mood disorders, and the potential for suicide. In addition, youth with anxiety disorders are at risk for failing to meet specific developmental tasks necessary for adult functioning, such as completing school, achieving financial independence, separating from the family of origin, and becoming gainfully employed. Thus studies of clinical samples must be directed toward examining prognostic factors, especially in children who have or have not received treatment, to determine whether early interventions can revise these deleterious pathways. It is only relatively recently that studies examining the efficacy of prescriptive psychosocial treatment protocols have begun to appear in the literature (e.g., Albano, Marten, et al., 1995; Kearney & Silverman, 1990; Kendall, 1994; March, Mulle, & Herbel, 1994; Ollendick, 1995), and cognitive-behavioral treatments appear to be effective for the majority of youths with anxiety disorders (Kazdin & Weisz, 1998; Ollendick & King, 1998). However, the long-term effectiveness of psychosocial treatments for anxiety disorders in youths remains largely unexplored. Similarly, research regarding both the short- and long-term effectiveness of pharmacological agents for anxiety in youths are just emerging in controlled clinical trials (e.g., RUPP Anxiety Study Group, 2001). Studies are just now underway evaluating the relative efficacy of cognitive-behavioral therapy, pharmacotherapy, and their combination in youths presenting with anxiety disorders (Albano & Kendall, 2002). Overall, questions regarding the prognosis for children with these disorders remain unanswered.

The continual study of developmental variations and influences will remain central to our further understanding of the nature of these disorders in youths. Elucidating the nature and mechanisms underlying certain vulnerability pathways, such as inhibited temperament, environmental, and familial factors, will no doubt occupy the attention of researchers for years to come. Several compelling etiological models have been reviewed in this chapter. Contemporary theorists point toward an integrated model, encompassing biological vulnerabilities, psychological constructs, as well as conditioning and environmental factors (see Barlow, 2002; Chorpita & Barlow, 2001; Hope, 1996). The continued study of the interaction between biological and psychological factors in children and adolescents should continue to provide insights into the nature and correlates of these disorders. Again, longitudinal studies are needed to explicate the interaction of factors within these etiological models. Moreover, studies are needed to examine the long-term implications of enduring and fixed factors, such as family environment or developmental disability, for course and prognosis.

REFERENCES

Abe, K., & Masui, T. (1981). Age–sex trends of phobic and anxiety symptoms in adolescents. *British Journal of Psychiatry, 138*, 297–302.

Achenbach, T. M. (1980). DSM-III in light of empirical research on the classification of child psychopathology. *Journal of the American Academy of Child Psychiatry, 19*, 395–412.

Achenbach, T. M. (1988). Integrating assessment and taxonomy. In M. Rutter, A. H. Tuma, & I. S. Lann (Eds.), *Assessment and diagnosis in child psychopathology*. New York: Guilford Press.

Achenbach, T. M. (1991). *Manual for the Child Behavior Checklist/4–18 and 1991 Profile*. Burlington: University of Vermont, Department of Psychiatry.

Achenbach, T. M. (1993). Implications of multiaxial empirically based assessment for behavior therapy with children. *Behavior Therapy, 24*, 91–116.

Achenbach, T. M., & Edelbrock, C. (1983). *Manual for the Child Behavior Checklist and Revised Child Behavior Profile*. Burlington: University of Vermont, Department of Psychiatry.

Achenbach, T. M., Howell, C. T., McConaughy, S. H., & Stanger, C. (1995). Six-year predictors of problems in a national sample of children and youth: I. Cross-informant syndromes. *Journal of the American Academy of Child and Adolescent Psychiatry, 34*, 336–347.

Agras, W. S., Chapin, H. N., & Oliveau, D. C. (1972). The natural history of phobias: Course and prognosis. *Archives of General Psychiatry, 26*, 315–317.

Ahadi, S. A., Rothbart, M. K., & Ye, R. (1993). Children's temperament in the US and China: Similarities and differences. *European Journal of Personality, 7*, 359–377.

Ahlawat, K. S. (1986). Cross-cultural comparison of anxiety for Jordanian and U.S. high school students. In C. D. Spielberger & R. Diaz-Guerrero (Eds.), *Cross cultural anxiety* (Vol. 3, pp. 93–112). Washington, DC: Hemisphere/Harper & Row.

Albano, A. M. (1995). Treatment of social anxiety in adolescents. *Cognitive and Behavioral Practice, 2*, 271–298.

Albano, A. M., Causey, D., & Carter, B. (2001). Fear and anxiety in children. In C. E. Walker & M. C. Roberts (Eds.), *Handbook of clinical child psychology* (3rd ed., pp. 291–316). New York: Wiley.

Albano, A. M., Chorpita, B. F., DiBartolo, P. M., & Barlow, D. H. (1995). *Comorbidity of DSM-III-R anxiety disorders in children and adolescents*. Unpublished manuscript, State University of New York at Albany.

Albano, A. M., & Detweiler, M. F. (2001). The developmental and clinical impact of social anxiety and social phobia in children and adolescents. In S. G. Hofmann & P. M. DiBartolo (Eds.), *Social phobia and social anxiety: An integration* (pp. 162–178). New York: Plenum Press.

Albano, A. M., DiBartolo, P. M., Heimberg, R. G., & Barlow, D. H. (1995). Children and adolescents: Assessment and treatment. In R. G. Heimberg, M. R. Liebowitz, D. A. Hope, & F. R. Schneier (Eds.), *Social phobia: Diagnosis, assessment, and treatment* (pp. 387–425). New York: Guilford Press.

Albano, A. M., & Kendall, P. C. (2002). Cognitive behavioral therapy for children and adolescents with anxiety disorders: Clinical research advances. *International Review of Psychiatry, 14*, 128–133.

Albano, A. M., Logsdon-Conradsen, S., & Barlow, D. H. (1999, March). Verbal interactions of social phobic adolescents and their parents: Evidence for the FEAR effect. In M. Patterson & S. Tracey (Chairs), *Social phobia in youth*. Symposium conducted at the annual meeting of the Anxiety Disorders Association of America, San Diego, CA.

Albano, A. M., Marten, P. A., Holt, C. S., Heimberg, R. G., & Barlow, D. H. (1995). Cognitive-behavioral group treatment for adolescent social phobia: A preliminary study. *Journal of Nervous and Mental Disease, 183*, 685–692.

Albano, A. M., Mitchell, W. B., Zarate, R., & Barlow, D. H. (1992, July). *Applied tension and positive mood induction in the treatment of specific phobia of blood*. Paper presented at the Fourth World Congress of Behavior Therapy, Queensland, Australia.

Alessi, N. E., & Magen, J. (1988). Panic disorder in psychiatrically hospitalized children. *American Journal of Psychiatry, 145*, 1450–1452.

Alessi, N. E., Robbins, D. R., & Dilsaver, S. C. (1987). Panic and depressive disorders among psychiatrically hospitalized adolescents. *Psychiatry Research, 20*, 275–283.

Alloy, L. B., Kelly, K. A., Mineka, S., & Clements, C. M. (1990). Comorbidity of anxiety and depressive disorders: A helplessness–hopelessness perspective. In J. D. Maser & C. R. Cloninger (Eds.), *Comorbidity of mood and anxiety disorders* (pp. 499–543). Washington, DC: American Psychiatric Press.

Alnæs, R., & Torgersen, S. (1990). Parental representation in patients with major depression, anxiety disorder and mixed conditions. *Acta Psychiatrica Scandinavica, 80*, 518–522.

American Psychiatric Association. (1952). *Diagnostic and statistical manual of mental disorders*. Washington, DC: Author.

American Psychiatric Association. (1968). *Diagnostic and statistical manual of mental disorders* (2nd ed.). Washington, DC: Author.

American Psychiatric Association. (1980). *Diagnostic and statistical manual of mental disorders* (3rd ed.). Washington, DC: Author.

American Psychiatric Association. (1987). *Diagnostic and statistical manual of mental disorders* (3rd ed., rev.). Washington, DC: Author.

American Psychiatric Association. (1994). *Diagnostic and statistical manual of mental disorders* (4th ed.). Washington, DC: Author.

Anderson, D. J., Williams, S., McGee, R., & Silva, P. A. (1987). DSM-III disorders in preadolescent children: Prevalence in a large sample from the general population. *Archives of General Psychiatry, 44*, 69–76.

Angold, A., & Costello, E. J. (1995). Developmental epidemiology. *Epidemiological Review, 17*, 74–82.

Antony, M. (1994). *Heterogeneity among specific phobia subtypes in DSM-IV*. Unpublished doctoral dissertation, State University of New York at Albany.

Ballenger, J. C., Carek, D. J., Steele, J. J., & Cornish-McTighe, D. (1989). Three cases of panic disorder with agoraphobia in children. *American Journal of Psychiatry, 146*, 922–924.

Barlow, D.H. (2000). Unraveling the mysteries of anxiety and its disorders from the perspective of emotion theory. *American Psychologist, 55*(11), 1245–1263.

Barlow, D. H. (2002). *Anxiety and its disorders: The nature and treatment of anxiety and panic* (2nd ed.). New York: Guilford Press.

Barlow, D. H., Chorpita, B. F., & Turovsky, J. (1996). Fear, panic, anxiety, and the disorders of emotion. In D. A. Hope (Ed.), *Nebraska Symposium on Motivation: Vol. 43. Integrated views of motivation and emotion* (pp. 251–328). Lincoln: University of Nebraska Press.

Barlow, D. H., & Durand, V. M. (1995). *Abnormal psychology: An integrative approach*. Pacific Grove, CA: Brooks/Cole.

Barrett, P. M., Dadds, M. R., Rapee, R. M., & Ryan, S. (1994, November). *Effectiveness of group treatment for anxious children and their parents*. Paper presented at the 28th Annual Convention of the Association for Advancement of Behavior Therapy, San Diego, CA.

Barrett, P. M., Rapee, R. M., & Dadds, M. R. (1993, November). *Cognitive and family processes in childhood anxiety*. Paper presented at the 27th Annual Convention of the Association for Advancement of Behavior Therapy, Atlanta, GA.

Barrett, P. M., Rapee, R. M., Dadds, M. M., & Ryan, S. M. (1996). Family enhancement of cognitive style in anxious and aggressive children. *Journal of Abnormal Child Psychology, 24*, 187–203.

Barrios, B. A., & Hartmann, D. P. (1997). Fears and anxieties. In E. J. Mash & L. G. Terdal (Eds.), *Behavioral assessment of childhood disorders* (3rd ed., pp. 230–327). New York: Guilford Press.

Barrios, B. A., & O'Dell, S. L. (1998). Fears and anxieties. In E. J. Mash & R. A. Barkley (Eds.), *Treatment of childhood disorders* (pp. 249–337). New York: Guilford Press.

Bauer, D. H. (1976). An exploratory study of developmental changes in children's fears. *Journal of Child Psychology and Psychiatry, 17*, 69–74.

Beidel, D. C. (1991). Social phobia and overanxious disorder in school-age children. *Journal of the American Academy of Child and Adolescent Psychiatry, 30*, 545–552.

Beidel, D. C., & Morris, T. L. (1993). Avoidant disorder of childhood and social phobia. *Child and Adolescent Psychiatric Clinics of North America, 2*, 623–638.

Beidel, D. C., & Morris, T. L. (1995). Social phobia. In J. S. March (Ed.), *Anxiety disorders in children and adolescents* (pp. 181–211). New York: Guilford Press.

Beidel, D. C., & Turner, S. M. (1988). Comorbidity of test anxiety and other anxiety disorders in children. *Journal of Abnormal Child Psychology, 16*, 275–287.

Beidel, D. C., Turner, S. M., & Morris, T. L. (1999). Psychopathology of childhood social phobia. *Journal of the American Academy of Child and Adolescent Psychiatry, 38*, 643–650.

Beitchman, J. H., Wekerle, C., & Hood, J. (1987). Diagnostic continuity from preschool to middle childhood. *Journal of the American Academy of Child and Adolescent Psychiatry, 26*, 694–699.

Bell-Dolan, D., & Brazeal, T. J. (1993). Separation anxiety disorder, overanxious disorder, and school refusal. *Child and Adolescent Psychiatric Clinics of North America, 2*, 563–580.

Bell-Dolan, D., Last, C. G., & Strauss, C. C. (1990). Symptoms of anxiety disorders in normal children. *Journal of the American Academy of Child and Adolescent Psychiatry, 29*, 759–765.

Benjamin, R. S., Costello, E. J., & Warren, M. (1990). Anxiety disorders in a pediatric sample. *Journal of Anxiety Disorders, 4*, 293–316.

Berg, C., Rapoport, J. L., Whitaker, A., Davies, M., Leonard, H., Swedo, S., Braiman, S., & Lenane, M. (1989). Childhood obsessive compulsive disorder: A two-year prospective follow-up of a community sample. *Journal of the American Academy of Child and Adolescent Psychiatry, 28*, 528–533.

Berkson, J. (1946). Limitations of the application of fourfold table analysis to hospital data. *Biometrics, 2*, 47–53.

Bernstein, G. A., & Borchardt, C. M. (1991). Anxiety disorders of childhood and adolescence: A critical review. *Journal of the American Academy of Child and Adolescent Psychiatry, 30*, 519–532.

Bernstein, G. A., & Garfinkel, B. D. (1986). School phobia: The overlap of affective and anxiety disorders. *Journal of the American Academy of Child and Adolescent Psychiatry, 25,* 70–74.

Biederman, J., Rosenbaum, J. F., Bolduc, E. A., Faraone, S. V., & Hirshfeld, D. R. (1991). A high risk study of young children of parents with panic disorder and agoraphobia with and without comorbid major depression. *Psychiatry Research,* 37, 333–348.

Biederman, J., Rosenbaum, J. F., Bolduc-Murphy, E. A., Faraone, S. V., Chaloff, J., Hirshfeld, D. R., & Kagan, J. (1993a). A three year follow-up of children with and without behavioral inhibition. *Journal of the American Academy of Child and Adolescent Psychiatry, 32,* 814–821.

Biederman, J., Rosenbaum, J. F., Bolduc-Murphy, E. A., Faraone, S., Chaloff, J., Hirshfeld, D. R., & Kagan, J. (1993b). Behavioral inhibition as a temperamental risk factor for anxiety disorders. *Child and Adolescent Psychiatric Clinics of North America, 2,* 667–684.

Biederman, J., Rosenbaum, J. F., Hirshfeld, D. R., Faraone, S. V., Bolduc, E. A., Gersten, M., Meminger, S. R., Kagan, J., Snidman, N., & Reznick, J. S. (1990). Psychiatric correlates of behavioral inhibition in young children of parents with and without psychiatric disorders. *Archives of General Psychiatry, 47,* 21–26.

Bird, H. R., Gould, M. S., Yager, T., Staghezza, B., & Canino, G. (1989). Risk factors for maladjustment in Puerto Rican children. *Journal of the American Academy of Child and Adolescent Psychiatry, 28,* 847–850.

Birmaher, B., Brent, D. A., Chiappetta, L., Bridge, J. Monga, S., & Baugher, M. (1999). Psychometric properties of the Screen for Child Anxiety Related Emotional Disorders (SCARED): A replication study. *Journal of the American Academy of Child and Adolescent Psychiatry, 38,* 1230–1236.

Birmaher, B., Khetarpal, S., Brent, D. A., Cully, M., Balach, L., Kaufman, J., & McKenzie-Neer, S. (1997). The Screen for Child Anxiety Related Emotional Disorders (SCARED): Scale construction and psychometric characteristics. *Journal of the American Academy of Child and Adolescent Psychiatry, 36,* 545–553.

Black, B. (1995). Separation anxiety disorder and panic disorder. In J. S. March (Ed.), *Anxiety disorders in children and adolescents* (pp. 212–234). New York: Guilford Press.

Black, B., & Robbins, D. R. (1990). Panic disorder in children and adolescents. *Journal of the American Academy of Child and Adolescent Psychiatry, 29,* 36–44.

Bouton, M. E., Mineka, S., & Barlow, D. H. (2001). A modern learning-theory perspective on the etiology of panic disorder. *Psychological Review, 108,* 4–32.

Bowen, R. C., Offord, D. R., & Boyle, M. H. (1990). The prevalence of overanxious disorder and separation anxiety disorder: Results from the Ontario Child Health Study. *Journal of the American Academy of Child and Adolescent Psychiatry, 29,* 753–758.

Bowlby, J. (1969). *Attachment and loss: Vol. 1. Attachment.* New York: Basic Books.

Bowlby, J. (1973). *Attachment and loss: Vol. 2. Separation: Anxiety and anger.* New York: Basic Books.

Bradley, S. J., & Hood, J. (1993). Psychiatrically referred adolescents with panic attacks: Presenting symptoms, stressors, and comorbidity. *Journal of the American Academy of Child and Adolescent Psychiatry, 32,* 826–829.

Brady, E. U., & Kendall, P. C. (1992). Comorbidity of anxiety and depression in children and adolescents. *Psychological Bulletin, 111,* 244–255.

Breier, A., Charney, D. S., & Heninger, G. R. (1986). Agoraphobia and panic attacks: Development, diagnostic stability, and course of illness. *Archives of General Psychiatry, 43,* 1029–1036.

Brown, D. R., Eaton, W. W., & Sussman, L. (1990). Racial differences in prevalence of phobic disorders. *Journal of Nervous and Mental Disease, 178,* 434–441.

Brown, T. A., & Barlow, D. H. (1992). Comorbidity among anxiety disorders: Implications for treatment and DSM-IV. *Journal of Consulting and Clinical Psychology, 60,* 835–844.

Brown, T. A., & Barlow, D. H. (2002). Classification of anxiety and mood disorders. In D. H. Barlow, *Anxiety and its disorders: The nature and treatment of anxiety and panic* (2nd ed., pp. 292–327). New York: Guilford Press.

Brown, T. A., Chorpita, B. F., & Barlow, D. H. (1998). Structural relationships among dimensions of the DSM-IV anxiety and mood disorders and dimensions of negative affect, positive affect, and autonomic arousal. *Journal of Abnormal Psychology, 107,* 179–192.

Burke, A. E., & Silverman, W. K. (1987). The prescriptive treatment of school refusal. *Clinical Psychology Review, 7,* 353–362.

Butler, G., & Mathews, A. (1983). Cognitive processes in anxiety. *Advances in Behavior Research and Therapy, 5,* 51–62.

Cantwell, D. P., & Baker, L. (1988). Issues in the classification of child and adolescent psychopathology. *Journal of the American Academy of Child and Adolescent Psychiatry, 27,* 521–533.

Cantwell, D. P., & Baker, L. (1989). Stability and natural history of DSM-III childhood diagnoses. *Journal of the American Academy of Child and Adolescent Psychiatry, 29,* 691–700.

Caron, C., & Rutter, M. (1991). Comorbidity in child psychopathology: Concepts, issues and research strategies. *Journal of Child Psychology and Psychiatry, 32,* 1063–1080.

Chorpita, B. F. (2001). Control and the development of negative emotions. In M. W. Vasey & M. R. Dadds (Eds.), *The developmental psychopathology of anxiety* (pp. 112–142). New York: Oxford University Press.

Chorpita, B. F. (2002). The tripartite model and dimensions of anxiety and depression: An examination of structure in a large school sample. *Journal of Abnormal Child Psychology, 30,* 177–190.

Chorpita, B. F., Albano, A. M., & Barlow, D. H. (1998). The structure of negative emotions in a clinical sample of children and adolescents. *Journal of Abnormal Psychology, 107,* 74–85.

Chorpita, B. F., & Barlow, D. H. (1998). The development of anxiety: The role of control in the early environment. *Psychological Bulletin, 124,* 3–21.

Chorpita, B. F., Brown, T. A., & Barlow, D. H. (1998). Perceived control as a mediator of family environment in etiological models of childhood anxiety. *Behavior Therapy, 29,* 457–476.

Chorpita, B. F., & Daleiden, E. L. (in press). Tripartite dimensions of emotion in a child clinical sample: Measurement strategies and implications for clinical utility. *Journal of Consulting and Clinical Psychology.*

Chorpita, B. F., Plummer, C. P., & Moffitt, C. (2000). Relations of tripartite dimensions of emotion to childhood anxiety and mood disorders. *Journal of Abnormal Child Psychology, 28,* 299–310.

Clark, L. A., & Watson, D. (1991). Tripartite model of anxiety and depression: Psychometric evidence and taxonomic implications. *Journal of Abnormal Psychology, 100*, 316–336.

Cobham, V. E., Dadds, M. R., & Spence, S. H. (1998). The role of parental anxiety in the treatment of childhood anxiety. *Journal of Consulting and Clinical Psychology, 66*, 893–905.

Cole, D. A., Peeke, L. G., Martin, J. M., Truglio, R., & Ceroczynski, D. (1998). A longitudinal look at the relation between depression and anxiety in children and adolescents. *Journal of Consulting and Clinical Psychology, 66*, 451–460.

Compton, S. N., Nelson, A. H., & March, J. S. (2000). Social phobia and separation anxiety symptoms in community and clinical samples of children and adolescents. *Journal of the American Academy of Child and Adolescent Psychiatry, 39*, 1040–1046.

Costello, E. J. (1989). Child psychiatric disorders and their correlates: A primary care pediatric sample. *Journal of the American Academy of Child and Adolescent Psychiatry, 28*, 851–855.

Costello, E. J., & Angold, A. (1995). Epidemiology in anxiety disorders in children and adolescents. In J. S. March (Ed.), *Anxiety disorders in children and adolescents* (pp. 109–124). New York: Guilford Press.

Costello, E. J., Farmer, E. M. Z., Angold, A., Burns, B. J., & Erkanli, A. (1997). Psychiatric disorders among American Indian and white youth in Appalachia: The Great Smoky Mountain Study. *American Journal of Public Health, 87*, 827–832.

Costello, E. J., Keeler, G. P., & Angold, A. (2001). Poverty, race/ethnicity, and psychiatric disorder: A study of rural children. *American Journal of Public Health, 91*, 1494–1498.

Costello, E. J., Stouthamer-Loever, M., & DeRosier, M. (1993). Continuity and change in psychopathology from childhood to adolescence. Paper presented at the Annual Meeting of the Society for Research in Child and Adolescent Psychopathology, Sante Fe, New Mexico. From: Costello, E. J., & Angold, A. (1995). Epidemiology. In J. S. March (Ed.), *Anxiety disorders in children and adolescents* (pp. 109–124). New York: Guilford Press.

Craske, M. E., Poulton, R., Tsao, J. C. I., & Plotkin, D. (2001). Paths to panic disorder/agoraphobia: An exploratory analysis from age 3 to 21 in an unselected birth cohort. *Journal of the American Academy of Child and Adolescent Psychology, 40*, 556–563.

Dadds, M. R., Heard, P. M., & Rapee, R. M. (1992). The role of family intervention in the treatment of child anxiety disorders: Some preliminary findings. *Behaviour Change, 9*, 171–177.

Daleiden, E. L. (1998). Childhood anxiety and memory functioning: A comparison of systemic and processing accounts. *Journal of Experimental Child Psychology, 68*, 216–235.

Derryberry, D., & Reed, M. A. (1996). Regulatory processes and the development of cognitive representations. *Journal of Research in Personality, 29*, 59–84.

Dierker, L., Albano, A. M., Clarke, G. N., Heimberg, R. G., Kendall, P. C., Merikangas, K. R., Lewinsohn, P. M., Offord, D. R., Kessler, R., & Kupfer, D. J. (2001). Screening for anxiety and depression in early adolescence. *Journal of the American Academy of Child and Adolescent Psychiatry, 40*, 929–936.

DiNardo, P. A., O'Brien, G. T., Barlow, D. H., Waddell, M. T., & Blanchard, E. B. (1983). Reliability of DSM-III anxiety disorders using a new structured interview. *Archives of General Psychiatry, 22*, 1070–1078.

Dinges, N. G., & Duong-Tran, Q. (1993). Stressful life events and co-occurring depression, substance abuse, and suicidality among American Indian and Alaskan Native adolescents. *Culture, Medicine, and Psychiatry, 16*, 487–502.

Dweck, C., & Wortman, C. (1982). Learned helplessness, anxiety, and achievement. In H. Krone & L. Laux (Eds.), *Achievement, stress and anxiety* (pp. 93–125). New York: Hemisphere.

Eaves, L. J., Silberg, J. L., Maes, H. H., Simonoff, E., Pickles, A., Rutter, M., Neale, M. C., Reynolds, C. A., Erikson, M. T., Heath, A. C., Loeber, R., Truett, K. R., Hewitt, J. K. (1997). Genetics and developmental psychopathology: 2. The main effects of genes and environment on behavioral problems in the Virginia Twin Study of Adolescent Behavioral Development. *Journal of Child Psychology and Psychiatry, 38*, 965–980.

Ehiobuche, I. (1988). Obsessive–compulsive neurosis in relation to parental child rearing patterns amongst Greek, Italian, and Anglo-Australian subjects. *Acta Psychiatrica Scandinavica, 78*, 115–120.

Ehlers, A. (1993). Somatic symptoms and panic attacks: A retrospective study of learning experiences. *Behaviour Research and Therapy, 31*, 269–278.

Eisen, A. R., & Engler, L. B. (1995). Chronic anxiety. In A. R. Eisen, C. A. Kearney, & C. A. Schaefer (Eds.), *Clinical handbook of anxiety disorders in children and adolescents*. Northvale, NJ: Aronson.

Eisen, A. R., & Kearney, C. A. (1995). *Practitioner's guide to treating fear and anxiety in children and adolescents: A cognitive-behavioral approach* (pp. 223–250). Northvale, NJ: Aronson.

Eley, T. C. (2001). Contributions of behavioral genetics research: Quantifying genetic, shared environmental and nonshared environmental influences. In M. W. Vasey & M. R. Dadds (Eds.), *The developmental psychopathology of anxiety* (pp. 45–59). New York: Oxford University Press.

Eley, T. C., & Stevenson, J. (1999a). Using genetic analyses to clarify the distinction between depressive and anxious symptoms in children. *Journal of Abnormal Child Psychology, 27*, 105–114.

Eley, T. C., & Stevenson, J. (1999b). Exploring the covariation between anxiety and depression symptoms: A genetic analysis of the effects of age and sex. *Journal of Child Psychology and Psychiatry, 40*, 1273–1282.

Essau, C. A., Conradt, J., & Petermann, F. (1999). Frequency of panic attacks and panic disorder in adolescents. *Depression and Anxiety, 9*, 19–26.

Essau, C. A., Conradt, J., & Petermann, F. (2000). Frequency, comorbidity, and psychosocial impairment of specific phobia in adolescents. *Journal of Clinical Child Psychology, 29*, 221–231.

Feehan, M., McGee, R., & Williams, S.M. (1993). Mental health disorders from age 15 to age 18 years. *Journal of the American Academy of Child and Adolescent Psychiatry, 32*, 1118–1126.

Ferdinand, R, F., & Verhulst, F. C. (1995). Psychopathology from adolescence into young adulthood: An 8-year follow-up study. *American Journal of Psychiatry, 152*, 586–594.

Flament, M., Koby, E., Rapoport, J., Berg, C., Zahn, T., Cox, C., Denckla, M., & Lenane, M. (1990). Childhood obsessive–compulsive disorder: a prospective follow-up study. *Journal of Child Psychology and Psychiatry, 31*, 363–380.

Flament, M. F., Whitaker, A., Rapoport, J. L., Davies, M., Zeremba-Berg, C., Kalikow, K. S., Sceery, W., & Shaffer, D. (1988). Obsessive compulsive disorder in adolescence: An epidemiological study. *Journal of the American Academy of Child and Adolescent Psychiatry, 27*, 764–771.

Fonesca, A. C., Yule, W., & Erol, N. (1994). Cross-cultural issues. In T. H. Ollendick, N. J. King, & W. Yule (Eds.), *International handbook of phobic and anxiety disorders in children and adolescents* (pp. 67–84). New York: Plenum Press.

Forthofer, M., Kessler, R., Story, A., & Gotlib, I. (1996). The effects of psychiatric disorders on the probability and timing of first marriage. *Journal of Health and Social Behavior, 37*, 121–132.

Fowles, D. C. (1995). A motivational theory of psychopathology. In W. D. Spaulding (Ed.), *Nebraska Symposium on Motivation: Vol. 41. Integrated views of motivation, cognition, and emotion* (pp. 181–238). Lincoln: University of Nebraska Press.

Frances, A., Widiger, T., & Fyer, M. R. (1990). The influence of classification methods on comorbidity. In D. Maser & C. D. Cloninger (Eds.), *Comorbidity of anxiety and mood disorders*. Washington, DC: American Psychiatric Association Press.

Francis, G., Last, C. G., & Strauss, C. C. (1987). Expression of separation anxiety disorder: The roles of age and gender. *Child Psychiatry and Human Development, 18*, 82–89.

Francis, G., Last, C. G., & Strauss, C. C. (1992). Avoidant disorder and social phobia in children and adolescents. *Journal of the American Academy of Child and Adolescent Psychiatry, 31*, 1086–1089.

Freud, A. (1965). *Normality and pathology in childhood: Assessment of development*. New York: International Universities Press.

Freud, S. (1955). Analysis of a phobia in a five-year-old boy. In J. Strachey (Ed. and Trans.), *The standard edition of the complete psychological works of Sigmund Freud* (Vol. 10, pp. 3–149). London: Hogarth Press. (Original work published 1909)

Friedman, S., & Paradis, C. M. (1991). African-American patients with panic disorder and agoraphobia. *Journal of Anxiety Disorders, 5*, 35–41.

Geller, D. A., Biederman, J., Faraone, S. V., Bellordre, C. A., Kim, G. S., Hagermoser, L., Cradock, K., Frazier, J., & Coffey, B. J. (2001). Disentangling chronological age from age of onset in children and adolescents with obsessive–compulsive disorder. *International Journal of Neuropsychopharmacology, 4*, 169–178.

Gerlsma, C., Emmelkamp, P. M. G., & Arrindell, W. A. (1990). Anxiety, depression, and perception of early parenting: A meta-analysis. *Clinical Psychology Review, 10*, 251–277.

Gerull, F. C., & Rapee, R. M. (2002). Mother knows best: The effects of maternal modelling on the acquisition of fear and avoidance behaviour in toddlers. *Behaviour Research and Therapy, 40*, 279–287.

Ginsburg, G. S., & Silverman, W. K. (2000). Gender role orientation and fearfulness in children with anxiety disorders. *Journal of Anxiety Disorders, 14*, 57–67.

Gittelman, R., & Klein, D. F. (1985). Childhood separation anxiety and adult agoraphobia. In A. H. Tuma & J. Maser (Eds.), *Anxiety and the anxiety disorders* (pp. 389–402). Hillsdale, NJ: Erlbaum.

Gray, J. A. (1982). *The neuropsychology of anxiety*. New York: Oxford University Press.

Gray, J. A., & McNaughton, N. (1996). The neuropsychology of anxiety: A reprise. In D. A. Hope (Ed.), *Nebraska Symposium on Motivation: Vol. 43. Perspectives on anxiety, panic, and fear* (pp. 61–134). Lincoln: University of Nebraska Press.

Guida, F. V., & Ludlow, L. H. (1989). A cross cultural study of test anxiety. *Journal of Cross-Cultural Psychology, 20*, 178–190.

Gurley, D., Cohen, P., Pine, D. S., & Brook, J. (1996). Discriminating anxiety an depression in youth: A role for diagnostic criteria. *Journal of Affective Disorders, 39*, 191–200.

Hampe, E., Noble, H., Miller, L. C., & Barrett, O. L. (1973). Phobic children one and two years posttreatment. *Journal of Abnormal Psychology, 82*, 446–453.

Harris, B. (1979). Whatever happened to Little Albert? *American Psychologist, 34*, 151–160.

Hayward, C., Killen, J. D., Hammer, L. D., Litt, I. F., Wilson, D. M., Simmonds, B., & Taylor, C. B. (1992). Pubertal stage and panic attack history in sixth- and seventh-grade girls. *American Journal of Psychiatry, 149*, 1239–1243.

Hebb, D. O. (1946). On the nature of fear. *Psychological Review, 53*, 259–276.

Hinshaw, S. P. (1992). Externalizing behavior problems and academic underachievement in childhood and adolescence: Causal relationships and underlying mechanisms. *Psychological Bulletin, 111*, 127–155.

Hirshfeld, D. R., Rosenbaum, J. F., Biederman, J., Bolduc, E. A., Faraone, S. V., Snidman, N., Reznick, J. S., & Kagan, J. (1992). Stable behavioral inhibition and its association with anxiety disorders. *Journal of the American Academy of Child and Adolescent Psychiatry, 31*, 103–111.

Hodges, K., McKnew, D., Cytryn, L., Stern, L., & Kline, J. (1982). The Child Assessment Schedule (CAS) diagnostic interview: A report on the reliability and validity. *Journal of the American Academy of Child Psychiatry, 21*, 486–473.

Hofmann, S., Albano, A. M., Heimberg, R. G., Tracey, S., Chorpita, B. F., & Barlow, D. H. (1999). Subtypes of social phobia in adolescents. *Depression and Anxiety, 9*, 8–15.

Hope, D.A. (Ed.). (1996). *Nebraska Symposium on Motivation: Vol. 43. Perspectives on anxiety, panic, and fear*. Lincoln: University of Nebraska Press.

Hudson, J. L., & Rapee, R. M. (2001). Parent–child interactions and anxiety disorders: An observational study. *Behaviour Research and Therapy, 39*, 1411–1427.

Ialongo, N., Edelsohn, G., Werthamer-Larsson, L., Crockett, L., & Kellam, S. (1994). The significance of self-reported anxious symptoms in first-grade children. *Journal of Abnormal Child Psychology, 22*, 441–455.

Ialongo, N., Edelsohn, G., Werthamer-Larsson, L., Crockett, L., & Kellam, S. (1995). The significance of self-reported anxious symptoms in first grade children: prediction to anxious symptoms and adaptive functioning in fifth grade. *Journal of Child Psychology and Psychiatry, 36*, 427–437.

Johnson, J. G., Cohen, P., Pine, D. S., Klein, D. F., Kasen, S., & Brook, J. S. (2000). Association between cigarette smoking and anxiety disorders during adolescence and early adulthood. *Journal of the American Medical Association, 284*, 2348–2351.

Joiner, T. E., Catanzaro, S. J., & Laurent, J. (1996). Tripartite structure of positive and negative affect, depression, and anxiety in child and adolescent psychiatric inpatients. *Journal of Abnormal Psychology*, *105*, 401–409.

Jones, M. C. (1924a). The elimination of children's fears. *Journal of Experimental Psychology*, *1*, 383–390.

Jones, M. C. (1924b). A laboratory study of fear: The case of Peter. *Pedagogical Seminar*, *31*, 308–315.

Kagan, J. (1997). Temperament and the reactions to unfamiliarity. *Child Development*, *68*, 139–143.

Kagan, J., Reznick, J. S., & Gibbons, J. (1989). Inhibited and uninhibited types of children. *Child Development*, *60*, 838–845.

Kagan, J., Reznick, J. S., & Snidman, N. (1987). The physiology and psychology of behavioral inhibition. *Child Development*, *58*, 1459–1473.

Kagan, J., Reznick, J. S., & Snidman, N. (1988). Biological bases of childhood shyness. *Science*, *240*, 167–171.

Kaplow, J. B., Curran, P. J., Angold, A., & Costello, E. J. (2001). The prospective relation between dimensions of anxiety and the initiation of adolescent alcohol abuse. *Journal of Clinical Child Psychology*, *30*, 316–326.

Karno, M., Golding, J. M., Sorenson, S. B., & Burnam, M. A. (1988). The epidemiology of obsessive–compulsive disorder in five U.S. communities. *Archives of General Psychiatry*, *45*, 1094–1099.

Kashani, J. H., & Orvaschel, H. (1988). Anxiety disorders in midadolescence: A community sample. *American Journal of Psychiatry*, *145*, 960–964.

Kashani, J. H., Orvaschel, H., Rosenberg, T. K., & Reid, J. C. (1989). Psychopathology in a community sample of children and adolescents: A developmental perspective. *Journal of the American Academy of Child and Adolescent Psychiatry*, *28*, 701–706.

Kazdin, A. E., & Weisz, J. R. (1998). Identifying and developing empirically supported child and adolescent treatments. *Journal of Consulting and Clinical Psychology*, *66*, 19–36.

Kearney, C. A. (1995). School refusal behavior. In A. R. Eisen, C. A. Kearney, & C. A. Schaefer (Eds.), *Clinical handbook of anxiety disorders in children and adolescents* (pp. 19–52). Northvale, NJ: Aronson.

Kearney, C.A. (2001). *School refusal behavior in youth: A functional approach to assessment and treatment*. Washington, DC: American Psychological Association.

Kearney, C. A., & Albano, A. M. (2000). *When children refuse school: Therapist's manual*. San Antonio, TX: Psychological Corporation.

Kearney, C. A., Albano, A. M., Eisen, A. R., Allan, W. D., & Barlow, D. H. (1997). The phenomenology of panic disorder in youngsters: An empirical study of a clinical sample. *Journal of Anxiety Disorders*, *11*, 49–62.

Kearney, C. A., & Allan, W. D. (1995). Panic disorder with or without agoraphobia. In A. R. Eisen, C. A. Kearney, & C. A. Schaefer (Eds.), *Clinical handbook of anxiety disorders in children and adolescents* (pp. 251–281). Northvale, NJ: Aronson.

Kearney, C. A., Eisen, A. E., & Schaefer, C. A. (1995). General issues underlying the diagnosis and treatment of child and adolescent anxiety disorders. In A. R. Eisen, C. A. Kearney, & C. A. Schaefer (Eds.), *Clinical handbook of anxiety disorders in children and adolescents* (pp. 3–15). Northvale, NJ: Aronson.

Kearney, C. A., Eisen, A. E., & Silverman, W. K. (1995). The legend and myth of school phobia. *School Psychology Quarterly*, *10*, 65–85.

Kearney, C. A., & Silverman, W. K. (1990). A preliminary analysis of a functional model of assessment and treatment of school refusal behavior. *Behavior Modification*, *14*, 340–366.

Kearney, C. A., & Silverman, W. K. (1992). Let's not push the "panic" button: A critical analysis of panic and panic disorder in adolescents. *Clinical Psychology Review*, *12*, 293–305.

Kearney, C. A., & Silverman, W. K. (1993). Measuring the function of school refusal behavior: The School Refusal Assessment Scale. *Journal of Clinical Child Psychology*, *22*, 85–96.

Kearney, C. A., & Silverman, W. K. (1996). *The evolution and reconciliation of taxonomic strategies for school refusal behavior. Clinical Psychology: Science and Practice*, *3*, 339–354.

Keller, M. B., & Baker, L. A. (1992). The clinical course of panic disorder and depression. *Journal of Clinical Psychiatry*, *53*(Suppl. 3), 5–8.

Keller, M. B., Lavori, P., Wunder, J., Beardslee, W. R., Schwartz, C. E., & Roth, J. (1992). Chronic course of anxiety disorders in children and adolescents. *Journal of the American Academy of Child and Adolescent Psychiatry*, *31*, 595–599.

Kendall, P. C. (1992). Childhood coping: Avoiding a lifetime of anxiety. *Behavioural Change*, *9*, 1–8.

Kendall, P. C. (1994). Treating anxiety disorders in children: Results of a randomized clinical trial. *Journal of Consulting and Clinical Psychology*, *62*, 100–110.

Kendall, P. C., & Warman, M. J. (1996). Anxiety disorders in youth: Diagnostic consistency across DSM-III-R and DSM-IV. *Journal of Anxiety Disorders*, *10*, 453–463.

Kendler, K. S., Neale, M. C., Kessler, R. C., Heath, A. C., & Eaves, L. J. (1992). Major depression and generalized anxiety disorder: Same genes, (partly) different environments? *Archives of General Psychiatry*, *49*, 716–722.

Kessler, R. C., Foster, C. L., Saunders, W. B., & Stang, P. E. (1995). Social consequences of psychiatric disorders, I: Educational attainment. *American Journal of Psychiatry*, *152*, 1026–1032.

Kessler, R. C., & Frank, R. G. (1997). The impact of psychiatric disorders on work loss days. *Psychological Medicine*, 27, 861–873.

Kessler, R. C., McGonagle, K., Zhao, S., Nelson, C. B., Hughes, M., Eshleman, S., Wittchen, H.-U., & Kendler, K. S. (1994). Lifetime and 12-month prevalence of DSM-III-R psychiatric disorders in the United States. *Archives of General Psychiatry*, *51*, 8–19.

King, N. J. (1993). Simple and social phobias. In T. H. Ollendick & R. J. Prinz (Eds.), *Advances in clinical child psychology* (Vol. 15, pp. 305–341). New York: Plenum Press.

King, N. J., Hamilton, D. I., & Ollendick, T. H. (1988). *Children's phobias: A behavioural perspective*. Chichester, England: Wiley.

Klein, R. G. (1995). Anxiety disorders. In M. Rutter, E. Taylor, & L. Hersov (Eds.), *Child and adolescent psychiatry: Modern approaches* (3rd ed., pp. 351–374). Oxford: Blackwell Scientific.

La Greca, A. M. (2001). Friends or foes?: Peer influences on anxiety among adolescents. In W. K. Silverman & P. Treffers (Eds.), *Anxiety disorders in children and adolescents* (pp. 159–186). New York Cambridge University Press.

La Greca, A. M., & Lopez, N. (1998). Social anxiety among adolescents: linkages with peer relations and friendships. *Journal of Abnormal Child Psychology*, *26*, 83–94.

Lapouse, R., & Monk, M. A. (1958). An epidemiologic study of behavior characteristics in children. *American Journal of Public Health, 48*, 1134–1144.

Lapouse, R., & Monk, M. A. (1959). Fears and worries in a representative sample of children. *American Journal of Orthopsychiatry, 29*, 803–818.

Last, C. G. (1989). Anxiety disorders of childhood or adolescence. In C. G. Last & M. Hersen (Eds.), *Handbook of child psychiatric diagnosis* (pp. 156–169). New York: Wiley.

Last, C. G. (1991). Somatic complaints in anxiety disordered children. *Journal of Anxiety Disorders, 5*, 125–138.

Last, C. G., & Francis, G. (1988). School phobia. In B. B. Lahey & A. E. Kazdin (Eds.), *Advances in clinical child psychology* (Vol. 11, pp. 193–222). New York: Plenum Press.

Last, C. G., Francis, G., Hersen, M., Kazdin, A. E., & Strauss, C. C. (1987). Separation anxiety and school phobia: A comparison using DSM-III criteria. *American Journal of Psychiatry, 144*, 653–657.

Last, C. G., Francis, G., & Strauss, C. C. (1989). Assessing fears in anxiety-disordered children with the Revised Fear Survey Schedule for Children (FSSC-R). *Journal of Clinical Child Psychology, 18*, 137–141.

Last, C. G., Hansen, C., & Franco, N. (1997). Anxious children in adulthood: A prospective study of adjustment. *Journal of the American Academy of Child and Adolescent Psychiatry, 36*, 645–652.

Last, C. G., Hersen, M., Kazdin, A. E., Finkelstein, R., & Strauss, C. C. (1987). Comparison of DSM-III separation anxiety and overanxious disorders: Demographic characteristics and patterns of comorbidity. *Journal of the American Academy of Child and Adolescent Psychiatry, 26*, 527–531.

Last, C. G., Hersen, M., Kazdin, A., Orvaschel, H., & Perrin, S. (1991). Anxiety disorders in children and their families. *Archives of General Psychiatry, 48*, 928–934.

Last, C. G., & Perrin, S. (1993). Anxiety disorders in African-American and white children. *Journal of Abnormal Child Psychology, 21*, 153–164.

Last, C. G., Perrin, S., Hersen, M., & Kazdin, A. E. (1992). DSM-III-R anxiety disorders in children: Sociodemographic and clinical characteristics. *Journal of the American Academy of Child and Adolescent Psychiatry, 31*, 1070–1076.

Last, C. G., Perrin, S., Hersen, M., & Kazdin, A. E. (1996). A prospective study of childhood anxiety-disorders. *Journal of the American Academy of Child and Adolescent Psychiatry, 35*, 1502–1510.

Last, C. G., & Strauss, C. C. (1989a). Panic disorder in children and adolescents. *Journal of Anxiety Disorders, 3*, 87–95.

Last, C. G., & Strauss, C. C. (1989b). Obsessive–compulsive disorder in childhood. *Journal of Anxiety Disorders, 3*, 295–302.

Last, C. G., & Strauss, C. C. (1990). School refusal in anxiety-disordered children and adolescents. *Journal of the American Academy of Child and Adolescent Psychiatry, 29*, 31–35.

Last, C. G., Strauss, C. C., & Francis, G. (1987). Comorbidity among childhood anxiety disorders. *Journal of Nervous and Mental Disease, 175*, 726–730.

Leonard, H. L., Goldberger, E. L., Rapoport, J. L., Cheslow, D. L., & Swedo, S. E. (1990). Childhood rituals: Normal development or obsessive compulsive symptoms? *Journal of the American Academy of Child and Adolescent Psychiatry, 29*, 17–23.

Leonard, H. L., & Rapoport, J. (1991). Obsessive–compulsive disorder. In J. M. Wiener (Ed.), *Textbook of child and adolescent psychiatry* (pp. 323–329). Washington, DC: American Psychiatric Press.

Leonard, H. L., Swedo, S., Lenane, M. C., Rettew, D. C., Hamburger, S. D., Bartko, J. J., & Rapoport, J. L. (1993). A 2- to 7-year follow-up study of 54 obsessive–compulsive children and adolescents. *Archives of General Psychiatry, 50*, 429–439.

Lewinsohn, P. M., Gotlib, I. H., Lewinsohn, M., Seeley, J. R., & Allen, N. B. (1998). Gender differences in anxiety disorders and anxiety symptoms in adolescents. *Journal of Abnormal Psychology, 107*, 109–117.

Lewinsohn, P. M., Hops, H., Roberts, R. E., Seeley, J. R., & Andrews, J. A. (1993). Adolescent psychopathology: I. Prevalence and incidence of depression and other DSM-III-R disorders in high school students. *Journal of Abnormal Psychology, 102*, 133–144.

Lewinsohn, P. M., Zinbarg, R., Seeley, J. R., Lewinsohn, M., & Sack, W. H. (1997). Lifetime comorbidity among anxiety disorders and between anxiety disorders and other mental disorders in adolescents. *Journal of Anxiety Disorders, 11*, 377–394.

Liddell, A., & Lyons, M. (1978). Thunderstorm phobias. *Behaviour Research and Therapy, 16*, 306–308.

Lillienfeld, S. O., Waldman, I. D., & Israel, A. C. (1994). A critical examination of the use of the term and concept of *comorbidity* in psychopathology research. *Clinical Psychology: Science and Practice, 1*, 71–83.

Livingston, R., Taylor, J. L., & Crawford, S. L. (1988). A study of somatic complaints and psychiatric diagnosis in children. *Journal of the American Academy of Child and Adolescent Psychiatry, 27*, 185–187.

Lonigan, C., Carey, M. & Finch, A. J. (1994). Anxiety and depression in children: Negative affectivity and the utility of self-reports. *Journal of Consulting and Clinical Psychology, 62*, 1000–1008.

Lonigan, C. J., Hooe, E. S., David, C. F., & Kistner, J. A. (1999). Positive and negative affectivity in children: Confirmatory factor analysis of a two-factor model and its relation to symptoms of anxiety and depression. *Journal of Consulting and Clinical Psychology, 67*, 374–386.

Lonigan, C. J., & Phillips, B. M. (2001). Temperamental influences on the development of anxiety disorders. In M. W. Vasey & M. R. Dadds (Eds.), *The developmental psychopathology of anxiety* (pp. 60–91). New York: Oxford University Press.

Macaulay, J. L., & Kleinknecht, R. A. (1989). Panic and panic attacks in adolescents. *Journal of Anxiety Disorders, 3*, 221–241.

MacFarlane, J., Allen, L., & Honzik, M. (1954). *A developmental study of the behavior problems of normal children between twenty-one months and fourteen years*. Berkeley: University of California Press.

Mackinaw-Koons, B., & Vasey, M.W. (2000). Considering sex differences in anxiety and its disorders across the lifespan: A construct validation approach. *Applied and Preventive Psychology, 9*, 191–209.

Maggini, C., Ampollini, P., Gariboldi, S., Cella, P.L., Peqlizza, L., & Marchesi, C. (2001). The Parma high school epidemiological survey: Obsessive compulsive symptoms. *Acta Psychiatrica Scandinavica, 103*, 441–446.

Manassis, K., & Kalman, E. (1990). Anorexia resulting from fear of vomiting in four adolescent girls. *Canadian Journal of Psychiatry, 35*, 548–550.

March, J. S., & Albano, A. M. (2002). Anxiety disorders in children and adolescents. In D. J. Stein & E. Hollander (Eds.), *Textbook of anxiety disorders* (pp. 415–427). Washington, DC: American Psychiatric Press.

March, J. S., Leonard, H. L., & Swedo, S. E. (1995). Obsessive–compulsive disorder. In J. S. March (Ed.), *Anxiety disorders in children and adolescents* (pp. 251–275). New York: Guilford Press.

March, J. S., Mulle, K., & Herbel, B. (1994). Behavioral psychotherapy for children and adolescents with obsessive-compulsive disorder: An open trial of a new protocol driven treatment package. *Journal of the American Academy of Child and Adolescent Psychiatry, 33*, 333–341.

March, J. S., Parker, J. D. A., Sullivan, K., Stallings, P., & Conners, C. (1997). The Multidimensional Anxiety Scale for Children (MASC): Factor structure, reliability, and validity. *Journal of the American Academy of Child and Adolescent Psychiatry, 36*, 554–565.

March, J. S., & Sullivan, K. (1999). Test–retest reliability of the Multidimensional Anxiety Scale for Children. *Journal of Anxiety Disorders, 13*, 349–358.

Marks, I. M. (1988). Blood–injury phobia: A review. *American Journal of Psychiatry, 145*, 1207–1213.

Marks, I. M., & Gelder, M. G. (1966). Different ages of onset in varieties of phobia. *American Journal of Psychiatry, 123*, 218–221.

Masi, G., Favilla, L, Mucci, M., & Millepiedi, S. (2000a). Depressive comorbidity in children and adolescents with generalized anxiety disorder. *Child Psychiatry and Human Development, 30*, 205–215.

Masi, G., Favilla, L, Mucci, M., & Millepiedi, S. (2000b). Panic disorder in clinically referred children and adolescents. *Child Psychiatry and Human Development, 31*, 139–151.

McClure, E. B., Brennan, P. A., Hammen, C., & Le Brocque, R. M. (2001). Parental anxiety disorders, child anxiety disorders, and the perceived parent–child relationship in an Australian high-risk sample. *Journal of Abnormal Child Psychology, 29*, 1–10.

McGee, R., Fehan, M., Williams, S., Partridge, F., Silva, P. A., & Kelly, J. (1990). DSM-III disorders in a large sample of adolescents. *Journal of the American Academy of Child and Adolescent Psychiatry*, 29, 611–619.

McNally, R. J. (1996). Cognitive bias in the anxiety disorders. In D. A. Hope (Ed.), Nebraska Symposium on Motivation: Vol. 43. Perspectives on anxiety, panic, and fear. Lincoln: Nebraska University Press.

Messer, S. C., & Beidel, D. C. (1994). Psychosocial correlates of childhood anxiety disorders. *Journal of the American Academy of Child and Adolescent Psychiatry, 33*, 975–983.

Miller, L. C. (1983). Fears and anxieties in children. In C. E. Walker & M. D. Roberts (Eds.), *Handbook of clinical child psychology* (pp. 337–380). New York: Wiley.

Miller, L. C., Barrett, C. L., Hampe, E., & Noble, H. (1972). Factor structure of childhood fears. *Journal of Consulting and Clinical Psychology, 39*, 264–268.

Mineka, S. (1985). Animal models of anxiety-based disorders: Their usefulness and limitations. In A. H. Tuma & J. D. Maser (Eds.), *Anxiety and the anxiety disorders* (pp. 199–244). Hillsdale, NJ: Erlbaum.

Mineka, S., Watson, D. W., & Clark, L. A. (1998). Psychopathology: Comorbidity of anxiety and unipolar mood disorders. *Annual Review of Psychology, 49*, 377–412.

Moreau, D., & Follett, C. (1993). Panic disorder in children and adolescents. *Child and Adolescent Psychiatric Clinics of North America, 2*, 581–602.

Moreau, D., & Weissman, M. M. (1992). Panic disorder in children and adolescents: A review. *American Journal of Psychiatry, 149*, 1306–1314.

Moreau, D., Weissman, M. M., & Warner, V. (1989). Panic disorder in children at high risk for depression. *American Journal of Psychiatry, 146*, 1059–1060.

Muris, P., Meesters, C., Merckelbach, H., Sermon, A., & Zwakhalen, S. (1998). Worry in normal children. *Journal of the American Academy of Child and Adolescent Psychiatry, 37*, 703–710.

Muris, P., Merckelbach, H., Mayer, B., & Prins, E. (2001). How serious are common childhood fears? *Behaviour Research and Therapy, 38*, 217–228.

Muris, P., Merckelbach, H., Mayer, B., van Brakel, A., Thissen, S., Moulaert, V., & Gadet, B. (1998). The Screen for Child Anxiety Related Emotional Disorders (SCARED) and traditional childhood anxiety measures. *Journal of Behavior Therapy and Experimental Psychiatry, 29*, 327–339.

Neal, A. M., Lilly, R. S., & Zakis, S. (1993). What are African American children afraid of?: A preliminary study. *Journal of Anxiety Disorders, 7*, 129–139.

Neal, A. M., & Turner, S. M. (1991). Anxiety disorders research with African Americans: Current status. *Psychological Bulletin, 109*, 400–410.

Nelles, W. B., & Barlow, D. H. (1988). Do children panic? *Clinical Psychology Review, 8*, 359–372.

Nelson, E. C., Grant, J. D., Bucholz, K. K., Glowinski, A., Madden, P. A. F., Reich, W., & Heath, A. C. (2000). Social phobia in a population-based female adolescent twin sample: Comorbidity and associated suicide-related symptoms. *Psychological Medicine, 30*, 797–804.

Nielsen, T. A., Laberge, L., Paquet, J., Tremblay, R. E., Vitaro, F., & Montplaisir, J. (2000). Development of disturbing dreams during adolescence and their relation to anxiety symptoms. *Sleep, 23*, 727–736.

Nolen-Hoeksema, S. (1987). Sex differences in unipolar depression. *Psychological Bulletin, 101*, 259–282.

Ollendick, T. H. (1979). Fear reduction techniques with children. In M. Hersen, R. M. Eisler, & P. M. Miller (Eds.), *Progress in behavior modification* (Vol. 8, pp. 127–168). New York: Academic Press.

Ollendick, T. H. (1983a). Fear in children and adolescents: Normative data. *Behaviour Research and Therapy, 23*, 465–467.

Ollendick, T. H. (1983b). Reliability and validity of the Revised Fear Survey Schedule for Children (FSSC-R). *Behaviour Research and Therapy, 21*, 685–692.

Ollendick, T. H. (1995). Cognitive-behavioral treatment of panic disorder with agoraphobia in adolescents: A multiple baseline design analysis. *Behavior Therapy, 26*, 517–531.

Ollendick, T. H., & Huntzinger, R. M. (1990). Separation anxiety disorder in childhood. In M. Hersen & C. G. Last (Eds.), *Handbook of child and adult psychopathology: A longitudinal perspective* (pp. 133–149). New York: Pergamon Press.

Ollendick, T. H., & King, N. J. (1991). Origins of childhood fears: An evaluation of Rachman's theory of fear acquisition. *Behaviour Research and Therapy, 29*, 117– 123.

Ollendick, T. H., & King, N. J. (1998). Empirically supported treatments for children with phobic and anxiety disorders. *Journal of Clinical Child Psychology, 27*, 156–167.

Ollendick, T. H., Matson, J., & Helsel, W. J. (1985). Fears in children and adolescents: Normative data. *Behaviour Research and Therapy*, *23*, 465–467.

Ollendick, T. H., Mattis, S. G., & King, N. J. (1994). Panic in children and adolescents: A review. *Journal of Child Psychology and Psychiatry*, *35*, 113–134.

Ollendick, T. H., & Mayer, J. A. (1984). School phobia. In S. M. Turner (Ed.), *Behavioral theories and treatment of anxiety* (pp. 367–411). New York: Plenum Press.

Orvaschel, H. (1988). Structured and semistructured interviews for children. In C. J. Kestenbaum & D. T. Williams (Eds.), *Handbook of clinical assessment of children and adolescents* (Vol. 1, pp. 31–42). New York: New York University Press.

Orvaschel, H., & Weissman, M. M. (1986). Epidemiology of anxiety disorders in children: A review. In R. Gittelman (Ed.), *Anxiety disorders of childhood* (pp. 58–72). New York: Guilford Press.

Öst, L.-G. (1987). Age of onset of different phobias. *Journal of Abnormal Psychology*, *96*, 223–229.

Otto, M. W., Pollack, M. H., Maki, K. M., Gould, R. A., Worthington, J. J., III, Smoller, J. W., & Rosenbaum, J. F. (2001). Childhood history of anxiety disorders among adults with social phobia: Rates, correlates, and comparisons with patients with panic disorder. *Depression and Anxiety*, *14*, 209–213.

Parker, G. (1979). Parental characteristics in relation to depressive disorders. *British Journal of Psychiatry*, *134*, 138–147.

Parker, G. (1981). Parental representation of patients with anxiety neurosis. *Acta Psychiatrica Scandinavica*, *63*, 33–36.

Parker, G. (1983). *Parental overprotection: A risk factor in psychosocial development*. New York: Grune & Stratton.

Pawlak, C., Pascual-Sanchez, T., Rae, P., Fischer, W., & Ladame, F. (1999). Anxiety disorders, comorbidity, and suicide attempts in adolescence: A preliminary investigation. *European Psychiatry*, *14*, 132–136.

Perrin, S., & Last, C. G. (1997). Worrisome thoughts in children referred for anxiety disorder. *Journal of Clinical Child Psychology*, *26*, 181–189.

Phillips, L., Draguns, J. G., & Bartlett, D. P. (1975). Classification of behavior disorders. In N. Hobbs (Ed.), *Issues in the classification of children*. San Francisco: Jossey-Bass.

Pine, D. S. (1994). Child–adult anxiety disorders. *Journal of the American Academy of Child and Adolescent Psychiatry*, *33*, 280–281.

Pine, D. S., Cohen, P., Gurley, D., Brook, J., & Ma, Y. (1998). The risk for early-adulthood anxiety and depressive disorders in adolescents with anxiety and depressive disorders. *Archives of General Psychiatry*, *55*, 56–64.

Pine, D. S., Klein, R. G., Coplan, J. D., Papp, L. A., Hoven, C. W., Martinez, J., Kovalenko, P., Mandell, D. J., Moreau, D., Klein, D. F., & Gorman, J. M. (2000). Differential carbon dioxide sensitivity in childhood anxiety disorders and nonill comparison group. *Archives of General Psychiatry*, *57*, 960–967.

Pollack, M. H., Otto, M. W., Rosenbaum, J. F., & Sachs, G. S. (1992). Personality disorders in patients with panic disorder: Association with childhood anxiety disorders, early trauma, comorbidity, and chronicity. *Comprehensive Psychiatry*, *33*, 78–83.

Rapee, R. M. (1997). Potential role of childrearing practices in the development of anxiety and depression. *Clinical Psychology Review*, *17*, 47–67.

Rapee, R. M. (2001). The development of generalized anxiety. In M. W. Vasey & M. R. Dadds (Eds.), *The developmental psychopathology of anxiety* (pp. 481–503). New York: Oxford University Press.

Rapoport, J. L., Elkins, R., Langer, D. H., Sceery, W., Buchsbaum, M. S., Gillin, J. C., Murphy, D. L., Zahn, T. P., Lake, R., Ludlow, C., & Mendelson, W. (1981). Childhood obsessive–compulsive disorder. *American Journal of Psychiatry*, *138*, 1545–1554.

Riddle, M. A., Scahill, L., King, R., Hardin, M., Towbin, K. E., Ort, S. I., Leckman, J. F., & Cohen, D. J. (1990). Obsessive compulsive disorder in children and adolescents: Phenomenology and family history. *Journal of the American Academy of Child and Adolescent Psychiatry*, *29*, 766–772.

Rosenbaum, J. F., Biederman, J., Bolduc, E. A., Hirshfeld, D. R., Faraone, S. V., & Kagan, J. (1992). Comorbidity of parental anxiety disorders as risk for childhood-onset anxiety in inhibited children. *American Journal of Psychiatry*, *149*, 475–481.

Rosenbaum, J. F., Biederman, J., Gersten, M., Hirshfeld, D. R., Meminger, S. R., Herman, J. B., Kagan, J., Reznick, J. S., & Snidman, N. (1988). Behavioral inhibition in children of parents with panic disorder and agoraphobia: A controlled study. *Archives of General Psychiatry*, *45*, 463–470.

Rosenbaum, J. F., Biederman, J., Hirshfeld, D. R., Bolduc, E. A., & Chaloff, J. (1991). Behavioral inhibition in children: A possible precursor to panic disorder or social phobia. *Journal of Clinical Psychiatry*, *52*(Suppl. 5), 5–9.

Rosenbaum, J. F., Biederman, J., Hirshfeld, D. R., Bolduc, E. A., Faraone, S. V., Kagan, J., Snidman, N., & Reznick, J. S. (1991). Further evidence of an association between behavioral inhibition and anxiety disorders: Results from a family study of children from a non-clinical sample. *Journal of Psychiatric Research*, *25*, 49–65.

RUPP (Research Units in Pediatric Psychopharmacology) Anxiety Study Group (2001). Fluvoxamine for the treatment of anxiety disorders in children and adolescents. *New England Journal of Medicine*, *344*, 1279–1285.

Rutter, M., Tizard, J., & Whitmore, K. (Eds.). (1970). *Education, health and behaviour*. London: Longmans, Green.

Rutter, M., & Tuma, A. H. (1988). Diagnosis and classification: Some outstanding issues. In M. Rutter, A. H. Tuma, & I. S. Lann (Eds.), *Assessment and diagnosis in child psychopathology* (pp. 437–452). New York: Guilford Press.

Sanderson, W. C., Rapee, R. M., & Barlow, D. H. (1989). The influence of an illusion of control on panic attacks induced via inhalation of 5.5% carbon-dioxide enriched air. *Archives of General Psychiatry*, *46*, 157–164.

Sarason, S. B., Davidson, K. S., Lightfall, F. F., Waite, R. R., & Ruebush, B. K. (1960). *Anxiety in elementary school children*. New York: Wiley.

Scherer, M. W., & Nakamura, C. Y. (1968). A Fear Survey Schedule for Children (FSS-FC): A factor analytic comparison with manifest anxiety (CMAS). *Behaviour Research and Therapy*, *6*, 173–182.

Schniering, C. A., Hudson, J. L., & Rapee, R. M. (2000). Issues in the diagnosis and assessment of anxiety disorders in children and adolescents. *Clinical Psychology Review*, *20*, 453–478.

Shaffer, D., Fisher, P., Dulcan, M. K., Davis, D., Piacentini, J., Schwab-Stone, M., Lahey, B., Bourdon, K., Jensen, P., Bird, H., Canino, G., & Regier, D. (1996). The NIMH Diagnostic Interview Schedule for Children, Version 2.3. (DISC 2.3): Description, acceptability, prevalence rates, and performance in the MECA study. *Journal of the American Academy of Child and Adolescent Psychiatry, 49*, 865–877.

Silove, D., Parker, G., Hadzi-Pavlovic, D., Manicavasagar, V., & Blaszczynski, A. (1991). Parental representations of patients with panic disorder and generalized anxiety disorder. *British Journal of Psychiatry, 159*, 835–841.

Silverman, W. K., & Ginsburg, G. S. (1995). Specific phobia and generalized anxiety disorder. In J. S. March (Ed.), *Anxiety disorders in children and adolescents* (pp. 151–180). New York: Guilford Press.

Silverman, W. K., La Greca, A., & Wasserstein, S. (1995). What do children worry about?: Worries and their relation to anxiety. *Child Development, 66*, 671–686.

Silverman, W. K., & Rabian, B. (1993). Simple phobias. *Child and Adolescent Psychiatric Clinics of North America, 2*, 603–622.

Smith, P., Perrin, S., Yule, W., & Rabe-Hesketh, S. (2001). War exposure and maternal reactions in the psychological adjustment of children from Bosnia–Hercegovina. *Journal of Child Psychology and Psychiatry, 42*, 395–404.

Solyom, L., Silberfeld, M., & Solyom, C. (1976). Maternal overprotection in the aetiology of agoraphobia. *Canadian Psychiatric Association Journal, 21*, 109–113.

Sonntag, H., Wittchen, H. U., Hofler, M., Kessler, R. C., & Stein, M. B. (2000). Are social fears and DSM-IV social anxiety disorder associated with smoking and nicotine dependence in adolescents and young adults? *European Psychiatry, 15*, 67–74.

Spence, S. H., Donovan, C., & Brechman-Toussaint, M. (1999). Social skills, social outcomes, and cognitive features of childhood social phobia. *Journal of Abnormal Psychology, 108*, 211–221.

Spence, S. H., Rapee, R., McDonald, C., & Ingram, M. (2001). The structure of anxiety symptoms among preschoolers. *Behaviour Research and Therapy, 39*, 1293–1316.

Spielberger, C. D. (1973). *Manual for the State–Trait Anxiety Inventory for Children*. Palo Alto, CA: Consulting Psychologists Press.

Spielberger, C. D., & Diaz-Guerrero, R. (Eds.). (1986). *Cross cultural anxiety* (Vol. 3). Washington, DC: Hemisphere/Harper & Row.

Spielberger, C. D., Diaz-Guerrero, R., & Strelau, J. (Eds.). (1990). *Cross cultural anxiety* (Vol. 4). Washington, DC: Hemisphere/Harper & Row.

Stark, K. D., & Laurent, J. (2001). Joint factor analysis of the Children's Depression Inventory and the Revised Children's Manifest Anxiety Scale. *Journal of Clinical Child Psychology, 30*, 552–567.

Stevenson, J., Batten, N., & Cherner, M. (1992). Fears and fearfulness in children and adolescents: A genetic analysis of twin data. *Journal of Child Psychology and Psychiatry, 33*, 977–985.

Strauss, C. C. (1990). Anxiety disorders of childhood and adolescence. *School Psychology Review, 19*, 142–157.

Strauss, C. C., Frame, C., & Forehand, R. (1987). Psychosocial impairment associated with anxiety in children. *Journal of Clinical Child Psychology, 16*, 235–239.

Strauss, C. C., & Last, C. G. (1993). Social and simple phobias in children. *Journal of Anxiety Disorders, 7*, 141–152.

Strauss, C. C., Last, C. G., Hersen, M., & Kazdin, A. E. (1988). Association between anxiety and depression in children and adolescents with anxiety disorders. *Journal of Abnormal Child Psychology, 16*, 57–68.

Strauss, C. C., Lease, C. A., Last, C. G., & Francis, G. (1988). Overanxious disorder: An examination of developmental differences. *Journal of Abnormal Child Psychology, 16*, 433–443.

Strauss, J., Birmaher, B., Bridge, J., Axelson, D., Chiappetta, L., Brent, D., & Ryan, N. (2000). Anxiety disorders in suicidal youth. *Canadian Journal of Psychiatry, 45*, 739–745.

Suomi, S. J. (1984). The development of affect in rhesus monkeys. In N. Fox & R. Davidson (Eds.), *The psychobiology of affective development*. Hillsdale, NJ: Erlbaum.

Swedo, S. E., Rapoport, J. L., Leonard, H., Lenane, M., & Cheslow, D. (1989). Obsessive–compulsive disorder in children and adolescents: Clinical phenomenology of 70 consecutive cases. *Archives of General Psychiatry, 46*, 335–341.

Thapar, A., & McGuffin, P. (1994). A twin study of depressive symptoms in childhood. *British Journal of Psychiatry, 165*, 259–265.

Thapar, A., & McGuffin, P. (1997). Anxiety and depressive symptoms in childhood: A genetic study of comorbidity. *Journal of Child Psychology and Psychiatry, 38*, 651–656.

Thyer, B. A., Neese, R. M., Cameron, O. G., & Curtis, G. C. (1985). Agoraphobia: A test of the separation anxiety hypothesis. *Behaviour Research and Therapy, 23*, 75–78.

Thyer, B. A., Neese, R. M., Curtis, G. C., & Cameron, O. G. (1986). Panic disorder: A test of the separation anxiety hypothesis. *Behaviour Research and Therapy, 24*, 209–211.

Thyer, B. A., Parrish, R. T., Curtis, G. C., Nesse, R. M., & Cameron, O. G. (1985). Ages of onset of DSM-III anxiety disorders. *Comprehensive Psychiatry, 26*, 113–122.

Topolski, T. D., Hewitt, J. K., Eaves, L. J., Silberg, J. L., Meyer, J. M., Rutter, M., Pickles, A., & Simonoff, E. (1997). Genetic and environmental influences on child reports of manifest anxiety and symptoms of separation anxiety and overanxious disorders: A community-based twin study. *Behavior Genetics, 27*, 15–28.

Torgersen, S. (1983). Genetic factors in anxiety disorders. *Archives of General Psychiatry, 40*, 1085–1089.

Tracey, S. A., Chorpita, B. F., Douban, J., & Barlow, D. H. (1997). Empirical evaluation of DSM-IV generalized anxiety disorder criteria for children and adolescents. *Journal of Clinical Child Psychology, 26*, 404–414.

Tuma, J. (1989). Mental health services for children: The state of the art. *American Psychologist, 44*, 188–199.

Turner, S. M., Beidel, D. C., & Costello, A. (1987). Psychopathology in the offspring of anxiety disorders patients. *Journal of Consulting and Clinical Psychology, 55*, 229–235.

Valez, C. N., Johnson, J., & Cohen, P. (1989). A longitudinal analysis of selected risk factors for childhood psychopathology. *Journal of the American Academy of Child and Adolescent Psychiatry, 28*, 861–864.

Valleni-Basile, L. A., Garrison, C. Z., Jackson, K. L., Waller, J. L., McKeown, R. E., Addy, C. L., & Cuffe, S. P. (1994). Frequency of obsessive–compulsive disorder in a community sample of young adolescents. *Journal of the American Academy of Child and Adolescent Psychiatry, 33*, 782–791.

van der Molen, G. M., van den Hout, M. A., van Dieren, A. C., & Greiz, E. (1989). Childhood separation anxiety and adult-onset panic disorders. *Journal of Anxiety Disorders, 3*, 97–106.

Vasey, M. W. (1995). Social anxiety disorders. In A. R. Eisen, C. A. Kearney, & C. A. Schaefer (Eds.), *Clinical handbook of anxiety disorders in children and adolescents* (pp. 131–168). Northvale, NJ: Aronson.

Vasey, M. W., Crnic, K. A., & Carter, W. G. (1994). Worry in childhood: A developmental perspective. *Cognitive Therapy and Research, 18*, 529–549.

Vasey, M. W., & Dadds, M. R. (Eds.). (2001). *The developmental psychopathology of anxiety*. New York: Oxford University Press.

Vasey, M. W., Daleiden, E. L., Williams, L. L., & Brown, L. M. (1995). Biased attention in childhood anxiety disorders: A preliminary study. *Journal of Abnormal Child Psychology, 23*, 267–279.

Velting, O. N., & Albano, A. M. (2001). Current trends in the understanding and treatment of social phobia in youth. *Journal of Child Psychology and Psychiatry, 42*, 127–140.

Verhulst, F. C., & Akkerhuis, G. W. (1988). Persistence and change in behavioral and emotional problems reported by parents of children aged 4–14. *Acta Psychiatrica Scandinavica* Suppl. 339, 77.

Verhulst, F. C., Akkerhuis, G. W., & Althaus, M. (1985). Mental health in Dutch children: II. The prevalence of psychiatric disorder and the relationship between measures. *Acta Psychiatrica Scandinavica*, Suppl. 324, 72.

Verhulst, F. C., van der Ende, J., Ferdinand, R. F., & Kasius, M. C. (1997). The prevalence of DSM-III-R diagnoses in a national sample of Dutch adolescents. *Archives of General Psychiatry*, 54, 329–336.

Vitiello, A. B., Behar, D., Wolfson, S., & Delaney, M. A. (1987). Panic disorder in prepubertal children [Letter]. *American Journal of Psychiatry, 144*, 525–526.

Vitiello, A. B., Behar, D., Wolfson, S., & McLeer, S. V. (1990). Diagnosis of panic disorder in prepubertal children. *Journal of the American Academy of Child and Adolescent Psychiatry, 29*, 782–784.

Warren, R., & Zgourides, G. (1988). Panic attacks in high school students: Implications for prevention and intervention. *Phobia Practice and Research Journal, 1*, 97–113.

Watson, D., Clark, L. A., & Harkness, A. R. (1994). Structures of personality and their relevance to psychopathology. *Journal of Abnormal Psychology, 103*, 346–353.

Watson, J. B., & Rayner, P. (1920). Conditioned emotional reactions. *Journal of Experimental Psychology, 3*, 1–14.

Weems, C. F., Silverman, W. K., & La Greca, A. M. (2000). What do youth referred for anxiety problems worry about?: Worry and its relation to anxiety and anxiety disorders in children and adolescents. *Journal of Abnormal Child Psychology, 28*, 63–72.

Weisz, J. R., Suwanlert, S., Chaiyasit, W., Weiss, B., Achenbach, T. M., & Walter, B. R. (1987). Epidemiology of behavioral and emotional problems among Thai and American children. *Journal of the American Academy of Child and Adolescent Psychiatry, 26*, 890–897.

Werry, J. S., & Quay, H. C. (1971). The prevalence of behavior symptoms in younger elementary school children. *American Journal of Orthopsychiatry, 41*, 136–143.

Wewetzer, C., Jans, T., Muller, B., Neudorfl, A., Bucherl, U., Remschmidt, H., Warnke, A., & Herpertz-Dahlmann, B. (2001). Long-term outcome and prognosis of obsessive–compulsive disorder with onset in childhood or adolescence. *European Child and Adolescent Psychiatry, 10*, 37–46.

Whitaker, A., Johnson, J., Shaffer, D., Rapoport, J., Kalikow, K., Walsh, B. T., Davies, M., Braiman, S., & Dolinsky, A. (1990). Uncommon troubles in young people: Prevalence estimates of selected psychiatric disorders in a nonreferred adolescent population. *Archives of General Psychiatry, 47*, 487–496.

Wilson, D. J., Chibaiwa, D., Majoni, C., Masukume, C., & Nkoma, E. (1990). Reliability and factorial validity of the Revised Children's Manifest Anxiety Scale in Zimbabwe. *Personality and Individual Differences, 11*, 365–369.

Wittchen, H., Stein, M., & Kessler, R. (1999). Social fears and social phobia in a community sample of adolescents and young adults: Prevalence, risk factors, and comorbidity. *Psychological Medicine*, 29, 309–323.

Wolff, R. (1989). Obsessive–compulsive disorder. In C. G. Last & M. Hersen (Eds.), *Handbook of child psychiatric diagnosis* (pp. 191–208). New York: Wiley.

Woodward, L. J., & Ferguson, D. M. (2001). Life course outcomes of young people with anxiety disorders in adolescence. *Journal of the American Academy of Child and Adolescent Psychiatry, 40*, 1086–1093.

Zahn-Wexler, C., Klimes-Dougan, B., & Slattery, M. J. (2000). Internalizing problems of childhood and adolescence: Prospects, pitfalls, and progress in understanding the development of anxiety and depression. *Developmental Psychopathology, 12*, 443–466.

Zimbardo, P., & Radl, S. (1981). The shy child. New York: McGraw Hill.

Zohar, A. H., Ratzoni, G., Pauls, D. L., Apter, A., Bleich, A., Kron, S., Rappaport, M., Weizman, A., & Cohen, D. J. (1992). An epidemiological study of obsessive–compulsive disorder and related disorders in Israeli adolescents. *Journal of the American Academy of Child and Adolescent Psychiatry, 31*, 1057–1061.

CHAPTER SEVEN

Childhood Posttraumatic Stress Disorder

Kenneth E. Fletcher

The unpredictable nature of many catastrophic events makes it difficult to determine the number of children each year who are exposed to traumatic events. Between 6% and 7% of the U.S. population is exposed annually to extreme stressors, ranging from natural disasters to driving accidents to crime to acts of terrorism (Norris, 1988). Many of the victims of these disasters are children. In 2000, an estimated 99,630 children ages 14 and under were treated in hospital emergency rooms for burn-related injuries (National Safe Kids Campaign, 2002), and approximately 879,000 children were found to have suffered from maltreatment, according to statistics collected by the National Clearinghouse on child Abuse and Neglect (2002). In 2000, persons ages 12–24 were subjected to violent victimization at rates higher than individuals of all other ages (Perkins, 1997), and in 1999, 12% of homicide victims were under the age of 18 (U.S. Department of Justice Bureau of Justice Statistics, 2002). In the same year, 894,000 children and adolescents 20 years old or younger were injured in motor vehicle accidents (U.S. Department of Transportation, 1993). Clearly, a good many children can be expected to encounter hazardous circumstances at least once before their childhood ends (Saigh, Yasik, Sack, & Koplewicz, 1999). In fact, in a recent survey of over 1,400 children and adolescents, it was found that one-quarter experienced one high-magnitude traumatic event by age 16 and 6% had experienced such an event within the past 3 months (Costello, Erkanli, Fairbank, & Angold, 2002).

Unfortunately, the likelihood of being exposed to calamitous events seems to be accelerating with the pace of modern life. Television and the rest of the mass media bring explosive disasters into the family living room with an immediacy that can be difficult to avoid. This was evident as far back as January 18, 1986, when children watched the *Challenger* space shuttle explosion live on television (Terr et al., 1999). The devastating effects of the Oklahoma City bombing of April 19, 1995, were broadcast across the country, causing distress in children and adolescents living far away from the disaster (Pfefferbaum, Seale, et al., 2000). When children in San Francisco were asked to draw their reactions to the World Trade Center and Pentagon tragedies of September 11, 2001, which occurred over 3,000 miles away, each and every one of them produced disturbingly graphic pictures of planes flying into towers while people jumped from the windows (Terr, 2001).

Exposure to traumatic events in childhood can have dire and long-lasting consequences, not only for traumatized children but for society as well. Green (1985) has suggested that "failure to master the trauma of childhood creates a continual need to repeat and reenact them during adult life" (p. 146), and others who have studied the subject agree (Pynoos & Eth, 1985b). There is evidence that childhood trauma is linked to later drug abuse, juvenile delinquency, and criminal behavior (Burgess, Hartman, & McCormack, 1987). Abused children may be more inclined than nonabused children to grow up to be abusing parents (Frederick, 1985a; Green, 1985). Childhood trauma also appears to be implicated in debilitating adult anxiety disorders (Faravelli, Webb, Ambonetti, Fonnesu, & Sessarego, 1985), dissociative experiences (Chu & Dill, 1990), borderline personality disorder (Herman, Perry, & van der Kolk, 1989), multiple personality disorder (now known as dissociative identity disorder) (Kluft, 1985), and adult psychiatric disturbance in general (Carmen, Rieker, & Mills, 1984).

Unfortunately, the predominant view as late as 15 years ago was that children are generally little affected by the worst of experiences, and then not for very long (Burt, 1943; Coromina, 1943; Freud & Burlingham, 1943; Garmezy & Rutter, 1985; Harrison, Davenport, & McDermott, 1967; Rigamer, 1986). This view prevailed despite evidence from other observers—and sometimes even from supporters of the dominant view (e.g., Burt, 1943)—that children respond to severe stress with behaviors that would today be recognized as symptomatic of posttraumatic stress (Brander, 1943; Lacey, 1972; Terr, 1979). This chapter reviews the literature on children's responses to traumatic circumstances in the light of current research on the subject. First, as preparation for this discussion, the evolution of the concept of posttraumatic stress must briefly be considered.

EVOLUTION OF THE CONCEPT OF POSTTRAUMATIC STRESS

The notion that traumatic events can lead to psychological disturbance is not a new idea (Kinzie & Goetz, 1996). Odysseus, by Homer's account, suffered from flashbacks (vivid reliving of the traumatic experience) and "survivor's guilt" (guilt over having survived when others did not) after fighting in the Trojan War (Figley, 1993). During the U.S. Civil War, combat-related stress reactions were recognized, but they were referred to as "nostalgia" (Ursano, Fullerton, & McCaughey, 1994) or "melancholia" (Figley, 1993). Posttraumatic stress reactions have been discussed in the literature under various names over the course of the past century (Foa, Steketee, & Rothbaum, 1989)—names such as "nervous shock" (Page, 1885), "shell shock" (Myers, 1940), "physioneurosis" (Kardiner, 1941), "traumatophobia" (Rado, 1942), and "war neurosis" (Grinker & Spiegel, 1945). Regardless of the name used, these accounts have reported similar reactions among survivors of catastrophic events: increased fearfulness and anxiety, fear of repetition of the stressful events, increased arousal and hypervigilance for other potentially threatening events, uncontrollable remembering of the original stressful events, efforts to forget about those events, avoidance of reminders of the events, social withdrawal, and a flattening of affect that sometimes leads to a sense of numbness. These symptoms still represent the core symptoms of posttraumatic stress disorder (PTSD) listed in current psychiatric taxonomies, such as the fourth edition of the *Diagnostic and Statistical Manual of Mental Disorders* (DSM-IV; American Psychiatric Association, 1994; see Table 7.1).

The current diagnostic category of PTSD represents a relatively recent conceptualization of traumatic stress reactions. It was first described in 1980 in DSM-III (American Psychiatric Association, 1980). The concept of PTSD at that time represented a radical departure from earlier conceptions of typical stress reactions.

Concepts of Stress Reactions Prior to DSM-III

Traditional Psychoanalytic Conceptualization

Prior to DSM-III, the predominant view of traumatic stress reactions was based on the traditional psychoanalytic explanation. Freud argued that traumatization occurs when the ego's "stimulus barrier" is overwhelmed by a flood of unmanageable stimuli from external stressors; the breaking of the stimulus barrier disrupts the organism's functioning (Freud, 1920/1955; Brett, 1993; Wilson, 1994). In general, the removal of the external stressor is expected to lead to quick restoration of the organism's functioning. However, Freud did note that unmanageable stimuli can at times become so extreme as to overpower an individual's coping mechanisms, which leads to a sense of overwhelming helplessness. At this point the individual is thought to regress and begin resorting to a primitive defense, the repetition compulsion, in an attempt to gain mastery over the traumatic experiences by compulsively repeating them in dreams, memories, and re-

TABLE 7.1. DSM-IV Diagnostic Criteria for, and Other Features of, Posttraumatic Stress Disorder (PTSD)

A. The person has been exposed to a traumatic event in which both of the following were present:

(1) the person experienced, witnessed, or was confronted with an event or events that involved actual or threatened death or serious injury, or a threat to the physical integrity of self or others
(2) the person's response involved intense fear, helplessness, or horror. **Note**: In children, this may be expressed instead by disorganized or agitated behavior.

B. The traumatic event is persistently reexperienced in one (or more) of the following ways:

(1) recurrent and intrusive distressing recollections of the event, including images, thoughts, or perceptions. **Note**: In young children, repetitive play may occur in which themes or aspects of the trauma are expressed.
(2) recurrent distressing dreams of the event. **Note**: In children, there may be frightening dreams without recognizable content.
(3) acting or feeling as if the traumatic event were recurring (includes a sense of reliving the experience, illusions, hallucinations, and dissociative flashback episodes, including those that occur on awakening or when intoxicated). **Note**: In young children, trauma-specific reenactment may occur.
(4) intense psychological distress at exposure to internal or external cues that symbolize or resemble an aspect of the traumatic event
(5) physiological reactivity on exposure to internal or external cues that symbolize or resemble an aspect of the traumatic event

C. Persistent avoidance of stimuli associated with the trauma and numbing of general responsiveness (not present before the trauma), as indicated by three (or more) of the following:

(1) efforts to avoid thoughts, feelings, or conversations associated with the trauma
(2) efforts to avoid activities, places, or people that arouse recollections of the trauma
(3) inability to recall an important aspect of the trauma
(4) markedly diminished interest or participation in significant activities
(5) feelings of detachment or estrangement from others
(6) restricted range of affect (e.g., unable to have loving feelings)
(7) sense of a foreshortened future (e.g., does not expect to have a career, marriage, children, or a normal life span)

D. Persistent symptoms of increased arousal (not present before the trauma), as indicated by two (or more) of the following:

(1) difficulty falling or staying asleep
(2) irritability or outbursts of anger
(3) difficulty concentrating
(4) hypervigilance
(5) exaggerated startle response

E. Duration of the disturbance (symptoms in Criteria B, C, and D) is more than 1 month.

F. The disturbance causes clinically significant distress or impairment in social, occupational, or other important areas of functioning.

Specify if:
Acute: if duration of symptoms is less than 3 months
Chronic: if duration of symptoms is 3 months or more

Specify if:
With Delayed Onset: if onset of symptoms is at least 6 months after the stressor

Associated descriptive features and mental disorders. Individuals with Posttraumatic Stress Disorder may describe painful guilt feelings about surviving when others did not survive or about the things they had to do to survive. Phobic avoidance of situations or activities that resemble or symbolize the original trauma may interfere with interpersonal relationships. . . . The following associated constellation of symptoms may occur and are more commonly seen in association with an interpersonal stressor (e.g., childhood sexual or physical abuse, domestic battering, being taken hostage, incarceration as a prisoner of war or in a concentration camp, torture): impaired affect modulation; self-destructive and impulsive behavior; dissociative symptoms; somatic complaints; feelings of

(*continued*)

Table 7.1. *(Continued)*

ineffectiveness, shame, despair, or hopelessness; feeling permanently damaged; a loss of previously sustained beliefs; hostility; social withdrawal; feeling constantly threatened; impaired relationships with others; or a change from the individual's previous personality characteristics.

There may be increased risk of Panic Disorder, Agoraphobia, Obsessive–Compulsive Disorder, Social Phobia, Specific Phobia, Major Depressive Disorder, Somatization Disorder, and Substance-Related Disorders. It is not known to what extent these disorders precede or follow the onset of Posttraumatic Stress Disorder.

Age-specific features. In younger children, distressing dreams of the event may, within several weeks, change into generalized nightmares of monsters, of rescuing others, or of threats to self or others. Young children usually do not have the sense that they are reliving the past; rather, the reliving of the trauma may occur through repetitive play (e.g., a child who was involved in a serious automobile accident repeatedly reenacts car crashes with toy cars). Because it may be difficult for children to report diminished interest in significant activities and constriction of affect, these symptoms should be carefully evaluated with reports from parents, teachers, and other observers. In children, the sense of a foreshortened future may be evidenced by the belief that life will be too short to include becoming an adult. There may also be "omen formation"—that is, belief in an ability to foresee future untoward events. Children may also exhibit various physical symptoms, such as stomachaches and headaches.

Note. From American Psychiatric Association (1994, pp. 425, 426, 427–428).

enactments (Freud, 1939/1964). When symptoms do not abate with time and distance from the trauma, the traditional psychoanalytic explanation is that current stress has revived infantile conflicts, which are the real cause of "traumatic neuroses" (Brett, 1993). In this way, traditional psychoanalytic theory ascribes enduring traumatic reactions to premorbid characteristics of the victim rather than to the threatening characteristics of the stressor.

Classification in DSM-I

The predominance of the psychoanalytic view of traumatic reactions was reflected in the American Psychiatric Association's DSM-I in 1952. The DSM-I classification of reactions to traumatic stress was termed "gross stress reaction," a transient, situational personality disorder. This classification was intended to cover acute responses to "intolerable stress" that "clear rapidly" when treated promptly, unless the condition progresses to a more chronic, "neurotic" disorder.

A Regression in DSM-II

By the time DSM-II was published (American Psychiatric Association, 1968), the definition of traumatic stress responses had undergone a puzzling regression. The "gross stress reaction" of DSM-I was reclassified in the second edition as "adjustment reaction of adult life," a condition about which DSM-II was strangely silent. This condition was defined only by three inadequate examples; no discussion of the symptomatology was included (Wilson, 1994). It may not be a coincidence that DSM-II was published at the height of the Vietnam War, at a time when both the military and the federal government argued vehemently against the possibility of long-term adverse psychological consequences to participation in the war.

PTSD in DSM-III and Beyond

The political debate about posttraumatic responses to Vietnam lasted over a decade. During that time, several mental health professionals began collecting case histories and research data on posttraumatic reactions to a variety of extremely stressful events—the Vietnam War (Figley, 1978), Hiroshima (Lifton, 1967), the Holocaust (Ettinger, 1961), and other disasters (Gleser, Green, & Winget, 1981). The data collected eventually led to the codification of PTSD in DSM-III (American Psychiatric Association, 1980; see also Blank, 1993; Saigh & Bremner, 1999; Scurfield, 1993).

The Definition of PTSD in DSM-III

The diagnostic definition of PTSD in DSM-III was ground-breaking for several reasons (Wilson, 1994). One innovation was the clustering of symptoms into three criteria that became the foundation of the definition of PTSD in all later editions. The first criterion of DSM-III, Criterion A, may have represented the most radical change from the previously predominant conceptualization of traumatic stress responses. For a diagnosis of PTSD to be considered, Criterion A required that an individual be exposed to "a recognizable stressor that would be expected to evoke significant symptoms of distress in almost all individuals." This requirement implied that, contrary to previous formulations of stress reactions, PTSD was to be considered a normal reaction to abnormal circumstances. In line with this position, DSM-III indicated that the intensity and scope of an individual's reactions can be expected to be directly related to the intensity and duration of the individual's exposure to the stressor. Moreover, removing the stressor was no longer taken as a guarantee that symptoms would abate. DSM-III explicitly stated that symptoms might last indefinitely. Thus, with the publication of the DSM-III definition of PTSD, traumatic stress reactions were no longer considered the result of the weakened nature of the victim; rather, they were seen as caused by the unusually threatening nature of the stressor.

Refinement in DSM-IV

The original description of PTSD contained in DSM-III has been refined in subsequent editions, but the current conceptualization contained in DSM-IV (American Psychiatric Association, 1994) is not as radically different from the definition given in DSM-III as that definition was different from earlier versions. According to the current definition of PTSD in DSM-IV (see Table 7.1), survivors of traumatic stress tend to experience unbidden dreams, memories, feelings, and behaviors that are reminiscent of the original traumatic experience (Criterion B). They tend to lose all sense of security, begin to anticipate further trouble, and become overaroused and easily startled (Criterion D). In an attempt to modulate the overwhelming feelings evoked by the recurring memories of the trauma, survivors often make an effort to avoid all thoughts and reminders of the trauma; they may also try to "turn off" their feelings, leading to flat affect, a sense of emotional numbness, and social withdrawal (Criterion C).

Alternate Definitions of PTSD

Other sources question current DSM-IV criteria for PTSD. Some argue, for example, that the requirement of three symptoms of denial or avoidance may be too restrictive (Green, 1993a)—particularly for children (Schwarz & Kowalski, 1991b), because it can be more difficult to assess symptoms of denial and numbing in children than in adults. French researchers, studying the impact on first- and third-grade children of a school hostage-taking incident in Paris, defined subclinical PTSD as DSM-IV criteria minus one symptom of Criterion C (avoidance) and one of Criterion D (overarousal). They found that whereas 7 (26.9%) of 26 children met full criteria for PTSD at some time during the 18-month follow-up period, 13 (50%) met criteria for subclinical PTSD while never fully attaining full criteria for PTSD diagnosis (Vila, Porsche, & Mouren-Simeoni, 1999). Moreover, 3 of the 7 who eventually met criteria for PTSD originally met criteria only for subclinical PTSD. It has been argued that the symptom lists for PTSD in DSM-IV and the 10th revision of the *International Classification of Diseases* (ICD-10) may not be inclusive enough (Keane, 1993), especially when the reactions of children are considered (Armsworth & Holaday, 1993). Others question the utility of any diagnostic criteria. They argue that it may be more fruitful to study PTSD as a continuous variable than a dichotomous one, as required by both DSM-IV and ICD-10 (Keane, 1993; Putnam, 1998).

HISTORICAL OVERVIEW OF THE STUDY OF CHILDREN'S STRESS REACTIONS

The stress reactions of adults have been studied much more frequently than have those of children. Some of the earliest accounts of children's stress reactions originated during World War II (Brander, 1943; Burt, 1943; Coromina, 1943; Freud & Burlingham, 1943). However, these accounts remained relatively infrequent during the war, and came to be made with even less frequency during the first 25–30 years after the war's end. Research on children's reactions to traumatic events did not begin in earnest until the publication of DSM-III in 1980, and children's reactions were not specifically mentioned in DSM until the revised third edition, DSM-III-R, was published (American Psychiatric Association, 1987).

Early Evidence

The first detailed evidence of child-specific posttraumatic reactions in children began to appear in the 1970s and 1980s, primarily from anecdotal sources (Eth & Pynoos, 1985a; Frederick, 1985a,

1986; Galante & Foa, 1986; Gislason & Call, 1982; Lacey, 1972; Newman, 1976; Rigamer, 1986; Senior, Gladstone, & Narcome, 1982; Terr, 1979, 1981a, 1981b, 1983a, 1983b, 1985a, 1985b). Very few attempts were made in the 1970s to systematically assess children's posttraumatic distress (Elmer, 1977; Milgram & Milgram, 1976; Milne, 1977; Ziv & Israeli, 1973), and these studies tended to assess only general outcomes (such as anxiety), rather than PTSD-specific symptomatology. Few reports at this time considered comparison groups, and those that did did not always choose appropriate comparison groups. Perhaps as a consequence of all these factors, the collective results of these studies were contradictory and generally inconclusive.

The Children of Chowchilla

The culmination of the early anecdotal literature can be found in the work of Terr (1979, 1983b, 1991), who has written extensively about the responses of school children in Chowchilla, California, to a 1976 kidnapping and subsequent 27-hour imprisonment, buried underground. Terr (1979) conducted detailed interviews with 23 of the 26 kidnapped children (6 boys and 17 girls, between the ages of 5 and 14 years) within 6–10 months after the kidnapping. Her report was among the first to analyze the responses of children to traumatic events in terms of contemporary conceptions of what she herself referred to as "posttraumatic symptomatology" (Terr, 1979).

Terr realized that many of the responses found in the children of Chowchilla were strikingly similar to those found in traumatized adults. Like adults, for example, the children reexperienced their kidnapping in dreams; also like adults, they avoided thoughts and reminders of their kidnapping. On the other hand, the children also reacted in child-specific ways. Unlike adults, for instance, the Chowchilla children did not appear to hallucinate or have flashback experiences of reliving the experience, nor did they exhibit any signs of affective numbing. In contrast with the tendency of traumatized adults to forget important aspects of their traumatic experience, no Chowchilla child, even 4 years after the event, forgot anything about the kidnapping (Terr, 1983b).

Children tended to relive their trauma through behavioral reenactments of significant parts of the experience, through retelling of the event, and through trauma-inspired play, wherein they played kidnapping or bus-driving games. The children of Chowchilla also suffered from misperceptions and/or hallucinations during and after the kidnapping, declining school performance, dreams of personal death, anniversary reactions (i.e., anniversaries of the kidnapping triggered increased symptomatology), pessimism about the future, and omen formation (the belief that events that occurred before the trauma foretold its occurrence). The children's fears seemed to become progressively generalized over time, too, changing from fears associated specifically with kidnapping to more general fears of everyday events.

Children's Reactions to an Australian Bushfire

More systematic research began to appear in the 1980s (Blom, 1986; Elizur & Kaffman, 1982; Gomes-Schwartz, Horowitz, & Sauzier, 1985; Saigh, 1985; Sirles, Smith, & Kusama, 1989). Despite the increased sophistication of the research, however, most studies remained primarily descriptive, lacked appropriate control or comparison groups, and depended upon reports from adults (parents or teachers) rather than the children themselves. Furthermore, either nonstandardized assessments were used, or standardized measures were used that were designed to assess general conditions (such as anxiety, depression, fear, or self-esteem), rather than PTSD-specific responses. Despite these limitations, the overall results of these studies, combined with anecdotal observations, provided substantial support for the notion that children can respond to traumatic experiences in a manner similar to that of traumatized adults.

The research by McFarlane (1987a; McFarlane, Policansky, & Irwin, 1987) into the psychological impact of a 1983 Australian bushfire on 808 children (427 boys and 381 girls) aged 8–12 is one of the best examples of the research of this period. One advantage of this study was its large sample size. Another advantage of the study was the existence of an equally large age- and sex-matched comparison group of 734 children from schools unaffected by the bushfire. Furthermore, assessments were repeated over several time periods: at 2, 8, and 26 months after the disaster.

Unfortunately, the results of the McFarlane study were diluted by important methodological limitations. For example, although the children's reactions were assessed via standardized measures (Rutter & Graham, 1967; Rutter, Tizard, & Whitmore, 1970), these measured only general behavioral problems and did not directly measure posttraumatic symptomatology—a problem noted by the authors themselves (McFarlane et al., 1987, p. 737). McFarlane (1987a) did ask about specific symptoms of posttraumatic stress at 8 months and at 26 months, but only four symptoms were assessed: having dreams or nightmares about the fire, playing games or painting pictures about the fire, getting upset at reminders, and talking about the fire. Over half of the children (53% at 8 months and 57% at 26 months) were reported by parents to have one or more of these behaviors. Parents reported that 8 months after the children were exposed to the bushfire, 35% of them still got upset at reminders, and after 26 months the proportion increased to 46%. Forty-three percent of exposed children were reported to talk about their traumatic experiences after 8 months, whereas 36% did so after 26 months. Fewer parents reported that their children played games related to the fire (13% after 8 months and 10% after 26 months), or that their children dreamed about the fire (13% after 8 months and 18% after 26 months). The comparison group does not appear to have been administered the PTSD items, perhaps because of the direct reference to exposure to the fire in those questions; as a consequence, the incidence rates for the four PTSD symptoms were not compared with rates in the comparison children.

Another difficulty with this study was its reliance on parent and teacher reports. This difficulty was compounded by the fact that parent and teacher reports generally did not agree—a lack of agreement that is common in child research (Achenbach, McConaughy, & Howell, 1987; Thabet & Vostanis, 2000). Teachers, for example, at both 8 and 26 months after the fire, reported that fewer than 30% of the children exposed to the bushfire displayed one of more of the PTSD symptoms. Parents, on the other hand, reported that more than 50% of the children had at least one symptom at both time periods.

Children's Responses to a School Shooting

Despite the limitations imposed on childhood trauma research by such factors as the unpredictability of catastrophic events, the reluctance of children and their families to discuss their traumatic experiences, and difficulties in defining and recruiting comparison groups, research has become increasingly rigorous since the mid-1980s (Clarke, Sack, & Goff, 1993; Deblinger, McLeer, Atkins, Ralphe, & Foa, 1989; Earls, Smith, Reich, & Jung, 1988; Famularo, Kinsherff, & Fenton, 1990; Green et al., 1991; Jones & Ribbe, 1991; Kinzie, Sack, Angell, Manson, & Rath, 1986; Kiser, Heston, Millsap, & Pruitt, 1991; Malmquist, 1986; Pfefferbaum, 1997; Pynoos & Nader, 1988; Realmuto et al., 1992; Saigh, 1989, 1991; Saigh, Yasik, Sack, & Koplewicz, 1999; Schwarz & Kowalski, 1991a, 1991b). Studies in the past 15 years have generally focused on the assessment of specific PTSD symptomatology, and many of them have used newly developed standardized measures. Larger sample sizes have become more common as well. Furthermore, an increasing number of studies have begun comparing the symptomatology of traumatized children with that of nontraumatized children.

School shootings have captured the national attention over the past 10 years as the frequency of their occurrence increases, and as the media gives them more coverage. On April 21, 1999, the nation watched in horror as two young gunmen in Colorado shot to death several of their schoolmates at Columbine High School and then took their own lives. The emphasis has been on healing rather than research in the aftermath of Columbine, so information about the impact of the tragedy is only slowly coming to light. However, one of the first and best of the rigorous research studies of the past 15 years concerned the impact of a school shooting. In the mid-1980s, a sniper fired repeatedly into a school's playground over a period of several hours, killing one child and one passer-by, and wounding 13 children. Pynoos et al. (1987) interviewed 159 of the children who attended that school in the aftermath of the shooting, using a version of Frederick's (1985b) adult PTSD Reaction Index (PTSD-RI) modified for children, which has since become the most frequently used instrument for assessing childhood posttraumatic stress symptomatology. The 53 children who had been at school during the attack reported higher incidence of all PTSD symptoms—except for fear of recurrence of the event and feelings of guilt—than did the 106 children who had not been at school that day. A dose effect was also demonstrated, with those closer to the shooting evidencing greater symptomatology.

When the children's answers to the 16 PTSD-RI interview questions were factor-analyzed, three factors that accounted for 50% of the variance were extracted. The first factor encompassed symptoms of two DSM-IV criteria: Criterion B, reexperiencing the trauma, and Criterion C, avoidance of reminders of the trauma or affective numbing. The second factor was defined by symptoms of DSM-IV Criterion D, overarousal (specifically, fears of recurrence, jumpiness and exaggerated startle response, and upset or fear at thoughts of the shooting). The final factor included other symptoms of overarousal (sleep disturbance and difficulty concentrating). Feelings of guilt did not meet the criterion for inclusion in any factor. Items in the first and third factors were always present among children with severe reactions, and they were least likely to be found among children with mild or no reactions. These results provide firm support for the application of DSM-IV criteria for PTSD to traumatized children.

Fourteen months after the school shooting, 100 of the 159 children originally interviewed by Pynoos et al. (1987) were reinterviewed with similar results (Nader, Pynoos, Fairbanks, & Frederick, 1990). Proximity to the shooting scene continued to be closely related to the severity of response. Fourteen months after the disaster, 19 children who had been on the playground during the sniper attack remained more symptomatic than 81 children who had not been on the playground. PTSD symptomatology at 14 months was also strongly associated with the intensity of the children's original reactions to the shooting. The majority of the children who had been on the playground during the shooting reported being afraid and being upset when thinking about the shooting. They continued to report more intrusive thoughts about the shooting and more fear of a recurrence of the incident, as well as more jumpiness, sleep disturbance, and somatic complaints, than children who had not been on the playground that day. Their distress was increased by the expectations—of themselves as well as of others—that they should already have recovered, now that more than a year had passed since the shooting.

PREVALENCE/INCIDENCE OF POSTTRAUMATIC STRESS RESPONSES IN CHILDREN

Epidemiology

Large epidemiological studies of the prevalence of PTSD among adults have been conducted over the past decade and a half (Breslau, Davis, Andreski, & Peterson, 1991; Davidson, Hughes, Blazer, & George, 1991; Heltzer, Robins, & McEvoy, 1987; Kulka et al., 1990; Norris, 1992). Fewer studies have systematically assessed the extent and severity of PTSD symptomatology in large samples of children exposed to traumatic stressors. One study investigated the reactions of 5,687 young Americans between the ages of 9 and 19 to Hurricane Hugo (Shannon, Lonigan, Finch, & Taylor, 1994; Lonigan, Shannon, Finch, Daugherty, & Taylor, 1991). Fifty-one percent of the children were girls. Ethnic origins were as follows: 67.3% European, 25.8% African, 3.6% Asian, 1.4% Hispanic, and 1.9% "other." PTSD was assessed with the PTSD-RI (Frederick, 1985b; Pynoos et al., 1987), which was modified to allow conservative judgments to be drawn about DSM-III-R caseness for PTSD.[1] Overall, 5.4% of the children (308) met Criteria A through D of DSM-III-R for PTSD. More girls (6.9%) than boys (3.8%) met all of these criteria for PTSD. No significant differences emerged as a function of race (African Americans, 6.3%; all other ethnic groups, 5.1%). School-age children (aged 9–12 years) were more likely to meet all PTSD criteria (9.2%) than were older children (4.2% of those between 13 and 15 years, and 3.1% of those between 16 and 19 years).

After a fire in a chicken-processing plant in North Carolina, 1,019 fourth- to ninth-grade students in the community were surveyed, and 11.9% were found to meet DSM-III-R criteria for PTSD (March, Amaya-Jackson, Terry, & Costanzo, 1997). In another study, 67% of 937 college students reported at least one traumatic event in their lifetime (Bernat, Ronfeldt, Calhoun, & Arias, 1998). Of these, 12% met criteria for PTSD diagnosis within the week previous to their assessment for the study. Of 490 adolescents assessed in the southeastern United States, 3% of girls and 1% of boys met DSM-IV criteria for PTSD (Cuffe et al., 1998). Of 1,618 children aged 6–18 randomly selected from five different public sectors of care, 3.5% of children or youths seeking alcohol or drug care were diagnosed with PTSD, as were 3.1% of those in the juvenile justice system, 3% of those using mental health services, 2.8% of those identified with serious mental health problems at school, and 1.7% of those in the child welfare system (Garland et al., 2001).

Meta-Analysis

DSM-IV Criteria

Most research to date confirms the general conclusion that the diagnostic symptom clusters of DSM-IV apply to traumatized children of all ages, from preschool through adolescence, as well as they do to traumatized adults (Saigh, Yasik, Sack, & Koplewicz, 1999). The symptom incidence rates summarized in Table 7.2 indicate that an average of 36% of children exposed to traumatic events are diagnosed with PTSD (based on 2,697 children from 34 samples; Fletcher, 1994), whereas an average of 24% of traumatized adults are diagnosed with PTSD (based on 3,495 adults from 5 samples described in den Velde et al., 1993; Kilpatrick & Resnick, 1993; and Smith & North, 1993). Similar results were found in a unique study of the reactions of both children (5–14 years old) and adults to the same event, a school shooting (Schwarz & Kowalski, 1991a, 1991b). Using a modified form of the PTSD-RI (Pynoos et al., 1987), the researchers found that children were at least as likely as adults to be diagnosed with PTSD. Using a moderate rating method, they found that 27% of children versus 19% of adults met DSM-III-R criteria for PTSD—not a significant difference.

On average, incidence rates for all DSM-IV symptoms of PTSD among traumatized children are higher than 20% (see Table 7.2), with the exception of a pessimistic outlook on the future (16%) and an inability to remember parts of the trauma (12%). Seven of the 11 highest-ranked DSM-IV symptoms for children of all ages (excluding rates based on 50 or fewer children) are symptoms of Criterion B, reexperiencing the trauma: feeling or showing distress at reminders of the trauma (51%); reenactment of significant parts of the event, such as gestures, actions, and sounds (40%); feeling as if the event were being relived (39%); intrusive memories of the events (34%); bad dreams about the events (31%); trauma-specific fears (31%); and talking excessively about the events (31%). Also included among the 11 symptoms with the highest incidence rates in Table 7.2 are three symptoms of the DSM-IV avoidance/numbing criterion (Criterion C): affective numbing (47%); loss of interest in previously important activities (36%); avoidance of reminders of the events (32%). One symptom of the DSM-IV overarousal criterion (Criterion D) is included among the 11 most reported childhood symptoms: difficulty concentrating (41%).

Associated Symptoms

Several clinicians and researchers have suggested that traumatized children are likely to present with other symptomatic responses in addition to those included in DSM-IV and ICD-10 (Saigh, Yasik, Sack, & Koplewicz, 1999). Incidence rates for 14 of these possible associated symptoms are listed in Table 7.2. Half of these rates are greater than 20%: those for dissociative response (48%), guilt (43%), generalized anxiety or fears (39%), low self-esteem (34%), omen formation (26%), depression (25%), and separation anxiety (23%). The least likely associated symptoms to be observed among traumatized children are self-destructive behavior (9%), panic attacks (8%), eating problems (7%), a warped time perspective (4%), and sleepwalking (1%).

It is important to remember that the incidence rates given above do not reflect the potential mediating and moderating influences of other factors on these rates. Thus, for example, if we disregard any factor other than exposure to a traumatic event, aggressive or antisocial behavior is observed in traumatized children 18% of the time, on average. Regressive behavior is observed 13% of the time. However, if these rates are viewed in terms of the age of the children, we find that both aggressive or antisocial behavior and regressive behavior seem to occur most frequently among preschoolers, and that the incidence of each kind of behavior decreases with age (see Table 7.2). The influence of such factors as age and type of stressor on symptom incidence rates is discussed in more detail in later sections of this chapter.

Associated Disorders

Alternate and comorbid diagnoses among traumatized children have yet to be studied in any depth (Saigh, Yasik, Sack, & Koplewicz, 1999). One alternate diagnosis has received some attention, however: attention-deficit/hyperactivity disorder (ADHD). Overall, the incidence rates average 13% for ADHD (see Table 7.2). At the moment it is unclear whether the reported difficulties of children with concentration, hyperactivity, and oppositional behavior are the consequences of traumatic experiences or are symptoms of preexisting disorders such as ADHD or oppositional defiant disorder. This may be particularly true when the traumatic experience is of a protracted or physically abusive nature. In such cases it is possible, as Famularo, Kinscherff, and Fenton (1992) point out, that the "difficult" behaviors associated with these diagnoses may have played a role in provoking the physical abuse, and that any similar symptoms

TABLE 7.2. Incidence Rates of Posttraumatic Stress Responses among Children and Adults

	Average incidence rates				
	Children[a]				
Symptoms	All ages	Preschool	School	Teen	Adults[b]
DSM-IV criteria and symptoms					
B. Reexperiencing (1 required)	88%		92%		44%
B1. Intrusive memories	34%		46%	64%	45%
B1. Posttraumatic play	23%	39%	14%		
B1. Daydreaming about the event	48%[c]		26%[c]		
B1. Talkativeness about the event	31%		31%		
B2. Bad dreams	31%	69%[d]	23%	30%[c]	36%
B3. Reliving the event	39%		40%	40%[c]	29%
B3. Reenactment of the event	40%[d]		54%[c]		
B4. Reminders are distressing	51%	89%[c]	42%	50%[c]	26%
B. Trauma-specific fears	31%	31%	35%	18%	45%
B5. Somatic complaints	23%	15%	37%	16%[c]	45%
C. Avoidance/numbness (three required)	46%		30%[d]		31%
C. Numbness	47%	65%[c]	44%	62%[c]	23%
C1. Efforts to forget about the event	24%		25%	46%[c]	46%
C2. Avoidance of reminders	32%	81%[c]	36%	32%[c]	33%
C3. Inability to recall parts of event	12%		0%[c]	36%[c]	27%
C4. Loss of interest in activities	36%		42%	32%[c]	28%
C5./C6. Detachment or withdrawal	25%	30%	33%	24%[d]	34%
C7. Pessimism about the future	16%		35%	8%[c]	61%
D. OVERAROUSAL (2 required)	66%		55%[d]		43%
D1. Difficulty sleeping	29%	27%[c]	32%	28%[d]	52%
D2. Irritability	23%	28%	14%	16%	29%
D3. Difficulty concentrating	41%	19%[c]	57%	20%[d]	41%
D4. Hypervigilance	25%	24%[c]	34%	44%[c]	27%
D5. Exaggerated startle response	28%		37%	32%[c]	38%
Diagnosis of PTSD	36%	39%[d]	33%	27%	24%
Associated symptoms or diagnoses					
Generalized anxiety	39%	57%	52%	14%[c]	38%
Separation anxiety	23%	36%	16%	4%	
Panic	8%		19%[d]	0%[c]	18%
Depression	25%	34%[d]	22%	22%[c]	14%
Guilt	43%		33%		15%
Regressive behavior	13%	17%	11%	4%	
Aggressive or antisocial behavior	18%	30%	12%	4%	35%
Low self-esteem	34%		53%[c]		
Dissociative response	48%[d]		49%[c]	48%[c]	16%
Self-destructive behavior	9%	1%[d]	15%[c]		
Eating problems	7%		14%		
Omen formation	26%		30%[d]		
Warped time perspective	4%		4%		
Sleepwalking	1%		1%		
Adjustment disorder	20%		14%[d]		
ADHD	13%		34%[d]		

Note. Percentages based on total $n \geq 100$ unless otherwise noted.

[a]Data from Fletcher (1994). Preschool ≤ 7; school = 6–12; teen = 12+.

[b]Data from Crocq et al. (1993); den Velde et al. (1993); Harel, Kahana, and Wilson (1993); Kilpatrick and Resnick (1993); Smith and North (1993); Weisaeth and Eitinger (1993).

[c]n = 11–49.

[d]n = 50–99.

stemming from the PTSD represent an overlap with a preexisting condition. On the other hand, more recent research has found no association between a diagnosis of ADHD and either exposure to traumatic events or diagnosis of PTSD (Wozniak et al., 1999). At the same time, because of the overlap in symptomatology between the two diagnoseis, it is advisable to carefully consider the need for differential diagnoses even among such obviously traumatized children as those who have been sexually abused (Weinstein, Staffelbach, & Biaggio, 2000).

DEVELOPMENTAL COURSE AND PROGNOSIS

Longitudinal research is beginning to provide a general outline of the developmental course and prognosis of childhood PTSD with the passage of time. In general, findings from follow-up studies of children's responses to single-occurrence, nonabusive stressors suggest that symptomatology peaks within the first year after the traumatic experience (Becker, Weine, Vojvoda, & McGlashan, 1999; Blom, 1986; Nader et al., 1990; Pfefferbaum, Gurwitch, et al., 2000), although a sizable number of children and adolescents are still symptomatic years later (Green et al., 1991, 1994; Terr, 1983b; Tyano et al., 1996; Winje & Ulvik, 1998; Yule et al., 2000). In one of the best-designed longitudinal studies, 217 survivors who had been children and adolescents at the time of the sinking of the ship *Jupiter* in Greek waters were intensively interviewed 5–8 years after the disaster, and their experiences were compared to a control group of 87 friends who had attended school with the survivors at the time of the sinking (Yule et al., 2000). Of the 217 survivors, 111 (51.7%) had developed PTSD at some time during the follow-up period, compared to 3.4% (3 of 87) of the control group.

It is interesting to note that not all of those who developed PTSD did so within the first 6 months following the disaster. In fact, 10% (11) did not develop PTSD until more than 6 months later. Onset of PTSD for two of these cases was within the first year, at 7 and 10 months.

> In four cases onset was at the anniversary of the trauma, and in one more case onset was soon after, at 15 months. There were four other cases where onset was still further delayed, at 21, 39, 55, and 60 months after the disaster. In all these cases there was some symptomatology prior to onset of PTSD, either symptoms of post-traumatic stress symptoms below diagnostic threshold, and/or another syndrome such as panic disorder. In two of the four cases of very delayed onset there was no clear trigger preceding the increase of post-traumatic stress symptomatology to above diagnostic threshold, and in the other two there were triggers: death of a cousin in one case, and travelling through a train tunnel in the other. It might have been expected that in these cases of very delayed onset, the PTSD that did develop would be transitory, but this was generally not the case. In the three cases of most delayed onset . . . , the disorder persisted for between 2 and 3 years and was still present at the time of follow-up. (Yule et al., 2000, p. 507)

Duration of PTSD was also examined in this study. Of the 111 who developed PTSD at some time during the follow-up period, the disorder lasted for less than 1 year in 30.1% of them; it lasted for 1–2 years for 16.4% of them, between 2 and 3 years for 12.6%, between 3 and 5 years for 14.4%, and for more than 5 years for 26.1%. This study makes it clear that the developmental course and prognosis of childhood PTSD after exposure to single-occurrence, nonabusive stressors are not straightforward matters.

The researchers also reported on risk factors for developing PTSD and for prolonged duration of PTSD upon its development (Udwin, Boyle, Yule, Bolton, & O'Ryan, 2000). Initial analyses looked at the association between outcomes and (1) a large number of predisaster variables, (2) objective and subjective factors associated with the events surrounding the sinking of the ship and the recovery, (3) variables related to the immediate aftermath of the sinking, and (4) scores from later follow-up screening questionnaires. Of these variables, 24 were found in bivariate analyses to be significantly associated with whether or not survivors ever developed PTSD.

Females were more likely to develop PTSD. Predisaster learning problems, school refusal, truancy, contact with mental health professionals, and violence at home were each associated with later PTSD diagnosis. Being a poor swimmer or a nonswimmer, being in the water during the disaster, being trapped, being injured, and seeing blood were individually associated with PTSD diagnosis. Fearing they might die, thinking they might not escape, and feeling panicked were also associated with later PTSD. Amnesia immediately after the disaster, and feelings of fear or guilt afterward, were likewise associated with developing PTSD—as were greater anxiety, more reported depression, higher scores on a measure of PTSD symptomatology (the Impact of Events Scale), less social support, less use of coping measures, and experiences of other stressful life events.

When all 24 of the significant bivariate risk factors were entered into a multivariate logistic regression analysis, 6 of them emerged as significant predictors of later PTSD. These included seeing blood during the disaster event, being trapped during the disaster, thinking they might not escape, feelings of panic and fear during the disaster, and high anxiety 5 months after the disaster. A similar analysis suggested that once PTSD developed, the existence of poor predisaster social relationships, predisaster medical problems, and higher depression 5 months after the disaster each served as a risk factor for increased duration of the disorder (Udwin et al., 2000).

No large-scale longitudinal studies have yet been conducted that examine the development and course of PTSD when repeated, multiple, or abusive stressors are experienced. Studies of children who have lived through war conditions do suggest outcomes similar to those associated with single-occurrence, nonabusive stressors, at least during the first year after trauma (Becker et al., 1999; Thabet & Vostanis, 2000); some survivors still experience PTSD symptomatology years later (Husain et al., 1998; Kinzie, Sack, Angell, Clarke, & Ben, 1989; Kinzie et al., 1986). However, when it comes to other types of repeated, multiple, and especially abusive stressors, incidence rates appear to remain uniformly high, regardless of the amount of time elapsed since the children were last exposed to the stressors (Elizur & Kaffman, 1982; Mannarino, Cohen, Smith, & Moore-Motily, 1991; Stuber, Nader, Yasuda, Pynoos, & Cohen, 1991). In fact, retrospective studies of adults who were sexually abused as children indicate that symptomatology can persist well into adulthood (Beitchman et al., 1992; Cahill, Llewelyn, & Pearson, 1991).

THE CONTEXT OF PTSD: A WORKING MODEL

Not everyone exposed to events "outside the range of usual human experience and that would be markedly distressing to almost everyone" (Criterion A, DSM-III-R; American Psychiatric Association, 1987) will react to the experience with symptoms of traumatic stress. DSM-IV reports prevalence rates for PTSD ranging from 3% to 58% among people exposed to traumatic events (American Psychiatric Association, 1994), and, as noted earlier, incidence rates for PTSD average 36% among children exposed to traumatic events and 24% among adults (see Table 7.2). This hardly amounts to a one-to-one correspondence between exposure to terrible circumstances and the subsequent development of PTSD. Individual reactions to disaster and catastrophe differ even among people who have been exposed to the same traumatic events.

As demonstrated by the examination of risk factors for developing PTSD after the sinking of the *Jupiter* (Udwin et al., 2000), in order to gain a more complete understanding of the etiology of PTSD, the contribution of other factors besides the traumatic experience itself must be considered. Figure 7.1 illustrates one approach to delineating the process whereby multiple factors are considered to contribute to the development of PTSD. The model depicted in Figure 7.1 is a working model, created in part to facilitate this chapter's discussion of childhood PTSD. Similar models, however, have been suggested by others (Green, Wilson, & Lindy, 1985; La Greca, Silverman, Vernberg, & Prinstein, 1996; Ursano et al., 1994). The factors considered important to the etiology of PTSD in the working model in Figure 7.1 include, in addition to the characteristics of the traumatic event itself (its nature, cause, severity, duration, etc.), cognitive, emotional, psychobiological, and behavioral responses to the traumatic event; individual characteristics of the survivor (biological vulnerabilities, age, gender, developmental stage, coping skills, etc.); and characteristics of the social environment (family support and cohesion, socioeconomic status [SES], community support, etc.). The model of the context for the development of PTSD, as delineated in Figure 7.1, will serve as a framework for the following discussion of the factors that current research indicates can contribute to the etiology of PTSD in children.

THE TRAUMATIC EVENT

Although PTSD cannot be diagnosed unless someone has first been exposed to a traumatic event, this criterion may be the least understood

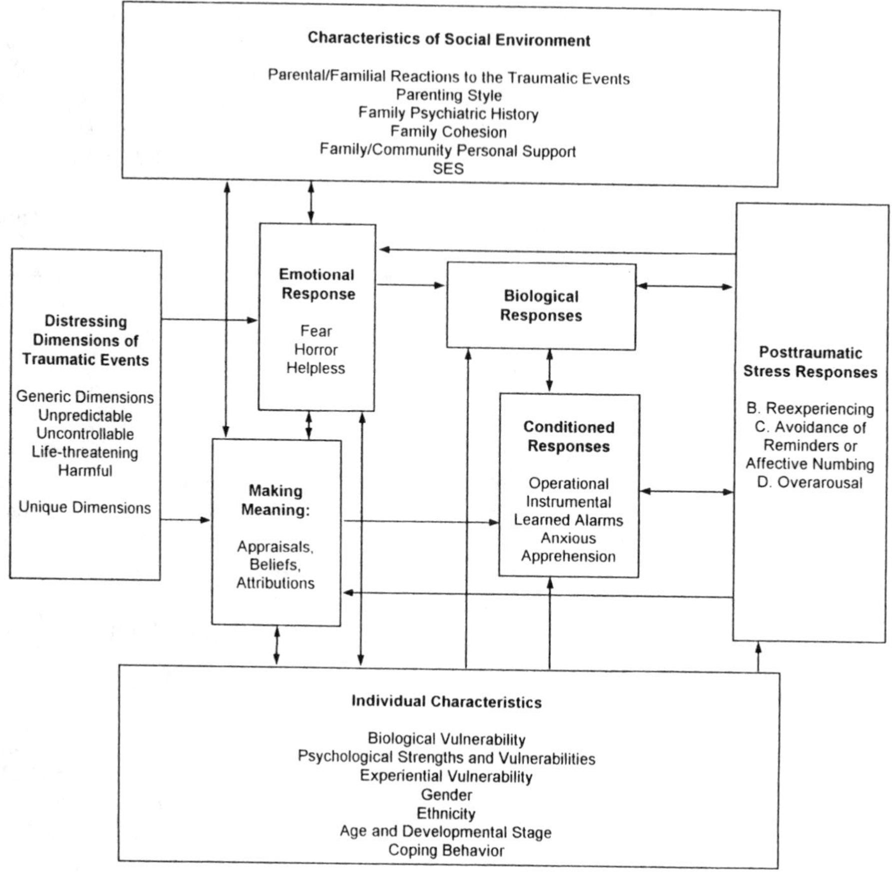

FIGURE 7.1. A working model of the context for the development of childhood PTSD.

of the DSM-IV diagnostic criteria for PTSD. Unfortunately, there are presently few guidelines for systematically defining the types of events that are to be considered "outside the range of usual human experience and that would be markedly distressing to almost anyone" (Criterion A, DSM-III-R). The current version of Criterion A in DSM-IV attempts to define traumatic events more narrowly as those that involve "actual or threatened death or serious injury, or a threat to the physical integrity of self or others" (see Table 7.1). However, events that qualify as traumatic according to DSM-IV standards can still differ greatly from one another. The health and well-being of children around the world are placed in jeopardy each year by such diverse traumatic events as motor vehicle accidents (Stallard, Velleman, Langsford, & Baldwin, 2001), natural disasters (Earls et al., 1988; Green et al., 1991; Goenjian et al., 2001; La Greca et al., 1996), fires (Jones & Ribbe, 1991), lightning strikes (Dollinger, 1985), dog bites to the face followed by surgery (Gislason & Call, 1982), life-threatening illnesses (Stoddard, Norman, & Murphy, 1989; Stuber et al., 1991; Walker, Harris, Baker, Kelly, & Houghton, 1999), war (Dyregrov, Gupta, Gjestad, & Mukanoheli, 2000; Hadi & Llabre, 1998; Thabet & Vostanis, 2000), interparental conflict and domestic violence (Jouriles, Murphy, & O'Leary, 1989; Lehmann, 2000; McCloskey & Walker, 2000), school shootings (Schwarz & Kowalski, 1991a), terrorist attacks (Pfefferbaum, Nixon, Tucker, et al., 1999), physical abuse (Adam, Everett, & O'Neal, 1992), and sexual abuse (Gomes-Schwartz, Horowitz, Cardelli, & Sauzier, 1990)—to name but a few of the possible calamities that can befall children (Saigh, Yasik, Sack, & Koplewicz, 1999). Differences clearly exist among such diverse types of traumatic events, and such differences are likely to contribute to the course of each child's individual posttraumatic reactions to those events. The ability to delineate these differences would presumably allow us to improve our understanding of the relationship between the kind of stressful experience and the resulting type of reaction.

Stressful Dimensions of Events

Inherent Stressfulness of Events

One approach to categorizing stressful events attempts to rank events according to their inherent stressfulness. Milgram (1989), for instance, has suggested that the following categories represent increasing degrees of stressfulness: upsetting, even painful, but not life-threatening events (e.g., breaking an arm); severe family disruptions (e.g., divorce); family misfortune (e.g., death through illness); personal misfortune (e.g., abuse); catastrophic group misfortune associated with natural disasters; and catastrophic group misfortune associated with human-made disasters. There are several problems with this approach to categorizing stressful events. One problem is that predefined categories and stressful events are not always easy to match. It is difficult to understand where, for example, the witnessing of domestic violence would fit in Milgram's typology. Another limitation of this approach is that it ultimately relies on subjective judgments of the amount of stressfulness associated with each category. Not everyone, for example, would rate abuse as a less stressful experience than exposure to a natural disaster, as seems to be implied by Milgram's typology.

Generic Stressful Dimensions of Events

Another approach to the categorization of stressful events proposes to shift the focus away from a priori categories of events ranked by their purported inherent levels of stressfulness, to characteristics or dimensions of events that are thought to increase their stressfulness (e.g., Green et al., 1985; Green, 1993b). From this perspective, the more an event can be characterized in terms of different traumatizing dimensions, the more stressful it can be considered to be. DSM-IV (see Table 7.1) lists several dimensions that are clearly associated with the increased stressfulness of any event: death, injury, or possible loss of physical integrity. The sudden occurrence and unexpectedness of events constitute another dimension thought to contribute to the stressfulness of events. Proximity to the traumatic events has also been found to be associated with higher levels of posttraumatic stress. Children who were on the playground during a sniper attack, for instance, displayed a greater incidence of PTSD symptomatology than did children inside the school but not on the playground; and children at school, whether on the playground or not, displayed higher rates than children not at school that day (Nader et al., 1990; Pynoos et al., 1987; Pynoos & Nader, 1989). Children and adolescents exposed in some way to the Oklahoma City bombing reported more symptoms of PTSD than those who had minimal exposure to the bombing (Pfefferbaum, Nixon, Krug, et al., 1999).

Other dimensions of events that appear to be associated with increased traumatization have been documented in the literature. Traumatic events that are ongoing or chronic lead to different, and generally more severe, outcomes than do nonabusive events of short duration (as discussed below and in Famularo et al., 1990; Green, 1985; Kiser et al., 1988; Terr, 1991). Events that are perceived as uncontrollable (by children and/or by their parents) appear to lead to worse stress reactions afterwards (Weigel, Wertlieb, & Feldstein, 1989). The more personal the impact of the traumatic events, the worse a child's reactions. For instance, children who were exposed to more damage to their homes in Hurricane Hugo were also more likely to have symptoms of PTSD afterward (Shannon et al., 1994). Separations from the family during a crisis can have devastating consequences (Crawshaw, 1963; Faravelli et al., 1985; Freud & Burlingham, 1943; Friedman & Linn, 1957; van der Kolk, 1987; Yule & Williams, 1990), as can the death or injury of a parent or sibling (Pfefferbaum, Nixon, Krug, et al., 1999). Social stigmatization of victims can also worsen reactions to traumatic events (Ayalon, 1982; Frederick, 1986; Nir, 1985). Many of the dimensions of stressors that have been suggested by the literature to be associated with increased stressfulness of events are listed in Table 7.3.[2]

Unique Stressful Dimensions of Events

The generic dimensions discussed above are those that might be found in nearly all stressful events. It is important to remember, however, that every traumatic event can be characterized not only by generic dimensions of distress, but also by its own uniquely stressful dimensions.

TABLE 7.3. Generic Distressing Dimensions of Traumatic Events for Children

General experience
Death, especially of someone related to the child or that the child knows
Injury, especially of the child or someone the child knows
Viewing wounded or bleeding persons
Viewing corpses
Suddenness and unexpectedness of the events
Perceived uncontrollability of the events
Duration and frequency of exposure to the events
The events were among a series of different stressors experienced
The events are liable to recur
The events had human rather than natural causes
Adverse consequences of the events are long-lasting
Adverse consequences of the events are irreversible
Personal impact on the child
Child was affected directly rather than as part of a group experience
Child perceived the events as a personal threat
Child was a primary rather than a secondary survivor (one who was not the immediate target of the stressor, such as a child of a Holocaust survivor or a Vietnam veteran)
Child experienced subjective loss as a consequence of the events (such as the loss of a pet)
Events involved moral conflicts for the child
Stigmatization is associated with exposure to the events
Impact on the child's family and home
Child perceived the events as a threat to family or friends
The event originated within the family
Child was dislocated from the home
Child was separated from parents or family

Children with cancer, for instance, are more likely than children exposed to other traumatic events to experience feelings of estrangement and social isolation, resulting in part from the stigma of their disease and in part from the side effects of therapy (e.g., loss of hair, prolonged absences from school; Nir, 1985). Children in war-torn countries may be more likely to have their social development inhibited, due partly to the greater sanctioning of violence in their social environment and partly to their fear of others (Arroyo & Eth, 1985; Ayalon, 1982; Kinzie et al., 1986). Although uniquely stressful dimensions are not discussed any further in this chapter, their contribution to the development of PTSD in children to traumatic events should always be considered (see Figure 7.1).

Responses to Two Types of Stressors

Average incidence rates of DSM-IV PTSD symptoms, and associated symptoms, are listed in Table 7.4 according to a two-part classification of traumatic events based on a tripartite typology suggested by Terr (1991). A two-part, rather than tripartite, classification was necessitated because of limitations imposed by the available empirical literature; however, as the following discussion demonstrates, even this simple typology is capable of illustrating the differential impact that types of stressors can have on children's traumatic stress reactions. The two categories of stressors referred to in Table 7.4 are defined as follows: (1) acute, nonabusive stressors, which encompass traumatic events (other than physical or sexual abuse) that occur only once (disasters such as floods, fires, transportation accidents, etc.); and (2) chronic or abusive stressors, which encompass ongoing or multiple stressors (such as war, chronic illness, repeated surgeries, etc.) and/or incidents of physical or sexual abuse, whether of single or repeated occurrence.

Stress Reactions That Are Similar for Acute, Nonabusive Stressors and Chronic or Abusive Stressors

Some stress reactions appear likely to be observed among children, regardless of the type of stressor involved. The incidence rates in Table 7.4 (disregarding those responses whose rates are based on sample sizes of less than 50 children), for example, indicate that regardless of the type of stressor involved, trauma-specific fears are equally likely to develop (30% for acute, nonabusive stressors and 33% for chronic or abusive stressors), as are difficulties sleeping (29% for acute and 30% for chronic stressors), aggressive or antisocial behavior (17% for acute and 20% for chronic stressors), and eating problems (5% for acute and 8% for chronic stressors). Children exposed to both types of stressors are also equally likely to be diagnosed with PTSD (36% each).

Symptoms Observed More Frequently after Exposure to Chronic or Abusive Stressors

Incidence rates of most of the symptoms associated with PTSD listed in Table 7.4 differ according to the type of stressor involved. Quite a few

TABLE 7.4. Incidence Rates of Children's Posttraumatic Stress Responses to Acute, Nonabusive Stressors and to Chronic or Abusive Stressors

Symptoms	Type of stressor: Acute, nonabusive	Type of stressor: Chronic or abusive
DSM-IV criteria and symptoms		
B. Reexperiencing (one required)	92%[a]	86%
B1. Intrusive memories	38%	27%
B1. Posttraumatic play	13%	40%
B1. Daydreaming about the event	26%[b]	
B1. Talkativeness about the event	31%	
B2. Bad dreams	23%	61%
B3. Reliving the event	30%	67%[b]
B3. Reenactment of the event	54%[b]	33%[b]
B4. Reminders are distressing	51%	74%[a]
B. Trauma-specific fears	30%	33%
B5. Somatic complaints	31%	15%
C. Avoidance/numbness (three required)	30%[a]	54%
C. Numbness	42%	56%
C1. Efforts to forget about the event	17%	55%
C2. Avoidance of reminders	22%	57%
C3. Inability to recall parts of event	9%	34%[b]
C4. Loss of interest in activities	42%	29%
C5./C6. Detachment or withdrawal	40%	14%
C7. Pessimism about the future	12%	35%[a]
D. Overarousal (two required)	55%[a]	71%
D1. Difficulty sleeping	29%	30%
D2. Irritability	20%	35%
D3. Difficulty concentrating	52%	24%
D4. Hypervigilance	31%	15%
D5. Exaggerated startle response	24%	48%
Diagnosis of PTSD	36%	36%
Associated symptoms or diagnoses		
Generalized anxiety	55%	26%
Separation anxiety	45%	35%
Panic	35%[b]	6%
Depression	10%	28%
Guilt	32%	59%[a]
Regressive behavior	6%	22%
Aggressive or antisocial behavior	17%	20%
Low self-esteem		34%
Dissociative response	31%[b]	100%[b]
Self-destructive behavior		9%
Eating problems	5%	8%
Omen formation	30%[a]	0%[b]
Warped time perspective	13%	0%[b]
Sleepwalking	1%	3%[b]
Adjustment disorder	16%[b]	21%
ADHD	22%[b]	11%

Note. Percentages based on total $n \geq 100$ unless otherwise noted. Data from Fletcher (1994).

[a] n = 50–99.

[b] n = 11–49.

symptoms, for instance, seem more likely to be observed among child survivors of chronic or abusive stressors than among child survivors of acute, nonabusive stressors. Children exposed to chronic or abusive stressors more often meet the DSM-IV Criterion C of three or more symptoms of avoidance or numbing (54% vs. 30%). Survivors of chronic or abusive stressors respond more frequently than do survivors of acute, nonabusive stressors by actively avoiding reminders of the traumatic events (57% vs. 22%), numbing of affect (56% vs. 42%), actively trying to forget about the events (55% vs. 17%), and engaging in regressive behavior (22% vs. 6%). Child survivors of chronic or abusive stressors are also more often distressed by reminders of their experiences (74% vs. 51%). They avoid reminders so much that they are more likely than survivors of acute, nonabusive stressors to reexperience their traumas in bad dreams (61% vs. 23%). Children exposed to enduring or abusive stressors are more likely to meet the DSM-IV Criterion D of two symptoms of overarousal (71% vs. 55%), too. Arousal in survivors of chronic or abusive stress is revealed more often by symptoms of exaggerated startle response (48% vs. 24%) and general irritability (35% vs. 20%). Negative affect is also more closely associated with chronic or abusive stress: feelings of guilt (59% vs. 32%), a pessimistic attitude toward the future (35% vs. 12%), and depression (28% vs. 10%).

Inappropriate sexual behavior may be the most frequently reported symptom of sexual abuse (Kendall-Tackett, Williams, & Finkelhor, 1993). Such behavior would appear to be an example of a trauma-specific symptom; however, some researchers have suggested that inappropriate sexual behaviors among sexually abused children might be considered a form of posttraumatic play. The incidence rates for posttraumatic play included in Table 7.4 for chronic or sexual stressors are based on this premise, in which case rates are higher (40%) than they are for nonsexualized posttraumatic play among children exposed to acute, nonabusive stressors (13%). It is worthwhile noting that although inappropriately sexualized behavior and play does occur frequently among sexually abused children, it cannot be assumed that such behavior provides incontrovertible evidence of sexual abuse, nor can its absence be taken as final proof that sexual abuse has not taken place.

Symptoms Observed More Frequently after Exposure to Acute, Nonabusive Stressors

Some symptoms of PTSD seem to be more likely to be observed among children exposed to acute, nonabusive stressors than among those exposed to chronic or abusive stressors. Most of these differences, as might be expected, seem to be related either to the chronicity of the event or its abusive nature. Those subjected to chronic stressors, for example, are forced over time to come to some kind of accommodation with their traumas. As discussed above, many survivors of chronic or abusive stressors seem to accomplish this by avoiding reminders, numbing of affect, and resorting to denial or dissociation. Survivors of single-occurrence stressors, on the other hand, are not forced to come to terms with the traumatic disruption of their lives in the way that survivors of more enduring stressors seem to be. Those exposed to acute, nonabusive stressors, in fact, appear to have a more difficult time putting the experience out of their minds. Thus they more frequently report intrusive memories (38% vs. 27%; see Table 7.4). Less frequent avoidance of reminders of the traumatic events, coupled with more frequent occurrence of intrusive memories, may be associated with greater incidence of hypervigilance (31% vs. 15%) when acute rather than chronic stressors are involved. Children exposed to acute, nonabusive stressors are also more likely to report symptoms of anxiety, ranging from generalized anxiety (55% vs. 26%) to difficulties concentrating (52% vs. 24%) to separation anxiety (45% vs. 35%). They are also more likely to suffer from somatic complaints (31% vs. 15%), to show decreased interest in previously important activities (42% vs. 29%), and to become socially withdrawn (40% vs. 14%).

EMOTIONAL REACTIONS

DSM-IV (see Table 7.1) requires that an emotional reaction of horror, fear, or helplessness accompany exposure to traumatic circumstances. Many children exposed to traumatic events do report feelings of distress (39%, on average; Fletcher, 1994). Research is beginning to show that children's emotional reactions to traumatic events can have a major impact on the development and course of PTSD afterward. Children's emotional reactions to Hurricane Hugo were found to be associated with the level of symptomatology afterwards (Shannon et al., 1994): Children who reported feeling sad, worried, scared, alone, or angry during the hurricane were most likely to display the full range of PTSD symptomatology. In fact, children's emotional reactions during the hurricane were more strongly associated with PTSD than was the actual damage sustained by children's households as a consequence of the hurricane.

The amount of fear experienced by young children (4–9 years of age) due to exposure to normative stressors was found to be associated with the level of posttraumatic stress in another study (Rossman, Bingham, & Emde, 1997). When college students were asked to describe the most stressful experience in their lives and their reactions to it, the more emotional reactions such as fear, anger, shame, guilt, or emotional numbing they reported, the more symptoms of posttraumatic stress they reported currently experiencing (Bernat et al., 1998). Their emotional reactions were significantly associated with symptoms of PTSD even after other risk factors were taken into account, such as the students' gender, the number of lifetime stressful events they had experienced, the perceived life threat of their most stressful experience, and whether or not someone else was seriously injured or killed, among other factors. Children's level of fear at the time of a physical injury was also significantly correlated with PTSD symptomatology (Aaron, Zaglul, & Emery, 1999). Recall, too, that feelings of fear and panic during the sinking of the *Jupiter* were particularly important risk factors for developing PTSD as a consequence of the experience (Udwin et al., 2000). Studies such as these suggest that children's emotional reactions to their traumatic experiences should be taken into account when investigators are assessing their potential for posttraumatic stress reactions.

MAKING MEANING: APPRAISALS, BELIEFS, AND ATTRIBUTIONS

The association between exposure to a traumatic event and extreme emotional response is usually mediated by an assessment of the traumatic event's meaning. Feelings of horror and fear follow upon appraisals of the potential threat and harmfulness of traumatic events. Feelings of helplessness and hopelessness develop after exposure to events that call into question a person's basic assumptions about the essential predictability, controllability, safety, and security of everyday life. The indirect path from trauma to emotional response via assessment of the meaning of the event is illustrated in Figure 7.1 by an arrow from traumatic event to assessment of meaning, followed by an arrow from meaning to emotional response.

Several theorists have suggested that posttraumatic responses represent a survivor's attempt to accommodate to and assimilate experiences that challenge the survivor's whole world view (e.g., Chemtob, Roitblat, Hamada, Carlson, & Twentyman, 1988; Epstein, 1990; Foa, Steketee, & Rothbaum, 1989; Horowitz, 1976a, 1976b; Janoff-Bulman, 1989; McCann & Pearlman, 1990a, 1990b; Norris & Kaniasty, 1991; Roth, Lebowitz, & DeRosa, 1997). Before Freud published his conceptualization of traumatic stress, Pierre Janet suggested that thoughts and memories of traumatic events intrusively recurred to survivors because they were too emotionally threatening to be integrated into their existing memory systems (van der Kolk, Brown, & van der Hart, 1989). In Janet's view, traumatic memories split off from normal memory and become dissociated from normal consciousness, but they continue to have an unconscious impact on an individual's feelings and behavior. Similarly, Horowitz (1976a, 1976b) has argued that traumatic events represent information that is unacceptable to a survivor's conceptual system, and therefore is not capable of being integrated into the system; at the same time, however, the conceptual system is compelled to process this unacceptable information somehow. Coming to terms with traumatic experience may require the survivor to restructure his or her conceptual system, to allow the traumatic experience to be accommodated and then assimilated into a restructured understanding of the world and the survivor's place in it.

Appraisals

"Appraisals" are evaluations people make about the importance and meaning of events in terms of their own personal health and safety (Lazarus & Folkman, 1984). Foa et al. (1989) suggest that theories of cognitive appraisal must be considered, in addition to a strictly behavioral approach, when one is attempting to explain PTSD symptomatology. Peterson and Seligman (1983), for example, have attempted to apply the theory of learned helplessness to an understanding of traumatization, suggesting that those who experience an aversive situation must appraise the situation as inescapable and unpredictable before a sense of helplessness can develop. Some theorists (Chemtob et al., 1988; Foa et al., 1989) have proposed that fear structures are created in a person's cognitive network after exposure to particularly aversive events. Fear structures are "programs for escape or avoidance behavior" (Foa et al., 1989, p. 166) that encompass at least three different kinds of information: information about the aversive situation, interpretative information about the meaning of the situation, and procedures for responding to the situation.

In the model of the context for the development of PTSD illustrated in Figure 7.1, appraisals are considered to mediate a child's emotional reactions to traumatic events. If an event is not perceived as threatening by a child, for instance, feelings of fear do not arise, and neither do symptoms of PTSD. Children younger than 8 years and 5 months who lived at Three Mile Island, for example, were unable to recognize the danger that the nuclear accident posed to them and their families; perhaps as a consequence, their concerns about the consequences of the nuclear accident were "vague and undifferentiated" (Handford et al., 1986, p. 351). Similar results have been found among children born within a year before or after the Chernobyl nuclear plant catastrophe (Bromet et al., 2000). On the other hand, children who thought they might not escape the sinking of the *Jupiter* were more likely to develop PTSD afterward (Udwin et al., 2000).

Beliefs

Some theorists (Epstein, 1990; Janoff-Bulman, 1989; McCann & Pearlman, 1990a, 1990b; Norris & Kaniasty, 1991; Roth et al., 1997) contend that stressful events become traumatic when they shatter certain basic beliefs that people normally hold about themselves and the world in which they live. Stressors can be traumatic if they pose overwhelming threats to a person's beliefs about the safety and security of the world, the certainty, orderliness, predictability, and controllability of the world, the person's sense of mastery and general self-esteem, or the trustworthiness of important others. An association has been found between PTSD symptomatology and such basic beliefs held by adults exposed to combat in Vietnam (Fletcher, 1988) and violent crime (Norris & Kaniasty, 1991). Few studies of children's beliefs have been made to date. Sexually abused children, however, have been found to report that they believe that the world is a dangerous place in which to live, that it is not responsive to their control, and that adults are not worthy of trust (Wolfe, Gentile, & Wolfe, 1989; Wolfe, Gentile, Michienzi, Sas, & Wolfe, 1991).

A Factor Analysis of Beliefs

Skidmore and Fletcher (1997) created the World View Survey to assess 50 beliefs associated with the basic assumptions thought to be affected by traumatic experience (Epstein, 1990; Janoff-Bulman, 1989)—as well as potentially positive beliefs, such as that it is good to be alive or that, having lived through traumatic experiences, one now feels capable of handling anything (Joseph, Williams, & Yule, 1993). Factor analysis produced nine factors, and a second-order factor analysis suggested that the nine factors fell under two superordinate factors.

The first higher-order factor comprised six of the original factors, all of which were related to the basic assumptions put forth by Epstein (1990) and Janoff-Bulman (1989): (1) Anxious Uncertainty (exemplified by beliefs such as "Life does not seem to make much sense any more"); (2) Inadequacy (e.g., "I am a jinx"); (3) Dangerous World (e.g., "The world is a dangerous place to live"); (4) Self-Abnegation (e.g., "Sometimes I think I am not a very good person"); (5) Lack of Control (e.g., "I feel like I have control over my life"—if disagreed with); and (6) Poor Attachment (e.g., "It is easy for me to make friends"—if disagreed with). The second higher-order factor comprised four of the original factors, most of which consisted of beliefs originally intended to indicate positive beliefs, but which correlations with PTSD symptoms indicated should be scored in a negative direction: (1) Poor Ego-Strength (e.g., "Since I have lived through some bad times, I have a better idea of what is important to me and what is not"); (2) Poor Attachment; (3) Lack of Personal Empowerment (e.g., "I feel like nothing can keep me from getting what I want out of life any more"); and (4) Negative Outlook (e.g., "Nowadays I feel like every new day I am alive is a gift"). Poor Attachment loaded on both higher-order factors.

Lifetime exposure to stressful events and current symptoms of PTSD were both correlated with all six of the factors associated with the first higher-order factor, but with none of the other factors. Thus the first six factors were clearly associated with traumatic experience and were considered scales of trauma-reactive beliefs. The remaining scales were considered simply measures of negative beliefs that did not have a direct association with traumatic experience. Responses of the college students to the scales of the World View Survey were compared to the responses of adolescent inpatient psychiatric patients, most of whom were diagnosed with PTSD. The adolescents scored significantly higher on all of the scales except Poor Ego-Strength and Negative Outlook.

Foreshortened Future

One belief or attitude that has been assessed among children with some frequency is the so-called "sense of foreshortened future." This is a pessimistic attitude about the future—a belief that one's life can end at any moment, and that therefore the future can be neither anticipated nor planned for. Terr (1991) has suggested that a negative attitude about the future will be relatively prevalent, regardless of the type of stressor encountered. Contrary to Terr's hypothesis, however, a pessimistic attitude about the future does not seem to be as prevalent among children exposed to acute, nonabusive stressors (12% on average—see Table 7.4; see also Ajdukovic, 1998; Green et al., 1991; Jones & Ribbe, 1991; Schwarz & Kowalski, 1991a; Terr, 1979) as it is among children exposed to more extreme chronic or abusive stressors (35% on average; Kinzie et al., 1986; Kiser et al., 1988; Zamvil, Wechsler, Frank, & Docherty, 1991). This illustrates the differential impact that stressor characteristics can have upon beliefs.

When researchers examined children's estimates of future negative events (which would seem to be characteristic of a pessimistic attitude about the future), the results showed that, contrary to expectations, children diagnosed with PTSD were no different from children in the control groups in their estimations (Dalgleish et al., 2000). All of the children, regardless of PTSD status, rated physically threatening events as more likely to happen to others than to themselves. Unlike the control groups, the group with PTSD also rated socially threatening events to be more likely to happen to others as well.

Attributions

Attribution theory is founded on the assumption that people try to make sense of their experience (Veronen & Kilpatrick, 1983). Explanations for unpredictable, uncontrollable, and aversive events can be attributed to either internal or external causes, to stable or unstable conditions over time, and to either specific or more global conditions (Abramson, Seligman, & Teasdale, 1978). Guilt or self-blame (an internal attribution of cause) has been found to be associated with children's traumatic experiences (see Tables 7.2 and 7.4; see also Kinzie et al., 1986; Pynoos et al., 1987; Realmuto et al., 1992; Schwarz & Kowalski, 1991a; Udwin et al., 2000; Wolfe et al., 1989, 1991). Internal causal attributions for negative experiences made by adolescents involved in the *Jupiter* ship disaster related to greater PTSD symptomatology 1 year after the disaster (Joseph, Brewin, Yule, & Williams, 1993). A pessimistic attitude about the future (discussed above) is an example of an attribution of continued (stable) insecurity and safety into the future. Global attributions of causality ("all adults are untrustworthy" vs. "just the adult who abused is untrustworthy") also seem to be associated with traumatization, at least in sexually abused children (Wolfe et al., 1989, 1991).

NEUROBIOLOGICAL CHANGES

There is mounting evidence that exposure to extreme stressors is associated with changes in brain structure and function among adults (Bremner, Southwick, & Charney, 1999; Glaser, 2000; Karr-Morse & Wiley, 1997; van der Kolk & Sporta, 1993; Yehuda, 1998). Animal models help explain how this might occur.

> Animals exposed to severe stress . . . show acute increases in stress-related neurotransmitters and neuropeptides, the chemical messengers of the brain, including corticotropin releasing factor (CRF), norepinephrine, serotonin, dopamine, endogenous benzodiazepines, and endogenous opiates. . . . Each of these neurotransmitters and neuropeptides have specific sites, or receptors, located on neurons to which they bind in order to exert their effects, which are also affected by stress, leading to changes in receptor number or affinity (the "stickiness" of binding to neurotransmitters and neuropeptides). Alterations in neurotransmitters and neuroreceptors result in changes in neuronal function in specific brain areas which are involved in the structure of neurons in these regions, which can lead to changes in function. These effects combine to alter the neuronal inter-connections, which result in long-term changes in brain "circuits" involved in the stress response. (Bremner et al., 1999, p. 103)

Although most research in this area has involved adults, some recent research points to similar changes among traumatized children and adolescents. Goenjian et al. (1996) found a blunted cortisol response to the dexamethasone suppression test among Armenian adolescents who developed PTSD after the earthquake of 1988. At the age of 2, infants raised in the extreme deprivation of Romanian orphanages had significantly lower levels of morning cortisol than home-raised children (Carlson & Earls, 1997). Levels of cortisol among girls 6–7 years old who had been abused within the last year were found to be lower than levels in control subjects (King, Mandansky, King, Fletcher, & Brewer, 2001). Decreased platelet adrenergic receptors were found in a group of abused children diagnosed with PTSD, suggesting down-regulation of peripheral adrenergic receptors in response to higher levels of catecholamines (Perry, 1994). An increased orthostatic heart rate response was also found among these children. Maltreated children (mean age = 10.4 years) diagnosed with PTSD were found to excrete greater concentrations of urinary dopamine, urinary free cortisol, norepinephrine, and epinephrine than either nontraumatized children diagnosed with overanxious disorder or healthy controls (De Bellis, Baum, et al., 1999). Moreover, concentrations of urinary catecholamine and urinary free cortisol were positively correlated with duration of the PTSD trauma and severity of PTSD symptoms in this study. These results differ from findings of lower urinary cortisol levels in adults with PTSD (Yehuda et al., 1995). The authors suggest that this difference might indicate an immaturity of adaptation of the hypothalamic–pituitary–adrenal (HPA) axis among severely maltreated children.

In a study using single-voxel proton magnetic resonance spectroscopy, the ratio of *N*-acetylaspartate to creatine (a marker of neuronal integrity) was found to be significantly lower in maltreated children and adolescents with PTSD than among healthy matched comparison subjects, suggesting that childhood PTSD may alter anterior cingulate neuronal metabolism (De Bellis, Keshavan, Spencer, & Hall, 2000). An anatomical magnetic resonance imaging scan showed maltreated children with PTSD to have smaller intracranial and cerebral volumes than matched controls (De Bellis, Keshavan, et al., 1999). Brain volume correlated positively with age of onset of PTSD and negatively with duration of the abuse. The authors suggest that the brain size changes might have resulted from their early traumatic experiences, and could therefore be related to greater catecholamine concentrations and raised cortisol levels. As the authors also point out, since brain size is correlated with measures of IQ, these results imply possible impairments to the cognitive functioning of severely traumatized children.

CONDITIONED RESPONSES

Cognitive-behavioral theorists note that many aspects of PTSD symptomatology can be explained by various models of learning, including traditional stimulus–response theories (Keane, Fairbank, Caddell, Zimering, & Bender, 1985; Foa et al., 1989) and more recently devised information-processing and cognitive network models (Foa et al., 1989; Pittman, 1988; Yates & Nasby, 1993). Mowrer's (1960) two-factor theory of learning, for example, has been used to explain how survivors of extreme stressors become aversively conditioned to a wide variety of cues (Keane, Fairbank, et al., 1985). Both classical and instrumental conditioning are considered to come into play. First, previously neutral stimuli become associated with extremely stressful events, and the neutral stimuli assume aversive properties as a consequence. The previously unconditioned stimulus (UCS) becomes a conditioned stimulus (CS) for fear responses. Pairing the new CS with a new neutral stimulus can also make the neutral stimulus aversive, through the process of higher-order conditioning. The process of stimulus generalization also helps increase the number and variety of aversive stimuli, by making other stimuli that are similar to already aversive stimuli aversive as well. The second stage of this process occurs when a traumatized individual learns to respond to aversive situations with avoidance or withdrawal, which can lead to a decrease in anxiety. In this way, Mowrer's two-factor theory provides a means of explaining the acquisition of fear and avoidance responses. The theory, however, has been criticized for its inability to account for symptoms of reexperiencing and overarousal (Foa et al., 1989; Mineka, 1979; Jones & Barlow, 1990).

Learned Alarms

Jones and Barlow (1990) have suggested that symptoms of reexperiencing and overarousal can be accounted for by conditioned responses (CRs) to internal or external cues that have become associated with traumatic experiences. Fearful responses to the original traumatic events are considered "true alarms," and the CRs to cues associated with the original events are considered "learned alarms."

> [T]rue alarms are regarded as a fear response that occurs when an individual is faced with a life-threatening event, particularly a severe one. . . . Learned alarms are seen as conditioned responses to either interoceptive or external cues. . . . PTSD . . . may reflect in part the conditioning that occurs upon activation of true alarms (i.e., evocation of fear and accompanying increases in a variety of physiological response systems that would support escape [flight] behavior under life threatening conditions). Such a response is adaptive in situations such as combat or rape and is a protective mechanism often necessary for survival. . . . For patients with PTSD in response to single or repeated true alarms, fear likely has become associated with both internal and external cues associated with the initial event. (Jones & Barlow, 1990, pp. 318–319)

The consistent finding that the severity of the stressor is associated with PTSD symptomatology suggests that extreme stressors serve as true alarms. The tendency of trauma survivors to react strongly to both external and internal cues related to the original trauma suggests that learned alarms play a large role in the etiology of PTSD as well.

Anxious Apprehension and Reexperiencing

According to Jones and Barlow (1990),

> the crucial step to pathology is the development of anxious apprehension about learned alarms. It is only this process, with its strong cognitive components such as distorted processing of information along with marked negative affect, that can account for the downward spiral of symptomatology associated with PTSD. This downward spiral would include the unremitting re-experiencing of learned alarms and associated traumatic memories, as well as the pattern of affective instability associated with alternate numbing and exacerbation of negative emotions and the occasional delayed emotional experience of PTSD symptomatology. (p. 319)

From this view, learned alarms lead to anxious apprehension and reexperiencing of the traumatic experience. This is perhaps especially likely to be the case when the circumstances surrounding the traumatic experience are perceived to be unpredictable and uncontrollable.

> Thus, if the vulnerabilities described above line up correctly, an individual will experience the overwhelming true alarm and subsequent learned alarms as unpredictable, uncontrollable aversive events. The individual will react to these events with chronic overarousal and additional cognitive symptoms of hypervigilance to trauma related cues . . . , accompanied by attention narrowing. . . . Since the original alarm contained strong arousal based components, the existing chronic overarousal combined with a hypervigilance to arousal that might signal the beginning of a future alarm would insure a succession of learned alarms and associated traumatic memories. (Jones & Barlow, 1990, p. 319)

The aversiveness can become emotionally overwhelming, which leads to avoidance of cues associated with the trauma. Unfortunately, due to the processes of stimulus generalization and higher-order conditioning described above, associated cues can be difficult to avoid. As a consequence, traumatized individuals become inclined to withdraw from the world, numb their affective responses, and sometimes resort to dissociation. However, they are rarely able to avoid intrusive memories of their traumatic experiences for long. As a result, the characteristic "phasing" found in PTSD begins—an alternation between reexperiencing and avoiding trauma-related memories and cues.

INDIVIDUAL CHARACTERISTICS

A child's stress reactions can be moderated at any stage of the process illustrated in Figure 7.1 by characteristics of both the individual child and the child's social environment. The meaning of the traumatic experience, for instance, will vary according to the capacity of the individual and his or her social environment to make sense of it. Similarly, a child's emotional repertoire can affect his or her capacity for emotional response. These and other moderating influences of the characteristics of the individual child and his or her social environment are considered in more detail below.

Biological Vulnerability

Family and twin studies have provided some evidence of familial predispositions to anxiety disorders (Jones & Barlow, 1990). It has been suggested that there may be genetic vulnerabilities, such as HPA axis reactivity, that might increase a person's chance of developing PTSD once exposed to traumatic events (True & Pitman, 1999). However, only a few studies have explored the association between PTSD in adults and family psychiatric history, and none have done so for children. Davidson, Swartz, Storck, Krishnan, and Hammett (1985) found that "sixty-six percent of [adult] PTSD probands gave a family history positive for psychiatric illness" (p. 91), compared to 79% of relatives of adult probands with depression and 93% for adult probands with generalized anxiety disorder. Foy, Resnick, Sipprelle, and Carroll (1987) found that 48% of one sample of Vietnam combat veterans with PTSD, and 71% of another sample, had family histories of psychopathology. On the other hand, these authors also found that 38% of combat veterans without PTSD in one sample, and 50% in the other, also had family histories of psychopathology. Support for a biological predisposition to PTSD is therefore only tentative at this point.

Jones and Barlow (1990) "postulate that the genetic component may be a predisposition to a diffuse stress responsivity reflected as chronic autonomic overarousal or noradrenergic lability" (p. 314), and they argue that research indicating differences in resting heart rate between combat veterans with PTSD and nonmilitary controls provides some evidence for this position. Evidence from the literature on resiliency among children exposed to extreme stressors indicates that temperament plays an important role in a child's ability to adapt successfully to stress (Wertlieb, Weigel, Springer, & Feldstein, 1987). Werner and Smith (1982) found that resilient children were more likely to be characterized as outgoing, positive in mood, and adaptable to change as infants. Wyman, Cowen, Work, and Parker (1991) found that among fourth- to sixth-grade children exposed to four or more stressors in their lives, stress-resilient children were more likely to have been perceived by their parents as easy-going rather than difficult as infants. Higher intelligence may also mitigate some of the effects of traumatic stress (Masten et al., 1988; Silva et al., 2000; Werner & Smith, 1982).

Psychological Strengths and Vulnerabilities

Self-Efficacy and Locus of Control

Because traumatic experiences are often characterized as unpredictable and uncontrollable events, issues surrounding personal control often emerge among traumatized individuals. It has been suggested that personal experience of mastery, self-efficacy, or control in aversive situations prior to a traumatic experience can attenuate the negative effects of such experience (Bandura, Taylor, Williams, Mefford, & Barchas, 1985; Foa et al., 1989; Foa, Zinbarg, & Rothbaum, 1992; Luthar, 1991; Miller, 1979; Mineka, 1979; Mineka & Kihlstrom, 1978; Weigel et al., 1989). Rotter (1966) has argued that individuals can be characterized according to whether or not they believe they have control over their environment. Those who believe they have control are said to exercise an internal locus of control. Those who consider themselves controlled by the environment, on the other hand, are said to have an external locus of control. Moran and Eckenrode (1992) found that maltreated female adolescents who demonstrated external locus of control and low self-esteem reported the highest levels of depression, whereas those with an internal locus of control and high self-esteem reported levels of depression that were close to levels of control subjects with similar personality profiles. Unfortunately, it is not clear whether these associations are due to predisposing personality characteristics, or whether they are the outcome of exposure to extreme stressors that are outside the control of the individuals involved. One prospective study of factors ameliorating risk in children (Seifer, Sameroff, Baldwin, & Baldwin, 1992) found that low external locus of control and unknown or undifferentiated locus of control (Connell, 1985; Peterson & Seligman, 1983), but not high internal locus of control, were associated with positive changes in functioning from 4 to 13 years of age—a finding that replicated earlier results reported by Weigel et al. (1989).

History of Psychiatric Problems

It is possible that a history of emotional or psychiatric problems can potentiate adverse posttraumatic stress responses. Prior developmental and psychiatric problems, for example, have been found to be associated with more PTSD symptomatology among sexually abused children (Davis et al., 2000). Earls et al. (1988) found that children most likely to be adversely affected 1 year after a disastrous flood were those with preexisting disorders. Shannon et al. (1994) found a positive association between trait anxiety and posttraumatic stress symptomatology among children exposed to Hurricane Hugo, leading them to suggest that a pretrauma history of anxiety may contribute to vulnerability to traumatic experiences. Children who had had predisaster contact with mental health professionals were more likely to develop PTSD after the sinking of the *Jupiter* (Udwin et al., 2000). On the other hand, McLeer, Deblinger, Atkins, Foa, and Ralphe (1988) found no significant association between symptomatology and trait anxiety when sexual abuse was involved. The difference, of course, may be due to the greater traumatization associated with sexual abuse. A tendency to low trait anxiety might be less helpful in moderating a child's reactions to the more overwhelming experience of sexual abuse.

Experiential Vulnerability

Considerable evidence has accumulated that a history of stressful life events is associated with higher levels of PTSD in children when they are later exposed to traumatic stressors (Conte & Schuerman, 1987; Kiser et al., 1988; Mannarino, Cohen, & Berman, 1994; Seifer et al., 1992; Wolfe, Jaffe, Wilson, & Zak, 1985). Early stressful experiences need not always sensitize a child to later trauma, however. The child's reactions to early stress experiences may be more important to the development of PTSD than exposure to such experiences per se may be (Rutter, 1983). As discussed previously, past experience of mastering threatening experiences may help steel the child against later traumatization due to stressful circumstances. Weigel et al. (1989), for example, found that perceptions of control served to moderate the effects of exposure to stressful events among school-age children.

Gender Differences

Rutter (1983) suggested that boys may be more vulnerable to stress than girls, but he was summarizing exposure to stressors that today would generally be considered less than traumatizing (such as hospitalization, birth of a sibling, and parental divorce). Milgram and Milgram (1976) did find that 6 months after the Yom Kippur War, fifth- and sixth-grade boys in Israel reported higher levels of anxiety than did girls. Other studies, however, have not found boys more often symptomatic than girls. Some have found no differences between boys and girls (Aaron et al., 1999; Earls et al., 1988; McFarlane, 1987a; Nader et al., 1990; Pynoos et al., 1987; Silva et al., 2000; Vila et al., 2001).

Most studies, however, have found higher incidence of PTSD among girls immediately after traumatic exposure and at later follow-ups (Adam et al., 1992; Ajdukovic, 1998; Curle & Williams, 1996; Goenjian et al., 1995; Green et al., 1991; Lonigan et al., 1991; Pfefferbaum, Nixon, Krug, et al., 1999; Shannon et al., 1994; Stallard et al., 2001; Udwin et al., 2000; Vernberg, La Greca, Silverman, & Prinstein, 1996; Yule et al., 2000; Zhao et al., 2001). In particular, girls appear to report more symptoms of intrusion (Vila et al., 1999; Winje & Ulvik, 1998), depression (Winje & Ulvik, 1998), and anxiety (Bolton et al., 2000; Vila et al., 1999). Goenjian et al. (2001) found that girls' feelings of fear, horror, and helplessness in response to the devastation of Hurricane Mitch were significantly higher than those of boys. Furthermore, although bivariate analysis indicated that girls reported more symptoms of PTSD than boys, multivariate analyses indicated that gender differences disappeared once subjective reactions were considered. This raises the question of whether or not girls experience higher levels of traumatic reactions because they experience more fear, horror, and helplessness during the disaster than do boys. Interestingly, school-age and adolescent girls exposed to Hurricane Hugo also reported higher levels of PTSD symptomatology than did boys, and these girls were more likely to report being distressed by the hurricane, feeling upset by thoughts of the hurricane, fearing its recurrence, isolating themselves, avoiding reminders of the hurricane, avoiding feelings about it, affective numbing, increased startle response, somatic complaints, and feelings of guilt (Lonigan et al., 1991; Shannon et al., 1994).

Gender-related differences may be related to specific types of posttraumatic stress reactions. Jaffe, Wolfe, Wilson, and Zak (1986) reported the items on the Child Behavior Checklist (Achenbach & Edelbrock, 1981) that distinguished between children from violent families and children from nonviolent families. Their results suggest that girls may react (at least to violence in the home) primarily with internalizing behavior problems (e.g., clinging, worrying, sullenness), whereas boys react with both internalizing and externalizing behavior problems (e.g., arguing, hyperactivity, cruelty, impulsivity, hot temper). Similar results were obtained by Kiser et al. (1988), who found that sexually abused girls between the ages of 2 and 6 years tended to feel sad and depressed, whereas sexually abused boys the same age tended to act enraged and aggressive. Blom (1986) found that after a school accident boys showed more sleep disturbances, fighting, and fears; girls showed more startle reactions, asked more questions, and appeared to think about the disaster more often than boys. Girls may be more likely not only to seek social support after a traumatic experience, but to receive such support from important others (Milgram & Toubiana, 1996).

The time of assessment may also make a difference in gender-related symptomatology. Sexually abused preschool boys tended to withdraw immediately after their abuse was revealed, whereas girls were more withdrawn a year later (Kiser et al., 1988). Posttraumatic stress symptomatology in response to a nuclear waste disaster decreased over time for boys while increasing for girls (Korol, Green, & Gleser, 1999). Boys displaced during wartime in Bosnia showed more symptoms of anxiety, overarousal, and intrusive thoughts than girls during initial assessments, but 8 months later girls were more symptomatic than boys in these areas (Stein et al., 1999).

Ethnic and Cultural Variations

Reactions to Acute, Nonabusive Stressors

Perhaps due to the difficulty of recruiting large enough samples of traumatized children from any background, investigation of ethnic and cultural variations in children's posttraumatic responses has been slow to develop (Beals et al., 1997; DeJong, Emmett, & Hervada, 1982; Duclos et al., 1998; Frederick, 1988; Hjern, Angel, & Höjer, 1991; Jones, Dauphinais, Sack., & Somervell, 1997; La Greca et al., 1996; Lindholm & Willey, 1986; Pierce & Pierce, 1984). Two large studies have examined differences in ethnic reactions to one type of acute, nonabusive stressors—hurricanes. As described earlier in the chapter, Shannon et al. (1994) assessed the reactions of 5,687 youths aged 9–19 who lived through Hurricane Hugo. The majority of these children were European American (67.3%); 25.8% were African American; 3.6% were Asian American; 1.4% were Hispanic American; and 1.9% were from "other minority" groups. Because of the small numbers of non-African American minorities in this sample, the researchers chose to analyze differences among three ethnic groups: European Americans, African Americans, and non-African American minorities. Even after statistical controls for severity of the traumatic experience and levels of trait anxiety, African American children reported symptoms related to Criteria A through D of DSM-III-R in greater proportions than the other children. Nevertheless, there was no significant difference between the proportions of African American (6.3%) and all other children (5.1%) who met the core criteria for PTSD, A through D.

On the other hand, when La Greca et al. (1996) examined the reactions of 442 fifth-, sixth-, and seventh-graders to Hurricane Andrew, ethnic differences in reactions were very clear. European American children made up 45.7% of the sample; Hispanic Americans and African American children each constituted 23.5% of the sample; and Asian Americans constituted 3.4%. In this study, Hispanic American and African American children reported equivalent levels of posttraumatic stress, levels which were about half a standard deviation higher than those of European American children. At the same time, the African American and Hispanic American children were less likely to show improvements in their PTSD symptomatology over time. The authors note, "These ethnic differences in PTSD reporting may be related to other variables associated with minority status, such as the limited availability of financial resources" (p. 721), but the reasons for the differences remain unclear.

Reactions to Chronic or Abusive Stressors

Sexual Abuse. Rao, DiClemente, and Ponton (1992) compared the medical records of four groups of American children—69 of Asian, 80 of African, children, 80 of Hispanic, and 80 of European origin—who had been referred to a clinic for sexual abuse. The four ethnic groups differed on several potentially important demographic variables. The Asian American and Hispanic American children tended to be older than the African American and European American children when they were referred to the sexual abuse clinic, even though the groups did not differ in the amount of time elapsed between last episode and presentation at the clinic. Those of Asian descent were more likely to be living with both parents at the time of evaluation; those of African descent were the least likely to be living with both parents; and those of European and Hispanic descent were in between the two extremes. Asian Americans were also less than half as likely as the other children to be living in a single-parent family. On the other hand, Asian American primary caretakers were half as likely as primary caretakers of the other groups to spontaneously report their children's abuse to authorities; they were also the least likely to believe their children's report of abuse. The most extreme forms of sexual abuse (vaginal or anal penetration) were less likely to have occurred among Asian Americans (36.4%) and European Americans (36.4%) than among Hispanic Americans (50.0%) and African Americans (58.4%).

Sexual acting out was least likely to be found among children of Asian descent (1.4% vs. 15.0% among those of African, 17.5% among those of European, and 13.8% among those of Hispanic descent). Asian American children were also the least likely to display anger (8.7%, vs. 21.3% among African Americans, 22.5% among European Americans, and 20.0% among Hispanic Americans). Urinary symptoms were least frequently observed among Asian American children (2.9%) and most frequently among European American children (17.5%), with African Americans (10.0%) and Hispanic Americans (6.3%) in between the two extremes. Suicidal ideation or attempts, on the other hand, occurred most frequently among those of Asian origin (21.7%, vs. 11.3% among those of African, 15.0% among those of European, and 10.0% among those of Hispanic origin).

War and Concentration Camp. Kinzie and his colleagues (Kinzie et al., 1986, 1989) assessed symptoms of PTSD among young Cambodian refugees living in the United States who had lived in concentration camps during the Pol Pot regime when they were of school age. Of 40 children (25 boys and 15 girls), 46.5% (19) met DSM-III-R criteria for PTSD 5–6 years after leaving the camps (Kinzie et al., 1989). Three years later, 48% (13) of the 27 young Cambodians who took part in a follow-up study also met criteria for PTSD (Kinzie et al., 1989), with 8 of them meeting criteria at both time periods. Avoidant behaviors were the most commonly reported symptoms, which (according to the authors of the study) may have reflected in part a cultural tendency to cope by passively accepting adversity. The incidence of depressive disorders was also high at both time periods (53% at Time 1 and 41% at Time 2), and its presence was strongly associated with the presence of PTSD. Fifteen percent of the children reported entertaining suicidal thoughts. Few incidents of antisocial or acting-out behaviors were observed. The children viewed school positively—an attitude that may have been due to their cultural value of scholarship. Those children living with a family member appeared to function better than did others living without a family member at Time 1 (Kinzie et al., 1986) but not at follow-up 3 years later (Kinzie et al., 1989).

In another study of PTSD among 46 Cambodian refugees (36 males and 10 females) in the United States 10 years after their traumatization as children and adolescents under the Pol Pot regime (Realmuto et al., 1992), 37% met DSM-III-R criteria for PTSD. Many more missed meeting the criteria because they displayed too few symptoms of overarousal. PTSD symptomatology was not significantly associated with depressive mood, anxiety, or dissociation in this sample of young people aged 12–23 years old.

On the whole, children of non-European descent may present with more severe symptomatology than children of other ethnic backgrounds when exposed to acute, nonabusive stressors. Cultural differences become more complex when chronic or abusive stressors are involved. However, much more study of cross-cultural differences in response to traumatic experience is required before any definite conclusions can be drawn concerning the differential impact of trauma on children of different cultural backgrounds.

Developmental Differences

Although most research to date confirms that the diagnostic symptom clusters of DSM-IV apply as well to traumatized children of all ages (from preschool through adolescence) as they do to traumatized adults, the manifestation of posttraumatic stress responses in children may differ according to age and level of development (Pynoos, Steinberg, & Wraith, 1995). In other words, not only may the symptomatology of children differ from that of adults, but it may also differ among children of different ages. A child's age and level of cognitive, emotional, and social development can have a significant impact on each stage in the development of PTSD. Preschool children, for example, may be less capable than school-age and adolescent children of appraising a technological disaster as threatening (Gathercole, 1998; Green et al., 1991; Handford et al., 1986). Younger children were the least likely to understand the implications of the Oklahoma City bombing, and they were the most likely to be confused, providing the highest number of incorrect facts concerning the bombing (Allen, Dlugokinski, Cohen, & Walker, 1999).

Even the assessment of posttraumatic stress responses in children younger than 4 years old presents its own particular set of challenges (Scheeringa, Zeanah, Drell, & Larrieu, 1995; Scheeringa, Peebles, Cook, & Zeanah, 2001; Zero to Three/National Center for Clinical Infant Programs, 1994). The emotional repertoire of younger children may be more limited than that of older children, too (Cicchetti, 1989; Cole & Putnam, 1992). Young children's previous experience with stressful events, especially with mastering such events, is also likely to be more limited than is the case for older children (Rutter, 1983); as a consequence, the coping options available to younger children are probably more limited than those available to older children (Rossman, 1992). The younger a child, the more likely his or her traumatic reactions are to depend upon the traumatic reactions of others, especially parents (Cohen & Mannarino, 1996b; Cornely & Bromet, 1986; Famularo, Fenton, Kinscherff, Ayoub, & Barnum, 1994; McFarlane, 1987b).

The incidence rates for symptoms of PTSD listed in Table 7.2 provide a general indication of the kinds of differences in symptom presentation that might be found among adults and among children of three different age groups: preschoolers (approximately 6 years or younger), school-age children (5–13 years of age), and adolescents (12–13 and older). Unfortunately, most of the rates for preschoolers and adolescents in Table 7.2 are based on small samples of children. The following discussion of the influence of age and developmental stage on the etiology of PTSD therefore focuses more on the differences between adults and children of all ages than on differences among the three age groups of children.

Reactions to Overwhelming Stimuli: Developmental Differences

Theorists have begun to apply developmental theory to the understanding of children's posttraumatic stress reactions (Cicchetti, 1989; Cole & Putnam, 1992; Fish-Murray, Koby, & van der Kolk, 1987; Kagan, 1983; Maccoby, 1983; Pynoos & Eth, 1985b; Pynoos et al., 1995; Rutter, 1983), and several relevant principles have emerged from the literature. For example, because younger children have less control over their own physiological and emotional functioning than do older children, distressing events are more likely to overwhelm them and lead to disorganized behavior than is the case for older children (American Psychiatric Association, 1994; Cicchetti, 1989; Cole & Putnam, 1992; Maccoby, 1983; Pynoos & Eth, 1985b). Traumatized children certainly seem more likely to be distressed by reminders of traumatic events (51% for all ages; see Table 7.2) than are traumatized adults (26%). Furthermore, regressive behaviors—indicative of feelings of being overwhelmed—appear to be reported on average most frequently among preschoolers (17%; see Table 7.2), less frequently among school-age children (11%), and least frequently among adolescents (4%). Affective numbing may be another reaction to feelings of being overwhelmed and helpless, which would help explain the greater incidence of numbing among traumatized children of all ages (47%; see Table 7.2) than among traumatized adults (23%).

The use of dissociation as a coping mechanism is thought to begin at about 2 years of age and to decline with age (Cole & Putnam, 1992). Children of all ages certainly appear to present with dissociative responses more frequently (48%; see Table 7.2) than do adults (16%), although this difference in incidence rates may be due to the small samples used to estimate children's rates, combined with a more liberal definition of dissociation used to estimate children's rates. Nevertheless, in the light of developmental theory (Cole & Putnam, 1992), incidence rates as high as those in Table 7.2 do suggest that children's dissociative responses to trauma are worthy of closer study than they have so far received.

Social Development, Growth of Identity, and Traumatic Reactions

Preschoolers, by necessity, rely a great deal on parental support in times of stress (Pynoos & Eth, 1985b). A child's dependence on parental support decreases with age, as the possibility of peer support develops during the school years, and self-reliance increases during adolescence (Cole & Putnam, 1992; Pynoos & Eth, 1985b; Rossman,

1992). This developmental progression is reflected in a decrease with age in the incidence of separation anxiety after traumatization: from 36% among traumatized preschoolers to 16% among school-age children to 4% among adolescents (see Table 7.2). Similarly, Rossman (1992) found that children aged 6–7 years were more likely to seek caregiver assistance in times of distress than were children aged 8–12 years. Rossman suggests that the older children's decreased dependence on caregiver assistance is a consequence of the children's growing use of social comparison during school years, in conjunction with their growing awareness of the negative effects dependence on adults has on evaluations of self-competence, which also begin to emerge at this time (Cole & Putnam, 1992; Maccoby, 1983). At the same time, the egocentricity of younger children (Piaget & Inhelder, 1969) can lead them to feel more responsible for their traumatic experiences than is the actual case. This might contribute to a greater incidence of guilt feelings among traumatized children (43%; see Table 7.2) than among traumatized adults (15%).

Cognitive Development and Reaction to Stress

Before children attain the Piagetian stage of operational thinking between the ages of 7 and 11, their understanding of the world depends more on fantasy and play than is later the case (Fish-Murray et al., 1987; Piaget & Inhelder, 1969; Rossman, 1992). As a consequence, preschoolers appear likely to try to come to terms with traumatic experience by engaging in posttraumatic play more frequently (39%; see Table 7.2) than do school-age children (14%). Younger children's memory may also be more visually and perceptually oriented than linguistically oriented (Fish-Murray et al., 1987; Gathercole, 1998; Pynoos & Eth, 1985b). This could imbue their reexperiences of traumatic events with a more vivid quality than the reexperiences of adults, which may be reflected in the higher incidence among children of feelings of reliving the traumatic events (39% vs. 29% among adults).

As a result of the greater flexibility of adults' cognitive systems (Fish-Murray et al., 1987; Pynoos & Eth, 1985b), adults may be more able than children to distance themselves from their reexperiences and view them as memories rather than actual experiences. Traumatized adults do on average report intrusive memories more frequently (45%; see Table 7.2) than do traumatized children (34%). Cognitive development may provide older children and adults with more control over their thoughts as well (Gathercole, 1998), and thus even though traumatized children may try to avoid reminders of their traumatic experiences as frequently (32%; see Table 7.2) as do traumatized adults (33%), adults try more often to forget about their traumas (46%) than do children (24%). Moreover, adults appear to succeed at forgetting parts of their traumatic experiences more often (27%; see Table 7.2) than do children (12%).

Adolescents and adults are also better able than younger children to appreciate the threat of traumatic events, and as a consequence they appear to have a greater understanding of their own increased vulnerability (Pynoos & Eth, 1985b). This would help explain the higher incidence of trauma-specific fears among traumatized adults (45%; see Table 7.2) than among traumatized children (31%). It would also help account for the much greater pessimism about the future expressed by adults (61%) than by children (16%). The consequent anxiety and overarousal could also contribute to a greater incidence of startle response in adults than in children (38% vs. 28%; see Table 7.2), as well as a greater incidence of panic in adults (18% vs. 8%).

Coping Behavior

Researchers are only slowly beginning to systematically investigate the coping processes of children exposed to traumatic experiences (Ayalon, 1982; Band, 1990; Compas, 1987; Curle & Williams, 1996; Curry & Russ, 1985; La Greca et al., 1996; Maccoby, 1983; Paardekooper, de Jong, & Hermanns, 1999; Rutter, 1983; Stallard et al., 2001; Wertlieb, Weigel, & Feldstein, 1987). Wertlieb, Weigel, and Feldstein (1987) have identified children's coping behaviors that (1) focus on the self, environment, or other; (2) serve to solve problems or manage emotion; or (3) are examples of the following coping styles: information seeking, support seeking, direct action, inhibition of action, or intrapsychic coping. Coping styles and strategies appear to be closely associated with age and developmental stage (Compas, 1987). In this regard, Rossman (1992) found age and gender differences in children's use of several strategies to regulate their emotional reactions to stressful situations. The use of self-calming behaviors (e.g., trying to calm oneself and relaxing when feeling bad) decreased with age, as did the use of self-distraction or avoidance behaviors (e.g., reading a book to take one's mind off a bad thing). Children 6–7 years old were more likely than children 8–12 years old to seek refuge in a caregiver (e.g., get a parent to help). Girls were more likely than boys to seek out a caregiver and to make use of peers (e.g., playing with a friend). Distress behaviors (e.g., crying or biting nails) were used more by girls at all ages, too, whereas boys' use of distress behaviors declined with age. On the other hand, girls' use of anger declined with age, whereas its use by boys declined between the ages of 8 and 9 years, only to increase again from 10 to 12 years.

Researchers are just beginning to examine the influence of coping behavior on the progress of PTSD. In one study the coping strategies of boys and girls between the ages of 7 and 18 years who were involved in motor vehicle accidents were examined in detail (Stallard et al., 2001). When 97 of these children and adolescents were assessed 6 weeks after their accidents, 36 (37.1%) were diagnosed with PTSD. When the coping skills of the children with and without PTSD were compared, no significant differences were found on the reported use of the active coping strategies of seeking social support, problem solving, and cognitive restructuring. The children with PTSD, however, were more likely to report using the avoidant, emotional coping strategies of social withdrawal, distraction, emotional regulation, and blaming others. The children with PTSD also reported using more kinds of strategies than those without PTSD. Children aged 7–9 years used more strategies than older children, as well. No gender differences were found, although an earlier study (Curle & Williams, 1996) found that girls reported using more coping strategies than boys. A logistic regression revealed that diagnosis of PTSD was associated with gender and the coping strategies of blaming others and social withdrawal. Those children who were still diagnosed with PTSD 8 months after their accidents reported being more likely to use strategies of distraction and social withdrawal. Among third- to fifth-grade children who survived Hurricane Andrew, positive coping, blaming others, showing anger, and social withdrawal were all associated with more symptoms of PTSD (La Greca et al., 1996). Sudanese refugee children aged 7–12 years reported resorting more than a comparison group of Ugandan children to strategies of emotional regulation, self-blame, cognitive reframing ("trying to see the good side of things"), and seeking social support (Paardekooper et al., 1999).

Interestingly, the most frequently reported coping behavior in all three of these studies was wishful thinking. The children without PTSD in the Stallard et al. (2001) study reported resorting to this coping strategy in times of trouble most often, too. In fact, there was no significant difference between the proportions of children with and without PTSD who used wishful thinking. However, the Sudanese refugee children did report using this strategy more often than the Ugandan children in the comparison group (Paardekooper et al., 1999). The results of these three studies can be compared so readily because all three made use of a measure of children's coping known as the Kidcope (Spirito, Stark, & Williams, 1988), which asks children to think about a specific situation and indicate which of 10 coping strategies they have used. In all three studies, the children who had been exposed to traumatic experiences resorted to more coping strategies than the comparison children. Although the Kidcope appears to be a useful standardized measure of children's coping, Stallard et al. (2001) have called attention to a conceptual confusion between some of these coping strategies and symptoms of PTSD. Social withdrawal, for example, is considered both a coping strategy and a symptom of avoidance. However, the measure does allow more careful consideration to be made of the impact of coping behaviors on the development and course of PTSD than they have heretofore received.

SOCIAL CHARACTERISTICS

Social Support

As noted earlier, the reaction of a child to trauma is often closely related to the reactions of the child's parents or other important adults, especially the mother (Ajdukovic, 1998; Bloch, Silber, & Perry, 1956; Cohen & Mannarino, 1996b; Crawshaw, 1963; Famularo et al., 1994; Flannery, 1990; Freud & Burlingham, 1943; Gislason & Call, 1982; Harrison et al., 1967; McFarlane, 1987b; Milgram & Toubiana, 1996; Newman, 1976; Silber, Perry, & Bloch, 1958; Winje & Ulvik, 1998), although this need not always be the case (Handford et al., 1986). Parents' reactions may be especially important for younger children (Crawshaw, 1963;

Freud & Burlingham, 1943; Holahan & Moos, 1987; Pynoos & Eth, 1985b). Stress-resilient children have been found to have close, positive relationships with their caregivers and to receive more support from both within and outside of the family (Ajdukovic, 1998; Holahan & Moos, 1987; Milgram & Toubiana, 1996; Seifer et al., 1992; Werner & Smith, 1982; Wyman et al., 1991, 1992). Sexually abused children who receive support from their mothers fare better after disclosure than do those whose mothers express disbelief or negative emotions toward their children (Conte & Schuerman, 1987; Everson, Hunter, Runyan, Edelsohn, & Coulter, 1989; Kendall-Tackett et al., 1993). The more social support children exposed to Hurricane Andrew reported receiving afterwards from parents and classmates, the fewer symptoms of PTSD they reported (La Greca et al., 1996). Similarly, the more social support children reported both prior to and after the sinking of the *Jupiter*, the less likely they were to develop PTSD; for those who did develop PTSD, the severity and duration of their posttraumatic stress symptomatology were reduced by such support (Udwin et al., 2000).

Parenting Style

A child's sense of competence and self-reliance appears to be encouraged in part by a flexible (Baumrind, 1971), warm, caring, and attentive parenting style (Maccoby & Martin, 1983). Rigid, coercive parenting, on the other hand, appears to reduce a child's sense of self-competence and self-esteem (Slater & Power, 1987). Posttraumatic stress reactions among displaced adolescents in Croatia were correlated with perceptions of a rejecting mother (Ajdukovic, 1998). Children whose parents provide positive, nurturant care and set limits in a constructive manner tend to be more stress-resilient than those whose parents are more rigid and less warm in their caregiving (Wyman et al., 1991, 1992). Palestinian children exposed to political violence, who perceived their mothers as very loving and caring but their fathers as not so, reported higher levels of PTSD (Punamaeki, Oouta, & El-Sarraj, 2001).

Family Discord versus Cohesion

Evidence is beginning to accumulate that family conflict (prior to, during, or after exposure to trauma) is associated with more severe symptoms of PTSD in children. Nir (1985) observed that parental discord can have a detrimental effect on children diagnosed with cancer. Stress-resilient children appear to come from more stable family environments than do less resilient children (Seifer et al., 1992; Wyman et al., 1991, 1992). In another study, adolescents with cancer who met criteria for lifetime PTSD saw their families as significantly more chaotic than those who did not have PTSD (Pelcovitz et al., 1998). After Hurricane Andrew, PTSD symptoms were more prevalent among children who reported high levels of parental conflict (Wasserstein & La Greca, 1998). The strongest predictor of PTSD symptomatology among children who lived through the Buffalo Creek flood was the parents' level of functioning and the home atmosphere (Green et al., 1991). Several writers have commented upon and documented the greater risk of psychosocial impairment among children from violent as compared to nonviolent families (Arroyo & Eth, 1985; Burgess et al., 1987; Jaffe et al., 1986; Walker & Greene, 1987; Wolfe et al., 1985; Wolfe, Zak, & Wilson, 1986). The act of witnessing family violence has been found to be associated in and of itself with PTSD, conduct problems, emotional problems, and deficits in social competence (Jouriles et al., 1989; Kiser et al., 1988; Lehmann, 2000; Martinez & Richters, 1993).

Other Characteristics of the Environment

Additional characteristics of the social environment are likely to contribute to the development of PTSD after traumatization. The level of family stress, the mobility of the family, and the psychiatric history of the family, for instance, have all been found to influence a child's stress reactions (Bloch et al., 1956; Felner, Gillespie, & Smith, 1985; Green, 1983; Masten et al., 1988; Nir, 1985; Silber et al., 1958; Vila et al., 2001). Felner et al. (1985) suggest that the composition of the family may also contribute to a child's reaction to trauma, in that children from single-parent families or reconstituted families may be more vulnerable than others.

Financial difficulties, too, have been found to be associated with symptoms of PTSD or general distress in children (Arroyo & Eth, 1985; Burgess et al., 1987; Elmer, 1977; Felner et al., 1985; Lonigan et al., 1991; Masten et al., 1988; Shannon et al., 1994; Vila et al., 2001). Low SES, in fact, may increase a child's chance of being exposed to traumatic events in the first place, especially violence in the community as well as in the home. Symptoms of PTSD have been observed in child witnesses to, and survivors of, community violence (Martinez & Richter, 1993).

Exposure to other stressors after living through a traumatic experience can also increase a child's risk for developing and prolonging the duration of PTSD symptomatology. Sudanese refugee children reported experiencing more daily stressors after relocating than did the Ugandan children in the comparison group (Paardekooper et al., 1999). These included such things as lack of clothing, poor sanitation, hunger, inability to pay school fees, worry about family members, and so on. Children of the *Jupiter* sinking who developed PTSD over the years afterward reported more exposure to other major life events during that time than did those who did not develop PTSD (Udwin et al., 2000). Children who reported more major life events after Hurricane Andrew reported more PTSD symptomatology 7 months after the disaster (La Greca et al., 1996).

TESTS OF SPECIFIC MODELS

Now that many of the potential risk factors for the development of PTSD after exposure to traumatic events have been identified, the next important step involves testing models such as the one discussed in this chapter. Udwin et al. (2000) tested such a model when examining the risk factors for developing PTSD after living through the sinking of the *Jupiter*. La Greca et al. (1996) explicitly tested a model similar to the one presented in this chapter. They found that in the final model, predisaster characteristics did not contribute to PTSD symptomatology 7 months after Hurricane Andrew. Characteristics of the children's hurricane experience accounted for the most variance in PTSD scores, with exposure variables reflecting life threat accounting for 15.1% of the variance, and exposure variables related to loss and disruption accounting for an additional 5%. Following that, ethnicity was found to account for 3% of the variance; major life events during the recovery period accounted for 3%; social support variables accounted for another 7%; and coping strategies accounted for an additional 6%. The complete model accounted for 39.1% of the total variance in PTSD symptomatology.

A few other researchers have also begun testing PTSD models. In one study, 937 college students were asked about the most stressful event in their lives (Bernat et al., 1998). The impact of various risk factors on current symptoms of PTSD was investigated via hierarchical regression analysis. The analysis determined that 7% of the variance in reports of symptoms could be accounted for by personal vulnerability factors, which in this case primarily consisted of the number of lifetime stressors reported (which accounted for 5% of the variance) and gender (which accounted for 2%, although this was not a significant effect in the final model). Objective dimensions of the most stressful event accounted for a total of a further 5% of the variance, with perceived threat to one's life accounting for 3% and the involvement of serious injury or death of someone else accounting for 2%. Interestingly, after these other factors were taken into account, actual injury to the self did not account for a significant amount of the variance. The experience of adverse emotions (such as fear, anger, shame or guilt) or emotional numbing in immediate reactions to the stressful event accounted for another 8% of the variance. The experience of physical reactions (e.g., dizziness, rapid heart rate, trembling or shaking, sweating, and nausea) following the stressful event accounted for a further 4% of the variance. Acute dissociative responses to the stressful event accounted for a final 3% of the variance. The complete model accounted for 30% of the variance in posttraumatic stress symptomatology.

Although these studies demonstrate the impact of various risk factors in the model—such as objective dimensions of stressful events, in concert with personal vulnerability factors and peritraumatic reactions immediately following the stressful event—on the development of posttraumatic symptomatology, the moderate amount of variance accounted for by the total model of risk factors for posttraumatic symptomatology also suggests that a good many factors remain unaccounted for. Moreover, the model-testing procedures used in these studies have relied on regression models, which do not fully take into account the complexity of a model (such as the one outlined in this chapter) that includes both moderating and mediating factors. One longitudinal study has examined a more complex theoretical model of this sort using path analysis. The problems and stresses that arose among 4,978 adolescents as a result of exposure to Hurricane Andrew were examined to determine their relationship to the occurrence of subsequent minor socially deviant behaviors thought to be indicative of traumatic responses to the hurricane and its aftermath—behaviors such as breaking things in anger, starting fist fights, and stealing from someone at school (Khoury et al., 1997).

The results indicated that among males, ethnicity did not play a role in either prehurricane or posthurricane deviant behavior. Among females, however, Hispanic or African descent was associated with higher levels of prehurricane deviant behavior. Prehurricane family support decreased posthurricane stress symptoms for females, but not for males. For both males and females, prehurricane family support was associated with decreased prehurricane deviant behavior. For females, it also decreased posthurricane stress symptoms, but it had no such effect for males. Prehurricane deviant behavior among males decreased posthurricane family support, but it had no such effect for females. Hurricane problems increased posthurricane stress symptoms for both males and females. Posthurricane stress symptoms were associated with decreased posthurricane family support for females but not for males. Posthurricane family support was associated with decreased posthurricane deviant behaviors for males and females, whereas posthurricane stress symptoms were associated with increased deviant behaviors for both males and females.

Collectively, these studies demonstrate the kinds of complexities that are involved in trying to determine the most appropriate model for explaining the onset and course of posttraumatic stress symptomatology among children and adolescents exposed to traumatic stressors.

CURRENT ISSUES AND FUTURE DIRECTIONS

It should be clear by this point that the last two decades of research on childhood traumatic stress reactions have demonstrated that children exposed to traumatic events can and do react in a manner very similar to that of traumatized adults. A substantial proportion of traumatized children, regardless of their age, exhibit behaviors symptomatic of the "core" DSM-IV symptoms of PTSD: reexperiencing the traumatic experience, avoidance of reminders of the experience or affective numbing, and overarousal. Furthermore, children have often been observed to respond to traumatic events with additional symptoms (e.g., guilt, depression, and generalized anxiety) that are also associated with PTSD in adults.

It should be equally clear at this point that our current understanding of childhood PTSD is far from complete. Future research must examine the etiology of childhood PTSD within a context that considers the impact of factors other than just exposure to traumatic events. Sufficient data are currently available to indicate that differences among stressful events themselves need to be considered more carefully in the future. Other factors that might influence the development of childhood PTSD are less well understood. We know next to nothing, for example, about how children make meaning out of their traumatic experience, and we are just beginning to examine how their emotional reactions to trauma can affect their posttraumatic responses. Physiological responses to childhood trauma are also little understood at the moment. Current research does provide enough evidence to tell us that we need to know more about the impact on PTSD of personal characteristics, such as gender, age, ethnicity, psychiatric history, sense of mastery, temperament, and coping skills. Little is known at the moment about the characteristics of a child's social environment that influence the development of PTSD.

Despite a growing body of research into children's reactions to extreme stressors, our contemporary understanding of childhood PTSD continues to rest on shaky methodological grounds. Better-designed research is required to shore up our present understanding of childhood PTSD. Larger samples are required. More comparisons must be made between the reactions of traumatized children and *comparable* nontraumatized children. Reports based on standardized assessment tools that ask PTSD-specific questions[3] must be gathered from multiple sources, including the children themselves. Assessments of potentially important symptoms other than those included in the DSM-IV diagnostic criteria should also be gathered (Armsworth & Holaday, 1993). Similarly, comorbid conditions deserve closer study. It is time, too, to begin testing models such as that presented in this chapter, to examine the impact of multiple risk factors on the etiology of PTSD in children.

Rigorous empirical studies of the effectiveness of different treatment approaches for childhood PTSD remain extremely rare (Cohen, 1998; Pfefferbaum, 1997). The four studies that have been conducted, though suffering from methodological limitations (Ruggiero, Morris, & Scotti, 2001), do provide preliminary evidence of the potential effectiveness of anxiety management techniques coupled with other cognitive-behavioral interventions (Cohen & Mannarino, 1996a, 1997; Deblinger, Lippman, & Steer, 1996; Goenjian et al., 1997; March, Amaya-Jackson, Murray, & Schulte, 1998). Another therapeutic approach to treating traumatized children that shows promise is based on exposure-based therapy (Albano, Miller, Côté, & Barlow, 1997; Saigh, Yasik, Oberfield, & Inamdar, 1999; Yule, 1998). More and better-designed research on effective treatment approaches for childhood PTSD is urgently needed.

In the final analysis, we have only just begun to grasp the process whereby exposure to traumatic events leads to PTSD in children. We know that children's symptoms of PTSD often look strikingly similar to those of adults. We know, too, that children frequently manifest PTSD symptomatology in an age-specific manner. This knowledge represents a substantial gain over the past two decades. Our accomplishments in this area should not allow us to become complacent, however. There is still much to learn about childhood PTSD. It is unclear, for example, why some children do not develop PTSD after exposure to traumatic events. The answer to that question could provide important clues about the kinds of treatment that would be most efficacious for those children who do develop PTSD. Because traumatic experience can seriously disrupt a child's development and lead to difficult problems later in life, it is incumbent upon us to seek a better understanding, based on firm methodological grounds, of the context within which childhood PTSD develops.

NOTES

1. The PTSD-RI was not designed to allow DSM criteria to be assessed, or a DSM diagnosis of PTSD to be made. Modifying the scale to allow this to be done can be problematic. One problem is related to the method used to dichotomize the 5-point Likert rating scales used to for each question on the PTSD-RI. One approach is to rate a symptom as present if that symptom is rated with one of the two highest ratings on the Likert scale. Another approach rates a symptom as present if any of the *three* highest ratings is marked on the scale. Estimates of incidence rates of a PTSD diagnosis will obviously differ according to which of these two approaches is chosen, with the first approach producing lower estimates (as demonstrated by Schwarz & Kowalski, 1991b). Evidence is accumulating that moderate levels of symptomatology immediately after exposure to traumatic events is strongly associated with later development of PTSD (La Greca et al., 1996). Shannon et al. (1994) and Lonigan et al. (1991) applied the first, more conservative approach.

2. Rating stressful events on each of the enumerated dimensions would allow for detailed comparisons between any kind of event. A scale for assessing these dimensions in stressful events, the Dimensions of Stressful Events Scale, is available from me.

3. Measures with good psychometric properties are beginning to appear. Those that appear to be particularly promising include an interview, the Children's PTSD Inventory (Saigh et al., 2000); a paper-and-pencil self-report, the Kiddie-Post-Traumatic Symptomatology scale (March et al., 1997); and another paper-and-pencil self-report, the Child's Reaction to Traumatic Events Scale (Jones, 1996). Four other interrelated instruments are available from me: a Childhood PTSD Interview suitable for paraprofessionals; a parent's version of the interview, a child's self-report (the When Bad Things Happen Scale), suitable for children with third-grade reading level or above; and a Parent's Report of the Child's Reactions to Stress paper-and-pencil scale (Fletcher, 1996). A child's version of the Clinician-Administered PTSD Scale for Children (Nader, Kriegler, Blake, & Pynoos, 1993) is a structured interview beginning to be used as well (Yule et al., 2000).

REFERENCES

Aaron, J., Zaglul, H., & Emery, R. E. (1999). Posttraumatic stress in children following acute physical injury. *Journal of Pediatric Psychology*, *24*, 335–343.

Abramson, L. Y., Seligman, M. E. P., & Teasdale, J. D. (1978). Learned helplessness in humans: Critique and reformulation. *Journal of Abnormal Psychology*, *87*, 49–94.

Achenbach, T., & Edelbrock, C. S. (1981). Behavior problems and competencies reported by parents of normal and disturbed children aged four through sixteen. *Monographs of the Society for Research in Child Development*, *46*(1, Serial No. 188).

Achenbach, T. M., McConaughy, S. H., & Howell, C. T. (1987). Child/adolescent behavioral and emotional problems: Implications of cross-informant correlations for situational specificity. *Psychological Bulletin*, *101*, 213–232.

Adam, B. S., Everett, B. L., & O'Neal, E. (1992). PTSD in physically and sexually abused psychiatrically hospitalized children. *Child Psychiatry and Human Development*, *23*, 3–8.

Ajdukovic, M. (1998). Displaced adolescents in Croatia: Sources of stress and posttraumatic stress reaction. *Adolescence*, *33*, 209–217.

Albano, A. M., Miller, P. P., Côté, G., & Barlow, D. H. (1997). Behavioral assessment and treatment of PTSD in prepubertal children: Attention to developmental factors and innovative strategies in the case study of a family. *Cognitive and Behavioral Practice*, *4*, 245–262.

Allen, S. F., Dlugokinski, E. L., Cohen, L. A., & Walker, J. L. (1999). Assessing the impact of a traumatic community event on children and assisting their healing. *Psychiatric Annals*, *29*, 93–98.

American Psychiatric Association. (1952). *Diagnostic and statistical manual of mental disorders*. Washington, DC: Author.

American Psychiatric Association. (1968). *Diagnostic and statistical manual of mental disorders* (2nd ed.). Washington, DC: Author.

American Psychiatric Association. (1980). *Diagnostic and statistical manual of mental disorders* (3rd ed.). Washington, DC: Author.

American Psychiatric Association. (1987). *Diagnostic and statistical manual of mental disorders* (3rd ed., rev.). Washington, DC: Author.

American Psychiatric Association. (1994). *Diagnostic and statistical manual of mental disorders* (4th ed.). Washington, DC: Author.

Armsworth, M. W., & Holaday, M. (1993). The effects of psychological trauma on children and adolescents. *Journal of Counseling and Development*, *72*, 49–56.

Arroyo, W., & Eth, S. (1985). Children traumatized by Central American warfare. In S. Eth & R. S. Pynoos (Eds.), *Post-traumatic stress disorder in children* (pp. 103–120). Washington, DC: American Psychiatric Press.

Ayalon, O. (1982). Children as hostages. *The Practitioner*, *226*, 1773–1781.

Band, E. B. (1990). Children's coping with diabetes: Understanding the role of cognitive development. *Journal of Paediatric Psychology*, *15*, 27–41.

Bandura, A., Taylor, C. B., Williams, S. L, Mefford, I. N., & Barchas, J. D. (1985). Catecholamine secretion as a function of perceived coping self-efficacy. *Journal of Consulting and Clinical Psychology*, *53*, 406–415.

Baumrind, D. (1971). Current patterns of parental authority. *Developmental Psychology Monographs*, *4*, 1–101.

Beals, J., Piasecki, J., Nelson, S., Jones, M., Keane, E., Dauphnais, P., Shirt, R. R., Sack, W. H., & Manson, S. M. (1997). Psychiatric disorder among American Indian adolescents: Prevalence in Northern American Plains youth. *Journal of the American Academy of Child and Adolescent Psychiatry*, *36*, 1252–1259.

Becker, D. E., Weine, S. M., Vojvoda, D., & McGlashan, T. H. (1999). Case series: PTSD symptoms in adolescent survivors of "ethnic cleansing." Results from a 1-year follow-up study. *Journal of the American Academy of Child and Adolescent Psychiatry*, *38*, 775–781.

Beitchman, J. H., Zucker, K. J., Hood, J. E., DaCosta, G. A., Akman, D., & Cassavia, E. (1992). A review of the long-term effects of child sexual abuse. *Child Abuse and Neglect*, *16*, 101–118.

Bernat, J. A., Ronfeldt, H. M., Calhoun, K. S., & Arias, I. (1998). Prevalence of traumatic events and peritraumatic predictors of posttraumatic stress symptoms in a non-clinical sample of college students. *Journal of Traumatic Stress*, *11*, 645–664.

Bloch, D. A., Silber, E., & Perry, S. E. (1956). Some factors in the emotional reaction of children to disaster. *American Journal of Psychiatry*, *113*, 416–422.

Blom, G. E. (1986). A school disaster: Intervention and research aspects. *Journal of the American Academy of Child Psychiatry*, *25*, 336–345.

Bolton, D., O'Ryan, D., Udwin, O., Boyle, S., & Yule, W. (2000). The long-term psychological effects of a disaster experienced in adolescence: II: General psychopathology. *Journal of Child Psychology and Psychiatry*, *41*, 513–523.

Brander, T. (1943). Psychiatric observations among Finnish children during the Russo-Finnish War of 1939–1940. *Nervous Child*, *2*, 313–319.

Bremner, J. D., Southwick, S. M., & Charney, D. S. (1999). The neurobioloy of posttraumatic stress disorder: An integration of animal and human research. In P. A. Saigh & J. D. Bremner (Eds.), *Posttraumatic stress disorder* (pp. 103–143). Needham Heights, MA: Allyn & Bacon.

Breslau, N., Davis, G. C., Andreski, P., & Peterson, E. (1991). Traumatic events and posttraumatic stress disorder in an urban population of young adults. *Archives of General Psychiatry*, *48*, 216–222.

Brett, E. A. (1993). Psychoanalytic contributions to a theory of traumatic stress. In J. P. Wilson & B. Raphael (Eds.), *International handbook of traumatic stress syndromes* (pp. 61–68). New York: Plenum Press.

Bromet, E. J., Goldgaber, D., Carlson, G., Panina, N., Golovakha, E., Gluzman, S. F., Gilbert, T., Gluzman, D., Lyubsky, S., & Schwartz, J. E. (2000). Children's well-being 11 years after the Chornobyl catastrophe. *Archives of General Psychiatry*, *57*, 563–571.

Burgess, A. W., Hartman, C. R., & McCormack, A. (1987). Abused to abuser: Antecedents of socially deviant behaviors. *American Journal of Psychiatry*, *144*, 1431–1436.

Burt, C. (1943). War neuroses in British children. *Nervous Child*, *2*, 324–337.

Cahill, C., Llewelyn, S. P., & Pearson, C. (1991). Long-term effects of sexual abuse which occurred in childhood: A review. *British Journal of Clinical Psychology*, *30*, 117–130.

Carlson, M., & Earls, F. (1997). Psychological and neuro-endrocrinological sequelae of early social deprivation in institutionalized children in Romania. *Annals of the New York Academy of Sciences*, *807*, 419–428.

Carmen, E., Rieker, P. P., & Mills, T. (1984). Victims of violence and psychiatric illness. *American Journal of Psychiatry*, *141*, 378–383.

Chemtob, C., Roitblat, H. C., Hamada, R. S., Carlson, J. G., & Twentyman, C. T. (1988). A cognitive action theory of post-traumatic stress disorder. *Journal of Anxiety Disorders*, *2*, 253–275.

Chu, J. A., & Dill, D. L. (1990). Dissociative symptoms in relation to childhood physical and sexual abuse. *American Journal of Psychiatry*, *147*, 887–892.

Cicchetti, D. (1989). How research on child maltreatment has informed the study of child development: Perspectives from developmental psychopathology. In D. Cicchetti & V. Carlson (Eds.), *Maltreatment: Theory and research on the causes and consequences of child abuse and neglect* (pp. 377–431). New York: Cambridge University Press.

Clarke, G., Sack, W. H., & Goff, B. (1993). Three forms of stress in Cambodian adolescent refugees. *Journal of Abnormal Child Psychology*, *21*, 65–77.

Cohen, J. (1998). Practice parameters for the assessment and treatment of children and adolescents with posttraumatic stress disorder. *Journal of the American Academy of Child and Adolescent Psychiatry*, 37(Suppl.), 4S-26S.

Cohen, J. A., & Mannarino, A. P. (1996a). A treatment outcome study for sexually abused preschool children: Initial findings. *Journal of the American Academy of Child and Adolescent Psychiatry*, *35*, 42–50.

Cohen, J. A., & Mannarino, A. P. (1996b). Factors that mediate treatment outcome of sexually abused preschool children. *Journal of the American Academy of Child and Adolescent Psychiatry*, 35, 1402–1410.

Cohen, J. A., & Mannarino, A. P. (1997). A treatment study for sexually abused preschool children: Outcome during a one-year follow-up. *Journal of the American Academy of Child and Adolescent Psychiatry, 36,* 1228–1235.

Cole, P. M., & Putnam, F. W. (1992). Effect of incest on self and social functioning: A developmental psychopathology perspective. *Journal of Consulting and Clinical Psychology, 60,* 174–184.

Compas, B. E. (1987). Coping with stress during childhood and adolescence. *Psychological Bulletin, 101,* 393–403.

Connell, J. P. (1985). A new multidimensional measure of children's perceptions of control. *Child Development, 56,* 1018–1041.

Conte, J. R., & Schuerman, J. R. (1987). Factors associated with an increased impact of child sexual abuse. *Child Abuse and Neglect, 11,* 201–211.

Cornely, P., & Bromet, E. (1986). Prevalence of behavior problems in three-year-old children living near Three Mile Island: A comparative analysis. *Journal of Child Psychology and Psychiatry, 27,* 489–498.

Coromina, J. (1943). Repercussions of the war on children as observed during the Spanish Civil War. *Nervous Child, 2,* 320–323.

Costello, E. J., Erkanli, A., Fairbank, J. A., & Angold, A. (2002). The prevalence of potentially traumatic events in childhood and adolescence. *Journal of Traumatic Stress, 15,* 99–112.

Crawshaw, R. (1963). Reactions to a disaster. *Archives of General Psychiatry, 9,* 157–162.

Crocq, M., Macher, J., Barros-Beck, J., Rosenberg, S. J., & Duval, F. (1993). Posttraumatic stress disorder in World War II prisoners of war from Alsace–Lorraine who survived captivity in the USSR. In J. P. Wilson & B. Raphael (Eds.), *International handbook of traumatic stress syndromes* (pp. 253–261). New York: Plenum Press.

Cuffe, S. P., Addy, C. L., Garrison, C. Z., Waller, J. L., Jackson, K. L., McKeown, R. E., & Chilappagari, S. (1998). Prevalence of PTSD in a community sample of older adolescents. *Journal of the American Academy of Child and Adolescent Psychiatry, 37,* 147–154.

Curle, C. E., & Williams, C. (1996). Post-traumatic stress reactions in children: Gender differences in the incidence of trauma reactions at two years and examination of factors influencing adjustment. *British Journal of Clinical Psychology, 35,* 297–309.

Curry, S. L., & Russ, S. W. (1985). Identifying coping strategies in children. *Journal of Clinical Child Psychology, 14,* 61–69.

Dalgleish, T., Moradi, A. Taghavi, R., Neshat-Doost, H., Yule, W., & Canterbury, R. (2000). Judgements about emotional events in children and adolescents with post-traumatic stress disorder and controls. *Journal of Child Psychology and Psychiatry, 41,* 981–988.

Davidson, J., Hughes, D. Blazer, D., & George, L. (1991). Post-traumatic stress disorder in the community: An epidemiological study. *Psychological Medicine, 21,* 713–722.

Davidson, J., Swartz, M., Storck, M., Krishnan, R. R., & Hammett, E. (1985). A diagnostic and family study of posttraumatic stress disorder. *American Journal of Psychiatry, 142,* 90–93.

Davis, W. B., Mooney, D., Racusin, R., Ford, J. D., Fleischer, A., & McHugo, G. J. (2000). Predicting post-traumatic stress after hospitalization for pediatric injury. *Journal of the American Academy of Child and Adolescent Psychiatry, 39,* 576–583.

De Bellis, M. D., Baum, A. S., Birmaher, B., Keshavan, M. S., Eccard, C. H., Boring, A. M., Jenkins, F. J., & Ryan, N. D. (1999). Developmental traumatology: Part I. Biological stress systems. *Biological Psychiatry, 45,* 1259–1270.

De Bellis, M. D., Keshavan, M. S., Clark. D. B., Casey, B. J., Giedd, J. N., Boring, A. M., Frustaci, K., & Ryan, N. D. (1999). Developmental traumatology: Part II. Brain development. *Biological Psychiatry, 45,* 1271–1284.

De Bellis, M. D., Keshavan, M. S., Spencer, S., & Hall, J. (2000). *N*-acetylaspartate concentration in the anterior cingulate of maltreated children and adolescents with PTSD. *American Journal of Psychiatry, 157,* 1175–1177.

Deblinger, E., Lippman, J., & Steer, R. (1996). Sexually abused children suffering posttraumatic stress symptoms: Initial treatment outcome findings. *Child Maltreatment, 1,* 310–321.

Deblinger, E., McLeer, S. V., Atkins, M. S., Ralphe, D., & Foa, E. (1989). Post-traumatic stress in sexually abused, physically abused, and nonabused children. *Child Abuse and Neglect, 13,* 403–408.

DeJong, A. R., Emmett, G. A., & Hervada, A. R. (1982). Sexual abuse of children: Sex-, race-, and age-dependent variations. *American Journal of Diseases of Children, 136,* 129–134.

den Velde, W. O., Falger, P. R. J., Hovens, J. E., de Groen, J. H. M., Lasschuit, L. J., Van Duijn, H., & Schouten, E. G. W. (1993). Posttraumatic stress disorder in Dutch resistance veterans from World War II. In J. P. Wilson & B. Raphael (Eds.), *International handbook of traumatic stress syndromes* (pp. 219–230). New York: Plenum Press.

Dollinger, S. J. (1985). Lightning-strike disaster among children. *British Journal of Medical Psychology, 58,* 375–383.

Duclos, C. W., Beals, J., Novins, D. K., Martin, C., Jewett, C. S., & Manson, S. M. (1998). Prevalence of common psychiatric disorders among American Indian adolescent detainees. *Journal of the American Academy of Child and Adolescent Psychiatry, 37,* 866–873.

Dyregrov, A., Gupta, L., Gjestad, R., & Mukanoheli, E. (2000). Trauma exposure and psychological reactions to genocide among Rwandan children. *Journal of Traumatic Stress, 13,* 3–21.

Earls, F., Smith, E., Reich, W., & Jung, K. G. (1988). Investigating psychopathological consequences of a disaster in children: A pilot study incorporating a structured diagnostic interview. *Journal of the American Academy of Child and Adolescent Psychiatry, 27,* 90–95.

Elizur, E., & Kaffman, M. (1982). Children's bereavement reactions following death of the father: II. *Journal of the American Academy of Child Psychiatry, 21,* 474–480.

Elmer, E. (1977). A follow-up study of traumatized children. *Pediatrics, 59,* 273–279.

Epstein, S. (1990). The self-concept, the traumatic neurosis, and the structure of personality. In D. Ozer, J. M. Healey, Jr., & A. J. Stewart (Eds.), *Perspectives on personality* (Vol. 3, pp. 63–98). Greenwich, CT: JAI Press.

Eth, S., & Pynoos, R. S. (Eds.). (1985). *Post-traumatic stress disorder in children.* Washington, DC: American Psychiatric Press.

Ettinger, L. (1961). Pathology of the concentration camp syndrome. *Archives of General Psychiatry, 5,* 371–379.

Everson, M. D., Hunter, W. M., Runyon, D. K., Edelsohn, G. A., & Coulter, M. L. (1989). Maternal support following disclosure of incest. *American Journal of Orthopsychiatry, 59,* 197–207.

Famularo, R., Fenton, T., Kinscherff, R., Ayoub, C., & Barnum, R. (1994). Maternal and child posttraumatic stress disorder in cases of child maltreatment. *Child Abuse and Neglect, 18,* 27–36.

Famularo, R., Kinscherff, R., & Fenton, T. (1990). Symptom differences in acute and chronic presentation of childhood post-traumatic stress disorder. *Child Abuse and Neglect, 14,* 439–444.

Famularo, R., Kinscherff, R., & Fenton, T. (1992). Psychiatric diagnosis of maltreated children: Preliminary findings. *Journal of the American Academy of Child and Adolescent Psychiatry, 31,* 863–867.

Faravelli, C., Webb, T., Ambonetti, A., Fonnesu, F., & Sessarego, A. (1985). Prevalence of traumatic early life events in 31 agoraphobic patients with panic attacks. *American Journal of Psychiatry, 142,* 1493–1494.

Felner, R. D., Gillespie, J. F., & Smith, R. (1985). Risk and vulnerability in childhood: A reappraisal. *Journal of Clinical Child Psychology, 14,* 2–4.

Figley, C. R. (Ed.). (1978). *Stress disorder among Vietnam veterans.* New York: Brunner/Mazel.

Figley, C. R. (1993). Foreword. In J. P. Wilson & B. Raphael (Eds.), *International handbook of traumatic stress syndromes* (pp. xvii–xx). New York: Plenum Press.

Fish-Murray, C. C., Koby, E. V., & van der Kolk, B. A. (1987). Evolving ideas: The effect of abuse on children's thought. In B. A. van der Kolk (Ed.), *Psychological trauma* (pp. 89–110). Washington, DC: American Psychiatric Press.

Flannery, R. B., Jr. (1990). Social support and psychological trauma: A methodological review. *Journal of Traumatic Stress, 3,* 593–611.

Fletcher, K. E. (1988). Belief systems, exposure to stress, and post-traumatic stress disorder in Vietnam veterans (Doctoral dissertation, University of Massachusetts at Amherst, 1988). *Dissertation Abstracts International, 49,* 1981B.

Fletcher, K. E. (1994). *What we know about children's posttraumatic stress responses: A meta-analysis of the empirical literature.* Unpublished manuscript, University of Massachusetts Medical Center, Worcester.

Fletcher, K. E. (1996, November). *Measuring school-aged children's PTSD: Preliminary psychometrics of four new measures.* Paper presented at the Twelfth Annual Meeting of the International Society for Traumatic Stress Studies, San Francisco.

Foa, E. B., Steketee, G., & Rothbaum, B. O. (1989). Behavioral/cognitive conceptualizations of post-traumatic stress disorder. *Behavior Therapy, 20,* 155–176.

Foa, E. B., Zinbarg, R., & Rothbaum, B. O. (1992). Uncontrollability and unpredictabiity in post-traumatic stress disorder: An animal model. *Psychological Bulletin, 112,* 218–238.

Foy, D. W., Resnick, H. S., Sipprelle, R. C., & Carroll, E. M. (1987). Premilitary, military, and postmilitary factors in the development of combat-related stress disorders. *The Behavior Therapist, 10,* 3–9.

Frederick, C. J. (1985a). Children traumatized by catastrophic situations. In S. Eth & R. S. Pynoos (Eds.), *Posttraumatic stress disorder in children* (pp. 73–99). Washington, DC: American Psychiatric Press.

Frederick, C. J. (1985b). Selected foci in the spectrum of posttraumatic stress disorders. In J. Laube & S. A. Murphy (Eds.), *Perspectives on disaster recovery* (pp. 110–130). East Norwalk, CT: Appleton-Century-Crofts.

Frederick, C. J. (1986). Post-traumatic stress disorder and child molestation. In A. W. Burgess & C. R. Hartman (Eds.), *Sexual exploitation of patients by health professionals* (pp. 133–142). New York: Praeger.

Frederick, C. J. (1988). Minority status and adolescent depression and/or suicide. In A. R. Stiffman & R. A. Feldman (Eds.), *Advances in adolescent mental health: Depression and suicide* (Vol. 3, pp. 159–169). Greenwich, CT: JAI Press.

Freud, A., & Burlingham, D. T. (1943). *War and children.* Westport, CT: Greenwood Press.

Freud, S. (1955). Beyond the pleasure principle. In J. Strachey (Ed. and Trans.), *The standard edition of the complete psychological works of Sigmund Freud* (Vol. 18, pp. 37–64). London: Hogarth Press. (Original work published 1920)

Freud, S. (1964). Moses and monotheism. In J. Strachey (Ed. and Trans.), *The standard edition of the complete psychological works of Sigmund Freud* (Vol. 23, pp. 3–137). London: Hogarth Press. (Original work published 1939)

Friedman, P., & Linn, L. (1957). Some psychiatric notes on the *Andrea Doria* disaster. *American Journal of Psychiatry, 14,* 426–432.

Galante, R., & Foa, D. (1986). An epidemiological study of psychic trauma and treatment effectiveness for children after a natural disaster. *Journal of the American Academy of Child Psychiatry, 25,* 357–363.

Garland, A. F., Hough, R. L., McCabe, K. M., Yeh, M., Wood, P. A., & Aarons, G. A. (2001). Prevalence of psychiatric disorders in youths across five sectors of care. *Journal of the American Academy of Child and Adolescent Psychiatry, 40,* 409–418.

Garmezy, N., & Rutter, M. (1985). Acute reactions to stress. In M. Rutter & L. Hersov (Eds.), *Child and adolescent psychiatry: Modern approaches* (2nd ed., pp. 152–176). Oxford: Blackwell.

Gathercole, S. E. (1998). The development of memory. *Journal of Child Psychology and Psychiatry, 39,* 3–27.

Gislason, I. L., & Call, J. D. (1982). Dog bite in infancy: Trauma and personality development. *Journal of the American Academy of Child Psychiatry, 21,* 203–207.

Glaser, D. (2000). Child abuse and neglect and the brain: A review. *Journal of Child Psychology and Psychiatry, 41,* 97–116.

Gleser, G., Green, B. L., & Winget, C. (1981). *Prolonged psychological effects of disaster: A study of Buffalo Creek.* New York: Academic Press.

Goenjian, A. K., Karayan, J., Pynoos, R. S., Minassian, D., Najarian, L. M., Steinberg, A. M., & Fairbanks, L. A. (1997). Outcome of psychotherapy among early adolescents after trauma. *American Journal of Psychiatry, 154,* 536–542.

Goenjian, A. K., Molina, L., Steinberg, A. M., Fairbanks, L. A., Alvarez, M. L., Goenjian, H. A., & Pynoos, R. S. (2001). Posttraumatic stress and depressive reactions among Nicaraguan adolescents after Hurricane Mitch. *American Journal of Psychiatry, 158,* 788–794.

Goenjian, A. K., Pynoos, R. S., Steinberg, A. M., Najarian, L. M., Asarnow, J. R., Karayan, I., Ghurabi, M., & Fairbanks, L. A. (1995). Psychiatric comorbidity in children after the 1988 earthquake in Armenia. *Journal of the American Academy of Child and Adolescent Psychiatry, 34,* 1174–1184.

Goenjian, A. K., Yehuda, R., Pynoos, R. S., Steinberg, A. M., Tashjian, M., Yang, R. K., Najarian, L. M., & Fairbanks, L. A. (1996). Basal cortisol, dexamethasone suppression of cortisol, and MHPG in adolescents after the 1988 earthquake in Armenia. *American Journal of Psychiatry, 153*, 929–934.

Gomes-Schwartz, B., Horowitz, J. M., Cardelli, A. P., & Sauzier, M. (1990). The aftermath of child sexual abuse: 18 months later. In B. Gomes-Schwartz, J. M. Horowitz, & A. P. Cardarelli (Eds.), *Child sexual abuse: The initial effects* (pp. 132–152). Newbury Park, CA: Sage.

Gomes-Schwartz, B., Horowitz, J. M., & Sauzier, M. (1985). Severity of emotional distress among sexually abused preschool, school-age, and adolescent children. *Hospital and Community Psychiatry, 36*, 503–508.

Green, A. H. (1983). Child abuse: Dimension of psychological trauma in abused children. *Journal of the American Academy of Child Psychiatry, 22*, 231–237.

Green, A. H. (1985). Children traumatized by physical abuse. In S. Eth & R. S. Pynoos (Eds.), *Post-traumatic stress disorder in children* (pp. 135–154). Washington, DC: American Psychiatric Press.

Green, B.L. (1993a). Disasters and posttraumatic stress disorder. In J. R. T. Davidson & E. B. Foa (Eds.), *Posttraumatic stress disorder: DSM-IV and beyond* (pp. 75–97). Washington, DC: American Psychiatric Press.

Green, B. L. (1993b). Identifying survivors at risk: Trauma and stressors across events. In J. P. Wilson & B. Raphael (Eds.), *International handbook of traumatic stress syndromes* (pp. 135–144). New York: Plenum Press.

Green, B. L., Grace, M. C., Vary, M. G., Kramer, T. L., Gleser, G. C., & Leonard, A. C. (1994). Children of disaster in the second decade: A 17-year follow-up of Buffalo Creek survivors. *Journal of the American Academy of Child and Adolescent Psychiatry, 33*, 71–79.

Green, B. L., Korol, M., Grace, M. C., Vary, M. G., Leonard, A. C., Gleser, G. C., & Smitson-Cohen, S. (1991). Children and disaster: Age, gender, and parental effects on PTSD symptoms. *Journal of the American Academy of Child and Adolescent Psychiatry, 30*, 945–951.

Green, B. L., Wilson, J. P., & Lindy, J. D. (1985). Conceptualizing post-traumatic stress disorder: A psychosocial framework. In C. R. Figley (Ed.), *Trauma and its wake* (Vol. 1, pp. 53–69). New York: Brunner/Mazel.

Grinker, R. R., & Spiegel, J. P. (1945). *Men under stress*. Philadelphia: Blakiston.

Hadi, F. A., & Llabre, M. M. (1998). The Gulf crisis experience of Kuwaiti children: Psychological and cognitive factors. *Journal of Traumatic Stress, 11*, 45–56.

Handford, H., Mayes, S. D., Mattison, R. E., Humphrey, F. J., Bagnoto, S., Bixler, E. O., & Kales, J. D. (1986). Child and parent reaction to the Three Mile Island nuclear accident. *Journal of the American Academy of Child Psychiatry, 25*, 346–356.

Harel, Z., Kahana, B., & Wilson, J. P. (1993). War and remembrance: The legacy of Pearl Harbor. In J. P. Wilson & B. Raphael (Eds.), *International handbook of traumatic stress syndomes* (pp. 263–274). New York: Plenum Press.

Harrison, S. I., Davenport, C. W., & McDermott, J. F. (1967). Children's reactions to bereavements: Adult confusions and misperceptions. *Archives of General Psychiatry, 17*, 593–597.

Heltzer, J., Robins, L., & McEvoy, L. (1987). Post-traumatic stress disorder in the general population: Findings of the Epidemiologic Catchment Area survey. *New England Journal of Medicine, 317*, 1630–1634.

Herman, J. L., Perry, J. C., & van der Kolk, B. A. (1989). Childhood trauma in borderline personality disorder. *American Journal of Psychiatry, 146*, 490–495.

Hjern, A., Angel, B., & Höjer, B. (1991). Persecution and behavior: A report from Chile. *Child Abuse and Neglect, 15*, 239–248.

Holahan, C. J., & Moos, R. H. (1987). Risk, resistance, and psychological distress: A longitudinal analysis with adults and children. *Journal of Abnormal Psychology, 96*, 3–13.

Horowitz, M. J. (1976a). *Stress response syndromes*. New York: Aronson.

Horowitz, M. J. (1976b). Psychological response to serious life events. In V. Hamilton & D. M. Warburton (Eds.), *Human stress and cognition* (pp. 235–263). New York: Wiley.

Hussain, S. A., Nair, J., Holcomb, W., Reid, J. C., Vargas, V., & Nair, S. S. (1998). Stress reactions of children and adolescents in war and siege conditions. *American Journal of Psychiatry, 155*, 1718–1719.

Jaffe, P., Wolfe, D., Wilson, S. K., & Zak, L. (1986). Family violence and child adjustment: A comparative analysis of girls' and boys' behavioral symptoms. *American Journal of Psychiatry, 143*, 74–77.

Janoff-Bulman, R. (1989). Assumptive worlds and the stress of traumatic events: Applications of the schema construct. *Social Cognition, 7*, 113–136.

Jones, J. C., & Barlow, D. H. (1990). The etiology of posttraumatic stress disorder. *Clinical Psychology Review, 10*, 299–328.

Jones, M. C., Dauphinais, P., Sack, W. H., & Somervell, P. D. (1997). Trauma-related symptomatology among American Indian adolescents. *Journal of Traumatic Stress, 10*, 163–173.

Jones, R. T. (1996). Psychometric review of Child's Reaction to Traumatic Events Scale (CRTES). In B. H. Stamm (Ed.), *Measurement of stress, trauma, and adaptation* (pp. 78–80). Lutherville, MD: Sidran Press.

Jones, R. T., & Ribbe, D. P. (1991). Child, adolescent, and adult victims of residential fire: Psychological consequences. *Behavior Modification, 15*, 560–580.

Joseph, S. A., Brewin, C. R., Yule, W., & Williams, R. (1993). Casusal attributions and post-traumatic stress in adolescents. *Journal of Child Psychology and Psychiatry, 34*, 247–253.

Joseph, S. A., Williams, R., & Yule, W. (1993). Changes in outlook following disaster: Development of a measure to assess positive and negative responses. *Journal of Traumatic Stress, 6*, 271–279.

Jouriles, E. N., Murphy, C. M., & O'Leary, D. (1989). Interspousal aggression, marital discord, and child problems. *Journal of Consulting and Clinical Psychology, 57*, 453–455.

Kagan, J. (1983). Stress and coping in early development. In N. Garmezy & M. Rutter (Eds.), *Stress, coping, and development in children* (pp. 191–216). New York: McGraw-Hill.

Kardiner, A. (1941). *The traumatic neuroses of war*. New York: Hoeber.

Karr-Morse, R., & Wiley, M. (1997). *Ghosts from the nursery: Tracing the roots of violence*. New York: Atlantic Monthly Press.

Keane, T. M. (1993). Symptomatology of Vietnam veterans with posttraumatic stress disorder. In J. R. T. Davidson & E. B. Foa (Eds.), *Posttraumatic stress disorder: DSM-IV and beyond* (pp. 99–111). Washington, DC: American Psychiatric Press.

Keane, T. M., Fairbank, J. A., Caddell, J. M., Zimering, R. T., & Bender, M. E. (1985). A behavioral approach to assessing and treating post-traumatic stress disorder in

Vietnam veterans. In C. R. Figley (Ed.), *Trauma and its wake* (Vol. 1, pp. 257–294). New York: Brunner/Mazel.

Kendall-Tackett, K. A., Williams, L. M., & Finkelhor, D. (1993). Impact of sexual abuse on children: A review and synthesis of recent empirical studies. *Psychological Bulletin, 113*, 164–180.

Khoury, E. L., Warheit, G. J., Hargrove, M. C., Zimmerman, R. S., Vega, W. A., & Gil, A. G. (1997). The impact of Hurricane Andrew on deviant behavior among a multiracial/ethnic sample of adolescents in Dade County, Florida: A longitudinal analysis. *Journal of Traumatic Stress, 10*, 71–91.

Kilpatrick, D., & Resnick, H. (1993). PTSD associated with exposure to criminal victimization in clinical and community populations. In J. Davidson & E. Foa (Eds.), *Posttraumatic stress disorder:DSM-IV and beyond* (pp. 99–111). Washington, DC: American Psychiatric Press.

King, J., Mandansky, D., King, S., Fletcher, K. E., & Brewer, J. (2001). Early sexual abuse and low cortisol. *Psychiatry and Clinical Neurosciences, 55*, 71–74.

Kinzie, J. D., & Goetz, R. R. (1996). A century of controversy surrounding posttraumatic stress-spectrum syndromes: The impact on DSM-III and DSM-IV. *Journal of Traumatic Stress, 9*, 159–179.

Kinzie, J. D., Sack, W. H., Angell, R. H., Clarke, G., & Ben, R. (1989). A three-year follow-up of Cambodian young people traumatized as children. *Journal of the American Academy of Child and Adolescent Psychiatry, 28*, 501–504.

Kinzie, J. D., Sack, W. H., Angell, R. H., Manson, S., & Rath, B. (1986). The psychiatric effects of massive trauma on Cambodian children: I. The children. *Journal of the American Academy of Child Psychiatry, 25*, 370–376.

Kiser, L. J., Ackerman, B. J., Brown, E., Edwards, N. B., McColgan, E., Pugh, R., & Pruitt, D. B. (1988). Posttraumatic stress disorder in young children: A reaction to purported sexual abuse. *Journal of the American Academy of Child Adolescent Psychiatry, 27*, 645–649.

Kiser, L. J., Heston, J., Millsap, P. A., & Pruitt, D. B. (1991). Physical and sexual abuse in childhood: Relationship with post-traumatic stress disorder. *Journal of the American Academy of Child and Adolescent Psychiatry, 30*, 776–783.

Kluft, R. P. (1985). *Childhood antecedents of multiple personality.* Washington, DC: American Psychiatric Press.

Korol, M., Green, B. L., & Gleser, G. C. (1999). Children's responses to a nuclear waste disaster: PTSD symptoms and outcome prediction. *Journal of the American Academy of Child and Adolescent Psychiatry, 38*, 368–375.

Kulka, R. A., Schlenger, W. E., Fairbank, J. A., Hough, R. L., Jordan, B. K., Marmar, C. R., & Weiss, D. S. (1990). *Trauma and the Vietnam War generation: Report of the findings from the National Vietnam Veterans Readjustment Study.* New York: Brunner/Mazel.

Lacey, G. N. (1972). Observations on Aberfan. *Journal of Psychosomatic Research, 16*, 257–260.

La Greca, A. M., Silverman, W. K., Vernberg, E. M., & Prinstein, M. J. (1996). Symptoms of posttraumatic stress in children after Hurricane Andrew: A prospective study. *Journal of Consulting and Clinical Psychology, 64*, 712–723.

Lazarus, R. S., & Folkman, S. (1984). *Stress, appraisal and coping.* New York: Springer.

Lehmann, P. (2000). Posttraumatic stress disorder (PTSD) and child witnesses to mother-assault: A summary and review. *Children and Youth Services Review, 22*, 275–306.

Lifton, R. J. (1967). *Death in life: Survivors of Hiroshima.* New York: Random House.

Lindholm, K. J., & Willey, R. (1986). Ethnic differences in child abuse and sexual abuse. *Hispanic Journal of Behavioral Sciences, 8*, 111–125.

Lonigan, C. J., Shannon, M. P., Finch, A. J., Jr., Daugherty, T. K., & Taylor, C. M. (1991). Children's reactions to a natural disaster: Symptom severity and degree of exposure. *Advances in Behaviour Research and Therapy, 13*, 135–154.

Luthar, S. S. (1991). Vulnerability and resilience: A study of high risk adolescents. *Child Development, 62*, 600–616.

Maccoby, E. E. (1983). Social-emotional development and response to stressors. In N. Garmezy & M. Rutter (Eds.), *Stress, coping, and development in children* (pp. 217–234). New York: McGraw-Hill.

Maccoby, E. E., & Martin, J. A. (1983). Socialization in the context of the family: Parent–child interaction. In P. H. Mussen (Series Ed.) & E. M. Hetherington (Vol. Ed.), *Handbook of child psychology: Vol. 4.* Socialization, personality, and social development (4th ed., pp. 1–101). New York: Wiley.

Malmquist, C. P. (1986). Children who witness parental murder: Posttraumatic aspects. *Journal of the American Academy of Child Psychiatry, 25*, 320–325.

Mannarino, A. P., Cohen, J. A., & Berman, S. R. (1994). The relationship between preabuse factors and psychological symptomatology in sexually abused girls. *Child Abuse and Neglect, 18*, 63–71.

Mannarino, A. P., Cohen, J. A., Smith, J. A., & Moore-Motily, S. (1991). Six- and twelve-month follow-up of sexually abused girls. *Journal of Interpersonal Violence, 6*, 494–511.

March, J. S., Amaya-Jackson, L., Murray, M. C., & Schulte, A. (1998). Cognitive-behavioral psychotherapy for children and adolescents with posttraumatic stress disorder after a single-incident stressor. *Journal of the American Academy of Child and Adolescent Psychiatry, 37*, 585–593.

March, J. S., Amaya-Jackson, L., Terry, R., & Costanzo, P. (1997). Posttraumatic symptomatology in children and adolescents after an industrial fire. *Journal of the American Academy of Child Psychiatry, 36*, 1080–1088.

Martinez, P., & Richters, J. E. (1993). The NIMH Community Violence Project: II. Children's distress symptoms associated with violence exposure. *Psychiatry, 56*, 22–35.

Masten, A. S., Garmezy, N., Tellegen, A., Pellegrini, D. S., Larkin, K., & Larsen, A. (1988). Competence and stress in school children: The moderating effects of individual and family qualities. *Journal of Child Psychology and Psychiatry, 29*, 745–764.

McCann, I. L., & Pearlman, L. A. (1990a). *Through a glass darkly: Understanding and treating the adult trauma survivor through constructivist self-development theory.* New York: Brunner/Mazel.

McCann, I. L., & Pearlman, L. A. (1990b). Vicarious traumatization: A framework for understanding the psychological effects of working with victims. *Journal of Traumatic Stress, 3*, 131–149.

McCloskey, L. A., & Walker, M. (2000). Posttraumatic stress in children exposed to family violence and single-event trauma. *Journal of the American Academy of Child and Adolescent Psychiatry, 39*, 108–115.

McFarlane, A. C. (1987a). Posttraumatic phenomena in a longitudinal study of children following a natural disaster. *Journal of the American Academy of Child and Adolescent Psychiatry, 26*, 764–769.

McFarlane, A. C. (1987b). Family functioning and overprotection following a natural disaster: The longitudinal effects of post-traumatic morbidity. *Australian and New Zealand Journal of Psychiatry, 21*, 210–218.

McFarlane, A. C., Policansky, S., & Irwin, C. P. (1987). A longitudinal study of the psychological morbidity in children due to a natural disaster. *Psychological Medicine, 17*, 727–738.

McLeer, S. V., Deblinger, E., Atkins, M. S., Foa, E. B., & Ralphe, D. L. (1988). Post-traumatic stress disorder in sexually abused children. *Journal of the American Academy of Child and Adolescent Psychiatry*, 27, 650–654.

Milgram, N. A. (1989). Children under stress. In T. H. Ollendick & M. Hersen (Eds.), *Handbook of child psychopathology* (2nd ed., pp. 399–415). New York: Plenum Press.

Milgram, R. M., & Milgram, N. A. (1976). The effect of the Yom Kippur War on anxiety level in Israeli children. *Journal of Psychology, 94*, 107–113.

Milgram, N., & Toubiana, Y. H. (1996). Children's selective coping after a bus disaster: Confronting behavior and perceived support. *Journal of Traumatic Stress, 9*, 687–702.

Miller, S. M. (1979). Controllability and human stress: Method, evidence, and theory. *Behaviour Research and Therapy, 17*, 287–304.

Milne, G. (1977). Cyclone Tracy: II The effects on Darwin children. *Australian Psychologist, 12*, 55–62.

Mineka, S. (1979). The role of fear in theories of avoidance learning, flooding, and extinction. *Psychological Bulletin, 86*, 985–1010.

Mineka, S. M., & Kihlstrom, J. F. (1978). Unpredictable and uncontrollable events: A new perspective on experimental neurosis. *Journal of Abnormal Psychology, 87*, 256–271.

Moran, P. B., & Eckenrode, J. (1992). Protective personality characteristics among adolescent victims of maltreatment. *Child Abuse and Neglect, 16*, 743–754.

Mowrer, O. H. (1960). *Learning theory and behavior*. New York: Wiley.

Myers, C. S. (1940). *Shell shock in France, 1914–18*. Cambridge, England: Cambridge University Press.

Nader, K., Kriegler, J. A., Blake, D. D., & Pynoos, R. S. (1993). *Clinician-Administered PTSD Scale for Children (CAPS-C)*. Unpublished manuscript, UCLA Neuropsychiatric Institute and Hospital and the National Center for PTSD.

Nader, K., Pynoos, R., Fairbanks, L., & Frederick, C. (1990). Children's PTSD reactions one year after a sniper attack at their school. *American Journal of Psychiatry, 147*, 1526–1530.

National Clearinghouse on Child Abuse and Neglect. (2002). National Child Abuse and Neglect Data System (NCANDS) Summary of Key Findings from Calendar Year 2000. [Online]. Available: httpp://www.calib.com/nccanch/pubs/factsheets/canstats.cfm.

National Safe Kids Campaign. (2002). Injury facts: Burn injury. [Online]. Available:http://www.safekids.org/tier3_cd.cfm?content_item_id=1011&folder_id=540.

Newman, C. J. (1976). Children of disaster: Clinical observations at Buffalo Creek. *American Journal of Psychiatry, 133*, 306–312.

Nir, Y. (1985). Post-traumatic stress disorder in children with cancer. In S. Eth & R. S. Pynoos (Eds.), *Post-traumatic stress disorder in children* (pp. 123–132). Washington, DC: American Psychiatric Press.

Norris, F. H. (1988). *Toward establishing a database for the prospective study of traumatic stress*. Paper presented at the National Institute of Mental Health workshop Traumatic Stress: Defining Terms and Instruments, Uniformed Services University of the Health Sciences, Bethesda, MD.

Norris, F. H. (1992). Epidemiology of trauma: Frequency and impact of different potentially traumatic events on different demographic groups. *Journal of Consulting and Clinical Psychology, 60*, 409–418.

Norris, F. H., & Kaniasty, K. (1991). The psychological experience of crime: A test of the mediating role of beliefs in explaining the distress of victims. *Journal of Social and Clinical Psychology, 10*, 239–261.

Paardekooper, B., de Jong, J. T. V. M., & Hermanns, J. M. A. (1999). The psychological impact of war and the refugee situation on South Sudanese children in refugee camps in Northern Uganda: An exploratory study. *Journal of Child Psychology and Psychiatry, 40*, 529–536.

Page, H. (1885). *Injuries of the spine and spinal cord without apparent mechanical lesion*. London: Churchill.

Pelcovitz, D., Libov, B. G., Mandel, F., Kaplan, S., Weinblatt, M., & Septimus, A. (1998). Posttraumatic stress disorder and family functioning in adolescent cancer. *Journal of Traumatic Stress, 11*, 205–221.

Perkins, C. (1997). Age patterns of victims of serious violent crime. *Bureau of Justice Statistics special report* (Report NCJ-162031, U.S. Department of Justice Office of Justice Programs). Washington, DC: Author.

Perry, B. D. (1994). Neurobiological sequelae of childhood trauma: PTSD in children. In M. M. Murberg (Ed.), *Catecholamine function in posttraumatic stress disorder: Emerging concepts* (pp. 233–256). Washington, DC: American Psychiatric Press.

Peterson, C., & Seligman (1983). Learned helplessness and victimization. *Journal of Social Issues, 2*, 103–116.

Pfefferbaum, B. (1997). Posttraumatic stress disorder in children: A review of the past 10 years. *Journal of the American Academy of Child and Adolescent Psychiatry, 36*, 1503–1511.

Pfefferbaum, B., Gurwitch, R. H., McDonald, N. B., Leftwich, M. J. T., Sconzo, G. M., Messenbaugh, A. K., & Schultz, R. A. (2000). Posttraumatic stress among young children after the death of a friend or acquaintance in a terrorist bombing. *Psychiatric Services, 51*, 386–388.

Pfefferbaum, B., Nixon, S. J., Krug, R. S., Tivis, R. D., Moore, V. L., Brown, J. M., Pynoos, R. S., Foy, D., & Gurwich, R. H. (1999). Clinical needs assessment of middle and high school students following the 1995 Oklahoma City bombing. *American Journal of Psychiatry, 156*, 1069–1074.

Pfefferbaum, B., Nixon, S. J., Tucker, P. M., Tivis, R. D., Moore, V. L., Gurwitch, R. H., Pynoos, R. S., & Geis, H. K. (1999). Posttraumatic stress responses in bereaved children after the Oklahoma City bombing. *Journal of the American Academy of Child and Adolescent Psychiatry, 38*, 1372–1379.

Pfefferbaum, B., Seale, T. W., McDonald, N. B., Brandt, E. N., Jr., Rainwater, S. M., Maynard, B. T., Meierhoefer, B., & Miller, P. D. (2000). Posttraumatic stress two years after the Oklahoma City bombing in youths geographically distant from the explosion. *Psychiatry: Interpersonal & Biological Processes, 63*, 358–370.

Piaget, J., & Inhelder, B. (1969). *The psychology of the child*. New York: Basic Books.

Pierce, L. H., & Pierce, R. L. (1984). Race as a factor in the sexual abuse of children. *Social Work Research Abstracts, 20*, 9–14.

Pittman, R. K. (1988). Post-traumatic stress disorder, conditioning, and network theory. *Psychiatric Annual, 18,* 182–189.

Punamaeki, R., Oouta, S., & El-Sarraj, E. (2001). Resiliency factors predicting psychological adjustment after political violence among Palestinian children. *International Journal of Behavioral Development, 25,* 256–267.

Putnam, F. W. (1998). Trauma models of the effects of childhood maltreatment. *Journal of Aggression, Maltreatment, and Trauma, 2,* 51–66.

Pynoos, R. S., & Eth, S. (1985a). Children traumatized by witnessing acts of personal violence: Homicide, rape, or suicide behavior. In S. Eth & R. S. Pynoos (Eds.), *Posttraumatic stress disorder in children* (pp. 19–43). Washington, DC: American Psychiatric Press.

Pynoos, R. S., & Eth, S. (1985b). Developmental perspective on psychic trauma in childhood. In C. R. Figley (Ed.) *Trauma and its wake* (Vol. 1, pp. 36–52). New York: Brunner/Mazel.

Pynoos, R. S., Frederick, C., Nader, K., Arroyo, W., Steinberg, A., Eth, S., Nunez, F., & Fairbanks, L. (1987). Life threat and posttraumatic stress in school-age children. *Archives of General Psychiatry, 44,* 1057–1063.

Pynoos, R. S., & Nader, K. (1988). Children who witness the sexual assaults of their mothers. *Journal of the American Academy of Child and Adolescent Psychiatry, 27,* 567–572.

Pynoos, R. S., & Nader, K. (1989). Children's memory and proximity to violence. *Journal of the American Academy of Child and Adolescent Psychiatry, 28,* 236–241.

Pynoos, R. S., Steinberg, A. M., & Wraith, R. (1995). A developmental model of childhood traumatic stress. In D. Cicchetti & D. J. Cohen (Eds.), *Developmental psychopathology: Vol. 2. Risk, disorder, and adaptation* (pp. 72–95). New York: Wiley.

Rado, S. (1942). Pathodynamics and treatment of war neurosis (traumatophobia). *Psychosomatic Medicine, 42,* 363–368.

Rao, K., DiClemente, R. J., & Ponton, L. E. (1992). Child sexual abuse of Asians compared with other populations. *Journal of the American Academy of Child and Adolscent Psychiatry, 31,* 880–886.

Realmuto, G. M., Masten, A., Carole, L. F., Hubbard, J., Groteluschen, A., & Chhun, B. (1992). Adolescent survivors of massive childhood trauma in Cambodia: Life events and current symptoms. *Journal of Traumatic Stress, 4,* 589–599.

Rigamer, E. F. (1986). Psychological management of children in a national crisis. *Journal of the American Academy of Child Psychiatry, 25,* 364–369.

Rossman, B. B. R. (1992). School-age children's perceptions of coping with distress: Strategies for emotion regulation and the moderation of adjustment. *Journal of Child Psychology and Psychiatry, 33,* 1373–1397.

Rossman, B. B. R., Bingham, R. D., & Emde, R. N. (1997). Symptomatology and adaptive functioning for children exposed to normative stressors, dog attack, and parental violence. *Journal of the American Academy of Child and Adolescent Psychiatry, 36,* 1089–1097.

Roth, S., Lebowitz, L., & DeRosa, R. R. (1997). Thematic assessment of posttraumatic stress reactions. In J. P. Wilson & T. M. Keane (Eds.), *Assessing psychological trauma and PTSD* (pp. 512–528). New York: Guilford Press.

Rotter, J. B. (1966). Generalized expectancies for internal versus external control of reinforcement. *Psychological Monographs, 80*(1, Whole No. 609).

Ruggiero, K. J., Morris, T. L., & Scotti, J. R. (2001). Treatment for children with posttraumatic stress disorder: Current status and future directions. *Clinical Psychology: Science and Practice, 8,* 210–227.

Rutter, M. (1983). Stress, coping, and development: Some issues and questions. In N. Garmezy & M. Rutter (Eds.), *Stress, coping, and development in children* (pp. 1–41). New York: McGraw-Hill.

Rutter, M., & Graham, P. (1967). A children's behaviour questionnaire for completion by teachers: Preliminary findings. *Journal of Child Psychology and Psychiatry, 8,* 1–11.

Rutter, M., Tizard, J., & Whitmore, K. (1970). *Education, health, and behavior.* London: Longman.

Saigh, P. A. (1985). Adolescent anxiety following varying degrees of war exposure. *Journal of Clinical Child Psychology, 14,* 311–314.

Saigh, P. A. (1989). The development and validation of the Children's Posttraumatic Stress Disorder Inventory. *International Journal of Special Education, 4,* 75–84.

Saigh, P. A. (1991). The development of posttraumatic stress disorder following four different types of traumatization. *Behaviour Research and Therapy, 29,* 213–216.

Saigh, P. A., & Bremner, J. D. (1999). The history of posttraumatic stress disorder. In P. A. Saigh & J. D. Bremner (Eds.), *Posttraumatic stress disorder* (pp. 1–17). Needham Heights, MA: Allyn & Bacon.

Saigh, P. A., Yasik, A. E., Oberfield, R. A., Green, B. L., Halamandaris, P. V., Rubenstein, H., Nester, J., Resko, J., Hetz, B., & McHugh, M. (2000). The Children's PTSD Inventory: Development and reliability. *Journal of Traumatic Stress, 13,* 369–380.

Saigh, P. A., Yasik, A. E., Oberfield, R. A., & Inamdar, S. C. (1999). Behavioral assessment of child-adolescent posttraumatic stress disorder. In P. A. Saigh & J. D. Bremner (Eds.), *Posttraumatic stress disorder* (pp. 354–375). Needham Heights, MA: Allyn & Bacon.

Saigh, P. A., Yasik, A. E., Sack, W. H., & Koplewicz, H. S. (1999). Child–adolescent posttraumatic stress disorder: Prevalence, risk factors, and comorbidity. In P. A. Saigh & J. D. Bremner (Eds.), *Posttraumatic stress disorder* (pp. 18–43). Needham Heights, MA: Allyn & Bacon.

Scheeringa, M. S., Zeanah, C. H., Drell, M. J., & Larrieu, J. A. (1995). Two approaches to the diagnosis of posttraumatic stress disorder in infancy and early childhood. *Journal of the American Academy of Child and Adolescent Psychiatry, 34,* 191–200.

Scheeringa, M. S., Peebles, C. D., Cook, C. A., & Zeanah, C. H. (2001). Toward establishing procedural, criterion, and discriminant validity for PTSD in early childhood. *Journal of the American Academy of Child and Adolescent Psychiatry, 40,* 52–60.

Schwarz, E. D., & Kowalski, J. M. (1991a). Malignant memories: PTSD in children and adults after a school shooting. *Journal of the American Academy of Child and Adolescent Psychiatry, 30,* 936–944.

Schwarz, E. D., & Kowalski, J. M. (1991b). Posttraumatic stress disorder after a school shooting: Effects of symptom threshold selection and diagnosis by DSM-III, DSM-III-R, or proposed DSM-IV. *American Journal of Psychiatry, 148,* 592–597.

Scurfield, R. M. (1993). Posttraumatic stress disorder in Vietnam veterans. In J. P. Wilson & B. Raphael (Eds.), *International handbook of traumatic stress syndromes* (pp. 285–295). New York: Plenum Press.

Seifer, R., Sameroff, A. J., Baldwin, C. P., & Baldwin, A. (1992). Child and family factors that amerliorate risk between 4 and 13 years of age. *Journal of the American Academy of Child and Adolescent Psychiatry*, *31*, 893–903.

Senior, N., Gladstone, T., & Narcombe, B. (1982). Child snatching: A case report. *Journal of the American Academy of Child Psychiatry*, *21*, 893–903.

Shannon, M. P., Lonigan, C. J., Finch, A. J., Jr., & Taylor, C. M. (1994). Children exposed to disaster: I. Epidemiology of post-traumatic symptoms and symptom profiles. *Journal of the American Academy of Child and Adolescent Psychiatry*, *33*, 80–93.

Silber, E., Perry, S. E., & Bloch, D. A. (1958). Patterns of parent–child interaction in disaster. *Psychiatry*, *21*, 159–167.

Silva, R. R., Alpert, M., Munoz, D. M., Singh, S., Matzner, F., & Dummit, S. (2000). Stress and vulnerability to posttraumatic stress disorder in children and adolescents. *American Journal of Psychiatry*, *157*, 1229–1235.

Sirles, E. A., Smith, J. A., & Kusama, H. (1989). Psychiatric status of intrafamilial child sexual abuse victims. *Journal of the American Academy of Child and Adolescent Psychiatry*, *28*, 225–229.

Skidmore, G. L., & Fletcher, K. E. (1997, November). *Assessing trauma's impact on beliefs: The World View Survey.* Paper presented at the Thirteenth Annual Meeting of the International Society for Traumatic Stress Studies, Montreal.

Slater, M. A., & Power, T. G. (1987). Multidimensional assessment of parenting in single-parent families. In, J. P. Vincent (Ed.), *Advances in family intervention, assessment and theory* (Vol. 4, pp. 197–228). Greenwich, CT: JAI Press.

Smith, E. M., & North, C. S. (1993). Posttraumatic stress disorder in natural disasters and technological accidents. In J. P. Wilson & B. Raphael (Eds.), *International handbook of traumatic stress syndromes* (pp. 405–419). New York: Plenum Press.

Spirito, A., Stark, J., & Williams, C. (1988). Development of a brief coping checklist for use with pediatric populations. *Journal of Pediatric Psychology*, *13*, 555–574.

Stallard, P., Velleman, R., Langsford, J., & Baldwin, S. (2001). Coping and psychological distress in children involved in road traffic accidents. *British Journal of Clinical Psychology*, *40*, 197–208.

Stein, B., Comer, D., Gardner, W., & Kelleher, K. (1999). Prospective study of displaced children's symptoms in wartime Bosnia. *Social Psychiatry Psychiatric Epidemiology*, *34*, 464–469.

Stoddard, F. J., Norman, D. K., & Murphy, J. M. (1989). A diagnostic outcome study of children and adolescents with severe burns. *The Journal of Trauma*, *29*, 471–477.

Stuber, M. L., Nader, K., Yasuda, P., Pynoos, R. S., & Cohen, S. (1991). Stress response after pediatric bone marrow transplantation: Preliminary results of a prospective longitudinal study. *Journal of the American Academy of Child and Adolescent Psychiatry*, *30*, 952–957.

Terr, L. C. (1979). Children of Chowchilla: A study of psychic trauma. *Psychoanalytic Study of the Child*, *34*, 552–623.

Terr, L. C. (1981a). "Forbidden games": Post-traumatic child's play. *Journal of the American Academy of Child Psychiatry*, *20*, 741–760.

Terr, L. C. (1981b). Psychic trauma in children: Observations following the Chowchilla school-bus kidnapping. *American Journal of Psychiatry*, *138*, 14–19.

Terr, L. C. (1983a). Child snatching: A new epidemic of an ancient malady. *Pediatrics*, *103*, 151–156.

Terr, L. C. (1983b). Chowchilla revisited: The effects of psychic trauma four years after a school-bus kidnapping. *American Journal of Psychiatry*, *140*, 1543–1550.

Terr, L. C. (1985a). Children traumatized in small groups. In S. Eth & R. S. Pynoos (Eds.), *Post-traumatic stress disorder in children* (pp. 47–70). Washington, DC: American Psychiatric Press, Inc.

Terr, L. C. (1985b). Psychic trauma in children and adolescents. *Psychiatric Clinics of North America*, *8*, 815–835.

Terr, L. C. (1991). Childhood traumas: An outline and overview. *American Journal of Psychiatry*, *148*, 10–20.

Terr, L. C. (2001, October). *School-aged children's drawings of the September 11, 2001, disasters*. Paper presented at the Second Annual Conference of the Worcester Institute on Loss and Trauma, Worcester, MA.

Terr, L. C., Bloch, D. A., Michel, B. A., Shi, H., Reinhardt, J. A., & Metayer, S. (1999). Children's symptoms in the wake of *Challenger*: A field study of distant-traumatic effects and an outline of related conditions. *American Journal of Psychiatry*, *156*, 1536–1544.

Thabet, A. A. M., & Vostanis, P. (2000). Post traumatic stress disorder reactions in children of war: A longitudinal study. *Child Abuse and Neglect*, *24*, 291–298.

True, W. R., & Pitman, R. (1999). Genetics and posttraumatic stress disorder. In P. A. Saigh & J. D. Bremner (Eds.), *Posttraumatic stress disorder* (pp. 144–159). Needham Heights, MA: Allyn & Bacon.

Tyano, S., Iancu, I., Solomon, Z., Sever, J., Goldstein, I., Touviana, Y, & Bleich, A. (1996). Seven-year follow-up of child survivors of a bus–train collision. *Journal of the American Academy of Child and Adolescent Psychiatry*, *35*, 365–373.

Udwin, O., Boyle, S., Yule, W., Bolton, D., & O'Ryan, D. (2000). Risk factors for long-term psychological effects of a disaster experienced in adolescence: Predictors of post traumatic stress disorder. *Journal of Child Psychology and Psychiatry*, *41*, 969–979.

U.S. Department of Justice. (1994). *Juvenile victimization: 1987–1992* (Fact Sheet 17, Office of Juvenile Justice and Delinquency Prevention). Washington, DC: Author.

U.S. Department of Justice Bureau of Justice Statistics. (2002). Crime and victim statistics: Victim characteristics. [Online]. Available: http://www.ojp.usdoj.gov/bjs/cvict_v.htm.

U.S. Department of Transportation. (1993). *Traffic safety facts* (Report No. DOT HS 808 022, National Highway Traffic Safety Administration). Washington, DC: Author.

Ursano, R. J., Fullerton, C. S., & McCaughey, B. G. (1994). Trauma and disaster. In R. J. Ursano, B. G. McCaughey, & C. S. Fullerton (Eds.), *Individual and community responses to trauma and disaster* (pp. 3–27). New York: Cambridge University Press.

van der Kolk, B. A. (1987). The separation cry and the trauma response: Developmental issues in the psychobiology of attachment and separation. In B. A. van der Kolk (Ed.), *Psychological trauma* (pp. 31–62). Washington, DC: American Psychiatric Press, Inc.

van der Kolk, B. A., Brown, P., & van der Hart, O. (1989). Pierre Janet on post-traumatic stress. *Journal of Traumatic Stress*, *2*, 365–378.

van der Kolk, B. A., & Sporta, J. (1993). Biological response to psychic trauma. In J. P. Wilson & B. Raphael (Eds.), *International handbook of traumatic stress syndromes* (pp. 25–33). New York: Plenum Press.

Vernberg, E. M., La Greca, A. M., Silverman, W. K., & Prinstein, M. J. (1996). Prediction of posttraumatic stress symptoms in children after Hurricane Andrew. *Journal of Abnormal Psychology, 105*, 237–248.

Veronen, L. J., & Kilpatrick, D. G. (1983). Stress management for rape victims. In D. Meichenbaum & M. E. Jaremko (Eds.), *Stress reduction and prevention* (pp. 341–374). New York: Plenum Press.

Vila, G., Porche, L., & Mouren-Simeoni, M. (1999). An 18-month longitudinal study of posttraumatic disorders in children who were taken hostage in their school. *Psychosomatic Medicine, 61*, 746–754.

Vila, G., Witowski, P., Tondini, M. C., Perez-Diaz, F., Mouren-Simeoni, M. C., & Jouvent, R. (2001). A study of posttraumatic stress disorders in children who experienced an industrial disaster in the Briey region. *European Child and Adolescent Psychiatry, 10*, 10–18.

Walker, A. M., Harris, G., Baker, A., Kelly, D., & Houghton, J. (1999). Post-traumatic stress responses following liver transplantation in older children. *Journal of Child Psychology and Psychiatry, 40*, 363–374.

Walker, L. S., & Greene, J. W. (1987). Negative life events, psychosocial resources, and psychophysiological symptoms in adolescents. *Journal of Clinical Child Psychology, 16*, 29–36.

Wasserstein, S. B., & La Greca, A. M. (1998). Hurricane Andrew: Parent conflict as a moderator of children's adjustment. *Hispanic Journal of Behavioral Sciences, 20*, 212–224.

Weisaeth, L., & Eitinger, L. (1993). Posttraumatic stress phenomena: Common themes across wars, disasters, and traumatic events. In J. P. Wilson & B. Raphael (Eds.), *International handbook of traumatic stress syndromes* (pp. 69–77). New York: Plenum Press.

Weigel, C., Wertlieb, D., & Feldstein, M. (1989). Perceptions of control, competence, and contingency as influences on the stress–behavior symptom relation in school-age children. *Journal of Personality and Social Psychology, 56*, 456–464.

Weinstein, D., Staffelbach, D., & Biaggio, M. (2000). Attention-deficit hyperactivity disorder and posttraumatic stress disorder: Differential diagnosis in childhood sexual abuse. *Clinical Psychology Review, 20*, 359–378.

Werner, E. E., & Smith, R. S. (1982). *Vulnerable but invincible: A longitudinal study of resilient children and youth*. New York: McGraw-Hill.

Wertlieb, D., Weigel, C., & Feldstein, M. (1987). Measuring children's coping. *American Journal of Orthopsychiatry, 57*, 548–560.

Wertlieb, D., Weigel, C., Springer, T., & Feldstein, M. (1987). Temperament as a moderator of children's stressful experiences. *American Journal of Orthopsychiatry, 57*, 234–245.

Wilson, J. P. (1994). The historical evolution of PTSD diagnostic criteria: From Freud to DSM-IV. *Journal of Traumatic Stress, 7*, 681–698.

Winje, D., & Ulvik, A. (1998). Long-term outcome of trauma in children: The psychological consequences of a bus accident. *Journal of Child Psychology and Psychiatry, 39*, 635–642.

Wolfe, D. A., Jaffe, P., Wilson, S. K., & Zak, L. (1985). Children of battered women: The relation of child behavior to family violence and maternal stress. *Journal of Consulting and Clinical Psychology, 53*, 657–665.

Wolfe, D. A., Zak, L., & Wilson, S. (1986). Child witnesses to violence between parents: Critical issues in behavioral and social adjustment. *Journal of Abnormal Child Psychology, 14*, 95–104.

Wolfe, V. V., Gentile, C., Michienzi, T., Sas, L., & Wolfe, D. (1991). The Children's Impact of Traumatic Events Scale: A measure of post-sexual-abuse PTSD symptoms. *Behavioral Assessment, 13*, 359–383.

Wolfe, V. V., Gentile, C., & Wolfe, D. A. (1989). The impact of sexual abuse on children: A PTSD formulation. *Behavior Therapy, 20*, 215–228.

Wozniak, J., Crawford, M. H., Biederman, J., Faraone, S. V., Spencer, T. J., Taylor, A., & Blier, H. K. (1999). Antecedents and complications of trauma in boys with ADHD: Findings from a longitudinal study. *Journal of the American Academy of Child and Adolescent Psychiatry, 38*, 48–55.

Wyman, P. A., Cowen, E. L., Work, W. C., & Parker, G. R. (1991). Developmental and family milieu correlates of resilience in urban children who have experienced major life stress. *American Journal of Community Psychology, 19*, 405–426.

Wyman, P. A., Cowen, E. L., Work. W. C., Raoof, A., Gribble, P. A., Parker, G. R., & Wannon, M. (1992). Interviews with children who experienced major life stress: Family and child attributes that predict resilient outcomes. *Journal of the American Academy of Child and Adolescent Psychiatry, 31*, 904–910.

Yates, J. L., & Nasby, W. (1993). Dissociation, affect, and network models of memory: An integrative proposal. *Journal of Traumatic Stress, 6*, 305–326.

Yehuda, R. (1998). Psychoneuroendocrinology of post-traumatic stress disorder. *Psychoneuroendocrinology, 21*, 359–379.

Yehuda, R., Kahana, B., Binder-Brynes, K., Southwick, S., Mason, J., & Giller, E. (1995). Low urinary cortisol exretion in Holocaust survivors with post-traumatic stress disorder. *American Journal of Psychiatry, 152*, 982–986.

Yule, W. (1998). Posttraumatic stress disorder in children and its treatment. In T. W. Miller (Ed.), *Stressful life events* (2nd ed., pp. 219–243). Madison, CT: International Universities Press.

Yule, W., Bolton, D., Udwin, O., Boyle, S., O'Ryan, D., & Nurrish, J. (2000). The long-term psychological effects of a disaster experienced in adolescence: I: The incidence and course of PTSD. *Journal of Child Psychology and Psychiatry, 41*, 503–511.

Yule, W., & Williams, R. M. (1990). Post-traumatic stress reactions in children. *Journal of Traumatic Stress, 3*, 279–295.

Zamvil, L. S., Wechsler, V., Frank, A., & Docherty, J. P. (1991). *Post-traumatic stress disorder in hospitalized children and adolescents*. Unpublished manuscript, Nashua Brookside Hospital, Nashua, NH.

Zero to Three/National Center for Clinical Infant Programs. (1994). *Diagnostic classification of mental health and developmental disorders in infancy and early childhood. (Diagnostic classification: 0–3)*. Washington, DC: Author.

Zhao, C., Li, J., Wang, M., Fan, Q., Zhang, F., Zhang, H., & Wang, X. (2001). Prevalence and correlated factors of posttraumatic stress disorder in adolescents 17 months after earthquake. *Chinese Mental Health Journal, 15*, 145–147.

Ziv, A., & Israeli, R. (1973). Effects of bombardment on the manifest anxiety level of children living in kibbutzim. *Journal of Consulting and Clinical Psychology, 40*, 287–291.

CHAPTER
EIGHT

Social Withdrawal in Childhood

Kenneth H. Rubin
Kim B. Burgess
Amy E. Kennedy
Shannon L. Stewart

This chapter concerns a topic unlike most that appear in this volume. Social withdrawal is not a clinically defined behavioral, social, or emotional disorder in childhood. Indeed, some individuals appear perfectly content to pass the better parts of their lives removed from others. These individuals include those who spend their days and/or nights tending to their computers; designing homes, automobiles, or space modules; writing scripts, poems, lyrics, or book chapters; and so forth. Often these individuals have a distinct need for solitude. Conversely, there are individuals who avoid others when in social company and those who choose solitude to escape the initiation and maintenance of interpersonal relationships. Lastly, there are individuals who have little choice in the matter of solitude, because they are isolated or rejected by others in their social community. In the latter two cases, social solitude could hardly be construed as normal or as psychologically or socially adaptive. But the display of solitude per se is not the problem; rather, the central issue is that social withdrawal may reflect underlying difficulties of a social or emotional nature.

To some researchers, the expression of social withdrawal reflects particular temperamental and/or personality characteristics or traits (e.g., Fox, Henderson, Rubin, Calkins, & Schmidt, 2001; Kagan, 1989). Others view withdrawal as a behavioral index of a child's isolation or rejection by the peer group (e.g., Hymel, Bowker, & Woody, 1993; Parkhurst & Asher, 1992). Still others believe that social withdrawal in childhood, depending upon the age at which it is observed, reflects the lack of a social approach motive and a preference for object manipulation and construction over interpersonal exchange (Asendorpf, 1990, 1993). Finally, there are those who believe that social withdrawal is linked to psychological maladaptation, as it represents a behavioral expression of internalized thoughts and feelings of social anxiety or depression (Bell-Dolan, Reaven, & Peterson, 1993; Nilzon & Palmerus, 1998). As the reader may quickly surmise, then, social withdrawal is an extremely slippery construct that has defied precise meaning and understanding. It becomes immediately evident why there has not been general agreement among traditionally trained clinical psychologists concerning the relevance and significance of social withdrawal vis-à-vis the development and expression of psychologically abnormal emotions, thoughts, and behaviors in childhood.

Given the slippery nature of the phenomenon, a central purpose of this chapter is to provide some definitional clarity for social withdrawal. Such clarity is especially important, because social withdrawal appears to have many "faces" (Rubin, 1982; Rubin & Mills, 1988), and the multiple forms of social solitude typically expressed in childhood carry with them different psychological functions and meanings (Coplan, Rubin, Fox, Calkins, & Stewart, 1994; Rubin, Coplan, Fox, & Calkins, 1995). To make matters more confusing, the expression of different forms of solitude appears to have different meanings not only at different points in childhood, but also within different social contexts (Rubin, Burgess, & Hastings, 2002) and cultures (Chen et al., 1998; Chen, Rubin, Li, & Li, 1999).

A second purpose of this chapter is to examine factors that may lead to the consistent display of social withdrawal during childhood. Third, we consider the correlates and consequences of social withdrawal. These latter two goals are accomplished by referring to a developmental framework within which pathways to and from social withdrawal are described (see Figure 8.1; see also Rubin, LeMare, & Lollis, 1990; Rubin & Burgess, 2001; Rubin & Lollis, 1988).

Having outlined the goals of this chapter, we now provide a rationale for including a chapter on social withdrawal in a volume concerned with child psychopathology. Perhaps the best way to begin is to provide the reader with a sense of the intrapersonal, felt significance of being socially withdrawn. The following letter was one of many that arrived in the office of Kenneth H. Rubin shortly after a description of his program of longitudinal research was carried by the newspaper wire services in Canada.

> I am taking the liberty of writing to you regarding an article in the newspaper last evening entitled "Socially Withdrawn Children Studied." I am now 51 years of age but definitely can identify with the children described in the article. I just wish—oh how I wish, that in-depth studies were done regarding the severity of the problem in my formative years.
>
> I have been employed for 27 years in the same position (stenographer) but my personality problem has been a detriment to me in my adult years. I recall one instance in my third year of grade school when my teacher approached me after recess with the enquiry "Have you no one to play with? I have noticed you standing by yourself at recess for several days now." I recall replying and *LYING*—"Yes, I've friends." The teacher was observant and I give her credit for this. However, I wish, oh how I wish, something had been done about my isolation at the tender age of 7 or 8. It has been a long, lonely road.
>
> Again my apologies for taking the liberty of writing but I am so happy, so very, very happy, that help is in store for the self-isolated child. Thank you for listening to me.

This letter, as well as many others that have been received in response to media coverage of our research program, has brought us a "real-world" sense of what it means to be socially withdrawn. It has also motivated us to understand better why social withdrawal, its meaning, its origins, its concomitants, and its consequences have been relatively ignored by clinical child psychologists. We begin this chapter with a substantive discussion, not of social withdrawal, but rather of the significance of peer engagement and peer relationships for normal growth and development. By addressing issues pertaining to the significance of peer interaction, we can poignantly illustrate the experiences and benefits that the socially withdrawn child fails to accrue.

THE SIGNIFICANCE OF PEER INTERACTION FOR NORMAL DEVELOPMENT

Theoretical statements about the etiology and psychological significance of social withdrawal were practically nonexistent until the late 1980s. Instead, those searching for a theoretical raison d'être for their research had to rely on the writings of cognitive and personality developmentalists vis-à-vis the significance of peer interaction for normal social, emotional, and cognitive growth. Piaget (1932), for example, posited that peer interaction provides a unique cognitive and social-cognitive growth context for children. He focused specifically on the relevance of disagreements with age-mates and the opportunities for negotiation arising from disagreements. These naturally occurring differences of opinion were assumed to engender cognitive conflict that requires both intra- and interpersonal resolution in order for positive peer exchanges and experiences to occur. The resolution of interpersonal disputes was thought to result in a better understanding of others' thoughts and emotions, the broadening of one's social repertoire with which to solve inter-

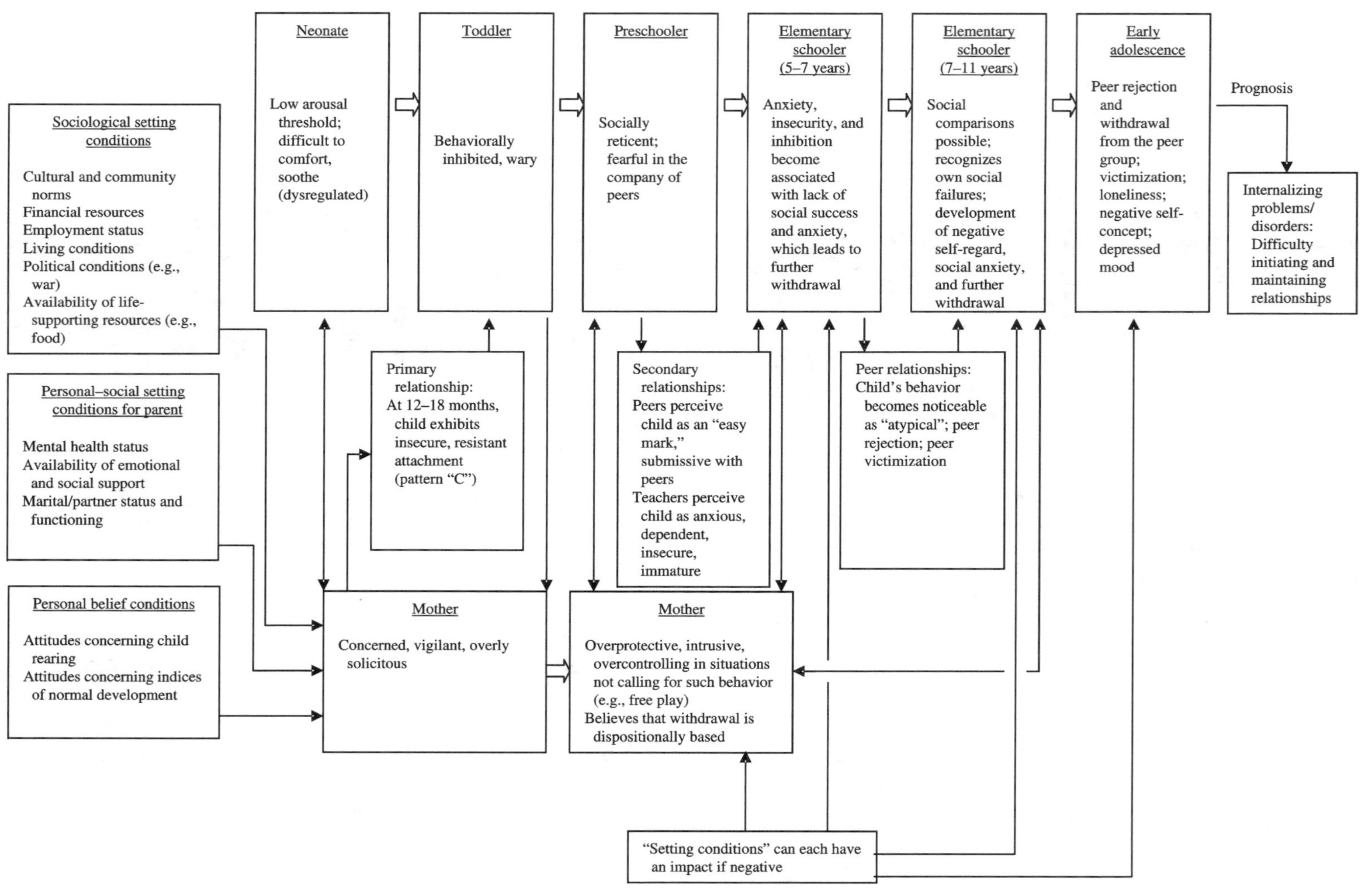

FIGURE 8.1. Pathways to and from social withdrawal.

personal disputes and misunderstandings, and the comprehension of cause–effect relations in social interaction.

Empirical support for these notions began to emerge in the 1970s, when researchers demonstrated that peer exchange, conversations, and interactions indeed produced intrapersonal cognitive conflict and a subsequent decline in egocentric thinking (e.g., Damon & Killen, 1982). Evidence was also offered for the associations among the *inability* to take perspective, the demonstration of maladaptive social behavior (e.g., Crick & Dodge, 1994), and the experience of qualitatively poor peer relationships (Chandler, 1973). Finally, researchers found that perspective-taking skills could be improved through peer interactions, particularly those experiences that involved role play. In turn, such improvement led to increases in prosocial behavior and to decreases in aggressive behavior (e.g., Iannotti, 1978; Selman & Schultz, 1990).

Given the brief review offered above, it appears reasonable to conclude that peer interaction influences the development of social cognition, and ultimately the expression of competent social behavior in the peer group. Peer interaction also allows children to understand the rules and norms of their peer subcultures. It is this understanding of norms and normative performance levels that engenders in the child an ability to evaluate his or her own competency levels against the perceived standards of the peer group. In addition to facilitating the development of social cognition, peer interaction enables the child to make self-evaluative judgments and to understand the self in relation to significant others.

This latter view concerning self-definition and identity was addressed almost 70 years ago in the writings of George Herbert Mead (1934). He suggested that exchanges among peers—whether experienced during cooperative or competitive activity, or during conflict or friendly discussion—enable a child to understand the self as both a subject and an object. Understanding that the self can be an object of others' perspectives gradually evolves into the conceptualization of a "generalized other" or an organized and coordinated perspective of the social group. In turn, recognition of the "generalized other" leads to the emergence of an organized sense of self.

Finally, the personality theorist Harry Stack Sullivan (1953) has provided an impetus for much current research concerning the significance of children's peer interactions. Sullivan suggested that the foundations of mutual respect, cooperation, and interpersonal sensitivity derive initially from children's peer and friendship relationships. Sullivan specifically emphasized the importance of "chumships," or special relationships, for the emergence of these concepts. Thus, once a child acquires an understanding of the concepts of equality, mutuality, and reciprocity from chums, these concepts can be applied more generally to other, less special peer relationships.

In summary, from these theoretical perspectives and the data supportive of them, it seems clear that peer interaction is essential for normal social-cognitive and socioemotional development. Peer interaction also influences children's understanding of the rules and norms of their peer subcultures (see Rubin, Bukowski, & Parker, 1998, for a recent review). It is this understanding of normative performance levels that engenders in a child an ability to evaluate his or her own competency against the perceived standards of the peer group. If peer interaction does lead to the development of social competencies and the understanding of the self in relation to others, it seems reasonable to think about the developmental consequences for those children who refrain from social interaction and avoid the company of their peers. It is this reasonable thought that drives much of the current research on social withdrawal.

DEFINING SOCIAL WITHDRAWAL IN CHILDHOOD

The child who interacts with peers at a less than normal rate is often referred to as "socially withdrawn." Similarly, the child who is observed or rated by others to spend more than an average amount of time alone is referred to as "socially withdrawn." In the past two decades, it has been commonplace to use the terms "social withdrawal," "social isolation," "inhibition," and "shyness" interchangeably to describe the behavioral expression of solitude. Although these constructs may be interrelated statistically and linked conceptually, they carry with them different psychological meanings. In this chapter, we distinguish among these terms of reference.

In 1993, Rubin and Asendorpf attempted to provide definitional clarity to the study of social withdrawal. They defined "inhibition" as the disposition to be wary and fearful when encountering *novel* (unfamiliar) situations. "Fearful shyness" was the term they used to describe inhibition in response to novel *social* situations. In middle childhood, shyness based on fear of novelty was said to be replaced by "self-conscious shyness," a phenomenon reflected by the display of inhibition in response to social-evaluative concerns. "Social isolation" refers to the expression of solitary behavior that results from being isolated (rejected) by the peer group. Finally, "social withdrawal" refers to the consistent display (across situations and over time) of all forms of solitary behavior when encountering familiar and/or unfamiliar peers. Social withdrawal therefore can be construed as isolating oneself *from* the peer group, whereas social isolation indicates isolation *by* the peer group (Rubin, Burgess, & Coplan, 2002).

To further complicate matters, in the early 1980s we inadvertently introduced confusion into the social withdrawal literature by using the terms "passive withdrawal" *and* "solitary-passive behavior." As it happens, these terms refer to different constructs! We (Rubin, Burgess, & Coplan, 2002) hope to create order from chaos by referring to "passive withdrawal" as the child's withdrawal *from* the peer group. Typically, the passive withdrawal construct is drawn from rating scale data (e.g., Revised Class Play [RCP], Pupil Evaluation Inventory [PEI]) and is represented by items such as "very shy," "feelings hurt easily," and "rather play alone than with others." The passive withdrawal construct may be contrasted with "active isolation," a term suggesting that the child is actively isolated *by* the peer group (i.e., rejected); this is represented by RCP or PEI items such as "often left out" and "can't get others to listen." "Solitary–passive withdrawal" is *observed* solitary behavior that involves exploratory and constructive activity. Solitary–passive withdrawal is actually not passive at all, given that it consists of active exploration and construction.

As we have noted earlier, there may be different motivations underlying withdrawal from the company of peers. For example, some children are more object- than person-oriented and thus prefer solitude to social activity. These children have been characterized as having a low social approach motive, but not necessarily a high avoidance motive (Asendorpf, 1990, 1991). When such children play alone during the preschool period, they are observed to engage in exploratory or constructive play (unfortunately labeled "solitary–*passive* play"; Rubin, 1982). Other children may wish to engage in social interaction but for some reason are compelled to avoid it. These children appear socially motivated, but for reasons to be noted later, they are wary, socially anxious, and fearful (Rubin & Asendorpf, 1993). When such children play alone during the preschool period, they are observed to engage in unoccupied and onlooker behaviors (labeled "reticence"; Coplan et al., 1994; Rubin, Coplan, et al., 1995). In both cases, social solitude may be displayed consistently over time and across contexts (Coplan & Rubin, 1998; Fox et al., 2001; Rubin et al., 2002).

To this constellation of constructs, one can now add "social phobia" or "social anxiety disorder." This phenomenon is marked by a fear of saying or doing things in public that will result in humiliation and embarrassment (Beidel & Turner, 1999). This latter construct is viewed as a clinical disorder in the *Diagnostic and Statistical Manual of Mental Disorders*, fourth edition (DSM-IV; American Psychiatric Association, 1994) and appears to have much in common with social withdrawal at the extreme.

In summary, regardless of motivational, dispositional, or emotional tendencies, it seems reasonable to suggest that refraining from peer interaction precludes children from taking advantage of the benefits of peer interchange described above. Social withdrawal, regardless of its "phenotypic face" or its dispositional, motivational, or emotional underpinnings, has been postulated to bring with it a number of developmental costs. Whether or not this conclusion is valid remains to be fully tested. In the following section, we review the relevant literature on clinical diagnosis and describe what the potential sequelae of social withdrawal might be. As the reader will note, however, there do appear to be different clinical diagnoses associated with the various forms of solitary behavior.

SOCIAL WITHDRAWAL AND CLINICAL DIAGNOSIS

Having defined the phenomenon of social withdrawal, having described the significance of peer interaction for normal growth and development, and having inferred that a lack of peer interaction should give rise for concern, it should not be surprising that the term "social withdrawal" is found in almost every textbook or review chapter on abnormal or clinical child psychology (e.g., Achenbach, 1995; Rutter, Taylor, & Hersov, 1994). It is also found on most standardized assessments of abnormal socioemotional functioning (e.g., Achenbach & Edelbrock, 1981). The phenomenon is consistently cited as evidence for an "overcontrolled disorder" (e.g., Lewis & Miller, 1990) or an internalizing problem (Achenbach & Edelbrock, 1981). In source after source, social withdrawal is contrasted with aggression as one of the two most frequently identified major dimensions of dysfunctional behavior in childhood (e.g., Achenbach, 1995).

Despite the apparent clinical significance of social withdrawal, the phenomenon is not well represented in formal diagnostic categories of childhood psychological disturbance. It is implicated as *symptomatic* of particular clinical and personality disorders in childhood and adolescence. These disorders include anxiety, phobias, major depression, schizophrenia, and avoidant personality.

Behavioral Inhibition, Shyness, Anxiety, and Phobic Disorders

"Behavioral inhibition" (BI) is a temperamental construct reflecting the tendency to be fearful and anxious during the toddler years, and socially wary and withdrawn in unfamiliar situations during the early school-age years (Calkins, Fox, & Marshall, 1996; Kagan, Reznick, Snidman, Gibbons, & Johnson, 1988). It has been argued that BI is a developmental precursor of social withdrawal in childhood and adolescence (Rubin, 1993; Rubin Burgess, & Coplan, 2002). Several researchers have suggested that BI represents a marker of anxiety and anxiety-proneness. For example, a positive relation exists between cortisol production in saliva and the demonstration of extremely inhibited behavior not only in the toddler period (Kagan, Reznick, & Snidman, 1987; Nachmias, Gunnar, Mangelsdorf, Parritz, & Buss, 1996), but also during early and middle childhood (Schmidt et al., 1997). The high cortisol levels of inhibited children may increase corticotropin-releasing hormone in the central nucleus of the amygdala, thereby exacerbating the social fearfulness response. Furthermore, high cortisol levels may predispose inhibited children to develop a cognitive working model to expect fear and anxiety when facing novelty. It is relevant to note that exaggerated autonomic responses to novelty are associated with internalizing problems such as anxiety.

Longitudinal data also suggest a link between BI in infancy and early childhood, and phobic and anxiety disorders in middle childhood (Hirshfeld et al., 1992). Children with BI evidence higher rates of phobic disorders (Biederman et al., 1993), and multiple anxiety disorders such as avoidant disorder, separation anxiety disorder, and agoraphobia (e.g., Rosenbaum et al., 1988), than do uninhibited children.

Recently, researchers relying on retrospective self-report of BI in samples of adolescents and young adults have demonstrated that childhood BI is associated at best with subclinical assessments of anxiety (Muris, Merckelbach, Wessel, & van de Ven, 1999). Yet adolescents and young adults who report retrospective BI appear to be at greater risk for social phobia than for generalized anxiety (Mick & Telch, 1998). Indeed, among teens reporting high BI, 22% evidenced social phobia—a risk factor four times greater than those who did not report childhood BI (Hayward, Killen, Kraemer, & Taylor Barr, 1998). It is important, however, to recognize that retrospective reports are methodologically less than optimal, especially when they are self-reports.

Childhood "shyness," a term that describes wariness in the face of unfamiliar others, is not generally associated with, or predictive of, an anxiety diagnosis in adolescence (Prior, Smart, Sanson, & Oberklaid, 2000). However, Prior et al. (2000) report that 42% of children who remain shy *throughout childhood* demonstrate anxiety in adolescence. These latter data are supported by a recent finding that persistent shyness, as assessed at ages 14, 20, 24, and 36 months, is associated with a broad-band assessment of internalizing problems (Schmitz et al., 1999).

Social Withdrawal and Internalizing Disorders

Social withdrawal becomes particularly significant as an index of psychopathology when categories of *adult* personality disorders are considered. A DSM-IV diagnosis of personality disorder is made when an individual's inflexible, long-lasting behavior pattern or personality style causes a high level of personal distress, as well as major problems in social situations or work functioning (American Psychiatric Association, 1994; Clark, Vorhies, & McEwan, 1994; Widiger, Trull, Clarkin, Sanderson, & Costa, 1994). Key symptomatology reflective of specific personality disorders incorporates many characteristics seen in childhood—specifically, timidity, seclusiveness, social withdrawal, or avoidance of social interaction.

From the outset, it is important to note that we do not know whether indices of social withdrawal in childhood are conceptually and empirically analogous to these same behavioral indices in later life. Similarly, whether the underlying motivations for these behaviors are the same is not yet known. For instance, some extremely withdrawn elementary school-age children are "loners" because they are fearful and socially anxious; others are "loners" because they are more object- than person-oriented. Nonetheless, these different motivations for social approach and avoidance discussed in the child personality literature may reflect vulnerabilities for particular adult personality disorders—specifically, schizoid and avoidant disorders.

Individuals with schizoid personality disorder are reserved, socially withdrawn, and seclusive (American Psychiatric Association, 1994; Joseph, 1992; Siever, 1981; Turkal, 1990). They prefer solitary work activities and hobbies, and lack warm, close relationships. These individuals have a profound defect in the ability to form social relationships (Millon, 1987). They are excessively introverted, and are particularly characterized by low warmth, low positive emotionality, and lack of gregariousness (Widiger et al., 1994). Not only do they have few relationships with others, but they also seem to have little desire for them (O'Brien, Trestman, & Siever, 1993). In addition, they often have poor social skills, lack a sense of humor, and seem detached from their environment. Emotionally, they appear flat, restricted, and cold, with little observable hostility when angry (American Psychiatric Association, 1994; Widiger et al., 1994).

Conversely, adult avoidant personality disorder is characterized by low self-esteem, fear of negative evaluation, and a pervasive behavioral, emotional, and cognitive avoidance of social interaction (American Psychiatric Association, 1994; Widiger, 2001). Key traits associated with this disorder include reticence in social relationships, avoidance of activities that require interpersonal contact, being overly sensitive to criticism, and fear of showing visible signs of anxiety in public (Stone, 1993). Individuals diagnosed with this particular personality disorder express a desire for affection, acceptance, and friendship; yet they often have few friends and share little intimacy with anyone. Fear of rejection plays a key role in distancing themselves from personal attachments. These avoidant individuals fail to enter into relationships unless the prospective partner provides unusually strong guarantees of uncritical acceptance (Millon, 1981; Millon & Everly, 1985).

Individuals with avoidant personality disorder are typically described as timid and withdrawn (Pilkonis, 1984; Turkal, 1990; Widiger & Sanderson, 1997). Hypervigilance tends to be their major coping mechanism. In addition, their nervousness often results in making companions uncomfortable, which may damage the quality of ongoing relationships and lead to rejection (Millon, 1981; Millon & Everly, 1985; Turkal, 1990). Avoidant individuals also cope by restricting the range of impinging environmental stimuli; hence they retreat from novel social experiences. This retreat inhibits the development of social self-efficacy for dealing with interpersonal situations (Costa & McCrae, 1985). Individuals diagnosed with avoidant personality disorder differ from those diagnosed with schizoid personality disorder, as the former group appears to be motivated to establish social relationships, whereas the latter group seems uninterested in doing so.

Social withdrawal is also implicated in the diagnosis of social phobia. Social phobia is an internalizing disorder that involves "a marked and persistent fear of social or performance situations in which embarrassment may occur" (American Psychiatric Association, 1994, p. 411). Thus withdrawal from social situations is mediated by fear of appraisal; in the case of social phobia, it is suggested that there is no approach–avoidance conflict, but simply an excessive motivation to avoid others. According to Millon (1996), those who have avoidant personality disorder withdraw as a function of felt insecurity in relating to others. Those with social phobia may be able to develop satisfying relationships with others, but refrain from interacting because of feelings of inadequacy, inferiority, and ineptitude. Importantly, there are no longitudinal or etiological data to indicate that avoidant personality disorder and social phobia derive from distinct developmental histories.

In summary, social withdrawal has been implicated in several diagnostic categories of *adult* personality disturbance. Furthermore, social withdrawal is viewed as symptomatic of anxiety disorders in childhood. Given the brief review offered above, it may be that the various forms of solitude and the motivations underlying these behavioral expressions vary from one disturbance to another. Thus we urge developmental and clinical researchers to address these possibilities in their future research agendas. Indeed, researchers should examine the developmental origins and course of disturbances that are associated with displays of solitude in children and adolescents. Relatedly, now is the time to begin research programs directed toward examining the etiology and developmental course of social withdrawal during childhood. To this end, we offer a developmental model in which the causes, concomitants, and consequences of childhood social withdrawal are highlighted. Given the different meanings of solitude in childhood, the model presented below allows for a conceptual intertwining of its various forms.

THE DEVELOPMENTAL COURSE OF CHILDHOOD SOCIAL WITHDRAWAL

Keeping with the goals of developmental psychopathology (Rutter & Sroufe, 2000), we have described a conceptual model of the origins and course of social withdrawal during childhood. This developmental model was first published in several sources (e.g., Rubin et al., 1990; Rubin, Hymel, Mills, & Rose-Krasnor, 1991) but has since undergone several iterations, given the ever-increasing empirical data base (Rubin & Burgess, 2001). Our model begins with the suggestion that individual differences in temperament set the stage for particular parental reactions that aid in the induction of (1) an insecure parent–child attachment relationship, and (2) a socially wary and withdrawn behavioral style. In turn, felt insecurity and behavioral wariness and solitude in social settings become associated with, and reflective and predictive of, markers of socioemotional maladaptation in childhood. Next we review the conceptual model and relevant empirical support.

Early Childhood: Etiological Perspectives on Social Withdrawal

Behavioral Inhibition

Why and how do children come to be socially withdrawn? Kagan and colleagues (e.g., Kagan, 1989; Kagan, Reznick, & Snidman, 1988) have argued that the pathway to social withdrawal begins with the dispositional or temperamental construct widely recognized as behavioral inhibition (BI). To Kagan and collaborators, some infants are genetically hard-wired with a physiology that biases them to be cautious, timid, and wary in unfamiliar social and nonsocial situations. These "inhibited" children differ from their uninhibited counterparts in ways that imply variability in the threshold of excitability of the amygdala and its projections to the cortex, hypothalamus, sympathetic nervous system, corpus striatum, and central gray (Kagan, Snidman, & Arcus, 1993).

Kagan has identified two dimensions of infant behavior that are predictive of later fearful and anxious behaviors in children: (1) frequency of motor activity, and (2) the display of negative affect. According to Kagan and Snidman (1991), the combined and consistent expression of infant motor arousal and negative affect is a function of elevated excitability in areas of the limbic system thought to be involved in fear responses. Infants who are easily and negatively aroused motorically and emotionally are likely to display BI in childhood (Kagan, Snidman, & Arcus, 1998).

Consistent with Kagan's argument that there is a physiological basis to social wariness and BI is the research of Fox and colleagues (e.g., Fox & Calkins, 1993; Fox et al., 2001). These researchers began by noting that adults exhibiting relatively greater electroencephalographic (EEG) activity in the right frontal lobe are more likely to express negative affect and rate emotional stimuli as negative (Jones & Fox, 1992). Moreover, adults diagnosed with unipolar depression, even in remission, are more likely to display right frontal EEG asymmetry compared to controls (Henriques & Davidson, 1990, 1991). Drawing from the adult literature on the psychophysiological underpinnings of emotion dysregulation, Fox and his collaborators have demonstrated that infants exhibiting right frontal EEG asymmetries are more likely to cry upon maternal separation, and to display signs of negative affect and fear of novelty (Davidson & Fox, 1989; Fox, Bell, & Jones, 1992) . Moreover, stable patterns of infant brain electrical activity predict temperamental fearfulness and BI in young children. For example, Calkins et al. (1996) recorded brain electrical activity of children at 9, 14, and 24 months and found that infants who displayed a pattern of stable right frontal EEG asymmetry across this 15-month period were more fearful, anxious, compliant, and behaviorally inhibited as toddlers than other infants. In addition, Fox, Calkins, and Bell (1994) have reported that negative reactivity and right frontal EEG asymmetry in response to mild stress predict the display of toddler BI.

These physiological data provide evidence that unique patterns of brain electrical activity may reflect increasing arousal of particular brain centers involved in the expression of fear and anxiety (LeDoux, 1989), and appear to reflect a particular underlying temperamental type. The functional role of hemispheric asymmetries in the regulation of emotion may be understood in terms of an underlying motivational structure to emotional behavior—specifically, the approach–withdrawal continuum. Infants exhibiting greater relative right frontal EEG asymmetry are more likely to withdraw from mild stress. Infants exhibiting the opposite pattern of activation are more likely to approach. It is argued that these patterns of frontal activation represent a dispositional characteristic underlying behavioral/temperamental responses to the environment. Also consistent with Kagan's findings is the report that infants who exhibit extreme degrees of motor arousal and negative affect in response to novelty display greater relative right frontal EEG activation, and are likely to be fearful and inhibited as toddlers (Fox & Calkins, 1993; Calkins et al., 1996).

Another physiological entity that distinguishes wary from nonwary infants and toddlers is "vagal tone," an index of respiratory sinus arrhythmia (RSA) that assesses the functional status or efficiency of the nervous system (Porges & Byrne, 1992), and that marks both general reactivity and the ability to regulate one's level of arousal. RSA comprises the high-frequency oscillations in heart period that are associated with the breathing cycle (Porges, 1995). Higher brain centers associated with emotions and cognitions can influence brainstem cardiorespiratory control centers and thus affect RSA, with a reduction in these measures under conditions of stress or effort (Berntson, Cacioppo, & Quigley, 1993). In the context of a neurobiological model of BI, high inhibition might be associated with low vagal tone and low heart period variability. Indeed, Kagan and colleagues found concurrent associations between low heart period (high heart rate) and increased BI as assessed in infancy and childhood (Kagan, Reznick, Clarke, Snidman, & Garcia-Coll, 1984; Kagan et al., 1988; Reznick et al., 1986). Anderson, Bohlin, and Hagekall (1999) reported similar relations between vagal tone and inhibition in a sample of Swedish toddlers. However, these findings have not been generally replicable across ages and samples (for a review, see Marshall & Stevenson-Hinde, 2001).

Lastly, the hypothalamic–pituitary–adrenocortical (HPA) axis is affected largely by stressful or aversive situations that involve novelty, uncertainty, and/or negative emotions (Levine, 1983). Infants with BI evidence significant increases in cortisol as a function of exposure to stressful social situations (Spangler & Schieche, 1998).

In conclusion, inhibited toddlers display greater reactivity in the sympathetic nervous system, greater muscle tension, and higher levels of salivary cortisol than do uninhibited children. Moreover, these children display elevated resting heart rates, higher basal cortisol readings, and greater pupil dilation. It is important to note, however, that human physiology is hardly immutable. Thus we suggest that BI in infancy and toddlerhood, and its physiological markers, may be altered or exacerbated through environmental means. For instance, we have suggested that a temperamentally inhibited infant may prove a challenge or stressor to his or her parents. Thus the interplay of endogenous, socialization, and early relationship factors may lead to a sense of felt insecurity, and ultimately to the chronic expression of social withdrawal. At the same time, we argue that changes in physiology may result from experiences that are interpreted by the child as nonstressful and as promoting a sense of felt security. We offer empirical substantiation for these premises below.

The above-described research pertains to the expression of BI and shyness, or wary, timid, and withdrawn behavior in the face of *novel* social and nonsocial circumstances. Whether or not shyness and BI are empirically related to social withdrawal, defined as the lack of peer interaction in both familiar *and* unfamiliar settings, is relatively unknown. Such links can and do make conceptual sense, but there are very few studies that support an association. We explore the limited literature in a subsequent section of this chapter.

Noteworthy is the fact that theorists who argue strongly for underlying biological and genetic components to the expression of social wariness and shyness do not generally suggest negative outcomes of a psychopathological nature for extremely shy or socially wary children. Also, these theorists have not typically provided a strong account for how environmental circumstances may influence and modify these biologically based traits. In other relevant theories, though, causal connections have been made between experiential, familial factors and the development of socially wary and withdrawn behaviors. We review one such theory below.

Attachment Relationships

According to attachment theorists, children develop an internalized model of the self in relation to others from the quality of their early parenting experiences (Bowlby, 1969). In the case of a secure parent–child relationship, the internal working model allows the child to feel confident and self-assured when introduced to novel settings. This sense of "felt security" fosters the child's active exploration of the social environment (Sroufe, 1983). Exploration of the social milieu allows the child to answer *other-directed* questions, such as "What are the properties of this other person?", "What is he or she like?", or "What can and does this person do?" (Rubin, Fein, & Vandenberg, 1983). Once these exploratory questions are answered, the child can address *self-directed* questions, such as "What can *I* do with this person?" Thus felt security is viewed as a central construct in socioemotional development; it enhances social exploration, which results in interactive peer play. Peer play, in turn, plays a significant role in the development of social competence (Rubin & Rose-Krasnor, 1992).

Children who develop insecure internal working models of social relationships, on the other hand, come to view the world as unpredictable, comfortless, and unresponsive (Sroufe, 1983). This insecure internal representation may lead some children to "shrink from their social worlds" (Bowlby, 1969, p. 208). Thus there may be a group of insecurely attached young children who refrain from exploring their social environments; this lack of exploration is likely to impede peer play and, as attachment theorists posit, may interfere with the development of social competence. It is the behavioral response of insecurity and anxiety-induced withdrawal from the peer culture that best conveys to us the meaning of "social withdrawal."

Linking Temperament and Attachment

As noted above, some newborns may be biologically predisposed to have a low threshold for the arousal of negative emotionality (e.g., Kagan et al., 1987). This temperamental trait may be aroused by an aversive stimulus and make these babies extremely difficult for their parents to comfort and soothe. Thus the interplay of endogenous, socialization, and early relationship factors may lead to the development of a sense of felt insecurity.

Support for our speculations about the relations between temperament and attachment derives from several recent sources. To begin with, approximately one-third of all children develop insecure internal working models of social relationships and come to view the world as unpredictable, comfortless, and unresponsive (Sroufe, 1983). That subgroup of insecurely attached young children who refrain from exploring their social environments have typically been classified as "resistant" or "C" babies. In novel settings, these infants maintain close proximity to the attachment figure; when the attachment figure (usually the mother) leaves the paradigmatic "Strange Situation" for a short period of time, "C" babies become disturbingly unsettled. Upon reunion with the attachment figure, these infants show ambivalence—angry, resistant behaviors interspersed with proximity, contact-seeking behaviors (e.g., Greenspan & Lieberman, 1988).

Direct evidence for a predictive relation between infant temperament and insecure "C" attachment status derives from several sources. Differences in irritability or reactivity in the neonatal period predict insecure attachment status (Miyake, Chen, & Campos, 1985). Meta-analyses have indicated that the temperamental characteristic of "proneness to distress" predicts the resistant behavior that partly defines insecure attachment status of the "C" variety (Goldsmith & Alansky, 1987). It is possible that irritability or proneness to distress presents as a significant stressor to parents, and as such influences the quality of mother–infant interactions and the quality of the attachment relationship (Izard, Haynes, Chisholm, & Baak, 1991). Thus the temperamental construct of "emotionality" (which comprises irritability and proneness to distress) could lay the basis for the development of qualitatively insecure attachment relationships. Support for this contention stems from the research of Izard, Porges, et al. (1991), who found that infant emotionality as well as infant resting-state cardiac activity (a physiological index of emotionality and emotion regulation) predicted insecure attachment status. More specific evidence for a connection between infant temperament and the particular classification of insecure attachment status derives from several sources. First, Thompson, Connell, and Bridges (1988) have reported that infant proneness to fear predicts distress to maternal separation. Such distress is usually allied with a "C" classification in the traditional attachment paradigm (Belsky & Rovine, 1987). The strongest support for a wariness–attachment link, however, stems from research demonstrating that infants who are dispositionally reactive to mildly stressful, novel social events are more likely to be classified as insecurely attached "C" babies than are their less reactive counterparts (Calkins & Fox, 1992; Fox & Calkins, 1993). Spangler and Schieche (1998) reported that of 16 "C" babies they identified, 15 were rated by mothers as showing BI.

Although support exists for a direct relation between temperament and insecure attachment, recent research indicates that this association is rather complex. It appears that when toddlers with BI are faced with novelty or social unfamiliarity, they become emotionally dysregulated; and this dysregulation seems to lead toddlers to retreat from unfamiliar adults and peers. That these youngsters become unsettled is supported by findings that confrontation with unfamiliarity brings increases in hypothalamic–pituitary–adrenocortical (HPA) activity (Spangler & Schieche, 1998). Interestingly, this relation between confrontation with unfamiliarity and increases in HPA activation has been reported for insecurely attached children in the Strange Situation (e.g., Gunnar, Mangelsdorf, Larson, & Hertsgaard, 1989; Nachmias et al., 1996). More to the point, "C" babies experience this increased HPA activity (Spangler & Schieche, 1998).

Attachment, Inhibition, and Social Withdrawal

The social behaviors of toddlers and preschoolers who have an insecure "C" attachment history are thought to be guided largely by fear of rejection. Conceptually, psychologists have predicted that when these insecurely attached children are placed in group settings with peers, they should attempt to avoid rejection through the demonstration of passive, adult-dependent behavior and withdrawal from social interaction (Renken, Egeland, Marvinney, Mangelsdorf, & Sroufe, 1989; Sroufe & Waters, 1977). Empirically, support for these conjectures derives from data indicating that infants who experience a "C" attachment relationship are more whiny, easily frustrated, and socially inhibited at 2 years of age than are their secure counterparts (Fox & Calkins, 1993; Matas, Arend, & Sroufe, 1978). "C" babies also tend to be less skilled in peer interaction as toddlers, and to be rated by their teachers as more dependent, helpless, tense, and fearful than their secure counterparts (Pastor, 1981).

Finally, Erickson, Sroufe, and Egeland (1985) have reported that "C" babies lack confidence and assertiveness at age 4 years. At 7 years, they are observed to be socially withdrawn (Renken et al., 1989). Additional support for both concurrent and predictive associations among insecure attachment, BI, and social withdrawal comes from more recent studies (e.g., Booth, Rose-Krasnor, McKinnon, & Rubin, 1994; Rubin, Booth, Rose-Krasnor, & Mills, 1995). Furthermore, among clinical samples of mothers with anxiety disorders, Manassis and colleagues reported that 65% of children aged 18 to 59 months exhibited BI (using Kagan's measures) and that 80% were insecurely attached (Strange Situation), although the authors did not distinguish between "A" (avoidant) babies and "C" babies (Manassis, Bradley, Goldberg, Hood, & Swinson, 1995).

It bears noting that insecure attachment relationships are also predicted by *maternal* behavior. For example, mothers of insecurely attached "C" babies are overinvolved and overcontrolling, compared to mothers of securely attached babies (Erickson et al., 1985). This particular finding will gain added relevance as the reader progresses through this chapter.

Inhibition and Social Reticence and Withdrawal in Early to Middle Childhood

Having developed a psychological profile of BI and insecure "C" attachment status, we suggest that such children may preclude themselves from the opportunities and outcomes associated with social exploration and peer play. BI during the toddler period, which is arguably a dispositional variable, has also been tied empirically to behavioral outcomes in early and middle childhood. First, investigators have consistently demonstrated that inhibited toddlers are likely to remain inhibited in the early and middle years of childhood (e.g., Broberg, Lamb, & Hwang, 1990; Burgess, Marshall, Rubin, & Fox, in press; Fox et al., 2001; Kagan, Gibbons, Johnson, Reznick, & Snidman, 1990; Kochanska & Radke-Yarrow, 1992; Rubin et al., 2002; Sanson, Pedlow, Cann, Prior, & Oberklaid, 1996; Scarpa, Raine, Venables, & Mednick, 1995). Nevertheless, this stability may be moderated by physiological factors. Marshall and Stevenson-Hinde (1998), for example, showed stability of socially inhibited behavior between ages 4.5 and 7 years, but only for those who had lower heart period (shorter interbeat intervals) at 4.5 years.

Importantly, there is now an empirically established link between BI assessed at age 2 years and social reticence assessed at age four. For example, we (Rubin et al. 2002) recently reported that toddler BI as assessed in the Kagan tradition (which involves the coding of latency to approach unfamiliar adults and toys, and proximity to the mother), together with social inhibition when observed in the company of another toddler, predicted anxious, wary, reticent behavior at age 4 years. Significantly, toddler inhibition only predicted preschoolers' reticence, but neither solitary–passive (constructive, exploratory) nor solitary–active behaviors. In a different longitudinal sample, we (Burgess et al., in press) found that toddlers with moderate or high BI (assessed via Kagan's traditional paradigm) displayed more reticent behaviors among unfamiliar peers at age 4 compared to uninhibited toddlers, thereby providing support for the stability of BI over time and across situations. Lastly, parental reports of their children's shy and withdrawn behaviors at age 4 also differentiated inhibited and uninhibited toddlers.

We contend that BI and reticence lead to the demonstration of social withdrawal during childhood, and that emotional and physiological functioning differs depending on the type of withdrawn behavior. Whereas nonsociable preschoolers who are proficient at regulating affect display constructive solitude, nonsociable preschoolers who are easily upset and difficult to soothe (emotionally dysregulated) display reticence among peers (Rubin, Coplan, et al., 1995). In addition, Fox and colleagues have indicated that socially reticent preschoolers display right frontal EEG asymmetry (Fox et al., 1995; Fox, Schmidt, Calkins, Rubin, & Coplan, 1996), but that such asymmetries are *not* associated with the frequent demonstration of quiet, solitary constructive activity. Fox and colleagues have also compared "continuously inhibited" children (high on social reticence at 48 months and high on BI earlier in life) and those children who changed inhibition status (low on social reticence at 48 months but high on BI earlier in life) over four time points: 9 months, 14 months, 24 months, and 48 months (Fox et al., 2001). Results indicated that children who were consistently inhibited displayed more internalizing difficulties at 48 months than those who were classified as continuously *un*inhibited and those who changed inhibition status. Furthermore, the children classified as consistently inhibited showed a pattern of relatively greater right frontal EEG activity at 9, 14, and 48 months compared to those children who changed inhibition status over the first 4 years of life. Children who were consistently *un*inhibited over the four time points displayed greater relative left frontal EEG asymmetry.

More recently, Schmidt has replicated the findings of Fox and colleagues in a separate sample (Schmidt et al., 1997); also, 7-year-old children who had been reticent at age 4 years were more likely to display right frontal EEG asymmetry (Schmidt, Fox, Schulkin, & Gold, 1999). In addition, Schmidt et al. (1997) have shown that reticence, but not other forms of solitude, is associated with the production of high morning basal cortisol, which again supports a physiology–reticence connection.

It is important to note that in all these studies early inhibition has been linked predictively to frequent demonstrations of inhibition and reticence in *unfamiliar* peer settings. This is a significant shortcoming, given that social withdrawal among *familiar* children is what appears most developmentally problematic (Asendorpf, 1993; Rubin & Mills, 1988; Rubin, Coplan, et al., 1995). Nevertheless, recent work by Coplan and colleagues does provide initial support for predictive and contemporaneous links between observed reticence among unfamiliar and familiar preschool-age peers (e.g., Coplan & Rubin, 1998; Coplan et al., 1994). Notably, both assessments of shyness/reticence among unfamiliar peers and reticence among familiar peers are associated with parent and teacher ratings of internalizing difficulties (Rubin, Coplan, et al., 1995). Moreover, in a recent study, we (Kennedy, Polak, Rubin, Fox, & Burgess, 2002) found that reticence, as displayed among unfamiliar peers at age 7, was associated predictively with both teacher ratings of anxious/withdrawn behavior and maternally reported withdrawn behavior at age 11. Lastly, Scarpa et al. (1995) found that BI, as assessed in the laboratory at age 3 years, predicted subsequent in-school social inhibition among Mauritian children at age 8 years; furthermore, teacher-rated inhibition remained stable from 8 to 11 years.

Thus evidence is emerging that the pathway to social withdrawal among familiar others has its origins in biologically based dispositional characteristics (assessed physiologically), the frequent demonstration of socially inhibited and reticent behaviors among unfamiliar peers, and the quality of the child's attachment relationship with the primary caregiver.

Stability, Correlates, and Consequences of Social Withdrawal

Thus far, we have examined etiological factors associated with the development of childhood social withdrawal. Next, we examine the correlates and consequences of withdrawal once it has been established as characteristic of the child's social repertoire. In our developmental model described elsewhere (Rubin & Burgess, 2001; Rubin et al., 1990; Rubin & Lollis, 1988), we argue that reluctance to explore novel, out-of-home settings impedes (1) possibilities of establishing normal social relationships; (2) the experience of normal social interactions; and (3) the development of social and cognitive skills that are supposedly encouraged by peer relationships and social play. Thus we predict a developmental sequence in which a socially inhibited, fearful, insecure child withdraws from the social world of peers; fails to develop those skills derived from peer interaction; and consequently becomes increasingly anxious and isolated from the peer group. We have also surmised that the recognition of social failure elicits thoughts and feelings of negative self-regard, which are continuously reinforced as the child develops an inadequate social repertoire to relate positively with peers.

Research on children's perceptions of their peers' social behaviors indicates that social withdrawal becomes more salient to the peer group with increasing age (Bukowski, 1990; Younger & Boyko, 1987; Younger & Daniels, 1992; Younger, Gentile, & Burgess, 1993). Given that deviation from age-normative social behavior is associated with the establishment of negative peer reputations, we have predicted that by middle to late childhood, social withdrawal and social anxiety become strongly associated with peer rejection and unpopularity. Finally, we have argued that the constellation of social withdrawal, social failure, negative self-regard, and peer rejection conspire in an insidious fashion to maintain and predict psychological problems of an internalizing nature, such as loneliness, depression, and feelings of insecurity within the peer group.

Stability of Social Withdrawal

The most extensive examination of the developmental course of social withdrawal emanates from the Waterloo Longitudinal Project (WLP), an ongoing study of an unselected sample of public school children. In this study, observed social withdrawal was stable from ages 5 to 9 years (Rubin, 1993; Rubin & Both, 1989), and peer assessments of withdrawal resulted in significant intercorrelations (all $p < .001$) between ages 7 and 10 years. Utilizing a categorical approach to identify extreme groups of socially withdrawn children (top 10–15%), the WLP revealed that across any 2-year period from ages 5 to 11 years, approximately two-thirds of them maintained their status (Rubin, 1993; Rubin, Chen, & Hymel, 1993). This latter finding supports Kagan and colleagues' contention (e.g., Kagan, 1989) that the developmental continuity of inhibition is strongest when the longitudinal sample contains children who represent behavioral extremes.

More recently, Ladd and Burgess (1999) examined the stability of social withdrawal from kindergarten to second grade, as assessed by teacher ratings. There was little support for stability of withdrawal among these young children; however, the withdrawn group was one standard deviation above the mean and not an extreme group, as was the case in the WLP or in Kagan's research. Like Ladd and Burgess (1999), Schneider, Richard, Younger, and Freeman (2000) did not find observed or parent-assessed social withdrawal to be too stable from ages 5 to 7 years. However, considerable stability was evidenced among extreme groups of withdrawn participants. Consistent with these latter findings and with those of the WLP, Schneider and colleagues have shown social withdrawal to be stable over a 3-year period during early adolescence. Once again, social withdrawal was found to be most highly stable across contexts and over time (fifth to eighth grades) for the subgroup of young adolescents who were the most withdrawn at the outset of the study (Schneider, Younger, Smith, & Freeman, 1998).

The relative stability reported in the WLP also bolsters earlier findings concerning the long-term stability of social withdrawal (Bronson, 1966; Kagan & Moss, 1962; Moskowitz, Schwartzman, & Ledingham, 1985). Although these studies vary considerably in time spans covered, developmental periods involved, kinds of methodology and measures employed, and types of social withdrawal, they show quite consistently that social withdrawal tends to persist across time.

Correlates of Social Withdrawal

The stability data just described are informative insofar as the prediction of solitary behavior is concerned. In our developmental model, however, we argue that social withdrawal reflects and predicts a negative quality of socioemotional life. The developmental course we have predicted for social withdrawal has received much support in recent years. For instance, during the preschool and primary grades, socially withdrawn children are less able to comprehend the perspectives of others (LeMare & Rubin, 1987), and are more likely than their more sociable age-mates to be adult-dependent and unassertive when faced with interpersonal dilemmas (Rubin, 1985; Rubin, Daniels-Beirness, & Bream, 1984). When they do attempt to assert themselves and gain compliance from their peers, they are more likely than their more sociable counterparts to be rebuffed (Rubin & Krasnor, 1986). Indeed, noncompliance to the requests of socially withdrawn children increases with age from early to middle childhood (Nelson, 2000; Stewart & Rubin, 1995). Among socially withdrawn children, moreover, the production of peer-directed requests become increasingly less assertive with age (Stewart & Rubin, 1995).

These latter findings are important for at least two reasons. First, the consistent and growing experience of failure in response to social initiatives suggests that a socially withdrawn child undergoes regular doses of rejection during peer interaction. Second, the experience of peer noncompliance probably carries with it negative emotional and cognitive burdens. In the face of consistent peer noncompliance, socially withdrawn children, unlike normal children, may begin to attribute their interactive failures to internal stable causes. Such an interpretation would be consistent with research demonstrating that some children perceive their social successes as unstable and externally caused, and their social failures as stable and internally caused (Goetz & Dweck, 1980; Hymel & Franke, 1985; Sobol & Earn, 1985). In the WLP, extremely withdrawn children were found to interpret social failure as caused by internal, stable causes (Rubin & Krasnor, 1986). Taken together, the experience of peer rebuff and the attribution of peer noncompliance to internal, dispositional causes suggests a feedback loop whereby the initially fearful and withdrawn youngster comes to believe that his or her social failures are dispositionally based; then these beliefs are strengthened by the increasing failure of the child's social initiatives. Ultimately, the child's behavioral reaction is to withdraw further from the peer milieu.

Consistent with these negative attributions is the finding that socially withdrawn children, from about 7 years of age onward, have negative self-perceptions of their social skills and social relationships (Asendorpf & van Aken, 1994; Hymel, Bowker, & Woody, 1993; Hymel, Rubin, Rowden, & LeMare, 1990; Morison & Masten, 1991; Parkhurst & Asher, 1992; Rubin, 1985; Rubin et al., 1993; Rubin, Hymel, & Mills, 1989). Moreover, with increasing age, social withdrawal becomes accompanied by feelings of loneliness and depression (Asendorpf, 1993; Bell-Dolan et al., 1993; Burgess & Younger, 2002; Rubin, Chen, et al., 1995; Rubin, Hymel, & Mills, 1989).

Finally, our model indicates that when socially withdrawn children become a salient and deviant group, they become rejected and actively isolated by their peers. Given the reality of peer rebuff during interactional encounters, it is not surprising that this postulate has been confirmed in numerous studies. Observational and peer assessments of social withdrawal have consistently been associated with sociometric measures of rejection from middle childhood onward (e.g., Boivin, Hymel, & Bukowski, 1995; French, 1988, 1990; Harrist, Zaia, Bates, Dodge, & Pettit, 1997; Hymel & Rubin, 1985; Ollendick, Greene, Weist, & Oswald, 1990; Rubin et al., 1993; Rubin, Hymel, & Mills, 1989). However, such relations are nonsignificant during early childhood, when social withdrawal is less atypical and less salient to the peer group (e.g., Hart et al., 2000; Ladd & Burgess, 1999).

Friendship and Social Withdrawal

It is one thing to be rejected by the peer group, but it is something else to lack friendships with others. "Friendship" refers to a voluntary, reciprocal, and mutually regulated relationship between a child and a peer. During childhood, friendships have been viewed as support systems that facilitate psychological and social development (Ladd, Kochenderfer, & Coleman, 1996).

Several indices have evolved to represent aspects of this relationship, including the size of a child's friendship network (i.e., number of mutual friendships), participation in a "very best" friendship, and quality of the friendships (see Rubin et al., 1998, for an extensive review). Unfortunately, a paucity of information exists with respect to shy/withdrawn children's friendships, and the data are limited for all ages and for all aspects of friendship.

Children with larger networks of mutual friends may receive higher levels of support; in turn, friendship network size may be associated with better psychological health (Ladd & Burgess, 2001). While one might expect that withdrawn children would have fewer mutual friendships than average children, because they seldom initiate exchanges with peers and respond to peers' initiations less often (Wanlass & Prinz, 1982), Ladd and Burgess (1999) found that young elementary school-age withdrawn children had as many mutual friends as their normative counterparts. The authors speculated that even though withdrawn children interact with peers less often than average children, they may still interact occasionally, and these encounters may be enough for them to nominate and be nominated as a friend. Note that this result was obtained among young children (ages 5–8), and that these withdrawn children were considered solitary–passive (asocial, uninterested) as opposed to reticent. More recently, we (Wojslawowicz, Burgess, Rubin, Rose-Krasnor, & Booth, 2002) found that extremely withdrawn preadolescents were as likely as their "control" age-mates to have a best friend. The prevalence in both cases was approximately 55%. Furthermore, of the shy/withdrawn children who had a best friend, 60% were able to maintain them over the entire school year. Thus, although they are typically noted as sociometrically rejected, withdrawn children do appear to have best friendships.

Being part of one very best friendship, especially a mutually positive one, may help children's adjustment (Hartup, 1997). But we have yet to discover whether friendship can buffer withdrawn children from such psychological difficulties as low self-esteem, loneliness, and depression. If friendships do buffer withdrawn children from negative psychological "outcomes," one would expect that only high-quality friendships would do so. Again, it remains an empirical question as to whether socially withdrawn children's friendships differ in quality from those of other children. We (Wojslawowicz et al., 2002) have indicated that the friends of extremely withdrawn children are more likely to be withdrawn too, compared to the friends of control and aggressive fifth-graders. Recently, Schneider (1999) observed that the friendships of withdrawn children (8–9 years old) were less competitive than those of control children. Furthermore, withdrawn children viewed their friendships as closer and more helpful than did their friends. These latter results raise an interesting question: Given that friendship is a dyadic construct, can a child's *perception* that the friendship *is* close or helpful be of psychological aid to that child, or is the *quality of the dyadic relationship* more psychologically significant for developmental outcomes? These are questions well worth exploring in future research.

Victimization and Social Withdrawal

Being victimized or bullied by peers implies that a child is regularly exposed to abusive interactions in the form of physical or verbal aggression. These negative events lead to fear of classmates, and ultimately to further withdrawal from peer interaction and possibly from school-related activities. During early childhood, socially withdrawn children do not seem to be victimized by their peers (Ladd & Burgess, 1999). By middle to late childhood, however, evidence reveals that peers do victimize them (Boivin et al., 1995; Hanish & Guerra, 2000; Wojslawowicz et al., 2002). Importantly, the best friends of withdrawn children are also more likely to be victimized by peers than are the best friends of control and aggressive preadolescents (Wojslawowicz et al., 2002). In this regard, withdrawn children may be involved in close relationships with others who are also victimized, thereby making the social quality of their individual and relationship "lives" less than optimal.

In summary, it would appear that many of the propositions in our developmental model have been confirmed. Social withdrawal in childhood *is* accompanied by intra- and interpersonal liabilities. By definition, socially withdrawn children do not interact as often as normal for their age cohort. Thus they make it difficult for themselves to master the skills derived from peer interactional experiences that appear necessary for "survival" in the peer group. The costs accompanying social withdrawal include being unassertive and unable to gain peer compliance; being rejected and victimized by peers; thinking poorly of one's social competence and relationships; feeling poorly about the self; and expressing loneliness. Clearly, social withdrawal can be taken as a "warning flag" for subsequent social and emotional problems of an internalizing nature.

Social Withdrawal as a Predictor of Maladaptation

The most extensive study of the predictive consequences of childhood social withdrawal has been the WLP (see Rubin, 1993, for a review). From the initial rounds of data analyses, observed passive withdrawal in kindergarten was found to predict self-reported feelings of depression, low general self-worth, and teacher-rated anxiety at age 11. Similar predictive correlations were found for observed passive withdrawal at age 7 years (Hymel et al., 1990; Rubin & Mills, 1988). These findings are noteworthy, because it would appear as if solitary play that is of a benign nature when observed during play sessions involving unfamiliar peers (passive solitude, or solitary constructive and exploratory activity) carries a very different meaning when observed among *familiar* peers.

Given that social withdrawal is contemporaneously associated with intrapersonal difficulties, and thus may be considered a behavioral reflection of these difficulties (anxiety, negative self-perceptions of social competence; e.g., Hymel, Bowker, & Woody, 1993; Rubin, 1993), it seemed reasonable in the WLP to examine how well the *constellation* of passive withdrawal, anxiety, and negative self-perceptions of social competence could predict later socioemotional difficulties. Data analyses revealed that this constellation, as assessed at 7 years, predicted lonely and depressive feelings at age 11 years (Rubin, Hymel, & Mills, 1989). It appears then that anxiety and withdrawal, in concert with negative thoughts about the self, ultimately predict subsequent negative affect—most notably, internalized feelings of loneliness and depression. In the final reports of the WLP findings, Rubin and colleagues (Rubin, 1993; Rubin, Chen, McDougall, Bowker, & McKinnon, 1995) indicated that a composite of observed social withdrawal (reticent and solitary–passive behaviors) and peer- and teacher-assessed passive/reticent withdrawal at age 7 years predicted adolescent (age 14 years) negative self-regard, loneliness, and feelings of a lack of integration and involvement in the family and peer group. This latter measure was construed as an assessment of felt security within the family and peer group. Furthermore, a composite of peer- and teacher-assessed passive/reticent withdrawal at age 11 years predicted negative self-perceptions of social competence, loneliness, and felt insecurities within the family and peer group (Rubin, Chen, et al., 1995). Thus the data again supported the premises of our developmental model.

Recently, other researchers have augmented or expanded the WLP findings. For example, Bowen, Vitaro, Kerr, and Pelletier (1995) found that kindergarten teacher ratings of anxious/withdrawn behavior and peer ratings of shyness were significant predictors of fifth-grade internalizing difficulties. Renshaw and Brown (1993) found that passive withdrawal at ages 9 to 12 years predicted loneliness assessed 1 year later. Also, Ollendick et al. (1990) reported that socially withdrawn fourth-graders were more likely to be perceived by peers as withdrawn and anxious, were more disliked by peers, received lower grades, and were more likely to have dropped out of school 5 years later than their well-adjusted counterparts. Boivin et al. (1995) found that social withdrawal (age 9) and peer rejection mediated by victimization led to depressed mood 2 years later. Morison and Masten (1991) indicated that children perceived by peers as withdrawn and isolated in middle childhood were more likely to think negatively about their social competencies and relationships in adolescence. Finally, Burgess and Younger (2002) found that shy/withdrawn adolescent males and females (ages 11–13) from a normative community sample had more negative self-perceptions, fewer positive self-perceptions, and higher levels of internalizing problems (such as depressive symptoms and somatic complaints) than did normative control and aggressive adolescents. Taken together, these recent investigations provide empirical support for the developmental pathway model (see Figure 8.1) regarding the consequences of social withdrawal.

Summary

In the present review, we have demonstrated that social withdrawal is (1) stable; (2) concurrently associated from early through late childhood with measures reflective of felt insecurity, negative self-perceptions, dependency, and social deference; (3) concurrently associated from middle childhood to early adolescence with peer rejection and victimization; and (4) predictive of internalizing difficulties by early adolescence.

Most samples described in our review have comprised groups of unselected school children. Furthermore, the "outcomes" of social withdrawal have not typically involved clinical assessments. This leaves open the question of whether clinical disorders can be predicted from *earlier* indices of social withdrawal and its concomitants. In one of the only published attempts to address this issue, Rubin (1993) administered the Children's Depression Inventory (CDI; Kovacs, 1980/1981) to 11-year-old WLP participants. Children whose CDI scores were one standard deviation or more above the mean for their age group were identified and constituted the top 8% of children in terms of depression scores. These children were then compared with their nondepressed schoolmates on indices of social and emotional well-being that had been assessed when they were 7 years of age. Follow-back discriminant-function analyses indicated that these children could *not* be distinguished from their normal counterparts on the basis of their popularity among peers at age 7 years. Furthermore, they were neither observed to be more aggressive in their free play, nor rated by their teachers as more hostile and aggressive. The depressed children *could* be distinguished from their normal counterparts, however, on the basis of observed social withdrawal, peer assessments of social withdrawal, and self-reported poor social competence. These results serve to support the developmental model we have proposed elsewhere, in which social withdrawal is described as a risk factor for the development of internalizing disorders (e.g., Rubin & Burgess, 2001; Rubin & Mills, 1991). Despite the initial support for this model, further longitudinal research is necessary before social withdrawal can be causally implicated in the development of maladaptation by adolescence and adulthood.

THE PARENTS OF SOCIALLY WITHDRAWN CHILDREN

Thus far, we have described etiological factors that may be responsible for the development of a socially withdrawn behavioral style in childhood—factors such as a child's dispositional characteristics and the quality of the parent–child relationship. We have also described the correlates and predictive consequences of childhood social withdrawal. Earlier, we have suggested that parents play a role in determining the course of social withdrawal in very *early* childhood. For example, mothers of insecurely attached "C" babies who appear to be on a trajectory toward social withdrawal are more overinvolved and overcontrolling than are mothers of securely attached babies (Erickson et al., 1985). Although this may be true, it would be rather ignorant to believe that once a child develops a given behavioral style, his or her peer group and the self-system take over and insidiously conspire to maintain and exacerbate the problems associated with social withdrawal. Although it *is* the case that socially withdrawn children (1) become increasingly salient to, and rejected by, peers with age, and (2) develop increasingly negative self-perceptions of their skills and relationships with age, it is also probable that the exigencies of being withdrawn filter back to the child's relationships and style of interaction with his or her parents (Burgess, Rubin, Cheah, & Nelson, 2001). Parents probably recognize the social insecurities and anxieties of their withdrawn child and respond in some fashion. In our developmental model, we propose that parental beliefs *and* parenting behaviors may maintain or exacerbate inhibited and withdrawn behavioral patterns.

Until recently, the scenario offered above was a relatively untested set of suppositions. Although an association between overprotective, overcontrolling, or overinvolved socialization strategies and social withdrawal in childhood has long been posited, it had seldom been directly investigated (e.g., Brunk & Henggeler, 1984; Hetherington & Martin, 1986). In this section of the chapter, we review the relevant literature on the connections among parenting beliefs, parenting behaviors, and social withdrawal.

Parenting Beliefs and Social Withdrawal in Childhood

In this chapter and elsewhere (e.g., Burgess, Rubin, Cheah, & Nelson, 2001; Rubin & Burgess, 2002), we have argued that once an inhibited behavioral style is established, parents may sense the child's anxieties and insecurities, and seek to improve the child's mastery of the environment through authoritarian direction or through actually solving the child's interpersonal and intrapersonal problems for him or her. Rubin, Mills, Hastings, and colleagues have addressed this possibility in a series of studies.

Rubin and Mills began with the notion that parenting behaviors are partly determined by parents' ideas about child behavior and development (Mills & Rubin, 1993a, 1993b; Rubin & Mills, 1992; Rubin, Mills, & Rose-Krasnor, 1989). Previous research has provided clear support for the notion that parents' behaviors are guided by (1) their values (Emmerich, 1969; Kohn, 1977; Stolz, 1967); (2) their beliefs about how children develop and how quickly they develop (e.g., Goodnow & Collins, 1990); (3) the methods they believe can promote optimal development (e.g., Maccoby & Martin, 1983); and (4) their attributions for the causes of their children's behaviors (e.g., Bugental & Shennun, 1984; Dix, Ruble, & Zambarano, 1989; Grusec & Kuczynski, 1980). To this end, parents' thoughts and feelings may indirectly affect children's social development by guiding parental behaviors (see Bugental & Goodnow, 1998, for an extensive review). These behaviors include not only the anticipatory or *proactive* strategies parents use to promote competent social behaviors, but also the *reactive* strategies they use to modify or eliminate unskilled and unacceptable behaviors in their children.

If the way parents think affects their sensitivity, and if their sensitivity contributes to children's socioemotional development, then it is quite possible that parents of socially withdrawn children differ from other parents in their patterns of cognition. Rubin, Mills, and Rose-Krasnor (1989) asked mothers of preschoolers to rate how important they felt it was for their children to develop a number of representative social skills (e.g., how to make friends); to what they attributed the development of these social skills (e.g., child-centered dispositional causes vs. external direct or indirect causes); and what they might do to aid in the development of such skills. In addition, the children were observed during classroom free play. Those preschoolers whose mothers indicated that the attainment of social skills was relatively unimportant were observed to cry more often when attempting to meet their social goals and to experience less social problem-solving success. These results are much like those reported in studies of the social problem-solving behaviors of socially withdrawn and reticent children (Nelson, 2000; Rubin & Krasnor, 1986; Stewart & Rubin, 1995). The children of mothers who believed that social skills emanate primarily from temperamental or dispositional factors were less socially assertive and successful during their peer exchanges. Finally, mothers who indicated that they would use high power-assertive strategies to socialize social skills (e.g., overcontrolling behaviors such as force, coercion, and strong commands) had children who were more likely to seek help from others, especially adults, and to use nonassertive social strategies to meet their own social goals. Teachers also rated these children as anxious, fearful, and withdrawn.

In a second study, Rubin and Mills (1990) used behavioral observations and teacher ratings to identify preschool children who were extremely anxious and withdrawn. Mothers of these children were compared with those of average children regarding their beliefs about the development of social skills and social withdrawal. Mothers were asked to rank, in order of importance, the most likely influences on the acquisition of a series of social skills (e.g., getting acquainted with someone new, resolving peer conflicts, getting accepted into an ongoing play group of unfamiliar peers, persuading other children to do what one wants). For each of the four social skills, mothers of anxious/withdrawn children placed significantly more importance on directive teaching than did the mothers of average children.

Rubin and Mills (1990) also presented the mothers of anxious/withdrawn children with stories of hypothetical incidents in which their own children behaved consistently in a socially withdrawn fashion. Following each story, mothers were asked how they would feel if their own children consistently acted this way, what attributions they would make about the causes of the behavior, and what they thought they would do to modify the behavior. The mothers of anxious/withdrawn children were more likely than mothers of average children to prefer using coercive strategies (e.g., directives) and less likely to prefer low power-assertive strategies (e.g., redirecting the child) and indirect or no response (e.g., seeking information from others, arranging opportunities for peer interaction, not responding) in reaction to their children's demonstration of socially withdrawn behavior. Mothers of anxious/withdrawn children were also more likely than mothers of average children to attribute the consistent display of social withdrawal to dispositional sources. Moreover, they expressed less puzzlement and more anger, disappointment, embarrassment, and guilt about their children's displays of withdrawal than did mothers of average children.

Together, the findings from these studies paint a consistent picture of mothers with socially withdrawn preschool children. The facts that these mothers placed greater importance on a directive approach to teaching social skills than did mothers of average children, and that they were more likely to choose controlling strategies for dealing with unskilled social behaviors, suggest that children with internalizing difficulties tend to have mothers who may be overinvolved. The causal attributions and emotional reactions of these mothers are also indicative of overinvolvement, and provide some tentative insights about why they may be overinvolved. These mothers were not only less tolerant of unskilled social behaviors than other mothers; they also felt more angry, disappointed, guilty, and embarrassed about these behaviors, and they were more inclined to blame them on a trait in their children.

This constellation of emotions and attributions suggests that mothers of withdrawn preschool-age children may regard their children as extensions of themselves and therefore consider their children's behavior as if it were their own. Moreover, the negative feelings reported by these mothers suggest that this overinvolvement has negative undercurrents. This dynamic is reminiscent of the pattern of anxious, overprotective parenting that has previously been linked to internalizing difficulties in children. Thus, in classic writings on parental overprotection or overcontrol, the phenomenon was described as constituting behaviors that interfere with or prevent the acquisition of independent and self-regulated behaviors (Levy, 1943; Parker, 1983). Overprotection typically involves the provision of help and physical comfort in situations where it is not required, as well as the intrusive restriction of independence (Anthony, 1970; Maccoby & Masters, 1970).

Although the data are consistent with the belief that socially withdrawn children are overcontrolled by their parents (e.g., Hetherington & Martin, 1986), it is important to remember that these studies concerned maternal *beliefs*, not behaviors; moreover, the mothers had socially withdrawn preschoolers. Whether the belief patterns described above extend to mothers of older or younger children is relatively unknown.

Relevant to these issues are two studies. In one study, Hastings and Rubin (1999) found that mothers whose toddlers were socially wary and inhibited believed 2 years hence that they would respond behaviorally to their children's social withdrawal with power assertion, especially if they had sons. Also, mothers of toddlers with BI who indicated a preference for an overprotective parenting style reported 2 years hence that they would respond with power assertion if their children behaved in a withdrawn fashion. In short, parents' beliefs about how they would react to their preschool children's displays of social withdrawal appear to be partially predicted by the characteristics of their children at age 2 years, as well as by their own earlier-expressed parenting preferences.

In the second relevant study, it was demonstrated that maternal beliefs change with increasing age of the withdrawn child. Mills and Rubin (1993b) found that mothers of extremely anxious/withdrawn elementary school-age children (5–9 years) described their affective reactions to the children's social withdrawal as involving *less* surprise and puzzlement than mothers of normal children indicated for their reactions. These data are themselves unsurprising, given the relative stability of withdrawal from the early to middle years of childhood. Moreover, although mothers of withdrawn elementary school-age children continued to attribute withdrawal to internal, personality traits of their children, they did *not* suggest that they would react to displays of withdrawal in a power-assertive manner (Mills & Rubin, 1993b). Perhaps these beliefs reflect parents' growing assumptions that dispositionally based behaviors become more difficult to change as children grow older; as such, it may make little sense to continue using direct means to control or change their children's withdrawn behavioral styles.

In summary, parental beliefs and cognitions reflect an intricate mix of causes and consequences of children's social behaviors. It may be that mothers of socially withdrawn preschool-age children are anxious and internalizing themselves, and transmit these problems to their children through an overinvolved pattern of parenting that creates a sense of felt insecurity. Indeed, preschool-age children of depressed mothers exhibit significantly more inhibited and anxious/withdrawn forms of play with both familiar and unfamiliar playmates than do children of nondepressed mothers (Kochanska, 1991; Rubin, Both, Zahn-Waxler, Cummings, & Wilkinson, 1991).

It may also be that mothers are very empathic with their children's extremely wary and reactive nature; empathy may result in the demonstration of *well-meant* overcontrol and overinvolvement. This reaction to their children's social characteristics may produce a mixture of defensive reactions (e.g., downplaying the importance of social skills) and negative emotions. For example, Thomasgard and Metz (1993) have suggested a model of maternal overprotection that is determined by such features as child and environmental or contextual factors. These authors have proposed that the child's role in either initiating or maintaining an overprotective relationship may derive from an inherent temperamental vulnerability (such as heightened emotional reactivity to the environment), and that this dispositional characteristic may elicit increased vigilance from the parent.

Thus it seems that children's social withdrawal may be a function of the interplay between maternal and child characteristics and the dialectic processes that are produced therein. Clearly, however, further developmental study of the relations between patterns of parenting and patterns of socioemotional adjustment is needed, in order to gain a better understanding of this interplay.

Parenting Behaviors and Social Withdrawal in Childhood

If parents' cognitions about the development of social competence and withdrawal influence their behaviors, then it would seem natural to expect that the socialization practices of parents whose children are withdrawn differ from those of parents whose children are socially competent and "normal." Two basic dimensions of parenting have been studied in this regard: "warmth/responsiveness" and "control/demandingness" (Baumrind, 1971; Maccoby & Martin, 1983). The dimension of warmth/responsiveness is an affective continuum of parenting, ranging from warm and sensitive behavior to cold or hostile behavior. The dimension of control/demandingness deals with issues of power assertion: At one end of the continuum are the frequent use of restrictive demands and high control, whereas at the opposite end of the continuum are frequent lack of supervision and low control. The interaction of the two continua constitutes a fourfold scheme that includes (1) "authoritative" parenting (high warmth, high control), (2) "authoritarian" parenting (low warmth, high control), (3) "indulgent/permissive" parenting (high warmth, low control), and (4) "indifferent/uninvolved" parenting (low warmth, low control) (Baumrind, 1971). To this fourfold schema one might add a fifth category; that is, the combination of excessive warmth and excessive control appears to constitute an "overprotective" style of parenting (Becker, 1964; Parker, Tupling, & Brown, 1979). Today overprotectiveness is encapsulated by the construct of "psychological control," a construct that refers broadly to the restriction of a child's autonomy (Barber, Olsen, & Shagle, 1994; Mills & Rubin, 1998). Psychologically controlling parents may attempt to direct every aspect of their children's lives, even in situations that ought to be unstructured, thereby leaving their children with few degrees of freedom.

Researchers have shown that children of authoritative parents are socially responsible and competent, friendly and cooperative with peers, and generally happy (Baumrind, 1967, 1971). This parenting style has been found to correlate contemporaneously and predictively with measures of moral reasoning and prosocial behavior in children, self-esteem (Hoffman, 1970; Yarrow, Waxler, & Scott, 1971), and academic achievement (Lamborn, Mounts, Steinberg, Dornbusch, & Darling, 1991; Steinberg, Lamborn, Dornbusch, & Darling, 1992). In contrast, Baumrind (1967) found that the parents of socially anxious, unhappy children who were insecure in the company of peers were more likely to demonstrate authoritarian socialization behaviors than the parents of more socially competent children. Relatedly, MacDonald and Parke (1984) found that boys perceived by teachers as socially withdrawn, as hesitant, and as spectators in the company of peers had fathers who were highly directive and less engaging or physically playful in their interactions with their sons. Their mothers were described as being less likely than mothers of nonwithdrawn sons to engage them in verbal exchange and interaction. The findings were less clear-cut for socially withdrawn daughters. In general, however, the researchers reported that during parent–child play, the parents of socially withdrawn children were less spontaneous, playful, and affectively positive than parents of more sociable children.

In a series of studies conducted about 50 years ago, it was consistently found that maternally reported overprotectiveness (excessive control and warmth) was associated with childhood submissiveness and dependency (Levy, 1943; Smith, 1958; Winder & Rau, 1962), whereby an overprotected child comes to allow the mother to think and act for him or her. More recently, Rubin and colleagues have found support for the contention that parental influence and control can maintain and exacerbate child inhibition and social withdrawal. We (Rubin, Hastings, Stewart, Henderson, & Chen, 1997) found that toddlers whose mothers perceived them as being socially wary, and who directed highly affectionate and intrusively controlling behaviors toward their children during a free-play situation, were more likely to demonstrate observed inhibited behaviors in the company of a same-age peer than those toddlers whose mothers perceived them to be socially wary but refrained from oversolicitous behavior. In a longitudinal investigation, we (Rubin, Burgess, & Hastings, 2002) found not only that toddler inhibition predicted socially reticent behavior at age 4 years, but also that maternal overcontrol was a significant moderator. For toddlers whose mothers were highly intrusive, inhibited behavior among peers predicted subsequent reticent behaviors; however, for toddlers whose mothers were not intrusively controlling, the relation between toddler inhibition and preschool reticence was nonsignificant. In a related study of reported rather than observed parenting styles, mothers' and fathers' perceptions of their toddlers as shy and inhibited at age 2 years were stable to age 4 years, and predicted a lack of parental encouragement of independence at age 4 years (Rubin, Nelson, Hastings, & Asendorpf, 1999). In a related study, Park, Belsky, Putnam, and Crnic (1997) found that the *stability* of inhibition among males (ages 2–3 years) was accompanied by inappropriately affectionate parenting.

Henderson and Rubin (1997) explored whether emotion-regulating processes, as measured physiologically, interacted with parental behavior to predict preschoolers' socially reticent behavior among peers. These researchers began with the premise that vagal tone (a marker of the tonic level of functioning of the parasympathetic nervous system, as described earlier) should be associated with the display of social behavior in the peer group. As noted earlier, children with low vagal tone have been found to be more inhibited in the presence of an adult stranger at age 2 years, and more reticent among peers at age 4 years. Henderson and Rubin (1997) reported that for preschoolers who showed low resting vagal tone, observed *and* reported maternal directive and critical behaviors were associated with children's reticent, wary, and anxious behaviors among peers. For children with high resting vagal tone, such maternal direction and criticism were not associated with behavioral reticence.

In a related study with a different sample, Rubin, Cheah, and Fox (2001) found that a highly directive and overly involved parenting style during mother–child free play was associated with the demonstration of socially reticent behavior among peers. Also, for emotionally dysregulated children, the lack of maternal direction during a potentially stressful problem-solving task predicted reticent behavior among peers. These latter findings strengthen the contention that children who tend to avoid social interaction have mothers who provide guidance and directives in an otherwise relaxed situation. Directiveness during goal-oriented tasks may be expected of parents (e.g., Kuczynski & Kochanska, 1995), but controlling the child's behavior in a pleasant, nonstressful, free-play environment is unnecessary. At the very least, such maternal behavior precludes the child from freely exploring the environment. The use of a highly directive parenting style during free play could suggest that the parent attempts to protect the child from stress or harm when neither is objectively present.

In a follow-up of these children at age 7 years, Cheah, Rubin, and Fox (1999) explored the influence of parenting and temperament at preschool age on the display of social solitude in middle childhood. In keeping with earlier research on the stability of socially withdrawn behavior, reticence at age 4 years significantly predicted reticent, socially anxious behaviors at age 7 years. Furthermore, mothers' displays of highly controlling and oversolicitous behaviors during a free-play session when children were 4 years old uniquely predicted behavioral reticence at age 7 years, beyond the initial level of reticence at age 4 years. Again, it appears that those mothers of reticent children who are overcontrolling and overinvolved (when it is unnecessary) exacerbate child reticence. Notably, this study revealed that such parenting behaviors make a contribution to reticence beyond the contribution of child temperament.

Another way in which parents of socially wary and withdrawn children vary from those of socially competent children is the extent to which affective interchanges are contingently responsive as well as psychologically derisive. Thus LaFreniere and Dumas (1992) found that mothers of anxious/withdrawn children (ages 2½–6 years) did not respond contingently to their children's displays of positive behavior and affect, but they did respond aversively to the children's negative behavior and negative affect. Among an older group of children, Mills and Rubin (1998) observed that, relative to mothers of normal children, mothers of extremely anxious/withdrawn children (aged 5–9 years) directed significantly more behavioral control statements to their children. Furthermore, mothers of anxious/withdrawn children used more psychological control statements, defined as devaluation statements or nonresponsiveness to the children.

Taken together, the extant data concerning the parenting behaviors and styles associated with social withdrawal focus clearly on at least two potential socialization contributors—psychological/behavioral control and overprotection. Parents who use high power-assertive strategies and who place many constraints on their children tend to rear shy, dependent children. Thus the issuance of parental commands, combined with constraints on exploration and independence, may hinder the development of competence in the social milieu. Restrictive control may also deprive the child of opportunities to interact with peers.

Of course, the developmental process is likely to involve bidirectional influences. Sensing their children's difficulties and perceived helplessness, some parents may try to support the children either by manipulating their social behaviors in a power-assertive, highly directive fashion (e.g., telling the children how to act or what to do) or by actually taking over for the children (e.g., intervening during object disputes, inviting a potential playmate to the home). For socially fearful and withdrawn children, the experience of parental overcontrol is likely to maintain or exacerbate rather than ameliorate their difficulties (see also Rapee, 1997, for a discussion of parental overcontrol and the development of social anxiety). Parental overdirectiveness will not allow a child to solve interpersonal problems on his or her own. It will also prevent the development of a belief system of social self-efficacy, and it probably perpetuates feelings of insecurity both within and outside of the family.

Note that the findings just described stem from very few data bases, and that the children in these studies varied widely with regard to age. Furthermore, the contexts within which parents of socially withdrawn children display overcontrol and overprotection have not been well specified. At this point, therefore, the socialization correlates and causes of social withdrawal are not well known. Parental or shared environmental effects seem to occur in early childhood, and unique peer group effects seem to increase with age. Another line of consideration pertains to the possibility that genetic factors shared by parents and their withdrawn children contribute to parenting styles, because both parents and children may have an underlying physiological predisposition that affects parental behaviors and affect. Thus the relative contributions or influences of shared environment and shared genetics have yet to be discovered. Clearly, these questions spur research that will garner much attention in the coming years.

EPIDEMIOLOGICAL FACTORS ASSOCIATED WITH SOCIAL WITHDRAWAL

Sex Differences

Information pertaining to sex differences in social withdrawal centers on two central issues: (1) differences in prevalence, and (2) differences in the correlates and outcomes of social withdrawal. With regard to prevalence, few researchers have reported sex differences in the extent to which children exhibit BI or social withdrawal. Data on parental ratings of early inhibition and/or shyness are equivocal. For example, Mathiesen and Tambs (1999) reported that parents rated their daughters as slightly more shy than sons at ages 18 and 30 months, but not later at 50 months. Others have found nonsignificant sex differences in observed and parent-rated BI and shyness at ages 2 and 4 years (Mullen, Snidman, & Kagan, 1993; Rowe & Plomin, 1977; Rubin et al., 1997, 1999; Simpson & Stevenson-Hinde, 1985).

Insofar as social withdrawal is concerned, researchers who have used peer ratings and nominations have not reported sex differences in preschool (Lemerise, 1997), middle childhood (Pekarik, Prinz, Leibert, Weintraub, & Neale, 1976), or late childhood (Rubin et al., 1993). Yet in early adolescence, some evidence indicates that girls self-report being shy more than boys (Crozier, 1995; Lazarus, 1982).

Although these latter findings cast some doubt on the notion that boys and girls do not differ in terms of how shy or socially withdrawn they are, some inconsistencies in the literature could be attributed to differences in the conceptualization of the constructs (i.e., shyness, inhibition, or social withdrawal), the age of the participants, the informant source, and method of assessment (i.e., self-reports, peer reports, parental ratings, or observations). It is also possible that gender differences in children's culturally based perceptions and schemas for shyness/withdrawal are related to these findings. For example, children tend to recall information about a hypothetical peer described as socially withdrawn when that peer is a girl, and the schema for withdrawal seems to be more accessible for girls than for boys (Bukowski, 1990).

Although the prevalence of inhibition, shyness, and social withdrawal may not vary between girls and boys, the correlates do. First, shy boys and shy girls appear to differ physiologically. Dettling, Gunnar, and Donzella (1999) reported that shyness in preschool-age boys, but not girls, was associated with increased cortisol level over the day at child care. Put another way, shy boys seem to feel greater stress as the day progresses in a social setting. Furthermore, Henderson, Fox, and Rubin (2001) found that negative reactivity at 9 months predicted displays of social wariness at age 4 years for boys, but not for girls. Second, researchers have indicated that boys' shy/withdrawn behavior is less accepted by their peers and teachers than that of shy girls is (Hinde, Stevenson-Hinde, & Tamplin, 1985; Moller, Hymel, & Rubin, 1992); furthermore, perhaps the type (e.g., reticence vs. solitary–passive behavior) or level (e.g., high, medium, or low) of withdrawal is relevant with regard to peer acceptance. For instance, whereas observed reticence in kindergarten-age children was negatively associated with social competence and academic achievement for both boys and girls, solitary–passive behavior was associated with ratings of internalizing problems and of social and academic maladjustment for boys only (Coplan, Gavinski-Molina, Lagacé-Séguin, & Wichmann, 2001).

Nelson's (2000) recent longitudinal report provides additional support for considering differential developmental patterns and sex differences for the withdrawn subtypes. Boys' displays of observed solitary–passive behavior at age 4 years were negatively associated with self-perceptions of maternal acceptance at 7 years of age, while the same was not true for girls who displayed frequent solitary–passive behavior. Furthermore, boys' solitary–passive withdrawal was concurrently associated with observed peer rejection, whereas the same did not hold true for girls. Solitary–passive behavior in early childhood has previously been thought to represent a "benign" type of solitude (e.g., Coplan et al., 1994; Rubin, 1982); however, these recent reports suggest that as early as the preschool period, some forms of social withdrawal may carry different psychological meanings for boys and girls.

Relatedly, Stevenson-Hinde and Glover (1996) found that mothers of young children who displayed high shyness (social reticence observed in home and laboratory settings) interacted more negatively with their children, regardless of sex. For children of moderate shyness, however, sex differences did emerge with regard to mother–child interactions. Specifically, mothers interacted more positively with moderately shy girls than with moderately shy boys. These data support earlier work in which parental responses to girls and boys varied with respect to socially withdrawn forms of behavior. For example, both Stevenson-Hinde (1989) and Engfer (1993) reported that the parents of inhibited/withdrawn toddler and preschool-age girls are warm, responsive, and sensitive. Yet the relations are in the opposite direction for boys: Parents of young withdrawn boys are cold, less affectionate, and less responsive than are parents of average children (see also Radke-Yarrow, Richters, & Wilson, 1988; Stevenson-Hinde & Hinde, 1986). Furthermore, insecurely attached ("C") boys, but not girls, are more likely than their secure counterparts to display passive, withdrawn behaviors in early and middle childhood (Renken et al., 1989). Although it is difficult to ascertain whether dispositional factors lead to different parental responses, or whether different parenting behavior leads to different social behavioral profiles for boys versus girls, the bottom line is that passive, inhibited, withdrawn boys and girls experience different socialization histories.

We have noted that both parents and peers respond differently to the demonstration of social withdrawal and shyness/reticence when boys versus girls exhibit them. It also appears as if the self-system is implicated in sex differences. During childhood and adolescence, socially withdrawn boys (but not girls) describe themselves as more lonely, as having poorer social skills, and as having lower self-esteem than their "average" peers (Morison & Masten, 1991; Rubin et al., 1993). Finally, Caspi, Elder, and Bem (1988) found that males who were shy in childhood married, became fathers, and established careers at a later age than their nonshy peers. In contrast, females who were shy in childhood did not marry or start families later than other women in the same cohort.

The different outcomes associated with social withdrawal for boys may be partly attributable to societal or cultural expectations; in Western societies, shyness/withdrawal appears to be less acceptable for boys than for girls (Sadker & Sadker, 1994). We review cultural differences next.

Culture

Thus far, we have described the developmental course of social withdrawal, its concomitants, and factors that influence its demonstration throughout childhood. We have also described some initial work that bears on the possibility of sex differences in inhibition, shyness, and withdrawal. Another important epidemiological factor is cultural variation. Almost every study described above has emanated from research laboratories in the Western world—countries like Australia (Sanson et al., 1996), Canada (e.g., Coplan et al., 2001; Rubin, Chen, et al., 1995), England (Stevenson-Hinde & Glover, 1996), Germany (Asendorpf & van Aken, 1994), Norway (Olweus, 1993), Sweden (Broberg et al., 1990), and the United States (Fox et al., 1996; Kagan, 1989). It is well known, however, that the evaluation of social behavior (e.g., inhibition, withdrawal) is influenced by cultural values and social conventions (Gresham, 1986). Consequently, adults view children's behaviors as normal or abnormal from the perspective of cultural norms and values. Whether or not parents seek professional help for their children is likely to be partially determined by cultural beliefs, values, perceptions, and norms.

Adults' judgments about child clinical problems differ markedly as a function of their cultural context. Prevailing social attitudes and values may help set thresholds for concerns about problematic child behaviors, emotions, and thoughts. For example, Weisz, Suwanlert, Chaiyasit, and Weiss (1988) compared the judgments of Thai and American parents, teachers, and clinical psychologists about two children—one with overcontrolled problems (e.g., shyness, fear), and one with undercontrolled problems (e.g., disobedience, fighting). Compared to Americans, Thais rated problems of both types as less serious, less worrisome, less likely to reflect personality traits, and more likely to improve with time. Cross-national differences in perceived seriousness were more pronounced for parents and teachers than for psychologists, suggesting that professional backgrounds and higher education may mitigate the effects of national belief systems.

In Western cultures, parents and peers view passive and reticent behaviors negatively. As already mentioned, individuals who display such behaviors are considered socially immature, fearful, and dependent. Unlike children in Western cultures, however, children in China are encouraged to be dependent, cautious, self-restrained, and behaviorally inhibited (Ho, 1986; Ho & Kang, 1984). Such behaviors are generally considered indices of accomplishment, mastery, and maturity (Feng, 1962; King & Bond, 1985). Similarly, shy, quiet children are described as well behaved. Researchers have consistently revealed that Chinese toddlers, children, adolescents, and adults are more inhibited, anxious, and sensitive than their North American counterparts (Chan & Eysenck, 1981; Chen et al., 1998; Gong, 1984; Watrous & Hsu, 1963). Sensitive, cautious, and inhibited behavior in children is highly praised and encouraged (Ho, 1986; Ho & Kang, 1984); it has been positively associated with competent/prosocial behavior, academic achievement, leadership, and peer acceptance concurrently and longitudinally in Chinese children (Chen et al., 1998; Chen, Rubin, & Li, 1995; Chen et al., 1999; Chen, Rubin, & Sun, 1992). Furthermore, the display of shy/sensitive behavior has been associated with maternal acceptance in samples of Chinese toddlers (Chen et al., 1998) and adolescents (Chen, Rubin, & Li, 1997), unlike in Western samples.

Whereas shy/inhibited behavior in Chinese samples has generally been associated with positive and adaptive outcomes, these associations might only be obtained within specific age groups and specific contexts. For example, Chen et al. (1995) found that peer-rated shyness/sensitivity was associated with peer acceptance, academic achievement, participation in school leadership, and teacher-assessed school competence at 8 and 10 years of age, but was not associated with the aforementioned positive outcomes at 12 years of age. By early adolescence, shyness/sensitivity was negatively associated with peer acceptance. Chen et al. (1995) also reported that indices of social isolation from the peer group (rejection) were associated with shyness/sensitivity at age 12, but not at ages 8 and 10, thereby giving some indication that shyness/sensitivity eventually becomes indicative of social maladjustment among Chinese preadolescents.

In a recent cross-cultural study of maternal beliefs, Cheah (2000) found that Chinese mothers reacted more strongly (with anger) to hypothetical vignettes of children's withdrawn behavior in the peer context than did European American mothers. She speculated that mothers perceive their children's withdrawal as a lack of cooperation, which would contradict the cultural expectation of collectivistic behaviors. These latter results suggest that the research program of Chen and colleagues (e.g., Chen et al., 1995, 1998, 1999) has focused primarily on reservedness in social company rather than on social withdrawal per se. In support of this contention, Hart et al. (2000) have recently revealed that teacher-rated social reticence is negatively associated with peer acceptance among young Chinese children.

Cross-cultural research on social withdrawal, shyness, and BI now extends beyond East–West comparisons. For instance, socially reticent/withdrawn behavior is associated with low peer acceptance among children in Argentina, Italy, and Russia (Attili, Vermigili, & Schneider, 1997; Hart et al., 2000; Schaughency, Vannatt, Langhinrichsen, Lally, & Seely, 1992). Also, Schneider, Attili, Vermigli, and Younger (1997) reported that Italian mothers respond more negatively to boys' than girls' demonstrations of social withdrawal.

In summary, the cultural milieu and societal values may have differential effects on the perception and treatment of wary and withdrawn behaviors. Given that the majority of the world's inhabitants do not reside in Western countries, the studies just described bear careful note. It would appear that the definitions of normality and psychological disorder described in the vast majority of texts may be culture-specific. Assuredly, this issue requires scrutiny—not only for the study of social withdrawal, but also for research on most other supposed behavioral anomalies in childhood. Relatedly, it would serve everyone's best interests not to generalize to other cultures Western culture-specific theories of the development of psychopathology.

A DEVELOPMENTAL PATHWAY TO CHILDHOOD SOCIAL WITHDRAWAL

Throughout this chapter, we have referred to a developmental model concerning the etiology, correlates, and outcomes of social withdrawal during childhood. As noted earlier, the pathway to the ontogeny of a socially withdrawn profile begins with newborns who are biologically predisposed to have a low threshold for arousal when confronted with social (or nonsocial) stimulation and novelty. This hyperarousal may make these babies extremely difficult to soothe and comfort. We propose that under some circumstances, parents may find these dispositional characteristics aversive and difficult to handle. Under conditions of stress and strain, parents may react to easily aroused and wary babies with the belief that the children are vulnerable and need protection. Such overprotective and oversolicitous parenting, in concert with the child dispositional factors of a low threshold for arousal and an inability to be easily soothed ("emotion dysregulation"; Rubin, Coplan, et al., 1995), are posited to predict the development of an insecure parent–infant attachment relationship. Thus, an interplay of endogenous, socialization, and early relationship factors as they coexist under an "umbrella" of negative setting conditions, such as stress and the lack of familial support, is suggested to lead to a sense of felt insecurity.

It is important to note that we believe an emotionally dysregulated infant will prove a significant challenge to parents, especially those who are experiencing stress in their lives. For instance, a lack of financial resources may create feelings of frustration, anger, and helplessness that can be translated into less optimal child-rearing styles, especially if the infant is perceived to be "difficult." Parents who are financially stressed are less nurturant, involved, child-centered, and consistent with their children than are less stressed parents (Conger, McCarty, Young, Lahey, & Kropp, 1984; Elder, Van Nguyen, & Caspi, 1985; Patterson, 1983, 1986). Parental marital/relationship discord and dissatisfaction are also stressors that may impede a sensitive response to children, especially temperamentally difficult infants. Like economic strain, parental relationship discord has been associated with insensitive, unresponsive parenting behaviors (Emery, 1982; Jouriles et al., 1991). Finally, parental psychopathology is a stressor related to the production of unresponsive, insensitive parenting. For example, maternal depression is associated with a lack of parental involvement, responsivity, spontaneity, and emotional support in child rearing (Downey & Coyne, 1990; Kochanska, Kuczynski, & Maguire, 1989; Zahn-Waxler et al., 1988). Given that depression is associated with maternal feelings of hopelessness and helplessness (Gurland, Yorkston, Frank, & Stone, 1967), the above-described pattern of parenting behaviors would not be a surprise if an infant were perceived as emotionally dysregulated.

Nevertheless, the effects of stress on parenting behaviors can be moderated or buffered by the availability of social support (Cohen & Wills, 1985; Compas, 1987; Crnic, Ragozin, Greenberg, Robinson, & Basham, 1983). It has been argued that supportive social networks are sources of emotional strength and of information that enhance feelings of competence to cope with stress, including those concerned with parenting. In summary, we propose that an emotionally dysregulated infant reared by unresponsive parents in a "high stress/low support" environment will develop an insecure attachment relationship with his or her primary caregiver.

We also propose that the infant's temperament, along with feelings of insecurity, guide him or her onto a trajectory toward BI. The consistent expression of BI precludes these children from experiencing the positive outcomes associated with social exploration and peer play. Thus we predict a developmental sequence in which an inhibited, fearful, insecure child withdraws from his or her social world of peers; fails to develop those skills derived from peer interaction; and consequently becomes increasingly anxious and isolated from the peer group.

As noted above, social reticence or withdrawal becomes increasingly salient to the peer group with age (Younger et al., 1993). This deviation from age-appropriate social norms is associated with the establishment of peer rejection; for example, by the middle to late childhood, social withdrawal and anxiety are as strongly correlated with peer rejection and unpopularity as aggression is (e.g., Rubin, Hymel, LeMare, & Rowden, 1989; Rubin et al., 1993).

Reluctance to explore and play cooperatively in their social environments is postulated to result in the development of an impoverished style of interpersonal negotiation skills. These children may make few attempts to direct the behaviors of peers, and when they do, it is likely that they will be met by peer rebuff (Nelson, 2000; Rubin & Rose-Krasnor, 1992; Stewart & Rubin, 1995). One outcome of social interactive failure and peer rejection probably will be the development of negative self-perceptions of social skills and peer relations (Boivin et al., 1995; Hymel, Woody, & Bowker, 1993; Nelson, 2000). Sensing the child's difficulties and perceived helplessness, the parents may try to direct their child's social behaviors in a power-assertive fashion by telling the child how to act or what to do, or by actually solving the child's interpersonal dilemmas for him or her. An overcontrolled or overinvolved parenting style then serves to maintain and exacerbate the socially withdrawn child's inter- and intrapersonal difficulties (e.g., Rubin et al., 2001, 2002).

In summary, we propose that social incompetence of an overcontrolled, withdrawn nature may be the product of an inhibited temperament, of an insecure parent–child relationship, of shared genetic vulnerabilities or traits with the parents, of overly directive and protective parenting, of family stress, and of the interactions among all of these factors. The consequences of this constellation of factors are the development of (1) negative thoughts and feelings about the self, (2) social anxiety, and (3) loneliness. If the establishment and maintenance of close interpersonal relationships are considered significant objectives that have not been met, another outcome may be depression.

It is very important to note that we do not view infant dispositional characteristics as necessarily leading to the pathway described above. A wary, fearful, inhibited temperament may be "deflected" toward the development of social competence by responsive and sensitive caregiving and by a relatively stress-free environment (Rubin et al., 1997, 2002). An inhibited, emotionally dysregulated temperament does not necessarily produce an incompetent, internalized, or overcontrolled behavioral style. On the other hand, parental overcontrol and overinvolvement, especially when accompanied by familial stress and lack of social support, can deflect a temperamentally easy-going infant toward a pathway of internalizing difficulties.

The developmental pathway we offer represents a useful heuristic for studying the etiology of social withdrawal. There are direct and indirect ways that dispositional characteristics, parent–child relationships, parenting styles, familial stress, and peer relationships might contribute to the development and maintenance of social withdrawal, its concomitants, and its outcomes. But the pathway must not be accepted as the only route to the development of social withdrawal. On an international level, we welcome our colleagues' support in providing alternative perspectives, as well as empirically derived information, on the developmental course of social withdrawal.

FUTURE DIRECTIONS

We have begun in this chapter by providing the reader with a raison d'être for considering social withdrawal to be a relevant topic for a volume on child psychopathology. In so doing, we have defined the phenomenon of interest and distinguished it from variables with which it is often confused—for example, inhibition, shyness, and isolation/rejection. Winding throughout the review has been a guiding developmental model that provides a framework for the literature reviewed. Also, it clearly specifies areas that require further examination.

The study of the developmental course of social withdrawal has garnered an enormous amount of attention in the past decade. A glance at the dates of the material cited in this chapter will attest to this fact. Much of the relevant work has been directed toward establishing the correlates and consequences of social withdrawal at different points in childhood and adolescence. However, the few longitudinal studies that exist in this regard must necessarily be replicated and/or extended if one seriously views social withdrawal as a risk factor for the development of psychopathology. Admittedly, the limited data do support this contention, but they are not conclusive.

Although we have suggested a number of etiological factors that conspire to produce a socially withdrawn profile in childhood, it is important to note that the supportive data have come from very few developmental laboratories. Again, further replication work is necessary. The extent to which dispositional factors, shared genetic traits, parenting styles, parent–child relationships, peer experiences, and gene × environment interactions predict the consistent display of socially withdrawn behavior in familiar peer contexts needs to be established well beyond the research in one or two laboratories. Moreover, the extent to which the developmental course of social withdrawal is similar or dissimilar for boys versus girls requires attention.

Finally, what we know about the developmental course of social withdrawal is constrained by the cultures in which we have studied the phenomenon. The large majority of the published literature is derived from studies conducted in North America and Western Europe. Consequently, virtually nothing is known about the developmental significance of social withdrawal in non-Western cultures. Clearly, additional cross-cultural work that falls along both East–West and North–South planes should be added to our research agenda. To this end, we have recently instigated the International Consortium for the Study of Social and Emotional Development, a consortium with researchers from such countries as Australia, Brazil, Canada, China, India, Italy, Korea, and the United States. This consortium has begun cross-replicated longitudinal studies of the developmental course of social competence, BI, and dysregulated temperament.

The bottom line is that a review of the literature on childhood social withdrawal undoubtedly has a place in this volume. Empirical work suggests that the quality of life for a socially withdrawn child on individual, family, and peer levels is less than pleasant. Withdrawn children are socially deferent, anxious, lonely, and insecure in the company of peers, as well as rejected by peers. They fail to exhibit age-appropriate interpersonal problem-solving skills, and they believe themselves to be deficient in social skills and social relationships. These characteristics do not augur well for socially withdrawn children. Whether or not the constellation of these factors leads inexorably to the development of psychopathology or clinical disorders is not yet known.

REFERENCES

Achenbach, T. M. (1995). Developmental issues in assessment, taxonomy, and diagnosis of child and adolescent psychopathology. In D. Cicchetti & D. J. Cohen (Eds.), *Developmental psychopathology* (Vol. 1, pp. 57–80). New York: Wiley.

Achenbach, T. M., & Edelbrock, C. (1981). Behavioral problems and competencies reported by parents of normal and disturbed children aged four through sixteen. *Monographs of the Society for Research in Child Development, 46*(1, Serial No. 188).

American Psychiatric Association. (1994). *Diagnostic and statistical manual of mental disorders* (4th ed.) Washington, DC: Author.

Anderson, K., Bohlin, G., & Hagekull, B. (1999). Early temperament and stranger wariness as predictors of social inhibition in 2 year olds. *British Journal of Developmental Psychology, 17*, 421–434.

Anthony, E. J. (1970). The behavior disorders of childhood. In P. H. Mussen (Ed.), *Carmichael's manual of child psychology* (Vol. 2, pp. 667–764). New York: Wiley.

Asendorpf, J. B. (1990). The development of inhibition during childhood: Evidence for situational specificity and a two-factor model. *Developmental Psychology, 26*, 721–730.

Asendorpf, J. B. (1991). Development of inhibited children's coping with unfamiliarity. *Child Development, 62*, 1460–1474.

Asendorpf, J. B. (1993). Beyond temperament: A two-factorial coping model of the development of inhibition during childhood. In K. H. Rubin & J. B. Asendorpf (Eds.), *Social withdrawal, inhibition and shyness in childhood* (pp. 265–289). Hillsdale, NJ: Erlbaum.

Asendorpf, J. B., & van Aken, M. A. G. (1994). Traits and relationship status: Stranger versus peer group inhibition and test intelligence versus peer group confidence as early predictors of later self-esteem. *Child Development, 65*, 1786–1798.

Attili, G., Vermigili, P., & Schneider, B. H. (1997). Peer acceptance and friendship patterns among Italian school children within a cross-cultural perspective. *International Journal of Behavioral Development, 21*, 277–288.

Barber, B. K., Olsen, J. E., & Shagle, S. C. (1994). Associations between parental psychological and behavioral control and youth internalized and externalized behaviors. *Child Development, 65*, 1120–1136.

Baumrind, D. (1967). Childcare practices anteceding three patterns of preschool behavior. *Genetic Psychology Monographs, 76*, 43–88.

Baumrind, D. (1971). Current patterns of parental authority. *Developmental Psychology Monographs, 4*, 1–101.

Becker, W. C. (1964). Consequences of different kinds of parental discipline. In L. W. Hoffman & M. L. Hoffman (Eds.), *Review of child development research* (Vol. 1, pp. 169–208). New York: Russell Sage.

Beidel, D. C., & Turner, S. M (1999). The natural course of shyness and related syndromes. In L.A. Schmidt & J. Schulkin (Eds.), *Extreme fear, shyness, and social phobia* (pp. 203–223). Oxford: Oxford University Press.

Bell-Dolan, D., Reaven, N. M, & Peterson, L. (1993). Depression and social functioning: A multidimensional study of linkages. *Journal of Clinical Child Psychology, 22*, 306–315.

Belsky, J., & Rovine, M. (1987). Temperament and attachment security in the strange situation: An empirical rapproachment. *Child Development, 58*, 787–795.

Berntson, G. G., Cacioppo, J. T., & Quigley, K. S. (1993). Respiratory sinus arrhythmia: Autonomic origins, physiological mechanisms, and psychophysiological implications. *Psychophysiology, 30*, 183–196.

Biederman, J., Rosenbaum, J. F., Bolduc-Murphy, E. A., Faraone, S. V., Chaloff, J., Hirshfeld, D. R., & Kagan, J. (1993). A 3-year follow-up of children with and without behavioral inhibition. *Journal of the American Academy of Child and Adolescent Psychiatry, 32*, 814–821.

Boivin, M., Hymel, S., & Bukowski, W. (1995). The roles of social withdrawal, peer rejection, and victimization by peers in predicting loneliness and depressed mood in childhood. *Development and Psychopathology, 7*, 765–785.

Booth, C. L., Rose-Krasnor, L., McKinnon, J., & Rubin, K. H. (1994). Predicting social adjustment in middle childhood: The role of preschool attachment security and maternal style. *Social Development, 3*, 189–204.

Bowen, F., Vitaro, F., Kerr, M., & Pelletier, D. (1995). Childhood internalizing problems: Prediction from kindergarten, effect of maternal overprotectiveness, and sex differences. *Development and Psychopathology, 7*, 481–498.

Bowlby, J. (1969). *Attachment and loss: Vol. 1. Attachment*. New York: Basic Books.

Broberg, A., Lamb, M. E., & Hwang, P. (1990). Inhibition: Its stability and correlates in sixteen-to-forty-month-old children. *Child Development, 61*, 1153–1163.

Bronson, W. C. (1966). Central orientations: A study of behavior organization from childhood to adolescence. *Child Development, 37*, 125–155.

Brunk, M. A., & Henggeler, S. W. (1984). Child influences on adult controls: An experimental investigation. *Developmental Psychology, 20*, 1074–1081.

Bugental, D., & Goodnow, J. J. (1998). Socialization processes. In W. Damon (Series Ed.) & N. Eisenberg (Vol. Ed.), *Handbook of child psychology: Vol. 3. Social, emotional, and personality development* (5th ed., pp. 389–462). New York: Wiley.

Bugental, D. B., & Shennun, W. A. (1984). "Difficult" children as elicitors and targets of adult communication patterns: An attributional-behavioral transactional analysis. *Monographs of the Society for Research in Child Development, 49*(Serial No. 205).

Bukowski, W. M. (1990). Age differences in children's memory of information about aggressive, socially withdrawn, and prosocial boys and girls. *Child Development, 61*, 1326–1334.

Burgess, K. B., Marshall, P. J., Rubin, K. H., & Fox, N. A. (in press). Infant attachment and temperament as predictors of subsequent externalizing problems and cardiac physiology. *Journal of Child Psychology and Psychiatry and Allied Disciplines*.

Burgess, K. B., Rubin, K. H., Cheah, C., & Nelson, L. (2001). Behavioral inhibition, social withdrawal, and parenting. In W. R. Crozier & L. Alden (Eds.), *International handbook of social anxiety: Concepts, research, and interventions relating to the self and shyness* (pp. 137–158). Sussex, UK: Wiley.

Burgess, K. B., & Younger, A. J. (2002). *Specificity of self and internalizing problems in socially withdrawn preadolescents*. Manuscript submitted for publication.

Calkins, S. D., & Fox, N. A. (1992). The relations among infant temperament, security of attachment, and behavioral inhibition at twenty-four months. *Child Development, 63*, 1456–1472.

Calkins, S. D., Fox, N. A., & Marshall, T. R. (1996). Behavioral and physiological antecedents of inhibition in infancy. *Child Development, 67*, 523–540.

Caspi, A., Elder, G. H., & Bem, D. J. (1988). Moving away from the world. Life-course patterns of shy children. *Developmental Psychology, 24*, 824–831.

Chan, J., & Eysenck, S. B. G. (1981, August). *National differences in personality: Hong Kong and England*. Paper presented at the joint IACCP-ICP Asian Regional Meeting, National Taiwan University, Taipei, Taiwan.

Chandler, M. (1973). Egocentrism and anti-social behavior: The assessment and training of social perspective-taking skills. *Developmental Psychology, 9*, 326–332.

Cheah, C. S. L. (2000). *Maternal proactive and reactive beliefs regarding preschoolers' social skills: A cross-cultural study of european american and mainland chinese mothers*. Unpublished doctoral dissertation, University of Maryland at College Park.

Cheah, C. S. L., Rubin, K. H., & Fox, N. A. (1999). *Predicting reticence at seven years: The influence of temperament and overprotective parenting at four years*. Poster presented at the biennial meeting of the Society for Research in Child Development, Albuquerque, NM.

Chen, X., Hastings, P. D., Rubin, K. H., Chen, H., Cen, G., & Stewart, S. L. (1998). Child-rearing practices and behavioral inhibition in Chinese and Canadian toddlers: A cross-cultural study. *Developmental Psychology, 34*, 677–686.

Chen, X., Rubin, K. H., & Li, Z. (1995). Social functioning and adjustment in Chinese children: A longitudinal study. *Developmental Psychology, 31*, 531–539.

Chen, X., Rubin, K. H., & Li, B. (1997). Maternal acceptance and social and school adjustment in Chinese children: A four-year longitudinal study. *Merrill–Palmer Quarterly, 43*, 663–681.

Chen, X., Rubin, K. H., Li, B., & Li, D. (1999). Adolescent outcomes of social functioning in Chinese children. *International Journal of Behavioural Development*, *23*, 199–223.

Chen, X., Rubin, K. H., & Sun, Y. (1992). Social reputation and peer relationships in Chinese and Canadian children: A cross-cultural study. *Child Development*, *63*, 1336–1343.

Clark, L. A., Vorhies, L., & McEwan, J. L. (1994). Personality disorder symptomatology from the five-factor model perspective. In P. T. Costa & T. A. Widiger (Eds.), *Personality disorders and the five-factor model of personality* (pp. 41–56). Washington, DC: American Psychological Association.

Cohen, S., & Wills, T. A. (1985). Stress, social support, and the buffering hypothesis. *Psychological Bulletin*, *98*, 310–357.

Compas, B. E. (1987). Coping with stress during childhood and adolescence. *Psychological Bulletin*, *101*, 393–403.

Conger, R. D., McCarty, J. A., Young, R. K., Lahey, B. B., & Kropp, J. P. (1984). Perception of child, child-rearing values, and emotional distress as mediating links between environmental stressors and observed maternal behavior. *Child Development*, *55*, 2234–2247.

Coplan, R. J., Gavinkski-Molina, M., Lagacé-Séguin, D. G., & Wichmann, C. (2001). When girls versus boys play alone: Nonsocial play and adjustments in kindergarten. *Developmental Psychology*, *37*, 464–474.

Coplan, R. J., & Rubin, K. H. (1998). Exploring and assessing nonsocial play in the preschool: The development and validation of the preschool play behavior scale. *Social Development*, *7*, 71–92.

Coplan, R. J., Rubin, K. H., Fox, N. A., Calkins, S. D., & Stewart, S. L. (1994). Being alone, playing alone, and acting alone: Distinguishing among reticience, and passive- and active-solitude in young children. *Child Development*, *65*, 129–137.

Costa, P. T., Jr., & McCrae, R. R. (1985). *The NEO Personality Inventory manual*. Odessa, FL: Psychological Assessment Resources.

Crick, N. R., & Dodge, K. A. (1994). A review and reformulation of social information-processing mechanisms in children's social adjustment. *Psychological Bulletin*, *115*, 74–101.

Crnic, K. A., Ragozin, A. S., Greenberg, M. T., Robinson, M. M., & Basham, R. B. (1983). Social interaction and developmental competence of pre-term and full term infants during the first year of life. *Child Development*, *54*, 1199–1210.

Crozier, W. R. (1995). Shyness and self-esteem in middle childhood. *British Journal of Educational Psychology*, *65*, 347–378.

Damon, W., & Killen, M. (1982). Peer interaction and the process of change in children's moral reasoning. *Merrill–Palmer Quarterly*, *28*, 347–378.

Davidson, R., & Fox, N. (1989). Frontal brain asymmetry predicts infants' response to maternal separation. *Journal of Abnormal Psychology*, *98*, 127–131.

Dettling, A. C., Gunnar, M. R., & Donzella, B. (1999). Cortisol levels of young children in full-day childcare centers: Relations with age and temperament. *Psychoneuroendocrinology*, *24*, 519–536.

Dix, T. H., Ruble, D. N., & Zambarano, R. J. (1989). Mothers' implicit theories of discipline: Child effects and the attribution process. *Child Development*, *60*, 1373–1391.

Downey, G., & Coyne, J. C. (1990). Children of depressed parents: An integrative review. *Psychological Bulletin*, *108*, 50–76.

Elder, G. H., Jr., Van Nguyen, T., & Caspi, A. (1985). Linking family hardship to children's lives. *Child Development*, *56*, 361–375.

Emery, R. (1982). Interparental conflict and the children of discord and divorce. *Psychological Bulletin*, *92*, 310–330.

Emmerich, W. (1969). The parental role: A functional–cognitive approach. *Monographs of the Society for Research in Child Development*, *34*(8, Serial No. 132).

Engfer, A. (1993). Antecedents and consequences of shyness in boys and girls: A 6-year longitudinal study. In K. H. Rubin & J. Asendorpf (Eds.), *Social withdrawal, inhibition, and shyness in childhood* (pp. 49–80). Hillsdale, NJ: Erlbaum.

Erickson, M. F., Sroufe, L. A., & Egeland, B. (1985). The relationship between quality of attachment and behavior problems in preschool in a high-risk sample. In I. Bretherton & E. Waters (Eds.), Growing points of attachment theory and research. *Monographs of the Society for Research in Child Development*, *50*(1–2, Serial No. 209), 147–166.

Feng, Y. L. (1962). *The spirit of Chinese philosophy* (E. R. Hughes, Trans.). London: Routledge & Kegan Paul.

Fox, N., Bell, M., & Jones, N. (1992). Individual differences in response to stress and cerebral asymmetry. *Developmental Neuropsychology*, *8*, 161–184.

Fox, N., & Calkins, S. (1993). Relations between temperament, attachment, and behavioral inhibition: Two possible pathways to extraversion and social withdrawal. In K. H. Rubin & J. Asendorpf (Eds.), *Social withdrawal, inhibition, and shyness in childhood* (pp. 81–100). Hillsdale, NJ: Erlbaum.

Fox, N. A., Calkins, S. D., & Bell, M. A. (1994). Neural plasticity and development in the first two years of life: Evidence from cognitive and socioemotional domains of research. *Development and Psychopathology*, *6*, 677–696.

Fox, N. A., Henderson, H. A., Rubin, K. H., Calkins, S. D., & Schmidt, L. A. (2001). Stability and instability of behavioral inhibition and exuberance: Psychophysiological and behavioral factors influencing change and continuity across the first four years of life. *Child Development*, *72*, 1–21.

Fox, N. A., Rubin, K. H., Calkins, S. D., Marshall, T. R., Coplan, R. J., Porges, S. W., Long, J., & Stewart, S. (1995). Frontal activation asymmetry and social competence at four years of age. *Child Development*, *66*, 1770–1784.

Fox, N. A., Schmidt, L. A., Calkins, S. D., Rubin, K. H., & Coplan, R.. J. (1996). The role of frontal activation in the regulation and dysregulation of social behavior during the preschool years. *Development and Psychopathology*, *8*, 89–102.

French, D. C. (1988). Heterogeneity of peer-rejected boys: Aggressive and nonaggressive subtypes. *Child Development*, *59*, 976–985.

French, D. C. (1990). Heterogeneity of peer-rejected girls. *Child Development*, *61*, 2028–2031.

Goetz, T., & Dweck, C. (1980). Learned helplessness in social situations. *Journal of Personality and Social Psychology*, *39*, 246–255.

Goldsmith, H. H., & Alansky, J. A. (1987). Maternal and infant temperamental predictors of attachment: A meta-analytic review. *Journal of Consulting and Clinical Psychology*, *55*, 805–816.

Gong, Y. (1984). Use of the Eysenck Personality Questionnaire in China. *Personality and Individual* Differences, 5, 431–438.

Goodnow, J. J., & Collins, A. W. (1990). *Development according to parents: The nature, sources, and consequences of parents' ideas*. Hove, England: Erlbaum.

Greenspan, S. I., & Lieberman, A. F. (1988). A clinical approach to attachment. In J. Belsky & T. Nezworski (Eds.), *Clinical implications of attachment* (pp. 387–424). Hillsdale, NJ: Erlbaum.

Gresham, F. M. (1986). Conceptual issues in the assessment of social competence in children. In P. S. Strain, M. J. Guralnick, & H. M. Walker (Eds.), *Children's social behavior: Development, assessment and modification* (pp. 143–179). New York: Academic Press.

Grusec, J. E., & Kuczynski, L. (1980). Directions of effect in socialization: A comparison of the parents vs. the child's behavior as determinants of disciplinary techniques. *Developmental Psychology, 16*, 1–9.

Gunnar, M. R., Mangelsdorf, S., Larson, M., & Hertsgaard, L. (1989). Attachment, temperament, and adrenocortical activity in infancy: A study of psychoendocrine regulation. *Developmental Psychology, 25*, 355–363.

Gurland, B., Yorkston, N., Frank, L., & Stone, A. (1967). *The structured and scaled interview to assess maladjustment* [Mimeographed booklet]. New York: New York State Psychiatric Institute, Division of Biometric Research, Department of Mental Hygiene.

Hanish, L. D., & Guerra, N. G. (2000). Predictors of peer victimization among urban youth. *Social Development, 9*, 521–543.

Harrist, A. W., Zaia, A. F., Bates, J. E., Dodge, K. A., & Pettit, G. S. (1997). Subtypes of social withdrawal in early childhood: Sociometric status and social-cognitive differences across four years. *Child Development, 68*, 278–294.

Hart, C. H., Yang, C., Nelson, L. J., Robinson, C. C., Olsen, J. A., Nelson, D. A., Porter, C. L., Jin S., Olsen, S. F., & Wu, P. (2000). Peer acceptance in early childhood and subtypes of socially withdrawn behaviour in China, Russia, and the United States. *International Journal of Behavioral Development*, 24, 73–81.

Hartup, W. W. (1997). Friendships and adaptation in the life course. *Psychological Bulletin, 121*, 355–370.

Hastings, P. D., & Rubin, K. H. (1999). Predicting mothers' beliefs about preschool-aged children's social behavior: Evidence for maternal attitudes moderating child effects. *Child Development, 70*, 722–741.

Hayward, C., Killen, J. D., Kraemer, H. C., & Taylor Barr, C. (1998). Linking self-reported childhood behavioral inhibition to adolescent social phobia. *Journal of the American Academy of Child and Adolescent Psychiatry, 12*, 1308–1316.

Henderson, H. A., Fox, N. A., & Rubin, K. H. (2001). Temperamental contributions to social behavior: The moderating role of frontal EEG asymmetry and gender. *Journal of the American Academy of Child and Adolescent Psychiatry, 40*, 68–74.

Henderson, H. A., & Rubin, K. H. (1997, April). *Internal and external correlates of self-regulation in preschool aged children*. Poster presented at the Biennial Meetings of the Society for Research in Child Development, Washington, DC.

Henriques, J., & Davidson, R. (1990). Regional brain electrical asymmetries discriminate between previously depressed and healthy control subjects. *Journal of Abnormal Psychology, 99*, 22–31.

Henriques, J., & Davidson, R. (1991). Left frontal hypoactivation in depression. *Journal of Abnormal Psychology, 100*, 535–545.

Hetherington, E. M., & Martin, B. (1986). Family factors and psychopathology in children. In H. C. Quay & J. S. Werry (Eds.), *Psychopathological disorders of childhood* (3rd ed., pp. 332–390). New York: Wiley.

Hinde, R. A., Stevenson-Hinde, J., & Tamplin, A. (1985). Characteristics of 3- to 4-year-olds assessed at home and their interactions in preschool. *Developmental Psychology, 21*, 130–140.

Hirshfeld, D. R., Rosenbaum, J. F., Biederman, J., Bolduc, E. A., Faraone, S. V., Snidman, N., Reznick, J. S., & Kagan, J. (1992). Stable behavioral inhibition and its association with anxiety disorder. *Journal of the American Academy of Child and Adolescent Psychiatry, 31*, 103–111.

Ho, D. Y. F. (1986). Chinese pattern of socialization: A critical review. In M. H. Bond (Ed.), *The psychology of Chinese people* (pp. 1–37). New York: Oxford University Press.

Ho, D. Y. F., & Kang, T. K. (1984). Intergenerational comparisons of child rearing attitudes and practices in Hong Kong. *Developmental Psychology, 20*, 1004–1016.

Hoffman, M. L. (1970). Moral development. In P. H. Mussen (Ed.), *Handbook of child psychology* (Vol. 2, pp. 261–359). New York: Wiley.

Hymel, S., Bowker, A., & Woody, E. (1993). Aggressive versus withdrawn unpopular children: Variations in peer and self-perceptions in multiple domains. *Child Development, 64*, 879–896.

Hymel, S., & Franke, S. (1985). Children's peer relations: Assessing self-perceptions. In B. H. Schneider, K. H. Rubin, & J. E. Ledingham (Eds.), *Children's peer relations: Issues in assessment and intervention* (pp. 75–91). New York: Springer-Verlag.

Hymel, S., & Rubin, K. H. (1985). Children with peer relationship and social skills problems: Conceptual, methodological, and developmental issues. In G. J. Whitehurst (Ed.), *Annals of child development* (Vol. 2, pp. 251–297). Greenwich, CT: JAI Press.

Hymel, S., Rubin, K. H., Rowden, L., & LeMare, L. (1990). A longitudinal study of sociometric status in middle and late childhood. *Child Development, 61*, 2004–2121.

Hymel, S., Woody, E., & Bowker, A. (1993). Social withdrawal in childhood: Considering the child's perspective. In K. H. Rubin & J. B. Asendorpf (Eds.), *Social withdrawal, inhibition and shyness in childhood* (pp. 237–262). Hillsdale, NJ: Erlbaum.

Iannotti, R. (1978). Effects of role-taking experiences on role-taking, empathy, altruism and aggression. *Developmental Psychology, 14*, 119–124.

Izard, C. E., Haynes, O. M., Chisholm, Y., & Baak, K. (1991). Emotional determinants of infant–mother attachment. *Child Development, 62*, 906–917.

Izard, C. E., Porges, S. W., Simons, R. F., Haynes, O. M., Parisi, M., Cohen, B., & Hyde, C. T. (1991). Infant cardiac activity: Developmental changes and relations with attachment. *Developmental Psychology, 27*, 432–439.

Jones, N., & Fox, N. (1992). Electroencephalogram asymmetry during emotionally evocative films and its relation to positive and negative affectivity. *Brain and Cognition, 20*, 280–299.

Joseph, L. (1992). *Character structure and the organization of the self.* New York: Columbia University Press.

Jouriles, E. N., Murphy, C. M., Farris, A. M., Smith, D. A., Richters, J. E., & Waters, E. (1991). Marital adjustment, parental disagreements about child rearing and behavior problems in boys: Increasing the specificity of the marital assessment. *Child Development*, *62*, 1424–1433.

Kagan, J. (1989). Temperamental contributions to social behavior. *American Psychologist*, *44*, 668–674.

Kagan, J., Gibbons, J. L., Johnson, M. O., Reznick, J. S., & Snidman, N. (1990). A temperamental disposition to the state of uncertainty. In J. Rolf, A. F. Masten, D. Cicchetti, K. H. Nuechterlein, & S. Weintraub (Eds.), *Risk and protective factors in the development of psychopathology* (pp. 164–178). New York: Cambridge University Press.

Kagan, J., & Moss, H. A. (1962). *Birth to maturity: A study of psychological development*. New York: Wiley.

Kagan, J., Reznick, J. S., Clarke, C., Snidman, N., & Garcia-Coll, C. (1984). Behavioral inhibition to the unfamiliar. *Child Development*, *55*, 2212–2225.

Kagan, J., Reznick, J. S., & Snidman, N. (1987). The physiology and psychology of behavioral inhibition in children. *Child Development*, *58*, 1459–1473.

Kagan, J., Reznick, J. S., & Snidman, N. (1988). Biological bases of childhood shyness. *Science*, *240*, 167–171.

Kagan, J., Reznick, J. S., Snidman, N., Gibbons, J., & Johnson, M. O. (1988). Childhood derivatives of inhibition and lack of inhibition to the unfamiliar. *Child Development*, *59*, 1580–1589.

Kagan, J., & Snidman, N. (1991). Infant predictors of inhibited and uninhibited profiles. *Psychological Science*, *2*, 40–44.

Kagan, J., Snidman, N., & Arcus, D. (1993). On the temperamental categories of inhibited and uninhibited children. In K. H. Rubin & J. Asendorpf (Eds.), *Social withdrawal, inhibition and shyness in childhood* (pp. 19–28). Hillsdale, NJ: Erlbaum.

Kagan J., Snidman, N., & Arcus, D. (1998). Childhood derivatives of high and low reactivity in infancy. *Child Development*, *69*, 1483–1493.

Kennedy, A. E., Polak, C. P., Rubin, K. H., Fox, N. A., & Burgess, K. B. (2002). *Physiological and social-behavioral predictors of internalizing difficulties from middle to late childhood*. Manuscript submitted for publication.

King, A. Y. C., & Bond, M. H. (1985). The Confucian paradigm of man: A sociological view. In W. S. Tseng & D. Y. H. Wu (Eds.), *Chinese culture and mental health* (pp. 29–45). New York: Academic Press.

Kochanska, G. (1991). Patterns of inhibition to the unfamiliar in children of normal and affectively ill mothers. *Child Development*, *62*, 250–263.

Kochanska, G., Kuczynski, L., & Maguire, L. (1989). Impact of diagnosed depression and self-reported mood on mothers' control strategies: A longitudinal study. *Journal of Child Psychology*, *17*, 493–511.

Kochanska, G., & Radke-Yarrow, M. (1992). Inhibition in toddlerhood and the dynamics of the child's interaction with an unfamiliar peer at age five. *Child Development*, *63*, 325–335.

Kohn, M. L. (1977). *Class and conformity: A study of values* (2nd ed.). Chicago: University of Chicago Press.

Kovacs, M. (1980/1981). Rating scales to assess depression in school-aged children. *Acta Paedopsychiatrica*, *46*, 305–315.

Kuczynski, L., & Kochanska, G. (1995). Function and content of maternal demands: Developmental significance of early demands for competent action. *Child Development*, *66*, 616–628.

LaFreniere, P., & Dumas, J. E (1992). A transactional analysis of early childhood anxiety and social withdrawal. *Development and Psychopathology*, *4*, 385–402.

Ladd, G. W., & Burgess, K. B. (1999). Charting the relationship trajectories of aggressive, withdrawn, and aggressive/withdrawn children during early grade school. *Child Development*, *70*, 910–929.

Ladd, G. W., & Burgess, K. B. (2001). Do relational risks and protective factors moderate the linkages between childhood aggression and early psychological and school adjustment? *Child Development*, *72*, 1579–1601.

Ladd, G. W., Kochendorfer, B. J., & Coleman, C. C. (1996). Friendship quality as a predictor of young children's early school adjustment. *Child Development*, *67*, 1103–1118.

Lamborn, S. D., Mounts, N. S., Steinberg, L., Dornbusch, S. M., & Darling, N. (1991). Patterns of competence and adjustment among adolescents from authoritative, authoritarian, indulgent, and neglectful families. *Child Development*, *62*, 1049–1065.

Lazarus, P. J. (1982). Incidence of shyness in elementary-school age children. *Psychological Reports*, *51*, 904–906.

LeDoux, J. (1989). Cognitive–emotional interactions in the brain. *Cognition and Emotion*, *4*, 267–274.

LeMare, L., & Rubin, K. H. (1987). Perspective-taking and peer interactions: Structural and developmental analyses. *Child Development*, *58*, 306–315.

Lemerise, E. A. (1997). Patterns of peer acceptance, social status, and social reputation in mixed-age preschool and primary classrooms. *Merrill–Palmer Quarterly*, *43*, 199–213.

Levine, S. (1983). A psychobiological approach to the ontogeny of coping. In N. Garmezy & M. Rutter (Eds.), *Stress, coping, and development in children* (pp. 107–131). Baltimore: Johns Hopkins University Press.

Levy, D. M. (1943). *Maternal overprotectiveness*. New York: Columbia University Press.

Lewis, M., & Miller, S. M. (1990). *Handbook of developmental psychopathology*. New York: Plenum Press.

Maccoby, E. E., & Martin, J. A. (1983). Socialization in the context of the family: Parent–child interaction. In P. H. Mussen (Series Ed.) & E. M. Hetherington (Vol. Ed.), *Handbook of child psychology: Vol. 4. Socialization, personality, and social development* (4th ed., pp. 1–101). New York: Wiley.

Maccoby, E. E., & Masters, J. C. (1970). Attachment and dependency. In P. H. Mussen (Ed.), *Carmichael's manual of child psychology* (Vol. 2, pp. 73–157). New York: Wiley.

MacDonald, K., & Parke, R. D. (1984). Bridging the gap: Parent–child play interaction and peer interactive competence. *Child Development*, *55*, 1265–1277.

Manassis, K., Bradley, S., Goldberg, S., Hood, J., & Swinson, B. (1995). Behavioural inhibition, attachment and anxiety in children of mothers with anxiety disorders. *Canadian Journal of Psychiatry*, *40*, 87–92.

Marshall, P. J., & Stevenson-Hinde, J. (1998). Behavioral inhibition, heart period, and respiratory sinus arrhythmia in young children. *Developmental Psychobiology*, *33*, 283–292.

Marshall, P. J., & Stevenson-Hinde, J. (2001). Behavioral inhibition: Physiological correlates. In W. Crozier & L. E. Alden (Eds.), *International handbook of social anxiety: concepts, research, and intervention relating to self and shyness* (pp. 53–76). New York: Wiley.

Matas, L., Arend, R. A., & Sroufe, L. A. (1978). The continuity of adaptation in the second year: Relationship between quality of attachment and later competence. *Child Development*, *49*, 547–556.

Mathiesen, K. S., & Tambs, K. (1999). The EAS Temperament Questionnaire: Factor structure, age trends, reliability, and stability in a Norwegian sample. *Journal of Child Psychology and Psychiatry*, *40*, 431–439.

Mead, G. (1934). *Mind, self and society*. Chicago: University of Chicago Press.
Mick, M. A. & Telch, M. J. (1998). Social anxiety and history of behavioral inhibition in young adults. *Journal of Anxiety Disorders*, *12*, 1–20.
Millon, T. (1981). *Disorders of personality: DSM-III*, Axis *II*. New York: Wiley.
Millon, T. (1987). *Manual for the MCMI II*. Minneapolis, MN: National Computer Systems.
Millon, T. (1996). *Personality and psychopathology: Building a clinical science. Selected papers of Theodore Millon*. New York: Wiley.
Millon, T., & Everly, G. S. (1985). *Personality and its disorders: A biological learning approach*. New York: Wiley.
Mills, R. S. L., & Rubin, K. H. (1993a). Parental ideas as influences on children's social competence. In S. Duck (Ed.), *Learning about relationships* (pp. 98–117). Newbury Park, CA: Sage.
Mills, R. S. L., & Rubin, K. H. (1993b). Socialization factors in the development of social withdrawal. In K. H. Rubin & J. Asendorpf (Eds.), *Social withdrawal, inhibition and shyness in childhood* (pp. 117–150). Hillsdale, NJ: Erlbaum.
Mills, R. S. L., & Rubin, K. H. (1998). Are behavioural and psychological control *both* differentially associated with childhood aggression and social withdrawal? *Canadian Journal of Behavioural Science*, *30*, 132–136.
Miyake, K., Chen, S., & Campos, J. (1985). Infant temperament, mother's mode of interactions, and attachment in Japan: An interim report. In I. Bretherton & E. Waters (Eds.), Growing points of attachment theory and research. *Monographs of the Society for Research in Child Development*, *50*(1–2, Serial No. 209), 276–297.
Moller, L., Hymel, S., & Rubin, K. H. (1992). Sex typing in play and popularity in middle childhood. *Sex Roles*, *26*, 331–353.
Morison, P., & Masten, A. (1991). Peer reputation in middle childhood as a predictor of adaptation in adolescence: A seven year follow-up. *Child Development*, *62*, 991–1007.
Moskowitz, D. S., Schwartzman, A. E., & Ledingham, J. E. (1985). Stability and change in aggression and withdrawal in middle childhood and early adolescence. *Journal of Abnormal Psychology*, *94*, 30–41.
Mullen, M., Snidman, N., & Kagan, J. (1993). Free-play behavior in inhibited and uninhibited children. *Infant* Behavior and Development, 16, 383–389.
Muris, P., Merckelbach, H., Wessel, I., & van de Ven, M. (1999). Psychopathological correlates of self-reported behavioural inhibition in normal children. *Behaviour Research and Therapy*, *37*, 575–584.
Nachmias, M., Gunnar, M., Mangelsdorf, S., Parritz, R. H., & Buss, K. (1996). Behavioral inhibition and stress reactivity: The moderating role of attachment security. *Child Development*, *67*, 508–522.
Nelson, L. J. (2000). *Social and nonsocial behaviors and peer acceptance: a longitudinal model of the development of self-perceptions in children ages 4 to 7 years*. Unpublished doctoral dissertation, University of Maryland at College Park.
Nilzon, K. R., & Palmerus, K. (1998). Anxiety and withdrawal of depressed 9–11 year olds three years later: A longitudinal study. *School Psychology International*, *19*, 341–349.
O'Brien, M. M., Trestman, R. L., & Siever, L. J. (1993). Cluster A personality disorders. In D. L. Dunner (Ed.), *Current psychiatric therapy* (pp. 65–82). Philadelphia: Harcourt Brace Jovanovich.
Ollendick, T. H., Greene, R. W., Weist, M. D., & Oswald, D. P. (1990). The predictive validity of teacher nominations: A five-year follow-up of at risk youth. *Journal of Abnormal Child Psychology*, *18*, 699–713.
Olweus, D. (1993). Victimization by peers: Antecedents and long-term outcomes. In K. H. Rubin & J. B. Asendorpf (Eds.), *Social withdrawal, inhibition and shyness in childhood* (pp. 315–341). Hillsdale, NJ: Erlbaum.
Park, S., Belsky, J., Putnam, S., & Crnic, K. (1997). Infant emotionality, parenting, and 3-year inhibtion: Exploring stability and lawful discontinuity in a male sample. *Journal of Abnormal Child Psychology*, *18*, 699–713.
Parker, G. (1983). *Parental overprotection: A risk factor in psychosocial development*. New York: Grune & Stratton.
Parker, G, Tupling, H., & Brown, L. B. (1979). A parental bonding instrument. *British Journal of Medical Psychology*, *52*, 1–10.
Parkhurst, J. T., & Asher, S. R. (1992). Peer rejection in middle school: Subgroup differences in behavior, loneliness, and interpersonal concerns. *Developmental Psychology*, *28*, 231–241.
Pastor, D. L. (1981). The quality of mother-infant attachment and its relationship to toddler's initial sociability with peers. *Developmental Psychology*, *17*, 323–335.
Patterson, G. R. (1983). Stress: A change agent for family process. In N. Garmezy & M. Rutter (Eds.), *Stress, coping, and development in children* (pp. 235–264). New York: McGraw-Hill.
Patterson, G. R. (1986). Maternal rejection: Determinant or product for deviant child behavior? In W. Hartup & Z. Rubin (Eds.), *Relationships and development* (pp. 73–94). Hillsdale, NJ: Erlbaum.
Pekarik, E., Prinz, R., Leibert, C., Weintraub, S., & Neale, J. (1976). The Pupil Evaluation Inventory: A sociometric technique for assessing children's social behavior. *Journal of Abnormal Child Psychology*, *4*, 83–97.
Piaget, J. (1932). *Six psychological studies*. New York: Random House.
Pilkonis, P. A. (1984). Avoidant and schizoid personality disorders. In H. E. Adams & P. B. Sutker (Eds.), *Comprehensive handbook of psychopathology* (pp. 479–494). New York: Plenum Press.
Porges, S. W. (1995). Cardiac vagal tone: A physiological index of stress. *Neuroscience and Biobehavioral Reviews*, *19*, 225–233.
Porges, S. W., & Byrne, E. A. (1992). Research methods for measurement of heart rate and respiration. *Biological Psychology*, *34*, 93–130.
Prior, M., Smart, D., Sanson, A., & Oberklaid, F. (2000). Does shy-inhibited temperament in childhood lead to anxiety problems in adolescence? *Journal of the American Academy of Child and Adolescent Psychiatry*, *39*, 461–468.
Radke-Yarrow, M., Richters, J., & Wilson, W. E. (1988). Child development in a network of relationships. In R. A. Hinde & J. Stevenson-Hinde (Eds.), *Relationships within families: Mutual influences* (pp. 48–67). Oxford: Clarendon Press.
Rapee, R. M. (1997). Potential role of childrearing practices in the development of anxiety and depression. *Clinical Psychology Review*, *17*, 47–67.
Renken, B., Egeland, B., Marvinney, D., Mangelsdorf, S., & Sroufe, L. (1989). Early childhood antecedents of aggression and passive-withdrawal in early elementary school. *Journal of Personality*, *57*, 257–281.
Renshaw, P. D., & Brown, P. J. (1993). Loneliness in middle

childhood: Concurrent and longitudinal predictors. *Child Development*, *64*, 1271–1284.

Reznick, J. S., Kagan, J., Snidman, N., Gersten, M., Baak, K., & Rosenberg, A. (1986). Inhibited and uninhibited behavior: A follow-up study. *Child Development*, *57*, 660–680.

Rosenbaum, J. F., Biederman, J., Gersten, M., Hirshfeld, D. R., Meminger, S. R., Herman, J. B., Kagan, J., Reznick, J. S., & Snidman, N. (1988). Behavioral inhibition in children of parents with panic disorder and agoraphobia: A controlled study. *Archives of General Psychiatry*, *45*, 463–470.

Rowe, D. C., & Plomin, R. (1977). Temperament in early childhood. *Journal of Personality Assessment*, *41*, 150–156.

Rubin, K. H. (1982). Non-social play in preschoolers: Necessary evil? *Child Development*, *53*, 651–657.

Rubin, K. H. (1985). Socially withdrawn children: An "at risk" population? In B. H. Schneider, K. H. Rubin, & J. E. Ledingham (Eds.), *Children's peer relations: Issues in assessment and intervention* (pp. 125–139). New York: Springer-Verlag.

Rubin, K. H. (1993). The Waterloo Longitudinal Project: Correlates and consequences of social withdrawal from childhood to adolescence. In K. H. Rubin & J. Asendorpf (Eds.), *Social withdrawal, inhibition and shyness in childhood* (pp. 291–314). Hillsdale, NJ: Erlbaum.

Rubin, K. H., & Asendorpf, J. (Eds.). (1993). *Social withdrawal inhibition, and shyness in childhood*. Hillsdale, NJ: Erlbaum.

Rubin, K. H., Booth, C., Rose-Krasnor, L., & Mills, R. S. L. (1995). Family relationships, peer relationships and social development: Conceptual and empirical analyses. In S. Shulman (Ed.), *Close relationships and socio-emotional development* (pp. 63–94). Norwood, NJ: Ablex.

Rubin, K. H., & Both, L. (1989). Iris pigmentation and sociability in childhood: A reexamination. *Developmental Psychobiology*, *22*, 717–726.

Rubin, K. H., Both, L., Zahn-Waxler, E. C., Cummings, M., & Wilkinson, M. (1991). Dyadic play behaviors of children of well and depressed mothers. *Development and Psychopathology*, *3*, 243–251.

Rubin, K. H., Bukowski, W., & Parker, J. (1998). Peer interactions, relationships, and groups. In W. Damon (Series Ed.) & N. Eisenberg (Vol. Ed.), *Handbook of child psychology: Vol. 3. Social, emotional, and personality development* (5th ed., pp. 619–700). New York: Wiley.

Rubin, K. H., & Burgess, K. B. (2001). Social withdrawal. In M. W. Vasey & M. R. Dadds (Eds.), *The developmental psychopathology of anxiety* (pp. 407–434). Oxford: Oxford University Press.

Rubin, K. H., & Burgess, K. B. (2002). Parents of aggressive and withdrawn children. In M. Bornstein (Ed.), *Handbook of parenting* (2nd ed., pp. 383–418). Mahwah, NJ: Erlbaum.

Rubin, K. H., Burgess, K. B., & Coplan, R. (2002). Social withdrawal and shyness. In P. K. Smith & C. Hart (Eds), *Handbook of childhood social development*. London, England: Blackwell.

Rubin, K. H., Burgess, K. B., & Hastings, P. D. (2002). Stability and social-behavioral consequences of toddlers' inhibited temperament and parenting behaviors. *Child Development*, *73*, 483–495.

Rubin, K. H., Cheah, C. S. L., & Fox, N. A. (2001). Emotion regulation, parenting and display of social reticence in preschoolers. *Early Education and Development*, *12*, 97–115.

Rubin, K. H., Chen, X., & Hymel, S. (1993). The socioemotional characteristics of extremely aggressive and extremely withdrawn children. *Merrill–Palmer Quarterly*, *39*, 518–534.

Rubin, K. H., Chen, X., McDougall, P., Bowker, A., & McKinnon, J. (1995). The Waterloo Longitudinal Project: Predicting adolescent internalizing and externalizing problems from early and mid-childhood. *Development and Psychopathology*, *7*, 751–764.

Rubin, K. H., Coplan, R. J., Fox, N. A., & Calkins, S. D. (1995). Emotionality, emotion regulation, and preschoolers' social adaptation. *Development and Psychopathology*, *7*, 49–62.

Rubin, K. H., Daniels-Beirness, T., & Bream, L. (1984). Social isolation and social problem solving: A longitudinal study. *Journal of Consulting and Clinical Psychology*, *52*, 17–25.

Rubin, K. H., Fein, G., & Vandenberg, B. (1983). Play. In P. H. Mussen (Series Ed.) & E. M. Hetherington (Vol. Ed.), *Handbook of child psychology: Vol. 4. Socialization, personality, and social development* (4th ed., pp. 693–774). New York: Wiley.

Rubin, K. H., Hastings, P. D., Stewart, S. L., Henderson, H. A., & Chen, X. (1997). The consistency and concomitants of inhibition: Some of the children, all of the time. *Child Development*, *68*, 467–483.

Rubin, K. H., Hymel, S., LeMare, L., & Rowden, L. (1989). Children experiencing social difficulties: Sociometric neglect reconsidered. *Canadian Journal of Behavioural Science*, *21*, 94–111.

Rubin, K. H., Hymel, S., & Mills, R. S. L. (1989). Sociability and social withdrawal in childhood: Stability and outcomes. *Journal of Personality*, *57*, 237–255.

Rubin, K. H., Hymel, S., Mills, R., & Rose-Krasnor, L. (1991). Conceptualizing different pathways to and from social isolation in childhood. In D. Cicchetti & S. Toth (Eds.), *Rochester Symposium on Developmental Psychopathology: Vol. 2. Internalizing and externalizing expressions of dysfunction* (pp. 91–122). Hillsdale, NJ: Erlbaum.

Rubin, K. H., LeMare, L. J., & Lollis, S. (1990). Social withdrawal in childhood: Developmental pathways to rejection. In S. R. Asher & J. D. Coie (Eds.), *Peer rejection in childhood* (pp. 217–249). New York: Cambridge University Press.

Rubin, K. H., & Lollis, S. (1988). Peer relationships, social skills, and infant attachment: A continuity model. In J. Belsky & T. Nezworski (Eds.), *Clinical implications of attachment* (pp. 167–221). Hillsdale, NJ: Erlbaum.

Rubin, K. H., & Mills, R. S. L. (1988). The many faces of social isolation in childhood. *Journal of Consulting and Clinical Psychology*, *56*, 916–924.

Rubin, K. H., & Mills, R. S. L. (1990). Maternal beliefs about adaptive and maladaptive social behaviors in normal, aggressive, and withdrawn preschoolers. *Journal of Abnormal Child Psychology*, *18*, 419–435.

Rubin, K. H., & Mills, R. S. L. (1991). Conceptualizing developmental pathways to internalizing disorders in childhood. *Canadian Journal of Behavioural Science*, *23*, 300–317.

Rubin, K. H., & Mills, R. S. L. (1992). Parents' thoughts about children's socially adaptive and maladaptive behaviors: Stability, change, and individual differences. In I. Sigel, J. Goodnow, & A. McGillicuddy-deLisi (Eds.), *Parental belief systems* (pp. 41–68). Hillsdale, NJ: Erlbaum.

Rubin, K. H., Mills, R. S. L., & Rose-Krasnor, L. (1989).

Maternal beliefs and children's social competence. In B. Schneider, G. Attili, J. Nadel, & R. Weissberg (Eds.), *Social competence in developmental perspective* (pp. 313–331). Dordrecht, The Netherlands: Kluwer.

Rubin, K. H., Nelson, L. J., Hastings, P., & Asendorpf, J. (1999). Transaction between parents' perceptions of their children's shyness and their parenting style. *International Journal of Behavioural Development*, *23*, 937–957.

Rubin, K. H., & Krasnor, L. (1986). Social cognitive and social behavioral perspectives on problem-solving. In M. Perlmutter (Ed.), *Minnesota Symposia on Child Psychology* (Vol. 18, pp. 1–68). Hillsdale,, NJ: Erlbaum.

Rubin, K. H., & Rose-Krasnor, L. (1992). Interpersonal problem-solving and social competence in children. In V. B. van Hasselt & M. Hersen (Eds.), *Handbook of social development: A lifespan perspective*. New York: Plenum Press.

Rutter, M., & Sroufe, L. A. (2000). Developmental psychopathology: Concepts and challenges. *Development and Psychopathology*, *12*, 265–296.

Rutter, M., Taylor, E., & Hersov, L. (Eds.). (1994). *Child and adolescent psychiatry: Modern approaches*. Oxford: Blackwell.

Sadker, M., & Sadker, D. (1994). *Failing at fairness: How America's schools cheat girls*. New York: Scribner.

Sanson, A., Pedlow, R., Cann, W., Prior, M., & Oberklaid, F. (1996). Shyness ratings: Stability and correlates in early childhood. *International Journal of Behavioural Development*, *19*, 705–724.

Scarpa, A., Raine, A., Venables, P. H., & Mednick, S.A. (1995). The stability of inhibited/inhibited temperament from ages 3 to 11 years in Mauritian children. *Journal of Abnormal Child Psychology*, *23*, 607–618.

Schaughency, E. A., Vannatta, K., Langhinrichsen, J., Lally, C. M. & Seely, J. (1992). Correlates of sociometric status in school children in Buenos Aires. *Journal of Abnormal Child Psychology*, *20*, 317–326.

Schmidt, L. A., Fox, N. A., Rubin, K. H., Sternberg, E. M., Gold, P. W., Craig, C., & Schulkin, J. (1997). Behavioral and neuroendocrine responses in shy children. *Developmental Psychobiology*, *30*, 127–140.

Schmidt, L. A., Fox, N. A., Schulkin, J., & Gold, P. W. (1999). Behavioral and psychophysiological correlates of self-presentation in temperamentally shy children. *Developmental Psychobiology*, *35*, 119–135.

Schneider, B. H. (1999). A multi-method exploration of the friendships of children considered socially withdrawn by their peers. *Journal of Abnormal Psychology*, *27*, 115–123.

Schneider, B. H., Attili, G., Vermigili, P., & Younger, A. (1997). A comparison of middle class English-Canadian and Italian mothers' beliefs about children's peer-directed aggression and social withdrawal. *International Journal of Behavioural Development*, *21*, 133–154.

Schneider, B. H., Richard, J. F., Younger, A. J., & Freeman, P. (2000). A longitudinal exploration of the continuity of children's social participation and social withdrawal across socioeconomic status levels and social settings. *European Journal of Social Psychology*, *30*, 497–519.

Schneider, B. H., Younger, A. J., Smith, T., & Freeman, P. (1998). A longitudinal exploration of the cross-context stability of social withdrawal in early adolescence. *Journal of Early Adolescence*, *18*, 734–396.

Selman, R. L., & Schultz, L. H. (1990). *Making a friend in youth: Developmental theory and pair therapy*. Chicago: University of Chicago Press.

Siever, L. J. (1981). Schizoid and schizotypal personality disorders. In J. R. Lion (Ed.), *Personality disorders: Diagnosis and management* (pp. 32–64). Baltimore: Williams & Wilkins.

Simpson, A. E., & Stevenson-Hinde, J. (1985). Temperamental characteristics of three- to four-year old boys and girls and child-family interactions. *Journal of Child Psychology and Psychiatry*, *26*, 43–53.

Smith, H. T. (1958). A comparison of interview and observation measures of mother behavior. *Journal of Abnormal and Social Psychology*, *57*, 278–282.

Sobol, M. P., & Earn, B. M. (1985). Assessment of children's attributions for social experiences: Implications for social skills training. In B. Schneider, K. H. Rubin, & J. E. Ledingham (Eds.), *Children's peer relationships: Issues in assessment and intervention* (pp. 93–110). New York: Springer-Verlag.

Spangler, G., & Schieche, M. (1998). Emotional and adrenocortical responses of infants to the Strange Situation: The differential function of emotional expression. *International Journal of Behavioural Development*, *22*, 681–706.

Sroufe, L. A. (1983). Infant–caregiver attachment and patterns of adaptation in preschool: The roots of maladaptation and competence. In M. Perlmutter (Ed.), *Minnesota Symposia on Child Psychology* (Vol. 16). Hillsdale, NJ: Erlbaum.

Sroufe, L. A., & Waters, E. (1977). Heart rate as a convergent measure in clinical and developmental research. *Merrill–Palmer Quarterly*, *23*, 3–25.

Steinberg, L., Lamborn, S. D., Dornbusch, S. M., & Darling, N. (1992). Impact of parenting practices on adolescent achievement: Authoritative parenting, school involvement and encouragement to succeed. *Child Development*, *63*, 1266–1281.

Stevenson-Hinde, J. (1989). Behavioral inhibition: Issues of context. In J. S. Reznick (Ed.), *Perspectives on behavioral inhibition* (pp. 125–138). Chicago: University of Chicago Press.

Stevenson-Hinde, J., & Glover, A. (1996). Shy girls and boys: A new look. *Journal of Child Psychology and Psychiatry*, *37*, 181–187.

Stevenson-Hinde, J., & Hinde, R. A. (1986). Changes in associations between characteristics and interactions. In R. Plomin & J. Dunn (Eds.), *The study of temperament: Changes, continuities, and challenges* (pp. 115–129). Hillsdale, NJ: Erlbaum.

Stewart, S. L., & Rubin, K. H. (1995). The social problem solving skills of anxious-withdrawn children. *Development and Psychopathology*, *7*, 323–336.

Stolz, L. M. (1967). *Influences* on parent behavior. Stanford, CA: Stanford University Press.

Stone, M. H. (1993). Cluster C personality disorders. In D. L. Dunner (Ed.), *Current psychiatric therapy*. Philadelphia: Harcourt Brace Jovanovich.

Sullivan, H. S. (1953). *The interpersonal theory of psychiatry*. New York: Norton.

Thomasgard, M., & Metz, W. P. (1993). Parental overprotection revisited. *Child Psychiatry and Human Development*, *24*, 67–80.

Thompson, R. A., Connell, J., & Bridges, L. J. (1988). Temperament, emotional and social interactive behavior in the strange situation: An analysis of attachment functioning. *Child Development*, *59*, 1102–1110.

Turkal, I. D. (1990). *The personality disorders: A psychological approach to clinical management*. New York: Pergamon Press.

Wanlass, R. L., & Prinz, R. J. (1982). Methodological issues in conceptualizing and treating childhood social isolation. *Psychological Bulletin*, *92*, 39–55.

Watrous, B. G., & Hsu, F. L. K. (1963). A Thematic Apperception Test study of Chinese, Hindu and American college students. In F. L. K. Hsu (Ed.), *Clan, caste, and club* (pp. 263–311). New York: Van Nostrand.

Weisz, J. R., Suwanlert, S., Chaiyasit, W., & Weiss, B. (1988). Thai and American perspectives on over- and undercontrolled child behavior problems: Exploring the threshold model among parents, teachers, and psychologists. *Journal of Consulting and Clinical Psychology*, *56*, 601–609.

Widiger, T. A. (2001). Social anxiety, social phobia, and avoidant personality. In W. R. Crozier & L. E. Alden (Eds.), *International* handbook of social anxiety (pp. 335–356). Chichester, England: Wiley.

Widiger, T. A., & Sanderson, C. J. (1997). Personality disorders. In A.Tasman, J. Kay, & J. A. Lieberman (Eds.), *Psychiatry* (Vol. 2, pp. 1291–1317). Philadelphia: Saunders.

Widiger, T. A., Trull, T. J., Clarkin, J. E., Sanderson, C., & Costa, P. T. (1994). A description of the DSM-III-R and DSM-IV personality disorders with the five-factor model of personality. In P. T. Costa (Ed.), *Personality disorders and the five-factor model of personality* (pp. 41–56). Washington, DC: American Psychological Association.

Winder, C. L., & Rau, L. (1962). Parental attitudes associated with social deviance in preadolescent boys. *Journal of Abnormal and Social Psychology*, *64*, 418–424.

Wojslawowicz, J. C., Burgess, K. B., Rubin, K. H., Rose-Krasnor, L., & Booth, C. (2002, August). The stability and quality of aggressive and shy/withdrawn children's best friendships. In K. B. Burgess & F. Vitaro (Chairs), *The qualities and functions of friendship in the case of shyness/withdrawal and aggression*. Symposium conducted at the biennial meeting of the International Society for the Study of Behavioural Development, Ottawa, Ontario, Canada.

Yarrow, M., Waxler, C., & Scott, P. M. (1971). Child effects on adult behavior. *Developmental Psychology*, *5*, 300–311.

Younger, A. J., & Boyko, K. A. (1987). Aggression and withdrawal as social schemas underlying children's peer perceptions. *Child Development*, *58*, 1094–1100.

Younger, A. J., & Daniels, T. (1992). Children's reasons for nominating their peers as withdrawn: Passive withdrawal versus active isolation. *Developmental Psychology*, *28*, 955–960.

Younger, A. J., Gentile, C., & Burgess, K. B. (1993). Chil-0dren's perceptions of social withdrawal: Changes across age. In K. H. Rubin & J. B. Asendorpf (Eds.), *Social withdrawal, inhibition and shyness in childhood* (pp. 215–235). Hillsdale, NJ: Erlbaum.

Zahn-Waxler, C., Mayfield, A., Radke-Yarrow, M., McKnew, D. H., Cytryn, L., & Davenport, D. (1988). A follow-up investigation of offspring of parents with bipolar disorder. *American Journal of Psychiatry*, *145*, 506–509.

IV

DEVELOPMENTAL AND LEARNING DISORDERS

CHAPTER NINE

Autistic Disorder

Laura Grofer Klinger
Geraldine Dawson
Peggy Renner

Autistic disorder is one of the pervasive developmental disorders, which are characterized by impairments in the development of reciprocal social and communication skills, abnormal language development, and a restricted repertoire of behaviors and interests. Autism seriously affects multiple domains, making it a challenging disorder to understand and to treat. When writing about her 2-year-old daughter with autism, Catherine Maurice (1993) described how autism affected all aspects of her daughter's development:

> It wasn't just that she didn't understand language. She didn't seem to be aware of her surroundings. She wasn't figuring out how her world worked, learning about keys that fit into doors, lamps that turned off because you pressed a switch, milk that lived in the refrigerator. . . . If she was focusing on anything, it was on minute particles of dust or hair that she now picked up from the rug, to study with intense concentration. Worse, she didn't seem to be picking up anyone's feelings. (pp. 32–33)

HISTORICAL CONTEXT

The term "autism" was coined by Bleuler in 1911 to describe individuals with schizophrenia who had a loss of contact with reality (Bleuler, 1911/1950). In the early 1940s, two men—Leo Kanner (1943) and Hans Asperger (1944/1991)—independently described children with disorders involving impaired social relationships, abnormal language, and restricted and repetitive interests. They believed that these children had a loss of contact with reality similar to that described by Bleuler, but without the concomitant diagnosis of schizophrenia.

In his initial report, Kanner (1943) presented case studies of 11 children whom he described as having an "extreme autistic aloneness" (p. 242). He noted that these children had an "inability to relate themselves in the ordinary way to people and situations from the beginning of life" (p. 242). In addition, he wrote that the syndrome led to language deviance characterized by delayed acquisition, echolalia, occasional mutism, pronoun reversals, and literalness. Finally, Kanner described these children as having an "obsessive desire for the maintenance of sameness" (p. 245), characterized by the development of elaborate routines and rituals. Because of their good rote memory and their normal physical appearance, Kanner concluded that these children were capable of achieving normal cognitive abilities.

In 1944, Asperger described a similar, but less severely impaired, group of four children that he diagnosed as having "autistic psychopathy." Similar to Kanner, Asperger described difficulties in social interaction including eye contact, affective expression, and conversational abilities. In contrast to Kanner's report, Asperger wrote about children who developed good language abilities by the time they entered school and often spoke pedantically like adults (Asperger, 1944/1991). Despite their good vocabularies and grammatical abilities, these children were impaired in their conversational skills and had unusual volume, tone, and flow of speech. Asperger commented on the high level of original thought displayed by these children and their tendency to become excessively preoccupied with a singular topic of interest. The diagnostic label of "Asperger syndrome" or "Asperger's disorder" has since been used to refer to this group of individuals.

Historically, it was believed that parents of children with autism were overly intellectual, were cold-hearted, and had a limited interest in other people, including their spouses and children (Kanner, 1943; Bettelheim, 1967). Bettelheim (1967) proposed that in response to rejecting parents, children with autism withdrew from social interaction and became self-sufficient. Until the mid-1970s, treatment regimens involved helping parents (usually mothers) to become less rejecting of their children. However, these initial hypotheses regarding the etiology of autism were not supported by empirical research conducted in the 1970s and 1980s. McAdoo and DeMyer (1978) and Koegel, Schreibman, O'Neill, and Burke (1983) administered the Minnesota Multiphasic Personality Inventory to parents of children with autism. Generally, these parents scored within the normal range on all of the personality measures. In addition, parents of children with autism and parents of children without disabilities reported similar levels of marital satisfaction and family cohesion.

Bernard Rimland (1964) and Eric Schopler (Schopler & Reichler, 1971) were among the first researchers to argue against the theory that parents were responsible for their children's autism. Rimland first proposed that the disorder is due to a neurological impairment. Schopler suggested that rather than treating the parents, the aim of therapists should be to involve parents as part of the treatment team working with their children.

DESCRIPTION OF THE DISORDER

Core Symptoms

Since the first edition of this book was published, research examining the early recognition of autistic symptomatology has flourished, and we are now able to identify several symptoms of autism that are present in the first 2 years of life (see Table 9.1). During the first few years of life, social, affective, communicative, and cognitive development are intrinsically linked, and any impairment in one area is likely to have negative consequences on the development of all the other areas as well. This connection between early-developing abilities has made it difficult, if not impossible, to ascertain whether autism results from a basic impairment in one or more specific areas. It is likely that there is no single primary deficit in autism, but rather a group of deficits affecting social, affective, linguistic, behavioral, and cognitive development. Although we review each of these domains of ability separately, it is important for the reader to realize that these abilities do not develop in isolation.

Social Abilities

Traditionally, autism has been considered to result from a primary deficit in socioemotional development that prevents children from interacting normally with others. In typical development,

TABLE 9.1. Early Symptoms of Autism

Social behavior	Typically develops	Behavior in children with autism[a]
Looking at faces	Birth	Less[b] at 12 months
Following person's gaze	6–9 months	Less at 18 months
Turning when name called	6–9 months	Less at 9 and 12 months
Showing objects to others	9–12 months	Less at 12 months
Pointing at interesting objects	9–12 months	Less at 12 and 18 months
Pointing to request	9–12 months	Not delayed at 18 months
Symbolic play	14 months	Absent at 18 months

[a]Data compiled from Baranek (1999), Baron-Cohen et al. (1996), and Osterling and Dawson (1994)—three studies comparing children with autism and children with typical development.
[b]"Less" indicates that this behavior was observed significantly less often in children with autism than in children with typical development at this chronological age.

the abilities to form attachment relationships, imitate another person, share a focus of attention with another person, understand another person's emotions, and engage in pretend play are all early-developing social abilities. In autism, these social abilities appear to be specifically impaired. However, recent research has revealed that these impairments may not be caused by an inability or complete lack of desire to interact with other people; rather, they may be due to impairments in understanding and responding to social information (cf. Dawson, Meltzoff, Osterling, Rinaldi, & Brown, 1998). The literature suggesting impairments in each of these early-developing socioemotional abilities is reviewed below.

Attachment. It was originally assumed that children with autism fail to bond with their parents. However, empirical evidence suggests that many children with autism do show differential responses to their caregivers as opposed to unfamiliar adults. Sigman and her colleagues (Sigman & Mundy, 1989; Sigman & Ungerer, 1984a) found that preschool-age children with autism directed more social behaviors and proximity seeking toward their caregivers than toward strangers following a brief separation. Moreover, Dissanayake and Crossley (1996) reported that proximity-seeking behaviors were similar in children with autism and children with Down syndrome.

Research has examined the quality of the attachment relationship between children with autism and their caregivers. Attachment quality is traditionally measured using Ainsworth's Strange Situation paradigm, in which secure attachment is demonstrated by the child's preference for social interaction with the mother versus a stranger (Ainsworth, Blehar, Waters, & Wall, 1978). Approximately 65% of normally developing middle-class American toddlers are classified as having a secure attachment relationship with their caregivers (Ainsworth, 1983). Capps, Sigman, and Mundy (1994) reported that all of the children with autism in their sample were classified as having an insecure attachment quality. Specifically, children with autism exhibited disoriented and disorganized behaviors directed toward their mothers. However, when the repetitive motor movements that are typically exhibited by individuals with autism were ignored (e.g., flapping, rocking, spinning), 40% of the children in their sample could be classified as being securely attached. Similarly, 50% of the children assessed by Rogers, Ozonoff, and Maslin-Cole (1993) were classified as having a secure attachment to their mothers. Thus secure attachment quality in autism approaches the rates seen in normally developing populations. Taken together, these findings suggest that autism does not result from a global impairment in the ability to form attachments, and that autism does not prevent the formation of attachment relationships (Dissanayake & Sigman, 2001). However, little is known about how attachment relationships develop over time in young children with autism, or whether impairments in understanding others leads to later abnormal attachment relationships (Dissanayake & Sigman, 2001).

Social Imitation. In normal development, imitation skills are present shortly after birth (Field, Woodson, Greenberg, & Cohen, 1982; Meltzoff & Moore, 1977). It has been hypothesized that early interactions involving mutual imitation facilitate infants' ability to understand the relationship between themselves and other people (Meltzoff & Gopnik, 1993; Stern, 1985). Young children with autism have specific impairments in their ability to imitate the movements of others, including body movements and actions with objects (Curcio, 1978; Dawson & Adams, 1984; Dawson, Meltzoff, Osterling, & Rinaldi, 1998; DeMyer et al., 1972; Sigman & Ungerer, 1984b; Stone, Ousley, & Littleford, 1997). Impairments have been found in both immediate and deferred imitation (Dawson, Meltzoff, Osterling, & Rinaldi, 1998) and have been associated with other social and language impairments displayed by children with autism. For example, poor imitation of body movements in 20-month-old (Charman et al., 2001) and 2-year-old (Stone et al., 1997) children with autism has been linked to later expressive language impairments. Based on this research, investigators (e.g., Dawson, 1991; Rogers & Pennington, 1991; Meltzoff & Gopnik, 1993) hypothesized that a failure to imitate may be a fundamental deficit in autism, interfering with the development of reciprocity, joint attention, and understanding of emotional states.

Even when children and adults with autism are capable of imitating another person, the imitation "style" seems awkward (Hobson & Lee, 1999; Loveland et al., 1994). For example, Hobson and Lee (1999) reported that 9- to 18-year-old individuals with autism could imitate novel actions with objects as well as language-age-matched persons with mental retardation. However, the participants with autism showed impairments in imitating the experimenter's action style (i.e., harsh or gentle movements) and in body orientation of the object (e.g., holding the object at the same angle to the body as modeled by the experimenter).

Although there is a general consensus that imitation skills are impaired in autism, the underlying reasons for these impairments continue to be debated. Recent theories have attributed imitation impairments either to motor praxis impairments in planning, sequencing, and executing intentional motor movements (Rogers, 1998a) or to difficulties in understanding the intersubjective experience of others, leading to impairments in matching the movements of self and others (Meltzoff & Gopnik, 1993; Hobson & Lee, 1999).

Joint Attention. Another mechanism by which infants gain an understanding of social information is the use of nonverbal behaviors, such as eye contact and gesture, to share a focus of attention with another person. "Joint attention" refers to the ability to "coordinate attention between interactive social partners with respect to objects or events in order to share an awareness of the objects or events" (Mundy, Sigman, Ungerer, & Sherman, 1986, p. 657). These early-developing abilities are considered important precursors to the development of spoken language (Bruner, 1975; Sugarman, 1984). Between 6 and 9 months of age, typically developing infants learn to share attention by looking between an object and a caregiver (Walden & Ogan, 1988). Later, between 9 and 12 months of age, infants learn that they can also share attention through the use of gesture (Hannan, 1987). Infants can both direct another's attention (through gestures such as pointing) and follow the gestures of others.

Impairments in using gaze and gesture as a means of sharing attention with others are among the first symptoms evident in autism. Through both home videotape studies (Osterling & Dawson, 1994) and prospective medical screening studies (Baron-Cohen et al., 1996), impairments in joint attention have been documented in 12- and 18-month-old children who later received a diagnosis of autism. Later, during the preschool years, deficits in joint attention (i.e., referential looking) have been shown to correctly diagnose 94% of children with autism compared to children with mental retardation (Mundy et al., 1986).

However, several researchers have found that the extent of impairment in joint attention behaviors in preschool-age children seems to be related to intellectual ability (Leekam & Moore, 2001; Mundy, Sigman, & Kasari, 1994). For example, Leekam and Moore (2001) reported a developmental effect for referential looking abilities in preschoolers with autism. In their study, 83% of preschoolers with an IQ above 70 followed an adult's gaze. However, only 25% of preschoolers with an IQ below 70 demonstrated gaze following. In contrast, developmentally delayed preschoolers were able to follow another person's gaze, regardless of their intellectual level. This study suggests that children with autism need a higher mental age or intellectual level than typically developing children in order to develop joint attention skills.

As with imitation impairments, there is a general consensus that joint attention skills are impaired in autism. However, the underlying mechanism for these impairments continues to be debated. Social theories of joint attention impairment suggest that children with autism fail to affectively share experiences with another person. Cognitive theories suggest that children with autism may have difficulty with attention orienting or with understanding another person's attentional focus (see Leekam & Moore, 2001, for a review of these theories).

Orienting to Social Stimuli. Several researchers have reported that persons with autism show decreased orienting to social stimuli. For example, in a study of home videotapes of toddlers' first-birthday parties, Osterling and Dawson (1994) found that toddlers with autism often failed to orient to social stimuli (faces, speech) in their environments. Dawson, Meltzoff, Osterling, Rinaldi, and Brown (1998) assessed experimentally whether, compared to receptive-language-mental-age-matched children with Down syndrome and with typical development, children with autism would fail to orient visually to naturally occurring social stimuli versus nonsocial stimuli. It was found that children with autism more frequently failed to orient to both social stimuli (name calling, clapping) and nonsocial stimuli (a rattle, a jack-in-the-box), but this failure was much more extreme for social stimuli. Similarly, Ruffman, Garnham, and Rideout (2001) reported that, compared to children with moderate learning disabilities, children with autism showed decreased anticipatory looking during a story task that involved human characters, but not during a story that involved nonsocial objects. Taken together, these results suggest that children with autism may exhibit a basic orienting impairment, especially for social stimuli.

This failure to attend to social stimuli has been hypothesized to contribute to the imitation and joint attention impairments described previously. For example, Swettenham et al. (1998) reported that 20-month-old children with autism spent more time shifting attention between two objects than between two people or between an object and a person. In contrast, developmentally delayed and typically developing toddlers showed the opposite pattern. Toth et al. (2001) further examined the relationship among social orienting, joint attention ability, and language ability in young children with autism. They reported a strong correlation between reduced social orienting abilities and poor joint attention. In addition, they found that social orienting and language ability were not related, even after they controlled for the relation between joint attention and language ability. This suggests a developmental model in which social orienting impairments may lead to joint attention impairments, which in turn lead to delayed language development

Face Perception. Face recognition abilities are essential for the development of interpersonal relationships. Indeed, typically developing infants recognize their mothers' faces within the first few days of life (Bushnell, Sai, & Mullen, 1989). There is increasing evidence that individuals with autism may be impaired in this very early-developing social ability. Several studies have documented face recognition impairments in older children, adolescents, and young adults with autism (e.g., Boucher & Lewis, 1992; Hauk, Fein, Maltby, Waterhouse, & Feinstein, 1999; Tantam, Monaghan, Nicholson, & Stirling, 1989; Teunisse & DeGelder, 1994). Boucher and Lewis (1992) found that children with autism were impaired in comparison to typically developing individuals on both a picture-matching task and a picture recognition task involving pictures of faces. However, they were not impaired on tasks using pictures of buildings; these results indicate that the impairment is specific to faces and is not one of generalized recognition memory. Klin et al. (1999) conducted one of the first face recognition studies in young children with autism and found impaired face recognition that was not related either to nonverbal or verbal delays or to impairments in spatial memory; this suggests that impairment in the processing of facial stimuli cannot be attributed to cognitive delays.

However, face-processing impairments have not been universally reported in the literature, and some studies have found evidence for intact face processing (Celani, Battacchi, & Arcidiacono, 1999; Davies, Bishop, Manstead, & Tantam, 1994). Interestingly, some studies showing intact face processing have reported an unusual approach to face perception. For example, Langdell (1978) reported that individuals with autism tend to focus on the mouth region of the face rather than the eyes. In comparison, typically developing individuals tend to focus on the eyes, not the mouth. Finally, several studies have found that individuals with autism did not show the typical decrement in face perception when shown inverted rather than upright faces (Hobson, Ouston, & Lee, 1988; Langdell, 1978). In reviewing this literature, Klin et al. (1999) proposed that these unusual processing styles may occur in older individuals with autism, who are able to complete face perception tasks accurately by using a compensatory strategy for face perception impairments.

The notion of an unusual face-processing style is supported by both electrophysiological and magnetic resonance imaging (MRI) studies of face processing in individuals with autism. Dawson and colleagues (Dawson, Carver, et al., 2002; McPartland, Dawson, Carver, & Panagiotides, 2001a, 2001b) recently conducted two electrophysiological studies of face processing. In the first study (Dawson, Carver, et al., 2002), 3- to 4-year-old children with autism-spectrum disorder, with developmental delay, and with typical development were presented with images of their mother's versus a stranger's face and of their favorite versus an unfamiliar toy. Typical and developmentally delayed children showed differential event-related potential (ERP) responses to their mothers' faces versus a stranger's face and to a favorite versus an unfamiliar toy. In contrast, children with autism failed to show a differential brain electrical response to their mothers' faces versus a stranger's face, but did show greater ERP to the unfamiliar versus the favorite toy. Their ERP patterns in response to toys were quite similar to those of the chronological-age-matched typical children (i.e., greater P400 and Nc amplitude at the lateral scalp locations in response to the unfamiliar toy).

In a second ERP study (McPartland et al., 2001a, 2001b), Dawson and colleagues found that high-functioning adolescents and adults with autism exhibited longer latency of the face-specific N170 ERP component relative to IQ-matched normal adolescents and adults, did not show a differential ERP response to upright versus inverted faces, and did not show the normal right-lateralized ERP consistently found in normal individuals. These studies suggest that in autism, the neural system related to face processing is less efficient (slower), lacks specificity to faces, and is abnormally represented in the brain.

Schultz et al. (2000) conducted a functional MRI (fMRI) study of face processing in autism and reported that individuals with autism used the region of the brain typically associated with the processing of objects (i.e., inferior temporal gyri) when they were shown pictures of faces. In contrast, they showed less brain activation of the brain region typically associated with face processing (i.e., fusiform gyrus). Although the evidence for face perception problems is compelling, more research needs to be conducted to determine how face perception problems are linked to the other social processing impairments in autism. For example, are face perception problems a causal factor or a consequence of a failure to attend to faces early in development (Carver & Dawson, 2002)?

Emotion Perception and Expression. Hobson (1989) proposed that individuals with autism have a core deficit in the perception and understanding of other people's emotions. This theory was supported by Weeks and Hobson's (1987) report that children with autism sorted a group of photographs according to the type of hat being worn rather than by facial expression. In contrast, chronological-age/Verbal-IQ-matched children with retardation sorted the photos on the basis of facial expression rather than type of hat. Other studies have found impaired performance when children with autism were asked to choose a picture displaying a specific emotional expression out of an array of pictures (e.g., Bormann-Kischkel, Vilsmeier, & Baude, 1995) or were asked to match pictures according to facial expression (Celani et al., 1999). These findings may be indicative of a face perception problem in general, or they may suggest that children with autism are insensitive to other people's facial expressions of emotion. However, this notion of a specific impairment in emotion perception has not been consistently supported in the literature, with a recent study showing that children with autism did not differ from a group of psychiatric controls (primarily children with attention-deficit/hyperactivity disorder [ADHD]) in their emotion recognition abilities (Buitelaar, van der Wees, Swaab-Barneveld, & van der Gaag, 1999). They reported that verbal memory and Performance IQ, not diagnosis, were the best predictors of emotion recognition abilities. In addition, Loveland et al. (1997) found no significant differences between individuals with autism and a mental-age-matched comparison group in ability to recognize emotions in videotape segments containing both verbal and nonverbal affective components. Taken together, recent studies have not supported the notion of a specific emotion recognition deficit in autism. However, as in the face perception literature, the conflicting results from the emotion perception literature may be linked to a compensatory strategy that is present in older, high-functioning individuals with autism.

It has also been hypothesized that individuals with autism are impaired in their ability to express their emotions. For example, Kasari, Sigman, Yirmiya, and Mundy (1993) reported that children with autism display unusual emotional expressions. In their study, children with autism were more likely to display negative affect and unusual blends of affective expressions. In contrast, Dawson, Hill, Spencer, Galpert, and Watson (1990) found that children with autism did not differ from receptive-language-mental-age-matched, normally developing children in the frequency or duration of smiles during a face-to-face interaction with their mothers. However, children with autism were much less likely to combine smiles with eye contact and were less likely to smile in response to their mothers' smiles. Dawson et al. (1990) suggested that children with autism have a specific impairment in their ability to engage in affective sharing experiences with another person.

Loveland et al. (1994) reported that producing affective expressions upon request is more difficult for persons with autism than for persons with Down syndrome with similar chronological age, mental age, and IQ scores. In this study, individuals with autism could perform rote copying of facial expressions, but had difficulty generating facial expressions without a model. However, this does not necessarily mean that individuals with autism are unable to produce spontaneous facial expressions; rather, they may have difficulty matching the verbal label to the corresponding emotional expression.

Symbolic Play. An important precursor to language development is the ability to engage in symbolic representation through pretend play. Normally, symbolic or pretend play gradually emerges between 12 and 22 months of age, with the majority of children achieving symbolic play by approximately 20 months of age (Riguet, Taylor, Benaroya, & Klein, 1981; Ungerer & Sigman, 1984). Symbolic play involves attributing animate characteristics to inanimate objects (e.g., pretending that a doll can speak) and using one object as if it were another (e.g., pretending that a block is a piece of fruit). In a prospective medical screening study, Baron-Cohen et al. (1996) reported that the absence of pretend play at 18 months of age was one of the earliest symptoms of autism. As children with autism develop language, their symbolic play increases (Amato, Barrow, & Domingo, 1999); however, their symbolic play remains delayed below the level expected from their language abilities (Amato et al., 1999; Riguet et al., 1981; Ungerer, 1989; Wing, 1978). Symbolic play can be elicited in structured situations (McDonough, Stahmer, Schreibman, & Thompson, 1997), but spontaneous symbolic play appears mechanical and repetitive without flexible, elaborate themes (Wing, 1978). Whether delayed symbolic play results from a metarepresentational impairment in understanding others (i.e., joint attention impairments) or is due to a more generalized cognitive deficit in symbolic thinking (i.e., executive function impairments) continues to be debated (see Charman, 1997, for a review).

Language and Communication Abilities

Given the significant impairments in early-developing social abilities that are considered to be precursors to language development (i.e., joint attention, symbolic play), it is not surprising that children with autism have significantly delayed and deviant language development. Historically, it was found that approximately 50% of individuals with autism remained mute throughout their lives (Rutter, 1978). However, with earlier diagnosis and intervention, this estimate is believed to be decreasing. Research has found that those children who develop gestural, nonverbal joint attention behaviors are more likely to develop language (Mundy, Sigman, & Kasari, 1990; Sigman & Ruskin, 1997).

Those individuals with autism who do learn to speak have deviant language, characterized by immediate or delayed echolalia (e.g., verbatim repetition of previously heard words or phrases), abnormal prosody (e.g., atypical rhythm, stress, intonation, and loudness) and pronoun reversal (e.g., use of "you" instead of "I" when referring to the self) (Cantwell, Baker, Rutter, & Mawhood, 1989; Kanner, 1943). Approximately 85% of children with autism who develop speech show immediate or delayed echolalia (Schuler & Prizant, 1985). Prizant and colleagues demonstrated that echolalia has many different communicative functions, including requesting, self-regulation, protesting, and affirmation; they have suggested that echolalia should be viewed as an effort to communicate rather than as meaningless utterances (Prizant & Rydell, 1984; Prizant, Schuler, Wetherby, & Rydell, 1997). Lee, Hobson, and Chiat (1994) examined pronoun usage among adolescents with autism and reported the tendency to refer to the examiner and to themselves by name rather than using personal pronouns. These findings suggest that although difficulties with personal pronouns may become less pronounced over time, they continue to exist throughout the life span.

Language impairments in autism are most pronounced in the pragmatic, or social, aspects of language use (see Tager-Flusberg, 1999, 2001, for reviews). Conversations by persons with autism are characterized by the use of irrelevant detail in conversations (e.g., providing dates and ages when discussing a particular event or person), perseveration, pedantic speaking on a particular topic of conversation, inappropriate shifts to a new topic, and ignoring of conversational initiations introduced by another person (Tager-Flusberg, 1999, 2001; Eales, 1993). Capps, Kehres, and Sigman (1998) found that children with autism exhibited difficulty in reciprocity during conversations, due to a lack of responsiveness to questions and comments. The children with autism also offered less spontaneous information than did children with other developmental delays matched on language ability. Eales (1993) has argued that these pragmatic impairments are due to impairments in understanding the intentions of another person during conversations. Similarly, Tager-Flusberg (1993, 1996) has hypothesized that persons with autism do not understand the speaker–listener discourse rules in conversations, because they are unable to take the listener's perspective into account. Their difficulty in understanding that others have a perspective different from their own manifests itself through abnormal pronoun use (e.g., saying "You want candy" when meaning "I want candy") and impairments in use of questions and statements (e.g., saying "Want cracker?" instead of stating "I want a cracker"). Difficulties with pragmatics or social aspects of language are also seen among highly verbal adults with autism (Lord & Paul, 1997).

In addition to pragmatic impairments, individuals with autism typically have difficulty in the semantic aspects of language. In a longitudinal study comparing preschool-age children with autism to a group of children with Down syndrome matched on expressive language age and chronological age, Tager-Flusberg (1989, 1993) reported that children with autism were not specifically impaired in their articulation abilities or acquisition of language structures (i.e., syntax and grammar). Children who acquired verbal language proceeded through the same sequence of grammatical development as typical children did, though they may have been delayed (Tager-Flusberg, 1999). However, they were impaired in how effectively they used the language skills that they had acquired. For example, although both groups used words in a variety of different ways and contexts (e.g., use of nouns, verbs, adjectives, etc.), the children with autism showed less variety in their choice of terms within each category. They did not appear to utilize the vocabulary that they had developed. In addition, the children with autism did not use their language to provide new information during a conversation or to elicit new information through the use of "wh-" questions (Tager-Flusberg, 1993, 1999). Such children seem to be lacking the curiosity necessary to utilize these types of information-gathering language skills (Koegel & Koegel, 1995).

In the area of language comprehension, persons with autism have been described as concrete and literal. They seem to have more difficulty understanding other people's language than they do learning the language structures necessary to produce language (Rapin, 1996). For example, Paul, Fischer, and Cohen (1988) reported that children with autism tended to rely on syntax rather than semantic content in their comprehension of language (e.g., relying on a word when determining the meaning of a sentence).

Repetitive Behaviors and Interests

Children with autism often engage in abnormal, ritualistic behaviors. In a review of the research in this area, Turner (1999a) has suggested that the repetitive behaviors in autism comprise two distinct categories of behaviors: lower-level behaviors that are characterized by repetitive motor movements, and higher-level or more complex behaviors that are characterized by insistence on following elaborate routines and circumscribed interests. In the area of repetitive motor movements, Volkmar, Cohen, and Paul (1986) found that parents of 50 children diagnosed with autism reported a variety of stereotyped movements, including rocking (65%), toe walking (57%), arm, hand, or finger flapping (52%), and whirling (50%). Such repetitive movements occur more often in younger and lower-functioning children with autism (Campbell et al., 1990; Wing, 1988; Wing & Gould, 1979). The more complex repetitive behaviors (elaborate routine and circumscribed interests) are observed in children with less severe levels of retardation and in persons with high-functioning autism. Elaborate routines include a complex series of motor movements, repeated rearranging or ordering of toys, and insistence on following the same sequence of events during everyday activities (e.g., driving routes, dressing routines, and food preferences). Intense, perseverative, circumscribed interests usually involve memorization of facts about a specific topic (e.g., the solar system, weather, U.S. presidents).

Lower-level repetitive motor behaviors and higher-level complex repetitive behaviors may have distinct developmental trajectories. For example, in a recent study of 40 high-functioning children with autism and Asperger syndrome, parental reports indicated a significant decrease in the severity of rigidity, stereotyped movements, and preoccupation with objects over time and an increase in circumscribed interests during the childhood years that leveled off in adolescence (South, Ozonoff, & McMahon, 2001).

Although these repetitive behaviors and interests have been considered to be a core component of autism since Kanner's early description of the disorder, relatively little research has been conducted to examine how specific these symptoms are to autism and whether these are early-developing "core" symptoms of autism (Charman & Swettenham, 2001; Turner, 1999a). Preference for sameness and distress over changes in routine are observed in young, typically developing children (Evans et al., 1997) and in individuals with a variety of clinical conditions (e.g., obsessive–compulsive disorder, Tourette syndrome, and mental retardation). Charman and Swettenham (2001) suggested that what may be unique to autism is the combination and severity of symptoms exhibited by individuals with autism. For example, Szatmari, Bartolucci, and Bremmer (1989) found that high-functioning individuals with autism displayed more repetitive and stereotyped behavior than did developmentally delayed individuals and a group of individuals receiving outpatient psychiatric services; this finding suggests that repetitive behaviors are not simply a result of the delayed development that often accompanies autism. However, more research is clearly needed on this issue.

More research is also needed to clarify the relationship between repetitive behaviors and the social and communication impairments that characterize autism. Studies examining the early symptoms of autism within the first year of life (e.g., Baron-Cohen et al., 1996; Osterling & Dawson, 1994; Robins, Fein, Barton, & Green, 2001) have consistently identified early social and communication impairments, but not repetitive movements or obsessive interests, as being core to the disorder. It has been hypothesized that repetitive behaviors may emerge as a coping strategy to help individuals with autism reduce high anxiety caused by an unpredictable and frightening social world (Baron-Cohen, 1989a). However, rates of stereotyped behaviors have been reported to decrease, not increase, during periods of social interaction (see Turner, 1999a, for a review). Alternatively, several researchers have hypothesized that the repetitive behaviors in autism may be related to the cognitive impairments in autism, including impaired central coherence, executive function, and abstraction abilities (i.e., Frith & Happe, 1994; Klinger, Lee, Bush, Klinger, & Crump, 2001; Ozonoff, Pennington, & Rogers, 1991; Turner, 1999a); however, whether repetitive behaviors cause the cognitive impairments or vice versa remains unclear.

Related Symptoms

Several behavioral problems—including self-injurious behavior, sleep disturbance, eating disturbance, and excessive anxiety—often occur in persons with autism.

Self-Injurious Behaviors

Behaviors such as head banging, finger or hand biting, head slapping, and hair pulling have been observed in persons with autism. When frustrated, persons with autism often have no verbal means of communicating their feelings and/or needs; as a result, they may engage in self-injurious behaviors as a way of expressing their frustration (Lainhart, 1999; Donnellan, Mirenda, Mesaros, & Fassbender, 1984). However, these behaviors may be more closely linked to the mental retardation that often accompanies autism than to autism per se (J. Dawson, Matson, & Cherry, 1998).

Sleep Disturbances

It is not uncommon for persons with autism to require less sleep than other family members, and parents often report that their children awake frequently during the night. Ruth Sullivan (1992) described her son, Joseph, at 2 years of age as being extremely hyperactive. She wrote, "It was as though his idle was stuck at rocket speed. He slept an average of three to four hours a night and screamed for the rest" (p. 247). Studies (Richdale, 1999; Patzold, Richdale, & Tonge, 1998; Richdale & Prior, 1995) have shown that between 44% and 83% of children with autism suffer from severe sleep problems, particularly before the age of 8. Commonly reported sleep problems include difficulty falling and staying asleep, as well as shortened night sleep and early morning waking. Although these sleep problems improve over time, older children continue to have difficulty falling asleep and tend to sleep less at night. While age seems to be a factor in sleep difficulties, the research to date suggests that intellectual functioning is unrelated. One limitation of the above-described studies is the reliance on parental reports as the sole source of information on sleep patterns. For example, a recent study by Schreck and Mulick (2000) found that although parents of children with autism verbally reported severe sleep difficulties in their children, parental behavioral ratings indicated similar quantities of sleep in children with autism, children with typical development, and children with mental retardation but without autism. More research is needed to clarify the nature of the sleep difficulties experienced by persons with autism.

Eating Disturbances

Eating disturbances are also frequently reported by parents, yet there is little research in this area. Eating disturbances during the early years of childhood are marked by unusual food preferences. Food preferences can be determined by the texture of the food (e.g., soft foods), the particular color of the food (e.g., brown), or a specific food taste (e.g., only one brand of a specific food). A 5-year-old boy we knew would only eat peanut butter and jam sandwiches if particular types of peanut butter and jam were used. Some children with autism may develop more ritualistic behaviors around mealtimes. For example, the 5-year-old just mentioned would also insist that the pieces of his sandwiches be cut into triangular shapes and the crusts removed. Eating problems typically do not subside during adulthood. Often adults with autism have to be supervised to ensure that they eat a well-balanced diet. For example, Powell, Hecimovic, and Christensen (1992) described a young man with autism who preferred foods with a soft texture: "He only eats steamed vegetables with a side dish of butterscotch pudding and half a banana for dinner" (p. 193).

Abnormal Fears and Response to Sensory Stimuli

Persons with autism often exhibit fearful responses to common everyday objects. Clinically, we have seen children with fears of vacuum cleaners, particular television commercials, elevators, blacktop, and clothing. These fears can cause many problems in daily living situations. The child who was afraid of blacktop refused to walk across parking lots, streets, and the school playground. Often these unusual fears appear related to abnormal sensory responses (Ornitz, 1989).

Children with autism often fail to respond to some sounds (such as their names being called) and overreact to other sounds (such as a siren in the distance). This lack of response to some sounds leads many parents of children with autism to believe that their children have hearing impairments. Similarly, individuals with autism often seem insensitive to pain, but at the same time they may have a hypersensitivity to clothing touching their skin. Ornitz (1989) has proposed that these disturbances result from an impaired ability to modulate sensory information, which is manifested in both under- and overreactivity and is present in all sensory systems. More research is needed to explain these symptoms of autism.

DEFINITIONAL AND DIAGNOSTIC ISSUES

As yet, there are no biological markers or medical tests for diagnosing autism. Therefore, the diagnosis of autism is based on behavioral symptoms and developmental history. As our understanding of autism has improved, the behavioral symptoms necessary for a diagnosis of autism have changed. The *Diagnostic and Statistical Manual of Mental Disorders*, fourth edition (DSM-IV; American Psychiatric Association, 1994) includes autistic disorder within the category of pervasive developmental disorders. As noted at the beginning of this chapter, pervasive developmental disorders are characterized by severe and pervasive impairments in reciprocal social interaction and communication, and by the presence of stereotyped behaviors, interests, and activities. Autistic disorder is the most prevalent of the pervasive developmental disorders and includes symptoms in all of the areas above. In addition, the onset of autism must be present by 3 years of age. Table 9.2 lists DSM-IV diagnostic criteria for autistic disorder.

Diagnostic Issues

Several different diagnostic instruments have been developed to aid clinicians in making accurate autism diagnoses. These instruments differ in terms of whether they provide a current or lifetime diagnosis, take into account symptom presentation within the context of developmental level, and differentiate between autism and the other pervasive developmental disorders. At present, none of the available instruments addresses all of these issues. It is beyond the scope of this chapter to review each of the autism diagnostic instruments, their validity and reliability, and their ability to address each of these diagnostic issues. However, a brief review of these issues and examples of instruments that address these issues is presented (see Table 9.3 for a partial listing of currently available diagnostic instruments and their ability to address these issues). See Lord (1997) and Klinger and Renner (2000) for more comprehensive reviews of this literature.

Current versus Lifetime Symptomatology

Diagnostic systems, such as the DSM-IV, assess whether symptom onset occurred prior to 3 years of age; thus retrospective report is required if the individual is beyond 3 years of age. Obtaining this information can be difficult when diagnosing an adolescent or adult when parental input is not available or parental memory is not accurate enough to report when the symptoms developed.

TABLE 9.2. DSM-IV Diagnostic Criteria for Autistic Disorder

A. A total of six (or more) items from (1), (2), and (3), with at least two from (1), and one each from (2) and (3):

(1) qualitative impairment in social interaction, as manifested by at least two of the following:
 (a) marked impairment in the use of multiple nonverbal behaviors such as eye-to-eye gaze, facial expression, body postures, and gestures to regulate social interaction
 (b) failure to develop peer relationships appropriate to developmental level
 (c) a lack of spontaneous seeking to share enjoyment, interests, or achievements with other people (e.g., by a lack of showing, bringing, or pointing out objects of interest)
 (d) lack of social or emotional reciprocity

(2) qualitative impairments in communication as manifested by at least one of the following:
 (a) delay in, or total lack of, the development of spoken language (not accompanied by an attempt to compensate through alternative modes of communication such as gesture or mime)
 (b) in individuals with adequate speech, marked impairment in the ability to initiate or sustain a conversation with others
 (c) stereotyped and repetitive use of language or idiosyncratic language
 (d) lack of varied, spontaneous make-believe play or social imitative play appropriate to developmental level

(3) restricted repetitive and stereotyped patterns of behavior, interests, and activities, as manifested by at least one of the following:
 (a) encompassing preoccupation with one or more stereotyped and restricted patterns of interest that is abnormal in either intensity or focus
 (b) apparently inflexible adherence to specific, nonfunctional routines or rituals
 (c) stereotyped and repetitive motor mannerisms (e.g., hand or finger flapping or twisting, or complex whole-body movements)
 (d) persistent preoccupation with parts of objects

B. Delays or abnormal functioning in at least one of the following areas, with onset prior to age 3 years: (1) social interaction, (2) language as used in social communication, (3) symbolic or imaginative play.

C. The disturbance is not better accounted for by Rett's Disorder or Childhood Disintegrative Disorder.

Note. From American Psychiatric Association (1994, pp. 70–71). Copyright 1994 by the American Psychiatric Association. Reprinted by permission.

Despite the possible difficulty in determining whether symptom onset began prior to 3 years of age, the criteria are consistent with recent research showing that symptoms are often present prior to 12 months of age (Baranek, 1999; Lord, 1995; Osterling & Dawson, 1994) or that, if symptoms appear following a period of normal development, this typically occurs between 16 and 24 months of age (Davidovitch, Glick, Holtzman, Tirosh, & Safir, 2000; Williams & Ozonoff, 2001; Williams, Ozonoff, & Landa, 2001). The Autism Diagnostic Interview—Revised (ADI-R; Lord, Rutter, & Le Couteur, 1994) is one of the few diagnostic instruments that allows for both a "current" and a "lifetime" diagnosis, which is important for establishing that symptoms were present before 3 years of age and for genetic studies of autism. The ADI-R is a standardized, semistructured, 1-hour parent interview designed to diagnose pervasive developmental disorders in children and adults with a mental age of 18 months and up. Caregivers are asked to describe their children's current behaviors and past behaviors, with a focus on the behaviors observed during their children's preschool years.

Symptom Presentation in the Context of Developmental Level

Because of the comorbidity between autism and mental retardation (see below), symptoms need to be interpreted within the context of developmental level or "mental age." Consider, for example, the DSM-IV criterion that pretend play skills must be delayed below the child's developmental level. Pretend play typically does not develop until 14–18 months of age; thus a child with a mental age of 1 year would not be expected to show any pretend play. In contrast, a child with a mental age of 18 months would be expected to show simple pretend play, such as holding a telephone up to his or her ear or feeding a doll. A

TABLE 9.3. Selected Assessment and Screening Instruments

Instrument and purpose	Age range	Current DSM-IV diagnosis	Lifetime diagnosis	Developmental level taken into account
Diagnosis				
Autism Diagnostic Interview—Revised (ADI-R; Lord, Rutter, & Le Couteur, 1994)	> 18 months[a]	Yes	Yes	Partially[b]
Augism Diagnostic Observation Scale—Generic (ADOS-G; Lord et al., 2000)	> 30 months[a]	Partially[c]	No	Yes
Screener				
Childhood Autism Rating Scale (Schopler, Reichler, De Vellis, & Daly, 1980)	> 36 months[a]	No	No	No
Early detection				
Checklist for Autism in Toddlers (CHAT; Baron-Cohen et al., 1996)	18 months	No	N/A	Yes
Modified Checklist for Autism in Toddlers (M-CHAT; Robins, Fein, Barton, & Green, 2001)	18–24 months	No	N/A	Yes
Pervasive Developmental Disorders Screening Test (PDDST; Siegel & Hayer, 1999)	0–36 months	No	N/A	Yes
Screening Tool for Autism in Two-Year-Olds (Stone, Coonrod, & Ousley, 2000)	24–35 months	No	N/A	Yes

[a]Mental age.
[b]Some questions are only administered if a child is within a specific age range.
[c]A supplemental parent interview about age of onset and repetitive behaviors is needed.

child with a mental age of 4 years should be able to engage in elaborate thematic play, such as pretending that dolls are having a party or setting up an elaborate army battle. The need to consider developmental level has resulted in diagnostic criteria that are most appropriate for elementary school-age children with autism and mild to moderate mental retardation (Lord, 1997). As a result, more errors are made in diagnoses of children who are extremely delayed, very young, or older and high-functioning.

Thus accurate use of the DSM-IV criteria depends on the clinician's knowledge of typical developmental milestones or use of an instrument that is sensitive to developmental level. At present, there is only one diagnostic instrument that was specifically developed to assess symptoms within the context of the child's developmental level: the Autism Diagnostic Observation Schedule—Generic (ADOS-G; Lord et al., 2000). The ADOS-G is a brief (30-minute), standardized, semistructured play session that consists of "planned social occasions;" these provide opportunities for the examiner to observe social interaction, communication, and imaginative play. It was developed to diagnose pervasive developmental disorders across a wide range of chronological and mental ages, and was normed on individuals ranging from 15 months through 40 years of age. The ADOS-G consists of four different modules, with each module appropriate for a different developmental stage and language level, ranging from nonverbal children to high-functioning adults and adolescents; the clinician chooses the module that is most similar to the individual's developmental level. However, the ADOS-G by itself does not provide sufficient information for a DSM-IV diagnosis of autism. A parental interview is needed to supplement the ADOS-G in order to obtain information about low-frequency behaviors (e.g., repetitive play) that may not be observed during a brief observation, and about the age of symptom onset if the individual is older than 36 months of age.

Ability to Differentiate among the Different DSM-IV Pervasive Developmental Disorders

Beginning with the publication of DSM-IV, several other pervasive developmental disorders have been differentiated from autism. These disorders include Asperger's disorder, Rett's disorder, childhood disintegrative disorder (CDD), and pervasive developmental disorder not otherwise specified (PDD-NOS). Each of these disorders is described below. Currently, none of the diagnostic instruments reliably differentiate among autistic disorder, Asperger's disorder, and PDD-NOS. It appears that although these disorders are considered distinct diagnoses in the DSM-IV, it is difficult to describe these differences adequately enough to produce a reliable and valid diagnostic instrument. Indeed, children often receive several different labels falling under the pervasive developmental disorder umbrella, depending on which clinician completed the evaluation and which diagnostic instrument was used.

Other Pervasive Developmental Disorders

Asperger's Disorder

Asperger (1944/1991) described a group of children with symptoms resembling Kanner's concept of autism, but without mental retardation or significant language delay. However, only within the last 10–15 years have researchers focused on Asperger syndrome as a distinct disorder. Tantam (1988) described the person with Asperger syndrome as "intelligent, a fluent but original language user, clumsy, an assiduous pursuer of idiosyncratic interests, and cut off from others by a subtle but pervasive oddity which obtrudes in every social situation" (p. 246). The majority of published studies have not used consistent diagnostic criteria for Asperger syndrome, making it difficult to make any definitive statements about the disorder. In general, researchers have agreed that the diagnosis of Asperger syndrome usually involves relatively intact intellectual and language functioning, accompanied by the impairments in reciprocal social interaction that are associated with autism. Moreover, individuals with Asperger syndrome have been characterized as having idiosyncratic interests that are often appropriate in content but always unusual in their intensity. Finally, several researchers have noted increased motor clumsiness among some individuals with Asperger syndrome (see Volkmar & Klin, 2001, and Klin, Volkmar, & Sparrow, 2000, for recent reviews).

DSM-IV defines Asperger's disorder as involving a severe and sustained impairment in social interaction, along with the development of restricted, repetitive behaviors and interests. In contrast to autistic disorder, DSM-IV stipulates that individuals with Asperger's disorder may not display clinically significant delays in language (e.g., single words must be used by age 2 years, and communicative phrases must be used by age 3 years), cognitive functioning, or adaptive behavior. If current or past behaviors are consistent with a DSM-IV diagnosis of autistic disorder, a diagnosis of Asperger's disorder cannot be given. This stringent criterion has made it quite difficult to diagnose Asperger's disorder using the DSM-IV (Miller & Ozonoff, 1997). Indeed, many clinicians and researchers do not follow DSM-IV criteria and diagnose Asperger syndrome when DSM-IV criteria for both autistic disorder and Asperger's disorder are met (i.e., language and cognitive development is not delayed, but there are at least 6 symptoms of autism).

More research is needed to clarify diagnostic criteria for Asperger's disorder as a distinct disorder from high-functioning autism. Ozonoff, South, and Miller (2000) compared a group of 23 children and adolescents with high-functioning autism and 12 children with Asperger's disorder defined by DSM-IV criteria. Although the group with autism was reported to have more severe symptoms during the preschool years and to have spent more time in special education, the two groups were remarkably similar in their current social and communicative behavior. Differences emerged in the area of repetitive behaviors: The group with autism showed an increased insistence on sameness, and the group with Asperger's disorder showed an increased rate of circumscribed interests. In addition, this study failed to replicate previous findings that individuals with Asperger's disorder have a higher Verbal than Performance IQ (see Klin & Volkmar, 1997, for a review), although the individuals with autism were more impaired in their verbal comprehension skills. Ozonoff and colleagues suggested that despite an early history of language delay and increased symptomatology, the group with autism had "caught up" to the group with Asperger's disorder by their teen years. Similarly, Gilchrist et al. (2001) found few differences between a group of adolescents with autism and a group of adolescents with Asperger syndrome, except that, consistent with differing developmental histories of language development, the latter group had better conversation skills. In fact, 80% of the group with Asperger syndrome met criteria for autism on the ADI-R. Clearly, more research is needed to determine whether these are indeed distinct disorders or whether the diagnoses differ primarily in degree of impairment. In addition, more research is needed to clarify the distinction between Asperger syndrome and other disorders, including schizoid personality disorder in childhood, nonverbal learning disability, and semantic–pragmatic processing disorder (Klin & Volkmar, 1997).

Recently, research has focused on describing the "strengths" in persons with Asperger syndrome and high-functioning autism, rather than simply focusing on the weaknesses. For example, there are several cognitive tasks (see the discussion below of central coherence tasks, such as block design and visual illusions) in which these individuals outperform typically developing individuals. Indeed, Baron-Cohen (2000) has proposed that the disorder should be viewed as a "difference" rather than a "disability." He argues that being more object-focused than people-focused is only a disability in a world that expects everyone to be social.

> For example, a child with Asperger syndrome/high-functioning autism who prefers to stay in the classroom poring over encyclopedias and rock collections during break time, when other children are outside playing together, could simply be seen as different, not disabled. It is not clear why the child with Asperger syndrome/high-functioning autism is seen as doing something less valuable than the other children. (p. 491)

Recent treatment approaches for Asperger syndrome also focus on emphasizing the areas of strengths shown by many individuals with this disorder (Ozonoff, Dawson, & McPartland, 2002).

Rett's Disorder

Rett's disorder is a progressive neurological disorder that begins within the first few years of life (see Van Acker, 1997, for a review). To date, this syndrome has only been diagnosed in females. DSM-IV defines Rett's disorder as involving a period of normal development for at least 5 months, followed by the loss of previously acquired skills. Although the disorder is typically described as having an onset following a period of normal development, early warning signs within the first year of life are often present. These early warning signs include mild hypotonia, tremulous neck movements, abnormal hand movements (excess hand waving, twisting of the wrists and arms), and abnormal language development (Van Acker, 1997). However, these early symptoms are mild and are not sufficient to alert the pediatrician or caregiver to the disorder until degeneration begins. DSM-IV defines deterioration as occurring in five different areas. First, although girls with Rett's disorder have a normal head circumference at birth, they show a deceleration of head growth between 5 and 48 months of age. Second, Rett's disorder involves a loss of purposeful hand movements between 5 and 30 months of age, and the subsequent development of characteristic stereotyped movements (such as hand wringing and hand washing). Third, a loss of social engagement occurs that resembles the social difficulties present in autism. Fourth, Rett's disorder is characterized by a poorly coordinated gait. Finally, the disorder involves severely impaired language development and is usually accompanied by severe or profound mental retardation. Associated symptoms often include facial grimacing, teeth grinding, breathing problems (e.g., hyperventilation, breath holding, and air swallowing), and seizure disorders. Following this initial phase of deterioration, a plateau phase begins (between approximately 2 and 10 years) in which there is an improvement in social functioning. During adolescence, a further deterioration in motor skills is often noted (Van Acker, 1997). This patern of symptom onset and plateau is quite different from the developmental pattern observed in autism. Whether Rett's disorder is truly a pervasive developmental disorder and whether it should be classified under this heading in the DSM-IV are controversial issues. Recent research has identified a possible X-linked gene mutation (methyl-CpG binding protein 2 gene) that may be responsible for Rett's disorder (Amir et al., 1999). If autism and Rett's disorder are similar disorders, it is hoped that this genetic breakthrough will increase our understanding of autism.

Childhood Disintegrative Disorder

CDD, also known as Heller syndrome, is characterized by an autistic-like condition that develops following at least a 2-year period of normal development (see Malhotra & Gupta, 1999, and Volkmar, Klin, Marans, & Cohen, 1997, for reviews). DSM-IV criteria define CDD as a clinically significant loss of previously acquired skills before the age of 10 years in at least two of the following areas: expressive or receptive language, social skills or adaptive behaviors, bowel or bladder control, play, and motor skills. Prior to this loss of skills, the child must exhibit age-appropriate social, communicative, and play skills. Following this disintegrative period, the behavioral symptoms are similar to those of autism. Volkmar and Rutter (1995) reported that compared to individuals with autism, individuals with CDD were more severely impaired, as evidenced by an increased incidence of mutism and IQ scores below 40.

In a review of the literature, Volkmar (1992) reported that the mean age of onset for CDD is 3.36 years with onset ranging from 1.2 to 9 years. He argued that this disorder is not simply a form of autism that is recognized later in life. In his study, children with autism who had developed limited speech and showed intact cognitive skills tended to receive a later diagnosis (after age 2 years). In contrast, the children diagnosed with CDD demonstrated a significant loss of previously acquired skills, and the majority had severe mental retardation. The majority of children reported in the literature (19 of 29 cases) spoke clearly in sentences prior to the onset of the disorder. It is unclear whether early symptoms predate the regression in CDD or if the symptom onset is sudden. It is also unclear whether CDD differs from autism with a history of language regression between 18 and 24 months (see the discussion of age of onset below). Volkmar et al. (1997) suggest that the diagnosis of CDD is only appropriate if a child was speaking in sentences prior to the regression. Also, they note that in addition to speech loss, CDD is typically accompanied by a regression in other areas, such as social functioning (99% of cases reported) and self-help skills (87% of cases reported). In contrast, autism with a history of language regression is not typically associated with a regression in these other areas.

Pervasive Developmental Disorder Not Otherwise Specified

DSM-IV includes a diagnosis of PDD-NOS for children who exhibit the symptoms of autism after the age of 3 years, or for children who show autistic symptomatology but do not have impairments in all three of the areas required for a diagnosis of autism (social interaction, communication, and repetitive behaviors or interests). The DSM-IV defines PDD-NOS as an appropriate diagnosis when a child has impairments in either social interaction, verbal and nonverbal communication skills, or stereotyped behaviors and interests. Volkmar, Shaffer, and First (2000) have recently expressed concern that this definition is too inclusive, as an impairment in one area of development is enough to be consistent with the DSM-IV diagnosis of PDD-NOS. They have argued that the diagnostic criteria should be changed to stipulate that impairments in reciprocal social interaction *must* be present, with additional impairments in either communication or restricted interests. This change would ensure that the diagnosis requires impairments in two areas of development, including impaired social interaction, which is considered a hallmark symptom of a pervasive developmental disorder.

In a review of the literature, Towbin (1997) listed four different situations in which a PDD-NOS diagnosis is given. First, this label is often used as a "default" diagnosis when inadequate information about symptom onset and presentation is available to make a definitive diagnosis. Second, the diagnosis is given to individuals whose symptoms are severe enough to be considered part of the "autism spectrum," but not sufficient to meet diagnostic criteria for autistic disorder. For example, several studies have found evidence for impaired social and communication abilities without the presence of stereotyped and repetitive behaviors in individuals diagnosed with PDD-NOS (see Charman & Swettenham, 2001, for a review). Third, PDD-NOS is diagnosed in individuals with a late age of onset (i.e., after 30 months) who do not meet criteria for CDD. Finally, PDD-NOS is used to describe conditions in which there is an early onset of impaired reciprocal social relationships that are not adequately described by our current diagnostic system. For example, Asperger syndrome would have fit within this category prior to its description as a separate disorder. Given the multiple meanings and uses of this diagnosis, it is difficult to make definitive statements about its nature, etiology, and symptom course.

Differential Diagnosis

Developmental Language Disorders

The differential diagnosis between autism and developmental language disorders (or the communication disorders, as DSM-IV calls them; e.g., expressive and mixed receptive–expressive language disorders, phonological disorder) may be difficult, especially in young children. However, Bartak, Rutter, and Cox (1975) and Cantwell et al. (1989) have documented that there are differences between these two types of disorders in terms of the type of language abnormalities, nonverbal communication, and social skills. Children with autism and developmental language disorders have similar delays in babbling, language acquisition, mean length of utterance, and grammatical complexity. However, children with autism show more deviant language development, including echolalia, pronoun reversal, stereotyped utterances, and metaphorical language. Also, children with autism are less likely to engage in spontaneous "chatting" conversation. Although articulation disorders are not common in verbal children with autism, children with developmental language disorders almost always show difficulties in articulation (Bishop, 1992). Compared to children with developmental language disorders, children with autism show significantly more impairments in nonverbal communication, including gesture and symbolic play (Bartak et al., 1975). Parents report that approximately 57% of children with developmental language disorders used gesture at home, whereas only 11% of children with autism are reported to use gesture. Both groups of children show delayed symbolic play development. Riguet et al. (1981) reported that symbolic play in children with autism is more delayed than would be expected by their delayed language development. Children with autism also show more difficulty in social interactions, including more gaze aversion, less group play, and more difficulty adapting to new situations (Bartak et al., 1975).

Mawhood, Howlin, and Rutter (2000) conducted a follow-up study on a group of young adults with autism and a group with developmental receptive language disorder who had been previously seen during their childhood years (Bartak et al., 1975; Cantwell et al., 1989). They found that the group with autism showed greater improvements in Verbal IQ than the group with receptive language disorder. This caused the two groups to look more similar than they had in childhood. However, the group with autism continued to show more deviant language (e.g., echolalia) and poorer conversational skills, suggesting that autism is a disorder of deviant and not simply delayed language. Of note is the fact that the group with language disorder showed problems with many different aspects of communication, not simply receptive language. For example, approximately 50% of this group had problems sustaining conversations, and 50% used abnormal prosody. These difficulties in the group with language disorder contributed to a greater difficulty in differentiating between the two groups in adulthood. However, the group with autism continued to show more impairments in social interactions and stereotyped behaviors than the group with language disorder (Howlin, Mawhood, & Rutter, 2000).

Research examining the distinction between high-functioning autism and semantic–pragmatic language disorder is less clear than the research differentiating between autism and receptive language disorder. Semantic–pragmatic language disorder (which is not a DSM diagnosis) is characterized by delayed speech development, intact articulation abilities, and difficulties using language appropriately in conversation, partially due to an overly literal understanding and use of language (Shields, Varley, Broks, & Simpson, 1996). Shields et al. (1996) compared elementary school-age children with typical development, phonological–syntactic disorder, semantic–pragmatic disorder, and autism on a variety of social cognition measures (i.e., theory-of-mind tasks, the Wechsler Comprehension subscale). Although the children with phonological–syntactic disorder did not differ from the typically developing children, both the children with autism and the children with semantic–pragmatic disorder were impaired on these tasks. These findings suggest that children with semantic–pragmatic disorder show the same degree of impaired social cognition as children with autism, and they call into question whether these are distinct diagnoses.

Childhood-Onset Schizophrenia

Autism and childhood-onset schizophrenia are considered separate disorders (see Asarnow & Asarnow, Chapter 10, this volume). In his original description of autism, Kanner (1943) made the following distinction between the two disorders: "While the schizophrenic tries to solve his problem by stepping out of a world of which he has been a part and with which he has been in touch, our children gradually compromise by extending cautious feelers into a world in which they have been total strangers from the beginning" (p. 249). Although both disorders are characterized by abnormal social interaction, childhood-onset schizophrenia is differentiated from autism by a later age of onset (i.e., it rarely occurs prior to 7 years), less impaired intellectual abilities, the presence of hallucinations and delusions, and the tendency to experience periods of remission and relapse (Green et al., 1984; Kolvin, 1971; Rutter, 1978). However, some high-functioning individuals with autism or Asperger syndrome may display behaviors that are mistakenly interpreted as evidence for schizophrenia (Konstantareas & Hewitt, 2001; Lainhart, 1999). For example, individuals with autism/Asperger syndrome often show a flat affect, often comment on the fact that they are not liked by others (typically a true rather than a paranoid statement), and may make tangential remarks that are due to concrete use of language and/or an obsessive interest. Volkmar and Cohen (1991) reviewed case records of 163 adolescents and adults with histories of autism, and reported only one concomitant diagnosis of schizophrenia. Thus the rate of schizophrenia among individuals with autism is approximately 0.6%, which is comparable to the rate of schizophrenia in the general population.

Comorbid Disorders

Mental Retardation. In a review of 13 studies conducted between 1966 and 1999, Fombonne (1999) reported that the comorbidity rate of autism and mental retardation (i.e., IQ below 70) ranged from 44% to 100%. Averaged across all studies, the rate of individuals without intellectual impairment was 25.4%, mild to moderate mental retardation was 23.2%, and severe to profound mental retardation was 55.5%. However, more recent estimates suggest that these figures may be too high and that the comorbidity between autism and mental retardation is between 40% (Baird et al., 2000) and 69% (Chakrabarti & Fombonne, 2001). The decline in the comorbidity between autism and mental retardation can be attributed to an increased diagnosis of autism in high-functioning individuals and the effectiveness of early intervention.

The fact that many children with autism have intact intellectual ability indicates that autism and mental retardation are distinct disorders. Compared to children with mental retardation of a comparable developmental level, children with autism display specific impairments in joint attention, motor imitation, symbolic play, and theory-of-mind abilities. Simple motor stereotypies (including self-injurious behaviors) are observed both in children with autism and in those with mental retardation, and appear to be a function of mental age rather than diagnosis (J. Dawson et al., 1998; Wing, 1978). In addition, individuals with autism tend to display a specific pattern of intellectual abilities, performing better on nonverbal visual–spatial tasks than on verbal tasks (Happe, 1994; Lockyer & Rutter, 1970). As a result, persons with autism tend to have higher Performance IQ scores than Verbal IQ scores.

Depression. Studies examining comorbid depression in individuals with a pervasive developmental disorder have reported rates ranging from 4% to 58% (Lainhart, 1999). Symptoms of comorbid depression include a worsening in behaviors, including agitation, social withdrawal and compulsions, and changes in sleep and appetite. Depression often occurs in high-functioning individuals during adolescence, when they develop a greater insight into their differences from others and a growing desire to have friendships (Kim, Szatmari, Bryson, Streiner, & Wilson, 2000).

Anxiety Disorders. The comorbid rate of anxiety disorders in autism ranges from 7% to 84%, with generalized anxiety disorder, agoraphobia, separation anxiety disorder, and simple phobia (now called specific phobia) being the most common diagnoses (Lainhart, 1999). Additionally, symptoms of obsessive–compulsive disorder are common (16–81%) in individuals with a pervasive developmental disorder with the rate of a comorbid diagnosis of pervasive developmental disorder and obsessive–compulsive disorder ranging from 1.5% to 29% (Lainhart, 1999). Kim et al. (2000) reported a greater incidence of anxiety disorders in adolescents with high-functioning autism and Asperger syndrome, compared to children from a community sample. However, it is often difficult to determine whether anxiety and obsessive–compulsive symptoms represent separate diagnoses or are part of the pervasive developmental disorder. Regardless of whether a secondary diagnosis is appropriate, these symptoms are amenable to medication and behavioral interventions in persons with autism.

Tic Disorders. Tic disorders occur more often in persons with autism than in the general population. For instance, in a recent large-scale study of 447 children and adolescents with pervasive developmental disorders, a comorbid rate of Tourette syndrome was observed in 6.5% of the participants with an additional 24.4% showing some tic behaviors that did not meet criteria for Tourette syndrome (Baron-Cohen, Scahill, Izaguirre, Hornsey, & Robertson, 1999). No differences in the frequency of comorbid Tourette syndrome were found across diagnostic categories of autism, Asperger syndrome, or other autism spectrum conditions. Taken together, this study suggests that greater than 30% of individuals with pervasive developmental disorders show some form of tics. It is possible that the high rate of tics observed in this study may be due to difficulties in distinguishing complex motor tics from the stereotypies and volitional vocal outbursts that occur in some persons with autism. In the absence of accurate self-report about whether the movements and sounds are volitional or not, it is difficult to know whether these are true tic disorders. However, family histories were strongly suggestive of a genetic component to these tics, as 78% of the children diagnosed with comorbid Tourette syndrome had a family history of tics and/or obsessive–compulsive disorder.

Seizure Disorders. The prevalence rate of seizure disorders in autism ranges from 11 to 39% (see Ballaban-Gil & Tuchman, 2000, for a review). Among persons with autism, seizure disorders are more common in individuals with comorbid mental retardation and in females. The age of seizure onset tends to occur either before 3 years of age or during puberty (11–14 years; Volkmar & Nelson, 1990). In addition, epileptiform abnormalities without evidence of clinical seizures is common in autism, with one study reporting electroencephalographic (EEG) abnormalities in 21% of 392 children who received sleep EEG recordings (Tuchman & Rapin, 1997).

DEVELOPMENTAL COURSE AND PROGNOSIS

Symptom Onset

Parental report suggests that there are two different patterns of symptom development in autism. The majority of parents report, in retrospect, that symptom onset occurred within the first year of life (Lord, 1995). Several studies examining the early symptoms of autism without relying on retrospective parent report have also found evidence for symptom onset prior to 18 months of age. For example, Osterling and Dawson (1994) reviewed home videotapes of first-birthday parties, and Baranek (1999) reviewed home videotapes of 9- to 12-month-old infants who later received a diagnosis of autism. Baron-Cohen et al. (1996) screened a population-based sample of more than 16,000 children at 18 months of age for symptoms of autism. Across all three studies, early symptoms identified include decreased looking at people's faces, a failure to turn when a child's name was called, failure to share interests with others by showing or pointing, and delayed pretend play (see Table 9.1). It is the combination of these symptoms, not a single symptom, that is indicative of autism. Although these symptoms are present during the first 18 months of life, autism is often not diagnosed until many months or years later, suggesting that parents and physicians may not notice these early symptoms. The fact that these symptoms represent a lack of skill development rather than the development of unusual behaviors may lead to the delay between symptom onset and diagnosis.

The second pattern of symptom development is characterized by a period of regression or loss of skills during the first 3 years of life. Estimates of the prevalence of this regression pattern in autism range from 20% to 47% (e.g., Davidovitch et al., 2000; Kurita, 1985; Lord, 1995). The average age of regression onset varies across studies ranging from 16 months (Williams & Ozonoff, 2001) to 24 months (Davidovitch et al., 2000). Regression has been reported in a variety of domains, including communication, social, cognitive, and self-help skills. However, the vast majority of cases in which a regression is reported involve a loss of previously acquired language development. Two recent studies investigated whether autistic symptoms were present before a period of regression. Using retrospective parent reports, both studies confirmed that approximately 50% of the children experiencing significant loss of skills after 12 months of age did show some preexisting delays (Williams & Ozonoff, 2001; Werner & Munson, 2001). There is considerable controversy about the relationship between symptom onset and developmental outcome, with some studies reporting that regression is associated with a poorer outcome, and other studies reporting no difference between children who experience an early onset of symptoms that continue through development and children who experience a regression period during development.

Symptom Profile Changes across the Life Span

Although impairments in social and communication skills, and the presence of restricted and repetitive behaviors, continue across the life span, the specific symptom presentation changes with development (Lord, 1997). For example, joint attention impairments in the use of eye contact and gestures have been identified as one of the earliest symptoms of autism (Baron-Cohen et al., 1996; Osterling & Dawson, 1994). However, Mundy et al. (1994) reported that the specific forms of joint attention impairments were related to mental age and IQ in young children with autism. Preschoolers with mental ages below 20 months demonstrated impairments in both gaze and gestural forms of joint attention. In contrast, preschoolers with mental ages above 20 months were impaired only in the gestural forms of joint attention. Similarly, the specific symptoms characterizing the restricted and repetitive behaviors and interests in persons with autism change with chronological and mental age. Repetitive motor movements (e.g., hand flapping) tend to occur more often in younger and lower-functioning children with autism, whereas intense, perseverative, circumscribed interests (e.g., obsessive interest in the weather) are common in older and higher-functioning individuals with autism (South et al., 2001; Wing, 1988).

Piven, Harper, Palmer, and Arndt (1996) compared parent reports of social skills, communication skills, and repetitive/ritualistic behaviors in adolescents and young adults with autism to retrospective parent reports of these behaviors at the age of 5 years. Improvements in social skills were reported in 82%, communication skills in 82% and repetitive/ritualistic behaviors in 55% of the 38 individuals. Because of this changing symptom presentation, it is difficult to formulate a list of necessary and sufficient diagnostic criteria that is valid across the life span. In fact, Piven, Harper, et al. (1996) reported that 13% of their sample no longer met diagnostic criteria for autism. Therefore, some professionals advocate the need for a lifetime history of symptoms in making an accurate diagnosis.

Prognosis

Overall, the existing longitudinal studies suggest that the prognosis for individuals with autism is poor with respect to academic achievement and independent living abilities. These studies pertain to individuals who probably have not received intensive early intervention, however. For many of those who do receive such intervention, the long-term prognosis may be more positive (see the discussion below on early intervention).

Kobayashi, Murata, and Yoshinaga (1992) conducted a large-scale follow-up study of 197 young adults with autism who had received therapeutic services during their childhood years. They reported that 27% of the individuals in their sample had achieved social independence (i.e., they were employed) or had a good chance for social independence (i.e., they were students at college or a technical school). The remaining 73% of their sample continued to need considerable supervision and were not employed. Only two individuals were living independently in an apartment. Approximately 47% of these young adults with autism had achieved sufficient language ability that allowed them to communicate verbally with others.

Both Gillberg and Steffenburg (1987) and Kobayashi et al. (1992) noted that a significant percentage (31–57%) of individuals with autism showed a deterioration in functioning or aggravation of symptoms during adolescence. This deterioration was characterized by increased hyperactivity, aggression, and ritualistic behavior, and by a loss of previously acquired language skills. Although some adolescents showed this deterioration concomitant with the onset of seizures, it was difficult to determine what precipitated the deterioration in the majority of cases. Interestingly, Kobayashi et al. (1992) noted that adolescence could also be a period of positive change. Approximately 43% of parents in their study reported that their children showed remarkable improvements during adolescence.

Across a number of studies, the two best predictors of favorable outcome in autism are nonretarded intellectual abilities (e.g., IQ greater than 70) and the development of some communicative speech prior to 5 years of age (Gillberg & Steffenburg, 1987; Howlin et al., 2000; Kobayashi et al., 1992; Mawhood et al., 2000; Szatmari, Bartolucci, Bremner, Bond, & Rich, 1989; Venter, Lord, & Schopler, 1992). However, the few studies examining outcome in high-functioning (i.e., without mental retardation) individuals continue to report difficulties in adolescence and throughout adulthood. In a review of the literature on outcome in high-functioning individuals with autism, Howlin (2000) reported that the proportion of individuals that were employed ranged from 5% to 44%, and that the proportion living independently ranged from 16% to 50%. Green, Gilchrist, Burton, and Cox (2000) examined adaptive behavior and social functioning in a group of 20 adolescents with Asperger syndrome. Even in this extremely high-functioning group (average IQ of 92), parental report indicated that only 50% of participants completed daily self-care activities independently, 15% used the telephone independently, 5% were able to plan their own routines, and none were involved in leisure activities outside the house. In addition, parents reported that their teenagers had extreme difficulties with social relationships: 90% of the group had difficulty making friends, and 85% had difficulty coping with teasing from peers.

Recent studies suggest that early intervention leads to a better prognosis, with increased likelihood of developing language, being placed in a regular education classroom, and higher IQ scores (Dawson & Osterling, 1997). As the diagnosis of autism can be made earlier than previously thought (e.g., by 2–3 years of age), it will be possible to implement earlier intervention services, which (let us hope) will lead to a brighter prognosis for persons with autism.

EPIDEMIOLOGY

Prevalence and Incidence

Pervasive developmental disorders are not as rare as previously believed. Historically, autism has been reported to occur in 4 to 5 cases per 10,000 persons (Lotter, 1966; Wing & Gould, 1979). Recent studies have indicated higher prevalence rates, however. Gillberg and Wing (1999) conducted a meta-analysis of 20 studies between 1966 and 1997; they noted that the prevalence rate for children born before 1970 was 4.7 cases per 10,000, whereas the prevalence rate for children born in 1970 or later was 11.2 per 10,000. In addition, they reported an estimated annual increase in autism diagnoses of 3.8% per year with studies from the 1990s reporting incidence rates ranging from 6 to 31 cases per 10,000. A recent population-based survey of 15,500 children between the ages of 2.5 and 6.5 years in Staffordshire, England reported rates as high as 16.8 per 10,000 for autism (Chakrabarti & Fombonne, 2001). Other studies combining all pervasive developmental disorders have found prevalence rates ranging from 16 per 10,000 (Fombonne, du Mazaubrun, Cans, & Grandjean, 1997) to 62.6 per 10,000 (Chakrabarti & Fombonne, 2001). Although evidence suggests that the prevalence of autism and other pervasive developmental disorders is rising, there continues to be much debate about whether this reflects a true increase, or whether this reflects improved awareness and better diagnostic tools for these disorders (especially in the detection of more high-functioning individuals with autism). Regardless of the reason, autism is clearly not as rare as previously believed.

Sex Differences

Autism occurs more frequently in males, with approximately three or four males for every one female with autism (Bryson, Clark, & Smith, 1988; Fombonne, 1999; Steffenburg & Gillberg, 1986; Volkmar, Szatmari, & Sparrow, 1993). Several researchers have reported that females with autism tend to receive lower scores on both verbal and nonverbal measures of intelligence (Bryson et al., 1988; Konstantareas, Homatidis, & Busch, 1989; Steffenburg & Gillberg, 1986; Volkmar et al., 1993). Volkmar et al. (1993) reported that proportionately more females with autism were in the severely retarded range (IQ below 35), and males with autism were 8.8 times more likely to have normal intellectual ability.

There have been conflicting reports about whether males and females differ in terms of severity of autistic symptomatology. A recent study comparing symptomatology on the ADI-R and the CARS found no differences in the symptoms of autism between males and females when they were matched on chronological and mental age (Pilowsky, Yirmiya, Shulman, & Dover, 1998). However, McLennan, Lord, and Schopler (1993) reported that among a group of high-functioning persons with autism (defined here as IQ greater than 60), parents rated males as more severely autistic than females, especially prior to 5 years of age. Taken together, these studies suggest that females with autism tend to be more severely retarded and thus display increased symptoms associated with autism. However, high-functioning females may show less severe forms of autism compared to high-functioning males.

Socioeconomic Status

Kanner's (1943) original sample consisted primarily of professional families from upper-income backgrounds. As a result, clinicians initially believed that autism was caused by cold, rejecting parents from wealthy families (Bettelheim, 1967). However, it is believed that earlier reports of increased rates of autism in families with upper socioeconomic status resulted from the fact that these families were most able to afford treatment services for their children. Empirical research has revealed that the socioeconomic distribution of families with autistic children is similar to the distribution within the general population (Fombonne, 1999; Schopler, Andrews, & Strupp, 1979; Steffenburg & Gillberg, 1986; Wing & Gould, 1979).

Cultural Factors

Autism is known to affect individuals throughout the world. Epidemiological research has been conducted in Canada (Bryson et al., 1988), England (Wing & Gould, 1979; Chakrabarti & Fombonne, 2001), France (Fombonne, du Mazaubrun, et al., 1997; Cialdella & Mamelle, 1989), Sweden (Steffenburg & Gillberg, 1986), Norway (Sponheim & Skjeldal, 1998), Iceland (Magnusson & Saemundsen, 2001), Japan (Honda, Shimizu, Misumi, Nimi, & Ohashi, 1996; Sugiyama & Abe, 1989), and Hong Kong (Chung, Luk, & Lee, 1990). Brief reports from Eastern Europe, including Russia (Lebedinskaya & Nikolskaya, 1993) and Croatia (Bujas-Petkovic, 1993) have been published. Across all of these studies, there is remarkable consistency in reports of autistic symptomatology, intellectual abilities, gender differences, and socioeconomic factors associated with autism. Thus, it seems that autism can be considered a universal disorder.

THEORETICAL FRAMEWORK: INFORMATION-PROCESSING AND NEUROPSYCHOLOGICAL PERSPECTIVES

Researchers have attempted to determine whether an underlying information-processing impairment or profile of impairments can explain some of the social, affective, and communicative impairments observed in individuals with autism. Over the last few years, research has focused on five different areas of possible information-processing impairments in autism: memory, theory of mind, executive function, attention, and abstraction. A brief review of each of these different areas follows. (See Table 9.4.)

Memory

Previous research examining memory functioning in persons with autism has yielded conflicting results. Several investigators have proposed that autism shares some similarity with an amnesic syndrome that results from combined damage to the hippocampus and amygdala (Bachevalier, 1994; Boucher, 1981; Boucher & Warrington, 1976; DeLong, 1992). Researchers have found some evidence of memory impairments in individuals with autism (e.g., Ameli, Courchesne, Lincoln, Kaufman, & Grillon, 1988; Boucher & Warrington, 1976). Other studies, however, have shown intact memory in persons with autism (Mottron, Morasse, & Belleville, 2001; Renner, Klinger, & Klinger, 2000; Bowler, Matthews, & Gardiner, 1997; Summers & Craik, 1994). This disparity in the literature may be explained partly by the level of cognitive functioning of the participants used in each study. Individuals with both autism and mental retardation have shown greater levels of impairment on memory tasks, while high-functioning individuals with autism have been relatively unimpaired on the same tasks. For example, Barth, Fein, and Waterhouse (1995) found that a group of children with both autism and mental retardation were more impaired on a visual recognition memory task than a group of children with mental retardation alone. In contrast, they found intact recognition memory abilities in a group of high-functioning children with autism. Similarly, Dawson and colleagues (Dawson, Meltzoff, Osterling, & Rinaldi, 1998; Dawson, Munson, et al., 2002) found that young children with autism were impaired on a delayed non-matching-to-sample task that assessed visual recognition memory. Thus it appears that young children with autism, or children with both autism and mental retardation, may have difficulty on tasks assessing recognition memory.

Other investigators finding that individuals with autism remember the same amount of information compared to controls have hypothesized that persons with autism may use different organizational strategies during encoding and retrieval. For example, Bowler et al. (1997) found that individuals with Asperger syndrome failed to use categorical information to aide in their retrieval during a free-recall task. Minshew and Goldstein (2001) also found that individuals with autism showed intact performance on simple memory tasks, but were impaired in their ability

TABLE 9.4. Profile of Information-Processing Abilities and Impairments in Pervasive Developmental Disorders

Cognitive function	Impaired ability	Intact ability
Memory	Encoding strategies	Auditory rote memory
Executive functions	Planning Flexibility Organization	Inhibition Set maintenance
Theory of mind	False belief Deception	None
Attention	Shifting attention Disengaging attention	Sustained attention Filtering Searching
Abstraction		
Central coherence	Global processing	Analytic processing
Automatic abstraction	Prototype formation	Rule-based learning Implicit memory
Reduced generalization	Common feature processing	Unique feature processing

to use strategies to organize memorization of more complex list-learning tasks. Similarly, Mottron et al. (2001) reported intact free recall in a group of high-functioning individuals with autism, but a failure to benefit from semantic cues during a cued-recall task. Renner et al. (2000) found an impaired primacy effect during a free-recall task with a group of high-functioning individuals with autism, although overall number of items remembered did not differ from that of typical controls. All of these studies support the notion that individuals with autism may not have overall memory impairment; instead, their poor performance may be due to a failure to organize information effectively in memory during encoding or retrieval. Furthermore, some individuals with autism, especially lower-functioning individuals, may have more basic recognition memory impairments.

Theory of Mind

The ability to understand that other people have beliefs, desires, and intentions that are different from one's own (i.e., a "theory of mind") emerges gradually from infancy and is firmly established by the age of 3 to 4 years (see Wellman, 1993, for a review). Baron-Cohen, Leslie, and Frith (1985) have hypothesized that children with autism have a specific impairment in their development of a theory of mind. Such an impairment in metarepresentation would explain the difficulties that children with autism have in social understanding and communication. In their seminal study, Baron-Cohen et al. (1985) compared theory-of-mind abilities in a group of children with autism, a group with Down syndrome, and a group with typical development. Children watched a puppet show in which a character, Sally, placed a toy in one location (e.g., a basket) and then left the room. While Sally was out of the room, the toy was moved to a different location (e.g., a box) by another puppet. Children were asked where Sally would look for the toy upon her return. In order to answer correctly (e.g., that Sally would look in the basket), children needed to understand that the puppet, Sally, had a belief that was different from their own. In this study, the majority of children with typical development and with Down syndrome answered the question correctly (85% and 86% of the time, respectively). In contrast, only 20% of the children with autism were able to predict the beliefs of others. In a later study, Baron-Cohen (1989a) reported that the 20% of children with autism who could successfully attribute a belief state to another person were impaired in more complex theory-of-mind tasks (e.g., predicting what one person thinks another person is thinking). Thus even those children who were able to understand another person's theory of mind at the level of a typically developing 4-year-old child were unable to show the level of understanding usually obtained by 7 years of age.

This general pattern of results has been replicated across tasks (i.e., tasks measuring deception, the ability to distinguish appearance from reality, descriptions of the functions of the brain, and knowledge that thoughts can be deciphered by the direction of eye gaze), chronological age, intelligence levels, and different pervasive developmental disorders (e.g., Baron-Cohen, 1989b; Baron-Cohen, Jolliffe, Mortimore, & Robertson, 1997; Ozonoff et al., 1991; Sicotte & Stemberger, 1999; Sodian & Frith, 1992). (See Baron-Cohen, 2001, for a review of findings with different kinds of tasks). In addition, Ozonoff and McEvoy (1994) reported that nonretarded adolescents with autism did not show improvements in theory of mind across a 3-year interval, suggesting that this may be a lifelong impairment.

However, theory-of-mind task performance has been significantly correlated with verbal mental age and Verbal IQ in persons with autism, indicating that this skill may be delayed rather than absent in autism (Happe, 1995; Ozonoff & McEvoy, 1994). The notion of delay rather than deviance is supported by research documenting that some persons with mental retardation may also have delayed theory-of-mind abilities (Yirmiya, Erel, Shaked, & Solomonica-Levi, 1998; Yirmiya, Solomonica-Levi, Shulman, & Pilowsky, 1996). However, Happe (1995) refuted the notion of simple developmental delay by showing that persons with autism needed a higher verbal mental age to pass theory-of-mind tasks than did typically developing children. She hypothesized that the children with autism needed higher vocabulary skills to pass these tasks because they used more verbally mediated, effortful processes than normally developing children. That is, although they could pass the tasks, they were not able to use the same early-developing processes used by typical children. It has been hypothesized that impairments in joint attention skills (Mundy & Sigman, 1989; Mundy, Sigman, & Kasari, 1993) and imitation skills (Meltzoff & Gopnik, 1993) may lead to difficulties in solving theory-of-mind tasks through the same processes used by typically developing children.

Executive Function

A number of researchers have documented that persons with autism have a core deficit in their ability to perform executive function tasks (Ozonoff & Jensen, 1999; Ciesielski & Harris, 1997; Ozonoff, 1995; Ozonoff & McEvoy, 1994). "Executive functions" are cognitive functions thought to involve the ability to maintain an appropriate problem-solving set in order to attain a future goal. These functions include planning, impulse control, inhibition of irrelevant responses, and working memory. Ozonoff et al. (1991) found that a group of nonretarded children and adolescents with autism were less successful on two different executive function tasks (the Tower of Hanoi and the Wisconsin Card Sorting Test) than a learning-disabled control group matched for chronological age and IQ. After 3 years, Ozonoff and McEvoy (1994) conducted a follow-up study with this same group of subjects. They reported that whereas the learning-disabled control group showed improvements on the executive function tasks, the autistic group did not show any improvement with development. These findings support the notion that executive function impairments may represent a lifelong deficit in autism.

Executive function deficits are not specific to autism and have been reported in other disorders, including schizophrenia and ADHD (see Pennington & Welsh, 1995, for a review of executive function impairments in these disorders, and Barkley, 1997, for ADHD). Recent research has begun to examine whether the profile of executive function impairments differs across diagnostic groups. Specifically, Ozonoff and Jensen (1999) compared individuals with autism and ADHD on three different executive function tasks measuring flexibility (Wisconsin Card Sorting Test), planning (Tower of Hanoi), and inhibition (Stroop Color–Word Test). Individuals with autism and individuals with ADHD showed two distinct information-processing profiles of strengths and weaknesses. Individuals with autism had difficulties with flexibility and planning, whereas inhibition was intact. In contrast, individuals with ADHD showed impairments in inhibition, while demonstrating intact flexibility and planning.

Although executive function impairments have been consistently documented in high-functioning and older children with autism (e.g., see Turner, 1999b), results are less consistent for preschoolers with autism. One recent study failed to find executive function deficits on eight different tasks in preschoolers with autism compared to developmentally delayed children (Griffith, Pennington, Wehner, & Rogers, 1999). These results can be interpreted in two ways. First, the tasks developed for young children with autism may not be tapping into the same skills as tasks used for older children and adults with autism.

Indeed, planning and flexible thinking skills are not considered to be well developed in typically developing preschool-age children. Alternatively, executive function impairments may not be an early-developing feature of autism; instead, they may develop as a result of other, more basic impairments in cognitive or social skills. This interpretation was supported by McEvoy, Rogers, and Pennington's (1993) finding that executive function impairments in preschoolers with autism were related to measure of joint attention and social interaction.

Attention Orienting

As noted earlier, clinical observations of individuals with autism highlight their tendency to be virtually unresponsive to some attention-getting stimuli (e.g., hearing their names being called) and to be overly focused on other stimuli (e.g., watching their fingers). Research supports these observations and suggests that individuals with autism have a profile of strengths and weaknesses in their attention skills. Specifically, research has shown that children and adults with high-functioning autism have an intact ability to focus and sustain their attention (Casey, Gordon, Mannheim, & Rumsey, 1993; Pascualvaca, Fantie, Papageorgiou, & Mirsky, 1998), but are impaired in their ability to orient their attention. Orienting consists of two components: the ability to disengage from the current location, and the subsequent ability to shift attention to a new location (Posner, 1980). Impairments in both disengaging and rapidly shifting attention have been demonstrated in high-functioning persons with autism (e.g., Casey et al., 1993; Townsend, Courchesne, & Egaas, 1996). Townsend, Harris, and Courchesne (1996) found that individuals with autism and cerebellar damage were slow to respond when given a short time to process information (100 milliseconds), but showed intact performance when given a longer processing time (800 milliseconds). The authors concluded that individuals with autism are slower to orient their attention. It is unclear which underlying processes (i.e., disengaging or shifting) are responsible for the slowing of attention allocation in individuals with autism. A recent study (Landry & Bryson, 1999) found that young children with autism have difficulties with disengaging their attention rather than shifting their attention. However, more research is needed to clarify this issue.

Abstraction Impairments

Several researchers have hypothesized that individuals with autism have an impaired ability to abstract information from their environment, leading to difficulties with generalization. That is, they have difficulty abstracting information within a single stimulus array and across experiences. Frith and Happe (Frith, 1989; Frith & Happe, 1994) proposed that persons with autism have a preference for processing parts of a stimulus rather than the whole stimulus. They described this preference as an impairment in the ability to "draw together diverse information to construct higher level meaning in context" (Frith & Happe, 1994, p. 121) and coined the term "weak central coherence" to describe this phenomenon. Support for the notion of weak central coherence comes from research demonstrating that persons with autism excel on tasks requiring the ability to perceive parts of stimuli rather than the whole (e.g., block design, embedded figures, and visual illusion tasks). In addition, Happe (1997) reported impairments on a task requiring the ability to abstract a concept from its context. Specifically, individuals with autism were impaired on a homograph test in which participants were asked to read words that could only be pronounced correctly if the sentence context was abstracted (e.g., "tear" could be pronounced "tear" in a woman's dress or "tear" in her eye). However, these findings have not been consistently replicated (Brian & Bryson, 1996; Mottron, Burack, Stauder, & Robaey, 1999).

Klinger and colleagues (Klinger & Dawson, 1995, 2001; Klinger et al., 2001; Klinger & Renner, 2000) have proposed that persons with autism are impaired in their ability to abstract or synthesize information automatically across multiple experiences. In other words, they are impaired in their implicit learning skills. "Implicit learning" is an automatic information-processing skill defined as the "acquisition of knowledge that takes place largely independently of conscious attempts to learn and largely in the absence of explicit knowledge about what was acquired" (Reber, 1993). This type of automatic or implicit learning is an early-developing skill that is present within the first few months of life (Gomez & Gerken, 1999; Saffran, Aslin, & Newport, 1996; Strauss, 1979; Younger, 1985). For example, 10-month-old infants have shown the ability to abstract information across experiences to form a prototype or summary image of previous information (Strauss, 1979; Younger, 1985). The notion of an impaired ability to abstract information automatically across experiences is supported by research demonstrating that persons with autism are impaired in their prototype formation ability (Klinger & Dawson, 1995, 2001). Klinger and Dawson reported that children with autism employed a rule-based approach to categorization, but did not abstract a prototype image across category exemplars. According to these authors, this finding supports the notion that autism is characterized by an early-developing information-processing impairment in the ability to integrate information across experiences. Implicit learning has been hypothesized to underlie young children's ability to understand the complex, unspoken rules that govern social interaction and language development (Gomez & Gerkin, 1999; Lewicki & Hill, 1987; Reber, 1993; Saffran et al., 1996; Saffran, Newport, Aslin, Tunick, & Barrueco, 1997). Therefore, Klinger et al. (2001) have proposed that these implicit or automatic learning impairments may be related to the social and language impairments that characterize autism. Furthermore, they have hypothesized that the repetitive behaviors and restricted interests characteristic of autism may be an attempt to make their environment one that is more predictable and relies on fewer implicit learning requirements. However, Klinger and Dawson (2001) reported that prototype impairments were not specific to autism and were also reported in children with Down syndrome. Therefore, more research is needed to examine whether automatic or implicit learning is specifically impaired in persons with autism.

Plaisted (2001) has theorized that impairments in central coherence and prototype formation may be explained by a perceptual process (i.e., "reduced generalization") in which individuals with autism focus on features that are unique rather than common to a situation or stimulus. This theory suggests that tasks requiring perceptual processing of unique features (e.g., central coherence tasks, such as an embedded figures task) should be easier for persons with autism. Although this theory focuses on an abnormal perceptual process in autism, it predicts that there will be resulting impairments in abstraction abilities. For example, this type of perceptual processing should lead to the development of narrowly defined categories rather than more generalized, abstract categories, and should thus produce prototype impairments.

Although they are intriguing, abstraction theories of autism have not received the overwhelming empirical validation received by executive function, theory-of-mind, and attention-orienting theories of autism. Future work is needed to examine how specific these findings are to autism and whether they are related to the behavioral symptoms of autism.

Summary

Two general conclusions can be derived from these findings that offer clues to the biological underpinnings of autism. First, individuals with autism show impairments in a wide range of domains, including theory of mind, attention, memory, executive functions, and abstraction abilities. Thus it is probable that brain dysfunction in autism involves a distributed brain system rather than one specific brain locus. Second, in most domains, impairments are not found across the board; some functions are spared. These findings suggest that autism is restricted to dysfunction of some brain systems and not others. Future research is needed that links these information-processing findings to underlying brain functioning (e.g., through the use of fMRI). In addition, further research is needed to determine whether these information-processing styles are linked to the social and language impairments and repetitive behaviors that characterize autism.

ETIOLOGY

Genetic Factors

The results of both family and twin studies suggest that genetic factors play a role in the etiology of autism and other pervasive developmental disorders (see Rutter, 2000, for a review). Across several epidemiological studies, the frequency of autism in siblings of autistic children is estimated to be between 2.2% and 4.5% (Szatmari, 1999; Jorde et al., 1991). This is approximately 15 to 30 times greater than the prevalence of autism in the general population, using a base rate of 15 per 10,000. If the entire range of pervasive developmental disorders is examined, the prevalence rate in siblings is even higher, approximately 6% (Szatmari, 1999).

Twin Studies

Epidemiological same-sex twin studies have reported concordance rates for monozygotic twins ranging from 36% to 91%, with a 0–5% concordance rate for dizygotic twins (Bailey, Le Couteur, Gottesman, & Bolton, 1995; Folstein & Rutter, 1977; Rutter et al., 1990; Steffenburg et al., 1989). The fact that these studies showed a much higher concordance rate among monozygotic twins strongly suggests a genetic component for autism. In addition, several studies examining the risk of autism in relatives have reported that approximately 0.18% of second-degree relatives and 0.12% of third-degree relatives had autism (DeLong & Dwyer, 1988; Jorde et al., 1991; Pickles et al., 1995; Szatmari et al., 1995). The much lower risk estimates for second- and third-degree relatives than for siblings of autistic probands suggest that several genes may play a factor in the development of autism, due to less genetic overlap in distant relatives (Pickles et al., 1995). It is estimated that autism involves 5–10 genes and possibly more (Pickles et al., 1995; Risch et al., 1999).

The Broader Autism Phenotype

Within the past few years, much research has been devoted to defining a broader autism phenotype. The term "broader autism phenotype" refers to the idea that relatives of persons with autism may not have the disorder itself, but express a "lesser variant" resulting from shared genes (Baron-Cohen & Hammer, 1997). Typically, this phenotype is defined as having difficulties in one or more of the three areas (social skills, communication skills, repetitive behaviors) that characterize autism. In a recent large-scale study, Pickles et al. (2000) reported that 178 out of 2,360 (7.5%) relatives of persons with autism fit the description of the broader autism phenotype. In comparison, only 20 out of 735 (2.5%) relatives of individuals with Down syndrome fit this description. In addition, Bolton et al. (1994) reported that 12% of siblings of children with autism fell into the broader phenotype category, as compared to 2% of siblings of children with Down syndrome. These studies add support to the notion that this spectrum of disorders is inherited.

Other studies have investigated the notion of a broader cognitive or information-processing phenotype, in which relatives of individuals with autism display some of the cognitive impairments that characterize autism (language delays, theory of mind, central coherence, etc.). The research examining a broader cognitive phenotype in siblings of children with autism has been mixed (see Bauminger & Yirmiya, 2001, for a review). Developmental disorders of speech, language, or reading have been reported in approximately 15–25% of siblings of children with autism (Baird & August, 1985; Bartak et al., 1975; Bolton & Rutter, 1990). However, other studies have reported no differences in overall IQ scores between siblings of children with autism and siblings of children with other developmental disorders (Folstein et al., 1999), or evidence of higher IQ scores in the siblings of children with autism (Fombonne, Bolton, Prior, Jordan, & Rutter, 1997; Szatmari et al., 1993). Increased rates of executive dysfunction have been reported in siblings of individuals with autism—including more difficulties with set shifting, planning, and verbal fluency—compared to siblings of developmentally delayed and typical controls (Hughes, Plumet, & Leboyer, 1999).

Researchers have also examined whether parents of children with autism showed a broader cognitive phenotype. Folstein et al. (1999) found that parents of children with autism (24%) reported an increased history of language-related difficulties (e.g., late onset of phrase speech, articulation difficulties, trouble learning to read or spell), compared to parents of children with Down syndrome (12%). They suggested that these difficulties may be distinct from those for social relating in the broader autistic spectrum. Baron-Cohen and Hammer (1997), testing the cognitive phenotype in parents of individuals with Asperger syndrome, reported evidence for theory-of-mind and central coherence impairments. Similarly, recent studies suggest that fathers of boys with autism show problems with weak central coherence, evident in both cognitive task performance and preferences for detail-focused activities (Briskman, Happe, & Frith, 2001; Happe, Briskman, & Frith, 2001). Taken together, there is evidence that the information-processing strengths and weaknesses characteristic of autism (see Table 9.4) may also be apparent in first-degree relatives.

In addition to familial aggregation of cognitive anomalies associated with autism, recent research has been devoted to the question of distinguishing personality or psychological traits in families of autistic individuals. One study examining 1,654 first-, second-, and third-degree relatives of children with autism compared to 746 relatives of children with Down syndrome found that obsessive–compulsive disorder and motor tics were significantly more common in first-degree relatives of children with autism (Bolton, Pickles, Murphy, & Rutter, 1998). Moreover, this increased rate of obsessive–compulsive disorder was related to social and communication impairments in the relatives of children with autism. Although mood disorders also tended to aggregate in these families, these disorders were not linked to the broader autism phenotype (i.e., social and communicative impairments; Bolton et al., 1998). Another study examining the personality traits of relatives of persons with autism found increased symptoms of anxiety, impulsiveness, aloofness, shyness, oversensitivity, irritability and eccentricity (Murphy et al., 2000). The understanding of the broader autism phenotype is crucial in linkage studies, as researchers must know whom to classify as an affected relative in the search for genes leading to the susceptibility of autism.

Bailey, Phillips, and Rutter (1996) have proposed a "two-hit mechanism," in which one set of causal factors predisposes a person to the broad array of cognitive–social difficulties characterizing the broader phenotype, and another, separate set of causal factors is involved in the transition to the more serious disorder of autism. This second set of causal factors could be either an additional genetic abnormality or an environmental event (e.g., a prenatal insult).

Genetic Linkage Studies

Several genetic linkage studies have been conducted (Alarcon et al., 2002; Ashley-Koch et al., 1999; Bailey, 1998; Barrett et al., 1999; Bradford et al., 2001; Buxbaum et al., 2001; International Molecular Genetic Study of Autism Consortium, 1998; Liu, 2001; Philippe et al., 1999; Risch et al., 1999). Candidate autism susceptibility regions include chromosomes 1p, 2q, 7q, 13q, 16p, and 19q. Linkage signals have generally been small and findings have not been well replicated across studies. An exception is chromosome 7, with three different groups reporting positive results (Ashley-Koch et al., 1999; Barrett et al., 1999; International Molecular Genetic Study of Autism Consortium, 1998).

In summary, it appears that there is no single gene that can account for the autism syndrome. Rather, there appear to be multiple genes involved; each one is a risk factor for a component of this complex syndrome, and various groupings of these genes result in parts of or the entire syndrome (Folstein et al., 1999). Susceptibility genes may have effects on a continually distributed phenotype. If this is the case, then gene discovery will require the development of quantitative (i.e., dimensional) measures of core components of the autism syndrome (Dawson, Webb, et al., 2002).

Prenatal and Perinatal Risk Factors

Numerous researchers have examined the relationship between pre- and perinatal complications and autism. In a review of the literature, Tsai (1987) concluded that increased maternal age (greater than 35 years), bleeding after the first trimester, use of prescription medication, and meconium in the amniotic fluid were seen more frequently in children with autism than in siblings or normally developing control children. However, these findings were not supported by Lord, Mulloy, Wendelboe, and Schopler (1991) in their study of high-functioning (IQ greater than 50) children with autism. In this study, there was a slight increase in the rate of prenatal difficulties in children with autism compared to their siblings, but this increase was not as large as indicated by previous research. In a more recent study, Bolton et al. (1997) found that both individuals with autism and individuals with Down syndrome experienced more obstetrical complications than their unaffected siblings. These results suggest that pre- and perinatal complications may be more closely associated with mental retardation than with autism per se. The only two factors that were more common in children with autism were (1) gestational age greater than 42 weeks; and (2) the tendency of such a child with autism to be either first-born, or fourth- or later-born. However, birth order findings may be coincidental after one takes into account the possibility that many parents stop having children after the birth of a disabled child (Jones & Szatmari, 1988; Lord et al., 1991; Piven et al., 1993).

Biochemical Findings

No specific biochemical markers for autism have been identified. Researchers have examined serotonin, dopamine, norepinephrine, and brain opioids in individuals with autism, but they have found inconsistent results (see Koenig, Tsatsanis, & Volkmar, 2001, for a review). The lack of consistent results may stem from methodological differences in whether peripheral or central levels of neurotransmitter were measured, from the lack of careful control for level of mental retardation, and from the relatively small samples that have been studied. It is important for additional work to continue in this area to isolate possible biochemical markers. A brief review of the research findings to date is provided below.

Serotonin

The neurotransmitter serotonin has been linked to the behavioral–physiological processes of sleep, pain and sensory perception, motor function, appetite, learning, and memory (Volkmar & Anderson, 1989). In addition, serotonin has been implicated in early brain development and plasticity (Azmitia & Whitaker-Azmitia, 1997; Lauder, 1993). The most consistent biochemical finding related to autism has been that between 25% and 50% of individuals with autism are hyperserotonemic; that is, their peripheral blood platelet levels are in the upper 5% of levels found in the normal population (Leboyer et al., 1999; McBride et al., 1998). Research examining the mechanism for hyperserotonemia has indicated that there may be an increased level of platelet uptake or platelet storage of serotonin (Marazziti et al., 2000; Katsui, Okuda, Usuda, & Koizumi, 1986; Rotman, Caplan, & Szekely, 1980). Leboyer et al. (1999) found that 51% of mothers, 45% of fathers, and 87% of siblings of individuals with autism also showed elevated levels of serotonin. Further research is needed to identify the link between increased serotonin levels and the behavioral symptoms of autism.

Dopamine

The neurotransmitter dopamine has been linked to the presence of stereotyped and repetitive behavior. Theoretically, increased levels of dopamine may play a role in the stereotyped and repetitive behaviors that characterize autism. This theory has received mixed support. Garreau et al. (1980) found elevated levels of urinary homovanillic acid, a metabolite of dopamine (Garreau et al., 1980). However, more recent studies have failed to replicate this finding (see Anderson & Hoshino, 1997, for a review), providing no evidence for elevated dopamine in persons with autism.

Norepinephrine

Norepinephrine, a neurotransmitter and a hormone, is influential in respiratory and cardiac function, attention, arousal, memory, anxiety, and movement (Volkmar & Anderson, 1989). Because of the increased arousal and anxiety symptoms associated with autism, there has been considerable interest in the possible link between autism and levels of norepinephrine. However, research examining peripheral and central amounts of norepinephrine and its metabolite, 3-methoxy-4-hydroxyphenylglycol, has not found consistent evidence in support of abnormal levels of norepinephrine in persons with autism (Gillberg, Svennerholm, & Hamilton-Hellberg, 1983; Young et al., 1981; Minderaa, Anderson, Volkmar, Akkerhuis, & Cohen, 1994).

Endogenous Opioids

Endogenous opioid peptides (endorphins) have been implicated in the regulation of pain perception, social and emotional behaviors, and motor activity (Panksepp & Sahley, 1987). Panksepp and colleagues (Panksepp, 1979; Panksepp & Sahley, 1987) proposed that self-injurious behaviors, social deficits, and cognitive impairments in autism may be linked to an elevation in endogenous opioids. However, studies have yielded mixed results, with some researchers finding evidence of increased endorphin levels in individuals with autism (Tordjman et al., 1997), and others finding lowered levels of endorphins (e.g., Leboyer et al., 1994; Sandman, Barron, Chicz-Demet, & Demet, 1990). The literature is complicated by the specific aspects of the endorphin system examined. For example, Leboyer et al. (1999) reported elevated levels in one specific endorphin system (C-terminally directed endorphins) in both individuals with autism and their mothers compared to typical controls, and decreased levels in another endorphin system (N-terminally directed endorphins). Further research is clearly needed to verify whether there is a relationship between autism and elevated endogenous opioids.

Immunizations

Wakefield et al. (1998) hypothesized that the growing prevalence of autism is related to increased immunizations among young children. Specifically, they hypothesized that autism, particularly when regression is present, is related to the measles, mumps, and rubella (MMR) vaccines that are given in a combined injection or in quick succession. This hypothesis has created much concern among parents and has decreased the rates of children receiving the MMR vaccine. However, recent research has not supported a link between autism and the MMR vaccine. Taylor et al. (1999) found that among 498 children with a pervasive developmental disorder, there was no evidence of increased diagnosis in those children who received vaccinations during the second year of life (1987 birth cohort); there was also no difference between age at diagnosis among children vaccinated before 18 months of age, vaccinated after 18 months of age, and never vaccinated. In addition, although regression occurred in approximately a third of the children, it was not related to age at vaccination. Similarly, Dales, Hammer, and Smith (2001) conducted a retrospective study of MMR vaccination rates by the age of 24 months and autism diagnosis rates among children born in 1980–1994 who were enrolled in California kindergarten classes (600–1,900 children per birth year). A marked increase in autism diagnoses was noted among this sample, from a rate of 4.4 cases per 10,000 in the 1980 cohort to a rate of 20.8 cases per 10,000 in the 1994 cohort. However, this increase was not related to increases in MMR vaccinations, which were relatively stable during this same time period. These data do not support an association between MMR immunizations and autism.

Neuroanatomical Findings

Several promising findings have been reported by researchers examining possible neuroanatomical abnormalities in autism. These findings are from studies using structural imaging techniques, brain autopsies, and animal models of autism. In general, neuroanatomical studies support the notion that autism is linked to a combination of brain enlargement in some areas and brain reduction in other areas (see Koenig et al., 2001, for a review). Although these findings may seem to contradict each other, taken together they suggest a single theory about the underlying cause of autism. That is, autism may be caused by abnormal cell growth during the early stages of prenatal and postnatal brain development. In normal brain development, neurons proliferate and become interconnected, gradually decreasing in size and number once certain connections become more heavily utilized than others. It is this process of neuronal growth and pruning that seems to be abnormal in autism, leaving some areas of the brain with too many neurons and other areas with too few neurons (Minshew, 1996). Research has suggested abnormalities in several areas of the brain: the cerebral cortex, the cerebellum, the limbic system, and the corpus callosum. In addition, some researchers have reported an overall brain enlargement rather than localization to a specific area. Evidence for abnormalities in each of these areas is now reviewed.

Brain Volume

Using MRI, several investigators have found evidence for brain enlargement in individuals with autism compared to age- and Performance-IQ-matched comparison groups (Filipek et al., 1992; Piven et al., 1995). In a follow-up study, Piven, Arndt, Bailey, and Andreasen (1996) reported that this enlargement was specific to occipital, parietal, and temporal regions, but not the frontal lobe. Imaging findings of increased brain volume are consistent with autopsy studies finding increased brain weight (Bailey et al., 1998; Bauman & Kemper, 1994). These findings are supported by the theory that autism is linked to abnormal neuronal migration and pruning during brain development.

Cerebral Cortex

Several studies have used MRI scans to examine malformations in the cerebral cortex of individuals with autism. Piven et al. (1990) reported cortical malformations in 7 of their 13 high-functioning autistic subjects. These abnormalities included polymicrogyria, macrogyria, and schizencephaly, and were located in a variety of different brain locations in both hemispheres. The authors believed that these malformations resulted from a defect in the migration of neurons to the cerebral cortex during the first 6 months of prenatal development. However, these abnormalities could result either from early-onset developmental brain malformations or from late-onset progressive atrophy.

Findings of brain enlargement specific to the occipital, parietal, and temporal regions (Piven, Arndt, et al., 1996) suggest that these particular areas of the cerebral cortex may be involved in autism. However, other investigators have reported conflicting findings. Courchesne, Press, and Yeung-Courchesne (1993) reported a reduced, not enlarged, volume in the parietal lobes in 43% (9 out of 23 individuals with autism). More research is needed to identify whether specific cortical areas are abnormal in autism.

Cerebellum

Support for abnormalities in the cerebellum of persons with autism comes from both MRI and autopsy studies. Courchesne, Yeung-Courchesne, Press, Hesselink, and Jernigan (1988) conducted MRI scans on 18 persons with autism ranging in age from 6 to 30 years. They reported that, compared to a group of nonautistic persons with normal MRI scans, 14 of the individuals with autism displayed hypoplasia of cerebellar vermal lobules VI and VII. In addition, no abnormalities were evident in the pons or the midbrain, suggesting that cerebellar hypoplasia is not associated with anatomical abnormalities of the major input and output pathways to the cerebellum (Hsu, Yeung-Courchesne, Courchesne, & Press, 1991). The authors speculated that cerebellar hypoplasia may result from maldevelopment within the cerebellum rather than an atrophy following a period of normal development. If neural output from the cerebellum is damaged as a result of this maldevelopment, there may be subsequent abnormal development and functioning in neuronal systems that are directly connected to the cerebellum—including systems regulating attention, sensory modulation, autonomic activity, and motor and behavior initiation (Courchesne et al., 1988). These systems have been implicated in the etiology of autism. Although promising, these results have not been consistently replicated (Garber & Ritvo, 1992; Kleiman, Neff, & Rosman, 1992), and more recent research suggests that there may be a link between cerebellar hypoplasia and low IQ rather than autism per se (Courchesne et al., 1994; Filipek, 1995).

Consistent with some MRI studies, autism studies have revealed Purkinje and granule cell loss in the neocerebellum of individuals with autism (Bauman & Kemper, 1985, 1996; Ritvo et al., 1986). In addition, a recent brain tissue study (Fatemi, Stary, Halt, & Realmuto, 2001) revealed decreased amounts of two proteins (Reelin and Bcl-2) in the cerebellum. Interestingly, these proteins have been implicated in cell migration and pruning, suggesting a possible biochemical marker for the structural abnormalities observed in autism.

Limbic System

The social skill impairments in autism have been theorized to reflect abnormal functioning in the limbic system. Bachevalier (1991, 1994) proposed an animal model for childhood autism, purporting that monkeys with lesions in the medial temporal lobe (e.g., the amygdala and hippocampus) show autistic-like behaviors—including failure to develop normal social relationships, blank facial expressions, poor body language, lack of eye contact, and motor stereotypies. Interestingly, when specific lesions were made in either the amygdala or the hippocampus, persistent disturbances in social interactions were only noted in the monkeys with lesions in the amygdala (Bachevalier, 1994). However, the most severe autistic-like behaviors were observed in monkeys with combined damage to both the amygdala and hippocampus. This finding suggests that less severe forms of autism may result from damage to the amygdala, whereas more severe forms of autism including mental retardation may require damage to both the amygdala and the hippocampus.

There is some empirical support for limbic system abnormalities in persons with autism. Autopsy studies have revealed reduced neuronal cell size and increased cell-packing density in limbic structures (e.g., the hippocampus and amygdale; Bauman & Kemper, 1988). However, MRI studies have not found any evidence of abnormalities in the hippocampus (Piven, Bailey, Ranson, & Arndt, 1998; Saitoh, Courchesne, Egaas, Lincoln, & Schreibman, 1995).

Corpus Callosum

Several studies have found evidence of reduced size of the corpus callosum in persons with autism (Egaas, Courchesne, & Saitoh, 1995; Piven, Bailey, Ranson, & Arndt, 1997). These findings suggest that there may be a link between autism and impaired communication between brain hemispheres.

Summary

Although the neuroanatomical findings often contradict each other, there is overwhelming evidence that autism is linked to abnormalities in brain development, leading some regions of the brain to be overdeveloped and others to be underdeveloped. In general, studies of the cerebral cortex have supported a theory of brain enlargement, while studies of subcortical structures have supported a theory of brain reduction. This suggests that there may be abnormal connections between subcortical and cortical pathways in persons with autism (Koenig et al., 2001). More research is needed to identify the specific pathways that are impaired, as well as the specific prenatal and postnatal neuronal migration systems that are involved.

Cortical Electroencephalographic Findings

Cortical EEG studies have supported the notion that hemispheric laterality is abnormal in autism. Studies examining brain activity during the administration of cognitive tasks have found that, compared to chronological-age-matched, normally developing controls, individuals with autism showed atypical patterns of hemispheric activation during language and motor imitation tasks, characterized by greater right- than left-hemisphere activation (Dawson, Warrenburg, & Fuller, 1982, 1983). A study examining brain activity during an alert resting state found that children with autism showed less inter- and intrahemispheric asymmetry than either normally developing or mentally retarded children (Cantor, Thatcher, Hrybyk, & Kaye, 1986). They interpreted this finding as evidence for diminished cortical differentiation in autism. In a study using EEG to measure brain activity in groups of autistic and developmentally matched normal children, Dawson and her colleagues (Dawson, Klinger, Panagiotides, Lewy, & Castelloe, 1995) found that the children with autism exhibited reduced EEG power in the frontal and temporal regions, but not in the parietal region. Differences were more prominent in the left than the right hemisphere.

EEG studies have also been used to examine abnormal social behavior in autism. Dawson et al. (1995) examined EEGs in subgroups of children with autism that were defined by the children's social behavior. One group was described as having a passive interaction style in which they rarely initiated social interaction. The other group was less impaired, actively approaching and engaging in social interaction. The children with the most social impairments (i.e., the passive group) demonstrated increased brain activity in the frontal region, compared to normally developing children matched on both chronological age and receptive language mental age. The autistic children with more developed social skills did not show this difference in brain activity. This is one of the first findings of biological differences that are linked to social skills impairments in autism.

FUTURE DIRECTIONS

Biological Research

Since the first edition of this book was published, research examining the genetic underpinnings of autism has expanded greatly. Our knowledge about the behavioral and cognitive symptoms of autism that are present in first-degree relatives has also increased. With newer, more sophisticated genetic methods, such as linkage analysis and quantitative trait locus analysis, we are hopeful that the specific autism susceptibility genes will be uncovered in the next decade. In addition, techniques for measuring brain anatomy and brain function, including fMRI and improved positron emission tomography (PET) methods, hold promise for increasing our understanding of the neurofunctional basis of this disorder. For example, the use of fMRI in conjunction with information-processing tasks will clarify whether individuals with autism are using the same brain regions for information processing as typically developing individuals are using.

Finally, there is a growing body of evidence that persons with autism have more difficulty processing social information than nonsocial information (cf. Dawson, Meltzoff, Osterling, Rinaldi, & Brown, 1998). For example, persons with autism are much less likely to orient to social than nonsocial stimuli; they have more difficulty imitating body actions than toy actions; they have more difficulty with the social aspects of language (pragmatics) than the more formal aspects (syntax); and so on. Future research is needed to clarify the biological underpinnings of these findings and to determine whether autism involves a dysfunction of a brain system that is specialized for social cognition.

Developing a Theoretical Framework Linking Biological, Information-Processing, and Behavioral Factors in Autism

An understanding of information-processing impairments in autism will aid in our understanding of the underlying neurofunctional abnormalities that cause autism and of the behavioral symptoms that characterize autism (Gillberg, 1999; Ozonoff, 1997; Rutter, 1999). Figure 9.1 illustrates a proposed theoretical framework to explain the relations among the biological abnormalities, cognitive processing impairments, and behavioral symptoms of autism. In this proposed framework, the behavioral symptoms of autism (i.e., social skills impairments, communication impairments, and repetitive behaviors) result from underlying information-processing impairments that are caused by neurofunctional abnormalities related to underlying genetic susceptibility for autism. Historically, researchers have focused on pieces of the proposed model, with little research examining the model in its entirety. For example, Townsend, Courchesne, and Egaas (1996) examined the link between abnormal cerebellar structure and attention orienting in autism, and found that individuals with autism and cerebellar damage were slow to respond when given a short time to process information. This research provides evidence that there is a link between information-processing impairments (i.e., slowed attention orienting) and underlying neuroanatomical abnormalities (i.e., MRI evidence of cerebellar abnormalities) in some persons with autism. However, the next link—that between attention-orienting impairments and social, language, and repetitive behavior impairments in a group of individuals with cerebellar damage—has not been examined.

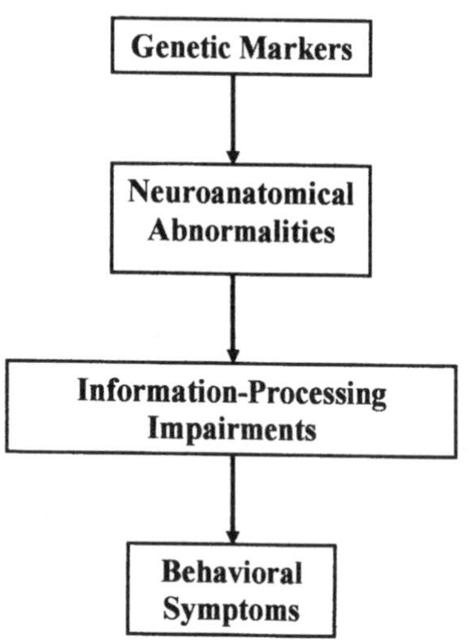

FIGURE 9.1. Theoretical link among biology, cognition, and behavior in autism.

Conversely, Klinger et al. (2001) examined the relationship between information-processing impairments and behavioral symptoms of autism, but have not directly examined the relation between underlying biological abnormalities and information-processing impairments. In their study, they found that abstraction impairments (i.e., implicit learning) were related to increased parental report of repetitive behaviors and social skills deficits in a group of children with autism (see Figure 9.2). Based on research tying implicit learning to basal ganglial and striatal functioning (Lieberman, 2000; Ashby, Alfonso-Reese, Turken, & Waldron, 1998), they hypothesized that abnormal basal ganglia functioning may underlie implicit learning impairments in autism, and that the behavioral symptoms of autism are caused by these implicit learning impairments. However, they did not directly examine the link between neurobiological abnormalities and behavioral symptomatology.

As our technological ability to measure brain functioning (e.g., through fMRI, EEG, and PET) improves, and as our research methodology for measuring information processing in young children improves, a goal of future research will be to measure brain functioning, information processing, and behavioral symptoms within a single sample of individuals with autism. This type of research is essential to understanding how the biological, cognitive, and behavioral components of autism are related. With this knowledge, improved treatment techniques that directly link biological abnormalities, information-processing strengths and weaknesses, and behavioral symptoms can be developed.

Identifying Subtypes

There is increasing evidence that autism is not a single disorder, but instead is a diagnostic label used to describe several different disorders that share some overlapping behavioral symptoms. For example, Rapin (1996) found evidence of discontinuity in functioning levels of a large sample of children with pervasive developmental disorders and concluded that there exists two distinct subgroups. Based on a large-scale epidemiological study, Wing and Gould (1979) proposed that there are three subgroups of autism. Focusing on variations in social behavior, Wing and Gould (1979) characterized the three groups as (1) "aloof/withdrawn," (2) "passive," and (3) "actively social-but-odd." Castelloe and Dawson

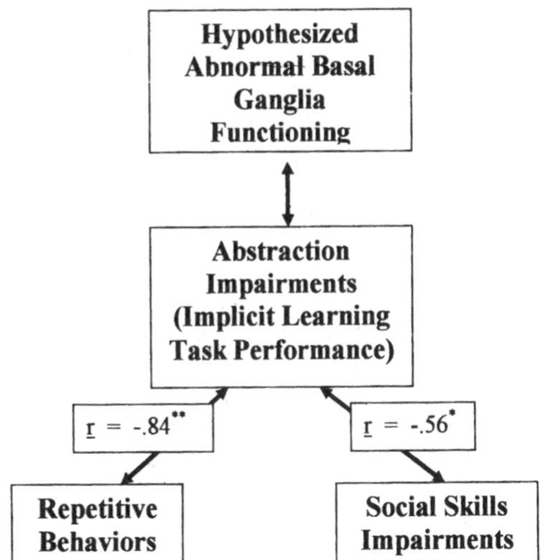

FIGURE 9.2. Example of a theory linking biology, cognition, and behavior in autism. Data from Klinger, Lee, Bush, Klinger, and Crump (2001). $^{*}p < .10$; $^{**}p < .05$; $n = 12$.

(1993) validated this subgroup classification system by demonstrating the existence of clusters of cognitive, language, and social symptoms as predicted by Wing and Gould (1979). In addition, Dawson et al. (1995) found that children classified as passive versus active-but-odd showed distinct patterns of EEG activity. More research is needed to identify behavioral, information-processing, and biological markers of different autism subtypes. Until subtypes have been identified, it is likely that investigators will continue to produce conflicting findings that are partially due to the different subtypes present in their specific studies. This heterogeneity among research participants will continue to make it difficult to identify information-processing and biological profiles that characterize persons with autism.

Early Diagnosis

Parents of children with autism often report that they were concerned about their children's development prior to 1 year of age and expressed this concern to their pediatricians by 18 months of age (Siegel, Pilner, Eschler, & Elliot, 1988). However, on average, a diagnosis of autism is not given until 4 years of age (Siegel et al., 1988). Recent research has increased our knowledge of the early social symptoms that characterize autism in the first 2 years of life. Research also suggests that the earlier the intervention, the better the outcome in terms of language development and placement in a regular education classroom (Dawson & Osterling, 1997). As our knowledge of the early symptoms of autism has increased, there has been an increased emphasis on the development of screening instruments to detect these symptoms in infants and toddlers (see Filipek et al., 1999).

Several instruments have been developed for use in primary care medical settings to screen for early symptoms of autism (see Table 9.3 for a list of recently developed screening instruments). Both the Modified Checklist for Autism in Toddlers (M-CHAT; Robins et al., 2001) and the Pervasive Developmental Disorders Screening Test (PDDST; Siegel & Hayer, 1999) are parent report checklists, while the Checklist for Autism in Toddlers (CHAT; Baron-Cohen et al., 1996) involves a combined parent report and professional observation. Each of these instruments incorporates the early diagnostic markers identified within the first few years of life—including deficits in eye gaze, pointing, and pretend play, as well as additional symptoms that are commonly reported by parents of young children.

These instruments are still in their early stages of development, with varied data regarding their validity and reliability. The CHAT was examined in a large-scale longitudinal population-based study of more than 16,000 children (Baird et al., 2000), producing disappointing results (sensitivity of 20% and positive predictive validity of 26.3%). The M-CHAT, a new adaptation of the CHAT, has been examined in a sample of 1,122 children seen for a pediatrician checkup and 171 high-risk children seen for an early intervention screen. Initial results are more promising than those for the original CHAT (sensitivity of 95%; positive predictive validity of 64%), although there are no longitudinal data on whether these diagnoses are valid across time. The PDDST is unique, in that different versions of the instrument have been designed for fast screening in a variety of settings (primary care clinics, developmental clinics, and autism specialty clinics). Using the primary care version of the PDDST, Siegel and Hayer (1999) reported promising results with a sample of 577 children—260 with a pervasive developmental disorder, 120 with some other developmental disorder, and 197 high-risk children due to low birthweight (sensitivity of 85%, specificity of 71%). As with the M-CHAT, no data are yet available on the long-term accuracy of these diagnoses.

Thus, although recent research suggests the possibility of developing accurate early screening instruments for autism within a primary care setting, none of the instruments has received enough validation for anyone to recommend its widespread clinical use. The next step for researchers in this field is to directly compare the accuracy of these instruments, in order to determine which leads to the most accurate screening. Although this work is still in the early stages, it is likely that detection of autism during the first 2 years of life will be possible in the very near future. As early detection becomes more likely, investigators will increasingly focus on the development of methods for early intervention.

Early Intervention

Rutter (1999) has noted that there is a two-way interplay between research and clinical practice, with each influencing the development of the other. Indeed, this type of interplay is seen in the recent emphasis on early intervention for young children with autism. The focus on early intervention has developed from research findings in biological, cognitive, and clinical domains. In the area of basic biological research, there is a growing literature indicating that brain development begins prenatally and continues during the first few postnatal years. This research suggests that there is a sensitive period in which early interventions may have a profound effect on the developing nervous system and result in improved behavioral outcomes for children with autism (see Dawson, Ashman, & Carver, 2001, for a review). In the area of cognitive research, recent evidence of early-developing information-processing impairments suggests that early intervention is needed either to prevent or to reduce the subsequent development of behavioral symptoms of autism (see Rogers, 1998b, for a review of early intervention techniques that address specific information-processing impairments in autism). Finally, support for early intervention also comes from clinical research identifying the early symptoms of autism and diagnostic instruments that are sensitive to these symptoms. As a result of all three sets of findings, there is an increasing demand for interventions designed for toddlers and preschoolers.

Because of the devastating nature of the disorder, parents have shown a willingness to try any possible treatment approach, and there is much controversy over which treatment approach is the most effective (e.g., Gresham & MacMillan, 1997a, 1997b; Smith & Lovaas, 1997). Bristol et al. (1996) have listed six different methodological issues that need to be addressed in order to determine which treatment approach is the most effective. Specifically, they have argued that treatment outcome research needs to (1) directly compare treatment approaches; (2) use random assignment to treatment conditions; (3) use standard treatment protocols; (4) use outside evaluators to measure treatment efficacy; (5) include an assessment of treatment integrity; and (6) use longitudinal designs to measure both immediate and long-term treatment effectiveness. Unfortunately, the majority of treatment outcome studies have failed to address all of these issues, leading to difficulty in determining whether one program is more effective than another (see Gresham & MacMillan, 1997a, for an example of how a failure to address these issues may mitigate promising treatment findings). Clearly, future research needs to be conducted that critically examines the effectiveness of different research programs.

In the absence of data that directly compare early intervention approaches, several investigators have described key components that are common across different treatment programs (Dawson & Osterling, 1997; Rogers, 1998b). In a review of eight different university-based intervention programs for children with autism in the United States, Dawson and Osterling (1997) reported that the majority of these intervention programs have demonstrated effectiveness, as measured by the fact that approximately 50% of children who received intervention services were placed in regular education elementary school classrooms (Anderson, Campbell, & Cannon, 1994; Handleman & Harris, 1994; Lord & Schopler, 1994; Lovaas, 1987; McClannahan & Krantz, 1994; McGee, Daly, & Jacobs, 1994; Rogers & DiLalla, 1991; Strain & Cordisco, 1994). Across these programs, IQ score improvements ranging from 19 to 30 points were noted, with an average IQ gain of 23 points. Investigators did not report whether a positive response to intervention was related to specific child characteristics, such as IQ or language ability. It should be noted, however, that the average Full Scale IQ of children participating in the programs fell in the moderately mentally retarded range, and that all children scored in the mentally retarded range (70 or below) at the beginning of intervention.

Thus, despite having autism and considerable mental delay, approximately half of the children responded very positively to early intervention, and all children reportedly made substantial gains.

Dawson and Osterling (1997) have identified several elements common to effective early intervention programs for children with autism:

1. A curriculum focusing on the areas of attention and compliance, motor imitation, communication, appropriate use of toys, and social skills.
2. Highly structured teaching environments with a low student-to-staff ratio.
3. Systematic strategies for generalizing newly acquired skills to a wide range of situations.
4. Maintenance of predictability and routine in the daily schedule.
5. A functional approach to problem behaviors (Donnellan et al., 1984).
6. A focus on skills needed for successful transitions from the early intervention program to the regular preschool or kindergarten classroom.
7. A high level of family involvement.

Dawson and Osterling (1997) have argued that there is a serious gap between the state of our knowledge of early intervention methods for children with autism and the methods actually used in most public school systems. Treatment approaches that are effective in a university-based research setting may not be readily transferable to a school-based setting, in which there is less opportunity for ongoing training of therapists and fewer resources to ensure treatment integrity (Gresham & MacMillan, 1997a). Future goals for intervention research include developing effective treatment programs that can be utilized in a community setting, and enabling researchers to become more effective communicators of our current knowledge to parents, teachers, and other service providers.

CONCLUSIONS

The past 15 years have witnessed substantial progress in our understanding and treatment of young children with autism. In particular, important strides have been made in our understanding of autism in the areas of genetic and neurofunctional abnormalities, early recognition/diagnosis, and information-processing impairments. In the past few years, there has been a proliferation of research examining the genetic and neurofunctional abnormalities in autism. As a result, our understanding of the biological underpinnings of autism has also increased significantly. We hope that the underlying genetics of autism will be uncovered in the next decade. In the area of early recognition/diagnosis, we are now able to identify the symptoms of autism that begin during the first 2 years of life. In the next decade, researchers will focus on refining early screening instruments appropriate for the first 2 years of life, so that pediatricians and other health care professionals are able to recognize symptoms of autism and refer children for diagnostic evaluations. In addition, cognitive studies have increased our understanding of the wide range of information-processing impairments and abilities shown by individuals with autism, and have yielded evidence of distinct neuropsychological profiles in persons with autism. The development of cognitive tests that are appropriate for very young children with autism are likely to yield new insights into the neuropsychology of autism. When combined with our ability to detect autism at an early age, subgroup identification may lead to more individualized treatment strategies. Finally, future research is needed to identify the links among underlying neurofunctional abnormalities, information-processing impairments, and behavioral symptoms of autism.

ACKNOWLEDGMENTS

We wish to thank Lea Karatheodoris for her endless hours assisting with library research, typing references, and reading drafts of this chapter. In addition, we would like to thank the children with autism and their families who have eagerly participated in research and provided the clinical insights that we have described in this chapter. Preparation of this chapter was supported by a program project grant cofunded by the National Institute of Child Health and Human Development (NICHD) and the National Institute on Deafness and Communication Disability (NIDCD) (Grant No. PO1HD34565), which is part of the NICHD/NIDCD Collaborative Program of Excellence in Autism.

REFERENCES

Ainsworth, M. D. (1983). Patterns of infant–mother attachment as related to maternal care: Their early history and their contribution to continuity. In D. Magnusson &

V. Allen (Eds.), *Human development: An interactional perspective* (pp. 35–55). New York: Academic Press.

Ainsworth, M. D., Blehar, M. D., Waters, E., & Wall, S. (1978). *Patterns of attachment: A psychological study of the Strange Situation.* Hillsdale, NJ: Erlbaum.

Alarcon, M., Canto, R. M., Liu, J., Gilliam, T. C., the Autism Genetic Resource Exchange Consortium, & Geschwind, D. H. (2002). Evidence for a language quantitative trait locus on chromosome 7q in multiplex families. *American Journal of Human Genetics, 70,* 60–71.

Amato, J., Barrow, M., & Domingo, R. (1999). Symbolic play behavior in very young verbal and nonverbal children with autism. *Infant–Toddler Intervention, 9,* 185–194.

Ameli, R., Courchesne, E., Lincoln, A., Kaufman, A. S., & Grillon, C. (1988). Visual memory processes in high-functioning individuals with autism. *Journal of Autism and Developmental Disorders, 18,* 601–615.

American Psychiatric Association. (1994). *Diagnostic and statistical manual of mental disorders* (4th ed.). Washington, DC: Author.

Amir, R. E., Van den Veyver, I. B., Wan, M., Tran, C. Q., Francke, U., & Zoghbi, H. Y. (1999), Rett syndrome is caused by mutations in X-linked MECP2, encoding methyl-CpG-binding protein 2. *Nature Genetics, 23,* 185–188.

Anderson, G. M., & Hoshino, Y. (1997). Neurochemical studies of autism.. In D. J. Cohen & F. R. Volkmar (Eds.), *Handbook of autism and pervasive developmental disorders* (2nd ed., pp. 325–343). New York: Wiley.

Anderson, S. R., Campbell, S., & Cannon, B. O. (1994). The May Center for early childhood education. In S. Harris & J. Handleman (Eds.), *Preschool education programs for children with autism* (pp. 15–36). Austin, TX: Pro-Ed.

Ashby, F. G., Alfonso-Reese, L. A., Turken, U., & Waldron, E. M. (1998). A neuropsychological theory of multiple systems in category learning. *Psychological Review, 105,* 442–481.

Ashley-Koch, A., Wolpert, C. M., Menold, M. M., Zaeem, L., Basu, S., Donnelly, S. L., Ravan, S. A., Powell, C. M., Qumsiyeh, M. B., Aylsworth, A. S., Vance, J. M., Gilbert, J. R., Wright, H. H., Abramson, R. K., Delong, G. R., Cuccaro, M. L., Pericak-Vance, M. A. J. (1999). Genetic studies of autistic disorder and chromosome 7. *Genomics, 61,* 227–236.

Asperger, H. (1991). "Autistic psychopathy" in childhood. In U. Frith (Ed. and Trans.), *Autism and Asperger syndrome* (pp. 37–92). Cambridge, England: Cambridge University Press. (Original work published 1944)

Azmitia, E., & Whitaker-Azmitia, P. (1997). Development and adult plasticity of serotonergic neurons and their target cells. In H. Baumbgartener & M. Goethert (Eds.), *Serotonergic neurons and 5-HT receptors in the central nervous system* (pp. 1–39). New York: Springer.

Bachevalier, J. (1991). An animal model for childhood autism: Memory loss and socioemotional disturbances following neonatal damage to the limbic system in monkeys. In C. A. Tamminga & S. C. Schulz (Eds.), *Advances in neuropsychiatry and psychopharmacology: Vol. 1. Schizophrenia research* (pp. 129–140). New York: Raven Press.

Bachevalier, J. (1994). Medial temporal lobe structures and autism: A review of clinical and experimental findings. *Neuropsychologia, 32,* 627–648.

Bailey, A. (1998). A full genome screen for autism with evidence for linkage to a region on chromosome 7q. *Human Molecular Genetics, 7,* 571–578.

Bailey, A., Le Couteur, A., Gottesman, I., & Bolton, P. (1995). Autism as a strongly genetic disorder: Evidence from a British twin study. *Psychological Medicine, 25,* 63–77.

Bailey, A., Luthert, P., Dean, A., Harding, Janota, I., Montgomery, M., Rutter, M., & Lantos, P. (1998). A clinicopathological study of autism. *Brain, 121,* 889–905.

Bailey, A., Phillips, W., & Rutter, M. (1996). Autism: Towards an integration of clinical, genetic and neuropsychological and neurobiological perspectives. *Journal of Child Psychology and Psychiatry, 37,* 89–126.

Baird, G., Charman, T., Baron-Cohen, S., Cox, A., Swettenham, J., Wheelwright, S., Drew, A., & Kemal, L. (2000). A screening instrument for autism at 18 months of age: A six-year follow-up study. *Journal of the American Academy of Child and Adolescent Psychiatry, 39,* 694–702.

Baird, T. D., & August, G. J. (1985). Familial heterogeneity in infantile autism. *Journal of Autism and Developmental Disorders, 15,* 315–321.

Ballaban-Gil, K., & Tuchman, R. (2000). Epilepsy and epileptiform EEG: Association with autism and language disorders. *Mental Retardation and Developmental Disabilities Research Reviews, 6,* 300–308.

Baranek, G. T. (1999). Autism during infancy: A retrospective video analysis of sensory–motor and social behaviors. *Journal of Autism and Developmental Disorders, 29,* 213–224.

Barkley, R. A. (1997). *ADHD and the nature of self-control.* New York: Guilford Press.

Baron-Cohen, S. (1989a). The autistic child's theory of mind: A case of specific developmental delay. *Journal of Child Psychology and Psychiatry, 30,* 285–297.

Baron-Cohen, S. (1989b). Are autistic children behaviorists?: An examination of their mental–physical and appearance–reality distinctions. *Journal of Autism and Developmental Disorders, 19,* 579–600.

Baron-Cohen, S. (2000). Is Asperger syndrome/high-functioning autism necessarily a disability? *Development and Psychopathology, 12,* 489–500.

Baron-Cohen, S. (2001). Theory of mind and autism: A review. *International Review of Research in Mental Retardation, 23,* 169–184.

Baron-Cohen, S., Cox, A., Baird, G., Swettenham, J., Nightingale, N., Morgan, K., Drew, A., & Charman, T. (1996). Psychological markers in the detection of autism in infancy in a large population. *British Journal of Psychiatry, 168,* 158–163.

Baron-Cohen, S., & Hammer, J. (1997). Parents of children with Asperger syndrome: What is the cognitive phenotype? *Journal of Cognitive Neuroscience, 9,* 548–554.

Baron-Cohen, S., Jolliffe, T., Mortimore, C., & Robertson, M. (1997). Another advanced test of theory of mind: Evidence from very high functioning adults with autism or Asperger syndrome. *Journal of Child Psychology and Psychiatry, 38,* 813–822.

Baron-Cohen, S., Leslie, A. M., & Frith, U. (1985). Does the autistic child have a "theory of mind"? *Cognition, 21,* 37–46.

Baron-Cohen, S., Scahill, V. L., Izaguirre, J., Hornsey, H., & Robertson, M. M. (1999). The prevalence of Gilles de le Tourette syndrome in children and adolescents with autism: A large scale study. *Psychological Medicine, 29,* 1151–1159.

Barrett, S., Beck, J., Bernier, R., Bisson, E., Braun, T., Casavant, T., Childress, D., Folstein, S., Garcia, M., Gardiner, M., Gilman, S., Haines, J., Hopkins, K., Landa, R., Meyer, N., Mullane, J., Nishimura, D., Palmer, P.,

Piven, J., Purdy, J., Santangelo, S., Searby, C., Sheffiled, V., Singleton, J., Slager, S., Struchen, T., Svenson, S., Vieland, V., Wang, K., & Winklosky, B. (1999). An autosomal genomic screen for autism. *American Journal of Medical Genetics, 88*, 609–615.

Bartak, L., Rutter, M. L., & Cox, A. (1975). A comparative study of infantile autism and specific developmental language disorder: I. The children. *British Journal of Psychiatry, 126*, 127–145.

Barth, C., Fein, D., & Waterhouse, L. (1995). Delayed match-to-simple performance in autistic children. *Developmental Neuropsychology, 11*, 53–69.

Bauman, M., & Kemper, T. (1985). Histoanatomic observations of the brain in early infantile autism. *Neurology, 35*, 866–874.

Bauman, M., & Kemper, T. (1988). Limbic and cerebellar abnormalities: Consistent findings in infantile autism. *Journal of Neuropathology and Experimental Neurology, 47*, 369.

Bauman, M., & Kemper, T. L. (1994). Neuroanatomic observations of the brain in autism. In M. L. Bauman & T. L. Kemper (Eds.), *The neurobiology of autism* (pp. 119–145). Baltimore: Johns Hopkins University Press.

Bauman, M., & Kemper, T. L. (1996). Observations on the Purkinje cells in the cerebellar vermis in autism. *Journal of Neuropathology and Experimental Neurology, 55*, 613.

Bauminger, N., & Yirmiya, N. (2001). The functioning and well-being of siblings of children with autism: Behavioral-genetic and familial contributions. In J. A. Burack, T. Charman, N. Yirmiya, & P. R. Zelazo (Eds.), *The development of autism: Perspectives from theory and research* (pp. 61– 80). Mahwah, NJ: Erlbaum.

Bettelheim, B. (1967). *The empty fortress: Infantile autism and the birth of self*. New York: Free Press.

Bishop, D. V. (1992). The underlying nature of specific language impairment. *Journal of Child Psychology and Psychiatry, 33*, 3–66.

Bleuler, E. (1950). *Dementia praecox or a group within the schizophrenias* (J. Zinkin, Trans.). New York: International Universities Press. (Original work published 1911)

Bolton, P., Macdonald, H., Pickles, A., Rios, P., Goode, S., Crowson, M., Bailey, A., & Rutter, M. (1994). A case–control family history study of autism. *Journal of Child Psychology and Psychiatry, 35*, 877–900.

Bolton, P., Murphy, M., Macdonald, H., Whitlock, B., Pickles, A., & Rutter, M. (1997). Obstetric complications in autism: Consequences or causes of the condition? *Journal of the American Academy of Child and Adolescent Psychiatry, 36*, 272–281.

Bolton, P., Pickles, A., Murphy, M., & Rutter, M. (1998). Autism, affective and other psychiatric disorders: Patterns of familial aggregation. *Psychological Medicine, 28*, 385–395.

Bolton, P., & Rutter, M. (1990). Genetic influences in autism. *International Review of Psychiatry, 2*, 67–80.

Bormann-Kischkel, C., Vilsmeier, M., & Baude, B. (1995). The development of emotional concepts in autism. *Journal of Child Psychology and Psychiatry, 36*, 1245–1259.

Boucher, J. (1981). Immediate free recall in early childhood autism: Another point of behavioral similarity with amnesic syndrome. *British Journal of Psychology, 72*, 211–215.

Boucher, J., & Lewis, V. (1992). Unfamiliar face recognition in relatively able autistic children. *Journal of Child Psychology and Psychiatry, 33*, 843–859.

Boucher, J., & Warrington, E. K. (1976). Memory deficits in early infantile autism: Some similarities to the amnesic syndrome. *British Journal of Psychology, 67*, 73–87.

Bowler, D. M., Matthews, N. J., & Gardiner, J. M. (1997). Asperger's syndrome and memory: Similarity to autism but not amnesia. *Neuropsychologia, 35*, 65–70.

Bradford, Y., Haines, J., Hutcheson, H., Gardiner, M., Braun, T., Sheffield, V., Cassavant, T., Huang, W., Wang, K., Vieland, V., Folstein, S., Santangelo, S., & Piven, J. (2001). Incorporating language phenotypes strengthens evidence of linkage to autism. *American Journal of Medical Genetics, 105*, 539–547.

Briskman, J., Happe, F., & Frith, U. (2001). Exploring the cognitive phenotype of autism: Weak "central coherence" in parents and siblings of children with autism. II. Real-life skills and preferences. *Journal of Child Psychology and Psychiatry, 42*, 309–317.

Bristol, M. M., Cohen, D. J., Costello, E. J., Denckla, M., Eckberg, T. J., Kallen, R., Kraemer, H. C., Lord, C., Maurer, R., McIlvane, W. J., Minshew, N., Sigman, M., & Spence, M. A. (1996). State of the science in autism: Report to the National Institutes of Health. *Journal of Autism and Developmental Disorders, 26*, 121–154.

Bruner, J. (1975). From communication to language: A psychological perspective. *Cognition, 3*, 255–287.

Bryson, S. E., Clark, B. S., & Smith, I. M. (1988). First report of a Canadian epidemiological study of autistic syndromes. *Journal of Child Psychology and Psychiatry, 29*, 433–445.

Buitelaar, J. K., van der Wees, M., Swaab-Barneveld, H., & van der Gaag, R. J. (1999). Verbal memory and Performance IQ predict theory of mind and emotion recognition ability in children with autistic spectrum disorders and psychiatric control children. *Journal of Child Psychology and Psychiatry, 40*, 869–881.

Bujas-Petkovic, Z. (1993). The three-dimensional modeling ability of a boy with autism [Letter to the editor]. *Journal of Autism and Developmental Disorders, 23*, 569–571.

Bushnell, I. W. R., Sai, F., & Mullin, J. T. (1989). Neonatal recognition of the mother's face. *British Journal of Developmental Psychology, 7*, 3–15.

Buxbaum, J. D., Silverman, J. M., Smith, C. J., Kilifarski, M., Reichert, J., Hollander, E., Lawlor, B. A., Fitzgerald, M., Greenberg, D. A., & Davis, K. L. (2001). Evidence for a susceptibility gene for autism on chromosome 2 and for genetic heterogeneity. *American Journal of Human Genetics, 68*, 1514–1520.

Campbell, M., Locascio, J., Choroco, M., & Spencer, E. K., Malone, R. P., Kafantaris, V., & Overall, J. E. (1990). Stereotypies and tardive dyskinesia: Abnormal movements in autistic children. *Psychopharmacology Bulletin, 26*(2), 260–266.

Cantor, D. S., Thatcher, R. W., Hrybyk, M., & Kaye, H. (1986). Computerized EEG analyses of autistic children. *Journal of Autism and Developmental Disorders, 16*, 169–188.

Cantwell, D. P., Baker, L., Rutter, M., & Mawhood, L. (1989). Infantile autism and developmental receptive dysphasia: A comparative follow-up into middle childhood. *Journal of Autism and Developmental Disorders, 19*, 19–31.

Capps, L., Kehres, J., & Sigman, M. (1998). Conversational abilities among children with autism and children with developmental delays. *Autism, 2*, 325–344.

Capps, L., Sigman, M., & Mundy, P. (1994). Attachment security in children with autism. *Development and Psychopathology, 6*, 249–261.

Carver, L., & Dawson, G. (2002). Evidence for an early impairment in neural systems for face recognition in autism. *Molecular Psychiatry*, 1: Supplement 2, 18–20.

Casey, B. J., Gordon, C. T., Mannheim, G. B., & Rumsey, J. M. (1993). Dysfunctional attention in autistic savants. *Journal of Clinical and Experimental Neuropsychology, 15*, 933–946.

Castelloe, P., & Dawson, G. (1993). Subclassification of children with autism and pervasive developmental disorder: A questionnaire based on Wing's subgrouping scheme. *Journal of Autism and Developmental Disorders, 23*, 229–241.

Celani, G., Battacchi, M. W., & Arcidiacono, L. (1999). The understanding of the emotional meaning of facial expressions in people with autism. *Journal of Autism and Developmental Disorders, 29*, 57–66.

Chakrabarti, S., & Fombonne, E. (2001). Pervasive developmental disorders in preschool children. *Journal of the American Medical Association, 285*, 3093–3099.

Charman, T. (1997). The relationship between joint attention and pretend play in autism. *Development and Psychopathology, 9*, 1–16.

Charman, T., Baron-Cohen, S., Swettenham, J., Baird, G., Cox, A., & Drew, A. (2001). Testing joint attention, imitation, and play as infancy precursors to language and theory of mind. *Cognitive Development,. 15*, 481–498.

Charman, T., & Swettenham, J. (2001). Repetitive behaviors and social-communicative impairments in autism: Implications for developmental theory and diagnosis. In J. A. Burack, T. Charman, N. Yirmiya, & P. R. Zelazo (Eds.), *The development of autism: Perspectives from theory and research* (pp. 325–345). Mahwah, NJ: Erlbaum.

Chung, S. Y., Luk, S. L., & Lee, P. W. H. (1990). A follow-up study of infantile autism in Hong Kong. *Journal of Autism and Developmental Disorders, 20*, 221–232.

Cialdella, P., & Mamelle, N. (1989). An epidemiological study of infantile autism in a French department (Rhone): A research note. *Journal of Child Psychology and Psychiatry, 30*, 165–175.

Ciesielski, K. T., & Harris, R. J. (1997). Factors related to performance failure on executive tasks in autism. *Child Neuropsychology, 3*, 1–12.

Courchesne, E., Press, G. A., & Yeung-Courchesne, R. (1993). Parietal lobe abnormalities detected with magnetic resonance in patients with infantile autism. *American Journal of Roentgenology, 160*, 387–393.

Courchesne, E., Townsend, J. P., Akshoomoff, N. A., Yeung-Courchesne, R., Press, G. A., Murakami, J. W., Lincoln, A. J., James, H. E., Saitoh, O., Egaas, B., Haas, R. H., & Schreibman, L. (1994). A new finding: Impairment in shifting attention in autistic and cerebellar patients. In H. Broman & J. Grafman (Eds.), *Atypical cognitive deficits in developmental disorders: Implications for brain function* (pp. 101–137). Hillsdale, NJ: Erlbaum.

Courchesne, E., Yeung-Courchesne, R., Press, G. A., Hesselink, J. R., & Jernigan, T. L. (1988). Hypoplasia of cerebellar vermal lobules VI and VII in autism. *New England Journal of Medicine, 318*, 1349–1354.

Curcio, F. (1978). Sensorimotor functioning and communication in mute autistic children. *Journal of Autism and Childhood Schizophrenia, 2*, 264–287.

Dales, L., Hammer, S. J., & Smith, N. J. (2001). Time trends in autism and in MMR immunization coverage in California. *Journal of the American Medical Association, 285*, 1183–1185.

Davidovitch, M., Glick, L., Holtzman, G., Tirosh, E., & Safir, M. P. (2000). Developmental regression in autism: Maternal perception. *Journal of Autism and Developmental Disorders, 30*, 113–119.

Davies, S., Bishop, D., Manstead, A. S. R., & Tantam, D. (1994). Face perception in children with autism and Asperger's syndrome. *Journal of Child Psychology and Psychiatry, 35*, 1033–1057.

Dawson, G. (1991). A psychobiological perspective on the early social-emotional development of children with autism. In D. Cicchetti & S. L. Toth (Eds.), *Rochester Symposium on Developmental Psychopathology* (Vol. 3, pp. 207–234). Rochester, NY: University of Rochester Press.

Dawson, G., & Adams, A. (1984). Imitation and social responsiveness in autistic children. *Journal of Abnormal Child Psychology, 12*, 209–225.

Dawson, G., Ashman, S., & Carver (2001). The role of early experience in shaping behavioral and brain development and its implications for social policy. *Development and Psychopathology, 12*, 695–712.

Dawson, G., Carver, L., Meltzoff, A., Panagiotides, H., McPartland, J., & Webb, S. (2002). Neural correlates of face recognition in young children with autism spectrum disorder, developmental delay, and typical development. *Child Development, 73*, 700–717.

Dawson, G., Hill, D., Spencer, A., Galpert, L., & Watson, L. (1990). Affective exchanges between young autistic children and their mothers. *Journal of Abnormal Child Psychology, 18*, 335–345.

Dawson, G., Klinger, L. G., Panagiotides, H., Lewy, A., & Castelloe, P. (1995). Subgroups of autistic children based on social behavior display distinct patterns of brain activity. *Journal of Abnormal Child Psychology, 23*, 569–583.

Dawson, G., Meltzoff, A. N., Osterling, J., & Rinaldi, J. (1998). Neuropsychological correlates of early symptoms of autism. *Child Development, 69*, 1276–1285.

Dawson, G., Meltzoff, A. N., Osterling, J., Rinaldi, J., & Brown, E. (1998). Children with autism fail to orient to naturally occurring social stimuli. *Journal of Autism and Developmental Disorders, 28*, 479–485.

Dawson, G., Munson, J., Estes, A., Osterling, J., McPartland, J., Toth, K., Carver, L., & Abbott, R. (2002). Neurocognitive function and joint attention ability in young children with autism spectrum disorder. *Child Development, 73*, 345–358.

Dawson, G., & Osterling, J. (1997). Early intervention in autism. In M. J. Guralnick (Ed.), *The effectiveness of early intervention* (pp. 307–326). Baltimore: Brookes.

Dawson, G., Warrenburg, S., & Fuller, P. (1982). Cerebral lateralization in individuals diagnosed as autistic in early childhood. *Brain and Language, 15*, 353–368.

Dawson, G., Warrenburg, S., & Fuller, P. (1983). Hemisphere functioning and motor imitation in autistic persons. *Brain and Cognition, 2*, 346–354.

Dawson, G., Webb, S., Schellenberg, G. D., Aylward, E., Richards, T., Dager, S., & Friedman, S. (2002). Defining the broader phenotype of autism: Genetic, brain, and behavioral perspectives. *Development and Psychopathology, 14*, 581–611.

Dawson, J., Matson, J., & Cherry, K. (1998). An analysis of maladaptive behaviors in persons with autism, PDD-NOS, and mental retardation. *Research in Developmental Disabilities, 19*, 439–448.

DeLong, G. R. (1992). Autism, amnesia, hippocampus, and learning. *Neuroscience Behavior Review, 16*, 63–70.

DeLong, G. R., & Dwyer, J. (1988). Correlation of family

history with specific autistic subgroups: Asperger's syndrome and bipolar affective disease. *Journal of Autism and Developmental Disorders*, *18*, 593–600.

DeMyer, M. K., Alpern, G., Barton, S., DeMyer, W. E., Churchill, D. W., Hingtgen, N. J., Bryson, C. Q., Pontius, W., & Kimberlin, C. (1972). Imitation in autistic, early schizophrenic, and nonpsychotic subnormal children. *Journal of Autism and Childhood Schizophrenia*, *2*, 264–287.

Dissanayake, C., & Crossley, S. A. (1996). Proximity and social behaviors in autism: Evidence for attachment. *Journal of Child Psychology and Psychiatry*, *37*, 149–156.

Dissanayake, C., & Sigman, M. (2001). Attachment and emotional responsiveness in children with autism. *International Review of Research in Mental Retardation*, *23*, 239–266.

Donnellan, A. M., Mirenda, P. L., Mesaros, R. A., & Fassbender, L. L. (1984). Analyzing the communicative functions of aberrant behavior. *Journal of the Association for Persons with Severe Handicaps*, *9*, 201–212.

Eales, M. J. (1993). Pragmatic impairments in adults with childhood diagnoses of autism or developmental receptive language disorder. *Journal of Autism and Developmental Disorders*, *23*, 593–617.

Egaas, B., Courchesne, E., & Saitoh, O. (1995). Reduced size of corpus callosum in autism. *Archives of Neurology*, *52*, 794–801.

Evans, D., Leckman, J., Carter, A., Reznick, S., Henshaw, D., King, R., & Pauls, D. (1997). Ritual, habit, and perfectionism: The prevalence and development of compulsive-like behavior in normal young children. *Child Development*, *68*, 58–68.

Fatemi, S. H., Stary, J. M., Halt, A. R., & Realmuto, G. M. (2001). Dysregulation of Reelin and Bcl-2 proteins in autistic cerebellum. *Journal of Autism and Developmental Disorders*, *31*, 529–535.

Field, T. M., Woodson, R., Greenberg, R., & Cohen, D. (1982). Discrimination and imitation of facial expressions by neonates. *Science*, *218*, 179–181.

Filipek, P. A. (1995). Quantitative magnetic resonance imaging in autism: The cerebellar vermis. *Current Opinions in Neurology*, *8*, 134–138.

Filipek, P. A., Accardo, P. J., Baranek, G. T., Cook, E. H., Dawson, G., Gordon, B., Gravel. J. S., Johnson, C. P., Kallen, R. J., Levy, S. E., Minshew, N. J., Prizant, B. M., Rapin, I., Rogers, S. J., Stone, W. L., Teplin, S., Tuchman, R. F., & Volkmar, F. R. (1999). The screening and diagnosis of autistic spectrum disorders. *Journal of Autism and Developmental Disorders*, *29*, 439–484.

Filipek, P. A., Richelme, C., Kennedy, D. N., Rademacher, J., Pitcher, D. A., Zidel, S., & Caviness, V. A. (1992). Morphometric analysis of the brain in developmental language disorders and autism. *Annals of Neurology*, *32*, 475.

Folstein, S. E., & Rutter, M. (1977). Infantile autism: A genetic study of 21 twin pairs. *Journal of Child Psychology and Psychiatry*, *18*, 297–321.

Folstein, S. E., Santangelo, S. L., Gilman, S. E., Piven, J., Landa, R., Lainhart, J., Hein, J., & Wzorek, M. (1999). Predictors of cognitive test patterns in autism families. *Journal of Child Psychology and Psychiatry*, *40*, 1117–1128.

Fombonne, E. (1999). The epidemiology of autism: A review. *Psychological Medicine*, *29*, 769–786.

Fombonne, E., Bolton, P., Prior, J., Jordan, H., & Rutter, M. (1997). A family study of autism: Cognitive patterns and levels in parents and siblings. *Journal of Child Psychology and Psychiatry*, *38*, 667–683.

Fombonne, E., du Mazaubrun, C., Cans, C., & Grandjean, H. (1997). Autism and associated medical disorders in a French epidemiological survey. *Journal of the American Academy of Child and Adolescent Psychiatry*, *36*, 1561–1569.

Frith, U. (1989). *Autism: Explaining the enigma*. Oxford: Blackwell.

Frith, U., & Happe, F. (1994). Autism: Beyond "theory of mind." *Cognition*, *50*, 115–132.

Garber, H. J., & Ritvo, E. R. (1992). Magnetic resonance imaging of the posterior fossa in autistic adults. *American Journal of Psychiatry*, *149*, 245–247.

Garreau, B., Barthelemy, C., Domenech, J., Sauvage, D., Num, J. P., Lelord, G., & Callaway, E. (1980). Disturbances in dopamine metabolism in autistic children: Results of clinical tests and urinary dosages of homovanillic acid (HVA). *Acta Psychiatrica Belgica*, *80*, 249–265.

Gilchrist, A., Green, J., Cox, A., Burton, D., Rutter, M., & Le Couteur, A. (2001). Development and current functioning in adolescents with Asperger syndrome: A comparative study. *Journal of Child Psychology and Psychiatry*, *42*, 227–240.

Gillberg, C. (1999). Neurodevelopmental processes and psychological functioning in autism. *Development and Psychopathology*, *11*, 567–587.

Gillberg, C., & Steffenburg, S. (1987). Outcome and prognostic factors in infantile autism and similar conditions: A population-based study of 46 cases followed through puberty. *Journal of Autism and Developmental Disorders*, *17*, 273–287.

Gillberg, C., Svennerholm, L., & Hamilton-Hellberg, C. (1983). Childhood psychosis and monoamine metabolites in spinal fluid. *Journal of Autism and Developmental Disorders*, *13*, 383–396.

Gillberg, C., & Wing, L. (1999). Autism: Not an extremely rare disorder. *Acta Psychiatrica Scandinavica*, *99*, 399–406.

Gomez, R. L., & Gerken, L. (1999). Artificial grammar learning by one-year-olds leads to specific and abstract knowledge. *Cognition*, *70*, 109–135.

Green, J., Gilchrist, A., Burton, D., & Cox, A. (2000). Social and psychiatric functioning in adolescents with Asperger syndrome compared with conduct disorder. *Journal of Autism and Developmental Disorders*, *30*, 279–293.

Green, W. H., Campbell, M., Hardesty, A. S., Grega, D. M., Padron-Gayol, M., Shell, J., & Erlenmeyer-Kimling, I. (1984). A comparison of schizophrenia and autistic children. *Journal of the American Academy of Child Psychiatry*, *23*, 399–409.

Gresham, F. M., & MacMillan, D. L. (1997a). Autistic recovery?: An analysis and critique of the empirical evidence on the early intervention project. *Behavioral Disorders*, *22*, 185–201.

Gresham, F. M., & MacMillan, D. L. (1997b). Denial and defensiveness in the place of fact and reason: Rejoinder to Smith and Lovaas. *Behavioral Disorders*, *20*, 219–230.

Griffith, E. M., Pennington, B. F., Wehner, E. A., & Rogers, S. J. (1999). Executive function in young children with autism. *Child Development*, *70*, 817–832.

Handleman, J., & Harris, S. (1994). The Douglass Developmental Disabilities Center. In S. Harris & J. Handleman (Eds.), *Preschool education programs for children with autism* (pp. 71–86). Austin, TX: Pro-Ed.

Hannan, T. (1987). A cross-sequential assessment of the occurrences of pointing in 3- to 12-month-old human infants. *Infant Behavior and Development*, *10*, 11–22.

Happe, F. G. (1994). Wechsler IQ profile and theory of mind in autism: A research note. *Journal of Child Psychology and Psychiatry, 35,* 1461–1471.

Happe, F. G. (1995). The role of age and verbal ability in the theory of mind task performance of subjects with autism. *Child Development, 66,* 843–855.

Happe, F. G. (1997). Central coherence and theory of mind in autism: Reading homographs in context. *British Journal of Developmental Psychology, 15,* 1–12.

Happe, F. G., Briskman, J., & Frith, U. (2001). Exploring the cognitive phenotype of autism: Weak "central coherence" in parents and siblings of children with autism: I. Experimental tests. *Journal of Child Psychology and Psychiatry, 42,* 299–308.

Hauk, M., Fein, D., Maltby, N., Waterhouse, L., & Feinstein, C. (1999). Memory for faces in children with autism. *Child Neuropsychology, 4,* 187–198.

Hobson, R. P. (1989). Beyond cognition: A theory of autism. In G. Dawson (Ed.), *Autism: Nature, diagnosis, and treatment* (pp. 22–48). New York: Guilford Press.

Hobson, R. P., & Lee, A. (1999). Imitation and identification in autism. *Journal of Child Psychology and Psychiatry, 40,* 649–659.

Hobson, R. P., Ouston, J., & Lee, A. (1988). Emotion recognition in autism: Coordinating faces and voices. *Psychological Medicine, 18,* 911–923.

Honda, W., Shimizu, Y., Misumi, K., Nimi, M., & Ohashi, Y. (1996). Cumulative incidence and prevalence of childhood autism in children in Japan. *British Journal of Psychiatry, 169,* 228–235.

Howlin, P. (2000). Outcome in adult life for more able individuals with autism or Asperger syndrome. *Autism, 4,* 63–83.

Howlin, P., Mawhood, L., & Rutter, M. (2000). Autism and developmental receptive language disorder: A follow-up comparison in early adult life. II. Social, behavioral, and psychiatric outcomes. *Journal of Child Psychology and Psychiatry, 41,* 561–578.

Hsu, M., Yeung-Courchesne, R., Courchesne, E., & Press, G. A. (1991). Absence of magnetic resonance imaging evidence of pontine abnormality in infantile autism. *Archives of Neurology, 48,* 1160–1163.

Hughes, C., Plumet, M., & Leboyer, M. (1999). Towards a cognitive phenotype for autism: Increased prevalence of executive dysfunction and superior spatial span amongst siblings of children with autism. *Journal of Child Psychology and Psychiatry, 40,* 705–718.

International Molecular Genetic Study of Autism Consortium. (1998). A full genome screen for autism with evidence for linkage to a region on chromosome 7q. *Human Molecular Genetics, 7,* 571–578.

Jones, M., & Szatmari, P. (1988). Stoppage rules and genetic studies of autism. *Journal of Autism and Developmental Disorders, 18,* 31–40.

Jorde, L., Hasstedt, S., Ritvo, E., Mason-Brothers, A., Freeman, B., Pingree, C., McMahon, W. B., Peterson, B, Jenson, W. R., & Moll, A. (1991). Complex segregation analysis of autism. *American Journal of Human Genetics, 49,* 932–938.

Kanner, L. (1943). Autistic disturbances of affective contact. *Nervous Child, 2,* 217–250.

Kasari, C., Sigman, M., Yirmiya, N., & Mundy, P. (1993). Affective development and communication in children with autism. In A. P. Kaiser & D. B. Gray (Eds.), *Enhancing children's communication: Research foundations for intervention* (pp. 201–222). Baltimore: Brookes.

Katsui, T., Okuda, M., Usuda, S., & Koizumi, T. (1986). Kinetics of ^{3}H-serotonin uptake by platelets in infantile autism and developmental language disorder (including five pairs of twins). *Journal of Autism and Developmental Disorders, 16,* 69–76.

Kim, J. A., Szatmari, P., Bryson, S. E., Streiner, D. L., & Wilson, F. J. (2000). The prevalence of anxiety and mood problems among children with autism and Asperger syndrome. *Autism, 4,* 117–132.

Kleiman, M. D., Neff, S., & Rosman, N. P. (1992). The brain in infantile autism: Are posterior fossa structures abnormal? *Neurology, 42,* 753–760.

Klin, A., Sparrow, S. S., de Bildt, A., Cicchetti, D. V., Cohen, D. J., & Volkmar, F. R. (1999). A normed study of face recognition in autism and related disorders. *Journal of Autism and Developmental Disorders, 29,* 499–508.

Klin, A., & Volkmar, F. R. (1997). Asperger's syndrome. In D. J. Cohen & F. R. Volkmar (Eds.), *Handbook of autism and pervasive developmental disorders* (2nd ed., pp. 94–122). New York: Wiley.

Klin, A., Volkmar, F. R., & Sparrow, S. (Eds.). (2000). *Asperger syndrome.* New York: Guilford Press.

Klinger, L. G., & Dawson, G. (1995). A fresh look at categorization abilities in persons with autism. In E. Schopler & G. Mesibov (Eds.), *Learning and cognition in autism* (pp. 119–136). New York: Plenum Press.

Klinger, L. G., & Dawson, G. (2001). Prototype formation in autism. *Development and Psychopathology, 13,* 111–124.

Klinger, L. G., Lee, J. M., Bush, D., Klinger, M. R., & Crump, S. E. (2001, April). *Implicit learning in autism: Artificial grammar learning.* Paper presented at the biennial meeting of the Society for Research in Child Development, Minneapolis, MN.

Klinger, L. G., & Renner, P. (2000). Performance-based measures in autism: Implications for diagnosis, early detection, and identification of cognitive profiles. *Journal of Clinical Child Psychology, 29,* 479–492.

Kobayashi, R., Murata, T., & Yoshinaga, K. (1992). A follow-up study of 201 children with autism in Kyushu and Yamaguchi areas, Japan. *Journal of Autism and Developmental Disorders, 22,* 395–411.

Koegel, L. K., & Koegel, R. L. (1995). Motivating communication in children with autism. In E. Schopler & G. Mesibov (Eds.), *Learning and cognition in autism* (pp. 73–87). New York: Plenum Press.

Koegel, R. L., Schreibman, L., O'Neill, R. E., & Burke, J. C. (1983). The personality and family-interaction characteristics of parents of autistic children. *Journal of Consulting and Clinical Psychology, 51,* 683–692.

Koenig, K., Tsatsanis, K. D., & Volkmar, F. R. (2001). Neurobiology and genetics of autism: A developmental perspective. In J. A. Burack, T. Charman, N. Yirmiya, & P. R. Zelazo (Eds.), *The development of autism: Perspectives from theory and research* (pp. 81–101). Mahwah, NJ: Erlbaum.

Kolvin, I. (1971). Psychoses in childhood: A comparative study. In M. Rutter (Ed.), *Infantile autism: Concepts, characteristics, and treatment* (pp. 7–26). Edinburgh: Churchill Livingstone.

Konstantareas, M. M., & Hewitt, T. (2001). Autistic disorder and schizophrenia: Diagnostic overlaps. *Journal of Autism and Developmental Disorders, 31,* 19–28.

Konstantareas, M. M., Homatidis, S., & Busch, J. (1989). Cognitive, communication, and social differences between autistic boys and girls. *Journal of Applied Developmental Psychology, 10,* 411–424.

Kurita, H. (1985). Infantile autism with speech loss before the age of thirty months. *Journal of the American Academy of Child Psychiatry, 24,* 191–196.

Lainhart, J. (1999). Psychiatric problems in individuals with autism, their parents and siblings. *International Review of Psychiatry, 11,* 278–298.

Landry, R., & Bryson, S. E. (1999, April). *Impaired disengagement and its relationship to self-regulatory behavior in young children with autism.* Paper presented at the biennial meeting of the Society for Research in Child Development, Albuquerque, NM.

Langdell, T. (1978). Recognition of faces: An approach to the study of autism. *Journal of Child Psychology and Psychiatry, 19,* 255–268.

Lauder, J. (1993). Neurotramsmitters as growth regulatory signals: Role of receptors and second messengers. *Trends in Neurosciences, 16,* 233–240.

Lebedinskaya, K. S., & Nikolskaya, O. S. (1993). Brief report: Analysis of autism and its treatment in modern Russian defectology. *Journal of Autism and Developmental Disorders, 23,* 675–679.

Leboyer, M., Bouvard, M. P., Recasens, C., Philippe, A., Guilloud-Bataille, M., Bondoux, D., Tabuteau, F., Dugas, M., Panksepp, J., & Launay, J. M. (1994). Differences between plasma N- and C-terminally directed beta-endorphin immunoreactivity in infantile autism. *American Journal of Psychiatry, 151,* 1797–1801.

Leboyer, M., Philippe, A., Bouvard, M., Guilloud-Bataille, M., Bondoux, D., Tabuteau, F., Feingold, J., Mouren-Simeoni, M., & Launay, J. (1999). Whole blood serotonin and plasma beta-endorphin in autistic probands and their first degree relatives. *Biological Psychiatry, 45,* 158–163.

Lee, A., Hobson, R. P., & Chiat, S. (1994). I, you, me, and autism: An experimental study. *Journal of Autism and Developmental Disorders, 24,* 155–176.

Leekam, S., & Moore, C. (2001). The development of attention and joint attention in children with autism. In J. A. Burack, T. Charman, N. Yirmiya, & P. R. Zelazo (Eds.), *The development of autism: Perspectives from theory and research* (pp. 105–129). Mahwah, NJ: Erlbaum.

Lewicki, P., & Hill, T. (1987). Unconscious processes as explanations of behavior in cognitive, personality, and social psychology. *Personality and Social Psychology Bulletin, 13,* 355–362.

Lieberman, M.D. (2000). Intuition: A social cognitive neuroscience approach. *Psychological Bulletin, 126,* 109–137.

Liu, A. (2001). Genomewide screen for autism susceptibility loci . *American Journal of Human Genetics, 69,* 327–340.

Lockyer, L., & Rutter, M. (1970). A five to fifteen year follow-up study of infantile psychosis: IV. Patterns of cognitive ability. *British Journal of Social and Clinical Psychology, 9,* 152–163.

Lord, C. (1995). Follow-up of two-year-olds referred for possible autism. *Journal of Child Psychology and Psychiatry, 36,* 1365–1382.

Lord, C. (1997). Diagnostic instruments in autism spectrum disorders. In D. J. Cohen & F. R. Volkmar (Eds.), *Handbook of autism and pervasive developmental disorders* (2nd ed., pp. 460–483). New York: Wiley.

Lord, C., Mulloy, C., Wendelboe, M., & Schopler, E. (1991). Pre- and perinatal factors in high-functioning females and males with autism. *Journal of Autism and Developmental Disorders, 21,* 197–209.

Lord, C., & Paul, R. (1997). Language and communication in autism. In D. J. Cohen & F. R. Volkmar (Eds.), *Handbook of autism and pervasive developmental disorders* (2nd ed., pp. 195–225). New York: Wiley.

Lord, C., Risi, S., Lambrecht, L., Cook, E. H., Leventhal, B. L., DiLavore, P. C., Pickles, A., & Rutter, M. (2000). The Autism Diagnostic Observation Schedule—Generic: A standard measure of social and communication deficits associated with the spectrum of autism. *Journal of Autism and Developmental Disorders, 30,* 205–223.

Lord, C., Rutter, M., & Le Couteur, A. (1994). Autism Diagnostic Interview—Revised: A revised version of a diagnostic interview for caregivers of individuals with possible pervasive developmental disorders. *Journal of Autism and Developmental Disorders, 24,* 659–685.

Lord, C., & Schopler, E. (1994). TEACCH services for preschool children. In S. Harris & J. Handleman (Eds.), *Preschool education programs for children with autism* (pp. 87–106). Austin, TX: Pro-Ed.

Lotter, V. (1966). Epidemiology of autistic conditions in young children: I. Prevalence. *Social Psychiatry, 1,* 124–137.

Lovaas, I. (1987). Behavioral treatment and normal educational and intellectual functioning in young autistic children. *Journal of Consulting and Clinical Psychology, 55,* 3–9.

Loveland, K. A., Tunali-Kotoski, B., Chen, Y. R., Ortegon, J., Pearson, D. A., Brelsford, K. A., & Gibbs, M. C. (1997). Emotion recognition in autism: Verbal and nonverbal information. *Development and Psychopathology, 9,* 579–593.

Loveland, K. A., Tunali-Kotoski, B., Pearson, D. A., Brelsford, K. A., Ortegon, J., & Chen, R. (1994). Imitation and expression of facial affect in autism. *Development and Psychopathology, 6,* 433–444.

Magnusson, P., & Saemundsen, E. (2001). Prevalence of autism in Iceland. *Journal of Autism and Developmental Disorders, 31*(2), 153–163.

Malhotra, S., & Gupta, N. (1999). Childhood disintegrative disorder. *Journal of Autism and Developmental Disorders, 29,* 491–498.

Marazziti, D., Muratori, F., Cesari, A., Masala, I., Baroni, S., Giannaccini, G., Dell'Osso, L., Cosenza, A., Pfanner, P., & Cassano, G. (2000). Increased density of the platelet serotonin transporter in autism. *Pharmacopsychiatry, 33,* 165–168.

Maurice, C. (1993). *Let me hear your voice: A family's triumph over autism.* New York: Fawcett Columbine.

Mawhood, L., Howlin, P., & Rutter, M. (2000). Autism and developmental receptive language disorder: A comparative follow-up in early adult life. I. Cognitive and language outcomes. *Journal of Child Psychology and Psychiatry, 41,* 547–559.

McAdoo, W. G., & DeMyer, M. K. (1978). Personality characteristics of parents. In M. Rutter & E. Schopler (Eds.), *Autism: A reappraisal of concepts and treatment* (pp. 251–267). New York: Plenum Press.

McBride, P., Anderson, G., Hertzig, M., Snow, M., Thompson, S., Khait, V., Shapiro, T., & Cohen, D. J. (1998). Effects of diagnosis, race, and puberty on platelet serotonin levels in autism and mental retardation. *Journal of the American Academy of Child and Adolescent Psychiatry, 37,* 767–776.

McClannahan, L., & Krantz, P. (1994). The Princeton Child Development Institute. In S. Harris & J. Handleman (Eds.), *Preschool education programs for children with autism* (pp. 107–126). Austin, TX: Pro-Ed.

McDonough, L., Stahmer, A., Schreibman, L., & Thompson, S. J. (1997). Deficits, delays, and distractions: An evaluation of symbolic play and memory in children with autism. *Development and Psychopathology, 9*, 17–41.

McEvoy, R. E., Rogers, S. J., & Pennington, B. F. (1993). Executive function and social communication deficits in young autistic children. *Journal of Child Psychology and Psychiatry, 34*, 563–578.

McGee, G., Daly, T., & Jacobs, H. A. (1994). The Walden preschool. In S. Harris & J. Handleman (Eds.), *Preschool education programs for children with autism* (pp. 127–152). Austin, TX: Pro-Ed.

McLennan, J. D., Lord, C., & Schopler, E. (1993). Sex differences in higher functioning people with autism. *Journal of Autism and Developmental Disorders, 23*, 217–227.

McPartland, J., Dawson, G., Carver, L., & Panagiotides, H. (2001a, November). *Neural correlates of face perception in individuals with autism spectrum disorder.* Poster presented at the International Meeting for Autism Research, San Diego, CA.

McPartland, J., Dawson, G., Carver, L., & Panagiotides, H. (2001b, April). *Neural correlates of face perception in autism.* Poster presented at the biennial meeting of the Society for Research in Child Development, Minneapolis, MN.

Meltzoff, A. N., & Gopnik, A. (1993). The role of imitation in understanding persons and developing a theory of mind. In S. Baron-Cohen, H. Tager-Flusberg, & D. J. Cohen (Eds.), *Understanding other minds: Perspectives from autism* (pp. 335–366). Oxford: Oxford University Press.

Meltzoff, A. N., & Moore, M. K. (1977). Imitation of facial and manual gestures by human neonates. *Science, 198*, 75–78.

Miller, J. N., & Ozonoff, S. (1997). Did Asperger's cases have Asperger disorder?: A research note. *Journal of Child Psychology and Psychiatry, 38*, 247–251.

Minderaa, R. B., Anderson, G. M., Volkmar, F. R., Akkerhuis, G. W., & Cohen, D. J. (1994). Noradrenergic and adrenergic functioning in autism. *Biological Psychiatry, 36*, 237–241.

Minshew, N. J. (1996). Brief report: Brain mechanisms in autism: Functional and structural abnormalities. *Journal of Autism and Developmental Disorders, 26*, 205–209.

Minshew, N. J., & Goldstein, G. (2001). The pattern of intact and impaired memory functions in autism. *Journal of Child Psychology and Psychiatry, 42*, 1083–1094.

Mottron, L., Burack, J. A., Stauder, J. E. A., & Robaey, P. (1999). Perceptual processing among high-functioning persons with autism. *Journal of Child Psychology and Psychiatry, 40*, 203–211.

Mottron, L., Morasse, K., & Belleville, S. (2001). A study of memory functioning in individuals with autism. *Journal of Child Psychology and Psychiatry, 42*, 253–260.

Mundy, P., & Sigman, M. (1989). The theoretical implications of joint-attention deficits in autism. *Development and Psychopathology, 1*, 173–183.

Mundy, P., Sigman, M., & Kasari, C. (1990). A longitudinal study of joint attention and language development in autistic children. *Journal of Autism and Developmental Disorders, 20*, 115–128.

Mundy, P., Sigman, M., & Kasari, C. (1993). The theory of mind and joint-attention deficits in autism. In S. Baron-Cohen, H. Tager-Flusberg, & D. J. Cohen (Eds.), *Understanding other minds: Perspectives from autism* (pp. 181–203). Oxford: Oxford University Press.

Mundy, P., Sigman, M., & Kasari, C. (1994). Joint attention, developmental level, and symptom presentation in autism. *Development and Psychopathology, 6*, 389–401.

Mundy, P., Sigman, M., Ungerer, J., & Sherman, T. (1986). Defining the social deficits of autism: The contribution of nonverbal communication measures. *Journal of Child Psychology and Psychiatry, 27*, 657–669.

Murphy, M., Bolton, P., Pickles, A., Fombonne, E., Piven, J., & Rutter, M. (2000). Personality traits of the relatives of autistic probands. *Psychological Medicine, 30*, 1411–1424.

Ornitz, E. M. (1989). Autism at the interface between sensory and information processing. In G. Dawson (Ed.), *Autism: Nature, diagnosis, and treatment* (pp. 174–207). New York: Guilford Press.

Osterling, J., & Dawson, G. (1994). Early recognition of children with autism: A study of first birthday home videotapes. *Journal of Autism and Developmental Disorders, 24*, 247–257.

Ozonoff, S. (1995). Executive function impairments in autism. In E. Schopler & G. Mesibov (Eds.), *Learning and cognition in autism* (pp. 199–220). New York: Plenum Press.

Ozonoff, S. (1997). Causal mechanisms of autism: Unifying perspectives from an information processing framework. In D. J. Cohen & F. R. Volkmar (Eds.), *Handbook of autism and pervasive developmental disorders* (2nd ed., pp. 868–879). New York: Wiley.

Ozonoff, S., Dawson, G., & McPartland, J. (2002). *A parent's guide to Asperger syndrome and high-functioning autism: How to meet the challenges and help your child thrive.* New York: Guilford Press.

Ozonoff, S., & Jensen, J. (1999). Brief report: Specific executive function profiles in three neurodevelopmental disorders. *Journal of Autism and Developmental Disorders, 29*, 171–177.

Ozonoff, S., & McEvoy, R. (1994). A longitudinal study of executive function and theory of mind development in autism. *Development and Psychopathology, 6*, 415–431.

Ozonoff, S., Pennington, B. F., & Rogers, S. J. (1991). Executive function deficits in high-functioning autistic individuals: Relationship to theory of mind. *Journal of Child Psychology and Psychiatry, 32*, 1081–1105.

Ozonoff, S., South, M., & Miller, J. N. (2000). DSM-IV-defined Asperger syndrome: Cognitive, behavioral and early history differentiation from high-functioning autism. *Autism, 4*, 29–46.

Panksepp, J. (1979). A neurochemical theory of autism. *Trends in Neurosciences, 2*, 174–177.

Panksepp, J., & Sahley, T. L. (1987). Possible brain opioid involvement in disrupted social intent and language development of autism. In E. Schopler & G. B. Mesibov (Eds.), *Neurobiological issues in autism* (pp. 357–372). New York: Plenum Press.

Pascualvaca, D. M., Fantie, B. D., Papageorgiou, M., & Mirsky, A. F. (1998). Attentional capacities in children with autism: Is there a general deficit in shifting focus? *Journal of Autism and Developmental Disorders, 28*, 467–478.

Patzold, L., Richdale, A., & Tonge, B. (1998). An investigation into the sleep characteristics of children with autism and Asperger's disorder. *Journal of Pediatrics and Child Health, 34*, 528–533.

Paul, R., Fischer, M. L., & Cohen, D. J. (1988). Brief report: Sentence comprehension strategies in children with autism and specific language disorders. *Journal of Autism and Developmental Disorders, 18*, 669–677.

Pennington, B. F., & Welsh, M. (1995). Neuropsychology and developmental psychopathology. In D. Cicchetti &

D. J. Cohen (Eds.), *Handbook of developmental psychopathology* (pp. 254–290). Cambridge, England: Cambridge University Press.

Philippe, A., Martinez, M., Guilloudbataille, M., Gillberg, C., Rastam, M., Sponheim, E., Coleman, M., Zappella, M., Aschauer, H., Vanmalldergerme, L., Penet, C., Feingold, J., Brice, A., & Leboyer, M. (1999). Genome-wide scan for autism susceptibility genes. *Human Molecular Genetics, 8*, 805–812.

Pickles, A., Bolton, P., Macdonald, H., Bailey, A., Le Couteur, A., Sim, L., & Rutter, M. (1995). Latent class analysis of recurrence risks for complex phenotypes with selection and measurement error: A twin and family history study of autism. *American Journal of Human Genetics, 57*, 717–726.

Pickles, A., Starr, E., Kazak, S., Bolton, P., Papanikolaou, K., Bailey, A., Goodman, R., & Rutter, M. (2000). Variable expression of the autism broader phenotype: Findings from extended pedigrees. *Journal of Child Psychology and Psychiatry, 41*, 491–502.

Pilowsky, T., Yirmiya, N., Shulman, C., & Dover, R. (1998). The Autism Diagnostic Schedule—Revised and the Childhood Autism Rating Scale: Differences between diagnostic systems and comparison between genders. *Journal of Autism and Developmental Disorders, 28*, 143–151.

Piven, J., Arndt, S., Bailey, J., & Andreasen, N. (1996). Regional brain enlargement in autism: A magnetic resonance imaging study. *Journal of the American Academy of Child and Adolescent Psychiatry, 35*, 530–536.

Piven, J., Arndt, S., Bailey, J., Havercamp, S., Andreasen, N. C., & Palmer, P. (1995). An MRI study of brain size in autism. *American Journal of Psychiatry, 152*, 1145–1149.

Piven, J., Bailey, J., Ransom, B. J., & Arndt, S. (1997). An MRI study of the corpus callosum in autism. *American Journal of Psychiatry, 154*, 1051–1056.

Piven, J., Bailey, J., Ransom, B. J., & Arndt, S. (1998). No difference in hippocampus volume detected on magnetic resonance imaging in autistic individuals. *Journal of Autism and Developmental Disorders, 28*, 105–110.

Piven, J., Berthier, M. L., Starkstein, S. E., Nehme, E., Pearlson, G., & Folstein, S. (1990). Magnetic resonance imaging evidence for a defect of cerebral cortical development in autism. *American Journal of Psychiatry, 147*, 734–739.

Piven, J., Harper, J., Palmer, P., & Arndt, S. (1996). Course of behavioral change in autism: A retrospective study of high-IQ adolescents and adults. *Journal of the American Academy of Child and Adolescent Psychiatry, 35*, 523–529.

Piven, J., Simon, J., Chase, G., Wzorek, M., Landa, R., Gayle, J., & Folstein, S. (1993). The etiology of autism: Pre-, peri-, and neonatal factors. *Journal of the American Academy of Child and Adolescent Psychiatry, 32*, 1256–1263.

Plaisted, K. C. (2001). Reduced generalization in autism: An alternative to weak central coherence. In J. A. Burack, T. Charman, N. Yirmiya, & P. R. Zelazo (Eds.), *The development of autism: Perspectives from theory and research* (pp. 149–169). Mahwah, NJ: Erlbaum.

Posner, M. I. (1980). Orienting of attention. *Quarterly Journal of Experimental Psychology, 32*, 3–25.

Powell, T. H., Hecimovic, A., & Christensen, L. (1992). Meeting the unique needs of families. In D. E. Berkell (Ed.), *Autism: Identification, education, and treatment* (pp. 187–224). Hillsdale, NJ: Erlbaum.

Prizant, B. M., & Rydell, P. J. (1984). An analysis of the functions of delayed echolalia in autistic children. *Journal of Speech and Hearing Research, 27*, 183–192.

Prizant, B., Schuler, A. L., Wetherby, A., & Rydell, P. (1997). Enhancing language and communication development: Language approaches. In D. J. Cohen & F. R. Volkmar (Eds.), *Handbook of autism and pervasive developmental disorders* (2nd ed., pp. 572–605). New York: Wiley.

Rapin, I. (1996). *Pre-school children with inadequate communication: Developmental language disorder, autism and low IQ* (Clinics in Developmental Medicine No. 139). London: MacKeith Press.

Reber, A. S. (1993). *Implicit learning and tacit knowledge: An essay on the cognitive unconscious*. New York: Oxford Unniversity Press.

Renner, P., Klinger, L. G., & Klinger, M. R. (2000). Implicit and explicit memory in autism: Is autism an amnesic disorder? *Journal of Autism and Developmental Disorders, 30*, 511–522.

Richdale, A. (1999). Sleep problems in autism: Prevalence, cause and intervention. *Developmental Medicine and Child Neurology, 41*, 60–66.

Richdale, A., & Prior, M. (1995). The sleep/wake rhythm in children with autism. *European Child and Adolescent Psychiatry, 4*, 175–186.

Riguet, C., Taylor, N., Benaroya, S., & Klein, L. (1981). Symbolic play in autistic, Down's, and normal children of equivalent mental age. *Journal of Autism and Developmental Disorders, 11*, 439–448.

Rimland, B. (1964). *Infantile autism: The syndrome and its implications for a neural theory of behavior*. New York: Appleton-Century-Crofts.

Risch, N., Spiker, D., Lotspeich, L., Nouri, N., Hinds, D., Hallmayer, J., Kalaydjieva, L., McCague, P., Dimiceli, S., Pitts, T., Nguyen, L., Yang, J., Harper, C., Thorpe, D., Vermeer, S., Young, H., Hebert, J., Lin, A., Ferguson, J., Chiotti, C., Wieseslater, S., Rogers, T., Salmon, B., Nicholas, P., Petersen, P.B., Pingree, C., McMahon, W., Wong, D. L., Cavallisforza, L. L., Kraemer, H. C., & Myers, R. M. (1999). A genomic screen of autism: Evidence for a multilocus etiology. *American Journal of Genetics, 65*, 493–507.

Ritvo, E. R., Freeman, B. J., Scheibel, A. B., Duong, T., Robinson, H., Guthrie, D., & Ritvo, A. (1986). Lower Purkinje cell counts in the cerebella of four autistic subjects: Initial findings of the UCLA–NSAC autopsy research report. *American Journal of Psychiatry, 143*, 862–866.

Robins, D. L., Fein, D., Barton, M. L., & Green, J. A. (2001). The Modified Checklist for Autism in Toddlers: An initial study investigating the early detection of autism and pervasive developmental disorders. *Journal of Autism and Developmental Disorders, 31*, 131–144.

Rogers, S. J. (1998a). An examination of the imitation deficit in autism. In J. Nadel & G. Butterworth (Eds.), *Imitation in infancy* (pp. 254–283). Cambridge, England: Cambridge University Press.

Rogers, S. J. (1998b). Neuropsychology of autism in young children and its implications for early intervention. *Mental Retardation and Developmental Disabilities Research Reviews, 4*, 104–112.

Rogers, S. J., & DiLalla, D. L. (1991). A comparative study of the effects of a developmentally based instructional model on young children with autism and young children with other disorders of behavior and development. *Topics in Early Childhood Special Education, 11*, 29–47.

Rogers, S. J., Ozonoff, S., & Maslin-Cole, C. (1993). Developmental aspects of attachment behavior in young children with pervasive developmental disorders. *Journal of the American Academy of Child and Adolescent Psychiatry*, *32*, 1274–1282.

Rogers, S. J., & Pennington, B. F. (1991). A theoretical approach to deficits in infantile autism. *Development and Psychopathology*, *3*, 137–162.

Rotman, A., Caplan, R., & Szekely, G. A. (1980). Platelet uptake of serotonin in psychotic children. *Psychopharmacology*, *67*, 245–248.

Ruffman, T., Garnham, W., & Rideout, P. (2001). Social understanding in autism: Eye gaze as a measure of core insights. *Journal of Child Psychology and Psychiatry*, *42*, 1083–1094.

Rutter, M. (1978). Diagnosis and definition. In M. Rutter & E. Schopler (Eds.), *Autism: A reappraisal of concepts and treatment* (pp. 1–25). New York: Plenum Press.

Rutter, M. (1999). The Emanuel Miller Memorial Lecture 1998. Autism: Two way interplay between research and clinical work. *Journal of Child Psychology and Psychiatry*, *40*, 169–188.

Rutter, M. (2000). Genetic studies of autism: From the 1970's into the millennium. *Journal of Abnormal Child Psychology*, *28*, 3–14.

Rutter, M., Macdonald, H., Le Couteur, A., Harrington, R., Bolton, P., & Bailey, A. (1990). Genetic factors in child psychiatric disorders: II. Empirical findings. *Journal of Child Psychology and Psychiatry*, *31*, 39–83.

Saffran, J. R., Aslin, R. N., & Newport, E. L. (1996). Statistical learning by 8-month-old infants. *Science*, *274*, 1926–1928.

Saffran, J. R., Newport, E. L., Aslin, R. N., Tunick, R. A., & Barrueco, S. (1997). Incidental language learning: Listening (and learning) out of the corner of your ear. *Psychological Science*, *8*, 101–105.

Saitoh, O., Courchesne, E., Egaas, B., Lincoln, A. J., & Schreibman, L. (1995). Cross-sectional area of the posterior hippocampus in autistic patients with cerebellar and corpus callosum abnormalities. *Neurology*, *45*, 317–324.

Sandman, C. A., Barron, J. L., Chicz-DeMet, A., & DeMet, E. M. (1990). Plasma β-endorphin levels in patients with self-injurious behavior and stereotypy. *American Journal on Mental Retardation*, *95*, 84–92.

Schopler, E., Andrews, C. E., & Strupp, K. (1979). Do autistic children come from upper middle-class parents? *Journal of Autism and Developmental Disorders*, *9*, 139–152.

Schopler, E., & Reichler, R. (1971). Parents as co-therapists in the treatment of psychotic children. *Journal of Autism and Childhood Schizophrenia*, *1*, 87–102.

Schopler, E., Reichler, R., De Vellis, R., & Daly, K. (1980). Toward objective classification of childhood autism: Childhood Autism Rating Scale (CARS). *Journal of Autism and Developmental Disorders*, *10*, 91–103.

Schreck, K., & Mulick, J. (2000). Parental report of sleep problems in children with autism. *Journal of Autism and Developmental Disorders*, *30*, 127–135.

Schuler, A., & Prizant, B. (1985). Echolalia. In E. Schopler & G. Mesibov (Eds.), *Communication problems in autism* (pp. 163–184). New York: Plenum Press.

Schultz, R. T., Gauthier, I., Klin, A., Fulbright, R., K., Anderson, A. W., Volkmar, F., Skudlarski, P., Lacaddie, C., Cohen, D. J., & Gore, J. C. (2000). Abnormal ventral temporal cortical activity during face discrimination among individuals with autism and asperger syndrome. *Archives of General Psychiatry*, *57*, 331–340.

Shields, J., Varley, R., Broks, P., & Simpson, A. (1996). Social cognition in developmental language disorders and high-level autism. *Developmental Medicine and Child Neurology*, *38*, 487–495.

Sicotte, C., & Stemberger, R. M. T. (1999). Do children with PDD-NOS have a theory of mind? *Journal of Autism and Developmental Disorders*, *29*, 225–233.

Siegel, B., & Hayer, C. (1999). *Detection of autism in the 2nd and 3rd year: The Pervasive Developmental Disorders Screening Test (PDDST)*. Paper presented at the biennial meeting of the Society for Research in Child Development, Albuquerque, NM.

Siegel, B., Pilner, C., Eschler, J., & Elliott, G. R. (1988). How children with autism are diagnosed: Difficulties in identification of children with multiple developmental delays. *Journal of Developmental and Behavioral Pediatrics*, *9*, 199–204.

Sigman, M., & Mundy, P. (1989). Social attachments in autistic children. *Journal of the American Academy of Child and Adolescent Psychiatry*, *28*, 74–81.

Sigman, M., & Ruskin, E. (1997). *Joint attention in relation to language acquisition and social skills in children with autism*. Paper presented at the biennial meeting of the Society for Research in Child Development, Washington, D.C.

Sigman, M., & Ungerer, J. A. (1984a). Attachment behaviors in autistic children. *Journal of Autism and Developmental Disorders*, *14*, 231–244.

Sigman, M., & Ungerer, J. A. (1984b). Cognitive and language skills in autistic, mentally retarded, and normal children. *Developmental Psychology*, *20*, 293–302.

Sodian, B., & Frith, U. (1992). Deception and sabotage in autistic, retarded and normal children. *Journal of Child Psychology and Psychiatry*, *33*, 591–605.

Smith, T., & Lovaas, O. I. (1997). The UCLA Young Autism Project: A reply to Gresham and MacMillan. *Behavioral Disorders*, *22*, 202–218.

South, M., Ozonoff, S., & McMahon, W. M. (2001, April). *Repetitive behavior and cognitive functioning in high-functioning autism and Asperger's syndrome*. Paper presented at the biennial meeting of the Society for Research in Child Development, Minneapolis, MN.

Sponheim, E., & Skjeldal, O. (1998). Autism and related disorders: Epidemiological findings in a Norwegian study using ICD-10 diagnostic criteria. *Journal of Autism and Developmental Disorders*, *28*, 217–227.

Steffenburg, S., & Gillberg, C. (1986). Autism and autistic-like conditions in Swedish rural and urban areas: A population study. *British Journal of Psychiatry*, *149*, 81–87.

Steffenburg, S., Gillberg, C., Hellgren, L., Andersson, L., Gillberg, I. C., Jakobsson, G., & Bohman, M. (1989). A twin study of autism in Denmark, Finland, Iceland, Norway, and Sweden. *Journal of Child Psychology and Psychiatry*, *30*, 405–416.

Stern, D. N. (1985). *The interpersonal world of the infant*. New York: Basic Books.

Stone, W. L., Coonrod, E. E., & Ousley, O. Y. (2000). Brief report: Screening Tool for Autism in Two-Year-Olds (STAT). Development and preliminary data. *Journal of Autism and Developmental Disorders*, *30*, 607–612.

Stone, W. L., Ousley, O. Y., & Littleford, C. D. (1997). Motor imitation in young children with autism: What's the object? *Journal of Abnormal Child Psychology*, *25*, 475–485.

Strain, P. S., & Cordisco, L. K. (1994). LEAP preschool. In S. Harris & J. Handleman (Eds.), *Preschool education programs for children with autism* (pp. 225–244). Austin, TX: Pro-Ed.

Strauss, M. S. (1979). Abstraction of prototypical information by adults and 10-month-old infants. *Journal of Experimental Psychology: Human Learning and Memory, 5,* 616–632.

Sugarman, S. (1984). The development of preverbal communication. In R. Schiefelbusch & J. Pickar (Eds.), *The acquisition of communicative competence* (pp. 23–67). Baltimore: University Park Press.

Sugiyama, T., & Abe, T. (1989). The prevalence of autism in Nagoya, Japan: A total population study. *Journal of Autism and Developmental Disorders, 19,* 87–96.

Sullivan, R. C. (1992). Parent essays: Rain Man and Joseph. In E. Schopler & G. Mesibov (Eds.), *High-functioning individuals with autism* (pp. 243–250). New York: Plenum Press.

Summers, J., & Craik, F. (1994). The effects of subject-performed tasks on the memory performance of verbal autistic children. *Journal of Autism and Developmental Disorders, 24,* 773–783.

Swettenham, J., Baron-Cohen, S., Charman, T., Cox, A., Baird, G., Drew, A., Rees, L., & Wheelwright, S. (1998). The frequency and distribution of spontaneous attention shifts between social and nonsocial stimuli in autistic, typically developing, and nonautistic developmentally delayed infants. *Journal of Child Psychology and Psychiatry, 39,* 747–753.

Szatmari, P. (1999). Heterogeneity and the genetics of autism. *Journal of Psychiatry and Neuroscience, 24,* 159–165.

Szatmari, P., Bartolucci, G., & Bremner, R. (1989). Asperger's syndrome and autism: Comparison of early history and outcome. *Developmental Medicine and Child Neurology, 31,* 709–720.

Szatmari, P., Bartolucci, G., Bremner, R., Bond, S., & Rich, S. (1989). A follow-up study of high-functioning autistic children. *Journal of Autism and Developmental Disorders, 19,* 213–225.

Szatmari, P., Jones, M., Fisman, S., Tuff, L., Bartolucci, G., Mahoney, W., & Bryson, S. (1995). Parents and collateral relatives of children with pervasive developmental disorders: A family history study. *American Journal of Medical Genetics, 60,* 282–289.

Szatmari, P., Jones, M. B., Tuff, L., Bartolucci, G., Fisman, S., & Mahoney, W. (1993). Lack of cognitive impairment in first-degree relatives of children with pervasive developmental disorders. *Journal of the American Academy of Child and Adolescent Psychiatry, 32,* 1264–1273.

Tager-Flusberg, H. (1989). A psycholinguistic perspective on language development in the autistic child. In G. Dawson (Ed.), *Autism: Nature, diagnosis, and treatment* (pp. 92–115). New York: Guilford Press.

Tager-Flusberg, H. (1993). What language reveals about the understanding of minds in children with autism. In S. Baron-Cohen, H. Tager-Flusberg, & D. J. Cohen (Eds.), *Understanding other minds: Perspectives from autism* (pp. 138–157). Oxford: Oxford University Press.

Tager-Flusberg, H. (1996). Current theory and research on language and communication in autism. *Journal of Autism and Developmental Disorders, 26,* 169–172.

Tager-Flusberg, H. (1999). A psychological approach to understanding the social and language impairments in autism. *International Review of Psychiatry, 11,* 325–334.

Tager-Flusberg, H. (2001). Understanding the language and communicative impairments in autism. *International Review of Research in Mental Retardation, 23,* 185–205.

Tantam, D. (1988). Annotation: Asperger's syndrome. *Journal of Child Psychology and Psychiatry, 29,* 245–255.

Tantam, D., Monaghan, L., Nicholson, J., & Stirling, J. (1989). Autistic children's ability to interpret faces: A research note. *Journal of Child Psychology and Psychiatry, 30,* 623–630.

Taylor, E. N., Miller, E., Farrington, C. P., Petropoulos, M. C., Favot-Mayoud, I., Li, J., & Waight, P. A. (1999). Autism and measles, mumps, and rubella vaccine: No epidemiological evidence for a causal association. *Lancet, 353,* 2026–2029.

Teunisse, J. & DeGelder, B. (1994). Do autistics have a generalized face processing deficit? *International Journal of Neuroscience, 77,* 1–10.

Tordjman, S., Anderson, G. McBride, A., Hertzig, M. E., Snow, M. E., Hall, L. M., Thompson, S., & Ferrari, P. (1997). Plasma β-endorphin, adrenocorticotropic hormone, and cortisol in autism. *Journal of Child Psychology and Psychiatry, 38,* 705–715.

Toth, K., Dawson, G., Munson, J., Abbott, R., Estes, A., & Osterling, J. (2001, April). *Defining the early social attention impairments in autism: Social orienting, joint attention, and responses to emotions.* Paper presented at the biennial meeting of the Society for Research in Child Development, Minneapolis, MN.

Towbin, K. E. (1997). Pervasive developmental disorder not otherwise specified. In D. J. Cohen & F. R. Volkmar (Eds.), *Handbook of autism and pervasive developmental disorders* (2nd ed., pp. 123–147). New York: Wiley.

Townsend, J., Courchesne, E., & Egaas, B. (1996). Slowed orienting of covert visual-spatial attention in autism: Specific deficits associated with cerebellar and parietal abnormality. *Development and Psychopathology, 8,* 563–584.

Townsend, J., Harris, N. S., Courchesne, E. (1996). Visual attention abnormalities in autism: Delayed orienting to location. *Journal of the International Neuropsychological Society, 2,* 541–550.

Tsai, L. (1987). Pre-, peri-, and neonatal factors in autism. In E. Schopler & G. Mesibov (Eds.), *Neurobiological issues in autism* (pp. 179–189). New York: Plenum Press.

Tuchman, R. F., & Rapin, I. (1997). Regression in pervasive developmental disorders: Seizures and epileptiform electroencephalogram correlates. *Pediatrics, 88,* 1211–1218.

Turner, M. (1999a). Annotation: Repetitive behavior in autism: A review of psychological research. *Journal of Child Psychology and Psychiatry, 40,* 839–849.

Turner, M. (1999b). Generating novel ideas: Fluency performance in high-functioning and learning disabled individuals with autism. *Journal of Child Psychology and Psychiatry, 40,* 189–201.

Ungerer, J. (1989). The early development of autistic children: Implications for defining primary deficits. In G. Dawson (Ed.), *Autism: Nature, diagnosis, and treatment* (pp. 75–91). New York: Guilford Press.

Ungerer, J., & Sigman, M. (1984). The relation of play and sensorimotor behavior to language in the second year. *Child Development, 55,* 1448–1455.

Van Acker, R. (1997). Rett's syndrome: A pervasive developmental disorder. In D. J. Cohen & F. R. Volkmar (Eds.), *Handbook of autism and pervasive developmental disorders* (2nd ed., pp. 60–93). New York: Wiley.

Venter, A., Lord, C., & Schopler, E. (1992). A follow-up study of high-functioning autistic children. *Journal of Child Psychology and Psychiatry, 33,* 489–507.

Volkmar, F. R. (1992). Childhood disintegrative disorder: Issues for DSM-IV. *Journal of Autism and Developmental Disorders*, *22*, 625–642.

Volkmar, F. R., & Anderson, G. M. (1989). Neurochemical perspectives on infantile autism. In G. Dawson (Ed.), *Autism: Nature, diagnosis, and treatment* (pp. 208–224). New York: Guilford Press.

Volkmar, F. R., & Cohen, D. J. (1991). Comorbid association of autism and schizophrenia. *American Journal of Psychiatry*, *148*, 1705–1707.

Volkmar, F. R., Cohen, D. J., & Paul, R. (1986). An evaluation of DSM-III criteria for infantile autism. *Journal of the American Academy of Child Psychiatry*, *25*, 190–197.

Volkmar, F. R., & Klin, A. (2001). Asperger's disorder or high-functioning autism: Same or different? *International Review of Research in Mental Retardation*, *23*, 83–110.

Volkmar, F. R., Klin, A., Marans, W., & Cohen, D. J. (1997). Childhood disintegrative disorder. In D. J. Cohen & F. R. Volkmar (Eds.), *Handbook of autism and pervasive developmental disorders* (2nd ed., pp. 47–59). New York: Wiley.

Volkmar, F. R., & Nelson, D. S. (1990). Seizure disorders in autism. *Journal of the American Academy of Child and Adolescent Psychiatry*, *29*, 127–129.

Volkmar, F. R., & Rutter, M. (1995). Childhood disintegrative disorder: Results of the DSM-IV autism field trial. *Journal of the American Academy of Child and Adolescent Psychiatry*, *34*, 1092–1095.

Volkmar, F. R., Shaffer, D., & First, M. (2000). PDDNOS in DSM-IV. *Journal of Autism and Developmental Disorders*, *30*, 74–75.

Volkmar, F. R., Szatmari, P., & Sparrow, S. S. (1993). Sex differences in pervasive developmental disorders. *Journal of Autism and Developmental Disorders*, *23*, 579–591.

Wakefield, A. J., Murch, S. H., Anthony, A., Linnell, J., Casson, D. M., Malik, M., Berelowitz, M., Dhillon, A. P., Thomson, M. A.,, Harvey, P., Valentine, A., Davies, S. E., & Walker-Smith, J. A. (1998). Ileal-lymphoid-nodular hyperplasia, non-specific colitis, and pervasive developmental disorder in children. *Lancet*, *351*, 637–641.

Walden, T., & Ogan, T. (1988). The development of social referencing. *Child Development*, *59*, 1230–1240.

Weeks, S. J., & Hobson, R. P. (1987). The salience of facial expression for autistic children. *Journal of Child Psychology and Psychiatry*, *28*, 137–152.

Wellman, H. M. (1993). Early understanding of mind: The normal case. In S. Baron-Cohen, H. Tager-Flusberg, & D. J. Cohen (Eds.), *Understanding other minds: Perspectives from autism* (pp. 10–39). Oxford: Oxford University Press.

Werner, E. B., & Munson, J. A. (2001). *Regression in autism: A description and validation of the phenomenon using a parent report and home video tapes.* Paper presented at the biennial meeting of the Society for Research in Child Development, Minneapolis, MN.

Williams, B. J., & Ozonoff, S. (2001, April). *Parental report of the early development of autistic children who experience a regression*. Paper presented at the biennial meeting of the Society for Research in Child Development, Minneapolis, MN.

Williams, B. J., Ozonoff, S., & Landa, R. (2001). *Parental report of the early development of autistic children who experience a regression*. Manuscript submitted for publication.

Wing, L. (1978). Social, behavioral, and cognitive characteristics: An epidemiological approach. In M. Rutter & E. Schopler (Eds.), *Autism: A reappraisal of concepts and treatment* (pp. 27–46). New York, Plenum Press.

Wing, L. (1988). The continuum of autistic characteristics. In E. Schopler & G. Mesibov (Eds.), *Diagnosis and assessment in autism* (pp. 91–110). New York: Plenum Press.

Wing, L., & Gould, J. (1979). Severe impairments of social interaction and associated abnormalities in children: Epidemiology and classification. *Journal of Autism and Developmental Disorders*, *9*, 11–29.

World Health Organization. (1992). *International classification of diseases* (10th rev.). Geneva: Author.

Yirmiya, N., Erel, O., Shaked, M., & Solomonica-Levi, D. (1998). Meta-analyses comparing theory of mind abilities in individuals with autism, individuals with mental retardation, and normally developing individuals. *Psychological Bulletin*, *124*, 283–307.

Yirmiya, N., Solomonica-Levi, D., Shulman, C., & Pilowsky, T. (1996). Theory of mind abilities in individuals with autism, Down syndrome, and mental retardation of unknown etiology: The role of age and intelligence. *Journal of Child Psychology and Psychiatry*, *37*, 1003–1014.

Young, J. G., Cohen, D. J., Kavanagh, M. E., Landis, H. D., Shaywitz, B. A., & Maas, J. W. (1981). Cerebrospinal fluid, plasma, and urinary MHPG in children. *Life Sciences*, *28*, 2837–2845.

Younger, B. (1985). The segregation of items into categories by ten-month-old infants. *Child Development*, *56*, 1574–1583.

CHAPTER TEN

Childhood-Onset Schizophrenia

Joan Rosenbaum Asarnow
Robert F. Asarnow

This chapter focuses on schizophrenia with childhood onset. Schizophrenia is a psychotic disorder, or group of disorders, characterized by the presence of one or more of a series of key symptoms: bizarre delusions, mood-incongruent hallucinations, thought disorder, grossly disorganized or catatonic behavior, and flat or grossly inappropriate affect during an active phase of the illness, as well as significant impairment and/or deterioration. Consider, for example, the following description of a young girl with schizophrenia.

> Mary had always been a very shy child. She would become mute at times, had severe difficulties making friends, was frequently oppositional, and had occasional enuresis. By the time she reached roughly 10 years of age, Mary showed academic difficulties in addition to continuing social isolation. She became depressed, felt that the devil was trying to make her do bad things, believed that her teacher was trying to hurt her, and became preoccupied with germs. Her behavior became increasingly disorganized; she talked of killing herself, appeared disheveled, and ran in front of a moving car in an apparent suicide attempt.
>
> This episode precipitated an inpatient psychiatric evaluation, during which Mary continued to show bizarre behavior. She lapsed into periods of intense anxiety and had one episode of uncontrolled animal-like screaming. At other times she would stare blankly into space and was frequently mute. Although Mary's functioning improved during hospitalization and she returned to her family, throughout her childhood and adolescent years she was tormented by fears, hallucinations, the belief that others were out to get her, and occasional bouts of depression often accompanied by suicide attempts. She continued to be socially isolated and withdrawn, and to perform poorly at school. At age 17 (after several brief inpatient hospitalizations), Mary was admitted to a state hospital, where she remained until the age of 19. During this period her affect was increasingly flat, and her psychotic symptoms persisted. One week after discharge from the hospital, Mary went into her room, locked the door, and overdosed on her medications. She was found dead the next morning.

This girl's story underscores several features of early-onset schizophrenia. First, schizophrenia does occur in children, although most cases of schizophrenia have their onsets in late adolescence or early adulthood. Second, children with schizophrenia frequently continue to struggle with schizophrenic symptoms during adolescence and adulthood. Third, because childhood is a period when crucial psychosocial competencies are developing, early-onset schizophrenia has a powerful impact on developing academic and social competence. Finally, Mary's battle with schizophrenia underscores the pain and morbidity associated with this illness.

This chapter reviews the literature on childhood-onset schizophrenia. It emphasizes research conducted after 1980, when the major diagnostic classification systems—the current version of which are the *International Classification of Diseases*, 10th revision (ICD-10; World Health Organization [WHO], 1993) and the *Diagnostic and Statistical Manual of Mental Disorders*, fourth editions (DSM-IV; American Psychiatric Association [APA], 1994)—endorsed the practice of using the same criteria to diagnose schizophrenia in children and adults. Prior to that time, the construct of childhood-onset schizophrenia was used to denote a relatively heterogeneous group of children with adult-type schizophrenia, autism, and other psychotic conditions. This not only made comparisons with the adult literature difficult, but complicated cross-study comparisons due to variations in the proportion of various subtypes of "children with schizophrenia" across studies. Several excellent reviews are available of the earlier literature (Beitchman, 1985; Cantor, 1988; Fish, 1977; Fish & Ritvo, 1978; McClellan & Werry, 1992; Prior & Werry, 1986; Rutter, 1972; Tanguay & Asarnow, 1985).

Renewed interest in childhood-onset schizophrenia has been stimulated by several factors. First, research suggesting that childhood-onset schizophrenia may be a more severe and familial variant of the disorder has stimulated the hope that etiological pathways for the disorder may be more clearly discernible in childhood-onset than in later-onset schizophrenia (Karatekin & Asarnow, 1999; R. F. Asarnow et al., in press; Jacobsen & Rapoport, 1998). Second, because of their youth, findings on children with schizophrenia are less likely to be confounded by such factors as neuroleptic treatment, institutionalization, and years of dysfunction. Third, the emergence of "developmental psychopathology" as a scientific discipline, in conjunction with the findings yielded by studies of children at risk for schizophrenia, has stimulated interest in such developmental questions as the impact of age of onset on the development of schizophrenia (R. F. Asarnow et al., 2001; Brennan & Walker, 2001; Marenco & Weinberger, 2000).

BRIEF HISTORICAL CONTEXT

As noted above, the 20th century has witnessed major changes in the criteria employed to diagnose schizophrenia in childhood. Two leading factors contributed to the changes in diagnostic criteria. First, in the 1930s child psychiatry began to emerge as a medical subspecialty. Early child psychiatrists, when confronted with the broad group of psychotic children who presented clinically, began to question whether these children were suffering from developmentally earlier manifestations of the adult form of schizophrenia. Second, this period was characterized by multiple shifts in the definition of schizophrenia, as the field addressed the still unresolved problem of defining the boundaries of schizophrenia (Kendler, McGuire, Gruenberg, O'Hare, et al., 1993).

Cases of childhood psychosis, in the absence of apparent organic brain disease, have been reported for at least 200 years (Walk, 1964). Contemporaneous with the description of various psychotic symptoms in adult psychiatry, descriptions of psychotic symptoms in children began to appear in the psychiatric literature. For example, describing what would later be called a functional psychosis in a child, Conolly (1861–1862) noted that

> the occasional existence of a disordered state of mental faculties in children, not depending on any temporary condition of an inflammatory kind, or on recognized chronic disease, and not on the result of accident, and more resembling mania than imbecility, does not seem to have been noticed even by medical practitioners until somewhat recently and certainly has not attracted particular attention. (p. 395)

Early in the 20th century, De Sanctis (1906) described a group of children presenting with an illness that he termed "dementia praecosissima" and likened to Kraepelin's "dementia praecox." Kraepelin (1919/1971) and Bleuler (1911/1950) observed that dementia praecox could begin during childhood. Furthermore, Kraepelin (1919/1971) noted that because of difficulties in identifying the point in time when the disease begins, it is likely that only the most severe cases of schizophrenia are identified in children.

Prior to the 1930s, schizophrenia was diagnosed in children via standards similar to those applied with adult patients (Fish & Ritvo, 1979). However, child psychiatrists began to see children with a broad range of conditions and varying levels of retardation. These conditions included mental retardation, organic brain syndromes, developmental disabilities, infantile autism, and childhood-onset forms of schizophrenia. Early child psychiatrists struggled with the question of how best to diagnose and classify this broad range of children. Recognition that schizophrenic symptoms might be expressed somewhat differently in children, in conjunction with efforts to classify the broad range of psychotic children, led to the emergence of the construct of "childhood schizophrenia" in American child psychiatry.

Thus, paralleling the numerous shifts in the concept of "schizophrenia" in adult psychiatry, the term "childhood schizophrenia" began to be used to describe a relatively heterogeneous group of children with profound early-onset impairments. Complicating matters further, operational definitions and specific diagnostic criteria were not generally used during the 1930s. Instead, samples were characterized via brief case descriptions or a list of major symptoms (see Fish & Ritvo, 1979).

The broad construct of "childhood schizophrenia" included children who today would receive DSM-IV diagnoses of autistic disorder, pervasive developmental disorder (PDD), schizophrenia, and psychotic disorder not otherwise specified (NOS). This contributed to considerable variability in the criteria that different clinicians used to define the category. Moreover, the breadth of the construct resulted in considerable heterogeneity among children grouped under the broad rubric of "childhood schizophrenia," and associated differences in the characteristics of so-called "childhood schizophrenics" studied in various clinical centers. To illustrate, Potter (1933) offered the following criteria for making a diagnosis of schizophrenia in a prepubertal child:

1. A generalized retraction of interest from the environment.
2. Dereistic[1] thinking, feeling and acting.
3. Disturbances of thought, manifest through blocking, symbolization, condensation, perseveration, incoherence and diminution sometimes to the extent of mutism.
4. Defect in emotional rapport.
5. Diminution, rigidity and distortion of affect.
6. Alterations of behavior with either an increase of motility leading to incessant activity, or a diminution of motility, leading to complete immobility or bizarre behavior with a tendency to perseveration or stereotypy. (p. 1254)

Compared to current DSM-IV criteria, Potter's criteria would probably include a broader group of children—including those with DSM-IV-defined schizophrenia, those with schizotypal personality disorder (SPD), and some children with PDD and autism. Interestingly, a 30-year follow-up of Potter's cases revealed that most of these children showed schizophrenia in adulthood, as defined in the early 1960s (Bennett & Kline, 1966).

In contrast, the nine criteria for "schizophrenic syndrome of childhood" proposed by a British working party (Creak, 1964) were more similar to the current criteria for autism and PDD. To complicate matters further, Kanner's descriptions of "early infantile autism" overlapped with other clinicians' descriptions of "childhood schizophrenia." Kanner (1949) concluded:

1. Early infantile autism is a well-defined syndrome, which an experienced observer has little difficulty in recognizing in the course of the first two years of the life of the patient.
2. The basic nature of its manifestations is so intimately related to the basic nature of childhood schizophrenia as to be indistinguishable from it, especially from the cases with insidious onset.
3. Early infantile autism may, therefore, be looked upon as the earliest possible manifestation of childhood schizophrenia. As such, because of the age at the time of the withdrawal, it presents a clinical picture which has certain characteristics of its own, both at the start and in the course of later development.
4. I do not believe that there is any likelihood that early infantile autism will at any future time have to be separated from the schizophrenias, as was the case with Heller's disease.
5. Nosologically, therefore, the great importance of the group which I have described as [having] early infantile autism lies in the correction of the impression that a comparatively normal period of adjustment must precede the development of schizophrenia. It also confirms the observation, made of late by many authors, that childhood schizophrenia is not so rare as was believed as recently as twenty years ago. (pp. 419–420)

In the late 1940s and 1950s, many disturbed children who were given a diagnosis of schizophrenia would be considered by current standards to show only questionable borderline or no psychotic symptoms. This contributed to even greater heterogeneity among children classified as having schizophrenia.

Bender's (1956) concept of schizophrenia, for example, included young children who were mute and retarded (whose symptoms would today be viewed as autistic), and children with complex speech problems similar to those described by Potter. Bender distinguished between two groups of schizophrenic children on the basis of age at onset: (1) a "pseudo-defective group," similar to Kanner's children with early infantile autism whose age at onset was under 2 years; and (2) schizophrenic children with later onsets, who were described as showing more neurotic, paranoid, and sociopathic symptoms. Many of the children in the second, later-onset group were followed into adulthood and showed schizophrenia as defined in that period (Fish & Ritvo, 1979, p. 269).

The DSM-II (APA, 1968) concept of "childhood schizophrenia" reflects the influences of Kanner and Bender:

> This category is for cases in which schizophrenic symptoms appear before puberty. The condition may be manifested by autistic, atypical, and withdrawn behavior; failure to develop identity separate from the mother's; and general unevenness, gross immaturity and inadequacy in development. These developmental defects may result in mental retardation, which should also be diagnosed. (This category is for use in the United States and does not appear in ICD-8. It is equivalent to "Schizophrenic reaction, childhood type" in DSM-I.) (p. 35)

Kolvin's classic studies of psychotic children (Kolvin, Ounsted, Humphrey, & McNay, 1971) contributed to a major shift in the conceptualization of schizophrenia in children. Kolvin et al. (1971) identified a group of children with "late-onset psychosis" (onset between 5 and 15 years of age) who, like adults with schizophrenia, were characterized by hallucinations, delusions, and formal thought disorder. Alternatively, children with "infantile psychosis" (onset prior to 3 years of age) showed autistic symptoms but not the characteristic schizophrenic symptoms seen in the late-onset group. These data were complemented by Rutter, Greenfeld, and Lockyer's (1967) finding that autistic children followed into adulthood did not show schizophrenic symptoms. Rutter (1972) concluded:

> Childhood schizophrenia has tended to be used as a generic term to include an astonishingly heterogeneous mixture of disorders with little in common other than their severity, chronicity, and occurrence in childhood. To add to the difficulty, the term has been employed in widely divergent ways by different psychiatrists. Some make the diagnosis very frequently; others do so quite rarely. A host of different syndromes have been included in the general category of "childhood schizophrenia"—infantile autism, the atypical child, symbiotic psychosis, dementia praecosissima, dementia infantilis, schizophrenic syndrome of childhood, pseudo-psychopathic schizophrenia, and latent schizophrenia to name but a few. In addition, a collection of eponyms have been attached to different conditions—Kanner, Mahler, and Heller, for example, all have syndromes named after them. The diagnostic situation can only be described as chaotic. Clinicians from different centers use the same term to mean different conditions and different terms to mean the same condition. We must conclude that the term "childhood schizophrenia" has outlived its usefulness. (p. 315)

DSM-III, DSM-III-R, and DSM-IV (as well as ICD-9 and ICD-10) represent a shift toward pre-1930s diagnostic practices. Schizophrenia in children is diagnosed according to the same criteria applied with adults, though allowances are made for minor differences in the manifestations of symptoms during childhood.

DESCRIPTION OF THE DISORDER

Whereas the definition of schizophrenia in DSM-III (APA, 1980) marked a sharp narrowing of the concept, there have been relatively few changes in diagnostic criteria from DSM-III to DSM-III-R (APA, 1987) and DSM-IV.

Core Symptoms

As shown in Table 10.1, the DSM-IV criteria for schizophrenia specify (1) the minimal duration of characteristic psychotic symptoms, with the requirement that such symptoms be present for a significant portion of the time during a 1-month period (or less if successfully treated); and (2) the core symptoms of schizophrenia—namely, characteristic delusions, hallucinations, formal thought disorder, grossly disorganized behavior, and negative symptoms (flat affect and anhedonia) (see Criterion A, Table 10.1). Some core symptoms—such as bizarre delusions and characteristic hallucinations consisting of a running commentary on the person's behavior or thoughts or two or more conversing voices—are sufficient by themselves to meet the active symptom criterion, as

TABLE 10.1. Summary of DSM-IV Criteria for Schizophrenia

A. *Characteristic symptoms:* Two or more of the symptoms listed below must be present for a significant portion of time during a 1-month period (or less if successfully treated): (1) delusions[a] (2) hallucinations[a] (3) disorganized speech (e.g., frequent derailment or incoherence) (4) grossly disorganized or catatonic behavior (5) negative symptoms, *i.e.*, affective flattening, alogia, or avolition B. Social/occupational dysfunction.	C. *Duration:* Continuous signs of disturbance for at least 6 months. D. Disorder not attributable to Mood Disorder or Schizoaffective Disorder. E. Disorder not due to substance use or general medical condition. F. If there is a history of Pervasive Developmental Disorder, an additional diagnosis of Schizophrenia is given only if prominent delusions or hallucinations are also present for at least a month (or less if successfully treated).

Note. Adapted from American Psychiatric Association (1994, pp. 285–286). Copyright 1994 by the American Psychiatric Association. Adapted by permission.

[a]Only one Criterion A symptom is required if delusions are bizarre or hallucinations consist of a running commentary on the person's behavior or thoughts, or two or more conversing voices.

noted in the table. The other Criterion A symptoms are weighted less heavily, and two or more of these symptoms are required to meet the active symptom criterion. DSM-IV criteria also require deterioration in functioning or failure to achieve the expected level of social development (Criterion B, Table 10.1). The boundaries between schizophrenia and mood disorders, schizoaffective disorder, organic disorders, substance use disorders, and autism are also specified (Criteria D, E, and F, Table 10.1); and the duration of disturbance, prodromal features, and residual features are defined. Results from several independent studies, all of which feature the use of operational diagnostic criteria to derive clinical diagnoses, provide compelling evidence that schizophrenia can be reliably diagnosed in children via the same criteria used with adults (for a review, see Werry, 1992).

Related Symptoms

Children with schizophrenia often present with a number of other symptoms and problems. Common symptoms reported among samples of children with schizophrenia include depression, oppositional behavior, conduct problems, and suicidal tendencies (see R. F. Asarnow et al., 2001; Russell, 1994; Russell, Bott, & Sammons, 1989).

In considering the data on related symptoms, however, it is important to note that childhood-onset schizophrenia typically presents with insidious as opposed to acute onset. Although some children experience acute onsets of schizophrenia, the majority of children appear to have been chronically impaired or to show insidious onset patterns (J. R. Asarnow & Ben-Meir, 1988; Fish, 1977; Gordon, Frazier, et al., 1994; Green et al., 1984; Hollis, 1995; Kolvin, 1971). This frequent combination of insidious onset and premorbid impairments complicates precise identification of the disorder's point of onset, as well as interpretation of "premorbid" or "comorbid" symptoms. How, for example, should one interpret the frequent presentation of symptoms of attention-deficit/hyperactivity disorder (ADHD) prior to and during schizophrenic episodes? Should the ADHD be viewed as a precursor state, an early manifestation of the schizophrenic illness, or a co-occurring condition? Future work is needed to address these issues.

DEFINITIONAL AND DIAGNOSTIC ISSUES

Developmental Issues

DSM-III, DSM-III-R, and DSM-IV employ comparable diagnostic criteria across age. This would appear to facilitate comparisons of child, adolescent, and adult onset cases, as well as analyses of continuities between childhood and adulthood. However, it is also possible that distinct developmental differences exist in the expression of the disorder. Indeed, current data suggest that hallucinations, delusions, and formal thought disorder are rare or difficult to diagnose prior to 7 years of age (for a review, see Caplan, 1994). The use of the same criteria across different ages may mask developmental trends. Furthermore, the use of criteria that are not adjusted to account for developmental trends is likely to result in the exclusion of some children who show early signs of the syndrome, but develop full-blown adult-type schizophrenia at a developmentally later stage (Fish, 1977, 1987).

Diagnosticians also confront age-specific problems in deriving diagnoses. For example, distinguishing between pathological symptoms such as delusions and imaginative fantasies typical during childhood can present diagnostic dilemmas. Because young children have more immature language and cognitive development, there are also frequent limitations in children's abilities to describe their experiences (for reviews, see Cantor, 1988; Edgell & Kolvin, 1972; Garralda, 1984a, 1984b; Russell et al., 1989).

The Boundaries of the Schizophrenia Spectrum

Further work is needed to clarify the boundaries of the schizophrenia spectrum in childhood. For example, research conducted by Rapoport and colleagues has highlighted the need to distinguish between children with schizophrenia and a subgroup of children with atypical psychosis, also labeled "multidimensionally impaired disorder" (Gordon, Frazier, et al., 1994; Jacobsen & Rapoport, 1998). These children meet DSM-IV criteria for psychotic disorder NOS, with symptoms including psychosis, poor affect regulation, and difficulty with attention and impulse control. Using clinical and test data, the authors distinguished children with multidimensionally impaired disorder from children with ADHD and schizophrenia, and concluded that the problems shown by the multidimensionally impaired group of children appeared to fall within the schizophrenia spectrum. However, these children had earlier cognitive and behavioral difficulties, and an earlier age of onset of psychotic symptoms, compared to the group with schizophrenia. Results of a 2- to 8-year follow-up study further revealed that half of these children later developed more specifically defined psychiatric disorders (schizoaffective, bipolar, and major depressive disorders), all involving mood episodes. The other half of the group was characterized by disruptive behavior disorders, with most being in remission from their psychotic symptoms. Based on this follow-up study, the authors concluded that we can distinguish children and adolescents with atypical psychotic disorders from children with schizophrenia, and that indeed this is a critical distinction. Psychotic symptoms in the multidimensionally impaired group appear to improve over time, though these children may go on to develop other serious difficulties. Chronic neuroleptic treatment may be inappropriate for children with these atypical psychoses (Jacobsen & Rapoport, 1998).

There is also a need to clarify the boundaries among schizophrenia, mood disorders, and schizoaffective disorder in youths. Results of existing studies highlight the limits of cross-sectional diagnoses and point to the importance of longitudinal diagnoses and careful patient monitoring over time in order to clarify this issue. Notably, based on results of their longitudinal study of children presenting with schizophrenia, Werry, McClellan, and colleagues (Werry, McClellan, & Chard, 1991; McClellan et al., 2001) have emphasized the difficulties in differentiating between youths who will continue to present with schizophrenia and those who will develop bipolar illness. The difficulties in differentiating between schizophrenia and mood disorders are further highlighted by the substantial subgroup of youths who initially present with schizophrenia and later show a more schizoaffective course (J. R. Asarnow, Tompson, & Goldstein, 1994; Eggers, 1989).

Finally, research on children presenting with schizotypal disorders highlights the similarities between children with schizophrenia and SPD (see J. R. Asarnow, Tompson, & Goldstein, 1994). Although it is clearly the case that not all of these children will develop full-blown schizophrenic syndromes, results of a follow-up of 12 youths presenting with DSM-III-defined schizotypal disorders revealed that continuing schizophrenia-spectrum disorders were the most common outcomes for these children, with 92%, 75%, and 80% of the sample meeting criteria for SPD, schizophrenia, or schizoaffective disorder during the first, second, and third years after initial assessment respectively. SPD was the most common follow-up diagnosis—67% in year 1, and 50% in years 2 and 3. One child developed full-blown schizophrenia during the third year of the follow-up, representing 10% of the sample. Schizoaffective disorder was diagnosed in 25% of the sample during years 1 and 2, and 20% of the sample in year 3. Over the course of the 3-year follow-up interval, 3 children presented with atypical bipolar disorder, representing 25% of the sample overall. This again underscores the overlap between the symptoms observed in bipolar disorder and syndromes considered to fall within the schizophrenia spectrum.

EPIDEMIOLOGY

Prevalence/Incidence

Most cases of schizophrenia have their onsets during late adolescence and early adulthood (Bleuler, 1911/1950; Kraepelin, 1919/1971; Riecher et al., 1991; Remschmidt, 1993; Weinberger, 1987). Schizophrenia is relatively rare in childhood and increases in frequency with adolescence (Beitchman, 1985; Burd & Kerbeshian, 1987; Remschmidt, 1993). The relative rarity of schizophrenia with childhood onset has resulted in limited epidemiological data on rates of schizophrenia in the general juvenile population. Results from a study conducted in North Dakota suggest a prevalence rate for DSM-III-defined schizophrenia of 0.19 per 10,000 children between 2 and 12 years of age (Burd & Kerbeshian, 1987), and Remschmidt, Schulz, Martin, Warnke, and Trott (1994) have suggested that roughly 1 child in 10,000 can be expected to develop schizophrenia. Because rates of a disorder may vary across communities with different characteristics (e.g., rural vs. urban, different ethnic makeups), these prevalence figures must be viewed as highly tentative until more representative data become available.

Sex Differences

Consistent with the adult literature documenting a predominance of males among early-onset cases, extant literature suggests an excess of males among childhood-onset cases, with current estimates suggesting male-to-female ratios in the range of 2:1 to 5:1 (Green, Padron-Gayol, Hardesty, & Bassiri, 1992; Hafner, Hambrecht, Loffler, Munk-Jorgenson, & Reichler-Rossier, 1998; Hollis, 1995; Kallman & Roth, 1956; Remschmidt et al., 1994; Russell et al., 1989; Volkmar, Cohen, Hoshino, Rende, & Rhea, 1988). The ratio of males to females appears to become more even in adolescence (Hollis, 1995; Remschmidt et al., 1994). It has been suggested that the excess of males in younger age groups may reflect a biological vulnerability in young males, similar to that seen in their higher rates of neurological disorders (Fish & Ritvo, 1979; Lewine, 1988). This apparent variation in the age-of-onset distributions for males and females could also reflect etiological differences across gender (e.g., greater vulnerability to viral infection in one gender).

Socioeconomic Factors

Epidemiological studies of adult schizophrenia have indicated an excess of schizophrenic cases among lower socioeconomic groups (Bromet & Fennig, 1999; Dohrenwend, Shrout, Link, & Skodol, 1987). It remains unclear, however, whether the association between schizophrenia and socioeconomic status is a consequence of the disorder, such that individuals suffering with the illness drift to lower socioeconomic levels because of the social dysfunction associated with the illness; or, alternatively, whether this association reflects causal factors. With respect to childhood-onset schizophrenia, results have been equivocal across studies. Extant studies have also employed clinic patients with associated referral biases, underscoring the need for further research to clarify this issue (for a review, see Werry, 1992).

Cultural Variations

Results from the WHO Collaborative Study on Determinants of Outcome of Severe Mental Disorders (Sartorius, Jablensky, Ernberg, Leff, & Gulbinat, 1987) indicate highly similar symptom profiles and incidence rates for schizophrenia across different countries and cultures. The WHO study employed carefully developed transculturally standardized diagnostic instruments and included individuals between 15 and 54 years of age. Thus, while some adolescents were included in this sample, the majority of the sample consisted of adults. Epidemiological studies with child and adolescent populations are needed to determine whether similar patterns will be detected among younger age groups. Another finding from the WHO study that merits examination with younger samples is the more favorable course and outcomes observed among patients in "developing" as opposed to "developed" countries (Leff et al., 1991; Sartorius et al., 1987). The more favorable outcome among individuals in developing countries was evident on measures of both clinical symptoms (e.g., remission, number of episodes) and measures of social functioning.

THEORETICAL FRAMEWORK

Most current etiological models of schizophrenia adopt a vulnerability–stress model. This framework has proven useful as a general guide to research, because it emphasizes the joint contribution of genetic predisposition and stressful life events to the development and recurrence of schizophrenia (see, e.g., Brennan & Walker, 2001; Cannon, 1998; Nuechterlein, 1987; Walker & Diforio, 1997; Zubin & Spring, 1977). These multifactorial models that emphasize interactions among biology, behavior, and environments have generally replaced the single-factor models that posited constitutional or environmental "causes" of schizophrenia. This shift toward multifactorial transactional models was stimulated by research underscoring the likely complexity and diversity of the etiological pathways to schizophrenia. For example, as shown in the vulnerability–stress model of childhood-onset schizophrenia presented in Figure 10.1, genetic risk factors are hypothesized to lead to central nervous system (CNS) dysfunction and impairments in attention and information processing. These individual characteristics are thought to interact with environmental stressors and protective factors to influence the likelihood that any individual will develop schizophrenia at various developmental stages.

As will be discussed in the sections on etiological factors that follow, however, the general vulnerability–stress model lacks specificity as to the indices of vulnerability or stress that are relevant to the disorder. Thus this model is generally offered as a heuristic device for integrating existing knowledge and organizing research, rather than as a formal hypothetico-deductive system. Three central constructs that are emphasized across various vulnerability–stress models are as follows:

"Vulnerability factors" refer to characteristics that predispose an individual to develop the disorder, and are assumed to be present in individuals at risk for the disorder and to constitute enduring characteristics of individuals who suffer from schizophrenic episodes. Both constitutional and environmental vulnerability factors have been posited, such as genetic factors, CNS damage resulting from obstetrical and birth complications, inadequate learning opportunities, and exposure to deviant family communication patterns. Some vulnerability factors may be specific to schizophrenia, whereas others may be associated with general risk for psychiatric disorder. To turn to Figure 10.1, whereas genetic loading for schizophrenia might represent a specific risk factor for schizophrenia, malnutrition might represent a nongenetic biological factor that might be associated with increased risk for psychiatric disorder in general.

"Stressors" are hypothesized to lead to an increased likelihood of a schizophrenic episode. Stressors may include major life events (e.g., death of a parent), as well as more chronic stressors, strains, and hassles. Major life change events that were acute at one point in time (e.g., death of a parent) may also become more chronic as time progresses (e.g., living in a home with a bereaved parent).

"Protective factors" refer to characteristics of the individual or environment that are associated with a reduced risk of an episode among individuals at risk. Possible protective factors that have been suggested in the literature include intelligence, social support, social competence, and healthy family communication (see J. R. Asarnow & Goldstein, 1986). Because one has to determine whether an individual is truly at risk before one can evaluate whether that individual has been protected from an illness, it is often difficult to identify protective factors. However, if one could identify a "true" and modifiable protective factor, this would have major implications for the development of primary and secondary prevention strategies.

Hypotheses concerning the ways in which vulnerability factors, stressors, and protective factors interact vary across models. Whereas some models postulate additive relationships in which posited factors are presumed to act relatively independently, transactional models emphasize person × environment interactions over time. Transactional models thus focus on the question of how genetically transmitted predispositions are expressed at various developmental stages and interact with caregiving environments to determine whether individuals develop schizophrenia as well as their levels of psychosocial functioning. (For more extensive discussion, see R. F. Asarnow, Asarnow, & Strandburg, 1989; J. R. Asarnow & Goldstein, 1986; Brennan & Walker, 2001; MacKain, Liberman, & Corrigan, 1994; Nuech-

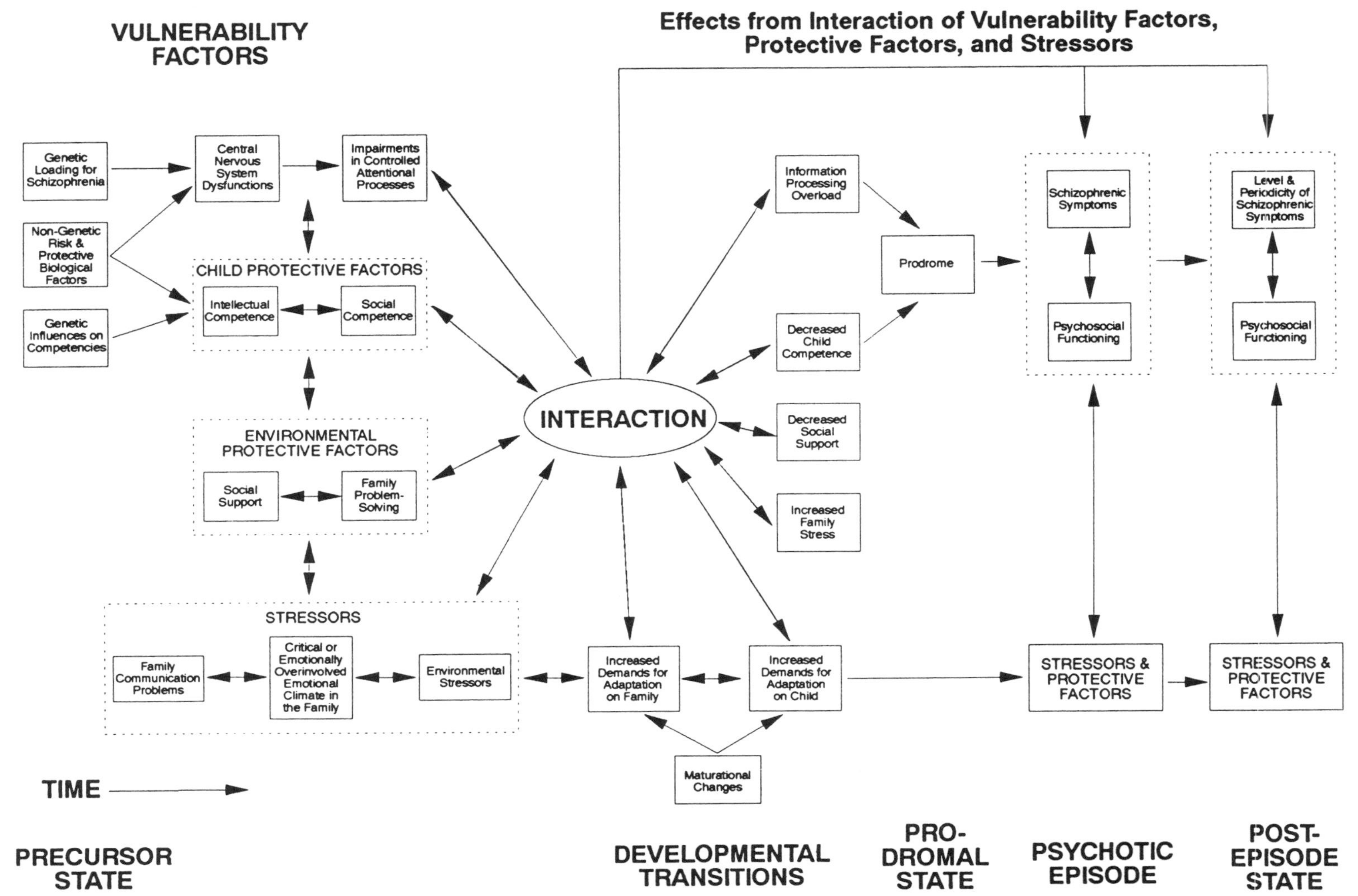

FIGURE 10.1. Vulnerability–stress model of childhood-onset schizophrenia.

terlein, 1987; Sameroff, 1990; Walker & Diforio, 1997).

Figure 10.1, which depicts a multifactorial vulnerability–stress model of childhood-onset schizophrenia (R. F. Asarnow et al., 1989), is an example of a transactional model. Variations in symptomatic behavior and psychosocial functioning are hypothesized to result from the interaction among enduring psychobiological vulnerabilities, environmental and biological stressors, and the moderating effects of individual competencies and individual and family coping responses. The model posits that a predisposition to schizophrenia is genetically transmitted. However, schizophrenic episodes are hypothesized to occur only among vulnerable individuals who are exposed to certain levels and types of stressors. Individuals with the greatest loading on vulnerability factors, the least effective coping responses and competencies, and the greatest exposure to stress are viewed as most likely to develop schizophrenic episodes and to have the most malignant outcomes. Alternatively, lower loadings on vulnerability factors, more effective coping responses and competencies, and lower levels of stress exposure are hypothesized to lead to more favorable outcomes.

Similar to other models proposed for adult schizophrenia (e.g., see Nuechterlein, 1987), the model presented in Figure 10.1 emphasizes developmental pathways by following a time line from left to right, beginning with genetic predisposition and progressing to precursor states, developmental transitions, prodromal states, psychotic episodes, and postpsychotic states. Schizophrenic episodes as well as postpsychotic states are conceptualized as including clinical symptoms and levels of social adaptation and school functioning.

Based on the existing literature, the model attempts to specify some hypotheses regarding personal vulnerability factors, significant stressors, and protective factors that may mitigate the effects of vulnerabilities and/or stressors. The literature with respect to these factors is reviewed next.

ETIOLOGIES

Despite the increased complexity of current theoretical frameworks and the major advances in our knowledge about schizophrenia, the causes of this illness (or set of illnesses) are still unknown. With respect to childhood-onset cases, efforts to understand etiology must further address the fact that children suffering from schizophrenia are clearly atypical among the larger group of schizophrenic patients by virtue of their early onset. Four major hypotheses have been offered to account for the atypical early onset among childhood cases:

1. Childhood-onset schizophrenia represents a particularly severe and chronic form of the illness, with the very early childhood onset reflecting a more severe biological disposition to the illness (Fish, 1977).
2. Childhood- and later-onset schizophrenia represent different illnesses.
3. The atypically early onset characteristic of childhood cases is associated with the presence of potentiating factors, such as severe psychosocial and/or biological stressors.
4. Childhood onset has no particular etiological significance; thus childhood-onset cases represent cases at the early end of the age-of-onset distribution, and early- and later-onset schizophrenia represent the same illness or illnesses with similar levels of clinical and etiological heterogeneity.

In the sections below, we review extant evidence with respect to major types of etiological factors in the context of these hypotheses regarding the significance of childhood onset.

Biological Factors

Increasing support for the view that schizophrenia is a primary brain disease has been stimulated by numerous studies documenting CNS dysfunction among persons with schizophrenia, as well as the dramatic improvements in outcome associated with neuroleptic medication (Weinberger, 1987). Two important facts, however, need to be addressed in any attempt to understand the nature of the CNS dysfunction in schizophrenia. First, there is no unitary brain lesion found in all patients with schizophrenia. Second, the brain lesions found in some of these patients are not unique or specific to schizophrenia "because other disorders that are associated with pathology in similar brain areas usually do not present as schizophrenia" (Weinberger, 1987, p. 661).

The Neurodevelopmental Model

In an elegant analysis, Weinberger (1987, p. 660) proposed a "neurodevelopmental model" of schizophrenia to account for the following three "inescapable clinical 'facts' about schizophrenia": (1) Most cases of schizophrenia have their onsets in late adolescence or early adulthood; (2) stress has been found to be associated with both onset and relapse; and (3) neuroleptic medications have dramatically improved outcome in many patients. As proposed by Weinberger, the neurodevelopmental model suggests that the neuropathology in schizophrenia involves a fixed brain lesion involving the limbic system and prefrontal cortex that occurs early in life, substantially prior to the onset of psychotic symptoms, and is "clinically silent" until a certain level of normal maturation is complete among the neural systems mediating the schizophrenic psychosis. The role of stress in precipitating clinical symptoms is proposed to be associated with normal maturational features of dopaminergic neural systems, specifically dopaminergic mechanisms involved in the activation of the prefrontal cortex. These mechanisms may constitute a key part of normal responses to stress. Consequently, the clinical decompensation often seen following stress among individuals with schizophrenia may reflect a breakdown in the normal physiological response to stress (Weinberger, 1987).

Despite the fact that childhood- and early-adolescent-onset schizophrenia is atypical by virtue of the early onset, several findings are consistent with aspects of Weinberger's neurodevelopmental model. First, the view that schizophrenia is a neurodevelopmental disorder associated with early-occurring neural pathology derives some support from accumulating data demonstrating that children with schizophrenia tend to manifest neurobehavioral, behavioral, and social impairments well in advance of the first onset of psychotic symptoms. For example, retrospective studies of children with schizophrenia have revealed a number of impairments in premorbid functioning (Schaeffer & Ross, 2002). Based on a retrospective review of prior records for youths with schizophrenia, Watkins, Asarnow, and Tanguay (1988) reported that during infancy and early childhood, their language acquisition is slow (particularly for expressive language) and their gross motor functioning is impaired. Somewhat later there are impairments in fine motor coordination. These findings are consistent with Hollis's (1995) report that the premorbid histories of children with schizophrenia were characterized by specific impairments of language production and comprehension, as well as motor impairments. These neurobehavioral impairments may be early manifestations of the brain lesions posited by neurodevelopmental models. As noted above, in Weinberger's neurodevelopmental model, hypothesized brain lesions are thought to be "clinically silent" at early developmental stages. Results from studies of schizophrenic children, as well as studies of children at risk for schizophrenia, suggest that the lesions may be "silent" only in the sense that they do not immediately produce active psychotic symptoms (for reviews, see R. F. Asarnow, Brown, & Strandburg, 1995; Watkins et al., 1988; J. R. Asarnow, 1988). It is worth noting that expressive language and motor skills are subserved by structures in the frontal lobes. It is in these areas that many of the early brain lesions are also found (Weinberger, 1987).

Difficulties with social behavior have also been noted in the early childhood histories of children who developed schizophrenia. Notably, Watkins et al. (1988) found that these children were characterized as showing a lack of social responsiveness during infancy, and problems with extreme mood lability, inappropriate clinging, and unexplained rage reactions during early childhood. J. R. Asarnow et al. (1994) found that children with schizophrenia were characterized by lower levels of premorbid adjustment than were a comparison group of children with major depression. Children with schizophrenia showed particularly poor levels of premorbid functioning in the areas of peer relationships, scholastic performance, school adaptation, and interests. Similarly, Hollis (1995) found that when compared to nonpsychotic psychiatric controls, children with schizophrenia showed more premorbid social impairments.

The Dopamine Hypothesis

The hypothesis that dopamine is involved in the pathogenesis of schizophrenia in adults is supported by several sources of evidence (see Carlsson, 1987; Sawa & Snyder, 2002). Most notably, the efficacy of phenothiazines and related drugs in controlling psychotic symptoms is correlated with the extent to which they block dopaminergic transmission. Alternatively, drugs such as amphetamine or L-DOPA that produce excessive release of dopamine have been found to be associated with the intensification of psychotic disorders. As Carlsson (1987) points out, however, it may "be more appropriate to speak of a dopamine hypothesis of psychosis" (p. 223) as opposed to schizophrenia, because these drugs appear to affect psychotic conditions other than schizophrenia, and some patients with schizophrenia show a poor response to pharmacological treatment.

Advances in basic knowledge regarding dopaminergic systems have underscored the complexity of dopaminergic mechanisms and suggested multiple alternative hypotheses concerning the nature of the dysfunction in schizophrenia. For example, problems could arise due to dopaminergic hyperfunction, an imbalance between dopaminergic systems and other systems, or a variety of subtle dopaminergic dysfunctions (Carlsson, 1987). Dopaminergic neurons, however, "play a crucial role in the modulation of mental, motor, endocrine, and autonomic functions and appear to be involved in the functional integration of recent cortical with older subcortical functions" (Carlsson, 1987, p. 233). More recent neurochemical hypotheses have emphasized the cortical amino acid neurotransmitter systems, such as GABA and glutamate (see Weinberger, 1997).

The Evidence on Biological Factors

In this section we review family studies, genetic factors, brain pathology, and neurocognition in childhood-onset schizophrenia.

Family Studies and Genetic Factors

There is strong evidence for an aggregation of schizophrenia and SPD, and limited or mixed evidence for the aggregation of paranoid, schizoid, and avoidant personality disorders (Kendler & Diehl, 1993; Kendler, 1997; Levinson & Mowry, 1991), in first-degree relatives of patients with adult-onset schizophrenia. Twin and adoption studies suggest that genetic factors are important in the etiology of schizophrenia (Kendler & Diehl, 1993). Some early data suggested a twofold increase in the aggregation of schizophrenic disorders among the first-degree relatives of children with schizophrenia, as compared to adults with schizophrenia (Fish, 1977; Kallman & Roth, 1956; Kolvin, 1971). It should be noted, however, that these early studies did not include modern features, such as "blind" assessments of relatives (which minimize the risk of biased diagnoses arising from knowledge of a proband's diagnostic status), control groups, structured diagnostic assessments, and operational diagnostic criteria. Consequently, results from early studies require confirmation in research using more stringent experimental procedures.

Modern family study methods, including the features cited above, were employed in a recent study of the first-degree relatives of probands with childhood-onset schizophrenia. The UCLA Family Study (R. F. Asarnow et al., 2001) tested the hypothesis that childhood-onset schizophrenia is a variant of adult-onset schizophrenia by determining whether first-degree relatives of probands with childhood-onset schizophrenia, like first-degree relatives of probands with adult-onset schizophrenia, have an increased risk for schizophrenia, SPD, and paranoid personality disorder. The aggregation of schizophrenia and schizophrenia-spectrum personality disorders in the first-degree relatives of probands with childhood-onset schizophrenia (n = 148) was compared to that in the first-degree relatives of probands with ADHD (n = 368) and community control (n = 206) probands; structured diagnostic interviews were used to make DSM-III-R diagnoses. Diagnoses of relatives were made by investigators who were unaware of proband diagnoses. A diagnostic hierarchy developed by Kendler, McGuire, Gruenberg, O'Hare, et al. (1993) was employed to permit comparison of the results of this study to modern family studies of probands with adult-onset schizophrenia.

Table 10.2 presents the lifetime morbid risk (a statistic that takes into account how much of the period of risk an individual has lived through) for schizophrenia-spectrum disorders and three other personality disorders in the parents and siblings of the three proband groups. There was an increased lifetime morbid risk for schizophrenia and SPD in parents of probands with childhood-onset schizophrenia, compared with parents of probands with ADHD and community control probands. The parents of probands with childhood-onset schizophrenia who were diagnosed as having schizophrenia themselves had an early age of first onset of schizophrenia (20.8 years). Risk for avoidant personality disorder was also increased in the parents of probands with childhood-onset schizophrenia, compared with parents of community controls. The psychiatric disorders that do and do not aggregate in the parents of probands with childhood-onset schizophrenia are remarkably similar to the disorders that do and do not aggregate in parents of probands with adult-onset schizophrenia in modern family studies. This provides strong evidence for

TABLE 10.2. Morbid Risk for Schizophrenia-Spectrum Disorders and Three Other Personality Disorders as Determined by Life-Table Analysis, in Parents and Siblings of Three Groups of Child Probands

	Parents						Siblings					
	Proband diagnosis			Log-rank tests between pairs of groups			Proband diagnosis			Log-rank tests between pairs of groups		
	Community control (n = 122)	ADHD (n = 223)	Schiz. (n = 102)	Schiz. vs. CC	Schiz. vs. ADHD	ADHD vs. CC	Community control (n = 84)	ADHD (n = 145)	Schiz. (n = 46)	Schiz. vs. CC	Schiz. vs. ADHD	ADHD vs. CC
1. Schizophrenia	0%	0.45% (± .45)	4.95% (± 2.16)	$\chi^2 = 6.15^a$	$\chi^2 = 7.68^a$	$\chi^2 = 0.54$	0%	0%	0%	—	—	—
2. Schizoaffective (depressed)	0%	0%	1.04% (± 1.04)	$\chi^2 = 1.27$	$\chi^2 = 2.31$	—	0%	0%	3.45% (± 3.39)	$\chi^2 = 0.62$	$\chi^2 = 1.10$	—
3. Schizotypal personality disorder	0%	0.9% (± 0.63)	4.21% (± 2.06)	$\chi^2 = 5.21^a$	$\chi^2 = 3.91^a$	$\chi^2 = 1.1$	5.88% (± 5.71)	6.82% (± 4.51)	9.01% (± 6.47)	$\chi^2 = 0.14$	$\chi^2 = .001$	$\chi^2 = 0.28$
4. Schizophreniform and atypical psychosis	0%	0.93% (± 0.66)	0%	—	$\chi^2 = 0.83$	$\chi^2 = 1.13$	0%	0%	0%	—	—	—
5. Paranoid personality disorder	0.82% (± 0.82)	3.21% (± 0.19)	4.4% (± 2.15)	$\chi^2 = 2.89$	$\chi^2 = 0.26$	$\chi^2 = 1.94$	0%	0%	13.33% (± 8.78)	$\chi^2 = 1.53$	$\chi^2 = 1.93$	—
Narrow spectrum = Σ 1–5[d]	0.82% (± 0.82)	5.4% (± 1.52)	13.86% (± 3.44)	$\chi^2 = 14.96^c$	$\chi^2 = 6.76^b$	$\chi^2 = 4.52^a$	5.88% (± 5.71)	6.82% (± 4.51)	23.79% (± 9.79)	$\chi^2 = 1.64$	$\chi^2 = 1.06$	$\chi^2 = 0.28$
Avoidant personality disorder	1.67% (± 1.17)	4.76% (± 1.47)	9.41% (± 3.17)	$\chi^2 = 6.40^a$	$\chi^2 = 2.23$	$\chi^2 = 2.08$	3.45% (± 3.39)	8.52% (± 5.07)	13.16% (± 8.90)	$\chi^2 = 0.22$	$\chi^2 = 0.08$	$\chi^2 = 0.29$
Schizoid personality disorder	0.83% (± 0.82)	0.47% (± 0.47)	2.3% (± 1.61)	$\chi^2 = 0.76$	$\chi^2 = 2.05$	$\chi^2 = 0.16$	0%	0%	7.69% (± 7.39)	$\chi^2 = 0.84$	$\chi^2 = 1.08$	—
Borderline personality disorder	1.69% (± 1.19)	2.0% (± 0.99)	2.60% (± 1.81)	$\chi^2 = 0.18$	$\chi^2 = 0.09$	$\chi^2 = 0.03$	0%	9.52% (± 6.41)	13.22% (± 9.21)	$\chi^2 = 1.71$	$\chi^2 = 0.05$	$\chi^2 = 1.37$

Note. Includes subjects directly interviewed and subjects diagnosed via family history. Numbers in parentheses are .95 confidence interval. From R. F. Asarnow et al. (2001, pp. 584–585). Copyright 2001 by the American Medical Association. Reprinted by permission.

[a] $p < .05$.

[b] $p < .01$

[c] $p < .001$.

[d] Narrow spectrum includes schizophrenia, schizoaffective disorder (depressed), schizotypal and paranoid personality disorder, and schizophreniform and atypical psychosis.

the continuity of childhood-onset and adult-onset schizophrenia.

The relative risk (ratio of risk for relatives of probands with childhood-onset schizophrenia vs. relatives of community control probands) for schizophrenia in the parents of probands with childhood-onset schizophrenia is 17. Relative risk is less sensitive to variations in diagnostic procedures and criteria than raw prevalence rates are. This is considerably greater than the six- and threefold relative risk for schizophrenia observed in parents in studies of "classic" and second-generation adult-onset schizophrenia. The three- to sixfold increase in the aggregation of schizophrenia in parents of probands with childhood-onset schizophrenia compared to published rates in parents of probands with adult-onset schizophrenia suggests that childhood-onset schizophrenia may be a more familial, possibly more genetic, form of schizophrenia than adult-onset schizophrenia. Parallel results are reported for a number of genetically transmitted disorders where early onset of disorder is associated with a heavy genetic loading for the disease. These findings are consistent with Rosenthal's (1970) suggestion that preadolescent schizophrenia may represent a more virulent form of adult schizophrenia with virtually complete penetrance.

A non-"blind" study of first-degree relatives conducted at the Child Psychiatry Branch of the National Institute of Mental Health (NIMH) (Lenane, Nicolson, Bedwell, & Rapoport, 1999) also found what appeared to be high rates of schizophrenia-spectrum disorders in relatives of probands with childhood-onset schizophrenia. The rates of schizophrenia-spectrum disorders in 126 first-degree relatives of 45 patients with childhood-onset schizophrenia were examined via structured diagnostic interviews. Using the same diagnostic hierarchy developed by Kendler's group that was used in the UCLA study, the investigators obtained the following rates: schizophrenia (3%), schizoaffective disorder (1%), either SPD or paranoid personality disorder (24%), and schizoid or avoidant personality disorder (7%). Forty-two percent of the 45 probands had at least one relative with a schizophrenia-spectrum diagnosis.

In addition to schizophrenia-spectrum disorders, certain personality traits have been hypothesized to reflect genetic liability to schizophrenia. The UCLA Family Study (Subotnik et al., 2002) examined Minnesota Multiphasic Personality Inventory (MMPI) scores for 50 parents of probands with childhood-onset schizophrenia, 153 parents of probands with ADHD, and 168 parents of community comparison probands. Only valid profiles of nonpsychotic biological parents were examined. The mean scores for the standard MMPI scales were in the nonpathological range for all three groups of parents. However, parents of schizophrenia probands were significantly higher on scale *Sc* than parents of community comparison children. The *Sc* scale was developed to identify patients diagnosed with schizophrenia. It includes items tapping psychotic symptoms, social alienation, sexual concerns, difficulties with impulse control and concentration, and a variety of fears and dissatisfactions. Mothers of probands with schizophrenia and probands with ADHD shared some "neurotic" personality characteristics. Twin studies with a nonclinical sample have shown scale *Sc* to have moderately high heritability; adoption studies have shown that this scale taps personality traits associated with a genetic predisposition to schizophrenia; and high-risk studies have shown that this scale can distinguish individuals with a genetic predisposition to schizophrenia from controls.

Certain neurocognitive impairments have been hypothesized to index genetic liability for schizophrenia. This hypothesis was tested (R. F. Asarnow et al., in press) by comparing parents of probands with childhood-onset schizophrenia (n = 79) to parents of probands with ADHD (n = 190) and parents of control children (n = 115) on three neurocognitive tasks shown in prior research to detect impairments in patients with adult-onset schizophrenia and with ADHD, as well as in relatives of patients with adult-onset schizophrenia. Parents were excluded from the study if they had diagnoses of psychosis. On both the Degraded Stimulus Continuous Performance Test and the Trail Making Test, parents of probands with childhood-onset schizophrenia performed significantly worse than parents of community controls and probands with ADHD, who did not differ significantly from each other. When rigorous cutoff scores derived from a logistic regression analysis were used, a combination of scores on the three neurocognitive tests identified 20% of mothers and fathers of probands with childhood-onset schizophrenia, compared to 0% of the mothers or fathers of community control probands. There was diagnostic specificity of the neurocognitive impairments. For mothers of probands, a combination of neurocognitive scores identified 11.4% of mothers in the childhood-onset schizophrenia group versus 0% of mothers in the ADHD group. For fathers of probands, a cutoff identifying 2.5% of fathers in the ADHD group classified 16% of fathers in the childhood-onset schizophrenia group. There were no significant neurocognitive differences between parents of probands with ADHD and parents of community control probands. Receiver operated characteristic curves revealed that the use of the procedure described here produced a level of diagnostic accuracy in the parents of the probands with childhood-onset schizophrenia that was sufficient for use in genetic linkage studies.

Chromosomal Anomalies

Chromosomal anomalies—either deletions of genes, translocations, or excessive repetition of genes—are found in a number of developmental and neuropsychiatric disorders. Detection of chromosomal anomalies can help identify chromosomal locations of genes that convey susceptibility for various disorders. There is an increased frequency (2%) of microdeletions of chromosome 22q11 in patients with adult-onset schizophrenia. Microdeletions of chromosome 22q11 are also found in patients with velocardiofacial syndrome. In patients with childhood-onset schizophrenia, the rate of 22q11 deletions (6.4%) is greater than in the general population and in samples with adult-onset schizophrenia (Usiskin et al., 1999).

The NIMH study of childhood-onset schizophrenia identified one case with a translocation (Gordon, Krasnewich, White, Lenane, & Rapoport, 1994; Jacobsen & Rapoport, 1998). This finding is interesting in relation to the literature indicating a variety of different cytogenetic anomalies among schizophrenic adults (for review, see DeLisi & Lovett, 1991; Sawa & Snyder, 2002). The translocation identified was an apparently balanced one involving chromosomes 1 and 7: 46,XY,t(1;7)(p22;q22).

Brain Imaging Studies

The neurodevelopmental model of schizophrenia was stimulated by observations of alterations in brain structures in adults with schizophrenia. These alterations are commonly believed to originate during fetal development. Although there have been relatively few *in vivo* studies of brain structures in patients with childhood-onset schizophrenia, many of the anomalies found in adult patients with schizophrenia are present in children with schizophrenia (for reviews, see Sowell, Toga, & Asarnow, 2000; Jacobsen & Rapoport, 1998).

There was postmortem evidence of brainstem abnormalities in the autopsied material of a man who died at 22 and had his first onset of schizophrenia at about 10 years of age (Casanova, Carosella, & Kleinman, 1990). Specific findings included central chromatolysis of neurons and mild gliosis in a restricted distribution of the brainstem and thalamus, and cell loss and cytoarchitectural disruption in the frontal lobes, prepyriform cortex, and entorhinal region. Casanova et al. (1990) suggest that these findings may reflect a "chronic derangement in the function of neurons of the rostral brainstem tegmental area and medial thalamus with secondary involvement of their terminal projection sites" (p. 313).

The Child Psychiatry Branch at NIMH has carried out seminal *in vivo* studies of brain structure in patients with childhood-onset schizophrenia, using structural magnetic resonance imaging (MRI). The NIMH group has found a 4% reduction in total cerebral volume in such patients (Rapoport et al., 1999; Kumra et al., 2000). This is consistent with the amount of reduction in total brain volume found in adults with schizophrenia (Lawrie & Abukmeil, 1998). The reduction in total brain volume was largely accounted for by reduced cortical gray matter. The UCLA group (Sowell et al., 2000) also found gray matter reductions in patients with schizophrenia.

Both the NIMH group (Kumra et al., 2000; Rapoport et al., 1997) and the UCLA group (Sowell et al., 2000; Levitt et al., 1999) found ventricular enlargements in patients with childhood-onset schizophrenia. The enlargements were predominantly in the posterior horns of the lateral ventricles (Sowell et al., 2000). There was a trend toward ventricular enlargement in a series of patients with childhood-onset schizophrenia or SPD studied at the University of New Mexico (Yeo et al., 1997). Schulz et al. (1983) described ventriculomegaly in adolescents with schizophrenia. Enlarged ventricles are perhaps the most consistently observed brain structure anomaly observed in adult patients with schizophrenia (Lawrie & Abukmeil, 1998).

In contrast to findings in adult patients, three cross-sectional volumetric studies found no reduction in mesial temporal lobe structures in children with schizophrenia (Jacobsen et al., 1996: Yeo et al., 1997; Levitt et al., 2001).

Statistical parametric mapping (a method of comparing gray matter, white matter, and cerebrospinal fluid in the entire brains of different groups) in patients with childhood-onset schizophrenia and controls revealed abnormalities in the midcallosum, posterior cingulate, caudate, and thalamus (Sowell et al., 2000). Callosal abnormalities had previously been detected via morphometric methods. After adjustment for decreased total cerebral volume, larger total, anterior, and posterior corpus callosum areas were found in children with schizophrenia (Jacobsen et al., 1997). These two studies suggest that in childhood-onset schizophrenia there may be white matter sparing in the context of decreased cortical volume.

There are also reductions in the volume of subcortical structures. After corrections for reduction in total brain volume, the volume of the vermis and the inferior posterior lobe of the cerebellum were reduced in patients with schizophrenia (Jacobsen et al., 1997).

Both the NIMH (Frazier et al., 1996) and UCLA (Blanton et al., 1999) groups have found volume increases in the basal ganglia. These increases are most likely related to neuroleptic exposure (Chakos et al., 1994).

Children with schizophrenia show greater changes in brain morphology over time than adults with schizophrenia do. When patients with childhood-onset schizophrenia and healthy subjects were rescanned at a 2-year follow-up, children with schizophrenia showed significantly greater decreases than healthy subjects in right temporal lobe, bilateral superior temporal gyrus and posterior superior temporal gyrus, right anterior superior temporal gyrus, and left hippocampal volumes over the follow-up interval (Jacobsen et al., 1998). There were greater increases in ventricular volume over the 2-year interval in the patients than in the controls (Rapoport et al., 1997).

A longitudinal analysis of the MRI scans of some of the patients with childhood-onset schizophrenia from the NIMH Child Psychiatry Branch cohort, using brain-mapping algorithms, detected striking anatomical profiles of accelerated gray matter loss. Surprisingly, there were dynamic changes, involving increasing amounts of cortex throughout adolescence, in which structures showed the greatest abnormalities over time.

> The earliest deficits were found in parietal brain regions, supporting visuospatial and associative thinking, where adult deficits are known to be mediated by environmental (nongenetic) factors. Over 5 years, these deficits progressed anteriorly into temporal lobes, engulfing sensorimotor and dorsolateral prefrontal cortices, and frontal eye fields. These emerging patterns correlated with psychotic symptom severity and mirrored the neuromotor, auditory, visual search, and frontal executive impairments in the disease. In temporal regions, gray matter loss was completely absent early in the disease but became pervasive later. Only the latest changes included dorsolateral prefrontal cortex and superior temporal gyri, deficit regions found consistently in adult studies. (Thompson et al., 2001, p. 11650)

Magnetic Resonance Spectroscopy

Magnetic resonance spectroscopy (MRS) is a new radiological technology that provides *in vivo* regional measures of brain chemistry. The UCLA group (Thomas et al., 1998) found a significant decrease in the ratio of *N*-acetylaspartase (NAA) to creatine (CR), a putative index of neuronal integrity, in frontal gray matter. In contrast, there were no differences in MRS spectra in occipital gray matter. Consistent with these results, the NIMH group (Bertolino et al., 1998) also found a decreased NAA/CR ratio exclusively in the prefrontal cortex and hippocampus of patients with childhood-onset schizophrenia. The reduction in this ratio in the prefrontal cortex and hippocampus was not simply a reflection of volume reductions in these areas. The NAA/CR ratios were not correlated with the volumes of these structures on MRI. The decreased NAA/CR ratio in frontal gray cortex and hippocampus may reflect decreased neuronal density.

More detailed *in vivo* studies of brain structure and neurochemistry in children with schizophrenia will further delimit when brain development in schizophrenia first goes awry by identifying specific brain anomalies associated with particular periods of brain development. One important clue emerging from the studies conducted to date is that childhood-onset schizophrenia appears to be associated with reductions in gray but not white matter. This finding, along with other data, point to deviations arising during fetal brain development. The neural circuits that are compromised appear to include both subcortical (cerebellum) and cortical (frontal gray) components. One of the most striking findings is the posterior-to-anterior cortical progression of reductions in brain volume observed over 5 years in children with schizophrenia. These neurodegenerative changes are much more extensive than have been observed in adults with schizophrenia over a comparable interval. Identifying the neurobiological processes that underlie the deviations in brain structures found in children with schizophrenia will provide important insights into the pathophysiology of schizophrenia.

Neurocognitive Studies

An important complement to brain imaging studies is an examination of neurocognitive functions that are sensitive to putative brain dysfunctions in schizophrenia. To delimit the nature of hypothesized CNS dysfunction, R. F. Asarnow et al. (1994) used a series of clinical neuropsychological and experimental tasks to link behavioral findings to putative CNS dysfunction. This was accomplished by using tasks that had been used to study patients with focal neuropathology and/or studies of brain electrical activity. One of the first findings to emerge from this research was that children with schizophrenia showed the same difficulties with attention and information processing that had been identified in adult schizophrenia. These children showed impairments on the span-of-apprehension task (R. F. Asarnow, Granholm, & Sherman, 1991; R. F. Asarnow & Sherman, 1984), an index of the speed of early visual information processing. When required to process larger arrays of visual information (5 and 10 letters vs. 1 and 3 letters), children with schizophrenia performed more poorly than children with DSM-III-defined attention deficit disorder and normal controls. The slope of the function relating the probability of target detection to array size was also steeper in children with schizophrenia, suggesting that the performance of such children is more disrupted when the amount of information they have to process is increased. Event-related potential data recorded during performance of the span-of-apprehension task indicated similar patterns of brain activity for both adults and children with schizophrenia (Strandburg, Marsh, Brown, Asarnow, & Guthrie, 1994). Individuals with childhood- or adult-onset schizophrenia produced less endogenous negative activity than did age-matched normal controls, which may reflect limitations in the processing resources available to carry out cognitive processing (R. F. Asarnow et al., 1994; Strandburg et al., 1994).

Thus, consistent with the hypothesis that schizophrenia in children and adults is associated with similar disease processes and dysfunctions, children with schizophrenia demonstrate an attention/information-processing deficit that has been shown to characterize schizophrenic adults. This deficit also shows some specificity to childhood-onset schizophrenia when compared to attention deficit disorder/ADHD, another childhood-onset disorder associated with attentional impairment. These findings assume particular significance when considered in relation to other research documenting that impairments on the span-of-apprehension task (1) remain relatively stable across changes in clinical state and characterize adult schizophrenic patients during periods of remission as well as during periods of disturbance; (2) show some specificity to schizophrenia in adults; and (3) show some degree of genetic influence. (For a review of span of apprehension in schizophrenia, see R. F. Asarnow et al., 1991.)

In a series of studies, R. F. Asarnow et al. (1994) have also analyzed the task demands and/or experimental conditions that are associated with the greatest and least neuropsychological impairment in children with schizophrenia. Results indicate the following:

1. Children with schizophrenia do not show impairments relative to normal controls on tasks assessing reception and comprehension of auditory stimuli, but do show impaired performance when required to attend to, remember, and respond to sequences of verbal and nonverbal stimuli that make extensive demands on processing capacity.
2. Children with schizophrenia show impairments on tests of visual perception, but only when memory demands are added to a task, so that a child is required to hold the sample stimulus in short-term memory prior to responding.
3. Impairments in visual–motor coordination and fine motor speed are found on tasks using the dominant hand, the nondominant hand, and both hands.
4. Similar to adults with schizophrenia, children with schizophrenia show impairments in executive functions—for example, allocating attention, as assessed on such tests as the Wisconsin Card Sorting Test (Grant & Berg, 1981), which requires a subject to sort cards varying along multiple dimensions into categories based on a sorting principle that the subject must discover.

5. Providing task-appropriate strategies or information to children with schizophrenia sometimes paradoxically impairs performance.
6. Children with schizophrenia show deficits in both verbal and spatial working memory, suggesting a limited allocation of resources to the central executive (Karatekin & Asarnow, 1998b).

Rather than pointing to unilateral focal brain disease, this pattern of results suggests that children with schizophrenia have difficulties on tasks that make extensive demands on information-processing resources, regardless of the hemisphere subserving the function(s) assessed by the task. This hypothesis focuses the search for a CNS substrate for schizophrenia on CNS structures involved in recruiting and controlling allocation of processing resources and the dynamic interaction between these structures.

Recent studies by Karatekin and Asarnow (1998a) further examined the role of limited processing resources and the allocation of processing resources in the neurocognitive impairments exhibited by children with schizophrenia. Children with schizophrenia were compared to children with ADHD and normal controls on tasks assessing parallel and serial visual search (Karatekin & Asarnow, 1998a). Parallel visual search is hypothesized to make minimal demands on processing resources. In contrast, serial search, particularly of large stimulus arrays when the target is absent, makes extensive demands on processing resources. Saccadic reaction times to the stimuli were recorded with a video-based eye monitor. As predicted, children with schizophrenia had a slower rate of serial search than normal controls, despite a normal rate of parallel search. This provides additional evidence that children with schizophrenia have limited processing resources and/or defective control allocation of processing resources. The children with ADHD also had slower rates of serial search and normal parallel search. Part of the slowing in serial search in children with ADHD was attributable to delayed initiation of search, as reflected in slow saccadic reaction time. In contrast, the children with schizophrenia had normal saccadic reaction times. These results suggest that low-level aspects of visual attention (i.e., coarse guidance of search, rate of parallel search, basic control of eye movements) are intact in children with schizophrenia. A subsequent study examined a higher-level aspect of visual attention, the "top-down" control of scene perception under minimal external constraints.

Exploratory eye movements to thematic pictures (e.g., a picture of fairy tale characters at a dining table) were examined in children with schizophrenia, children with ADHD, and normal controls (Karatekin & Asarnow, 1999) via a video monitoring system. Children were asked three questions that varied in amount of structure about each picture. Children with schizophrenia looked at fewer relevant, but *not* more irrelevant, regions than normal controls. They tended to stare more when asked to decide what was happening (global question), but not when asked to attend to specific regions (focal and counting questions). The fact that eye movement parameters of the children with schizophrenia did not differ from those of controls on the focal and counting questions argues against the possibility that the impairments on the global question were attributable to disturbances in oculomotor functioning, lack of motivation, or disengagement of attention. Moreover, this same group of children with schizophrenia had normal saccadic reaction times during both serial and parallel visual search. There was no evidence that the children with schizophrenia did not understand the gist of the pictures. It appears that the impairment of the children with schizophrenia is attributable to higher-order stages of scene perception, which involve actively testing, confirming, and modifying initial hypotheses about the pictures based on contextual cues. Taken collectively, the results of this study suggest that children with schizophrenia have an impairment in the top-down control of selective visual attention in the service of self-guided action. These are functions that are typically supported by the frontal lobes.

Environmental Stressors

The available data suggest that childhood-onset schizophrenia is a familial disorder. However, the observation that concordance rates for monozygotic twins are substantially less than 100% indicates that nongenetic factors also influence the likelihood of an individual's developing schizophrenia. Because the presence of psychiatric illness in a parent is likely to be associated with impaired parental role functioning, it is also likely that there are complex interactions between familial psychiatric disorder and environmental factors. Furthermore, if (as expected with adult schizophrenia) considerable genetic and etiological heterogeneity is identified in childhood-onset schizophrenia, some forms of the disorder may prove to be more closely linked to environmental stress than others.

Pregnancy and Birth Complications

Pregnancy and birth complications constitute one environmental factor that has been implicated as a potential etiological factor in schizophrenia. The difficulties of differentiating between the effects of child and environmental characteristics, however, are highlighted by Cantor's (1988) finding that although comparable rates of birth complications were observed among "schizophrenic" and control samples, a higher rate of "perinatal instability" was observed for males with schizophrenia than for control males. The category of "perinatal instability" included such difficulties as cyanotic episodes that could reflect vulnerability in the infant, thus highlighting the possibility that some children may be more vulnerable to pre- and/or perinatal complications. A recent examination of the birth records of 36 children with schizophrenia and 35 sibling comparison subjects revealed no significant differences between the two groups in rates of obstetrical complications (Nicolson et al., 1999). Patients with childhood-onset schizophrenia and obstetrical complications did not have an earlier age of onset of schizophrenia than patients without a history of obstetrical complications. Data indicating high rates of perinatal difficulties among adults with schizophrenia (for a review, see McNeil, 1988), as well as among high-risk children (of schizophrenic parents) who developed schizophrenia (Cannon, Barr, & Mednick, 1991; Parnas et al., 1982), highlight the need for further examination of pregnancy and birth complications and of their interaction with genetic liability in childhood-onset schizophrenia.

Data highlighting possible links between schizophrenia and prenatal exposure to viral infection further underscore the possible etiological role of such early environmental stressors. Notably, Mednick, Machon, Huttunen, and Bonett (1988) reported an elevated rate of adult schizophrenia among individuals who were exposed to a severe Type A2 influenza epidemic during their second trimester of gestation. Increased risk for schizophrenia was not found among individuals exposed to the epidemic during the first and third trimesters of gestation, suggesting that it is the *timing* of the stressor during a critical period of gestation that is associated with the increased risk for schizophrenia. Given the likely etiological heterogeneity of schizophrenia, Cannon et al. (1991) have suggested that "teratogenic agents such as viruses may be responsible for the fetal neural disturbances leading to schizophrenia in *some* cases" (p. 13; emphasis in original).

Psychosocial Stress

The role of psychosocial stress in the etiology of schizophrenia is clearest in studies of high-risk samples where the illness has not yet developed, because the occurrence of the schizophrenic illness is associated with significant psychosocial stress in families. Unfortunately, because childhood-onset schizophrenia is relatively rare, very few cases of this disorder have been described in the literature on children at risk for schizophrenia. However, Fish did describe two cases of childhood-onset schizophrenia, both independently diagnosed at 10 years of age (for a review, see Fish, 1987). Although this represents a very small sample, it merits note that these were the only children in the sample who were identified as having histories of physical abuse. These two children were also reared by mothers with schizophrenia and had the most severe signs of neurointegrative disorder or what Fish has termed "pandysmaturation," which is defined as a pattern of transient lags and disorganization of gross motor and/or visual motor development in conjunction with lags in physical growth. These descriptions highlight the likely interactions between genetic and environmental factors in the development of many children with schizophrenia.

Kallman and Roth (1956) examined the home environments of siblings and dizygotic twins of probands with childhood-onset schizophrenia. Disturbed rearing environments were somewhat more likely to be associated with schizophrenia-spectrum outcomes, but were also found in cases with healthy outcomes. Whereas roughly 82% of the homes of twins and siblings diagnosed as schizoid or schizophrenic were classified as "inadequate" based on the presence of at least one disturbed or inadequate parent, economic distress, or broken homes, 64.8% of all twins and siblings classified as "normal" also came from homes classified as "inadequate." The high level of difficulties described in these home environments may have been associated, however, with the fact that all of these homes contained a child with schizophrenia.

J. R. Asarnow and colleagues (for a review, see J. R. Asarnow, Tompson, & Goldstein, 1994) have conducted a series of studies aimed at describing the environments of children with schizophrenia and children with SPD. Although SPD is controversial in childhood, links between schizophrenia and SPD are suggested by research indicating elevated rates of SPD among the biological relatives of patients with schizophrenia (for a review, see Kendler, 1988), as well as by high-risk research suggesting that schizotypal symptoms such as social isolation and signs of thought disturbance may be early precursors of schizophrenia (for a review, see J. R. Asarnow, 1988). By including children with SPD in these studies, J. R. Asarnow and her colleagues sought to examine the broader schizophrenia spectrum, and possibly to evaluate predictors of the onset of schizophrenia among a group of children hypothesized to be at risk for full-blown schizophrenic disorders.

This work has addressed two general questions: (1) Are the family attributes that have been found to be associated with the onset and course of adult schizophrenia also observed in families of children with schizophrenia-spectrum disorders? (2) Are there specific family environmental attributes that are associated with schizophrenia spectrum disorders in childhood, and less common in families of children with other psychiatric disorders and families of children with no evidence of psychiatric disorder? Because both parents and children contribute to the quality of family interaction, this research has assessed both parent and child behaviors.

Communication quality was assessed with a measure of "communication deviance" (CD; Jones, 1977; Singer & Wynne, 1965), as well as a measure of communication scored from samples of direct family interaction (Tompson, Asarnow, Goldstein, & Miklowitz, 1990). CD refers to a confusing, unclear communication style that leads to a disruption in the focus of attention. Typically, CD is assessed via projective tests such as the Thematic Apperception Test (TAT) or the Rorschach, and is conceptualized as an interpersonal manifestation of thought and attentional disturbance. Prior research has demonstrated that parents of adults with schizophrenia tend to show higher levels of CD than to parents of patients with other disorders and parents of normal controls do. In addition, Goldstein (1987) found an increased risk for adult schizophrenia-spectrum disorders among disturbed but nonpsychotic adolescents whose parents scored high on the CD measure. Similar to these findings for adult schizophrenia, J. R. Asarnow, Goldstein, and Ben-Meir (1988) observed that parents of children with schizophrenia and SPD were more likely to score high on CD (assessed on the TAT) than were parents of children with depressive disorders. Children with schizophrenia and children with SPD from high-CD families showed the most severe impairments and the poorest attentional functioning, as indexed by the Freedom from Distractibility factor of the Wechsler Intelligence Scale for Children—Revised (a factor based on scores from the Arithmetic, Digit Span, and Coding subtests). This suggests that CD in parents may be associated with a particularly severe form of childhood schizophrenia-spectrum disorders, or perhaps may be associated with family interactional processes that exacerbate the severity of dysfunction. CD was also found among some parents of children with depression, but CD was not associated with differences in the severity of impairment or attentional functioning in this group, suggesting that the CD construct may have particular significance for the development of schizophrenic disorders.

In a second study (Tompson et al., 1990) assessing direct parent–child communication, no differences were identified between the communication styles of parents of children with schizophrenia-spectrum disorders and those of parents of children with major depression. Alternatively, children with schizophrenia-spectrum disorders showed significantly more communication problems than children with major depression did during the interaction task, particularly on codes assessing thought disorder and difficulties maintaining attention to task. Collectively, these findings raise the possibility that the children's presence during the interaction resulted in parents' increasing their efforts to communicate clearly as they responded to the attention and thought problems of their disturbed children.

The clinical and etiological significance of the CD findings merits exploration. One hypothesis that has been offered is that the high rate of CD identified among parents may be associated with the stress of living with a severely disturbed child with schizophrenia. Alternatively, it has been suggested that high CD may be a marker of subclinical or full-blown psychopathology in a relative. Goldstein et al. (1992), however, did not find a significant association between high CD and the presence of diagnosable psychiatric disorder among parents of adults with schizophrenia.

Another construct examined by J. R. Asarnow and colleagues is the affective quality of parent–child interactions. Observational measures of direct parent–child interaction, as well as the expressed emotion (EE) measure (which is obtained in a child's absence), were used. The EE measure assesses critical and emotionally over-involved attitudes of a parent toward a child. Numerous studies have shown that EE is a strong predictor of outcome among adults with schizophrenia (for reviews, see Cutting & Docherty, 2000; Leff, 1991; Leff & Vaughn, 1985; King, 2000; Rosenfarb, Goldstein, Mintz, & Nuechterlein, 1995; Winterseen & Rasmussen, 1997), and Goldstein (1987) reported that measures of EE obtained during adolescence were associated with an increased risk of schizophrenia-spectrum disorders in young adulthood.

In contrast to results with adult schizophrenia, rates of EE using the Five-Minute Speech Sample index were relatively low among parents of children with schizophrenia-spectrum disorders (23% vs. 44% in the most comparable adult sample) and did not differ significantly from rates of EE in a normal comparison group (J. R. Asarnow, Tompson, Hamilton, Goldstein, & Guthrie, 1994). High EE ratings among parents of children with schizophrenia-spectrum disorders tended to result from high scores on the criticism dimension rather than emotional overinvolvement. Interestingly, high EE was significantly more frequent among parents of depressed children than among parents of children with schizophrenia-spectrum disorders or normal controls (J. R. Asarnow, Tompson, Hamilton, et al., 1994; J. R. Asarnow, Tompson, Woo, & Cantwell, 2001)—a finding that is consistent with other reports indicating high rates of EE among parents of children with other nonschizophrenic disorders (Hibbs et al., 1991; Stubbe, Zahner, Goldstein, & Leckman, 1993).

Alternatively, on a direct family interaction task in which parents and children attempted to resolve an affectively charged family problem, parents of children with schizophrenia-spectrum disorders were significantly more likely to express harsh criticism toward the children than were parents of normal controls, or parents of depressed children (Hamilton, Asarnow, & Tompson, 1999). This again underscores the likely impact of children's behavior on the behavior of their parents.

In summary, results of studies of the family environments of children with schizophrenia-spectrum disorders underscore the stress and distress experienced by many of these families. Whereas children with these disorders tend to show difficulties with attention and thought disturbance during direct family interactions, their parents are likely to make harsh critical comments, perhaps in response to frustrations resulting from the children's tendency to drift off task and/or offer disorganized and peculiar ideas. Future research is needed to clarify the impact of family stress on the course of childhood-onset schizophrenia and SPD, and to clarify associations among family genetic and family environmental variables.

COMMON COMORBIDITIES

One observation that has received clear documentation is that many children with schizophrenia meet criteria for comorbid diagnoses. Despite uncertainties regarding how the presence of a comorbid condition should be viewed in the context of a diagnosis of schizophrenia, investigators who have used semistructured diagnostic interviews have tended to report high rates of codiagnoses among children with schizophrenia. To illustrate, Russell et al. (1989) found that 68% of their sample of schizophrenic children met criteria for another DSM-III diagnosis. The most common codiagnoses were conduct disorder or oppositional disorder (31%) and atypical depression or dysthymic disorder (37%). This high rate of depression codiagnoses, coupled with reports that some cases initially presenting with schizophrenia meet criteria for bipolar or schizoaffective disorders at follow-up (Eggers, 1989; Werry et al., 1991; Zeitlin, 1986), underscores the limitations of cross-sectional diagnoses based on evaluations conducted at a single point in time. In this context, it is important to recall that the boundaries of the schizophrenia spectrum are not resolved, and that some forms of schizoaffective disorder appear to be closely linked to schizophrenia (Kendler, 1988; Kendler, McGuire, Gruenberg, Spellman, & O'Hare, 1993).

Given earlier controversies regarding the association between autism and schizophrenia, it merits note that there does not appear to be an elevated risk of schizophrenia among samples of children with autism or other PDDs (Burd & Kerbeshian, 1987; Volkmar & Cohen, 1991), although there is occasional overlap between autistic and schizophrenic syndromes and symptoms over time (e.g., Konstantareas & Hewitt, 2001; Petty, Ornitz, Michelman, & Zimmerman, 1984).

TREATMENT AND SERVICE DELIVERY STRATEGIES

The major advances in genetics, the biological sciences, neurochemistry, and psychology have potential to lead to the development of more effective treatment and prevention strategies. As reviewed below, at present a number of pharmacological and psychosocial treatment strategies are used clinically, and some data are available on treatment effects. However, controlled treatment trials with youths suffering from schizophrenia are urgently needed. Given the relative rarity of childhood-onset schizophrenia, such studies will be expensive and will require multiple sites and extensive case-finding efforts. Despite the limitations of current data, to address the clinical needs of these youths, practice parameters have been developed by the American Academy of Child and Adolescent Psychiatry (McClellan et al., 2001). These practice parameters emphasize antipsychotic medications in combination with psychoeducational, psychotherapeutic, and social and educational support programs.

Pharmacological Treatment

Recent years have witnessed the completion of well-designed studies examining the efficacy of antipsychotic medications for the treatment of schizophrenia in youths. Current evidence is limited, however, and there is a need for additional clinical trials. Nevertheless, extent data do support a role for antipsychotic medication. In a randomized double-blind study with children, Spencer and Campbell (1994) found a significant advantage for haloperidol (1.5–3.5 mg/day or 0.02–0.12 mg/kg/day) relative to placebo. However, side effects were observed, the most common of which were sedation and parkinsonism. Similarly, results of a double-blind placebo-controlled trial of haloperidol (2–16 mg/day, mean 9.8 mg/day) versus loxapine (10–200 mg/day, mean 87.5 mg/day) with adolescents suffering from schizophrenia revealed that both antipsychotic medications were associated with reductions in schizophrenic symptoms, compared to placebo (Pool, Bloom, Mielke, Roniger, & Gallant, 1976). There was also a tendency for more severely ill adolescents to benefit more from the active drugs versus the placebo.

The safety and efficacy of atypical antipsychotics have also been evaluated in recent years. At present, there are over 15 studies that support the antipsychotic efficacy of clozapine in treating children and adolescents with schizophrenia (see Remschmidt, Fleischhaker, Henninghaisen, & Schulz, 2000), but only one of these studies used a randomized double-blind design (Kumra et al., 1996). Therefore, controlled clinical trials are needed to clarify short- and long-term efficacy (Campbell, Rapoport, & Simpson, 1999; Remschmidt et al., 2000). Because enthusiasm regarding clozapine is tempered by the risk of serious adverse effects, such as seizures, neutrophenia, granulocytopenia, myocarditis, and agranulocytosis, clozapine is not recommended as a first-line antipsychotic medication. Most patients are treated with at least two conventional antipsychotics prior to receiving a clozapine trial. When used, clozapine requires careful monitoring of hematological parameters and other adverse effects. Advantages of clozapine treatment for treatment-resistant schizophrenia in youths include (1) high antipsychotic efficacy during the acute episode; (2) more improvement in youths with chronic schizophrenia and a high rate of negative symptoms; and (3) fewer extrapyramidal adverse effects, leading to relatively good tolerability in comparison to typical antipsychotics (Remschmidt et al., 2000). Clozapine treatment can be beneficial in children and adolescents during acute schizophrenic episodes, particularly when treatment with conventional antipsychotics is associated with severe extrapyramidal side effects and/or predominant negative symptoms. Interested readers are referred to Remschmidt et al. (2000) and McClellan et al. (2001) for thorough reviews of clozapine treatment guidelines.

There are less systematic data on risperidone, another atypical antipsychotic with a similar profile to clozapine. Results of an open study found that risperidone treatment was associated with reductions in schizophrenic symptoms among

10 adolescents with schizophrenia, but a high rate of extrapyramidal side effects was observed (Armenteros, Whitaker, Welikson, Stedge, & Gorman, 1997).

Psychosocial Treatment

Although the literature contains rich clinical descriptions of psychosocial treatment strategies for children with schizophrenia (e.g., Campbell, 1978; Cantor, 1988; Fish, 1968; McClellan & Werry, 1992; Remschmidt et al., 1994), a recent search revealed no controlled trials of psychosocial interventions. Although medications may control psychotic symptoms for some children with schizophrenia, the need to supplement pharmacological treatment with special school programs, social skills training, family treatment, case management, and rehabilitation services is generally recognized in clinical practice. Psychosocial treatments for adults with schizophrenia may also have applicability for children and teenagers (see, e.g., Bellack & Mueser, 1984; Falloon et al., 1985; Hogarty et al., 1995; Kavanagh & Mueser, 2001; Leff et al., 1989; Liberman & Kopelowicz, 1995; Linszen et al., 1996; McFarlane et al., 1995; Schooler et al., 1997). Behavioral family treatment emphasizing training in communication and problem-solving skills, and social skills training emphasizing instruction and practice in such skills as maintaining appropriate eye contact and initiating conversations, would seem to have particular promise. Systematic evaluation of alternative psychosocial treatment strategies is clearly needed.

Prevention

The combination of results from studies of children at risk for schizophrenia, advances in knowledge regarding the prodromes and precursor states for schizophrenia, and improvements in treatments have led to efforts at preventing schizophrenia in adults. Recent studies have shown considerable promise. For example, McGorry et al. (in press) found that a 6-month preventive intervention targeted at patients considered to be at very high risk for development of a frank schizophrenic psychosis was associated with significantly fewer patients' developing a first episode of psychosis, as compared to needs-based supportive therapy. The preventive intervention involved low-dose risperidone and cognitive-behavioral therapy plus needs-based supportive therapy. For patients who adhered to risperidone treatment, the preventive intervention appeared to afford protection against progression to psychosis for 6 months after risperidone was discontinued. However, overall outcome for the two treatment groups (preventive intervention vs. needs-based supportive therapy) did not differ 6 months after treatment when an intent-to-treat analysis was used. McGlashan and colleagues have also initiated multisite prevention trials aimed at reducing the duration of untreated psychoses through early detection and treatment, using a combination of active outreach and community education, medication, psychosocial treatment, and family education. Preliminary results suggest reduction in the duration of untreated psychosis among patients after the early detection system was initiated (McGlashan, 1998; Johannessen et al., 2001).

These studies involved adults, and these preventive approaches have not yet been applied with youths. However, the promising findings from the adult literature suggest the value of extending these prevention strategies to children. Indeed, the fact that most children are in school and are seen for regular pediatric visits suggest that early identification of at-risk children is likely to be easier and less costly than it is for adults (for a review of primary care intervention strategies, see J. R. Asarnow, Jaycox, & Anderson, in press). On the other hand, the use of low-dose medications without a clear indication is potentially more dangerous and less acceptable for children, although concerns have also been raised about off-label use of medication as a first-line treatment for adults (McGorry et al., in press). Therefore, although research focusing on prevention clearly has merits in child populations, strategies will have to be developed to address ethical and developmental considerations.

Outcome and Prognostic Factors

Despite the crucial importance of data on longitudinal course and prognostic factors for providing optimal clinical care and establishing the validity of psychiatric syndromes, there are limited data on the course of childhood-onset schizophrenia. The time needed to complete longitudinal studies has also meant that most current outcome data are derived from samples collected during the pre-DSM-III period, when more modern assessment and diagnostic procedures were not available. With this caveat, we review results from studies of early-onset schizophrenia and related disorders.

The results obtained by Werry et al. (1991) present the poorest view of prognosis. Although 90% of the sample was receiving neuroleptic treatment, remission (defined as an absence of subsequent schizophrenic episodes) was observed in only 3% of the sample over the course of a 1- to 16-year follow-up interval (mean follow-up interval of roughly 5 years). Chronic schizophrenia or two or more schizophrenic episodes were observed in 90% of the sample; and 13% of the sample had died, all of whom were described as placing themselves in the lethal situation, although the question of whether these were clear suicides or delusion-driven accidents could not be resolved. Only 17% of the sample were full-time students or had full-time employment. The average Global Assessment of Functioning score was 40, reflecting a relatively severe level of impairment (major impairment in several areas or some impairment in reality testing or communication). Because Werry et al. (1991) used outcome diagnoses rather than admission diagnoses to classify their subjects, a number of youths with bipolar outcomes were excluded from the "schizophrenic sample." This probably led to a more pessimistic view of outcome than would have been observed had admission diagnoses been used to define the sample.

A better prognosis is suggested by Eggers (1989), who reported on 57 patients diagnosed with schizophrenia prior to 14 years of age. At a follow-up evaluation 6 to 40 years later (mean = 16 years), patients with schizophrenia and schizoaffective psychoses were examined separately. Within the sample of patients with schizophrenia, 27% were classified as in remission, 24% were described as showing slight defects, and 49% were described as showing severe defects. Because cross-national differences in practice patterns and other variables could influence results, it is important to note that the Werry et al. (1991; see also Werry & McClellan, 1992) study was conducted in New Zealand, and the Eggers (1978, 1989) study was conducted in Germany.

Outcome data from a sample of children diagnosed with schizophrenia between 7 and 14 years of age (J. R. Asarnow, Tompson, & Goldstein, 1994) are similar to those observed in the Eggers (1989) sample. Over the course of a 3- to 7-year follow-up, 61% of this sample showed continuing schizophrenia as they progressed through adolescence, and 67% showed continuing schizophrenia or schizoaffective disorder. When outcome was defined via global adjustment scores, there was considerable variability in outcomes: 56% of the sample showed improvement in functioning over the course of the follow-up, and the other 44% showed minimal improvement or a deteriorating course. Twenty-eight percent of the sample were classified as showing good outcomes. These youth had global adjustment scores of 60 or above at the final follow-up, indicating relatively good psychosocial adjustment.

Evidence for variability in outcome is also provided by results of Zeitlin's (1986) case record study. Whereas 50% (4 of 8) children diagnosed with schizophrenia between 8 and 15 years of age received diagnoses of schizophrenia as adults, the other half of this group received other diagnoses (bipolar disorder, $n = 3$; unspecified personality disorder with questions regarding possible schizophrenia, $n = 1$). Less variability in outcome was observed if children were characterized according to the presence versus absence of psychosis: 9 of the 10 children diagnosed with psychosis in childhood (90%) presented with psychoses as young adults. Eight of these children received diagnoses of schizophrenia as children, and the other two received childhood diagnoses of bipolar disorder. Underscoring the importance of looking at the developmental characteristics of the disorder was the finding that the two children with nonacute onsets of schizophrenia in childhood were both diagnosed with schizophrenia as adults, whereas four of the six children with schizophrenia with acute onsets of disorder received adult diagnoses other than schizophrenia. Depressed mood was also more common among children with schizophrenia receiving adult diagnoses of affective psychoses, as compared to children with schizophrenia receiving diagnoses of schizophrenia as adults. These data suggest the likely continuity for psychotic disorder between childhood and adulthood, but highlight the difficulties differentiating between schizophrenic and affective psychoses, as well as the potential importance of examining such clinical features as onset patterns and depressed mood.

In a similar follow-up study of adolescent-onset schizophrenia, Hollis (2000) examined outcomes for 93 patients with diagnoses of psychoses in childhood or adolescence and seen at the Maudsley Hospital in London. The average length of follow-up was 11.5 years, and the mean age at follow-up was 27.2 years (range 17–39 years). Results indicated high diagnostic stability for schizophrenia and affective psychosis, with more variation over time for schizoaffective and atypical psychoses. When compared to the other psychoses, schizophrenia was associated with significantly more severe impairment and symptomotology. Adolescents who presented with schizophrenia tended to have a chronic illness course and severe impairments in social relationships and independent living. Furthermore, adolescents with schizophrenia had significantly poorer educational achievement and spent significantly less time in employment.

Another approach to defining outcome is to examine degree of dysfunction as indicated by rehospitalization and out-of-home placement rates. Data are available on this issue based on telephone interviews conducted with families and caretakers of 18 children with schizophrenia or SPD. Children were first seen during psychiatric hospitalizations (J. R. Asarnow, Goldstein, Carlson, et al., 1988). Results indicated a high risk of out-of-home placement among children with schizophrenia and those with SPD, underscoring the continuing impairment observed in these children. Although all but two children were sent home at discharge from the hospital, within 13 months 57% of these children were placed out of their homes. Placement was usually in residential treatment centers for extended periods of time (range 560–730 days, with some children still in placement after 730 days) and precipitated by out-of-control behavior. Rehospitalization also occurred, with two children rehospitalized shortly after discharge due to safety concerns, and five additional children rehospitalized within 2.5 years of discharge. Reasons for rehospitalization were out-of-control behavior (four children) and suicide attempts (one child). One child in the sample died by suicide as a young adult, again underscoring the high risk of suicide among individuals suffering with schizophrenia.

Werry and McClellan (1992) and Eggers (1989) examined predictors of outcome. Results differed somewhat, depending on the outcome criterion (e.g., symptoms, social functioning), but abnormal premorbid adjustment predicted poor outcome in both samples. In addition, impairment after first admission was a predictor of outcome in the Werry and McClellan (1992) sample. Thus having a poor level of adjustment prior to the onset of schizophrenia, as well as a high level of impairment following the first admission for the illness, was associated with poorer outcome.

FUTURE DIRECTIONS

Major advances in our understanding of childhood-onset schizophrenia have been achieved since the 1930s. Notably, we currently have clear evidence that schizophrenia with childhood onset can be reliably diagnosed via the same criteria employed with adults, and that childhood-onset schizophrenia continues into adult life in many cases. Similarities between children and adults with schizophrenia in such diverse domains as genetics, brain imaging, neurocognition, thought disorder, treatment response, outcome, and family patterns suggests continuity between the childhood- and adult-onset forms of the disorder. Similar to findings with adults, considerable within-group variability is also observed among children with schizophrenia, underscoring the need to clarify the degree of clinical and etiological heterogeneity among these children. Finally, there appear to be important differences between childhood- and later-onset schizophrenia. In addition to the atypical early onset characteristic of childhood-onset cases, current findings suggest that these children may be characterized by particularly poor premorbid adjustment, increased family loading for schizophrenia-spectrum disorders, higher rates of insidious as opposed to acute onsets, greater loss of cortical gray matter over time, and possibly poorer outcomes.

The progress that has been achieved to date has allowed us to better treat and understand this devastating illness. Current data (1) support the view of schizophrenia as a primary brain disease with complex etiological pathways involving biological, environmental, and cultural factors; (2) provide some support for the view that childhood-onset cases may represent a particularly severe variant of schizophrenia, in which etiological pathways and the biological substrate for the disorder may be more clearly discernible; and (3) suggest that, like adult-onset schizophrenia, childhood-onset schizophrenia shows some degree of heterogeneity. As outlined in this chapter, future research is needed to clarify the causes, consequences, treatment, and prevention of schizophrenic disorders in children.

ACKNOWLEDGMENTS

Preparation of this chapter was facilitated by National Institute of Mental Health Grants No. MH46981-02 and No. MH45112-11, and by support from the Della Martin Foundation.

NOTE

1. "Mental activity in which fantasy runs on unhampered by logic and experience" (*Dorland's Illustrated Medical Dictionary*, 1985, p. 360).

REFERENCES

American Psychiatric Association (APA). (1968). *Diagnostic and statistical manual of mental disorders* (2nd ed). Washington, DC: Author.

American Psychiatric Association (APA). (1980). *Diagnostic and statistical manual of mental disorders* (3rd ed.). Washington, DC: Author.

American Psychiatric Association (APA). (1987). *Diagnostic and statistical manual of mental disorders* (3rd ed., rev.). Washington, DC: Author.

American Psychiatric Association (APA). (1994). *Diagnostic and statistical manual of mental disorders* (4th ed.). Washington, DC: Author.

Armenteros, J. L., Whitaker, A. H., Welikson, M., Stedge, D., & Gorman, J. (1997). Risperidone in adolescents with schizophrenia: An open pilot study. *Journal of the American Academy of Child and Adolescent Psychiatry, 36*, 694–700.

Asarnow, J. R. (1988). Children at risk for schizophrenia: Converging lines of evidence. *Schizophrenia Bulletin, 14*(4), 613–631.

Asarnow, J. R., Asarnow, R. F., Hornstein, N., & Russell, A. T. (1991). Childhood-onset schizophrenia: Developmental perspectives on schizophrenic disorders. In E. F. Walker (Ed.), *Schizophrenia: A life course developmental perspective* (pp. 95–122). New York: Academic Press.

Asarnow, J. R., & Ben-Meir, S. (1988). Children with schizophrenia spectrum and depressive disorders: A comparative study of onset patterns, premorbid adjustment, and severity of dysfunction. *Journal of Child Psychology and Psychiatry, 29*, 477–488.

Asarnow, J. R., & Goldstein, M. J. (1986). Schizophrenia during adolescence and early adulthood: A developmental perspective. *Clinical Psychology Review, 6*, 211–235.

Asarnow, J. R., Goldstein, M. J., & Ben-Meir, S. (1988). Parental communication deviance in childhood onset schizophrenia spectrum and depressive disorders. *Journal of Child Psychology and Psychiatry, 29*, 825–838.

Asarnow, J. R., Goldstein, M. J., Carlson, G. A., Perdue, S., Bates, S., & Keller, J. (1988). Child-onset depressive disorders: A follow-up study of rates of rehospitalization and out-of-home placement among child psychiatric inpatients. *Journal of Affective Disorders, 15*, 245–253.

Asarnow, J. R.. Jaycox, L., & Anderson, M. (in press). Depression among youth in primary care: Models for delivering mental health services. *Child and Adolescent Psychiatric Clinics of North America*.

Asarnow, J. R., Tompson, M., & Goldstein, M. J. (1994). Childhood-onset schizophrenia: A followup study. *Schizophrenia Bulletin, 20*, 599–618.

Asarnow, J. R., Tompson, M. C., Hamilton, E., Goldstein, M. J., & Guthrie, D. (1994). Family expressed emotion, childhood-onset depression, and childhood-onset schizophrenia spectrum disorders: Is expressed emotion a nonspecific correlate of child psychopathology or a specific risk factor for depression? *Journal of Abnormal Child Psychology, 22*, 129–146.

Asarnow, J. R., Tompson, M., Woo, S., & Cantwell, D. (2001). Expressed emotion: A risk factor for depression? *Journal of Abnormal Child Psychiatry, 29*, 573–583.

Asarnow, R. F., Asamen, J., Granholm, E., Sherman, T., Watkins, J., & Williams, M. (1994). Cognitive/neuropsychological studies of children with a schizophrenic disorder. *Schizophrenia Bulletin, 20*, 647–670.

Asarnow, R. F., Asarnow, J. R., & Strandberg, R. (1989). Schizophrenia: A developmental perspective. In D. Cicchetti (Ed.), *Rochester Symposium of Developmental Psychopathology: Vol. 4. The emergence of a discipline* (pp. 189–219). Hillsdale, NJ: Erlbaum.

Asarnow, R. F., Brown, W., & Strandburg, R. (1995). Children with a schizophrenic disorder: neurobehavioral studies. *European Archives of Psychiatry and Clinical Neuroscience, 245*, 70–79.

Asarnow, R. F., Granholm, E., & Sherman, T. (1991). Span of apprehension in schizophrenia. In S. R. Steinhauer, J. H. Gruzelier, & J. Zubin (Eds.), *Handbook of schizophrenia: Vol. 5. Neuropsychology, psychophysiology and information processing* (pp. 335–370). Amsterdam: Elsevier.

Asarnow, R. F. Nuechterlein, K. H., Fogelson, D., Subotnik, K. L., Payne, D. A., Russell, A. T., Asamen, J., Kuppinger, H., & Kendler, K. S. (2001). Schizophrenia and schizophrenia-spectrum personality disorders in the first-degree relatives of children with schizophrenia: The UCLA Family Study. *Archives of General Psychiatry*, 58, 581–588.

Asarnow, R. F., Nuechterlein, K. H., Subotinik, K. L., Fogelson, D. L., Torquato, R. D., Payne, D. L., Asamen, J., Mintz, J., & Guthrie, D. (in press). Neurocognitive impairments in non-psychotic parents of children with schizophrenia and attention deficit hyperactivity disorders: The UCLA Family Study. *Archives of General Psychiatry*.

Asarnow, R. F., & Sherman, T. (1984). Studies of visual information processing in schizophrenic children. *Child Development, 55*, 249–261.

Beitchman, J. H. (1985). Childhood schizophrenia: A review and comparison with adult-onset schizophrenia. *Psychiatric Clinics of North America, 8*, 793–814.

Bellack, A. S., & Mueser, K. T. (1984). A comprehensive treatment program for schizophrenia and chronic mental illness. *Community Mental Health Journal, 22*, 175–189.

Bender, L. (1956). Schizophrenia in childhood: Its recognition, description and treatment. *American Journal of Orthopsychiatry, 26*, 499–506.

Bennett, S., & Klein, H. R. (1966). Childhood schizophrenia: 30 years later. *American Journal of Psychiatry, 122*, 1121–1124.

Bertolino, A., Kumra, S., Callicott, J. H., Mattay, V. S., Lestz, R. M., Jacobsen, L., Barnett, I. S., Duyn, J. H., Frank, J. A., Rapoport, J. L., & Weinberger, D. R. (1998). Common pattern of cortical pathology in childhood-onset and adult-onset schizophrenia as identified by proton magnetic resonance spectroscopic imaging. *American Journal of Psychiatry, 155*, 1376–1383.

Blanton, R. E., Levitt, J., Thompson, P. M., Badrtalei, S., Capetillo-Cunliffe L., & Toga, A. W. (1999). Average 3-dimensional caudate surface representations in a case of juvenile-onset schizophrenia. *Archives of General Psychiatry, 53*, 617–624.

Bleuler, E. (1950). *Dementia praecox or the group of schizophrenias* (J. Zinkin, Trans). New York: International Universities Press. (Original work published 1911)

Brennan, P. A., & Walker, E. F. (2001). Vulnerability to schizophrenia: Risk factors in childhood and adolescence. In R. E. Ingram & J. M. Price Eds.), *Vulnerability to psychopathology: Risk across the lifespan* (pp. 329–354). New York: Guilford Press.

Bromet, E. J., & Fennig, S. (1999). Epidemiology and natural history of schizophrenia. *Biological Psychiatry, 46*, 871–881.

Burd, L., & Kerbeshian, J. (1987). A North Dakota prevalence study of schizophrenia presenting in childhood. *Journal of the American Academy of Child and Adolescent Psychiatry, 26*, 347–350.

Campbell, M. (1978). Use of drug treatment in infantile autism and childhood schizophrenia: A review. In M. A. Lipton, A. DiMascio, & K. F. Killam (Eds.), *Psychopharmacology: A generation of progress* (pp. 1451–1462). New York: Raven Press.

Campbell, M., Rapoport, J., & Simpson, G. M. (1999). Antipsychotics in children and adolescents. *Journal of the American Academy of Child and Adolescent Psychiatry, 38*, 537–545.

Cannon, T. D. (1998). Neurodevelopmental influences in the genesis and epigenesis of schizophrenia: An overview. *Applied and Preventive Psychology, 7*(1), 47–62.

Cannon, T. D., Barr, C. E., & Mednick, S. A. (1991). Genetic and perinatal factors in the etiology of schizophrenia. In E. F. Walker (Ed.), *Schizophrenia: A life course developmental perspective* (pp. 9–31). New York: Academic Press.

Cantor, S. (1988). *Childhood schizophrenia.* New York: Guilford Press.

Caplan, R. (1994). Communication deficits in childhood schizophrenia spectrum disorders. *Schizophrenia Bulletin, 20*, 671–684.

Carlsson, A. (1987). The dopamine hypothesis of schizophrenia 20 years later. In H. Hafner, W. F. Gattaz, & W. Janzarik (Eds.), *Search for the causes of schizophrenia* (Vol. 1, pp. 223–235). Berlin: Springer-Verlag.

Casanova, M. F., Carosella, N., & Kleinman, J. E. (1990). Neuropathological findings in a suspected case of childhood schizophrenia. *Journal of Neuropsychiatry and Clinical Neurosciences, 2*, 313–319.

Chakos, M. H., Lieberman, J. A., Bilder, R. M., Borenstein, M., Lerner, G., Borgets, B., Wu, H., Kinon, B., & Ashtari, M. (1994). Increase in caudate nuclei volumes of first-episode schizophrenic patients taking antipsychotic drugs. *American Journal of Psychiatry, 151*, 1430–1436.

Conolly, J. (1861–1862). Juvenile insanity. *American Journal of Insanity, 18*, 395–403.

Creak, M. (1964). Schizophrenia syndrome in childhood: Further progress report of a working party. *Developmental Medicine and Child Neurology, 6*, 530–535.

Cutting, L. P., & Docherty, N. M. (2000). Schizophrenia outpatients' perceptions of their parents: Is expressed emotion a factor? *Journal of Abnormal Psychology, 109*, 266–272.

Dohrenwend, B. P., Shrout, P. E., Link, B. G., & Skodol, A. E. (1987). Social and psychological risk factors for episodes of schizophrenia. In H. Hafner, W. F. Gattaz, & W. Janzarik (Eds.), *Search for the causes of schizophrenia* (Vol. 1, pp. 275–296). Berlin: Springer-Verlag.

DeLisi, L. E., & Lovett, M. (1991). The reverse genetic approach to the etiology of schizophrenia. In H. Hafner & W. F. Gattaz (Eds.), *Search for the causes of schizophrenia* (Vol. 2, pp. 144–170). Heidelberg, Germany: Springer-Verlag.

De Sanctis, S. (1906). Sopra alcuna varieta della demenza precoce. *Rivista Sperimentale di Freniatria e Medicina Legale delle Alienazioni Mentale*, pp. 141–165.

Edgell, H. G., & Kolvin, I. (1972). Childhood hallucinations. *Journal of Child Psychology and Psychiatry, 13*, 279–287.

Eggers, C. (1978). Course and prognosis in childhood schizophrenia. *Journal of Autism and Childhood Schizophrenia, 8*, 21–36.

Eggers, C. (1989). Schizoaffective disorders in childhood: A followup study. *Journal of Autism and Developmental Disorders, 19*, 327–342.

Falloon, I. R. H., Boyd, J. L., McGill, C. W., Williamson, M., Razani, J., Mos, H., Gilderman, A., & Simpson, G. (1985). Family management in the prevention of morbidity of schizophrenia: Clinical outcome of a two year longitudinal study. *Archives of General Psychiatry, 42*, 887–896.

Fish, B. (1968). Methodology in child psychopharmacology. In D. H. Efron, J. O. Cole, J. Levine, & J. R. Wittenborn (Eds.), *Psychopharmacology: Review of progress* (PHS Publication No. 1836, pp. 989–1001). Washington, DC: U.S. Government Printing Office.

Fish, B. (1977). Neurobiological antecedents of schizophrenia in children: Evidence for an inherited congenital neurointegrative deficit. *Archives of General Psychiatry, 34*, 1297–1313.

Fish, B. (1987). Infant predictors of the longitudinal course of schizophrenic development. *Schizophrenia Bulletin, 13*, 395–410.

Fish, B., & Ritvo, E. R. (1979). Psychoses of childhood. In J. D. Noshpitz (Ed.), *Basic handbook of child psychiatry* (Vol. 2, pp 249–304). New York: Basic Books.

Frazier, J. A., Giedd, J. N., Hamburger, S. D., Albus, K. E., Kaysen, D., Vaituzis, A. C., Rajapakse, J. C., Lenane, M. C., McKenna, K., Jacobsen, L. K., Gordon, C. T., Brier, A., & Rapoport, J. L. (1996). Brain anatomic magnetic resonance imaging in childhood-onset schizophrenia. *Archives of General Psychiatry, 53*, 617–624.

Garralda, M. E. (1984a). Hallucinations in children with conduct and emotional disorders: I. The clinical phenomena. *Psychological Medicine, 14*, 589–596.

Garralda, M. E. (1984b). Psychotic children with hallucinations. *British Journal of Psychiatry, 145*, 74–77.

Goldstein, M. J. (1987). The UCLA High Risk Project. *Schizophrenia Bulletin, 13*, 505–514.

Goldstein, M. J., Talovic, S. A., Nuechterlein, K. H., Fogelson, D. L., Subotnick, K., & Asarnow, R. (1992). Family interaction versus individual psychopathology: Do they indicate the same processes in the families of schizophrenics? *British Journal of Psychiatry, 161*, 97–102.

Gordon, C. T., Frazier, J. A., McKenna, K., Giedd, J., Zametkin, A., Zahn, T., Hommer, D., Hong, W., Kaysen, D., Albus, K. E., & Rapoport, J. L. (1994). Childhood-onset schizophrenia: An NIMH study in progress. *Schizophrenia Bulletin, 20*, 697–712.

Gordon, C. T., Krasnewich, D., White, B., Lenane, M., & Rapoport, J. L. (1994). Translocation involving chromosomes 1 and 7 in a boy with childhood-onset schizophrenia. *Journal of Autism and Developmental Disorders, 24*, 537–545.

Grant, D. A., & Berg, E. A. (1981). *Wisconsin Card Sorting Test.* Odessa, FL: Psychological Assessment Resources.

Green, W., Campbell, M., Hardesty, A., Grega, D., Padron-Gayol, M., Shell, J., & Erlenmeyer-Kimling, L. (1984). A comparison of schizophrenic and autistic children. *Journal of the American Academy of Child Psychiatry, 23*, 399–409.

Green, W., Padron-Gayol, M., Hardesty, A. S., & Bassiri, M. (1992). Schizophrenia with childhood onset: A phenomenological study of 38 cases. *Journal of the American Academy of Child and Adolescent Psychiatry, 35*, 968–976.

Hafner, H., Hambrecht, M., Loffler, W., Munk-Jorgenson, P., & Reichler-Rossier, A. (1998). Causes and consequences of the gender difference in age of onset of schizophrenia. *Schizophrenia Bulletin, 24*, 99–113.

Hamilton, E. B., Asarnow, J. R., & Tompson, M. (1999). Family interaction styles of children with depressive disorders, schizophrenia-spectrum disorders, and normal controls. *Family Process, 38*(4), 463–476.

Hibbs, E. D., Hamburger, S. D., Lenane, M., Rapoport, J. L., Kreusi, M. J. P., Keysor, C. S., & Goldstein, M. J. (1991). Determinants of expressed emotion in families of disturbed and normal children. *Journal of Child Psychology and Psychiatry, 32*, 757–770.

Hogarty, G. E., Kornblith, S. J., Greenwald, D., DiBarry, A. Cooley, S., Flesher, S., Reiss, D., Carter, M., & Ulrich, R. (1995). Personal therapy: A disorder-relevant psychotherapy for schizophrenia. *Schizophrenia Bulletin, 21*, 379–393.

Hollis, C. (1995). Child and adolescent (juvenile onset) schizophrenia: A case control study of premorbid developmental impairments. *British Journal of Psychiatry, 166*, 489–495.

Hollis, C. (2000). Adult outcomes of child- and adolescent-onset schizophrenia: Diagnostic stability and predictive validity. *American Journal of Psychiatry, 157*, 1652–1659.

Jacobsen, L. K., Giedd, J. N., Castellanos, F. X., Vaituzis, A. C., Hamburger, S. D., Kumra, S., Lenane, M. C., & Rapoport, J. L. (1998). Progressive reduction of temporal lobe structures in childhood-onset schizophrenia. *American Journal of Psychiatry, 155*, 678–685.

Jacobsen, L. K., Giedd, J. N., Rajapakse, J. C., Hamburger, S. D., Vaituzis, A. C., Frazier, J. A., Lenane, M. C., & Rapoport, J. L. (1997). Quantitative magnetic resonance imaging of the corpus callosum in childhood onset schizophrenia. *Psychiatry Research, 68*, 77–86.

Jacobsen, L. K., Giedd, J. N., Vaituzis, A. C., Hamburger, S. D., Rajapakse, J. C., Frazier, J. A., Kaysen, D., Lanane, M. C., McKenna, K., Gordon, C. T., & Rapoport, J. L. (1996). Temporal lobe morphology in childhood-onset schizophrenia. *American Journal of Psychiatry, 153*, 355–361.

Jacobsen, L. K., & Rapoport, J. L. (1998). Research update: Childhood-onset schizophrenia: Implications of clinical and neurobiological research. *Journal of Child Psychology and Psychiatry, 39*, 101–113.

Johannessen, J., McGlashan, T., Larsen, T. K., Horneland, M., Joa, I., Mardal, S., Kvebaek, R., Friis, S., Melle, I., Opjordsmoen, S., Simonsen, E., Ulrik, H., & Vaglum, P. (2001). Early detection strategies for untreated first-episode psychosis. *Schizophrenia Research, 51*, 39–46.

Jones, J. E. (1977). Patterns of transactional style deviance in the TAT's of parents of schizophrenics. *Family Process, 16*, 327–337.

Kallman, F. J., & Roth, B. (1956). Genetic aspects of preadolescent schizophrenia. *American Journal of Psychiatry, 112*, 599–606.

Kanner, L. (1949). Problems of nosology and psychodynamics of early infantile autism. *American Journal of Orthopsychiatry, 19*, 416–426.

Karatekin, C., & Asarnow, R. (1998a). Components of visual search in childhood-onset schizophrenia and attention-deficit/hyperactivity disorder. *Journal of Abnormal Child Psychology, 25*, 367–380.

Karatekin, C., & Asarnow, R. (1998b). Working memory in childhood-onset schizophrenia and attention-deficit/hyperactivity disorder. *Psychiatry Research, 80*, 165–176.

Karatekin, C., & Asarnow, R. (1999). Exploratory eye movements to pictures in childhood-onset schizophrenia and attention-deficit/hyperactivity disorder (ADHD). *Journal of Abnormal Child Psychology, 27*, 35–49.

Kavanagh, D. J., & Mueser, K. T. (2001). The future of cognitive and behavioral therapies in the prevention and early management of psychosis: Opportunities and risks. *Behavior Therapy, 32*, 693–724.

Kendler, K. S. (1988). The genetics of schizophrenia: An overview. In M. T. Tsuang & J. C. Simpson (Eds.), *Handbook of schizophrenia: Vol. 3. Nosology, epidemiology and genetics of schizophrenia* (pp. 437–462). Amsterdam: Elsevier.

Kendler, K. S., (1997). The genetic of schizophrenia. In H. I. Kaplan & B. J. Sadock (Eds.), *Comprehensive textbook of psychiatry* (pp. 321–357). Baltimore: Williams & Wilkins.

Kendler, K. S., & Diehl, S. R. (1993). The genetics of schizophrenia: A current, genetic epidemiologic perspective. *Schizophrenia Bulletin, 19*, 261–284.

Kendler, K. S., McGuire, M., Gruenberg, A. M., O'Hare, A., Spellman, M., & Walsh, D. (1993). The Roscommon Family Study: I. Methods, diagnosis of probands, and risk of schizophrenia in relatives. *Archives of General Psychiatry, 50*, 527–540.

Kendler, K. S., McGuire, M., Gruenberg, A. M., Spellman, M., & O'Hare, A. (1993). The Roscommon Family Study: II. The risk of nonschizophrenic nonaffective psychoses in relatives. *Archives of General Psychiatry, 50*, 645–652.

King, S. (2000). Is expressed emotion cause or effect in the mothers of schizophrenic young adults? *Schizophrenia Research, 45*(1–2), 65–78.

Kolvin, I. (1971). Psychoses in childhood: A comparative study. In M. Rutter (Ed.), *Infantile autism: Concepts, characteristics and treatment* (pp. 7–26). Edinburgh: Churchill Livingstone.

Kolvin, I., Ounsted, C., Humphrey, M., & McNay, A. (1971). Six studies in the childhood psychoses. *British Journal of Psychiatry, 118*, 385–395.

Konstantareas, M. M., & Hewitt, T. (2001). Autistic disorder and schizophrenia: Diagnostic overlaps. *Journal of Autism and Developmental Disorders, 31*, 19–28.

Kraepelin, E. (1971). *Dementia praecox and paraphrenia* (R. M. Barclay, Trans.; G. M. Robertson, Ed.). Huntington, NY: Krieger. (Original work published 1919)

Kumra, S., Frazier, J. A., Jacobsen, L. K., McKenna, K., Gordon, C. T., Lenane, M., Hamburger, S., Smith, A., Albus, K., Alaghband-Rad, J., & Rapoport, J. L. (1996). Childhood-onset schizophrenia: A double-blind clozapine–haloperidol comparison. *Archives of General Psychiatry, 53*, 1090–1097.

Kumra, S., Giedd, J. N., Vaituzis, A. C., Jacobsen, L. K., McKenne, K., & Bewell, J. (2000). Childhood-onset psychotic disorders: Magnetic resonance imaging of volumetric differences in brain structure. *American Journal of Psychiatry, 157*, 1467–1474.

Lawrie, S. M., & Abukmeil, S. S. (1998). Brain abnormality in schizophrenia: A systematic and quantitative review of volumetric magnetic resonance imaging studies. *Brain Journal of Psychiatry, 172,* 110–120.

Leff, J. P. (1991). Interaction of environment and personality in the course of schizophrenia. In H. Hafner & W. F. Gattaz (Eds.), *Search for the causes of schizophrenia* (Vol. 2, pp. 94–108). Berlin: Springer-Verlag.

Leff, J., P. Berkowitz, R., Shavit, N., Strachan, A., Glass, I., & Vaughn, C. (1989). A trial of family therapy v. a relatives group for schizophrenia. *British Journal of Psychiatry, 154,* 58–66.

Leff, J. P., Sartorius, N., Jablensky, A., Anker, M., Korten, A., Gulbinat, W., & Ernberg, G. (1991). The International Pilot Study of Schizophrenia: Five-year follow-up of findings. In H. Hafner & W. F. Gattaz (Eds.), *Search for the causes of schizophrenia* (Vol. 2, pp. 57–66). Berlin: Springer-Verlag.

Leff, J. P., & Vaughn, C. (1985). *Expressed emotion in families: Its significance for mental illness.* New York: Guilford Press.

Lenane, M. C., Nicolson, R., Bedwell, J., & Rapoport, J. L. (1999). Schizophrenia spectrum disorders in the relatives of patients with childhood-onset schizophrenia. *Schizophrenia Research, 36,* 92–104.

Levinson, D. F., & Mowry, B. J. (1991). Defining the schizophrenia spectrum: Issues for genetic linkage studies. *Schizophrenia Bulletin, 17,* 491–514.

Levitt, J. G., Blanton, R. E., Asarnow, R., Caplan, R., Capetillo-Cunliffe, L., Toga, A. W., & McCracken, J. (1999). Ventricular morphometry in childhood-onset schizophrenia. *Society for Neuroscience Abstracts, 25,* 489.

Levitt, J. G., Blanton, R. E., Caplan, R., Asarnow, R., Guthrie, D., Toga, A. W., Capetillo-Cunliffe, L., & McCracken, J. T. (2001). Medial temporal lobe in childhood-onset schizophrenia. *Psychiatry Research, 108,* 17–27.

Lewine, R. R. J. (1988). Gender in schizophrenia. In M. T. Tsuang & J. C. Simpson (Eds.), *Handbook of schizophrenia: Vol. 3. Nosology, epidemiology and genetics of schizophrenia* (pp. 379–397). Amsterdam: Elsevier.

Liberman, R. P., & Kopelowicz, A. (1995). Basic elements in biobehavioral treatment and rehabilitation of schizophrenia. *International Clinical Psychopharmacology, 9* (Suppl. 5), 51–58.

Linszen, D., Dingemans, P., Van Der Does, J. W., Nugter, A., Scholte, P., Lenior, R., & Goldstein, M. J. (1996). Treatment, expressed emotion and relapse in recent onset schizophrenic disorders. *Psychological Medicine, 26,* 333–342.

MacKain, S. J., Liberman, R. P., & Corrigan, P. W. (1994). Can coping and competence override stress and vulnerability in schizophrenia? In R. P. Liberman & J. Yager (Eds.), *Stress in psychiatric disorders* (pp. 53–82). New York: Springer.

Marenco, S., & Weinberger, D. R. (2000). The neurodevelopmental hypothesis of schizophrenia: Following a trail of evidence from cradle to grave. *Development and Psychopathology, 12,* 501–527.

McClellan, J. M., & Werry, J. S.(1992). Schizophrenia. *Psychiatric Clinics of North America, 15,* 131–148.

McClellan, J. M., Werry, J. S., Bernet, W., Arnold, V., Beitchman, J., Benson, S., Bukstein, O., Kinlan, J., Rue, D., & Shaw, J. (2001). Practice parameter for the assessment and treatment of children and adolescents with schizophrenia. *Journal of the American Academy of Child and Adolescent Psychiatry, 40*(7, Suppl.), 4S–23S.

McFarlane, W., Lukens, E., Link, B. Link, B., Dushay, R. et al. (1995). Multiple family groups and psychoeducation in the treatment of schizophrenia. *Archives of General Psychiatry 52,* 679–687.

McGlashan, T. (1998). Early detection and intervention of schizophrenia: rationale and research. *British Journal of Psychiatry, 172,* 3–6.

McGorry, P. D., Yung, A., Phillips, L., Yuen, H. P., Francey, S., Cosgrave, E., Germano, D., Bravin, J., Adlard, S., McDonald, T., Blair, A., & Jackson, H. (in press). A randomized controlled trial of interventions designed to reduce the risk of progression to first episode psychosis in a clinical sample with subthreshold symptoms. *Archives of General Psychiatry.*

McNeil, T. F. (1988). Obstetric factors and perinatal injuries. In M. T. Tsuang & J. C. Simpson (Eds.), *Handbook of schizophrenia: Vol. 3. Nosology, epidemiology and genetics* (pp. 319–344). Amsterdam: Elsevier.

Mednick, S. A., Machon, R. A., Huttunen, M. O., & Bonett, D. (1988). Adult schizophrenia following prenatal exposure to an influenza epidemic. *Archives of General Psychiatry, 45,* 189–192.

Nicolson, R., Malaspina, D., Giedd, J. N., Hamburger, S., Lenane, M., Bedwell, J., Fernandez, T., Berman, A., Susser, E., & Rapoport, J. L. (1999). Obstetrical complications and childhood-onset schizophrenia. *American Journal of Psychiatry, 156,* 1650–1652.

Nuechterlein, K. H. (1987).Vulnerability models for schizophrenia: State of the art. In H. Hafner, W. F. Gattaz & W. Janzarik (Eds.), *Search for the causes of schizophrenia* (Vol. 1, pp. 297–316). Berlin: Springer-Verlag.

Parnas, J., Schulsinger, F., Teasdale, T. W., Schulsinger, H., Feldman, P. M., & Mednick, S. A. (1982). Perinatal complications and clinical outcome within the schizophrenia spectrum. *British Journal of Psychiatry, 140,* 416–420.

Petty, L. P., Ornitz, E. M., Michelman, J. D., & Zimmerman, E. G. (1984). Autistic children who become schizophrenic. *Archives of General Psychiatry, 41,* 129–135.

Pool, D., Bloom, W., Mielke, D. H., Roniger, J. J., & Gallant, D. M. (1976). A controlled evaluation of Loxitane in seventy-five adolescents schizophrenic patients. *Current Therapeutic Research, 19,* 99–104.

Potter, H. W. (1933). Schizophrenia in children. *American Journal of Psychiatry, 12,* 1253–1270.

Prior, M., & Werry, J. S. (1986). Autism, schizophrenia, and allied disorders. In H. C. Quay & J. S. Werry (Eds.), *Psychopathological disorders of childhood* (3rd ed., pp. 156–210). New York: Wiley.

Rapoport, J. L., Giedd, J. N., Blumenthal, J., Hamburger, S., Jeffries, N., & Fernandez, T. (1999). Progressive cortical change during adoscence in childhood-onset schizophrenia: A longitudinal magnetic resonance imaging study. *Archives of General Psychiatry, 56,* 649–54.

Rapoport, J. L., Giedd, J. N., Kurma, S., Jacobsen, L., Smith, A., Lee, P., Nelson, J., & Hamburger, S. (1997). Childhood-onset schizophrenia: Progressive ventricular change during adolescence. *Archives of General Psychiarty, 54,* 897–903.

Remschmidt, H. E. (1993). Schizophrenic psychoses in children and adolescents. *Triangle, 32,* 15–24.

Remschmidt, H. E., Fleischhaker, Henninghaisen, K., & Schulz, E. (2000). Management of schizophrenia in children and adolescents: The role of clozapine. *Pediatric Drugs, 2,* 253–262.

Remschmidt, H. E., Schulz, E., Martin, M., Warnke, A., & Trott, G. (1994). Childhood-onset schizophrenia: History of the concept and recent studies. *Schizophrenia Bulletin, 20*, 727–746.

Riecher, A., Maurer, K., Loffler, W., Fatkenheuer, B., An Der Heiden, W., Munk-Jorgensen, P., Stromgren, E., & Hafner, H. (1991). Gender differences in age at onset and course of schizophrenic disorders: A contribution to the understanding of the disease? In H. Hafner & W. F. Gattaz (Eds.), *Search for the causes of schizophrenia* (Vol. 2, pp. 14–33). Berlin: Springer-Verlag.

Rosenfarb, I. S., Goldstein, M. J., Mintz, J., & Nuechterlein, K. H. (1995). Expressed emotion and subclinical psychopathology observable within the transactions between schizophrenic patients and their family members. *Journal of Abnormal Psychology, 104*, 259–267.

Rosenthal, D. (1970). *Genetic theory and abnormal behavior.* New York: McGraw-Hill.

Russell, A. T. (1994). The clinical presentation of childhood-onset schizophrenia. *Schizophrenia Bulletin, 20*, 631–646.

Russell, A. T., Bott, L., & Sammons, C. (1989). The phenomenology of schizophrenia occurring in childhood. *Journal of the American Academy of Child and Adolescent Psychiatry, 28*, 399–407.

Rutter, M. (1972). Childhood schizophrenia reconsidered. *Journal of Autism and Childhood Schizophrenia, 2*, 315–337.

Rutter, M., Greenfeld, D., & Lockyer, L. (1967). A five to fifteen year follow-up study of infantile psychosis: II. Social and behavioral outcome. *British Journal of Psychiatry, 113:* 1183–1199.

Sameroff, A. J. (1990). *Prevention of developmental psychopathology using the transactional model: Perspectives on host, risk agent, and environment interactions.* Paper presented at the first National Conference on Prevention Research, National Institute of Mental Health, Bethesda, MD.

Sartorius, N., Jablensky, A., Ernberg, G., Leff, J., & Gulbinat, W. (1987). Course of schizophrenia in different countries: Some results of a WHO international comparative 5-year follow-up study. In H. Hafner, W. F. Gattaz, & W. Janzarik (Eds.), *Search for the causes of schizophrenia* (Vol. 1, pp. 107–113). Berlin: Springer-Verlag.

Sawa, A., & Snyder, S. (2002). Schizophrenia: Diverse approaches to a complex disease. *Science, 296*, 692–695.

Schaeffer, J. L., & Ross, R. G. (2002). Childhood-onset schizophrenia: Premorbid and prodromal diagnostic and treatment histories. *Journal of the American Academy of Child and Adolescent Psychiatry, 41*, 538–545.

Schooler, N., Keith, S., Severe, J., Matthews, S., Bellack, A., Glick, I., Hargreaves, W., Kane, J., Ninan, P., Frances, A., Jacobs, M., Lieberman, J., Mance, R., Simpson, G., & Woerner, M. (1997). Relapse and rehospitalization during maintenance treatment of schizophrenia. *Archives of General Psychiatry, 54*, 453–463.

Schulz, S. C., Koller, M. M., Kishore, P. R., Hamer, R. M., Gehl, J. J., & Friedel, R. O. (1983). Ventricular enlargement in teenage patients with schizophrenia spectrum disorder. *American Journal of Psychiatry, 140*, 1592–1595.

Singer, M. T., & Wynne, L. C. (1965). Thought disorder and family relations of schizophrenics: IV. Results and implications. *Archives of General Psychiatry, 12*, 201–209.

Sowell, E. R., Levitt, J., Thompson, P. M., Holmes, C. J., Blanton, R. E., Kornsand, D. S., Caplan, R., McCracken, J., & Asarnow, R. F. (2000). Brain abnormalities in early onset schizophrenia spectrum disorder observed with statistical parametric mapping of structural magnetic resonance images. *American Journal of Psychiatry, 157*, 1475–1484.

Sowell, E. R., Toga, A., & Asarnow, R. F. (2000). Brain abnormalities observed in childhood-onset schizophrenia: A review of the structural magnetic resonance imaging literature. *Mental Retardation and Developmental Disabilities Research Reviews, 6*, 180–185.

Spencer, E. K., & Campbell, M. (1994). Schizophrenic children: Diagnosis, phenomenology and pharmacotherapy. *Schizophrenia Bulletin, 20*, 713–726.

Strandburg, R. J., Marsh, J. T., Brown, W. S., Asarnow, R. F., & Guthrie, D. (1994). Information processing deficits across childhood- and adult-onset schizophrenia: ERP correlates. *Schizophrenia Bulletin, 20*, 685–696.

Stubbe, D. E., Zahner, G., Goldstein, M. J., & Leckman, J. F. (1993). Diagnostic specificity of a brief measure of expressed emotion: A community study of children. *Journal of Child Psychology and Psychiatry, 34*, 139–154.

Subotnik, K. L., Asarnow, R. F., Nuechterlein, K. H., Fogelson, D. L., Gottesman, I. I., Thorpe, T. I., Payne, D. A., Giannini, C. A., Kuppinger, H. E., & Torquato, R. D. (2002). *MMPI vulnerability indicators for schizophrenia: UCLA Family Study findings for parents of offspring with childhood-onset schizophrenia or ADHD.* Manuscript submitted for publication.

Tanguay, P. E., & Asarnow, R. F. (1985). Schizophrenia in children. In A. J. Solnit, D. J. Cohen, & J. E. Schowalter (Eds.), *Psychiatry: Vol. 2. Child psychiatry* (pp. 1–10). Philadelphia: Lippincott.

Thomas, M. A., Yong, K., Levitt, J., Caplan, R., Curran, J., Asarnow, R., & McCracken, J. (1998). Preliminary study of frontal lobe [^{1}H]MR spectroscopy in childhood-onset schizophrenia. *Journal of Magnetic Resonance Imaging, 8*, 841–846.

Thompson, P. M., Vidal, C., Giedd, J. N., Gochman, P., Blumenthal, J., Nicolson, R., Toga, A. W., & Rapoport, J. L. (2001). Mapping adolescent brain change reveals dynamic wave of accelerated gray matter loss in very early-onset schizophrenia. *Proceedings of the National Academy of Sciences USA, 25*, 11650–11655.

Tompson, M. C., Asarnow, J. R., Goldstein, M. J., & Miklowitz, D. J. (1990). Thought disorder and communication problems in children with schizophrenia spectrum and depressive disorders and their parents. *Journal of Clinical Child Psychology, 19*, 159–168.

Usiskin, S. I., Nicolson, R., Krasnewich, D. M., Yan, W., Lenane, M., & Wudarsky, M. (1999). Velocardiofacial syndrome in childhood-onset schizophrenia. *Journal of the American Academy of Child and Adolescent Psychiatry, 38*, 1536–1543.

Volkmar, F. R., & Cohen, D. J. (1991). Comorbid association of autism and schizophrenia. *American Journal of Psychiatry, 148*, 1705–1707.

Volkmar, F. R., Cohen, D. J., Hoshino, Y., Rende, R. D., & Rhea, P. (1988). Phenomenology and classification of the childhood psychoses. *Psychological Medicine, 18*, 191–201.

Walk, A. (1964). The pre-history of child psychiatry. *British Journal of Psychiatry, 110*, 754–767.

Walker, E. F., & Diforio, D. (1997). Schizophrenia: A neural diathesis–stress model. *Psychological Review, 104*, 667–685.

Watkins, J. M., Asarnow, R. F., & Tanguay, P. (1988). Symptom development in childhood onset schizophrenia. *Journal of Child Psychology and Psychiatry, 29*, 865–878.

Weinberger, D. R. (1987). Implications of normal brain development for the pathogenesis of schizophrenia. *Archives of General Psychiatry, 44*, 660–669.

Weinberger, D. R. (1997). The biological basis of schizophrenia: New directions. *Journal of Clinical Psychiatry, 58*, 22–27.

Werry, J. S. (1992). Child and adolescent (early onset) schizophrenia: A review in light of DSM-III-R. *Journal of Autism and Developmental Disorders, 22*, 601–624.

Werry, J. S., & McClellan, J. M. (1992). Predicting outcome in child and adolescent (early onset) schizophrenia and bipolar disorder. *Journal of the American Academy of Child and Adolescent Psychiatry, 31*, 147–150.

Werry, J. S., McClellan, J. M., & Chard, L. (1991). Childhood and adolescent schizophrenia, bipolar, and schizoaffective disorders: A clinical and outcome study. *Journal of the American Academy of Child and Adolescent Psychiatry, 30*, 457–465.

Wintersteen, R. T., & Rasmussen, K. L. (1997). Fathers of persons with mental illness: A preliminary study of coping capacity and service needs. *Community Mental Health Journal, 33*, 401–413.

World Health Organization (WHO). (1993). *The ICD-10 classification of mental and behavioural disorders: Diagnostic criteria for research.* Geneva: Author.

Yeo, R. A., Hodde-Vargas, J., Hendren, R. L., Vargas, L. A., Brooks, W. M., Ford, C. C., Gangestad, S. W., & Hart, B. L. (1997). Brain abnormalities in schizophrenia-spectrum children: Implications for neurodevelopmental perspective. *Psychiatry Research: Neuroimaging Section, 76*, 1–13.

Zeitlin, H. (1986). *The natural history of psychiatric disorder in children* (Institute of Psychiatry, Maudsley Monograph No. 29). Oxford: Oxford University Press.

Zubin, J., & Spring, B. (1977). Vulnerability: A new view of schizophrenia. *Journal of Abnormal Psychology, 86*, 103–126.

CHAPTER ELEVEN

Mental Retardation (Intellectual Disabilities)

Robert M. Hodapp
Elisabeth M. Dykens

Mental retardation has historically been an area of intense interest to scientists, practitioners, and policy makers. Today as well, scientists are making important new discoveries, fostering hope that certain forms of mental retardation might be eliminated over the next few decades. Practitioners are excited by the participation of persons with mental retardation into the "mainstream," where these individuals are increasingly being treated as fully participating members of their societies. Policy makers too have contributed to this new era, passing laws that mandate educational and service rights, as well as an end to discrimination in employment and other areas.

To get a sense of just how far persons with mental retardation have advanced, some brief history is useful. Like the disciplines of social work, education, nursing, and medicine, the study and treatment of mental retardation essentially began in the mid-1800s (Scheerenberger, 1983). In the early 1850s, Samuel Gridley Howe founded the first public and Harvey Wilbur the first private training schools for persons with mental retardation in the United States. Quickly thereafter, facilities were started throughout the country; by 1890, 20 of these facilities were opened, in 15 states (Haskell, 1944). As originally operated, these facilities served as warm, humane "substitute families" for persons with mental retardation. These facilities—and the professionals who ran them—opened the way for the field's modern service delivery system.

In 1876, these training school directors met to form a society that was later to become the American Association on Mental Retardation (AAMR), the main organization for professionals working in mental retardation (Scheerenberger, 1983). Through its two journals, the *American Journal on Mental Retardation* and *Mental Retardation*, the AAMR has long promoted research, intervention, and social policy efforts on behalf of persons with mental retardation. As we describe below, the AAMR remains involved in many social and scientific debates.

In both earlier and present times, the study and treatment of mental retardation have constituted a multidisciplinary field, touching on numerous professions and perspectives that relate to individuals with mental retardation. In all these disciplines, research has been prominent, much of it related to new applications from the psychological and biological sciences. Such applications began early on, including Goddard's (1913a) studies employing the new Binet–Simon tests to examine residents at the Vineland (New Jersey) Training School in the years directly after the tests had been developed in France. Such "translations" of new developments to the population with mental retardation have always characterized the scientific study of mental retardation.

At the same time as the field has featured service, institutional, and scientific advances, many dark days have also occurred. Particularly important have been the many scandals and abuses first discovered in the 1960s (Blatt & Kaplan, 1966). In essence, the home-like training schools of the late 19th century often became the inhumane warehouses of the mid-20th century. Although less widespread, abuses have occurred in science and social policy as well, especially with regard to the "science" of eugenics (Dugdale, 1910; Goddard, 1913b) and the sterilization laws passed in California and other states during the 1920s (see Davies & Ecob, 1959).

This mixture of advances and abuses has led to the current situation, which can best be described as "monumental advances amidst monumental controversies." Advances have been made as we learn the causes, consequences, and cures (or at least management) of mental retardation, and most of this new knowledge has been gained over the past 40 years. It is startling to realize, for example, that the chromosomal cause of the most common genetic form of mental retardation—Down syndrome—was only discovered in 1959 (Lejeune, Gautier, & Turpin, 1959), or that the genetic basis of the second most common genetic form of mental retardation—fragile-X syndrome—was only understood in the late 1960s and early 1970s (see Dykens, Hodapp, & Leckman, 1994). Several hundred genetic causes of mental retardation have now been identified, and treatments for many seem likely over the next few decades. Similar advances have occurred in the biochemistry, psychology, and psychiatry of mental retardation.

But if the past decade has been an exciting time for those in mental retardation, so too has it been a contentious time. Debates continue as to the appropriate definition of mental retardation, the appropriate role of professionals as opposed to consumers (i.e., persons with mental retardation), and the best ways to study many aspects of behavior in these individuals. Such issues pit well-meaning persons against one another in ways that threaten progress.

To complicate matters further, we may be witnessing a renaming of the phenomenon itself. At its 2001 annual meeting, the AAMR decided to drop the term "mental retardation," though no replacement term was immediately agreed to. Several possibilities exist. Many European countries use the term "intellectual disability," and a major international journal is entitled the *Journal of Intellectual Disability Research*. In Great Britain, the term "learning disabilities" is often used for mental retardation, though the term has a totally different meaning in the United States. As this litany of contentious issues attests, research and intervention in mental retardation are in flux, and those involved are unsure or divided about many of the most basic issues.

This chapter describes the many issues and controversies that surround mental retardation. Although we express our opinions, our attempt throughout is to overview "the state of the art" in the mental retardation field. Such concerns range from definitional and diagnostic issues, to how one performs research, to how best one serves or supports persons with mental retardation.

WHAT IS MENTAL RETARDATION?

Core Features

When asked to describe a person with mental retardation, most people would probably speak of a person with Down syndrome, probably a boy. Some mention might be made that the problem first appears in childhood, and that the child learns at a slower rate, has deficient cognitive/mental processes, and is below normal in intelligence. Furthermore, most adults clearly differentiate "mental retardation" from "mental illness," where people talk of emotional instability, erratic behavior, and tenseness or anxiety (Caruso & Hodapp, 1988).

Although this description would be partially accurate, mental retardation is a much more complex phenomenon. For example, persons with mental retardation vary widely in their levels of functioning; in their abilities to function in school or at work; and in the degree to which they have concomitant emotional, physical, or medical conditions. The causes of mental retardation are also numerous, from the many genetic disorders to other pre-, peri-, and postnatal problems and insults.

At present, three major features are thought to characterize persons with mental retardation. First, these individuals have subnormal intellectual functioning. Defined as IQ scores below a certain level, this criterion highlights the intellectual nature of mental retardation. But intellectual deficits do not exist in a vacuum. A second important feature of mental retardation therefore involves deficits in adaptive behavior, or the ability to perform "daily activities required for personal and social self-sufficiency" (Sparrow, Balla, & Cicchetti, 1984, p. 6). Such abilities involve communicating one's needs to others; performing daily living skills, such as eating, dressing, grooming, and toileting; and being socialized to follow rules and to work and play with others. A third feature of mental retardation is that it begins early in life. Deficiencies caused by adult-onset degenerative diseases (e.g., Alzheimer disease) or adult-onset head trauma are not considered to be mental retardation.

Levels of Functioning

Lowered intelligence, impaired adaptive behaviors, and childhood onset give a basic sense of mental retardation, but these common features hide the wide variation from one person to another. For this reason, researchers have long described persons with mental retardation by their degree of intellectual impairment. This classification system designates persons with mental retardation as mildly, moderately, severely, or profoundly retarded.

"Mild mental retardation" (IQ = 55–70) constitutes the largest group of persons with mental retardation—possibly as many as 90%, according to the *Diagnostic and Statistical Manual of Mental Disorders*, fourth edition (DSM-IV; American Psychiatric Association [APA], 1994). These individuals appear similar to nonretarded individuals, and often blend into the nonretarded population in the years before and after formal schooling. As adults, some of these individuals hold jobs, marry, raise families, and are indistinguishable from nonretarded people; they may simply appear slow or need extra help in negotiating life's problems and tasks. More persons with mild mental retardation come from minority and low-socioeconomic-status (low-SES) backgrounds than would be expected from their numbers in the general population (Hodapp, 1994; Stromme & Magnus, 2000). This so-called "overrepresentation" of minority group members has been used to criticize measures of intelligence (see Reynolds & Brown, 1984), as well as to highlight the importance of both environmental–cultural (Ogbu, 1994) and genetic (Jensen, 1969) influences.

"Moderate mental retardation" (IQ = 40–54), the second most common level, refers to those persons with more intellectual and adaptive impairment. More of these individuals are diagnosed as having mental retardation during the preschool years. Many individuals with moderate mental retardation show one or more clear organic causes for their mental retardation. For example, many persons with Down syndrome and with fragile-X syndrome are at moderate levels of mental retardation. Although some persons with moderate mental retardation require few supportive services, most continue to require some help throughout life. In a study by Ross, Begab, Dondis, Giampiccolo, and Meyers (1985), for example, 20% of persons with IQs from 40 to 49 lived independently, while 60% were considered dependent and 20% totally dependent on others. In a similar way, some of these individuals held jobs in the outside work force as unskilled laborers, while others worked in supervised workshop programs.

"Severe mental retardation" (IQ = 20 or 25–39) refers to persons with more severe impairments. The majority of these individuals suffer from one or more organic causes of mental retardation. Many persons with severe mental retardation show concurrent physical or ambulatory problems, while others have respiratory, heart, or other co-occurring conditions. Most persons with severe mental retardation require some special assistance throughout their lives. Many live in supervised group homes or small regional facilities, and most work in either workshop or "pre-workshop" settings.

"Profound mental retardation" (IQ below 25 or 20) involves persons with the most severe levels of intellectual and adaptive impairments. These persons generally learn only the rudiments of communicative skills, and intensive training is required to teach them basic eating, grooming, toileting, and dressing behaviors. Persons with profound mental retardation require lifelong care and assistance. Almost all show organic causes for their mental retardation, and many have severe co-occurring conditions that sometimes lead to death during childhood or early adulthood. Some persons with profound mental retardation can perform preworkshop tasks, and most live in supervised group homes or small, specialized facilities.

Situational and Contextual Issues

Core features and levels of impairment highlight several issues that further complicate the picture of mental retardation. The first of these issues involves social system factors. As noted above, persons with mild mental retardation are often not diagnosed in the preschool years (Gruenberg, 1964). These individuals often become known to psychologists and social service workers during the school years (Larson et al., 2001).

Several reasons account for the school-based rise in the numbers of children considered to have mild mental retardation. Obviously, schools emphasize cognitive skills; when children are required to read, write, or perform arithmetic and other school subjects, their cognitive deficiencies become apparent. Their abilities are further challenged in junior high and high school, when more complex intellectual and academic tasks are required.

In addition, teachers have extensive experience in dealing with children of a particular age. Whereas a parent may not realize that the child is behind his or her age-mates intellectually, a primary or secondary school teacher has seen hundreds of 1st-, 4th-, or 10th-grade children. That teacher can identify and refer for testing children who have problems associated with mild mental retardation.

Such concerns have led to research into how, exactly, students come to be identified and diagnosed as having mental retardation. In the United States, this diagnostic process often begins when teacher concerns are expressed to so-called "student study teams" (SSTs; Del'Homme, Kasari, Forness, & Bagley, 1996). Such SSTs are generally multidisciplinary in nature, and are designed to help teachers to implement educational strategies that might head off further problems.

Once such problems appear more serious, however, referral is subsequently made for special education testing and diagnosis. At this point, one sees that schools often do not make decisions in line with AAMR, DSM-IV, or other formal diagnostic systems. In one study, for example, 35 children identified to SSTs had IQs below 75, but only 6 of these children (17%) were diagnosed as having mental retardation (MacMillan, Gresham, Siperstein, & Bocian, 1996). In contrast, the majority of children (19, or 54%) were diagnosed as having learning disabilities, even though few of these children (6 of 19) showed the large deficit in academic achievement (as measured by achievement tests) compared to aptitude (as measured by IQ tests) required for such a diagnosis. Probably due to the increased stigma of a diagnosis of mental retardation (as opposed to one of learning disabilities), school personnel may shy away from diagnosing children as having mental retardation. As MacMillan et al. (1996) note, their study supports the "position that mild mental retardation has all but ceased to exist as a diagnostic construct in the public schools" (p. 169). Such a conclusion may be somewhat extreme—particularly given that the study was conducted in California, where IQ testing is less often performed and where the SSTs did not have access to the researchers' IQ test data. Still, such findings do highlight some of the situational and contextual factors at play in diagnoses of mental retardation.

Again after the school years, persons with mild mental retardation often blend back into the larger population. Studies vary wildly in their prevalence rates, depending on when, where, and how they were conducted (see Kiely & Lubin, 1991, and Roeleveld, Zielhuis, & Gabreels, 1997, for discussions of epidemiology in mental retardation). However, such studies generally show low rates of mental retardation during the preschool years, gradual increases until a peak in early adolescence, and then gradual declines in the adult years. For the most part, this higher prevalence rate during the school years is due to the population with mild mental retardation; such individuals are most likely to be identified and diagnosed only during the school years (cf. Zigler & Hodapp, 1986).

In this sense, mental retardation is a social phenomenon that is influenced by schools and other social systems. Special educators even refer to "system-identified" samples, or persons with mental retardation who are identified through the school system (as opposed to by parents or physicians). Others decry the phenomenon of the so-called "6-hour retarded child"—the child who is considered to be mildly retarded while attending school, but not after school hours (or years). How system factors relate to mental retardation is a difficult, if not unresolvable, issue.

A second important complication involves the "overrepresentation" of minority and low-SES children within the retarded population (Artiles & Trent, 1994). Such overrepresentation seems due to the lower average IQ scores of African American and other minority groups, as well as to the generally lower scores of persons from lower-SES groups. Indeed, if minority or low-SES groups show an average IQ of, say, 90 or 85, then their entire "IQ curve" has been shifted to the left; many more individuals from these groups will therefore have IQ scores below 70, assuming that these groups also show standard deviations of approximately 15 points (i.e., as in the general population). Historically, such concern led the AAMR to change the IQ score criterion from below 85 to below 70 from 1961 to 1973 (Grossman, 1973). In addition, all definitions from the 1970s on have advocated the use of adaptive behavior as a central feature of mental retardation. The idea has been to ensure that persons with mental retardation truly do show intellectual and adaptive deficits. Yet even with these changes, the overrepresentation of minority and low-SES children continues, particularly among those children with mild mental retardation (MacMillan, Gresham, & Siperstein, 1993; Roeleveld et al., 1997).

DEFINITIONAL AND DIAGNOSTIC ISSUES

Definitions in mental retardation are complicated by the presence of two different professional groups that produce definitional and classificatory manuals. The first group, the APA (1994), currently considers mental retardation as the first of its "disorders usually first diagnosed in infancy, childhood, or adolescence." In addition, as noted in DSM-IV, mental retardation and personality disorders are listed along a separate axis to ensure "that consideration will be given to the possible presence of Personality Disorders and Mental Retardation that might otherwise be overlooked when attention is directed to the usually more florid Axis I disorders" (APA, 1994, p. 26).

The other main diagnostic and classification criteria are those presented by the AAMR. The AAMR has produced diagnostic manuals or revisions in 1959, 1961, 1973, 1977, and 1983 (see Grossman, 1983). In late 1992, the AAMR produced a revised definition of mental retardation (AAMR, 1992). This definition proposed sweeping definitional and classificatory changes from the organization's earlier manuals. We first describe two earlier sets of criteria (the 1983 AAMR and the 1987 DSM-III-R definitions). We then discuss the 1992 AAMR definition, as well as the APA's 1994 definition in DSM-IV. Finally, we provide an overview of the various definitions, and look ahead to the recently proposed revision of the AAMR manual.

The DSM-III-R and the 1983 AAMR Definitions

The criteria for a diagnosis of mental retardation promulgated in DSM-III-R (APA, 1987) are nearly identical to those provided in the AAMR's 1983 classification manual (Grossman, 1983). According to both manuals, mental retardation is characterized by three essential features: "(1) significantly subaverage general intellectual functioning, accompanied by (2) significant deficits or impairments in adaptive functioning, with (3) onset before the age of 18" (APA, 1987, p. 28).

Both the 1983 AAMR and the DSM-III-R criteria further specify the first two factors. "Significantly subaverage general intellectual functioning" is defined as an IQ score of 70 or below on the Wechsler Intelligence Scale for Children—Revised (WISC-R), the Stanford–Binet, the Kaufman Assessment Battery for Children (K-ABC), or some other individually administered psychometric test of intelligence. Deficits in adaptive behavior are defined as deficient functioning on the Vineland Adaptive Behavior Scales (Sparrow et al., 1984) or other adaptive behavior scales. If psychometric measures of adaptive behavior are lacking, "clinical judgment of general adaptation alone, the person's age and cultural background being taken into consideration, may suffice" (APA, 1987, p. 29).

The 1992 AAMR Definition

On the surface, the 1992 AAMR definition (AAMR, 1992) appears similar to the DSM-III-R and 1983 AAMR definitions. The definition reads as follows:

> Mental retardation refers to substantial limitations in present functioning. It is characterized by significantly subaverage intellectual functioning, existing concurrently with related limitations in two or more of the following applicable adaptive skill areas: communication, self-care, home living, social skills, community use, self-direction, health and safety, functional academics, leisure, and work. Mental retardation manifests before age 18. (p. 1)

In further specifying each of these criteria, the 1992 AAMR definition notes that "significantly subaverage" is equivalent to "IQ standard scores of approximately 70 or 75 and below" (p. 5). Although the exact meaning of this phrase remains unclear, most mental retardation researchers (e.g., MacMillan et al., 1993) have concluded that the 1992 definition essentially changes the IQ criterion from IQ below 70 to IQ below 75.

Similarly, the 1992 AAMR definition gives increasing weight to adaptive behavior. As opposed to general adaptive behavior deficits, the 1992

AAMR definition proposes 10 areas of adaptive behavior; the criteria for mental retardation are satisfied when the individual shows deficits in 2 or more of these 10 adaptive areas.

A third change in the 1992 AAMR definition involves levels of impairment. In an effort to conceptualize mental retardation more as an interaction between the person and the environment, the 1992 AAMR definition discards the categories of mental retardation based on levels of impairment; according to this system, individuals should no longer be considered to have mild, moderate, severe, or profound mental retardation. Instead, individuals are categorized in terms of their need for supportive services. Supportive services are specified as intermittent, limited, extensive, and pervasive; these levels of support are to be listed in each area of adaptive skills (AAMR, 1992, pp. 31–33).

The DSM-IV Definition

In contrast to earlier times, when the AAMR and APA definitions were virtually identical, the APA (1994) was faced with a difficult decision when providing its definition of mental retardation in DSM-IV. The AAMR's definitional manual was published in late 1992, and even before its publication the definition received harsh reviews (e.g., Jacobson & Mulick, 1992). Much of the criticism concerned the effects on practice—specifically, on diagnosis and classification—brought about by the 1992 AAMR definition. The critics decried the "political correctness" of this definition, noting that adherence to this system might have many unintended negative consequences. Should the APA make definitional changes in line with the controversial 1992 AAMR definition, or should it keep the definition more or less unchanged from DSM-III-R?

The resulting DSM-IV diagnostic criteria are in many ways a compromise. The DSM-IV definition (APA, 1994, p. 46) proposes the following three criteria of mental retardation:

A. Significantly subaverage intellectual functioning: an IQ of approximately 70 or below on an individually administered IQ test . . .
B. Concurrent deficits or impairment in present adaptive functioning (i.e., the person's effectiveness in meeting the standards expected for his or her age by his or her cultural group) in at least two of the following skill areas: communication, self-care, home living, social/interpersonal skills, use of community resources, self-direction, functional academic skills, work, leisure, health, and safety.
C. The onset is before age 18 years.

Thus DSM-IV retains the 1983 AAMR definition's IQ criterion of 70; the "approximately" refers to the small errors that occur in estimating any person's "true IQ" from a single testing (allowing the examiner some small leeway). At the same time, the DSM-IV system adopts the 1992 AAMR adaptive criterion of deficits in 2 of 11 adaptive domains—DSM-IV appears to consider as separate "health" and "safety," thus producing 11 as opposed to 10 adaptive domains (the 1992 AAMR definition combines the two). In addition, DSM-IV provides codes based on the "degree of severity reflecting level of intellectual impairment" (p. 46)—the mild, moderate, severe, and profound levels historically discussed in the study and treatment of mental retardation.

Overview of the Definitions of Mental Retardation

Of all the definitions of mental retardation discussed above (for convenience, we summarize the IQ and adaptive criteria from the two AAMR definitions and the DSM-IV in Table 11.1), the AAMR's 1992 definition has generated the most controversy. Much of this debate has centered on the IQ criterion. Most mental retardation workers feel that a change to "IQ standard scores of approximately 70 or 75 and below" effectively changes the IQ criterion to IQs below 75. Although a 5-point increase may seem small, the Gaussian (or bell curve) nature of the IQ distribution makes particularly important this "high-end" change in the definition of mental retardation. As MacMillan et al. (1993) note, "Small shifts in the upper limit have substantial consequences for the percentage of the population eligible to be diagnosed with mental retardation (Reschly, 1992). *Twice as many people are eligible* when the cutoff is 'IQ 75 and below' as when it is 'IQ 70 and below'" (p. 327; emphasis in original).

In a similar way, many critics have derided the changes in the adaptive behavior criterion. The 1992 AAMR definition proposes 10 areas of adaptive behavior, including such rarely tested areas as leisure, health and safety, community use, and self-direction. But factor-analytic studies of adaptive behavior have consistently revealed from two to seven factors of adaptive behavior, with a single

TABLE 11.1. Comparing the Main Definitions of Mental Retardation

Definition	IQ	Adaptive
1983 AAMR definition (Grossman, 1983)	"IQ 70 and below on standardized tests of intelligence" (can extend to IQ 75, "depending on the reliability of the intelligence test used")	"Significant limitations in meeting standards of maturation, learning, personal independence and/or social responsibility that are expected for his or her age level and cultural group, as determined by clinical assessment and, usually, standardized scales."
1992 AAMR definition (AAMR, 1992)	"IQ standard scores of approximately 70 or 75 and below"	"Limitations in two or more of the following applicable skill areas" (10 listed; see text)
DSM-IV definition (APA, 1994)	IQ standard scores of "approximately 70 or below"	"Concurrent deficits or impairments in present adaptive functioning . . . in at least two of the following areas" (11 listed; see text)

primary factor accounting for most of the variance (Harrison, 1987; McGrew & Bruininks, 1989). It thus seems inappropriate to test 10 (or 11) areas when little empirical support suggests that the construct has 10 separate domains.

A further problem is the absence of formal, psychometrically sound measures for several of these domains. For such areas as leisure, health and safety, and use of community resources, for example, it is unclear exactly how (or with which instrument) these domains are to be measured. The 1992 AAMR definition allows for clinical judgment to be used in these cases. In fairness, all other diagnostic manuals—including the 1987 DSM-III-R and the 1983 AAMR—allow the use of clinical judgment in the evaluation of adaptive deficiencies, but problems associated with clinical judgment would seem exacerbated when there are so many domains. Making things more difficult are the findings that many of these domains are not independent, and that many are new to clinicians and other social service personnel.

A final issue concerns the levels of impairment. In the 1992 AAMR definition, the authors have disposed of mild, moderate, severe, and profound mental retardation in favor of four levels of environmental supports (intermittent, limited, extensive, and pervasive). The authors' desire was to change the concept of mental retardation from an inherent characteristic of the individual to an interaction between the individual and the services needed by that individual. In this way, the "problem" of mental retardation is shared by the individual and that individual's environments.

Although the change is well-meaning, its effects remain unclear. Researchers and clinicians have long used levels of mental retardation as a way to characterize an individual's level of impairment. Such levels of intellectual impairment are sometimes, but not always, related to needed levels of support. Whereas persons with IQs in the moderate, severe, and profound ranges almost always need some supports, those with mild retardation vary widely in their adaptive abilities. For example, in their study of special education students as adults, Ross et al. (1985) found that whereas 64% of persons with mild mental retardation functioned independently, 24% and 12% were either partially or totally dependent on others, even though they were at identical intellectual levels. The move away from level of impairment to levels of support thus generates unnecessary confusion.

For both clinicians and researchers, then, the 1992 AAMR definition's lack of attention to basic psychometric issues is troubling (Gresham, MacMillan, & Siperstein, 1995). Many critics (e.g., Jacobson & Mulick, 1992; MacMillan et al., 1993) predicted that if the new AAMR definition were to be followed, it would lead to an increase in the size of the population with mental retardation, greater numbers of incorrect diagnoses, and increases in the overrepresentation of several minority groups. Jacobson and Mulick (1996) even led the American Psychological Association's Division 33 on mental retardation to adopt its own definition. Their definition was much closer to the DSM-III-R, 1983 AAMR, and DSM-IV definitions. Given that so many professionals and groups criticized the 1992 AAMR definition, its fate was in question from even before its formal publication in late 1992.

And what, in fact, has been the fate of the 1992 AAMR definition of mental retardation? With very few exceptions, researchers have ignored it. In published articles, one sees almost no research articles that use an IQ of 75 as the IQ cutoff, or that mention the 10 (or 11) hypothesized domains of adaptive behavior. Researchers similarly have continued to ignore subjects' "degrees of needed supports"—as opposed to their levels of impairment. Examining how subject groups were described from 1993 through 1997 in the *American Journal on Mental Retardation*, *Mental Retardation*, or *Education and Training in Mental Retardation*, Polloway, Smith, Chamberlain, Denning, and Smith (1999) found that 98.5% of articles employed the Grossman (1983) level-of-impairment descriptors (mild, moderate, severe, and profound mental retardation). Polloway et al. (1999) conclude that the "supports model" championed by the 1992 AAMR definition "has had no significant impact in terms of subject description in mental retardation research" (p. 203).

In a similar way, societal institutions mostly do not use the 1992 AAMR definition. In a survey of mental retardation guidelines used by the 50 states plus the District of Columbia, Denning, Chamberlain and Polloway (2000) found that 44 states continued using the 1983 AAMR manual for definition and classification, 4 reported use of the 1992 AAMR manual as the basis of their regulations, and 3 remaining states used neither model. Thus states, and the practitioners working within those states, also seem to be relying on the 1983 AAMR definition.

Even given these and other criticisms (e.g., Greenspan, 1997), the AAMR has recently begun revising the 1992 AAMR manual (Ad Hoc Committee on Terminology and Classification, 2001). Such revisions, which currently are only in the discussion stage, will continue to include the three diagnostic criteria of all earlier definitions: IQ, adaptive behavior, and onset before age 18. At the same time, the proposed AAMR definition will more fully emphasize the contexts in which functioning occurs, the need to consider cultural and linguistic diversity, and the ties of diagnosis and classification to interventions and supports (Ad Hoc Committee on Terminology and Classification, 2001). Although each emphasis seems fairly uncontroversial when stated in the abstract, it remains unclear how, specifically, the Ad Hoc Committee will define and classify persons with mental retardation. One can only hope that the many valid criticisms of the 1992 AAMR definition will have some impact on future formulations.

DEVELOPMENTAL COURSE AND PROGNOSIS

As noted earlier, DSM-IV considers mental retardation as a disorder that begins in childhood and persists in relatively stable form into adulthood. Although in general this characterization is accurate, several qualifications are necessary.

Stability of IQ

The first issue involves the stability of intelligence as measured by IQ tests. For children in general, IQ tests given in the infancy years do not predict later IQ. For example, the correlation is essentially 0 between Bayley Developmental Quotient scores (i.e., "infant IQs") when children are 1 year of age and IQ scores when children are 12 years old (Vernon, 1979). Yet by the time children are 4 years of age, the correlation with IQ 12 years later is .77; similar correlations—ranging from .70 to .90—occur when children are tested during middle to late childhood or adulthood, then again 6 or 12 years later.

For children with mental retardation, the picture is somewhat different in that even the youngest infants show IQ stability, particularly at the lower IQ levels. Infants with IQ scores below 50 on the Bayley test are likely to continue to have low IQs in their childhood and adult years (Maisto & German, 1986). Similarly, in a 5-year longitudinal study of children who had mild to moderate delays at age 3, Bernheimer and Keogh (1988) found very high correlations (.70 to .90) between early and later IQ. From a mean IQ of 67.1 at age 3, these children showed a mean IQ of 70.3 when tested 6 years later. Similarly, in a study of children tested at 4-year intervals, Silverstein (1982) also found high stability in average IQ, from 65.7 at age 11 to 64.0 at age 14. Such stability even continues on into adulthood. In the sole study of this issue, Ross et al. (1985) examined adults who had been in special education classes as children 35 years earlier. These researchers concluded that IQ scores "showed no meaningful increase over some 35 years" (p. 69).

But group stability over time does not imply that the IQ stays constant for every single individual. Many studies have found that individual

IQs can change up or down, and that most changes occur for children at or just above the mild mental retardation range (e.g., Goodman & Cameron, 1978). As a result, many persons who test in the mildly retarded range on first testing will show slightly higher IQs on second testing, thereby making it unclear who should and should not be diagnosed with mental retardation. Such IQ changes are not as often observed in children with moderate, severe, and profound mental retardation. As Bernheimer and Keogh (1988) note, "the predictive validity of developmental tests is related to level of performance early on, with less reliable prediction for the children within the higher developmental quotient range" (p. 541).

Type of Retardation

A second issue affecting the stability of IQ concerns the child's type of mental retardation. Although we discuss this issue in more detail below, children with different types of mental retardation vary in their trajectories of intellectual development as they get older. Children with Down syndrome decrease in IQ over time; these children continue to develop in intelligence, but they do so at slower and slower rates throughout the childhood years (see Hodapp, Evans, & Gray, 1999, for a review).

A similar problem occurs in fragile-X syndrome, but mainly in late middle childhood or the teen years. Thus boys with fragile-X syndrome show steady or near-steady IQs during the preschool period (Bailey, Hatton, & Skinner, 1998) and even until 10–15 years of age, at which point their development slows considerably (Dykens et al., 1989; Hodapp, Dykens, et al., 1990). In fragile-X syndrome, these slowings appear to be age-related; that is, boys of whatever IQ with this syndrome show these slowings during the 10- to 15-year age period, suggesting some link to pubertal development. Whatever the reason for such slowings, fragile-X and Down syndromes show that the specific type of mental retardation may affect rates of intellectual development as children get older.

Although less often examined, trajectories of adaptive behavior may also change based on a child's type of mental retardation. We (Dykens, Hodapp, & Evans, 1994) found that the Vineland adaptive behavior age-equivalent scores of children with Down syndrome "plateaued" during the middle childhood years (although a more recent longitudinal study did not find plateauing adaptive scores in 3- to 10-year-old children with Down syndrome; Hauser-Cram et al., 2001). Similar to findings for IQ (Gibson, 1966) and grammatical development (Fowler, 1988), children with Down syndrome as a group seem to make few advances in adaptive behavior between the ages of approximately 7 and 11 years, even as development occurs before and after these times. In fragile-X syndrome, the early teen years again seem implicated in the slowing of development. Dykens, Ort, et al. (1996) found that boys with fragile-X syndrome slowed in adaptive levels in the early teen years, even after they had been developing steadily (albeit at a slowed pace) until that time.

Mental retardation is, then, a relatively stable condition from childhood into adulthood, but a condition that is affected by a child's level of impairment and type of retardation. In addition, certain intensive early intervention programs—such as that mounted by the Abecedarian Project (Ramey & Ramey, 1992)—have been shown to boost IQ scores by approximately 10–15 points, although more family-centered, less "IQ-oriented" interventions seem more effective in promoting school and postschool achievement (e.g., Seitz, 1992). For many reasons, then, one's IQ score is not perfectly stable. Given that IQ is not perfectly stable, some individuals will go into and out of the mental retardation category. More IQ instability seems to occur among persons with mild mental retardation; persons with more severe levels of mental retardation show higher test–retest stability in IQ over the childhood and adulthood years. In addition, certain types of mental retardation show slowings or plateaus in intellectual and adaptive development, leading to greater impairments as these children get older.

EPIDEMIOLOGY

Prevalence

Depending on where one draws IQ and adaptive cutoff scores, the numbers of persons with mental retardation will vary widely. But even with a stable IQ criterion of 70 and below, the number of persons with mental retardation is open to debate. The standard view is that approximately 3% of the population has mental retardation. This 3% number is derived from adding the 2.28% of people with IQs two or more standard deviations below the population mean (i.e., IQs below 70, given a normal bell curve of intelligence) to some "extra" persons who will be described below. But this standard view makes several assumptions that seem, on the surface, unacceptable. Jane Mercer (1973), an early and leading proponent for a prevalence rate of only 1%, first described these four assumptions, and we discuss them below.

1. *IQ as the sole criterion of mental retardation*. A 3% prevalence rate implies that IQ is the sole criterion of mental retardation. But in all recent definitions of mental retardation, adaptive behavior is also highlighted. Terms such as "accompanied by significant limitations in adaptive functioning" (APA, 1994, p. 39) are common, highlighting that intellectual deficits by themselves, constitute only one of the diagnostic criteria. But adaptive behavior and IQ levels are not synonymous, particularly at mild levels of mental retardation. Especially for persons with mild mental retardation, some individuals will show IQ scores below 70 and have adaptive deficits, whereas others will show IQ scores below 70 and not have adaptive deficits. To the extent that IQ and adaptive behavior are not correlated, fewer and fewer children will be both intellectually and adaptively impaired.

2. *IQ stability*. Although IQ scores are relatively stable after infancy and for lower-IQ children, persons with mild mental retardation will often show increases from one testing to another. Such IQ changes seem more likely among children with mild mental retardation. As in the discussion of IQ as the sole criterion of mental retardation, the instability of IQ—particularly its likelihood of "regressing to the population mean" (i.e., going up) on second testings—makes it likely that fewer persons will be diagnosed with mental retardation.

3. *System issues*. A third issue relates to diagnostic practices. The "school-based" nature of diagnosis—again with children in the mild range of mental retardation—means that fewer children are identified during the preschool and after-school years. Indeed, even among children with severe and profound mental retardation, increasing prevalence rates appear until about the age of 15, mainly due to systems not identifying children at the earlier ages (Roeleveld et al., 1997). Again, prevalence rates are affected.

4. *Life expectancy*. A final issue relates to death rates. At the lower levels of functioning, death tends to occur at earlier ages. Earlier deaths occur especially in persons with profound mental retardation, particularly when these individuals have ambulatory or respiratory problems (Eyman & Miller, 1978). Several specific etiologies of mental retardation also seem prone to earlier deaths; for example, Down syndrome is characterized by a high prevalence of heart ailments, respiratory problems, leukemia, and early-onset Alzheimer disease (Pueschel, 1987). Although recent medical advances have lengthened the life expectancy of persons with Down syndrome into the late 50s, this span is still 20 or so years less than the life expectancies of persons without mental retardation. Similar to persons with Down syndrome, individuals with Prader–Willi syndrome (another genetic disorder of mental retardation) are prone to earlier deaths, due to the health complications related to the disorder's often-occurring extreme obesity (Dykens & Cassidy, 1996).

As a result of these four factors, the prevalence rates of mental retardation are generally below 3%. DSM-IV estimates the prevalence rate at approximately 1%. Although this rate may be slightly low, a 3% rate seems too high. In the few studies so far, rates of about 2% have often been found (Zigler & Hodapp, 1986), particularly when studies have examined every person in a town or region. Other studies, especially those employing registries or hospital records, have more often reported rates from below 1% to 1.5% (see Larson et al., 2001, for a review). These percentages include a rate of approximately 0.4% for individuals in the severe and profound ranges (Abramowicz & Richardson, 1975; Roeleveld et al., 1997; Stromme & Hagburg, 2000), along with wildly varying rates of individuals with mild mental retardation. But with the exception of prevalence rates for individuals with severe and profound mental retardation, all of these numbers depend on each individual study's specific diagnostic and case-finding procedures. Summarizing 43 prevalence studies performed from 1981 through 1995, Roeleveld et al. (1997) concluded that these studies reveal "an enormous gap in our knowledge about [mental retardation]. Many studies are hampered by imperfections in study methodology, and valid estimates of prevalence rates are scarce. There seems to be a strong need for standardization of definitions and research methods in this area" (p. 130).

Sex Differences

More males than females are found in the population with mental retardation (APA, 1994). In

Stromme and Hagberg's (2000) recent study, for example, males exceeded females by a ratio of 1.3:1, and other studies also show a 20–40% excess in males versus females. This overabundance of males can be seen at both the more severe and more mild levels of mental retardation, and across studies performed many years apart and with differing methodologies (Roeleveld et al., 1997).

Why such discrepancies exist is less clear. Some authors argue that the male central nervous system is more susceptible to a wide range of prenatal and postnatal insults (McLaren & Bryson, 1987); others contend that parents may differentially register their children, or that some other case-finding discrepancy accounts for at least some of this difference.

Another partial explanation involves sex-linked disorders, particularly fragile-X syndrome (Dykens, Hodapp, & Finucane, 2000). Fragile-X syndrome is now recognized as the second most common genetic disorder (after Down syndrome) and the most common hereditary disorder associated with mental retardation. That is, unlike Down syndrome, fragile-X syndrome is passed down from one generation to the next.

Although the gene for fragile-X syndrome (the FMR-1 gene) is located on the X chromosome, this syndrome does not follow a traditional X-linked inheritance pattern. About one-third to one-half of the females who carry and transmit the disorder are themselves affected, showing mild to moderate cognitive or emotional involvements. Furthermore, about 20% of males with the FMR-1 gene transmit the disorder but are themselves unaffected. Peculiarities of the FMR-1 gene account for some of this variable expression in males and females. Overall, though, more boys than girls are affected with fragile-X syndrome. It is partly due to the prevalence of fragile-X syndrome and other X-linked disorders that more males than females have mental retardation.

Socioeconomic and Ethnic Factors

As mentioned above, mental retardation is more prevalent among children who are of lower SES and who are from minority groups. Like many findings in mental retardation, however, the tie of mental retardation to low-SES and minority status is found primarily in children with mild mental retardation; children at more severe levels of mental retardation appear to occur about equally in different racial and socioeconomic groups.

This relationship between mild mental retardation and parental SES—and its highly correlated measure, parental IQ—was first noted in a classic study by Reed and Reed (1965). Studying several generations of families in Minnesota, Reed and Reed found that children of low-IQ parents tended to have lower IQs themselves, whereas children of higher-IQ parents generally had higher IQs (see also Broman, Nichols, Shaughnessy, & Kennedy, 1987). Such relations between mental retardation and SES have most recently been found in a Norwegian population study, in which Stromme and Magnus (2000) noted a higher prevalence both of mild mental retardation and of "unspecified" mental retardation (which is associated with mild mental retardation) in children of lower-SES parents. Both genetic and environmental factors probably account for such findings, but, again, reasonably strong relations exist between parental SES and IQ levels and children's IQs, particularly within the mild range of mental retardation.

The issue of mild mental retardation's association with race is more complicated. In many studies, average IQ levels for the African American population are lower than those found in the European American population. As a result, more African American children would be expected to be among the mildly retarded group; this indeed has been the general finding (MacMillan et al., 1993). Again, many environmental and cultural factors are involved, as is the possibility that tests may be biased in favor of children from European American, middle-class backgrounds. Concern over minority overrepresentation partly led to the AAMR's change in the IQ criterion from 85 to 70 in its 1973 manual (Grossman, 1973). The idea was that children with mental retardation should show significant intellectual deficits that co-occur with the children's problems in adaptive behavior.

In recent years, many school and mental retardation professionals have de-emphasized even further the importance of IQ in diagnostic decisions. California has gone furthest in this regard, mainly as a result of a well-known court case against the San Francisco school system. In this case, *Larry P. vs. Riles* (1979), parent advocates joined professionals such as Jane Mercer in arguing that African American children were being unfairly placed in special education classes on the basis of IQ test results. The plaintiffs further argued that IQ tests were biased against African American children, and that the use of these tests was the main reason for the overrepresentation of minority children in special education programs. Other professionals argued strongly against such sweeping generalizations. They noted that, considered alone, lower average IQ scores do not constitute evidence that tests are biased against minority group children. Furthermore, these professionals questioned whether IQ tests were the major reason why minorities are overrepresented in special education classes, especially given the fact that most children are not tested with psychometric instruments until they have already failed in school (Lambert, 1981). In spite of these arguments, the presiding judge in the *Larry P.* case, Judge Peckham ruled for the plaintiffs, holding that IQ tests are biased and should not be used in placement decisions for minority group children. California school systems now prohibit IQ tests in decisions to place minority group children in special education classes.

Regardless of one's views of the correctness of Judge Peckham's ruling, the *Larry P.* decision has produced several changes in diagnostic practice in California. Lambert (1981) notes that the judge's decision has led to fewer diagnoses of mild mental retardation in California's school systems; whereas 35,110 children were diagnosed as "educable mentally retarded" (the school term for mild retardation) in the 1973–1974 school year, only 19,370 were diagnosed as such in 1977–1978. More recent support for the "disappearing" (or at least shrinking) population of children with mild mental retardation is seen in the study by MacMillan et al. (1996; discussed above).

Furthermore, Prasse and Reschly (1986) note that school psychologists now give greater weight to tests of intellectual processing and of adaptive behavior. Ironically, the decision has not affected overrepresentation rates per se. Taylor (1990) notes that minority overrepresentation continues among the mildly retarded school population, particularly among California's African American children (MacMillan, Hendrick, & Watkins, 1988). Minority and SES factors in mild mental retardation remain difficult and unresolved.

THEORETICAL FRAMEWORKS

As with any population, different theoretical perspectives have been used to conceptualize individuals with mental retardation. We detail below several aspects of developmental approaches, then briefly discuss a few other prominent perspectives. Table 11.2 highlights the major theoretical approaches.

Developmental Approaches

Some of the greatest developmental thinkers of the 20th century were interested in mental retardation. Werner (1941) examined children with mental retardation in his early work at the Wayne State Training School outside Detroit; Piaget and Inhelder (1947; see also Inhelder, 1943/1968) examined thinking in children with retardation; and Vygotsky (Reiber & Carton, 1993) started the entire field of "defectology" in the Soviet Union during the late 1920s (Hodapp, 1998).

But a fully fledged "developmental approach" to mental retardation only began in the late 1960s. At that time, Zigler (1969) applied the sequences and structures found in nonretarded children to children with mental retardation. Zigler's focus was mainly on children with "familial mental retardation"—that is, children showing no obvious organic insult that caused their mental retardation. In recent years, however, developmental approaches have included newer work on families and other ecologies in which children develop (Hodapp, 1997a), and they have been applied to children with Down syndrome (Cicchetti & Beeghly, 1990), fragile-X syndrome (Dykens, Hodapp, & Leckman, 1994), and other organic conditions causing mental retardation. We now discuss three issues in these expanded approaches: sequences, cross-domain relations, and families.

Sequences

The most salient aspect of all developmental approaches concerns sequences of development. In Zigler's (1969) original approach, he proposed the "similar-sequence hypothesis"—the idea that children with mental retardation (particularly those with familial mental retardation) would proceed, in order, through the various cognitive sequences found in nonretarded children's development. Children with mental retardation were predicted to proceed from sensorimotor to preoperational to concrete operational to formal operational thought, and to proceed in order even through the substages of sensorimotor (e.g., Dunst, 1980) and other Piagetian stages. Whenever children without retardation proceed in invariant order, children with mental retardation too should traverse an identical sequence.

TABLE 11.2. Theoretical Frameworks Used in Mental Retardation

Framework	Main characteristics	Implications in mental retardation
Developmental		
Child issues	Use of normal development to inform us about populations with mental retardation Similar-sequence and similar-structure hypotheses Two-group approach and revisions	Sequences are used in curriculum; framework identifies important prerequisites and domains of development; populations with mental retardation tell us about nonretarded development; focus on development in persons with different types of mental retardation
Family issues	Family systems reactions to offspring with mental retardation Double ABCX model Stress-and-coping emphases	Interventions with all members and subsystems of families; identification of stressors and ameliorating factors
Eco-cultural	Relation of culture and disability Familial reactions based on cultural norms and expectations	Helps determine culturally sensitive interventions
Social role	Person with mental retardation plays a role in a social system Emphasis on system's relations to person	Highlights effects of school, social service, and other institutions; questions professional practice
Behaviorist	Behaviors due to history of environmental rewards, punishments Emphasis on how changes in environment lead to improved performance	Successfully teaches lowest-functioning individuals self-help skills; decreases maladaptive behaviors; teaches parents techniques to control behavior and teach new behaviors

With very few exceptions, the similar-sequence hypothesis has held true for children with mental retardation. Across many Piagetian and other cognitive and linguistic sequences, these children—like nonretarded children—have been found to develop in the same sequences. Such sequential development has been found in examinations of several sensorimotor concepts, affective responding, identity and equivalence conservation, seriation, transitivity, moral reasoning, comparison processes, time, space, relative thinking, role taking, mental imagery, geometric concepts, and classification and class inclusion (for a review of these studies, see Weisz & Zigler, 1979).

Furthermore, such similar sequences have been found to occur in children with familial and with various organic forms of mental retardation. For example, Cicchetti and Mans-Wagener (1987), Dunst (1990) and others have noted that the sensorimotor development of children with Down syndrome occurs in an identical order to sensorimotor development in nonretarded children. Children with Down syndrome also show identically ordered development in such areas as symbolic play (Beeghly, Weiss-Perry, & Cicchetti, 1990) and language (Fowler, 1988).

Cross-Domain Relations

The second tenet of Zigler's (1969) original developmental formulation concerned the so-called "similar-structure hypothesis"—that children with mental retardation have the same organization of intelligence as do nonretarded children. Hypothesized most directly for children with familial mental retardation, the similar structure hypothesis predicts that these children should perform similarly to nonretarded children when matched on overall mental age (MA) or other indices of overall mental functioning. Thus children with and without mental retardation who have the same MA should perform similarly on attentional, linguistic, information-processing, vocabulary, or other cognitive or linguistic tasks. Having no single "defect" or deficit causing their impaired intellectual functioning, children with familial mental retardation, like all groups of children, should demonstrate even or flat profiles from one domain to another.

For the most part, the similar-structure hypothesis has been supported, at least when children have familial mental retardation (Weisz, Yeates, & Zigler, 1982). These children may have some slight deficits in memory and learning set formation compared to MA-matched nonretarded children (Weiss, Weisz, & Bromfield, 1986), but the reasons for such possible deficits are unclear. Children with familial mental retardation may indeed have deficits in memory, learning set formation, or information-processing skills (Mundy & Kasari, 1990); conversely, these children's relatively poor performance may be due to the trouble these children have in staying motivated to perform what are often boring, repetitive tasks (Weisz, 1990). Yet these children perform similarly to MA-matched nonretarded children on Piagetian tasks, making the entire issue less clear-cut.

The picture for children with organic mental retardation is much clearer. Over many studies, children with organic mental retardation perform worse than do nonretarded MA-matched children (Weisz et al. 1982). In contrast to children with familial mental retardation, then, these children do appear to have one or more specific areas of deficit.

But researchers now realize that organic mental retardation is not a single entity, and that children with different etiologies differ in their behaviors. For example, children with Down syndrome demonstrate particular deficits in linguistic grammar relative to their abilities in other areas (Fowler, 1990). Boys with fragile-X syndrome perform reasonably well on holistic, Gestalt-like tasks and tasks tapping learned knowledge (i.e., achievement tasks). In contrast, these boys are particularly weak in sequential (or bit-by-bit) processing, by comparison either with their own abilities in other areas (Dykens, Hodapp, & Leckman, 1987) or with the abilities of children with Down syndrome of the same MAs (Hodapp et al., 1993).

The most startling etiology-based findings involve Williams syndrome. Williams syndrome is a rare disorder in which children have a particular, "elfin-like" facial appearance; these children are often talkative and outgoing (Udwin, Yule, & Martin, 1987). Bellugi, Wang, and Jernigan (1994) have noted that many of these children show particular, high-level abilities in language and language-like tasks, compared to MA-matched retarded or nonretarded children. These children show vocabulary levels that are several years ahead of their overall MAs (Bellugi, Marks, Birhle, & Sabo, 1988), and they can tell stories with high-level grammar, as well as with sound effects and other storytelling devices (Reilly, Klima, & Bellugi, 1990). Table 11.3 illustrates the storytelling and language skills of two representative children, one with Williams syndrome and one with Down syndrome (the children were of the same chronological ages, MAs, and IQs).

Two lessons arise from behavior in different organic syndromes of mental retardation.The first, obvious lesson involves the realization that children with different forms of mental retardation differ in their behavioral functioning. So far, specific types of mental retardation show different strengths and weaknesses in certain cognitive, linguistic, or adaptive skills (Dykens et al., 2000); some disorders show high susceptibilities to particular types of psychopathology (Dykens, 1995, 2000). Future research may need to emphasize the various *types* of mental retardation, as opposed to a single, all-encompassing entity of "mental retardation" per se.

A second lesson involves how children's abilities are organized across various domains. Contrary to Piaget's views of horizontally organized stages of development, both nonretarded and retarded children show unevenness from one developmental domain to the next. The extent of such unevenness, however, has caused considerable debate over the past 5 years. Indeed, until the middle to late 1990s, many researchers argued that findings in Williams syndrome supported Fodor's (1983) proposal that many domains (specifically language) are "modular," having little contact and interaction with other domains. Similarly, Gardner (1983) hypothesizes independent development in linguistic, musical, logical/mathematical, spatial, bodily/kinesthetic, and personal domains. Findings from children with Williams syndrome and from exceptional individual children (e.g., Curtiss, 1977; Yamada, 1990) also seemed to support such modular views of children's functioning.

More recently, however, various psycholinguists have more closely examined children with Williams syndrome. Their findings both support and refute prior claims. It does appear, for example, that children with Williams syndrome show relative strengths in language (particularly as opposed

TABLE 11.3. Comparison of Language and Storytelling in Williams Syndrome versus Down Syndrome

Child with Williams syndrome	Child with Down syndrome
Once upon a time there was this boy who had a dog and a frog. And it was nighttime. And there was a . . . bowl. And the boy and the dog looked in the . . . looked in the bowl. Then it was nighttime and time for the boy to go to bed. But, as the boy and the dog were sleeping, the frog climbed out. And, when it was morning [whispers], the frog was gone.	He looks in the bowl. He . . . sleep. Then the frog got away. He looked in the bowl . . . and it empty.

Note. Children responded to a picture book story about a boy and a dog, who lose and then find their pet frog. Quotes from Reilly, Klima, and Bellugi (1990, p. 377).

to their visual–spatial skills), although only 5% of these children have language that might be considered at age-appropriate levels, or "spared" (Bishop, 1999). But it is also probably the case that language is not "modular" in the sense meant by Fodor (1983) or Gardner (1983). Indeed, in a large-scale study of various aspects of cognition and language in children with Williams syndrome, Mervis, Morris, Bertrand, and Robinson (1999) found strong correlations (from .47 to .64) between various measures of short-term memory and grammatical levels.

Finally, as in several genetic disorders causing mental retardation, there appears to be a developmental process, such that relative strengths become stronger as a child ages (Hodapp & Dykens, 2001). In Williams syndrome, children may have slightly higher linguistic versus nonlinguistic abilities early on, but this pattern of "language over nonlanguage" becomes more pronounced at later ages (Bellugi, Mills, Jernigan, Hickok, & Galaburda, 1999; Paterson, Brown, Gsodl, Johnson, & Karmiloff-Smith, 1999). Similarly, boys with fragile-X syndrome—who show higher simultaneous (i.e., Gestalt) processing than sequential (step-by-step) processing even early on—become more pronounced in this profile as they get older (Hodapp et al., 1993). Such developmental patterns highlight the ways in which children's cognitive–linguistic strengths (and weaknesses) "emerge" with development, and the complicated ways in which children's already existing propensities might interact with particular environments to strengthen etiology-related profiles (Abbeduto, Evans, & Dolan, 2000).

Families and Ecologies

The past few years have seen a renewed interest in the families of children with mental retardation (e.g., Krauss, Simeonsson, & Ramey, 1989). Three major themes characterize this work.

New Perspectives. Family researchers have recently changed from "pathology-oriented" to "stress-and-coping-oriented" perspectives when examining families of children with mental retardation (Blacher & Hatton, 2001). To get an idea of this change, consider how in prior years many studies examined mothers and fathers to see whether they were more likely to be depressed or to suffer from other forms of psychopathology. Solnit and Stark (1961) noted how parents "mourn" the loss of the idealized (i.e., normal) infant; Drotar, Baskiewicz, Irvin, Kennell, and Klaus (1975) proposed three stages of maternal mourning (shock, depression/anger, emotional reorganization); and Gath (1977) noted that parents of children with Down syndrome were more likely to divorce. Even siblings were examined for the extent to which they suffered "role tensions" (Farber, 1959) and psychopathology (Lobato, 1983) compared to siblings of nonretarded children.

In recent years, the perspective has shifted from psychopathology to stress and coping (Hodapp, 2002). Using this perspective, researchers conceptualize the child with mental retardation as an "extra stressor" in the family system (e.g., Crnic, Friedrich, & Greenberg, 1983). As with all stressors, families and individual family members can be affected—sometimes negatively, but sometimes positively as well. Most importantly, the stress-and-coping perspective identifies factors that help parents cope. For example, among families raising a child with mental retardation, more affluent families cope better than poorer families (Farber, 1970); two-parent families cope better than single-parent families (Beckman, 1983); and women in better marriages cope better than those in more conflicted marriages (Beckman, 1983;

Friedrich, 1979). Though such findings may not be surprising, they do show the effects of various supports for families raising children with disabilities.

In addition to these more "demographic" variables, recent work has also begun to examine the nature of the coping strategies employed by parents. In their interviews of 27 families, Grant and Whittell (2000) found that several strategies were judged effective by parents in managing events and solving problems concerning their child or adult offspring with mental retardation. Parents reported that it was helpful for them to build on personal experience and expertise; to have a regular routine or structure; to have access to a trusted person to talk things over with; to set priorities; and to be able to choose from among a repertoire of coping strategies. In addition to heralding an important area for future research, understandings of such parental coping strategies have obvious clinical importance.

As such studies progress, it is also becoming obvious that mothers and fathers differ. Mothers request more social-emotional support, information about the children's condition, and help in child care (Bailey, Blasco, & Simeonsson, 1992), whereas fathers are more concerned about the financial costs of raising their children with mental retardation (Price-Bonham & Addison, 1978). Krauss (1993) finds that mothers are especially concerned about the "personal" costs of raising children with mental retardation (such things as changes in their relationship with their husbands, role restrictions, etc.), whereas fathers report more stress related to the children's temperament and their relationship to the children (such as feelings of being close to and reinforced by the children). Mothers are helped by supportive social networks, whereas fathers cope better when extended social networks provide a minimum amount of criticism (Frey, Greenberg, & Fewell, 1989). In addition, it appears that mothers (as opposed to fathers) more often rely on personal or religious beliefs (Grant & Whittell, 2000). Thus mothers and fathers may indeed differ in how they understand their children with mental retardation, which aspects of raising the children are stressful, and which personal or external factors best alleviate stress.

New Models. Just as researchers have changed from pathological to stress-and-coping perspectives, so too have they developed new models to understand these families (Blacher & Hatton, 2001). One of the most influential of these models is the "Double ABCX" model (Minnes, 1988). The Double ABCX model states that the crisis (or "X") of raising a child with mental retardation is a function of the specific characteristics of the child (the "stressor event," or A), mediated by the family's internal and external resources (B) and by the family's perceptions of the child (C). But this ABCX is not static: The child develops, familial resources may change, and so too may familial perceptions. Thus the "Double" of the Double ABCX model.

The Double ABCX model is a useful general framework for examining families of children with mental retardation. Consider, for example, the "developmental" aspects of familial reactions. Mothers of children with mental retardation have long been thought to undergo a "mourning process" in response to these children (Solnit & Stark, 1961). Based on this mourning model, researchers developed "stage models" of maternal mourning (cf. Blacher, 1984), emphasizing the time-bound nature of maternal reactions.

Increasingly, however, we have come to realize that a mother does not undergo a single reaction to parenting a child with mental retardation, but that many reactions occur at many times over the child's life. Wikler (1986) finds that mothers report extra stress when their children are entering puberty (11–15 years) and again when the children enter adulthood (20–21 years); others find a "pile-up" of stressors as the children get older (Minnes, 1988). To worsen matters, parents oftentimes have smaller social networks (Kazak & Marvin, 1984), and make less use of formal support services as the children get older (Suelzle & Keenan, 1981). Thus changes in a child and in the parents' perceptions of the child—that is, in the A (child) and C (perceptions) components of the Double ABCX model—affect parental and familial adaptation.

New Attention to Etiology. Children with different forms of mental retardation differ in their behavior (Dykens et al., 2000), and such differences may also affect family functioning. Specifically, it appears that families of children with Down syndrome are more often cohesive and harmonious (Mink, Nihira, & Meyers, 1983); these mothers also experience less stress and have larger and more satisfying social support networks (Goldberg, Marcovitch, MacGregor, & Lojkasek, 1986). Such differences occur even years later, when researchers compare adaptation in families of middle-aged adults with Down syndrome versus adults with other disorders. Seltzer, Krauss, and Tsunematsu (1993) have found that, compared to mothers of middle-aged individuals with other forms of mental retardation, mothers of middle-aged adults with Down syndrome report less conflicted family environments, more satisfaction with their social supports, and less stress and burden associated with caregiving. Compared to parents of children with other forms of mental retardation or with other disabilities, parents of children with Down syndrome may even feel more rewarded by their children (Hodapp, Ly, Fidler, & Ricci, 2001). The etiology of Down syndrome, then, seems to be helpful to parents and families.

But exactly why such "etiology-based" familial patterns occur remains unknown. To date, most researchers have attributed any advantage to families of children with Down syndrome to what might be called "associated characteristics" of the disorder. Thus Seltzer et al. (1993) note that Down syndrome is a common, well-known, and well-researched syndrome, with large and active parent organizations. In addition, as Down syndrome often occurs in children born to older mothers, the parents' age and SES (having spent more years in the work force) may also be causing any parent or family differences from parents and families of children with other developmental disabilities (Cahill & Glidden, 1996). Any or all of these variables that are associated with Down syndrome, then, may cause parents to feel less isolated and more supported.

A second, albeit not mutually exclusive, alternative concerns what might be called the "indirect effects" of Down syndrome (Hodapp, 1997b, 1999). That is, a specific genetic disorder causing mental retardation may predispose a child to show that disorder's "characteristic" behaviors (direct effects), but these behaviors in turn probably elicit specific reactions from others in the child's environment (indirect effects). In the case of Down syndrome, the behaviors in question probably relate to lower rates of severe psychopathology, as well as to more frequent displays of happy and sociable dispositions. Thus, compared to children with other types of mental retardation, children with Down syndrome generally show lower rates of maladaptive behavior/psychopathology (Dykens & Kasari, 1997; Meyers & Pueschel, 1991). Most studies also find that these children are considered by their parents to be happy and sociable (Carr, 1995; Hornby, 1996). Compared to retarded or nonretarded age-mates, children with Down syndrome even show more immature, "baby-like" faces, and such faces have been found to be associated with others' judgments that such children are warmer and more outgoing (Fidler & Hodapp, 1999). Indeed, then, children with Down syndrome themselves differ from other groups with mental retardation. Both child and "associated" characteristics, then, might lead to better adjustment by parents and families of children with Down syndrome.

Other Important Theoretical Orientations

Eco-Cultural Perspectives

Drawing upon anthropological and cross-cultural work with nonretarded children (Super & Harkness, 1986), several researchers have examined the "developmental niche" filled by a child with mental retardation (Gallimore, Keogh, & Bernheimer, 1999). Much of this work centers around the meaning of the child to the family, and how parental goals for the child fit with parents' goals for themselves, for other family members, and for the family as a whole.

For example, Gallimore, Weisner, Kaufman, and Bernheimer (1989) noted the "accommodations" made by different families of children with mental retardation. Some families set up their entire family systems to ensure that the children received maximal intellectual stimulation. In contrast, other families were much more concerned with the other, nonretarded children. In these families, the children with mental retardation were not felt to need extra stimulation, and more family-oriented goals were emphasized. Such a focus on accommodations, and on how such accommodations might change as a child develops, marks an important new focus within studies of children with mental retardation and their families (Gallimore et al., 1999).

Social Role Theory

In another perspective on mental retardation, the child with retardation is seen as merely fulfilling a social role. Indeed, to some (e.g., Mercer, 1992), the "social" nature of mental retardation is emphasized by the recent decrease in diagnoses of mild mental retardation.

Along with the rise in the social role perspective has been the view that the field is undergoing a "support revolution" (Schwartz, 1992). Some claim that developmental and biomedical orientations toward mental retardation have been replaced by this new support paradigm, which emphasizes the supports a given individual needs in order to play an age-appropriate role in the society. Although attempts to provide better, more individualized services are beneficial, the effect of other changes seems unclear. For instance, many segments of AAMR are now demanding representation of consumers—persons with mental retardation—on all boards, committees, and review panels. Such changes may not necessarily ensure adequate representation or input for all persons with mental retardation.

Behavioral Techniques

Behavioral techniques based on the writings of Skinner (1968), Foxx and Azrin (1974), and others have been successfully used in three different ways. First, behavior modification techniques have been effective in training adaptive behaviors to persons with mental retardation. Such behaviors as grooming, toileting, eating, and dressing have all been taught to individuals with profound and severe retardation. Behavioral techniques have also been successfully employed to stop maladaptive behaviors, such as hurting others or themselves. Overall, behavioral training has been impressive in increasing adaptive and decreasing maladaptive behaviors (Carr et al., 1999; Matson, 1990).

Second, behavioral techniques have been very helpful for parents. Parents of very impaired or difficult-to-control children are often at a loss about how to proceed. In many cases, behaviorists' clear schedules of rewards and punishments have helped parents elicit adaptive as opposed to maladaptive behaviors. Similarly, parents have been taught how to model desired behaviors, to break down complex tasks into smaller components, and to "chain together" these components (Baker & Brightman, 1997).

A third area of behavioral success involves vocational and prevocational training and work. When behavioral techniques are used to teach skills and token economies are employed to keep workers on task, many persons with mental retardation can now work successfully in supported work environments (Wehman, Sale, & Parent, 1992). Again, many of these individuals are very impaired, whereas others had shown maladaptive behaviors that previously made it impossible for them to be productive in a job setting.

ETIOLOGIES

Mental retardation results from many different causes. Some of these causes occur prenatally, as in all of the genetic disorders and accidents *in utero*. Other types of retardation are caused by perinatal insults, such as prematurity or anoxia at birth. Still other types of mental retardation occur as a result of meningitis, head trauma, or other "after-birth insults." In addition to the many different types of mental retardation that have one or more specific causes, many—perhaps the majority—of persons have mental retardation with no obvious pre-, peri-, or postnatal cause.

How are we to make sense of these many different etiologies? Historically, researchers have postulated what has come to be called the "two-group approach" to mental retardation. We briefly overview this approach, then describe recent advances in behavioral knowledge, particularly concerning persons with different genetic disorders that cause mental retardation.

The Two-Group Approach

Researchers and clinicians have historically described two distinct groups of persons with mental retardation (Zigler, 1967, 1969). The first group demonstrates a clear organic cause for their mental retardation; the second group shows mental retardation with no clear organic cause. This distinction between "organic" and "familial" (or "cultural–familial") forms of mental retardation has characterized work from the beginning of the 20th century onward (cf. Burack, 1990). Table 11.4 shows the two-group approach.

To start with the familial group, these individuals represent what is probably the single biggest mystery in mental retardation. Constituting one-half to two-thirds of all persons with mental retardation, these individuals show no cause for their mental retardation. Some researchers feel that persons with familial mental retardation do indeed have slight, hard-to-detect neurological problems that cause their lowered levels of intelligence (Baumeister & MacLean, 1979). Others feel that environmental deficits, or overstimulation, may cause familial mental retardation. Still others feel that these persons form the lower end of a Gaussian, bell-shaped curve of intelligence (e.g., Zigler, 1967).

At present, it appears that mental retardation in certain percentages of this familial group may be due to each of these factors. Thus, until a few

TABLE 11.4. The Two-Group Approach to Mental Retardation

	Organic	Cultural–familal
Definition	Individual shows a clear organic cause of mental retardation	Individual shows no obvious cause of retardation; sometimes another family member is also retarded
Characteristics	More prevalent at moderate, severe, and profound levels of retardation	More prevalent in mild mental retardation
	Equal or near-equal rates across all ethnic and SES levels	Higher rates within minority groups and low-SES groups
	More often associated with other physical disabilities	Few associated physical or medical disabilities
Causes[a]	Prenatal (genetic disorders, accidents *in utero*)	Polygenic (i.e., parents of low IQ)
	Perinatal (prematurity, anoxia)	Environmentally deprived
	Postnatal (head trauma, meningitis)	Undetected organic conditions

[a]Causes are suspected for cultural–familial mental retardation.

decades ago, most individuals with fragile-X syndrome would have been diagnosed as having mental retardation of unknown causes; indeed, the National Fragile X Foundation (1994, cited in Dykens et al., 2000) estimates that as many as 80% of those affected with that disorder may remain undiagnosed. Similarly, given that approximately 50% of the variation in IQ scores is due to the environment and that there is an association of family SES with mild mental retardation (Broman et al., 1987; Stromme & Magnus, 2000), low-SES environments (particularly the most impoverished) may indeed cause mental retardation in a portion of this group. Finally, behavior geneticists have now identified at least one of the many "polygenes" responsible for the 50% of IQ variation due to genetic factors. This gene is located on chromosome 6. One variant of that gene was found much more often in high-IQ children in two independent samples, and seems to account for approximately 2% of the variance in IQ (Chorney et al., 1998). Many different factors—operating separately or together—probably account for the intellectual disabilities in children with familial or cultural–familial mental retardation.

Regardless of cause, persons with familial mental retardation function predominantly at the mild level of retardation. As such, these are the individuals who blend into the larger population before and after the school years, and who are more likely to be from minority groups and low-SES backgrounds. In addition, these individuals are much more likely to have parents who are themselves low in intelligence. Thus the many controversies surrounding definition and supportive services are all present in discussions of familial mental retardation (Hodapp, 1994).

Persons in the second group, those with organic mental retardation, demonstrate one or more clear causes of their mental retardation. As noted above, such causes can occur pre-, peri-, or postnatally. In 1983, Grossman noted that there were over 200 organic causes of mental retardation (including all types). By the late 1990s, however, approximately 750 different genetic causes of mental retardation had been identified (Opitz, 1996), and other "organic but not genetic" causes (such as fetal alcohol syndrome) also exist. Table 11.5 presents several of the more prominent genetic forms of mental retardation.

Although persons with certain genetic conditions (Prader–Willi syndrome; some cases of Down syndrome and fragile-X syndrome) account for some (and possibly an increasing) percentage of persons with mild mental retardation (Rutter, Simonoff, & Plomin, 1996), virtually all persons with more severe levels of mental retardation show organic impairments. Using the latest, most sophisticated genetic and other tests for organicity, Stromme and Hagberg (2000) reported that a full 96% of their group with severe mental retardation showed one or more "biopathological" causes (only 4% of these children showed unspecified causes). In contrast, only 68% of children with mild mental retardation showed one or another organic cause, with 32% having unspecified causes. Thus the large majority of persons at more severe levels show a clear etiology for their mental retardation, whereas some sizable percentage at more mild levels do not.

Also related is the issue of the sheer number of persons at more severe levels of mental retardation. Indeed, relative to predictions from a normal or Gaussian curve of intelligence, there are simply too many persons with severe and profound mental retardation. This excess of individuals at the lower ranges of intelligence constitutes the "extra" persons that make up the hypothesized 3% prevalence rate of mental retardation discussed above (Dingman & Tarjan, 1960). This excess at the lowest levels is assumed to occur because of the many individuals who have various organic forms of mental retardation.

Differentiating Types of Organic Mental Retardation

As noted above, researchers are increasingly realizing that persons with different forms of organic mental retardation differ behaviorally. For example, many boys with fragile-X syndrome show cognitive profiles and trajectories differing from those of children with Down syndrome. Striking differences also occur in psychopathology between etiological groups (see the next section). Variable profiles, trajectories, and psychopathology highlight that it is overly simplistic to speak of "organic mental retardation" as if it were a single entity.

A better understanding of each particular syndrome's characteristic behaviors, or "behavioral phenotype," also helps refine both the timing and type of intervention efforts (e.g., Hodapp & Dykens, 1991). In fragile-X syndrome, for example, trajectories of IQ and adaptive behaviors underscore the importance of early intervention, while the syndrome's characteristic cognitive profile has led to a host of specific psychotherapeutic and educational recommendations (Dykens & Hodapp, 1997; Hodapp & Fidler, 1999). Detailed descriptions of behavioral phenotypes also help screen high-risk samples.

Behavioral research on genetic etiologies is also critical given recent revolutionary advances in molecular genetics. Technological advances in the so-called "new genetics" bring forth a demand for improved research that links genes to behavior (Dykens, 1995). For example, much of the variable and puzzling behavioral phenotype in fragile-X syndrome is attributed to the actual amount of protein produced by the FMR-1 gene. This type of genotype–phenotype work furthers our knowledge of gene function and may ultimately lead to innovative gene therapies (Anderson, 1994).

Despite the renewed importance of syndromic behavior, researchers interested in the behavior of persons with mental retardation have historically classified groups according to their level of impairment. Thus psychologists and special educators often compare children with mild mental retardation to those with severe or profound mental retardation; these workers rarely consider

TABLE 11.5. Prominent Genetic Forms of Mental Retardation

Disorder	Genetics	Prevalence	Prominent behavioral features
Down syndrome	95% involve trisomy 21	1–1.5/1,000 live births	Moderate mental retardation; slowing rate of development as child gets older; social strengths; weaknesses in grammar and speech
Fragile-X syndrome	Fragile site on X chromosome	0.73–0.92/1,000 live births	Moderate mental retardation; more males than females; for males, strength in simultaneous processing, weakness in sequential processing, slowed development from puberty; hyperactivity and autistic-like behaviors
Prader–Willi syndrome	Two-thirds involve deletions on chromosome 15; remainder involve maternal disomy	1/15,000 live births	Mild mental retardation; proneness to obesity, food foraging, and preoccupations; stubbornness and obsessive–compulsive behaviors

the causes of the children's retardation. In contrast, geneticists, pediatricians, and psychiatrists generally classify by etiology. These researchers examine persons with Down syndrome, fragile-X syndrome, or other causes of mental retardation.

We have described these orientations as two rarely overlapping "cultures" of behavioral research in mental retardation (Hodapp & Dykens, 1994). Both cultures study the behavior of persons with mental retardation, yet they differ in their technical languages, expertises, and journals. As a result, many workers in the genetic tradition do not often use sophisticated behavioral measures, or apply their findings to pertinent issues in the wider mental retardation field. Conversely, many behavioral researchers are unaware of revolutionary advances in genetics, and ignore the effects of etiology on their research designs and findings. The main features of these two cultures are summarized in Table 11.6.

To some extent, however, this situation may gradually be changing. Over the past decade, the amount of research devoted to children with several genetic disorders has grown greatly (Dykens & Hodapp, 2001). When the numbers of empirical articles on behavior from the 1980s versus the 1990s were compared, the numbers of articles on Williams syndrome increased from 10 to 81; on Prader–Willi syndrome, from 24 to 86; and on fragile-X syndrome, from 60 to 149. Even in Down syndrome, the sole etiology featuring a long-standing tradition of behavioral research, the amount of behavioral research almost doubled—from 607 to 1,140 articles—from the 1980s to the 1990s (Hodapp & Dykens, in press).

In addition to increased numbers of articles, such articles have produced striking increases in our knowledge of behavior in several syndromes. Developmental psycholinguists, for example, have increasingly come to understand the profile of high language abilities and low visual–spatial abilities in Williams syndrome (Mervis et al., 1999), finding connections and disconnections that inform discussions of modularity and cross-domain relations more generally. Similarly, there now exists a better appreciation of the increased abilities in visual versus auditory short-term memory in children with Down syndrome (Hodapp et al., 1999). Children with Down syndrome also show particular problems in linguistic grammar (Fowler, 1990), in articulation (Kumin, 1994), and in expressive (as opposed to receptive) language skills (Miller, 1999). Clinical psychologists have focused on such behaviors as obsessions and compulsions in Prader–Willi syndrome (Dykens, Leckman, & Cassidy, 1996) and

TABLE 11.6. The "Two Cultures" of Behavioral Research in Mental Retardation

Level-of-impairment-based	Etiology-based
Main characteristics	
Group by degree of disability	Group by etiology
Less regard for genetic etiology	De-emphasize degree of disability
Professions (with some overlap)	
Behavioral psychologists	Geneticists
Special educators	Genetic counselors
Clinical psychologists	Child psychiatrists
Social workers	Pediatricians
	Psychiatrists
Strengths	
Advances in behavioral measurement	Advances in molecular genetics
Weaknesses	
Often less aware of advances in genetics and molecular genetics	Often less sophisticated in behavioral measurement
Often less appreciation for impact of genetic etiology on research or intervention	Often less application of findings to pertinent issues in larger mental retardation field

anxiety and fears in Williams syndrome (Dykens, in press). In short, we now know much more about cognitive, linguistic, adaptive, and maladaptive behaviors in a few genetic disorders than we did even a decade ago.

At the same time, we could equally well describe the etiology glass as not half full, but half empty. Indeed, the exponential increase in knowledge still involves only a few syndromes, and it remains the case that not a single behavioral research article exists for many of the 750+ genetic disorders causing mental retardation. In addition, challenges remain in "bridging" the more medical/genetic and more behavioral cultures, in assessing the impact of mental retardation versus genetic status, and in accounting for between-syndrome similarities and differences (Dykens et al., 2000). More specific definitional and measurement issues inherent in phenotype research have also been outlined (Dykens, 1995, 2000). The issue of "dual diagnosis"—described below—also exemplifies this need for "cross-cultural" collaborations and more genetically informed research.

DUAL DIAGNOSIS

Early interests in psychopathology and mental retardation waned in the 1920s and were revisited in the late 1960s (Menolascino, 1970). Since that time, remarkable strides have been made in developing appropriate maladaptive behavior rating scales (Aman, 1991; Einfeld & Tonge, 1992), identifying advantages and limitations of psychiatric nosology in this population (Dykens, 2000; Sovner, 1986), and using research to fine-tune pharmacological and behavioral treatments (Menolascino & Fleisher, 1993; Rush & Frances, 2000). These accomplishments have helped in understanding the degree to which children with mental retardation can be "dually diagnosed"—that is, have both mental retardation and (other) psychiatric disorders.

As a result of these advances, we now know that children with mental retardation, compared to their nonretarded peers, display psychiatric disorders or behavioral and emotional problems at very high rates (Matson & Frame, 1986). Estimates of dual diagnoses among these children range from 10% (Jacobson, 1982) to 50% (Richardson, Katz, Koller, McLaren, & Rubinstein, 1979; Rutter, Tizard, Yule, Graham, & Whitmore, 1976). Although these estimates vary widely, they do indicate that psychiatric disorders are common among children with mental retardation (see also Bouras, 1999; Tonge, 1999).

In a similar way, persons with mental retardation show the full range of psychiatric disorders. Relative to nonretarded children, children with mental retardation often show more anxiety, depression, withdrawal, conduct problems, aggression, and self-injury. Persons diagnosed with mental retardation have also been shown to have most of the other major DSM diagnoses (Cullinan, Epstein, Matson, & Rosemier, 1984; Dykens & Volkmar, 1997; Dekry & Ehly, 1981; Volkmar, Burack, & Cohen, 1990). Table 11.7 gives a sampling of these findings (and of the wide variability across studies) for three diagnostic categories: schizophrenia/psychosis, depression, and attention-deficit hyperactivity disorder (ADHD).

But understanding dual diagnosis is also complicated by several major problems. First, studies vary widely in their methodologies. Some studies examine entire populations of persons with mental retardation, whereas others limit their examinations to clinic-based samples. Different approaches are used for assessing pathology, such as behavioral checklists, psychiatric nosology, or focusing on just one type of problem (e.g., psychoses or phobias). Such differences among studies make problematic any general, overall statements about dual diagnosis.

A second issue involves the "goodness of fit" between standard psychiatric nosology and persons with mental retardation (Dykens, 2000; Sovner, 1986). Many psychiatric categories are not easily applied to this population. For example, certain problems seem quite common in children with mental retardation, including temper tantrums, aggression, hyperactivity, and diminished responsiveness to others (Jacobson, 1982; Einfeld & Tonge, 1996). Although many of these behaviors can be quite severe and warrant intensive intervention, they may or may not be symptomatic of psychiatric illness. In addition, many children and adults with mental retardation have particular difficulty labeling and expressing internal states (Glick, 1998; Jacobson, 1990). As a result, clinicians may have particular difficulty accurately diagnosing "internalizing" psychiatric disorders (e.g., depression or anxiety) in persons with mental retardation.

Even when information is obtained from other informants, difficult issues arise. For example, checklists and diagnoses require judgments from

TABLE 11.7. Rates (%) of Three Diagnoses in Children and Adolescents with Heterogeneous Mental Retardation

Study	*n*	Method	Schizophrenia/ psychosis	Depression	ADHD
Gillberg et al. (1986)	149 adolescents	Behaviors	1.0	10.0	11.0
Gath & Gumley (1986)	154 children and adolescents	ICD		10.0	7.0
Reid (1980)[a]	60 children	ICD	8.3		15.0
Jacobson (1990)	42,479 children and adults	Records	6.0–7.0		
Grizenko et al. (1991)[a]	176 adolescents and adults	DSM	2.8/2.3	3.4	

Note. Data from Dykens and Hodapp (2001).
[a]Clinic or hospital sample.

parents, teachers, or clinicians as to when certain behaviors should be labeled as maladaptive or deviant. Some behaviors (such as hallucinations or delusions) are clearly deviant, regardless of the person's chronological age or MA. Other behaviors or emotions, however, may be quite consistent with a person's MA, yet are deviant from chronological age expectations. A 15-year-old with an MA of 2 or 3 may show fantasy–reality blurrings typical of "normal" preschoolers, or "terrible two" tantrums that reflect "normal" bids for increased separation and autonomy. Considering MA-based versus chronological-age-based expectations is thus an important aspect of making accurate diagnoses in this population.

These problems have recently been addressed by work that specifically examines psychopathology in populations with mental retardation. Dosen and Gielen (1993) have proposed alternative diagnostic criteria for such features as depression, and behavioral checklists are increasingly being normed on mentally retarded versus "normal" children (Aman & Singh, 1994; Einfeld & Tonge, 1992; Reiss, 1990). Such efforts allow for a better "fit" of psychopathology and mental retardation in the dual-diagnosis field.

But other advances are also needed. Researchers have yet to consider the effects of etiology on many of the dual-diagnosis prevalence rates or on other key findings emanating from the dual-diagnosis movement. As noted above, this lack of attention to etiology seems associated with the "level-of-impairment" bias in the larger mental retardation field. Yet many genetic syndromes do show salient patterns of maladaptive behavior and psychopathology. Two syndromes exemplify such syndrome-specific psychiatric and behavioral features.

Fragile-X Syndrome

Fragile-X syndrome results in a spectrum of learning and emotional problems in both males and females. Many individuals with the syndrome show characteristic cognitive profiles, as well as hyperactivity and attention deficits (see Dykens et al., 2000, for a review). Females are less often affected with mental retardation, whereas males are apt to be moderately affected, especially in the postpubertal years. These males may also manifest perseverative speech and behaviors, stereotypies, and tactile defensiveness.

Early case reports noted several boys with fragile-X syndrome who met DSM-III criteria for autism (August & Lockhart, 1984; Meryash, Szymanski, & Gerald, 1982). After in-depth studies of the behaviors shown by such boys, however, it now appears that only some—probably from 15% to 25%—have full-blown autism (McCabe, de la Cruz, & Clapp, 1999). Instead of full-blown autism, the behavior of most males with fragile-X syndrome is better described as falling along a continuum of social anxiety, shyness, social withdrawal, and mutual gaze aversion (Bregman, Leckman, & Ort, 1988; Cohen, Veitze, Sudhalter, Jenkins, & Brown, 1991; Reiss & Freund, 1990). In addition, attention deficits and hyperactivity are seen in the majority of both clinic-referred and nonreferred males (Baumgardner, Reiss, Freund, & Abrams, 1995).

For females with fragile-X syndrome, the clinical picture is more variable, though often somewhat less severe. These girls and women generally show similar albeit lesser problems with social anxiety, shyness, gaze aversion, and inattention (Lachiewicz & Dawson, 1994; Sobesky, Porter, Pennington, & Hagerman, 1995). Even compared to other mothers of children with disabilities, more mothers of these children show depressive features (Thompson et al., 1994), and relatively weak interpersonal skills are also often evident.

Over the past few years, studies have increasingly demonstrated that the degree of cognitive impairment in this disorder for both boys and girls relates to the extent of fragile-X protein (FMR-1P) produced (which in turn is due to the degree to which the trinucleotide cytosine-guanine-guanine repeat is methylated). Fully affected males with mental retardation produce no FMR-1P (Tassone et al., 1999); in contrast, males who produce some FMR-1P generally have higher IQs. A similar effect appears to be operating in girls with fragile-X syndrome. For both boys and girls, however, the amount of protein has yet to be linked to the presence or degree of maladaptive behavior/psychopathology.

Prader–Willi Syndrome

First identified in 1956 (Prader, Labhardt, & Willi, 1956), Prader–Willi syndrome is now known to be caused in one of several ways. Most cases of Prader–Willi syndrome are attributed to a paternally inherited deletion, or missing piece, on chromosome 15. But about 30% of cases are caused by a maternal disomy, in which both chromosome 15's come from the mother. In either case, genetic information is missing from the father. As we discuss below, these two causes of Prader–Willi syndrome show some differences in behavior.

Developmentally, Prader–Willi syndrome shows at least two distinct phases. Infants show hypotonia, feeding and sucking problems, and developmental delay. In striking contrast to this "failure-to-thrive" period, the second phase begins between 2 and 6 years of age and is characterized by hyperphagia, food preoccupations, and food seeking (Holm et al., 1993). Without proper dietary management, persons with the syndrome often become obese.

Maladaptive behaviors may also change as these children develop. Young children are typically described as pleasant, friendly, and affectionate (Cassidy, 1992). Although these features do not necessarily disappear, the beginning of hyperphagia is associated with the onset or worsening of many maladaptive behaviors. These problems include temper tantrums, impulsivity, stubbornness, underactivity, fatigue, food stealing, compulsions, and difficulties with peers. Indeed, from 70% to 95% of various samples show these problems (Dykens & Cassidy, 1999). Among adults with the syndrome, heightened vulnerabilities—even compared to those of other adults with mental retardation—have also been found for mood disorder (Beardsmore, Dorman, Cooper, & Webb, 1998) and for psychosis and thought disturbance (Clarke, 1998).

Other key aspects of maladaptive behavior are also gradually becoming known in Prader–Willi syndrome. Children, for example, show increases in maladaptive behavior with age, whereas adults may show a more variable course (Dykens, Hodapp, Walsh, & Nash, 1992a; Dykens & Cassidy, 1995). Weight does not appear related to intelligence (Dykens, Hodapp, Walsh, & Nash, 1992b), but it may be associated with psychopathology. Curiously, Dykens and Cassidy (1995) note that confused thinking, delusions, hallucinations, anxiety, fearfulness, and sadness appear more common in thinner than in heavier individuals; such findings may lead to a wider emphasis in interventions on issues other than weight loss.

Attention has also begun to focus on the obsessions and compulsions of these individuals. In one study comparing 91 children and adults with Prader–Willi syndrome to nonretarded persons diagnosed with obsessive–compulsive disorder (OCD), Dykens, Leckman, and Cassidy (1996) found few differences between the two groups. Like the nonretarded persons diagnosed with OCD, individuals with Prader–Willi syndrome showed high rates of non-food-related symptomatology, including such things as hoarding (58% of sample); need to tell, ask, or know (53%); excessive ordering and arranging (40%); repeating rituals (37%); and cleaning (24%). It also appears that at least some of these behaviors begin during the toddler and preschool period. Comparing three groups of 2- to 6-year-olds—typically developing children, Down syndrome, and Prader–Willi syndrome—Dimitropoulos, Feurer, Butler, and Thompson (2001) found higher rates of compulsive behaviors in the young children with Prader–Willi syndrome. Specific behaviors common in children with Prader–Willi syndrome (and much less common in the other two groups) included repeatedly removing and then replacing items (56.6% of sample); insisting on doing chores themselves (51.8%); arranging objects in certain patterns (45.8%); insisting on doing activities/chores at same time daily (43.4%); and picking at face/body to point of gouging skin (32.5%). Obsessions and compulsions are increasingly being appreciated as significant problems in individuals with Prader–Willi syndrome.

A final issue relates to the genetic status of persons with Prader–Willi syndrome. Recall that the disorder can involve either a deletion on the chromosome 15 contributed from the father, or receiving two chromosome 15's from the mother (called maternal "uniparental disomy," or UPD). Although it was earlier thought that the two groups were relatively similar behaviorally, it now appears that persons with the deletion (vs. UPD) form of Prader–Willi syndrome show more maladaptive behaviors (Dykens, Cassidy, & King, 1999). Persons with the deletions show a greater number of problem behaviors on the Child Behavior Checklist (Achenbach, 1991) and greater symptom-related distress on the Yale–Brown Obsessive–Compulsive Scale (Goodman et al., 1989).

Other behavioral differences also relate to the deletion–UPD distinction. Specifically, individuals with deletions seem slightly more cognitively impaired (Dykens et al., 1999), although the main differences may involve Verbal IQs (Roof et al., 2000). Even more curious is a recent finding related to jigsaw puzzles. For many years, high-level performance on jigsaw puzzles has been considered one of the "supportive" behavioral criteria for Prader–Willi syndrome (Holm et al., 1993). Recently, Dykens (2002) has found that a facility with jigsaw puzzles occurs in children with the deletion, but not the UPD, form of Prader–Willi syndrome. The children with deletions performed at levels well above those of same-age typically developing children; in this study, children with the deletion form of Prader-Willi syndrome were able to fit almost three times as many pieces into a puzzle in a 3-minute period as typically developing children were. Strangely, however, these same children with Prader–Willi syndrome did not perform as well as typically developing age-mates on such seemingly similar tasks as the WISC Block Design subtest or the K-ABC Triangles subtest. But such was not the case for children with UPD. On both jigsaw puzzles and visual–spatial IQ subtests, children with UPD showed fairly low levels of performance.

It appears, then, that certain syndromes have distinct maladaptive behaviors, yet there are far too many syndromes to presume that every single syndrome shows unique psychopathology. Furthermore, even though fragile-X and Prader–Willi syndromes share such maladaptive behaviors as perseveration, persons with each syndrome may perseverate in different ways (e.g., odd preoccupations in fragile-X syndrome, food obsessions in Prader–Willi). Future phenotypic research will need to identify how various syndromes are "the same but different" (Dykens, 1995). Clearly, considerable work remains to be done in these as well as in hundreds of lesser-known syndromes. This work needs to better describe maladaptive behavior and psychiatric illness within syndromes, to refine treatment, and to assess the "percentage of variance" attributed to general mental retardation as opposed to specific genetic status (Dykens, 2000).

Compared to earlier times, then, researchers and clinicians have advanced greatly in their understanding of dually diagnosed persons. Many of these advances involve views of psychopathology that are specifically related to persons with mental retardation. But other advances are also needed. Traditionally, the dual-diagnosis movement has not been etiologically based, leaving unanswered critical issues regarding syndrome-specific psychopathology, treatment, and outcome, as well as potential new understandings of gene–behavior relations.

CURRENT ISSUES AND FUTURE DIRECTIONS

Although many issues pervade the study and treatment of mental retardation, six deserve special notice. Working toward the solution of each will help advance the field of mental retardation for many years to come.

Defining and Classifying Persons with Mental Retardation

The upcoming revision of the 1992 AAMR definition extends what has recently been the hottest debate about mental retardation. By changing from a definition of IQ below 70 and adaptive deficits to one focusing on IQ "below 70 or 75" and deficits in 2 of 10 adaptive domains, the 1992 AAMR definition threatened to affect the number and characteristics of the retarded population. Given the controversial nature of the 1992 AAMR definition, it is perhaps understandable that neither researchers (Polloway et al., 1999) nor state regulations (Denning et al., 2000) have so far followed that manual's definition or classificatory criteria. How, exactly, the forthcoming AAMR definition addresses such issues will be closely watched by all professionals studying or serving persons with mental retardation.

In a larger sense, however, the debate over the 1992 definition—and its proposed revision—highlights mental retardation's many constituencies. Mental retardation concerns many different people: the affected individuals themselves; their families and advocates; policy makers; and special educators, social workers, physicians, group home personnel, geneticists and genetic counselors, psychologists and psychiatrists, and other professionals. All will benefit from a standard definition of mental retardation—from a definition that different professions (each with its unique perspectives, approaches, and needs) can apply to a common population to be studied and served.

Improving Service Delivery

Equally challenging are issues of service delivery. These issues mostly pertain to schools and residences. On the whole, great strides have been made in service delivery over the past 20–30 years. Persons with mental retardation now enjoy the right to a public school education, and in many cases, this schooling occurs in classrooms with nonretarded age-mates. Many children with mental retardation benefit from such contacts and experiences. In the postschool years, persons with mental retardation enjoy residential opportunities such as individual or shared apartments and group homes. Such homes allow adults with mental retardation to become part of their communities—to live among and interact with nonretarded peers. Such progress in "integrated" schooling and living settings, which do seem to benefit the large majority of persons with mental retardation (Freeman & Alkin, 2000), would have been unheard of only three decades ago.

Yet some retardation workers are concerned about exactly how normalization has been implemented. Zigler, Hodapp, and Edison (1990) note that there has often been more concern with where a person with mental retardation lives or is educated than with what happens within that setting. They decry the overemphasis on a "social address model" in mental retardation, on the single issue of the setting in which interactions occur. Instead, these authors note, we should pay more attention to what occurs *within* every setting, while providing a continuum of high-quality services for every person, regardless of age, etiology, or degree of impairment.

Describing Psychopathology and Serving Persons with Dual Diagnoses

A related issue concerns psychopathology. For many years, parents, advocates, and even researchers were loath to examine the tie between mental retardation and psychopathology. More recently, we have begun to realize that persons with mental retardation often do have various psychopathological conditions.

In order to make progress in describing psychopathology in this population, a joining of different fields seems necessary. It will not be enough simply to apply diagnoses—or even checklists—derived from nonretarded populations to persons with mental retardation. More attention will need to be given to how methodological/diagnostic concerns within populations with mental retardation complicate the dual-diagnosis issue (Dykens, 2000). A joining of different professionals and different perspectives seems mandatory if we are ever to truly understand and intervene with persons who show both mental retardation and psychopathological conditions.

Further concerns relate to the provision of the services themselves. In many ways, persons with mental retardation are a hidden group within our society, and residing in more typical settings has not always helped this state of affairs. Indeed, in reviewing the recent history of dual diagnosis, Jacobson (1999) argues that, even as persons with mental retardation take part more fully in normal, everyday life, too often those who have co-occurring emotional/behavioral disorders go unserved. Even when dually diagnosed persons are served, evaluations and treatments are performed by community mental health professionals who often have little experience and training in mental retardation. Jacobson (1999) concludes that "there are serious concerns about dual diagnosis services, their uneven accessibility and lack of resources" (p. 344).

Joining the Two Cultures of Behavioral Research

A fourth, more research-related issue involves the two cultures of behavioral research in mental retardation. Compared to the numerous advances in genetics, we know relatively little about the behaviors associated with many different genetic disorders. Even when we consider the enormous increase in the number of etiology-based behavioral articles in recent years (Dykens & Hodapp, 2001), the two cultures of mental retardation remain divided.

In order to research and intervene with persons with mental retardation, we must link psychologists, special educators, and others interested in behavior to geneticists, psychiatrists, and others interested in etiology. Granted, such collaborations will not always be easy to accomplish. In addition to turf issues, different professions have vast amounts of specialized knowledge and terms. To clinical geneticists, for example, it is commonplace to talk of cytogenetics and molecular genetics; fluorescent *in situ* hybridization; full versus partial mutation; deletion, disomy, and amplification; trisomy, translocation, and mosaicism. Psycholinguists have terms that are no less exotic; consider such examples as fast mapping, code switching, and the novel name–nameless category (N3C) principle. In short, even as they are becoming absolutely essential, interdisciplinary collaborations remain difficult (see Hodapp, 1998, for a fuller discussion).

Promoting Research in Several Additional Areas

Besides requiring greater cooperation and multidisciplinary approaches, future mental retardation research will need to become more comprehensive. We need to know more about behavioral functioning across a wide variety of areas. For example, we continue to know little about how persons with mental retardation attribute their successes or failures (to intrinsic or extrinsic factors, to skill or luck?). In addition to knowing little about attributions of persons with mental retardation themselves, we similarly know little about the attributions about these persons' successes or failures that are made by their mothers, fathers, siblings, teachers, or classmates. Similarly, with the exception of Alzheimer-related studies of Down syndrome, the field has only begun examining many issues of aging; the effects of sex/gender differences on a variety of behaviors; and the effects of various "ecologies" within which children with mental retardation live (although see Hauser-Cram et al., 2001). Also unclear is how each issue might change in relation to different genetic (or nongenetic) causes of mental retardation.

Why are there so many gaps in our knowledge of persons with mental retardation? Here we need to consider the field of mental retardation research and treatment more broadly. As presently constituted, the field is fairly large; to give one example, the field's two main journals—the *American Journal on Mental Retardation* and *Mental Retardation*—are received by over 11,000 subscribers (American Psychological Association, 1997). The large majority of these professionals are practitioners, including special educators, group home workers, regional center or institutional employees, and state-level administrators.

In contrast, the actual number of active researchers remains relatively small. Indeed, the main conference devoted exclusively to behavioral issues in mental retardation—the annual Gatlinburg Conference, sponsored by the National Institute of Child Health and Human Development—generally draws only about 150–200 persons. This number has remained relatively steady over the years, and the field struggles to entice newer investigators into mental retardation research. On a related matter, Baumeister (1997) has questioned whether behavioral (as opposed to biomedical) workers in mental retardation are getting their fair share of the federal funding pie.

Part of the problem here stems from the field's structure, part from the way the field is perceived. To this day, only a handful of programs exist that are exclusively devoted to doctoral-level training in mental retardation research. Partly as a result, mental retardation researchers are scattered widely across various university departments of education, psychology, child psychiatry, public health, and social work. And, although periodic reviews have considered the study of mental retardation to be a "Cinderella field" that will soon come into its own (see King, State, Shah, Davanzo, & Dykens, 1997, for the latest example), the widespread perception continues that studying people with disabilities is a lower, less interesting, less exciting calling. One thus sees that mental retardation is included within (but is not a highly prominent subarea of) psychiatry and child psychiatry, just as special education exists within (but is not prominent in) departments of education. One would hope that such perceptions might be changing, and that the recent work examining gene–brain–behavior connections might increase the field's status. For now, however, mental retardation research—while it may formally exist as part of many disciplines—is probably not a highly esteemed area of any.

Changing Populations with Mental Retardation

A final issue concerns who, exactly, will have mental retardation in the years to come. Although it is currently unclear whether future years will bring greater or lesser numbers of persons with mental retardation, the composition of that population will change dramatically. Already on the horizon are new discoveries that will lead to more precise genetic diagnoses *in utero* for many different genetic disorders. Similarly, gene therapies may someday cure many disorders, or at least greatly alleviate their effects.

But other forces may lead to greater numbers of persons with mental retardation. Newborn intensive care units now are able to save neonates weighing even below 750 grams (or 1 pound, 10 ounces), but such children often show cognitive impairments compared to full-term or even slightly heavier newborns even into the middle childhood years (Taylor, Klein, Minich, & Hack, 2000). In a similar way, the rise in pediatric AIDS and the epidemic of babies suffering from their mothers' substance misuse may well increase mental retardation prevalence rates in the years to come. Already we are seeing the effects of fetal alcohol syndrome; Streissguth et al. (1991) note that these children have lower IQs (mean = 68), often show ADHD and other attentional problems, and have difficulties in school and later life. Reviewing these issues, Baumeister, Kupstas, and Klindworth (1991) have spoken of "the new morbidity"; they stress that the population with mental retardation may differ radically from the retarded populations of earlier years.

We return, then, to the idea that recent work on mental retardation consists of "monumental advances amidst monumental controversies." The advances involve characterizations of development; attention to etiology; and new research in genetics, psychopathology, and many other areas. But the controversies also deserve mention, as definitional, service delivery, and "cultural" issues threaten to divide the field. Given an uncertain future in all of these areas, and a changing (possibly growing) population, only time will tell how well we advance in understanding and helping individuals with mental retardation.

REFERENCES

Abbeduto, L., Evans, J., & Dolan, T. (2001). Theoretical perspectives on language and communication in mental retardation and developmental disabilities. *Mental Retardation and Developmental Disabilities Research Reviews*, *7*, 45–55.

Abramowicz, H. K., & Richardson, S. (1975). Epidemiology of severe mental retardation in children: Community studies. *American Journal of Mental Deficiency*, *80*, 18–39.

Achenbach, T. M. (1991). *Manual for the Child Behavior Checklist/4–18 and 1991 Profile*. Burlington: University of Vermont, Department of Psychiatry.

Ad Hoc Committee on Terminology and Classification. (2001). Request for comments on proposed edition of *Mental retardation: Definition, classification, and systems of supports*. *AAMR News and Notes*, *14* (5), 1, 9–12.

Aman, M. G. (1991). *Assessing psychopathology and behavior problems in persons with mental retardation: A review of available instruments*. Rockville, MD: U.S. Department of Health and Human Services.

Aman, M. G., & Singh, N. N. (1994). *Aberrant Behavior Checklist—Community supplementary manual*. East Aurora, NY: Slosson Educational.

American Association on Mental Retardation (AAMR). (1992). *Mental retardation: Definition, classification, and systems of supports*. Washington, DC: Author.

American Psychiatric Association (APA). (1987). *Diagnostic and statistical manual* (3rd ed., rev.). Washington, DC: Author.

American Psychiatric Association (APA). (1994). *Diagnostic and statistical manual of mental disorders* (4th ed.). Washington, DC: Author.

American Psychological Association. (1997). *Journals in psychology: A resource listing for authors*. Washington, DC: Author.

Anderson, W. F. (1994). Gene therapy for genetic disorder. *Human Gene Therapy*, *5*, 281–282.

Artiles, A. J., & Trent, S. C. (1994). Overrepresentation of minority students in special education: A continuing debate. *Journal of Special Education*, *27*, 410–437.

August, G. J., & Lockhart, L. H. (1984). Familial autism and the fragile-X chromosome. *Journal of Autism and Developmental Disorders*, *14*, 197–204.

Bailey, D. B., Blasco, P., & Simeonson, R. (1992). Needs expressed by mothers and fathers of young children with disabilities. *American Journal on Mental Retardation*, *97*, 1–10.

Bailey, D. B., Hatton, D. D., & Skinner, M. (1998). Early developmental trajectories of males with fragile X syndrome. *American Journal on Mental Retardation*, *103*, 29–39.

Baker, B. L., & Brightman, A. J. (1997). *Steps to independence: Teaching everyday skills to children with special needs* (3rd ed.). Baltimore: Brookes.

Baumeister, A. A. (1997). Behavioral research: Boom or bust? In W.E. MacLean, Jr. (Ed.), *Ellis' handbook of mental deficiency: Psychological theory and research* (3rd ed., pp. 3–45). Mahwah, NJ: Erlbaum.

Baumeister, A. A., Kupstas, F. D., & Klindworth, L. M. (1991). The new morbidity: A national plan of action. *American Behavioral Scientist, 34*, 468–500.

Baumeister, A. A., & MacLean, W. (1979). Brain damage and mental retardation. In N. R. Ellis (Ed.), *Handbook of mental deficiency: Psychological theory and research* (2nd ed., pp. 197–230). Hillsdale, NJ: Erlbaum.

Baumgardner, T. L., Reiss, A. L., Freund, L. S., & Abrams, M. T. (1995). Specification of the neurobehavioral phenotype in males with fragile X syndrome. *Pediatrics, 95*, 744–752.

Beardsmore, A., Dorman, T., Cooper, S. A., & Webb, T. (1998). Affective psychosis and Prader–Willi syndrome. *Journal of Intellectual Disability Research, 42*, 463–471.

Beckman, P. (1983). Influence of selected child characteristics on stress in families of handicapped children. *American Journal of Mental Deficiency, 88*, 150–156.

Beeghly, M., Weiss-Perry, M., & Cicchetti, D. (1990). Beyond sensorimotor functioning: Early cognitive development and play development of children with Down syndrome. In D. Cicchetti & M. Beeghly (Eds.), *Children with Down Syndrome: A developmental approach* (pp. 329–368). New York: Cambridge University Press.

Bellugi, U., Marks, S., Bihrle, A., & Sabo, H. (1988). Dissociation between language and cognitive functions in Williams syndrome. In D. Bishop & K. Mogford (Eds.), *Language development in exceptional circumstances* (pp. 177–189).London: Churchill Livingstone.

Bellugi, U., Mills, D., Jernigan, T., Hickok, G., & Galaburda, A. (1999). Linking cognition, brain structure, and brain function in Williams syndrome. In H. Tager-Flusberg (Ed.), *Neurodevelopmental disorders* (pp. 111–136). Cambridge, MA: MIT Press.

Bellugi, U., Wang, P., & Jerrigan, T. (1994). Williams syndrome: An unusual neuropsychological profile. In S. H. Broman & J. Grafman (Eds.), *Atypical cognitive deficits in developmental disorders* (pp. 23–56). Hillsdale, NJ: Erlbaum

Bernheimer, C., & Keogh, B. (1988). Stability of cognitive performance of children with developmental delays. *American Journal of Mental Deficiency, 92*, 539–542.

Bishop, D. V. (1999). An innate basis for language? *Science, 286*, 2283–2284.

Blacher, J. (1984). Sequential stages of parental adjustment to the birth of the child with handicaps: Fact or artifact? *Mental Retardation, 22*, 55–68.

Blacher, J., & Hatton, C. (2001). Current perspectives on family research in mental retardation. *Current Opinion in Psychiatry, 14*, 477–482.

Blatt, B., & Kaplan, F. (1966). *Christmas in Purgatory*. Boston: Allyn & Bacon.

Bouras, N. (Ed.). (1999). *Psychiatric and behavioural disorders in developmental disabilities and mental retardation*. Cambridge, England: Cambridge University Press.

Bregman, J. D., Leckman, J. F., & Ort, S. I. (1988). Fragile X syndrome: Genetic predisposition to psychopathology. *Journal of Autism and Developmental Disorders, 18*, 343–354.

Broman, S., Nichols, P. L., Shaughnessy, P., & Kennedy, W. (1987). *Retardation in young children: A developmental study of cognitive deficit*. Hillsdale, NJ: Erlbaum.

Burack, J. A. (1990). Differentiating mental retardation: The two-group approach and beyond. In R. M. Hodapp, J. A. Burack, & E. Zigler (Eds.), *Issues in the developmental approach to mental retardation* (pp. 27–48). New York: Cambridge University Press.

Cahill, B. M., & Glidden, L. M. (1996). Influence of child diagnosis on family and parent functioning: Down syndrome versus other disabilities. *American Journal on Mental Retardation, 101*, 149–160.

Caruso, D. R., & Hodapp, R. M. (1988). Perceptions of mental retardation and mental illness. *American Journal on Mental Retardation, 93*, 118–124.

Carr, E. G., Horner, R. H., Turnbull, A. P., Marquis, J. G., McLaughlin, D. M., McAtee, M. L., Smith, C. E., Ryan, K. A., Ruef, M. B., Doolabh, A., & Braddock, D. (1999). *Positive behavior support for people with developmental disabilities: A research synthesis*. Washington, DC: American Association on Mental Retardation.

Carr, J. (1995). *Down's syndrome: Children growing up*. Cambridge, England: Cambridge University Press.

Cassidy, S. B. (Ed.). (1992). *Prader–Willi syndrome and other chromosome 15q deletion disorders*. New York: Springer-Verlag.

Chorney, M. J., Chorney, K., Seese, N., Owen, M. J., Daniels, J., McGuffin, P., Thompson, L. A., Detterman, D. K., Benbow, C., Lubinski, D., Eley, T., & Plomin, R. (1998). A quantitative trait locus associated with cognitive ability in children. *Psychological Science, 9*, 159–166.

Cicchetti, D., & Beeghly, M (Eds.). (1990). *Children with Down Syndrome: A developmental approach*. New York: Cambridge University Press.

Cicchetti, D., & Mans-Wagener, L. (1987). Sequences, stages, and structures in the organization of cognitive development in infants with Down Syndrome. In I. Uzgiris & J. McV. Hunt (Eds.), *Infant performance and experience: New findings with the Ordinal Scales* (pp. 281–310). Urbana: University of Illinois Press.

Clarke, D. (1998). Prader–Willi syndrome and psychotic symptoms: 2. A preliminary study of prevalence using the Psychopathology Assessment for Adults with Developmental Disability Checklist. *Journal of Intellectual Disability Research, 42*, 451–454.

Cohen, I. L., Vietze, P. M., Sudhalter, V., Jenkins, E. C., & Brown, W. T. (1991). Effects of age and communication level on eye contact in fragile X males and non-fragile X autistic males. *American Journal of Medical Genetics, 38*, 498–502.

Crnic, K., Friedrich, W., & Greenberg, M. (1983). Adaptation of families with mental retardation: A model of stress, coping, and family ecology. *American Journal of Mental Deficiency, 88*, 125–138.

Cullinan, D., Epstein, M. H., Matson, J. L., & Rosemier, R. A. (1984). Behavior problems of mentally retarded and nonretarded adolescent pupils. *School Psychology Review, 13*, 381–384.

Curtiss, S. (1977). *Genie: A psycholinguistic study of a modern-day "wild child."* New York: Academic Press.

Davies, S. P., & Ecob, K. C. (1959). The challenge to the schools. In S. P. Davies (Ed.), *The mentally retarded in society* (pp. 153–192). New York: Columbia University Press.

Dekry, S. J., & Ehly, S. W. (1981). Factor/cluster classification of profiles from Personality Inventory for Children in a school setting. *Psychological Reports, 48*, 843–846.

Del'Homme, M., Kasari, C., Forness, S. R., & Bagley, R. (1996). Prereferral intervention and students at-risk for emotional or behavioral disorders. *Education and Treatment of Children, 19,* 272–285.

Denning, C. B., Chamberlain, J. A., & Polloway, E. A. (2000). An evaluation of state guidelines for mental retardation: Focus on definition and classification practices. *Education and Training in Mental Retardation, 35,* 226–232.

Dimitropoulos, A., Feurer, I. D., Butler, M. G., & Thompson, T. (2001). Emergence of compulsive behavior and tantrums in children with Prader–Willi syndrome. *American Journal on Mental Retardation, 106,* 39–51.

Dingman, H. F., & Tarjan, G. (1960). Mental retardation and the normal distribution curve. *American Journal of Mental Deficiency, 64,* 991–994.

Dosen, A., & Gielen, J. M. (1993). Depression in persons with mental retardation: Assessment and diagnosis. In R. J. Fletcher & A. Dosen (Ed.), *Mental health aspects of mental retardation: Progress in assessment and treatment* (pp. 70–97). New York: Lexington Books.

Drotar, D., Baskiewicz, A., Irvin, N., Kennell, J., & Klaus, M. (1975). The adaptation of parents to the birth of an infant with congenital malformation: A hypothetical model. *Pediatrics, 56,* 710–717.

Dugdale, R. L. (1910). *The Jukes: A study in crime, pauperism, disease, and heredity.* New York: Putnam.

Dunst, C. J. (1980). *A clinical and educational manual for use with the Uzgiris and Hunt Scales of Infant Psychological Development.* Baltimore: University Park Press.

Dunst, C. J. (1990). Sensorimotor development of infants with Down syndrome. In D. Cicchetti & M. Beeghly (Eds.), *Children with Down Syndrome: A developmental approach* (pp. 180–230). New York: Cambridge University Press.

Dykens, E. M. (1995). Measuring behavioral phenotypes: Provocations from the "new genetics." *American Journal on Mental Retardation, 99,* 522–532.

Dykens, E. M. (2000). Psychopathology in children with intellectual disabilities. *Journal of Child Psychology and Psychiatry, 41,* 407–417.

Dykens, E. M. (in press). Anxiety, fears, and phobias in Williams syndrome. *Journal of Developmental Neuropsychology.*

Dykens, E. M. (2002). Are jigsaw puzzle skills "spared" in persons with Prader–Willi syndrome? *Journal of Child Psychology and Psychiatry, 43,* 343–352.

Dykens, E. M., & Cassidy, S. B. (1995). Correlates of maladaptive behavior in children and adults with Prader–Willi syndrome. *American Journal of Medical Genetics, 60,* 546–549.

Dykens, E. M., & Cassidy, S. B. (1996). Prader–Willi syndrome: Genetic, behavioral, and treatment issues. *Child and Adolescent Psychiatric Clinics of North America, 5,* 913–927.

Dykens, E. M., & Cassidy, S. B. (1999). Prader–Willi syndrome. In S. Goldstein & C. R. Reynolds (Eds.), *Handbook of neurodevelopmental and genetic disorders in children* (pp. 525–554). New York: Guilford Press.

Dykens, E. M., Cassidy, S. B., & King, B. H. (1999). Maladptive behavior differences in Prader–Willi syndrome associated with paternal deletion versus maternal uniparental disomy. *American Journal on Mental Retardation, 104,* 67–77.

Dykens, E. M., & Hodapp, R. M. (1997). Treatment issues in genetic mental retardation syndromes. *Professional Psychology: Research and Practice, 28*(3), 263–270.

Dykens, E. M., & Hodapp, R. M. (2001). Research in mental retardation: Toward an etiologic approach. *Journal of Child Psychology and Psychiatry, 42,* 49–71.

Dykens, E. M., Hodapp, R. M., & Evans, D. W. (1994). Profiles and development of adaptive behavior in males with fragile X syndrome. *Journal of Autism and Developmental Disorders, 23,* 135–145.

Dykens, E. M., Hodapp, R. M., & Finucane, B. M. (2000). *Genetics and mental retardation syndromes: A new look at behavior and interventions.* Baltimore: Brookes.

Dykens, E. M., Hodapp, R. M., & Leckman, J. F. (1987). Strengths and weaknesses in the intellectual functioning of males with fragile X syndrome. *American Journal of Mental Deficiency, 92,* 234–236.

Dykens, E. M., Hodapp, R. M., & Leckman, J. F. (1994). *Sage Series on Developmental Clinical Psychology and Psychiatry: No. 28. Behavior and development in fragile X syndrome.* Newbury Park, CA: Sage.

Dykens, E. M., Hodapp, R. M., Ort, S. I., Finucane, B., Shapiro, L., & Leckman, J. F. (1989). The trajectory of cognitive development in males with fragile X syndrome. *Journal of the American Academy of Child and Adolescent Psychiatry, 28,* 422–426.

Dykens, E. M., Hodapp, R. M., Walsh. K., & Nash, L. J. (1992a). Adaptive and maladaptive behavior in Prader–Willi syndrome. *Journal of the American Academy of Child and Adolescent Psychiatry, 31,* 1131–1136.

Dykens, E. M., Hodapp, R. M., Walsh, K., & Nash. L. J. (1992b). Profiles, correlates and trajectories of intelligence in Prader–Willi syndrome. *Journal of the American Academy of Child and Adolescent Psychiatry, 31,* 1125–1130.

Dykens, E. M., & Kasari, C. (1997). Maladaptive behavior in children with Prader–Willi syndrome, Down syndrome, and nonspecific mental retardation. *American Journal on Mental Retardation, 102,* 228–237.

Dykens, E. M., Leckman, J. F., & Cassidy, S. B. (1996). Obsessions and compulsions in Prader–Willi syndrome. *Journal of Child Psychology and Psychiatry, 37,* 995–1002.

Dykens, E. M., Ort, S., Cohen, I., Finucane, B., Spiridigliozzi, G., Lachiewicz, A., Reiss, A., Freund, L., Hagerman, R., & O'Connor, R. (1996). Trajectories and profiles of adaptive behavior in males with fragile X syndrome: Multicenter studies. *Journal of Autism and Developmental Disorders, 26,* 287–301.

Dykens, E. M., & Volkmar, F. R. (1997). Medical conditions associated with autism. In D. J. Cohen & F. R. Volkmar (Eds.), *Handbook of autism and pervasive developmental disorders* (2nd ed., pp. 388–407). New York: Wiley.

Einfeld, S. L., & Tonge, B. J. (1992). *Manual for the Developmental Behaviour Checklist: Primary carer version.* Randwick, Australia: School of Psychiatry, University of New South Wales.

Einfeld, S. L., & Tonge, B. J. (1996). Population prevalence of psychopathology in children and adolescents with intellectual disability: II. Epidemiological findings. *Journal of Intellectual Disability Research, 40,* 99–109.

Eyman, R. K., & Miller, C. A. (1978). A demographic overview of severe and profound mental retardation. In C. E. Meyers (Ed.), *Quality of life in severely and profoundly mentally retarded people* (pp. ix–xii). Washington, DC: American Association on Mental Deficiency.

Farber, B. (1959). The effects of the severely retarded child on the family system. *Monographs of the Society for Research in Child Development, 24,* No. 2.

Farber, B. (1970). Notes on sociological knowledge about families with mentally retarded children. In M. Schreiber (Ed.), *Social work and mental retardation* (pp. 118–124). New York: John Day.

Fidler, D. J., & Hodapp, R. M. (1999). Craniofacial maturity and perceived personality in children with Down syndrome. *American Journal on Mental Retardation, 104,* 410–421.

Fodor, J. (1983). *Modularity of mind: An essay on faculty psychology.* Cambridge, MA: MIT Press.

Fowler, A. (1988). Determinants of rate of language growth in children with Down syndrome. In L. Nadel (Ed.), *The psychobiology of Down syndrome* (pp. 217–245). Cambridge, MA: MIT Press.

Fowler, A. (1990). The development of language structure in children with Down syndrome. In D. Cicchetti & M. Beeghly (Eds.), *Children with Down Syndrome: A developmental approach* (pp. 302–328). New York: Cambridge University Press.

Foxx, R. M., & Azrin, N. H. (1974). *Toilet training the retarded: A rapid program for day and nighttime independent toileting.* Champaign, IL: Research Press.

Freeman, S. F. N., & Alkin, M. C. (2000). Academic and social attainments of children with mental retardation in general education and special education settings. *Remedial and Special Education, 21,* 3–18.

Frey, K., Greenberg, M., & Fewell, R. (1989). Stress and coping among parents of handicapped children: A multidimensional perspective. *American Journal on Mental Retardation, 94,* 240–249.

Friedrich, W. N. (1979). Predictors of coping behavior of mothers of handicapped children. *Journal of Consulting and Clinical Psychology, 47,* 1140–1141.

Gallimore, R., Keogh, B. K., & Bernheimer, L. P. (1999). The nature and long-term implications of early developmental delays: A summary of evidence from two longitudinal studies. *International Review of Research in Mental Retardation, 22,* 105–135.

Gallimore, R., Weisner, T., Kaufman, S., & Bernheimer, L. (1989). The social construction of eco-cultural niches: Family accommodation of developmentally delayed children. *American Journal on Mental Retardation, 94,* 216–230.

Gardner, H. (1983). *Frames of mind.* New York: Basic Books.

Gath, A. (1977). The impact of an abnormal child upon the parents. *British Journal of Psychiatry, 130,* 405–410.

Gath, A., & Gumley, D. (1986). Behaviour problems in retarded children with special reference to Down's syndrome. *British Journal of Psychiatry, 149,* 156–161.

Gibson, D. (1966). Early developmental staging as a prophecy index in Down's syndrome. *American Journal of Mental Deficiency, 70,* 825–828.

Gillberg, C., Persson, E., Grufman, M., & Themmer, U. (1986). Psychiatric disorders in mildly and severely mentally retarded urban children and adolescents: Epidemiological aspects. *British Journal of Psychiatry, 149,* 68–74.

Glick, M. (1998). A developmental approach to psychopathology in people with mild mental retardation. In J. A. Burack, R. M. Hodapp, & E. Zigler (Eds.), *Handbook of mental retardation and development* (pp. 563–580). New York: Cambridge University Press.

Goddard, H. H. (1913a). The improvability of feeble-minded children. *Journal of Psycho-Aesthenics, 17,* 121–126.

Goddard, H. H. (1913b). *The Kallikak family: A study in the heredity of feeble-mindedness.* New York: Macmillan.

Goldberg, S., Marcovitch, S., MacGregor, D., & Lojkasek, M. (1986). Family responses to developmentally delayed preschoolers: Etiology and the father's role. *American Journal on Mental Retardation, 90,* 610–617.

Goodman, J. F., & Cameron, J. (1978). The meaning of IQ constancy in young retarded children. *Journal of Genetic Psychology, 132,* 109–119.

Goodman, W. K., Price, L. H., Rasmussen, S. A., Mazure, C., Fleischmann, R. L., Hill, C. L., Heninger, G. R., & Charney, D. S. (1989). The Yale–Brown Obsessive–Compulsive Scale: Development, use and reliability. *Archives of General Psychiatry, 46,* 1006–1011.

Grant, G., & Whittell, B. (2000). Differentiating coping strategies in families with children or adults with intellectual disabilities: The relevance of gender, family composition, and the life span. *Journal of Applied Research in Intellectual Disabilities, 13,* 256–275.

Greenspan, S. (1997). Dead manual walking? Why the 1992 AAMR definition needs redoing. *Education and Training in Mental Retardation, 32,* 179–190.

Gresham, F. M., MacMillan, D. L., & Siperstein, G. N. (1995). Critical analysis of the 1992 AAMR definition: Implications for school psychology. *School Psychology Quarterly, 10,* 1–19.

Grizenko, N., Cvejic, H., Vida, S., & Sayegh, L. (1991). Behaviour problems in the mentally retarded. *Canadian Journal of Psychiatry, 36,* 712–717.

Grossman, H. (Ed.). (1973). *Manual on terminology and classification in mental retardation* (Special Publications Series No. 2). Washington, DC: American Association on Mental Deficiency.

Grossman, H. (Ed.). (1983). *Classification in mental retardation* (3rd rev.). Washington, DC: American Association on Mental Deficiency.

Gruenberg, E. (1964). Epidemiology. In H. A. Stevens & R. Heber (Eds.), *Mental retardation* (pp. 255–285). Chicago: University of Chicago Press.

Harrison, P. (1987). Research with adaptive behavior scales. *Journal of Special Education, 21,* 37–68.

Haskell, P. H. (1944). Mental deficiency over a hundred years. *American Journal of Psychiatry, 100,* 107–118.

Hauser-Cram, P., Warfield, M. E., Shonkoff, J. P., Krauss, M. W., Sayer, M. W., & Upshur, C. C. (2001). Children with disabilities: A longitudinal study of child development and family well-being. *Monographs of the Society for Research in Child Development, 66*(3, Serial No. 266).

Hodapp, R. M. (1994). Cultural–familial mental retardation. In R. Sternberg (Ed.), *Encyclopedia of intelligence* (pp. 711–717). New York: Macmillan.

Hodapp, R. M. (1997a). Developmental approaches to children with disabilities: New perspectives, populations, prospects. In S. S. Luthar, J. A. Burack, D. Cicchetti, & J. R. Weisz (Eds.), *Developmental psychopathology* (pp. 189–207). Cambridge, England: Cambridge University Press.

Hodapp, R. M. (1997b). Direct and indirect behavioral effects of different genetic disorders of mental retardation. *American Journal on Mental Retardation, 102,* 67–79.

Hodapp, R. M. (1998). *Development and disabilities.* Cambridge, England: Cambridge University Press.

Hodapp, R. M. (1999). Indirect effects of genetic mental retardation disorders: Theoretical and methodological issues. *International Review of Research in Mental Retardation, 22,* 27–50.

Hodapp, R. M. (2002). Parenting children with mental retardation. In M. Bornstein (Ed.), *Handbook of parenting: Vol. 1. How children influence parents* (2nd ed., pp. 355–381). Mahwah, NJ: Erlbaum.

Hodapp, R. M., & Dykens, E. M. (1991). Toward an etiology-specific strategy of early intervention with handicapped children. In K. Marfo (Ed.), *Early intervention in transition* (pp. 41–60). New York: Praeger.

Hodapp, R. M., & Dykens, E. M. (1994). The two cultures of behavioral research in mental retardation. *American Journal on Mental Retardation, 97*, 675–687.

Hodapp, R. M., & Dykens, E. M. (2001). Strengthening behavioral research on genetic mental retardation disorders. *American Journal on Mental Retardation, 106*, 4–15.

Hodapp, R. M., & Dykens, E. M. (in press). Studying behavioral phenotypes: Issues, benefits, challenges. In E. Emerson, C. Hatton, T. Parmenter, & T. Thompson (Eds.), *International handbook of applied research in intellectual disabilities*. New York: Wiley.

Hodapp, R. M., Dykens, E. M., Hagerman, R., Schreiner, R., Lachiewicz, A., & Leckman, J. F. (1990). Developmental implications of changing trajectories of IQ in males with fragile X syndrome. *Journal of the American Academy of Child and Adolescent Psychiatry, 29*, 214–219.

Hodapp, R. M., Evans, D. W., & Gray, F. L. (1999). Intellectual development in children with Down syndrome. In J. Rondal, J. Perera, & L. Nadel (Eds.), *Down syndrome: A review of current knowledge* (pp. 124–132). London: Whurr.

Hodapp, R. M., & Fidler, D. J. (1999). Special education and genetics: Connections for the 21st century. *Journal of Special Education, 33*, 130–137.

Hodapp, R. M., Leckman, J. F., Dykens, E. M., Sparrow, S., Zelinsky, D., & Ort, S. I. (1993). K-ABC profiles in children with fragile X syndrome, Down syndrome, and nonspecific mental retardation. *American Journal on Mental Retardation, 97*, 39–46.

Hodapp, R. M., Ly, T. M., Fidler, D. J., & Ricci, L. A. (2001). Less stress, more rewarding: Parenting children with Down syndrome. *Parenting: Science and Practice, 1*, 317–337.

Holm, V. A., Cassidy, S. B., Butler, M. G., Hanchett, J. M., Greenswag, L. R., Whitman, L., & Greenberg, F. (1993). Prader–Willi syndrome: Consensus diagnostic criteria. *Pediatrics, 91*, 398–402.

Hornby, G. (1996). Fathers' views of the effects on their families of children with Down syndrome. *Journal of Child and Family Studies, 4*, 103–117.

Inhelder, B. (1968). *The diagnosis of reasoning in the mentally retarded* (W. B. Stephens, Trans.). New York: John Day. (original work published 1943).

Jacobson, J. W. (1982). Problem behavior and psychiatric impairment within a developmentally delayed population: I. Behavior frequency. *Applied Research in Mental Retardation, 3*, 121–139.

Jacobson, J. W. (1990). Do some mental disorders occur less frequently among persons with mental retardation? *American Journal on Mental Retardation, 94*, 596–602.

Jacobson, J. W. (1999). Dual diagnosis services: History, progress and perspectives. In N. Bouras (Ed.), *Psychiatric and behavioural disorders in developmental disabilities and mental retardation* (pp. 329–358). Cambridge, England: Cambridge University Press.

Jacobson, J. W., & Mulick, J. (1992). A new definition of mental retardation or a new definition of practice? *Psychology in Mental Retardation and Developmental Disabilities, 18*, 9–14.

Jacobson, J. W., & Mulick, J. (Eds.). (1996). *Manual of diagnosis and professional practice in mental retardation*. Washington, DC: American Psychological Association.

Jensen, A. R. (1969). How much can we boost IQ and scholastic achievement? *Harvard Educational Review, 39*, 1–123.

Kazak, A., & Marvin, R. (1984). Differences, difficulties, and adaptation: Stress and social networks in families with a handicapped child. *Family Relations, 33*, 67–77.

Kiely, M., & Lubin, R. A. (1991). Epidemiological methods. In J.L. Matson & J.A. Mulick (Eds.), *Handbook of mental retardation* (2nd ed., pp. 586–602). New York: Pergamon Press.

King, B. T., State, M. W., Shah, B., Davanzo, P., & Dykens, E. M. (1997). Mental retardation: A review of the past 10 years. Part I. *Journal of the American Academy of Child and Adolescent Psychiatry, 36*, 1656–1663.

Krauss, M. W. (1993). Child-related and parenting stress: Similarities and differences between mothers and fathers of children with disabilities. *American Journal on Mental Retardation, 97*, 393–404.

Krauss, M. W., Simeonsson, R., & Ramey, S. L. (Eds.). (1989). Special issue on research on families. *American Journal on Mental Retardation, 94*(3).

Kumin, L. (1994). Intelligibility of speech in children with Down syndrome in natural settings: Parents' perspective. *Perceptual and Motor Skills, 78*, 307–313.

Lachiewicz, A. M., & Dawson, D. V. (1994). Behavior problems of young girls with fragile X syndrome. *American Journal of Medical Genetics, 51*, 364–369.

Lambert, N. M. (1981). Psychological evidence in *Larry P. v. Wilson Riles*: An evaluation by a witness for the defense. *American Psychologist, 36*, 937–952.

Larry P. v. Riles, Civil Action No. C-71-2270, 343F. Supp. 1306 (N.D. Cal. 1979).

Larson, S. A., Lakin, K. C., Anderson, L., Kwak, N., Lee, J. H., & Anderson, D. (2001). Prevalence of mental retardation and developmental disabilities: Estimates from the 1994/1995 National Health Interview Survey Disability Supplements. *American Journal on Mental Retardation, 106*, 231–252.

Lejeune, J., Gautier, M., & Turpin, R. (1959). Etudes des chromosomes somatiques de neuf enfants mongoliens. *Comptes Rendus de l'Academie des Sciences, 48*, 1721.

Lobato, D. (1983). Siblings of handicapped children: A review. *Journal of Autism and Developmental Disorders, 13*, 347–364.

MacMillan, D. L., Gresham, F. M., & Siperstein, G. N. (1993). Conceptual and psychometric concerns about the 1992 AAMR definition of mental retardation. *American Journal on Mental Retardation, 98*, 325–335.

MacMillan, D. L., Gresham, F. M., Siperstein, G. N., & Bocian, K. M. (1996). The labyrinth of IDEA: School decisions on referred students with subaverage general intelligence. *American Journal on Mental Retardation, 101*, 161–174.

MacMillan, D. L., Hendrick, I. G., & Watkins, A. (1988). Impact of *Diana*, *Larry P.*, and P.L. 94–142 on minority students. *Exceptional Children, 54*, 24–30.

Maisto, A. A., & German, M. L. (1986). Reliability, predictive validity, and interrelationships of early assessment indices used with developmentally delayed infants and children. *Journal of Clinical Child Psychology, 15*, 327–332.

Matson, J. L. (Ed.). (1990). *Handbook of behavior modification with the mentally retarded*. New York: Plenum Press.

Matson, J. L., & Frame, C.L. (1986). *Psychopathology among mentally retarded children and adolescents*. Beverly Hills, CA: Sage.

McCabe, E. R. B., de la Cruz, F., & Clapp, P. (1999). Workshop on fragile X: Future research directions. *American Journal of Medical Genetics*, *86*, 317–322.

McGrew, K., & Bruininks, R. (1989). Factor structure of adaptive behavior. *School Psychology Review*, *18*, 64–81.

McLaren, J., & Bryson, S. E. (1987). Review of recent epidemiological studies of mental retardation: Prevalence, associated disorders, and etiology. *American Journal on Mental Retardation*, *92*, 243–254.

Menolascino, F. J. (Ed.). (1970). *Psychiatric approaches to mental retardation*. New York: Basic Books.

Menolascino, F. J., & Fleisher, M. H. (1993). Mental health care in persons with mental retardation: Past, present and future. In R. J. Fletcher & A. Dosen (Eds.), *Mental health aspects of mental retardation: Progress in assessment and treatment* (pp. 18–41). New York: Lexington Books.

Mercer, J. (1973). *Labeling the mentally retarded: Clinical and social systems perspectives on mental retardation*. Berkeley: University of California Press.

Mercer, J. (1992). The impact of changing paradigms of disability on mental retardation in the year 2000. In L. Rowitz (Ed.), *Mental retardation in the year 2000* (pp. 15–38). New York: Springer-Verlag.

Mervis, C. B., Morris, C. A., Bertrand, J. M., & Robinson, B. F. (1999). Williams syndrome: Findings from an integrated program of research. In H. Tager-Flusberg (Ed.), *Neurodevelopmental disorders* (pp. 65–110). Cambridge, MA: MIT Press.

Meryash, D. L., Szymanski, L. S., & Gerald, P. (1982). Infantile autism associated with the fragile X syndrome. *Journal of Autism and Developmental Disorders*, *12*, 295–296.

Meyers, B. A., & Pueschel, S. M. (1991). Psychiatric disorders in persons with Down syndrome. *Journal of Nervous and Mental Disease*, *179*, 609–613.

Miller, J. (1999). Profiles of language development in children with Down syndrome. In J. F. Miller, M. Leddy, & L. A. Leavitt (Eds.), *Improving the communication of people with Down syndrome* (pp. 11–39). Baltimore: Brookes.

Mink, I., Nihira, C., & Meyers, C. (1983). Taxonomy of family life styles: I. Homes with TMR children. *American Journal of Mental Deficiency*, *87*, 484–497.

Minnes, P. (1988). Family stress associated with a developmentally handicapped child. *International Review of Research on Mental Retardation*, *15*, 195–226.

Mundy, P., & Kasari, C. (1990). The similar-structure hypothesis and differential rate of development in mental retardation. In R. M. Hodapp, J. A. Burack, & E. Zigler (Eds.), *Issues in the developmental approach to mental retardation* (pp. 71–92). New York: Cambridge University Press.

Ogbu, J. (1994). Culture and intelligence. In R. J. Sternberg (Ed.), *Encyclopedia of human intelligence* (pp. 328–338). New York: Macmillan.

Opitz, J. (1996, March). *Historiography of the causal analysis of mental retardation*. Speech to the 29th Annual Gatlinburg Conference on Research and Theory in Mental Retardation, Gatlinburg, TN.

Paterson, S. J., Brown, J. H., Gsodl, M. K., Johnson, M. H., & Karmiloff-Smith, A. (1999). Cognitive modularity and genetic disorders. *Science*, *286*, 2355–2358.

Piaget, J., & Inhelder, B. (1947). Diagnosis of mental operations and theory of intelligence. *American Journal of Mental Deficiency*, *51*, 401–406.

Polloway, E. A., Smith, J. D., Chamberlain, J., Denning, C. B., & Smith, T. E. C. (1999). Levels of deficits or supports in the classification of mental retardation: Implementation practices. *Education and Training in Mental Retardation*, *34*, 200–206.

Prader, A., Labhart, A., & Willi, H. (1956). Ein Syndrom von Adipositas, Kleinwuchs, Kryptorchismus and Oligophrenie nach myotonieartigem Zustand in Neugeborenenalter. *Schweizerische Medizinishe Wochenschrift*, *86*, 1260–1261.

Prasse, D. P., & Reschly, D. J. (1986). *Larry P.*: A case of segregation, testing, or program efficacy? *Exceptional Children*, *52*, 333–346.

Price-Bonham, S., & Addison, S. (1978). Families and mentally retarded children: Emphasis on the father. *The Family Coordinator*, *27*, 221–230.

Pueschel, S. (1987). Health concerns in persons with Down Syndrome. In S. Pueschel, C. Tingey, J. Rynders, A. Crocker, & D. Crutcher (Eds.), *New perspectives on Down Syndrome* (pp. 113–133). Baltimore: Brookes.

Ramey, C., & Ramey, S. L. (1992). Effective early intervention. *Mental Retardation*, *30*, 337–345.

Reed, E. W., & Reed, S. C. (1965). *Mental retardation: A family study*. Philadelphia: Saunders.

Reiber, R. W., & Carton, A. S. (Eds.). (1993). *The collected works of L. S. Vygotsky: Vol. 2. The fundamentals of defectology*. (J. Knox & C. B. Stephens, Trans). New York: Plenum Press.

Reid, A. H. (1980). Psychiatric disorders in mentally handicapped children: A clinical and follow-up study. *Journal of Mental Deficiency Research*, *24*, 287–298.

Reilly, J. S., Klima, E., & Bellugi, U. (1990). Once more with feeling: Affect and language in atypical populations. *Development and Psychopathology*, *2*, 367–391.

Reiss, A. L., & Freund, L. (1990). Fragile X syndrome, DSM-III-R and autism. *Journal of the American Academy of Child and Adolescent Psychiatry*, *29*, 885–891.

Reiss, S. (1990). *Reiss Scales for Children's Dual Diagnosis*. Orland Park, IL: International Diagnostic Systems.

Reschly, D. J. (1992). Mental retardation: Conceptual foundations, definitional criteria, and diagnostic operations. In S. R. Hynd & R. E. Mattison (Eds.), *Assessment and diagnosis of child and adolescent psychiatric disorders: Vol. 2. Developmental disorders* (pp. 23–67). Hillsdale, NJ: Erlbaum.

Reynolds, C. R., & Brown, R. T. (1984). *Perspectives on bias in mental testing*. New York: Wiley.

Richardson, S. A., Katz, M., Koller, H., McLaren, J., & Rubinstein, B. (1979). Some characteristics of a population of mentally retarded young adults in a British city: A basis for estimating some service needs. *Journal of Mental Deficiency Research*, *23*, 275–285.

Roeleveld, N., Zielhuis, G. A., & Gabreels, F. (1997). The prevalence of mental retardation: A critical review of recent literature. *Developmental Medicine and Child Neurology*, *39*, 125–132.

Roof, E., Stone, W., MacLean, W., Feurer, I. D., Thompson, T., & Butler, M. G. (2000). Intellectual characteristics of Prader–Willi syndrome: Comparison of genetic subtypes. *Journal of Intellectual Disability Research*, *44*, 25–30.

Ross, R. T., Begab, M. J., Dondis, E. H., Giampiccolo, J., & Meyers, C. E. (1985). *Lives of the retarded: A forty-year follow-up study*. Stanford, CA: Stanford University Press.

Rush, A. J., & Frances, A. (Eds.). (2000). Treatment of psychiatric and behavioral problems in mental retardation [Special issue]. *American Journal on Mental Retardation*, *105*(3).

Rutter, M., Simonoff, E., & Plomin, R. (1996). Genetic influences on mild mental retardation: Concepts, findings, and research implications. *Journal of Biosocial Science, 28*, 509–526.

Rutter, M., Tizard, J., Yule, W., Graham, P. & Whitmore, K. (1976). Research report: Isle of Wight Studies, 1964–1974. *Psychological Medicine, 6*, 313–332.

Scheerenberger, R. C. (1983). *A history of mental retardation*. Baltimore: Brookes.

Schwartz, D. (1992). *Crossing the river: Creating a conceptual revolution in community and disability*. Cambridge, MA: Brookline Books.

Seitz, V. (1992). Intervention programs for impoverished children: A comparison of educational and family support programs. *Annals of Child Development, 7*, 73–103.

Seltzer, M., Krauss, M. W., & Tsunematsu, N. (1993). Adults with Down syndrome and their aging mothers: Diagnostic group differences. *American Journal on Mental Retardation, 97*, 496–508.

Silverstein, A. B. (1982). Note on the constancy of IQ. *American Journal of Mental Deficiency, 87*, 227–228.

Skinner, B. F. (1968). *The technology of teaching*. New York: Appleton-Century-Crofts.

Sobesky, W. E., Porter, D., Pennington, B. F., & Hagerman, R. J. (1995). Dimensions of shyness in fragile X females. *Developmental Brain Dysfunction, 8*, 280–292.

Solnit, A., & Stark, M. (1961). Mourning and the birth of the defective child. *Psychoanalytic Study of the Child, 16*, 523–537.

Sovner, R. (1986). Limiting factors in the use of DSM-III criteria with mentally ill/mentally retarded persons. *Psychopharmacology Bulletin, 22*, 1055–1059.

Sparrow, S. S., Balla, D. A., & Cicchetti, D. V. (1984). *Vineland Adaptive Behavior Scales*. Circle Pines, MN: American Guidance Service.

Streissguth, A. P., Aase, J. M., Clarren, S. K., Randels, S. P., LaDue, R. A., & Smith, D. F. (1991). Fetal Alcohol Syndrome in adolescents and adults. *Journal of the American Medical Association, 265*, 1961–1967.

Stromme, P., & Hagberg, G. (2000). Aetiology in severe and mild mental retardation: A population-based study of Norwegian children. *Developmental Medicine and Child Neurology, 42*, 76–86.

Stromme, P., & Magnus, P. (2000). Correlations between socioeconomic status, IQ, and aetiology in mental retardation: A population-based study of Norwegian children. *Social Psychiatry and Psychiatric Epidemiology, 35*, 12–18.

Suelzle, M., & Keenan, V. (1981). Changes in family support networks over the life cycle of mentally retarded persons. *American Journal of Mental Deficiency, 86*, 267–274.

Super, C., & Harkness, S. (1986). The developmental niche: A conceptualization at the interface of child and culture. *International Journal of Behavioral Development, 9*, 545–569.

Tassone, F., Hagerman, R. J., Ikle, D., Dyer, P. N., Lampe, M., Willemsen, R., Oostra, B. A., & Taylor, A. K. (1999). FMRP expression as a potential prognostic indicator in fragile X syndrome. *American Journal of Medical Genetics, 84*, 250–261.

Taylor, H. G., Klein, N., Minich, N. M., & Hack, M. (2000). Middle-school-age outcomes of children with very low birthweight. *Child Development, 71*, 1495–1511.

Taylor, R. L. (1990). The *Larry P.* decision a decade later: Problems and future directions. *Mental Retardation, 28*(1), iii–vi.

Thompson, M. M., Gogeness, G. A., McClure, E., Clayton, R., Johnson, C., Hazelot, B., Cho, C. G., & Zellmer, V. T. (1994). Neurobehavioral characteristics of CGG amplification status in fragile X females. *American Journal of Medical Genetics, 54*, 378–383.

Tonge, B. J. (1999). Psychopathology of children with developmental disabilities. In N. Bouras (Ed.), *Psychiatric and behavioural disorders in developmental disabilities and mental retardation* (pp. 157–174). Cambridge, England: Cambridge University Press.

Udwin, O., Yule, W., & Martin, N. (1987). Cognitive abilities and behavioral characteristics of children with idiopathic infantile hypercalcaemia. *Journal of Child Psychology and Psychiatry, 28*, 297–309.

Vernon, P. (1979). *Intelligence: Heredity and environment*. San Francisco: Freeman.

Volkmar, F. R., Burack, J. A., & Cohen, D. J. (1990). Deviance and developmental approaches in the study of autism. In R. M. Hodapp, J. A. Burack, & E. Zigler (Eds.), *Issues in the developmental approach to mental retardation* (pp. 246–271). New York: Cambridge University Press.

Wehman, P., Sale, P., & Parent, W. S. (Eds.). (1992). *Supported employment: Strategies for integration of workers with disabilities*. Boston: Andover Medical.

Weiss, B., Weisz, J. R., & Bromfield, R. (1986). Performance of retarded and nonretarded persons on information-processing tasks: Further tests of the similar-structure hypothesis. *Psychological Bulletin, 90*, 153–178.

Weisz, J. R. (1990). Cultural-familial mental retardation: A developmental perspective on cognitive performance and "helpless" behavior. In R. M. Hodapp, J. A. Burack, & E. Zigler (Eds.), *Issues in the developmental approach to mental retardation* (pp. 137–168). New York: Cambridge University Press.

Weisz, J. R., Yeates, K., & Zigler, E. (1982). Piagetian evidence and the developmental-difference controversy. In E. Zigler & D. Balla (Eds.), *Mental retardation: The developmental-difference controversy* (pp. 213–276). Hillsdale, NJ: Erlbaum.

Weisz, J. R., & Zigler, E. (1979). Cognitive development in retarded and nonretarded persons: Piagetian tests of the similar sequence hypothesis. *Psychological Bulletin, 86*, 831–851.

Werner, H. (1941). Psychological processes investigating deficiencies in learning. *American Journal of Mental Deficiency, 43*, 233–235.

Wikler, L. (1986). Periodic stresses in families of mentally retarded children: An exploratory study. *American Journal of Mental Deficiency, 90*, 703–706.

Yamada, J. E. (1990). *Laura: A case for the modularity of language*. Cambridge, MA: MIT Press.

Zigler, E. (1967). Familial mental retardation: A continuing dilemma. *Science, 155*, 292–298.

Zigler, E. (1969). Developmental versus difference theories of retardation and the problem of motivation. *American Journal of Mental Deficiency, 73*, 536–556.

Zigler, E., & Hodapp, R. M. (1986). *Understanding* mental retardation. New York: Cambridge University Press.

Zigler, E., Hodapp, R. M., & Edison, M. (1990). From theory to practice in the care and education of retarded individuals. *American Journal on Mental Retardation, 95*, 1–12.

CHAPTER TWELVE

Learning Disabilities

G. Reid Lyon
Jack M. Fletcher
Marcia C. Barnes

Since learning disabilities (LDs) were federally designated as "handicapping conditions" in 1969, children identified with LDs now represent approximately one-half of all children receiving special education services in the United States (U.S. Department of Education, 1999). In the years since publication of the first edition of this chapter (Lyon, 1996b), progress has been made on understanding and treating LDs, especially in the area of reading. Here significant advances have been made in classification and definition issues (Fletcher et al., in press; Lyon et al., 2001), assessment practices (Fuchs & Fuchs, 1998; Speece & Case, 2001; Torgesen & Wagner, 1998; 2002), neurobiological correlates involving the brain (Eden & Zeffiro, 1998; Joseph, Noble, & Eden, 2001; Shaywitz et al., 2000), genetics (Grigorenko, 2001; Olson, Forsberg, Gayan, & DeFries, 1999; Wood & Grigorenko, 2001), and interventions (Felton & Brown, 1993; Foorman, Francis, Fletcher, Schatschneider, & Mehta, 1998; Fuchs et al., 2001; Lovett, Lacarenza, Borden, Frijters, Steinbach, DePalma, 2000; Lovett, Steinbach, & Frijters, 2000; Mathes, Howard, Allen, & Fuchs, 1998; Vellutino et al., 1996; Torgesen et al., 1999, 2001; Vaughn, Linan-Thompson, & Hickman-Davis, 2002). The advances in interventions are especially promising, as the research shows that reading disabilities are preventable in many children, and that intensive interventions can be effective with older children who have severe reading difficulties. Moreover, in the reading area, research is converging on a comprehensive model of the most common LD—dyslexia—that accounts for biological and environmental factors as well as for the effects of intervention, and is grounded in reading development theory (Grigorenko, 2001; Lyon et al., 2001; Rayner, Foorman, Perfetti, Pesetsky, & Seidenberg, 2002). Indeed, the same theory that explains how children develop reading skills explains why some fail, unifying research on LDs in reading and the normative development of reading ability. Given these advances for dyslexia, similar advances for other LDs cannot be far behind.

Within the context of this significant progress, the next section of this chapter reviews briefly the historical events that have molded the general field of LDs into its present form, with a focus on the origins of current policy-based definitions of LDs. Subsequent sections address in detail the core features of specific types of LDs. The reader should note from the outset that LDs do not constitute a homogeneous disorder. In fact, LDs by definition refer to deficits in one or more of several domains, including reading disabilities, mathematics disabilities, and disabilities of written expression. Since each type of LD is characterized by distinct definitional and diagnostic issues, as well as issues associated with heterogeneity, each is covered separately in this chapter. Thus, for each LD domain, a review of critical background information, constructs, and research and policy trends is provided. More specifically, a review of each major domain of LD is organized to address (1) a review of current definitional and diagnostic issues confronting each specific type of disability within the domain; (2) the epidemiology and developmental course of the disability; (3) core processes that have been identified for each disability; (4) a review of the neurobiological mechanisms hypothesized to cause and/or contribute to the specific type of LD, when any have been identified; and (5) intervention research. The chapter concludes with a brief review of current issues and a look toward the future.

HISTORY OF THE FIELD

A number of sources are available that provide overarching reviews of the field's scientific, social, and political history and development. These include works by Doris (1993), Fletcher and Morris (1986), Hallahan and Cruickshank (1973), Kavale and Forness (1985), Kavanagh and Truss (1988), Lyon et al. (2001), Myers and Hammill (1990), Morrison and Siegel (1991), Rutter (1982), Satz and Fletcher (1980), and Torgesen (1991). These works trace the origins of the field in a comprehensive and detailed fashion, and they should be consulted if one desires a more complete historical perspective on LDs. In general, these commentaries indicate that the field of LDs developed in response to two major needs.

First, the field is linked closely with the historical need to understand individual differences in learning and performance among children and adults displaying *specific* deficits in using spoken or written language, while maintaining integrity in general intellectual functioning. This unexpected pattern of strengths and *specific* weaknesses in learning was first noted and studied by physicians and psychologists, thus giving the field the biomedical and psychological orientation that has always characterized it. Second, the LD movement developed as an applied field of special education driven by social and political forces, and in response to the need to provide services to youngsters whose learning characteristics were not being adequately addressed by the educational system. Each of these historical contexts is reviewed briefly.

Learning Disabilities and the Study of Individual Differences

Gall's Influence

As Torgesen (1991) and Mann (1979) have pointed out, interest in the causes and outcomes of inter- and intraindividual differences in cognition and learning can be traced to early Greek civilization. However, the first work that had clear relevance to today's conceptualizations of LDs was conducted by Gall in the context of his work on disorders of spoken language in the early 19th century (Wiederholt, 1974). In describing the characteristics of one patient with brain damage, Gall recorded the following:

> In consequence of an attack of apoplexy, a soldier found it impossible to express in spoken language his feelings and ideas. His face bore no signs of a deranged intellect. His mind (*esprit*) found the answer to questions addressed to him and he carried out all he was told to do; shown an armchair and asked if he knew what it was, he answered by seating himself in it. He could not articulate on the spot a word pronounced for him to repeat; but a few moments later the word escaped from his lips as if voluntarily. . . . It was not his tongue, which was embarrassed; for he moved it with great agility and could pronounce quite well a large number of isolated words. His memory was not at fault, for he signified his anger at being unable to express himself concerning many things, which he wished to communicate. It was the faculty of speech, alone which was abolished. (quoted in Head, 1926, p. 11)

The relevance of Gall's observations to present conceptualizations of LDs was summarized by Hammill (1993). According to Hammill, Gall noted that some of his patients could not speak but could produce thoughts in writing, thus manifesting a pattern of relative strengths and weaknesses in oral and written language. In addition, Gall established that such patterns of strengths and weaknesses were a function of brain damage, and that brain damage could selectively impair one particular language capability but not affect others. Thus the clinical roots were established for the present-day observation that many children with LDs manifest "specific" deficits rather than pervasive or "generalized" deficits. Finally, Gall argued that it was essential to rule out other disabling conditions, such as mental retardation or deafness, that could impair a patient's performance. Within this context, the origins for the "exclusion" component of current definitions of LDs are evident.

Early Neurology and Acquired Language Disorders

A number of other medical professionals also began to observe and report on patients demonstrating intraindividual strengths and weaknesses that included specific deficits in linguistic, reading, and cognitive abilities. For example, Broca (1863, 1865) provided important observations that have served to build the foundation of the "specificity" hypothesis in learning disabilities. Broca (1865) reported that "expressive aphasia," or the inability to speak, resulted from selective (rather than diffuse) lesions to the anterior regions of the left hemisphere primarily localized in the second frontal convolution. The effects of a lesion to this area of the brain were highly consistent in right-handed individuals, and *did not* appear to affect receptive language ability (listening) or other, nonlanguage functions (e.g., visual perception, spatial awareness, etc.).

In a similar vein, Wernicke (1894) introduced the concept of a "disconnection syndrome" when he predicted that the aphasic syndrome termed "conduction aphasia" could result from a disconnection of the receptive (sensory) speech area from the motor speech zone by a punctate lesion in the left hemisphere. Wernicke's observations have also been relevant to theory building in LDs, since he reported that a complex function such as receptive language could be impaired within an individual who did not display other significant cognitive or linguistic dysfunctions. Thus the concept of intraindividual differences in information processing was born more than a century ago, primarily via observations and clinical studies with adults with specific brain damage.

In the latter 1800s and early 1900s, additional cases of unexpected cognitive and linguistic difficulties within the context of otherwise normal functioning were reported. These cases were unique, as they did not seem to have the same lesional basis as acquired disorders of language, occurring with impairment of sensory or motor functions. For example, Kussmaul (1877) described a patient who was unable to read despite having intact intellectual and perceptual skills. Additional reports by Hinshelwood (1895, 1900, 1917), Jackson (1906), Morgan (1896), and others (Bastian, 1898; Clairborne, 1906; Stephenson, 1905) distinguished a specific type of learning deficit characterized by an inability to read against a background of normal intelligence and adequate opportunity to learn. For example, Hinshelwood (1917) described one 10-year-old youngster as follows:

> The boy had been at school three years and had got on well with every subject except reading. He was apparently a bright and in every respect an intelligent boy. He had been learning music for a year and had made good progress in it. . . . In all departments of his studies where the instruction was oral he had made good progress, showing that his auditory memory was good. . . . He performs simple sums quite correctly, and his progress in arithmetic has been regarded as quite satisfactory. He has no difficulty in learning to write. His visual acuity is good. (pp. 46–47)

Thus, by the beginning of the 20th century, evidence from several sources contributed to a set of observations that defined a unique type of learning difficulty in adults *and* children—specific rather than general in presentation, and distinct from disorders associated with sensory handicaps and subaverage general intelligence. As Hynd and Willis (1988) have summarized, the most salient and reliable observations included the following: (1) The children had some form of congenital learning problem; (2) more male than female children were affected; (3) the disorder was heterogeneous with respect to the specific pattern and the severity of deficits; (4) the disorder might be related to a developmental process affecting primarily left-hemisphere central language processes; and (5) typical classroom instruction was not adequate in meeting the children's educational needs. More recent evidence has supported some of these observations, but many have not been validated, as is made evident in later discussions.

Orton and the Origins of Dyslexia

During the 1920s, Samuel Orton extended the study of reading disabilities with clinical studies designed to test the hypothesis that reading deficits were a function of a delay or failure of the left cerebral hemisphere to establish dominance for language functions. According to Orton (1928), children with reading disabilities tended to reverse letters such as "b/d" and "p/q," and words such as "saw/was" and "not/ton," because of the lack of left-hemispheric dominance for the processing of linguistic symbols.

As Torgesen (1991) pointed out, neither Orton's theory of reading disabilities nor his observation that reversals were symptomatic of the disorder have stood the test of time. However, Orton's (1928, 1937) writings were highly influential in stimulating research, mobilizing teacher and parent groups to bring attention to reading disorders and other LDs that had a deleterious impact on a child's academic, behavioral, and social development, and on the development of instructional techniques for teaching reading-disabled children. Moreover, Orton's influence on present-day conceptualizations of LDs can be seen indirectly in his early attempts to classify, within the same conceptual and etiological framework, a *range* of language and motor disabilities in addition to reading disabilities (Doris, 1993). More specifically, in 1937 Orton reported a number of cases of children of average to above-average intelligence who manifested (1) "developmental alexia," or difficulty learning to read; (2) "developmental agraphia," or significant difficulty in learning to write; (3) "developmental word deafness," or a specific deficit in verbal understanding within a context of normal auditory acuity; (4) "developmental motor aphasia," or motor speech delay; (5) abnormal clumsiness; and (6) stuttering. Orton (1937) was the first to stress that reading disabilities were manifested at the symbolic level, appeared to be related to cerebral dysfunction rather than a lesional defect as postulated by Hinshelwood, and did not co-occur strictly with low intelligence.

The Straussian Movement and the Concept of Cerebral Dysfunction

Whereas Orton's contributions are linked primarily to the development of scientific and clinical interest in reading disabilities (particularly dyslexia), it was the work of Strauss and Werner (1943) and their colleagues (Strauss & Lehtinen, 1947) during the period after World War II that led directly to the emergence of the more general category of LDs as a formally recognized field (Doris, 1993; Rutter, 1982; Torgesen, 1991). This work built on an earlier series of attempts to understand the behavioral difficulties of children who subsequently were described as hyperactive; in this series of clinical observations, children's overactivity, impulsivity, and concrete thinking were attributed to brain damage, in the absence of physical evidence for an injury to the brain. Strauss and Werner expanded this concept in research involving children with mental retardation. They were particularly interested in comparing the behavior of children whose retardation was associated with known brain damage to that of children whose retardation was not associated with neurological impairment, but was presumably familial in nature. Strauss and Lehtinen (1947) reported that children with mental retardation and brain injury manifested difficulties on tasks assessing figure–ground perception, attention, and concept formation in addition to hyperactivity, whereas non-brain-damaged children with mental retardation performed in a manner similar to children who were not retarded and were less likely to show behavioral overactivity. Within the context of these studies, Strauss's group subsequently observed patterns similar to those of children with mental retardation and brain injury in children with average intelligence, but behavioral and learning difficulties. They attributed to these children a syndrome they called "minimal brain injury" (MBI). From these studies, the concept of "minimal brain dysfunction" (MBD) emerged in the 1960s (Clements, 1966), with an emphasis on the Straussian thesis that MBI or MBD could be identified solely on the basis of behavioral signs even when physical and neurological examinations were normal:

> When no mental retardation exists, the presence of psychological disturbances can be discovered by the use of some of our qualitative tests for perceptual and cognitive disturbances. Although the . . . [physical] criteria may be negative, whereas the behavior of the child in question resembles that characteristic for brain injury, and even though the performances of the child on our tests are not strongly indicative of brain injury, it may still be reasonable to consider a diagnosis of brain injury. (Strauss & Lehtinen, 1947, p. 112)

The Straussian movement had a profound influence on the development of the field (Doris, 1993; Hallahan & Cruickshank, 1973; Kavale & Forness, 1985). In summarizing the influence of Strauss, Torgesen (1991, p. 12) pointed out that three concepts emerging from his work served to provide a rationale for the development of the field of LDs separately from other fields of education:

1. Individual differences in learning should be understood by examining the different ways that children approach learning tasks (the processes that aid or interfere with learning).
2. Educational procedures should be tailored to patterns of processing strengths and weaknesses in the individual child.
3. Children with deficient learning processes may be helped to learn normally if those processes

are strengthened, or if teaching methods that do not stress weak areas can be developed.

Likewise, Kavale and Forness (1985) reported that the research and writings of Strauss and his colleagues had a significant influence on the development of the LD paradigm—but through ideas that were more theoretical than those summarized by Torgesen (1991). The ideas included the following:

1. The locus of an LD is within the affected individual, and thus represents a medical (disease) model.
2. LDs are associated with (or caused by) neurological dysfunction.
3. The academic problems observed in children with LDs are related to psychological processing deficits, most notably in the perceptual–motor domain.
4. The academic failure of children with LDs occurs despite the presence of normal intelligence; that is, there is a discrepancy between IQ (average or above) and academic achievement (subaverage).
5. LDs cannot primarily be due to other handicapping conditions.

We would add to this list the idea that brain dysfunction can be identified solely through behavioral signs even in the absence of a history of neurological disease, and we would also note the linking of behavioral characteristics of hyperactivity with LDs. Strauss and Werner's writings had a tremendous impact on the thinking and careers of several behavioral scientists who, in the 1950s and 1960s, were studying children who failed to learn in school despite having normal intelligence.

Cruickshank, Myklebust, Johnson, and Kirk, and the Concept of LDs

Foremost among the behavioral scientists involved in the early conceptualization and study of LDs were William Cruickshank, Helmer Myklebust, Doris Johnson, and Samuel Kirk, all of whom propelled the field away from a focus on etiology toward an emphasis on learner characteristics and educational interventions to address learning deficits. For example, Cruickshank and his colleagues (Cruickshank, Bice, & Wallin, 1957; Cruickshank, Bentzen, Ratzburg, & Tannenhauser, 1961) were instrumental in studying and recommending modifications in classroom environments to reduce stimuli hypothesized to be distracting for children with learning and attention deficits. Likewise, Helmer Myklebust and Doris Johnson, working at Northwestern University, conducted numerous studies of the effects of different types of language and perceptual deficits on academic and social learning in children, and were among the first to develop well-designed intervention procedures for the remediation of disabilities in skills related to school learning (Johnson & Myklebust, 1967). However, it was Samuel Kirk who had the greatest influence on the formal recognition of LDs as handicapping conditions. In fact, it was Kirk who proposed the term "learning disabilities" in a 1963 conference devoted to exploring problems of perceptually handicapped children. Kirk (1963) stated:

> I have used the term "learning disabilities" to describe a group of children who have disorders in the development of language, speech, reading and associated communication skills needed for social interaction. In this group, I do not include children who have sensory handicaps such as blindness, because we have methods of managing and training the deaf and blind, I also excluded from this group children who have generalized mental retardation. (pp. 2–3)

Thus, by 1963, the new field of LDs was moving toward the formal designation of LDs as handicapping conditions. This movement was based largely on the arguments of Kirk and others that children with LDs were indeed different with respect to learning characteristics from children with mental retardation or emotional disturbance; that these learning characteristics resulted from intrinsic (i.e., neurobiological) rather than environmental factors; that LDs were "unexpected," given the children's strengths in other areas; and that children with LDs required specialized educational interventions. What is interesting is that the field received its initial momentum on the strength of clinical observation and advocacy. Only in the past 20 years has a systematic research base begun to emerge.

Learning Disabilities as an Applied Field Molded by Social and Political Forces

As has been noted, the creation of the applied special education category of LDs in the 1960s reflected a belief by physicians, behavioral scientists, educators, and parents that some children had learning handicaps that were not being addressed effectively by extant educational practices (Zigmond, 1993). More specifically, prior to the mid-1960s, children who displayed unusual learning characteristics in the context of average to above-average intelligence were disenfranchised from educational services, because their cognitive and educational characteristics did not correspond to any recognized categories of disability. This disenfranchisement successfully stimulated a socially and politically based advocacy movement designed to protect children from being underserved by our educational system (Lyon et al., 2001; Lyon & Moats, 1993; Moats & Lyon, 1993).

The fact that LDs were initially and formally identified as handicapping conditions on the basis of advocacy rather than systematic scientific inquiry is certainly not uncommon in either educational or public health domains. In fact, in the United States, the majority of scientific advances are typically stimulated by vocal critics of the educational or medical status quo. It is rare that a psychological condition, disease, or educational problem is afforded attention until political forces are mobilized by parents, patients, or other affected individuals expressing their concerns about their quality of life to their elected officials. Clearly, this was the case in the field of LDs, where parents and child advocates successfully lobbied Congress to enact legislation in 1969 via the Education of the Handicapped Act (P.L. 91-230). This law authorized research and training programs to address the needs of children with specific LDs (Doris, 1993).

The diagnostic concept of LDs gained significant momentum during the 1960s and 1970s. As Zigmond (1993) has explained, the proliferation of children diagnosed as having LDs during these two decades was related to multiple factors. First, the label of "LDs" was not a stigmatizing one. Parents and teachers were certainly more comfortable with the term than with etiologically based labels such as "brain injuries," "MBD," and "perceptual handicaps." Second, receiving a diagnosis of an LD did not imply low intelligence, behavioral difficulties, or sensory handicaps. Quite the contrary, children with LDs manifested difficulties in learning *despite* having average to above-average intelligence and intact hearing, vision, and emotional status. The fact that youngsters with LDs displayed robust intelligence gave parents and teachers hope that difficulties in learning to read, write, calculate, or reason mathematically could be surmounted if only the right set of instructional conditions and settings could be identified. Advocacy efforts fueled a series of consensus conferences, two of which are most noteworthy: one on MBI and the other on LDs. Both attempted to define the disabilities widely believed to hamper the educational behavioral performance of many children in schools under a single overarching concept.

Definition of MBD

In the 1960s, the twin strands of individual differences and applications through social and political advocacy joined together, initially through efforts to define this syndrome of unexpected behavioral difficulties and underachievement due to factors intrinsic to the child. The first significant effort involved the development of a definition of MBI in 1962. In a meeting organized by what is now the National Institute of Neurological Disorders and Stroke, along with the Easter Seals Society, a formal definition of a syndrome called "minimal brain dysfunction" was formulated:

> The term "minimal brain dysfunction syndrome" refers . . . to children of near average, average, or above average general intelligence with certain learning or behavioral disabilities ranging from mild to severe, which are associated with deviations of function of the central nervous system. These deviations may manifest themselves by various combinations of impairment in perception, conceptualization, language, memory, and control of attention, impulse, or motor function. (Clements, 1966, pp. 9–10)

This definition essentially substituted "dysfunction" for "injury," recognizing the etiological implications of terms like "injury." It identified children with MBD as heterogeneous, with both behavioral and learning difficulties. As we noted above, the definition stipulated that brain dysfunction could be identified solely on the basis of behavioral signs.

The definition of MBD was controversial from its initial formulation (Rutter, 1982; Satz & Fletcher, 1980). It was based on over half a century of careful clinical observation and research reports especially characteristic of neurology at the time. There was also empirical support from emergent and at the time, highly innovative psychophysiological methods by researchers led by Dykman, Ackerman, Clements, and Peters (1971). Educators, however, objected to the concept, because it seemed too oriented to a medical model and implied that psychologists and physicians would have to work in schools in order to make the diagnosis. Others found the concept fuzzy and too broad (Rutter, 1982; Satz & Fletcher, 1980). The latter concern was magnified in the 1970s with the development of checklists for MBD that included over 30 symptoms (Peters, Davis, Goolshy, & Clements, 1973). These symptoms ranged from difficulties with academic skills to aggressive, acting-out behavior. The syndrome thus seemed so broad that the treatment implications of identifying a child with MBD were unclear (Rutter, 1982; Satz & Fletcher, 1980).

When the third edition of the *Diagnostic and Statistical Manual of Mental Disorders* (DSM-III) was published by the American Psychiatric Association (1980), the concept of MBD was dropped, and the learning and behavioral characteristics were separately defined as "specific developmental disorders" and "attention deficit disorder" (ADD). This division was wise, as the classification problem that plagued those interested in MBI and MBD was the comorbidity of learning and attention disorders. Many children with LDs also meet criteria for attention-deficit/hyperactivity disorder (ADHD). However, they are separate types of disorders, both requiring intervention. Heritability, neurobiological correlates, and intervention needs are clearly different, so unifying them as a single syndrome did not facilitate research or practice (Fletcher, Shaywitz, & Shaywitz, 1999).

Recent efforts to redefine the concept of MBD as "atypical brain development" (Gilger & Kaplan, 2002) are not likely to prove useful, as indicating that brain development is atypical in children with these "unexplained" learning and behavioral difficulties is hardly new and almost tautologous, given the state of the evidence reviewed below. It is not much different than simply invoking "cerebral dysfunction" as an explanation of MBD or LDs. History shows that such broad, overarching concepts lead to clumping together of behaviors and learning characteristics that need to be better differentiated in order to facilitate intervention. As we show below, this is becoming increasingly possible in the area of LDs (and ADHD).

Federal Definition of LDs

Not surprisingly, the development of the definition of MBD led to reactions among educators and other professionals working in schools. In 1966, the U.S. Office of Education organized a meeting in which the participants formally defined Kirk's (1963) concept of "learning disability," as follows:

> The term "specific learning disability" means a disorder in one or more of the basic psychological processes involved in understanding or in using language, spoken or written, which may manifest itself in an imperfect ability to listen, speak, read, write, spell, or to do mathematical calculations. The term includes such conditions as perceptual handicaps, brain injury, minimal brain dysfunction, dyslexia, and developmental aphasia. The term does not include children who have learning disabilities, which are primarily the result of visual, hearing, or motor handicaps, or mental retardation, or emotional disturbance, or of environmental, cultural, or economic disadvantage (U.S. Office of Education, 1968, p. 34)

The resemblance of this 1966 definition of an LD to the 1962 definition of MBD (Clements, 1966) is striking. The notion of MBD as an "unexpected" disorder not attributable to mental deficiency, sensory disorders, emotional disturbance, or cultural or economic disturbance was retained, reflecting work over the previous 60 years. Etiological terms were dropped and replaced by educational descriptors. The implicit attribution to intrinsic factors within the child was retained as the definition was clearly intended to be inclusive of minimal brain dysfunction and other formulations derived from neurology and psychology (Doris, 1993; Rutter, 1982; Satz & Fletcher, 1980).

The most significant attribution for the pivotal importance of this definition is the fact that it continues as the federal definition of an LD. It has persisted through a series of parental and professional advocacy efforts that led to the provision of special education services for children with LDs. This occurred initially through the 1969 Learning Disabilities Act. The statutory definition of LDs in the 1969 Act then appeared in the Education for All Handicapped Children Act of 1975 (P.L. 94-142), and is currently reflected in the 1997 reauthorization of the Individuals with Disabilities Education Act (IDEA). This definition has persisted despite the fact that it does not specify any inclusionary criteria for LDs. It essentially says that LDs are heterogeneous and not due to low intelligence and other exclusionary conditions. In a sense, the disorders became legitimized and codified in public law mostly on the basis of what they were not.

The absence of inclusionary criteria became an immediate problem in 1975, with passage of P.L. 94-142 and the expectation that states would identify and serve children with LDs. In response to this problem, the U.S. Office of Education (1977) published recommendations for procedures for identifying LDs that included the notion of a discrepancy between IQ and achievement as a marker for LDs, as follows:

> . . . a severe discrepancy between achievement and intellectual ability in one or more of the areas: (1) oral expression; (2) listening comprehension; (3) written expression; (4) basic reading skill; (5) reading comprehension; (6) mathematics calculation; or (7) mathematic reasoning. The child may not be identified as having a specific learning disability if the discrepancy between ability and achievement is primarily the result of: (1) a visual, hearing, or motor handicap; (2) mental retardation; (3) emotional disturbance, or (4) environmental, cultural, or economic disadvantage. (p. G1082)

The use of IQ–achievement discrepancy as a marker for LDs has had a profound impact on how LDs are conceptualized. There was little research at the time validating an IQ–achievement discrepancy model, but researchers, practitioners, and the public continue to assume that such a discrepancy is a marker for specific types of LDs that are unexpected and categorically distinct from other forms of underachievement. Some researchers continue to use IQ–achievement discrepancy as a key aspect of the identification process (Kavale & Forness, 2000), despite the fact that, as we will discuss below, the evidence base for its validity as a central feature of LD classification is weak to nonexistent (Fletcher et al., in press; Lyon et al., 2001). But the impact of IQ–achievement discrepancy is clearly apparent in the regulations concerning LD identification in the 1992 and 1997 reauthorizations of IDEA. The statute has maintained the definition of LDs formulated in the 1966 meeting, while the regulations maintain the 1977 procedures. The most recent reauthorization includes the following regulatory recommendations:

> (a) A team may determine that a child has a specific learning disability if:
>
> (1) The child does not achieve commensurate with his or her age and ability levels in one or more of the areas listed in paragraph (a) (2) of this section, when provided with learning experiences appropriate for the child's age and ability levels; and
>
> (2) The team finds that a child has a severe discrepancy between achievement and intellectual ability in one or more of the following areas: (i) Oral expression; (ii) Listening comprehension; (iii) Written expression; (iv) Basic reading skill; (v) Reading comprehension; (vi) Mathematics calculation; or (vii) Mathematics reasoning. (U.S. Department of Education, 1999, p. 12457)

Other Definitions of LD

The federal definition of LDs has been widely critized (Fletcher et al., in press; Kavale & Forness, 1985; Kavale & Nye, 1981; Lyon, 1987, 1994a, 1994b; Lyon, Gray, Kavanagh, & Krasnegor, 1993; Lyon et al., 2001; Senf, 1981, 1986, 1987; Ysseldyke & Algozzine, 1983). As Torgesen (1991) has pointed out, this definition has at least four major problems that renders it ineffective:

1. It does not indicate clearly enough that LDs are a heterogeneous group of disorders.
2. It fails to recognize that LDs frequently persist and are manifested in adults as well as children.
3. It does not clearly specify that, whatever the cause of LDs, the "final common path" consists of inherent alterations in the way information is processed.
4. It does not adequately recognize that persons with other handicapping or environmental limitations may have an LD *concurrently* with these conditions.

Other formal attempts to tighten the federal definition of LDs have not fared appreciably better (Moats & Lyon, 1993), as can be seen in the revised definition produced by the National Joint Committee on Learning Disabilities (NJCLD, 1988) (see also Hammill, 1993; Hammill, Leigh, McNutt, & Larsen, 1981):

> *Learning disabilities* is a general term that refers to a heterogeneous group of disorders manifested by significant difficulty in the acquisition and use

of listening, speaking, reading, writing, reasoning, or mathematical abilities. These disorders are intrinsic to the individual, presumed to be due to central nervous system dysfunction, and may occur across the life span. Problems in self-regulatory behavior, social perception, and social interaction may exist with learning disabilities but do not by themselves constitute a learning disability. Although learning disabilities may occur concomitantly with other handicapping conditions (for example, sensory impairment, mental retardation, social and emotional disturbance) or with extrinsic influences (such as cultural differences, insufficient or inappropriate instruction), they are not the result of these conditions or influences. (p. 1)

Although the NJCLD definition addresses the issues of heterogeneity, persistence, intrinsic etiology, and comorbidity discussed by Torgesen (1991), it continues to reflect a vague and ambiguous description of multiple and heterogeneous disorders. These types of definitions cannot be easily operationalized or empirically validated, and do not provide clinicians, teachers, and researchers with useful information to enhance communication or improve predictions. There are no inclusionary criteria, and it is also a definition based on exclusion. Given this state of the field, many scholars have called for a moratorium on the development of broad definitions, and advocate definitions that only address LDs defined in terms of coherent and operational domains. As Stanovich (1993) has stated,

> Scientific investigations of some generically defined entity called "learning disability" simply make little sense given what we already know about heterogeneity across various learning domains. Research investigations must define groups specifically in terms of the domain of deficit (reading disability, arithmetic disability). The extent of co-occurrence of these dysfunctions then becomes an empirical question, not something decided a priori by definition practices. (p. 273)

It should be noted that both DSM-IV (American Psychiatric Association, 1994) and the *International Classification of Diseases*, 10th revision (ICD-10; World Health Organization, 1992) have in fact defined classified and coded learning disorders and specific developmental disorders of scholastic skills into specific deficit domains. For example, DSM-IV provides criteria for the diagnosis of "reading disorder" (315.00), while ICD-10 provides identification criteria under the term "specific reading disorder" (F81.0). DSM-IV and ICD-10 refer to disabilities in mathematics as "mathematics disorder" (315.1) and "specific disorder of arithmetical skills" (F81.2), respectively. Finally, disabilities involving written language skills are classified and coded by DSM-IV as "disorder of written expression" (315.2) and by ICD-10 as "specific spelling disorder" (F81.1). These definitions implicitly support the heterogeneity and exclusion components of most definitions. Interestingly, they also invoke IQ–achievement discrepancy as an inclusionary criterion. But they are essentially the same definitions applied to each domain, thus lacking any real specificity. The problems with the federal definition of LDs thus also apply to the DSM-IV and ICD-10 definitions.

Regardless of whether one approaches the task of defining LDs in a general fashion as has been traditionally done at the federal level, or whether one seeks to define domain-specific LDs (e.g., reading disability) as advocated by Stanovich (1993), the definitional process must be informed by, and constructed within, a classification system that ultimately has communicative and predictive power. The logic underlying the development of such a classification system is that identification, diagnosis, treatment, and prognosis cannot be addressed effectively until the heterogeneity across and within domain-specific LDs is accounted for, and until subgroups and subtypes are delineated that are theoretically meaningful, reliable, and valid. Of utmost importance is the validity of the three classification hypotheses implicit in most definitions of LDs. In the next section, we review evidence for the validity of the IQ–achievement discrepancy hypothesis and the exclusion hypothesis. Then we use a review of the heterogeneity hypothesis to discuss what we know about domain-specific LDs.

Summary

The field of LDs emerged from a genuine social and educational need. LDs constitute a diagnostic category that is viable in clinical practice, law, and policy. Historically, parents, educators, and other advocates for children have successfully negotiated a special education category subsuming LDs as a means of protecting of civil rights and procedural safeguards in law (Keogh, 1993; Lyon & Moats, 1993; Martin, 1993; Zigmond, 1993). In many respects, however, LDs became legitimized and codified in public law more for what they were not than what they were. Moreover, the concept of LDs is based on what is now a century of attempts to define it as an overarching classification applicable to a wide segment of childhood difficulties involving learning (and behavior). Only in the past 20 or so years have serious and systematic research efforts been deployed toward the task of understanding the causes, developmental course, treatment conditions, and long-term outcomes of LDs from a scientific perspective.

Unfortunately, as Lyon (1996b) stated in the first edition of this chapter, many of these efforts have not led to more precise definitions and interventions for those with LDs, despite significant research advances. These difficulties, and the reification of historically unsupported assumptions about LDs that have not stood up under scientific scrutiny, may well prevent us from implementing what we have learned from the significant advances in research that have occurred over the past 20 years. This is unfortunate. The groups of advocates who successfully implemented essential educational reforms legitimizing the concept of LDs and helped make a systematic research program possible may be hanging on to components of the definition that are outdated, indefensible, and not lined up with research. In doing so, they may be promulgating identification and intervention practices that are not effective, making it difficult to implement practices that have merged from research (Fletcher et al., in press; Lyon et al., 2001). These practices have the potential to ameliorate some of the adverse long-term outcomes often associated with LDs (Bruck, 1985; Francis, Shaywitz, Stuebing, Shaywitz, & Fletcher, 1996; Satz, Buka, Lipsitt, & Seidman, 1998; Spreen, 1989).

IQ–achievement discrepancy has achieved a prominent role as a component of the definition and classification of children with LDs. However, it is only one component of most definitions of LDs. Two other components, which involve the *heterogeneity* of LDs and the role of *exclusionary* factors, have been key components of almost every attempt to define or classify LDs and their historical antecedents. These components of different definitions are *hypotheses* about the classification of LDs. IQ–achievement discrepancy is essentially a hypothesis that children who are identified as having LDs can be differentiated from other poorly achieving children on variables not used to define either IQ or achievement (e.g., cognitive characteristics, response to intervention, prognosis). The heterogeneity hypothesis postulates that there are seven potentially overlapping subgroups of LDs. The exclusion hypothesis is that children defined as having LDs differ from children whose low achievement is expected because of such factors as mental retardation; sensory disorders; emotional disturbance; social, economic, and cultural disadvantage; and inadequate instruction.

To understand these issues, we first must provide a more thorough discussion of definitional and classification issues underlying the discrepancy, heterogeneity, and exclusion hypotheses. In doing so, we emphasize that we are not questioning the validity of the concept of LDs and that there is considerable evidence for the validity of this concept, even though some prominent hypotheses may lack validity. There is clear evidence from multiple sources that indicate that children with specific LDs can be differentiated from (1) typically achieving children; (2) children with other LDs (e.g., reading vs. math); and (3) children with other types of processing difficulties (e.g., ADHD). Moreover, different LDs vary in their neurobiological correlates and intervention needs, as well as their cognitive correlates (Fletcher et al., in press; Lyon et al., 2001; Morris, in press). More of this evidence will be reviewed below when we discuss different types of LDs involving reading, math, and written expression.

PROBLEMS WITH THE CONCEPT OF DISCREPANCY

A fundamental historical assumption underlying the construct of LDs is that the academic difficulties manifested by individuals with LDs are *unexpected*, given adequate intelligence, opportunities to learn, freedom from socioeconomic disadvantage or emotional difficulties, and strengths in other academic areas and adaptive functions. The assumption of "unexpected underachievement" has been commonly operationalized as an aptitude–achievement discrepancy, where aptitude is typically assessed via intelligence tests. It is based on the premise that individuals who display such a discrepancy are *qualitatively* different from individuals with low achievement and comparably low IQ scores (i.e., so-called "slow learners"). These differences are presumed to exist both in phenotypic variables, such as cognitive skills or response to intervention, and in genotypic variables, such as differences in the heritability of the disorders or their neurophysiological signatures (Fletcher et al., 1998, in press; Lyon et al., 2001; Siegel, 1992; Stanovich, 1993).

Recent studies of children with LDs in reading and other academic areas cast doubt on the utility and validity of the notion of discrepancy. This research has been most extensive in the area of reading, where it involves evaluations of (1) response to intervention; (2) cognitive characteristics; (3) development and prognosis of reading difficulties; and (4) neurobiological factors. In areas of the LD definition involving disorders of speech and language, math, and written expression, the evidence is less extensive, but is consistent with that from the reading research. In the reading area, the research occurs across the age range, including adults (Stuebing et al., 2002), and involves multiple approaches to definition of LDs in reading (word recognition, comprehension). Similar results occur when different measures of IQ are used (e.g., Verbal IQ, Performance IQ; Fletcher et al., 1994; Stanovich & Siegel, 1994). As we shall see, such convergence is not surprising, given the psychometric limitations inherent in attempts to utilize IQ–achievement discrepancy as a marker of LDs. In this section, we provide an overview of this research, first in reading and then in other areas of LDs. We conclude the section with a discussion of psychometric issues.

IQ–Achievement Discrepancy and Reading Disabilities

Response to Intervention

Several studies have examined the outcomes of reading interventions in relationship to different indices of IQ or IQ–achievement discrepancy. Aaron (1997) reviewed earlier studies that sometimes included comparisons of groups defined as having an IQ–achievement discrepancy and as low-achieving but having no such discrepancy. He found that both groups made little progress in their reading development, even with remedial placements. More recent studies have explicitly examined this hypothesis in remedial or prevention interventions and are summarized in Table 12.1. Table 12.1 shows that five of the six studies found no relation of intervention outcomes to IQ or IQ–achievement discrepancy. The exception was a remedial study of children with reading difficulties in grades 2–5 (Wise, Ring, & Olson, 2000). In this study, Full Scale IQ predicted about 5% of the variance in word-reading outcomes on one measure of word reading, but this effect was not apparent on other measures of word reading or assessments of phonological processing ability. Summarizing the results of their study, Vellutino, Scanlon, and Lyon (2000) concluded that "the IQ–achievement discrepancy does not reliably distinguish between disabled and non-disabled readers. . . . Neither does it distinguish between children who were found to be difficult to remediate and those who are readily remediated, prior to initiation of remediation, and it does not predict response to remediation" (p. 235). These findings are especially important in showing that IQ–achievement discrepancy is not specifically associated with those who respond to intervention.

TABLE 12.1. Intervention Studies Addressing the Relationships of Word Recognition Outcomes and IQ

Study	Relationship with word recognition outcomes? IQ	IQ–achievement discrepancy
1. Foorman et al. (1997)	No	—
2. Hatcher & Hulme (1999)	No	—
3. Torgesen et al. (2000)	No	—
4. Torgesen et al. (2001)	No	—
5. Vellutino et al. (2000)	No	No
6. Wise et al. (2000)	Yes[a]	—

[a]Only one of three outcome measures, 5% of variance.

Some of these studies found that levels of IQ predicted growth in reading comprehension ability (Wise et al., 2000; Hatcher & Hulme, 1999; Torgesen et al., 1999). However, keep in mind that the subtests making up a Verbal IQ scale are commonly found to represent a general verbal comprehension factor closely related to vocabulary (Fletcher et al., 1996; Sattler, 1993; Share, Jorm, MacLean, & Matthews, 1989). As vocabulary is a component of IQ and a robust correlate of reading comprehension skills (Torgesen & Wagner, 2002), it is not surprising that Verbal IQ predicts reading comprehension. The relevant construct, however, is not IQ but vocabulary (Sternberg & Grigorenko, 2002). Consider that if measures of phonological processing were included as IQ subtests, it is unlikely that any child with word recognition problems would meet an IQ–achievement discrepancy definition; such a child's IQ would, on average, be much lower with the phonological subtests than without them! Altogether, these results do not indicate that children defined as IQ- and achievement-discrepant versus low-achieving but nondiscrepant differ in response to intervention, or even that different interventions are needed.

Cognitive Correlates

There is a long history of research over the past 20 years addressing whether cognitive variables not used to define children as IQ–achievement discrepant versus low achieving differentiate the two groups described above. These studies, reviewed by Aaron (1997), Fletcher et al. (1998), Siegel (1992), and Stanovich (1991), find null to small but statistically significant differences between poorly reading children with IQ–achievement discrepancy and poorly reading children with no such discrepancy. However, the issue is not so much whether such groups of children are different, but how much they differ and whether the differences are meaningful. Two recent studies have attempted to address this issue through meta-analyses of the burgeoning research on the cognitive correlates of poor reading in groups variously defined as having IQ–achievement discrepancy and as low-achieving but nondiscrepant. The advantage of meta-analysis is that it moves the interpretation of the results of a large number of studies to an empirical basis, where the results are synthesized across the different studies.

In the first meta-analytic study, Hoskyn and Swanson (2000) coded 19 studies that met stringent IQ and achievement criteria. They computed effect sizes from studies in which cognitive skills were compared in poorly reading children who were all low-achieving but who differed in IQ. An effect size difference of 0 indicates complete overlap of the two groups. Effect sizes over 0.20 are considered small; those over 0.50 are considered medium; and those over 0.80 are considered large. Table 12.2 shows negligible to small differences on several measures of reading and phonological processing (range = –0.02 to –0.29), but larger differences on measures of vocabulary (0.55) and syntax (0.87). The authors concluded that most cognitive abilities assessed in the meta-analysis, especially those closely related to reading, showed considerable overlap between the two groups, leading them to question the validity of IQ–achievement discrepancy. This overlap occurred despite the attempt by Hoskyn and Swanson (2000) to select studies in which low achievement was associated with low IQ scores. Some studies included children with IQ scores in the deficient range.

TABLE 12.2. Representative Average Effect Sizes for Comparisons of Poorly Reading Children with and without IQ–Achievement Discrepancy

Construct	Effect size	95% confidence interval	
		Lower	Upper
Real-word reading	–0.02	–1.44	1.05[a]
Pseudoword reading	0.29	–0.50	1.01[a]
Phonological processing	0.27	–0.67	1.36[a]
Automaticity	0.05	–1.21	0.85[a]
Vocabulary	0.55		
Syntax	0.76		

Note. Data from Hoskyn and Swanson (2000).
[a]Interval includes 0.

In the second study, Stuebing et al. (2002) synthesized 46 studies that compared groups composed of poor readers who met explicit criteria for IQ–achievement discrepancy or for nondiscrepant low achievement. These studies were derived from a review of several hundred articles published from 1973 to 1998 that potentially addressed the validity of the IQ–achievement discrepancy hypothesis. The 46 studies met multiple criteria for inclusion and exclusion, but were more liberal than those examined by Hoskyn and Swanson (2000), especially in allowing IQ to range freely in both groups. The most important criteria required explicit discrepancy criteria to form the discrepant group, and an indication that the low-achieving, nondiscrepant group did not include individuals who might have IQ–achievement discrepancy or typical achievement in reading. Variables used to form groups were not used to estimate effect sizes in addressing validity, as the definitions ensured large group differences on group formation variables.

In addition to effect sizes in cognitive ability, Stuebing et al. (in press) also assessed achievement and behavior domains. Aggregated effect sizes were negligible for the behavior (–0.05; 95% confidence interval = –0.14, 0.05) and achievement domains (–0.12; 95% confidence interval = –0.16, –0.07). A small effect size difference was found for the cognitive ability domain (0.30; 95% confidence interval = 0.27, 0.34), showing high scores in the IQ- and achievement-discrepant group. As this group had IQ scores that were, on average, about one standard deviation higher than those of the group with nondiscrepant low achievement, the surprising finding is that the aggregated difference in cognitive ability was *only* 0.30 of a standard deviation! The effect sizes for the behavioral domain were homogeneous. However, effect sizes in the achievement and cognitive ability domains were heterogeneous and depended on what tasks were examined.

When the achievement domain was evaluated (Table 12.3), those tasks that involved word recognition, oral reading, and spelling showed small effect sizes, indicating poorer performance by the group with IQ–achievement discrepancy. Tasks involving reading comprehension, math, and writing yielded negligible effect sizes. The small effect sizes for the former measures may reflect their similarity to the types of tasks used to define poor reading in many of the studies, since many used word recognition as the measure of poor reading.

Table 12.4 summarizes effect sizes for tasks in the cognitive domain. As in the Hoskyns and Swanson (2000) meta-analysis, cognitive abilities closely related to reading did not differentiate the two groups with poor reading: phonological awareness (–0.13;95% confidence interval = –0.23, –0.02), rapid naming (–0.12;95% confidence interval = –0.30, 0.07), verbal memory (0.10;95% confidence interval = –0.01, 0.19), and vocabulary (0.10;95% confidence interval = –0.02, 0.22). Thus the core cognitive skills that research (see Torgesen & Wagner, 2002) has shown to underlie reading disability do not discriminate children with IQ–achievement discrepancy from children with low achievement but no such discrepancy. Not surprisingly, measures of IQ not used to define the groups demonstrated large effect sizes. Measures of cognitive skills involving spatial cognition and concept formation yielded small to medium effect sizes, the direction of both showing better performance by the IQ- and achievement-discrepant group. These tasks are similar to those used in many IQ tests.

Other analyses indicated that the size of the effects in different studies could be predicted by the IQ and reading tasks used to define the groups, indicating that sampling variation across studies explains the effect size differences that emerge across studies. Like Sternberg and Grigorenko (2002), Hoskyn and Swanson (2000), and others (Aaron, 1997; Siegel, 1992; Stanovich & Siegel, 1994), Stuebing et al. (2002) have concluded that LD classifications based on IQ–achievement discrepancy have at best weak validity. The difference is that this conclusion is based on an empirical synthesis of multiple studies—not a single study or review of studies.

TABLE 12.3. Representative Average Effect Sizes for Achievement Constructs

Construct	Effect size	95% confidence interval	
		Lower	Upper
Spelling	–0.31	–0.43	–0.18
Oral reading	–0.25	–0.42	–0.09
Real-word reading	–0.25	–0.39	–0.11
Pseudoword decoding	–0.23	–0.34	–0.12
Reading comprehension	–0.04	–0.17	0.08[a]
Mathematics concepts	0.03	–0.07	0.13[a]
Mathematics computations	0.06	–0.11	0.23[a]

Note. Data from Stuebing et al. (2002).
[a]Interval includes 0.

TABLE 12.4. Representative Average Effect Sizes for Cognitive Ability Constructs

Construct	Effect size	95% confidence interval	
		Lower	Upper
Phonological awareness	–0.13	–0.23	–0.02
Rapid naming	–0.12	–0.30	0.07[a]
Orthographic awareness	–0.10	–0.29	0.08[a]
Verbal short-term memory	0.10	–0.01	0.19[a]
Vocabulary/lexical	0.10	–0.02	0.22
Focused attention	0.16	0.04	0.28
Fine motor	0.26	0.11	0.40
Spatial	0.43	0.30	0.55
Perceptual–motor	0.47	0.31	0.62
Nonverbal short-term memory	0.47	0.17	0.77
Verbal IQ	0.60	0.49	0.72
Syntax	0.72	0.30	1.14
Nonverbal IQ	0.86	0.75	0.96
Full Scale IQ	1.01	0.81	1.21

Note. Data from Stuebing et al. (2002).
[a]Interval includes 0.

Development and Prognosis

There is little evidence that the long-term development of reading skills in children defined as IQ- and achievement-discrepant in reading is different from those defined as low-achieving but nondiscrepant. In an early study, Rutter and Yule (1975) reported that children in the former group showed more rapid development of academic skills than children in the latter group. However, the reading and spelling skills of the low-achieving but nondiscrepant children were lower at baseline. As children were not randomly assigned to the two groups, the greater advances may reflect regression to the mean.

In a subsequent study of a large longitudinal cohort in New Zealand, Share, McGee, and Silva (1989) attempted to replicate these findings, using similar definitions and alternative methodologies that would tease out the relationship of IQ and reading over time. They found no relationship of IQ and reading achievement within age bands of 7, 9, 11, and 13 years. Moreover, scores were not predictive of change in reading skills over time. Share et al. (1989) concluded that IQ is not a relevant explanatory variable for predicting the development of children with reading difficulties. Vellutino et al. (2000) summarized several studies showing that reading skills involving word recognition were only weakly correlated with IQ.

Francis et al. (1996) examined this question using data from the Connecticut Longitudinal Project, an epidemiological, population-based study that assessed reading skills yearly, beginning in grade 1 and continuing into adulthood (Shaywitz, S. E. Shaywitz, Fletcher, & Escobar, 1990; S. E. Shaywitz et al., 1992; Shaywitz et al., 1999). Children were defined as having IQ–achievement discrepancy or nondiscrepant low achievement in reading in grade 3. The growth of reading skills was compared using the yearly assessments of reading in grades 1–9. The results showed no differences between the two groups with reading difficulties in the rate of growth over time or the level of reading ability at any age despite the average 18-point higher IQ score characterizing the discrepant group. About half the children in the discrepant group received special education services. Fletcher et al. (in press) extended these findings through grade 12. Of particular importance was the finding that over 70% of those who read poorly in grade 3 read poorly in grade 12. Without adequate intervention, LDs in reading are chronic, lifelong conditions, regardless of how they are defined.

More recently, Flowers, Meyer, Lovato, Woods, and Felton (2001) analyzed the growth of word decoding, reading comprehension, phonological processing, and rapid naming abilities in children identified as having IQ–achievement discrepancy ($n = 51$) and as having nondiscrepant low achievement in reading ($n = 89$) in grade 3. These children were part of two epidemiologically derived samples (total $n = 515$), one drawn from the general population of a specific school district and the other from a grade 3 sample of children with extremely deficient reading. Although 76% of the discrepant group was identified as having LDs by the schools, compared with 10% of the nondiscrepant group, only 57% of the discrepant group received services. Using growth curve models similar to those used by Francis et al. (1996), these authors found no differences in level of attainment or growth over the 10-year interval. Poorly reading children remained below their peers on the measures of reading abilities as well as their cognitive correlates through grade 12.

In a study of the precursors of poor reading, Wristers, Francis, Foorman, Fletcher, and Swank (2002) used a sample of poorly reading children defined as either discrepant or nondiscrepant in grades 1 and 2. These groups were formed from a sample of over 900 children and compared on a variety of measures obtained up to four times yearly in kindergarten and grade 1. The measures included phonological awareness, rapid naming, vocabulary, perceptual skills, and reading ability. The results revealed almost no differences in growth or level of attainment in these skills prior to identification as disabled in reading. Thus the null results apparent for the developmental course of reading disabilities can be extended from kindergarten to grade 12, regardless of how children with poor reading are defined. The IQ–achievement discrepancy hypothesis accrues no validity from these longitudinal studies.

Neurobiological Factors

The IQ–achievement discrepancy hypothesis has been explicitly addressed in research on genetic factors in LDs, and implicitly in neuroimaging research. Pennington, Gilger, Olson, and DeFries (1992) used a large sample of monozygotic and diozygotic twins in which at least one member of each twin pair was classified with reading disability, and a set of control twins in which neither member of each pair was disabled in reading, to create a nondisabled group and three groups with reading disability: one with IQ–achievement discrepancy, one with no such discrepancy, and a mixed discrepant–nondiscrepant group. Pennington et al. found no evidence for differential genetic etiology based on type of definition. They also did not find evidence for significant differences in gender ratios, clinical correlates, and neuropsychological profiles.

It is possible that the Pennington et al. (1992) study was underpowered, as large samples are necessary to demonstrate differences in heritability. Wadsworth, Olson, Pennington, and DeFries (2000) evaluated genetic factors and their relation to reading disabilities by subdividing twin pairs with and without reading disabilities according to higher (≥100) and lower (≤100) IQ scores. Although the overall heritability of reading skills was .58, children with reading disabilities and lower IQ scores had a heritability estimate of .43, compared to .72 for the higher IQ group. These statistically and practically significant differences in heritability are nonetheless small. Wadsworth et al. (2000) required almost 400 pairs of twins in order to detect the difference. Wadsworth et al. further observed that the higher IQ scores could be related to more intractable, genetically based reading disabilities, despite strong environmental support for IQ and for learning to read. The children with reading disabilities and lower IQ scores may have had more pervasive deficiencies in cognitive development and reading that reflected broader environmental disadvantages. For example, children in the lower-IQ group had homes where there were fewer books and where mothers had fewer years of education. Wadsworth et al. (2000) concluded that excluding lower-IQ children from intervention or remediation because they did not meet an IQ–achievement discrepancy definition was appropriate, because environmental influences had more impact on reading disabilities in this group.

There are also studies of children with reading disabilities that utilize functional imaging methods, such as functional magnetic resonance imaging (fMRI) and magnetic source imaging (MSI); these studies are reviewed in detail in the section below on dyslexia. Although no study has a sample that is large enough to actually compare poorly reading children with and without IQ–achievement discrepancy, it is noteworthy that no studies include only those children with discrepancy. There is no evidence from these studies that these two groups of children have different neuroimaging profiles. In particular, studies that permit examination of individual brain activation profiles, especially MSI, show no differences in brain maps from poorly reading children with and without IQ–achievement discrepancy.

Conclusions: IQ–Achievement Discrepancy and Reading Disabilities

These results show that the IQ–achievement discrepancy hypothesis has at best weak validity for children with LDs in reading. These findings span multiple assessment domains. Most telling are the largely null results for relations of IQ and IQ–achievement discrepancy with intervention outcomes and prognosis. If IQ and IQ–achievement discrepancy are not related to these critically important domains, and in essence are not relevant for treatment planning, what is their relevance other than preservation of older concepts of LDs? Moreover, discrepancy definitions do not take into account of the changing demands of reading over time (Snowling, Bishop, & Stothard, 2000). Unfortunately, this pattern of null results continues as we turn to other forms of LDs.

IQ–Achievement Discrepancy and Speech–Language Disorders

The federal definition of LDs includes disorders of oral expression and listening comprehension. These disorders can also be represented as disorders of expressive and receptive language, which constitute a separate category in special education under IDEA. A consensus group convened by the National Institute of Deafness and Communication Disorders concluded that the practice of using IQ scores to identify children with these disorders was not supported by research and practice (Tager-Flusberg & Cooper, 1999). This conclusion was based on an emerging data base on the validity of "cognitive referencing," the term for discrepancy identification used in this area (Casby, 1992).

In this data base, the most convincing evidence came from an epidemiological study by Tomblin and Zhang (1999). The investigators used measures of nonverbal IQ and oral language ability to create three groups of children from a large epidemiological study: a group with no impairment; a group with specific language impairment (IQ > 87 and composite language skills < 1.25 standard deviations below age); and a group with general delay (IQ < 87 and composite language skills < 1.25 standard deviations below age). Comparisons of the three groups on different language measures showed consistent differences between the nonimpaired group and both language-impaired groups. However, differences between the two language-impaired groups were also apparent: "Children with general delay closely parallel the specifically language-impaired group except that the children with general delay were more impaired and noticeably poorer on the test involving comprehension of sentences (grammatical understanding)" (p. 367). Tomblin and Zhang (1999) questioned whether even this latter difference in grammatical understanding is specific to either group, noting that: "current diagnostic methods and standards for specific language impairment do not result in a group of children whose profiles of language achievement are unique" (p. 367).

IQ–Achievement Discrepancy and Math Disabilities

There are a few studies comparing children who meet an IQ–achievement discrepancy definition of math disabilities with those who meet a low-achievement definition, but not the discrepancy definition. Fletcher et al. (in press) compared these two groups of children, also ensuring that neither met definitions of reading disabilities, on cognitive variables involving attention, language, problem solving, concept formation, and visual–motor skills. The results showed that the discrepant group had higher performance levels on all variables. The group that had nondiscrepant low achievement in math was notably poorer in vocabulary despite average reading skills. The critical issue, as for reading disabilities, is not that the groups differ. Differences in level of performance are expected, because IQ tests are used to define the groups, one group has higher IQ scores, and IQ is moderately to highly correlated with each of the measures (e.g., vocabulary) used to evaluate the children. More important is the *pattern* (shape) of differences between the groups. Testing the profiles for differences in pattern did not yield a statistically significant difference, and the effect size was negligible (0.06). As we have shown in the reading area (Fletcher et al., 1998), eliminating variability due to the difference in vocabulary—a proxy for IQ in many studies—eliminates the differences in level of performance apparent between the two math groups. It is not likely that vocabulary has much to do with math, as word problems were not part of the definition—just paper-and-pencil computations. The differences appear to be a product of the definitions, and the correlates of poor math achievement do not appear to differ once the differences induced by the definition are taken into account. The differences in vocabulary between those with IQ–achievement discrepancy versus nondiscrepant low achievement in math versus reading most likely reflect the higher correlation of reading with vocabulary than math.

Psychometric Factors

Thus far, we have addressed the *validity* of the IQ–achievement discrepancy approach to identification. However, there are also well-known psychometric factors that raise questions about the *reliability* of any test-based model for identifying individual students with LDs, whether definitions based on IQ–achievement discrepancy or nondiscrepant low achievement are used. Although these problems have been well documented for various approaches to the estimation of discrepancy, many of the same issues will affect the use of a definition based on low achievement. These problems involve the measurement error of the tests, the unreliability of difference scores, and the use of cutoff points to subdivide a normal distribution.

It is well established that approaches to IQ–achievement discrepancy that are based on regression methods adjusting for the correlation of IQ and achievement are superior to other methods when two tests are involved (Bennett & Clarizio, 1988; Reynolds, 1984–1985). IQ and achievement test scores are moderately correlated, so the failure to adjust for this correlation leads to regression to the mean. Regression effects indicate that when individuals are chosen because of low performance on one test, they will, on average, have scores that are less extreme on the second test. The effect is that these individuals will score closer to the mean on the second test. This phenomenon results in overidentification of LDs at upper levels of IQ and underidentification at lower levels of IQ. A regression approach adjusts for the correlation of IQ and achievement, thus correcting this problem.

However, regression approaches have other problems. In addition to the influence of measurement error, difference scores are typically lower in reliability (Bereiter, 1967) than the measures used to compute the difference. The low reliability of difference scores can be exacerbated because it artificially constrains the variance in scores (Rogosa, 1995), as in the case when IQ and achievement scores are used to identify the lower-performing segment of the population.

A more significant problem involves the use of a cutoff point, particularly when the score is not criterion-referenced and the score distributions have been normalized. As we discuss for reading below, most studies have reported that reading achievement test scores are normal and continuous (Dobbins, 1988; Jorm, Share, Matthews, & Matthews, 1986; Rodgers, 1983; S. E. Shaywitz et al., 1992; Silva, McGee, & Williams, 1985). Setting any cutoff point in the absence of validation research is therefore inherently arbitrary. The problems emerge when the measurement error of the test is considered. Because of measurement error, any cutoff point will be associated with considerable instability in classifications. Scores will fluctuate around the cutoff point with repeat testing, even for a decision as transparently straightforward as demarcating low achievement or mental deficiency. This fluctuation is not a problem of repeat testing, nor is it a matter of selecting the ideal cutoff score. The problem is that no single score can perfectly capture a student's ability in a single domain.

Approaches in which a normal distribution is subdivided to create groups have also been widely criticized in the measurement literature (Cohen, 1983) when the intent has been to compare the resultant groups. This process imposes an arbitrary group structure on continuous distributions that are essentially dimensional in nature. Subdividing continuous distributions also artificially constrains the within-group variability and reduces the range of measurement. The process distorts the relative importance of the underlying dimensions to performance on other measures. The result is often reduced power in statistical comparisons, as well as specious results due to the failure to control fully for the correlation between the two dimensions being categorized.

These technical problems have been widely described in the literature on analysis of variance and regression. Other studies have specifically examined the stability of classifications of LDs. S. E. Shaywitz et al. (1992) found that definitions based on IQ–achievement discrepancy were especially unstable from grades 1 to 3, but were more stable from grades 3 to 5. However, this study did not examine definitions of low achievement. In a systematic study of this issue, Francis et al. (2002) used simulated data and actual data from the Connecticut Longitudinal Study to evaluate the stability of classifications based on definitions of IQ–achievement discrepancy and nondiscrepant low achievement. If the groups formed by either definition represented meaningful subdivisions of the achievement distribution, some degree of stability over time would be expected. The results of the simulations showed that groups formed by imposing cutoff points based on either definition of LDs were unstable over time, even when the simulations were designed with high reliability of measurement and to minimize individual change. Similar instability was apparent in longitudinal data from the Connecticut Longitudinal Study, where 39% of children designated as having LDs in grade 3 using different definitions changed group placement with repeated testing in grade 5. These results show that the practice of subdividing a normal distribution with arbitrary cutoff points leads to instability in group membership. Approaches to the identification of LDs that are based solely on test scores, and not linked to specific behavioral criteria, are not adequately reliable for decision making about individual children.

Conclusions: IQ–Achievement Discrepancy Hypothesis

The evidence reviewed above for children with reading difficulties suggests that the IQ–achievement discrepancy classification hypothesis lacks strong evidence for external validity across multiple domains. Data from other LD domains are sparse, but extant studies yield results like those in the reading area, showing that those differences that do emerge are products of how the groups are formed and not true markers of valid differences. The psychometric evidence shows that classifications based on cutoff points have problems with reliability. Thus this review suggests that the IQ–achievement discrepancy classification hypothesis has at best weak validity. Weak validity does not justify the prominence of concepts of aptitude and intelligence in public conceptions of LDs, or their role in federal regulations. The evidence most certainly does not justify the effort and expense expended by schools in giving IQ tests to address eligibility for special education in the LD category. The identification process for individual children is inherently arbitrary and unrelated to outcomes.

EXCLUSIONARY FACTORS

Stipulating that LDs are is not due to mental deficiency, sensory disorders, or cultural/linguistic diversity is reasonable, as children with these characteristics have different intervention needs. There are issues with distinctions between mental deficiency and LDs that make the precise demarcation unclear, but information beyond IQ tests is essential for identifying mental deficiency (MacMillan & Siperstein, 2002). Other exclusions stem from policy decisions that involve the need to avoid the mixing of special education and compensatory education funds, as well as the existence of other eligibility categories in IDEA to support children with special needs (e.g., mental retardation, emotional disturbance). The original exclusionary criteria were not meant to exclude children from placement, but to better classify each child's difficulties—on the assumption that when economic disadvantage, emotional disturbance, and inadequate instruction are the primary causes of underachievement, different interventions are needed.

In the other exclusionary areas, determining the primary "cause" when the evidence is largely behavioral has proven a difficult proposition. The cognitive correlates of academic difficulties in children with achievement deficiencies attributed to emotional disturbance; inadequate instruction; and cultural, social, and economic disadvantage do not appear to be different according to these putative causes. Moreover, the intervention needs, responses to interventions, or mechanisms whereby interventions work do not appear to vary according to these factors (Fletcher et al., in press; Lyon et al., 2001). As such, these distinctions are not strongly related to the types of intervention programs that are likely to be effective, especially in reading. Of particular concern is the idea that inadequate instruction precludes LDs, when in fact it may cause LDs. In this section, we examine specifically exclusion due to socioeconomic disadvantage and lack of opportunity for learning.

Social and Economic Disadvantage

Although all current definitions of LDs state that the academic deficits encompassed by the disorder cannot be attributed to economic disadvantage and cultural factors (including race or ethnicity), limited information exists regarding how race, ethnicity, and cultural background might influence school learning in general and the expression of different types of LDs in particular. However, it is encouraging to note that work being conducted by Frank Wood and his colleagues (Wood, Felton, Flowers, & Naylor, 1991) has begun to shed light on these issues. In a longitudinal study of specific LDs (in reading) within a random sample of 485 children selected in the first grade and followed through the third grade (55% European American, 45% African American), Wood et al. (1991) found that the effects of race were, in fact, important as well as highly complicated. For example, at the first-grade level, race did not appear to be an influential variable in reading development once vocabulary ability was accounted for. That is, once a child's age and level of vocabulary development were known, race did not provide any additional predictive power to forecasting first-grade reading scores. However, by the end of the third grade, race had become a significant predictive factor ($p = .001$) even when the most powerful predictors—first-grade reading scores—were also in the prediction equation. Specifically, by the end of the third grade, African American youngsters were having significantly greater difficulties learning to read.

In attempting to understand this race effect, Wood and his group assessed a number of additional demographic factors, including parental marital status, parental education, parental status as a welfare recipient, socioeconomic status (SES), the number of books in the home, and occupational status. Their findings were clear: The presence of any or all of these demographic variables in the prediction equation "did not remove the race effect from its potency as an independent predictor of third-grade reading" (Wood et al., 1991, p. 9).

A major issue is that many of the conditions that are excluded as potential influences on LDs interfere with the development of cognitive and linguistic skills that lead to the academic deficits that in turn lead to LDs (Lyon et al., 2001). Parents with reading problems, for example, many find it difficult to establish adequate home literacy practices because of the cumulative effects of their reading difficulties (Wadsworth et al., 2000). Children who grow up in economically disadvantaged environments are behind in language development when they enter school (Hart & Risley, 1995). This delay will interfere with the development of reading and math skills.

Moreover, interventions that address the early development of these skills seem to promote academic success in evaluative studies of Title I programs, as well as intervention studies in which alphabetic forms of instruction have been shown to be advantageous for economically disadvantaged children (Foorman et al., 1998; National Reading Panel, 2000). Thus the mechanisms and practices that promote reading success in advantaged populations appear to be similar to those that promote reading success and failure in disadvantaged populations. There is little evidence that the phenotypic representation of reading disabilities varies according to SES. Children at all SES levels appear to have reading problems predominantly (but not exclusively) because of word-level difficulties apparent in the beginning stages of reading development (Foorman et al., 1998; Wood, Flowers, Buchsbaum, & Tallal, 1991). In some children word-level difficulties may reflect a disadvantaged literacy environment, while other children exhibit these same word-level difficulties, although they have come from a more advantaged environment.

As Kavale (1988) and Lyon (1996a) have pointed out, the basis for excluding disadvantaged children from the LD category has more to do with how children are served than with empirical evidence demonstrating that characteristics of reading failure are different in groups with LDs versus economic disadvantage. Kavale (1988) has stated that "the culturally disadvantaged child is well served by various federally funded title programs, but these are usually mandated under guidelines and revisions different from special education. Specifically, the emphasis is on compensatory education while special education programs function as remedial programs" (p. 195). This often has the effect of eliminating economically disadvantaged children from special education services, with the exception of categories related to mental deficiency and emotional disturbance; economically disadvantaged children are disproportionately represented in these special education categories. Kavale (1988) has further stated that "since culturally disadvantaged children have been shown to exhibit the behavioral characteristics included as primary traits in definitions of LD, it is difficult to determine why the culturally disadvantaged group is categorically excluded from the LD classification. Yet, children from lower SES levels with LD-type behaviors have little chance for receiving LD diagnoses and treatment with an increased likelihood of being labeled retarded in spite of the fact that LD and CD [culturally disadvantaged] groups are not clearly identifiable as separate entities" (p. 205).

Lack of Opportunity

Exclusion based on opportunity to learn makes sense if there has been no effort to teach a child. But this notion is often expanded to include children whose instruction has not been adequate. Although children's failure to respond to appropriate instruction is a very strong indication of a disability, the cognitive problems associated with their LDs parallel those exhibited by children who do not respond to adequate instruction. The two types of children are equally disabled.

Of the different exclusionary criteria for LDs, instructional factors are the least frequently examined, but perhaps the most important. The opportunity-to-learn exclusion presumed that the field has a good understanding of what constitutes adequate instruction. At the time the federal definition was adopted, this was not the case. Recent consensus reports (Snow, Burns, & Griffin, 1998; National Reading Panel, 2000) make it clear that we do know a lot about teaching children to read. At least in reading, which accounts for most forms of LD, consideration of the students' response to high-quality intervention may need to become part of the definition of LDs (Gresham, in press; Fuchs & Fuchs, 1998). As the recent report of the National Reading Panel on disproportionate representation of minorities in special education has made clear (Donovon & Cross, 2002), why should the complex identification criteria and expensive due-process procedures of special education be used before an attempt is made to provide a powerful intervention early in a child's development? A child's failure to respond to high-quality intervention may be the best way to operationalize the notion of opportunity to learn. Excluding children on this basis is not logical.

Conclusions: Exclusionary Factors

For children with mental deficiency, sensory disorders, and emotional disturbance, there are other classifications in IDEA that can lead to services. For children who are deemed culturally, economically, or socially disadvantaged, compensatory education programs are available. What is there for children who develop academic difficulties because of poor instruction? Excluding such children does not seem a reasonable practice. Including them when they don't respond to high-quality instruction seems reasonable, but essential if "LDs" is to be more than a term for "instructional casualties."

Thus approaching the exclusion hypothesis from the perspective of classification research shows little evidence supporting exclusions based on economic disadvantage and lack of opportunity to learn. This reflects the difficulties of differentiating forms of low achievement that are presumably "specific" or "unexpected" from those than can be attributed to other causes, where low achievement is expected. This does not mean that the concept of LDs is not valid or that the exclusions should not be used, particularly since many children can be served under other categories in IDEA or other approaches to providing services (e.g., compensatory education). There may well be needs outside the academic area that are better addressed through identification for other categories or programs. These exclusions must be seen as policy-based determinations to facilitate service delivery and to avoid mixing of funds, not as classification factors that have strong validity. Exclusions due to inadequate instruction are not justifiable, as lack of instruction can essentially cause reading difficulties. Response to high-quality intervention may need to become part of the definition of LDs, especially given the weaknesses of psychometric approaches to the identification of individual children.

HETEROGENEITY

LDs are clearly domain-specific, meaning that disabilities involving reading, math, and written expression are different in terms of phenotypic descriptions and intervention needs. Although many children have more than one of these disorders, there are prototypes for subgroups of children with isolated disabilities in the domains of reading and math. The problem is that the categories in federal regulations do not line up well with the domains that have emerged from research. Moreover, this heterogeneity alone makes difficult the proposition that LDs can be subsumed under a single overarching conceptualization.

In discussing this issue, Fletcher et al. (in press) and Lyon et al. (2001) have noted that two of the categories in the federal definition, oral expression and listening comprehension, are addressed in the speech and language category. As such, the basis for duplication is not clear. Moreover, even if listening comprehension is not regarded as a component of receptive language, it closely parallels reading comprehension in children who do not show word-reading disabilities. In the other five areas (basic reading, reading comprehension, math calculations, math concepts, and written expression), the organization is not consistent with subgroups apparent in research.

Table 12.5 lists the LD subgroups that have been identified in research. These subgroups include three forms of reading disabilities, involving word recognition, comprehension, and fluency; two forms of math disabilities, depending on the presence or absence of word recognition difficulties; and disorders of written expression.

TABLE 12.5. Subgroups of LDs with Empirical Support

Reading disorder—word recognition
Reading disorder—comprehension
Reading disorder—fluency
Mathematics disorder
Reading–mathematics disorder
Disorders of written expression—handwriting, spelling, text generation (?)

The latter may be divided into disorders involving spelling, handwriting, and expression, but the research base is not presently adequate to support these distinctions. In this section, we discuss each of these disorders under the domains of reading, math, and written expression.

Prior to this discussion, it is important to recognize that many children have LDs in more than one domain. In addition, LDs often co-occur with disorders of attention (ADHD) (Barkley, 1998; Fletcher, Shaywitz, & Shaywitz, 1999; Shelton & Barkley, 1994). In the area of reading, the two types of disorders are distinct and separable (Lyon, 1994a, 1994b; Wood et al., 1991). For example, LDs involving basic reading are consistently associated with deficits in phonological awareness, whereas the effects of ADHD on cognitive functioning are variable, with primary deficits noted in executive functions (Barkley, 1997). Furthermore, ADHD appears relatively unrelated to phonological awareness tasks, which are strongly linked to word-level reading difficulties (Fletcher, Shaywitz, & Shaywitz, 1999; Shaywitz, Fletcher, & Shaywitz, 1994; Wood et al., 1991). In studies examining comorbidity of math disabilities and ADHD, the groups overlap more than groups with reading disabilities and ADHD do. This reflects the role of executive functions (strategy use, procedural learning) and working memory in both math disabilities and ADHD. But the disorders are separable on dimensions involving attention and behavior (Fletcher et al., 2002). Finally, disorders of written language and math are especially common in children defined with ADHD (Barkley, 1997). Nonetheless, reading problems are also common (Fletcher, Shaywitz, & Shaywitz, 1999). In most instances, these appear to be comorbid associations: A child with disabilities involving ADHD and a domain-specific LD appears like a child with ADHD in the behavioral lens, and like a child with an LD in the cognitive lens. However, when both forms of disability are apparent, the cognitive and academic deficits invariably appear more severe (Fletcher et al., in press).

A number of authors have also reported that children with reading disabilities present with co-occurring social-emotional difficulties (Bryan, Donahue, Pearl, & Sturm, 1981; Tallal, 1988). A majority of such social-emotional difficulties appear, in some clinical studies, to be secondary to difficulties in learning to read. For example, of the 93 adults in a clinic population with LDs, the majority of whom displayed reading problems, 36% had received counseling or psychotherapy for low self-esteem, social isolation, anxiety, depression, and frustration (Johnson & Blalock, 1987). Likewise, others (Bruck, 1986; Cooley & Ayers, 1988; Paris & Ika, 1989) have reported that many of the emotional problems displayed by readers with LDs reflect adjustment difficulties resulting from labeling or academic failure. However, a meta- analysis of the relationship between LDs and social skills found little evidence for specific deficits in children broadly defined as having LDs. Many of these studies were not well controlled for other factors related to social skills, such as ADHD and SES. The failure to specify the subgrouping of LDs into reading versus math disabilities is unfortunate, as there is evidence that children with math disabilities are more impaired than those with reading disorders, especially if other nonverbal processing skills are also impaired (Rourke, 1989, 1993). Other studies find that reading problems are associated with higher rates of internalizing and externalizing psychopathology, even in nonclinical samples (Willcutt & Pennington, 2000). In this later study, the comorbid association of reading disabilities and ADHD could explain much of this relationship. When ADHD was controlled for, externalizing disorders were no longer linked, but relationships with internalizing symptoms persisted, especially in girls with reading disabilities. Finally, recent large-scale clinical trials show that improving reading and math instruction in programs that provide positive behavioral support reduces subsequent behavioral difficulties in first-graders followed into middle school. The most significant path is from achievement to behavior, so poor achievement clearly leads to behavioral difficulties (Kellam, Rebok, Mayer, Ialongo, & Kalodner, 1994). Altogether, while we do not further emphasize the comorbidity issue, it should be kept in mind throughout the remainder of the chapter. These findings point out the significant need to identify and intervene early with those children who are at risk for academic failure, given the substantial social and emotional consequences that can occur if the disabilities are not remediated.

READING DISORDERS

The federal definition specifies two areas of reading disabilities: basic reading (word recognition) and reading comprehension. That difficulties with word recognition represent a specific form of LD in reading is well established (Shaywitz, 1996). Children can also clearly be identified with comprehension difficulties that do not involve the word recognition module (Oakhill & Yuill, 1996). Much more is known about the nature and causes of disabilities in word recognition, as less reading research has been devoted to studying how children understand what they read (Snow, 2002).

What are not addressed in the federal definition are difficulties that involve the automatization of word recognition skills and speed of reading connected text. These problems also occur in children with accurate word recognition skills. Unfortunately, less is known about fluency deficits in reading, despite recent development of hypotheses suggesting that deficiencies in reading fluency represent a separate subgroup of reading disabilities (Wolf & Bowers, 1999; Wolf, Bowers, & Biddle, 2001). In this section, we review evidence for subgroups with reading disabilities specific to word recognition, comprehension, and fluency.

Word Recognition Disability (Dyslexia)

Definitional Issues

Word-level reading disability (WLRD) is synonymous with "dyslexia," a form of LD that has been described throughout the 20th century as "word blindness," "visual agnosia for words," and "specific reading disability" (Doris, 1993). The evolution of the concept of "dyslexia" from a vague and general term to a synonym for WLRD provides an example of how definitions of LDs can move from exclusionary to inclusionary. As an example of an exclusionary definition, consider the definition formulated by the World Federation of Neurology in 1968:

> A disorder manifested by difficulties in learning to read despite conventional instruction, adequate

intelligence, and socio-economic opportunity. It is dependent upon fundamental cognitive disabilities, which are frequently of constitutional origin. (Critchley, 1970, p. 11)

In contrast, consider the following definition of dyslexia formulated by a research committee of the International Dyslexia Society (Lyon, 1995b; Shaywitz, 1996), which we have modified to be consistent with advances in research:

> Dyslexia is one of several distinct learning disabilities. It is a specific language-based disorder intrinsic to the person characterized by difficulties in the development of accurate and fluent single word decoding skills, usually associated with insufficient phonological processing and rapid naming abilities. These difficulties in single word decoding are often unexpected in relation to age and other cognitive and academic abilities; they are not the result of generalized developmental disability or sensory impairment. Dyslexia is manifest by variable difficulty with different forms of language, often including, in addition to problems reading, a conspicuous problem with acquiring proficiency in writing and spelling. Reading comprehension problems are common, reflecting word-decoding and fluency problems.

This definition identifies dyslexia as WLRD proximally caused by phonological processing problems. It is inclusionary because it specifies that children can be identified with dyslexia when they show problems decoding single words in isolation and have difficulties with phonological processing. In contrast to what we reported in the first edition of this chapter, measuring the constructs of word recognition and phonological processing can now be done with relative ease. The difficulty now faced is specifying the level of impairment that would constitute disability. Nonetheless, the definition is linked to intervention. Again in contrast to what we noted in the first edition of the chapter, it is established that treatments emphasizing the development of word recognition skills improve reading achievement in children, including those with dyslexia (National Reading Panel, 2000; Swanson, 1999). In addition, interventions that address the development of phonological processing skills prevent this type of reading problem (National Reading Panel, 2000; Snow et al., 1998). The concept of IQ–achievement discrepancy is not used as an inclusionary criterion. Indeed, IQ tests are not even required for identification. The definition differentiates dyslexia as an LD from mental retardation and sensory disorders.

Dyslexia is also most likely a dimensional disorder, and definitions must take into account the inherent arbitrariness of subdividing this dimension. Although some studies of children with LDs in reading have suggested that the distribution of achievement test scores is not normal, and have identified a natural breaking point (Miles & Haslum, 1986; Rutter & Yule, 1975; Wood & Grigorenko, 2001), most studies have reported that reading scores are normal and do not identify a natural subdivision (Dobbins, 1988; Jorm et al., 1986; Rodgers, 1983; S. E. Shaywitz et al., 1992; Silva et al., 1985). In the Rutter and Yule studies, the hump has been attributed to an inadequate ceiling on the reading test (van der Wissell & Zegers, 1985) and to the inclusion of a large number of brain-injured children with IQ scores in the deficient range (Fletcher et al., 1998). The studies by Miles and Haslum (1986) and Wood and Grigorenko (2001) do not provide enough details for evaluation. The other North American study (S. E. Shaywitz et al., 1992) used data from the Connecticut Longitudinal Study to ascertain whether a categorical or dimensional definition and model best described dyslexia or other LDS in reading. Shaywitz et al. (1992) obtained empirical evidence to support Stanovich's (1988) contention that dyslexia occurs along a continuum of reading ability.

These findings suggest that LDs in reading (e.g., dyslexia) operate like disorders such as hypertension and obesity that occur along a continuum (Shaywitz et al., 1994). Moreover, these findings indicate that dyslexia is not an all-or-none phenomenon, but rather occurs in degrees. These results are in line with the data showing no differences between poorly reading children with and without IQ–achievement discrepancy, and suggest that many more children may be affected with dyslexia than previously thought (see "Epidemiology," below).

The impact of these findings on clinical diagnostic practices and public policy could be substantial. For example, although limited resources may necessitate imposition of cutoff points for the provision of special education services, it must be recognized that such cutoff points are arbitrary and that many children in need of specialized interventions may be denied help (Lyon et al., 2001). As we have discussed in the section on IQ–achievement discrepancy, the absence of natural cutoff points or cutoff points that have not been validated is a major problem for any psychometric approach to identification. The utter failure to address this problem reflects the stranglehold of the IQ–achievement discrepancy model and the concept of "unexpectedness" in research on LDs.

Epidemiology

The prevalence of dyslexia has been estimated as high as 17.4% of the school-age population (Shaywitz et al., 1994), but reading disabilities in general have historically generated prevalence estimates of at least 10–15% of the school-age population (Benton & Pearl, 1978). These estimates are in the context of reports from the National Assessment of Educational Progress indicating that 38% of children in grade 4 read below the basic level of proficiency. Of course, as reading disabilities appear to be dimensional, prevalence depends on where the cutoff point is set, and criterion-related estimates of prevalence are not available.

Dyslexia is the most common form of LD. Lerner (1989) reported that 80% of all children served in special education programs have problems with reading, while Kavale and Reese (1992) found that over 90% of children in Iowa with the LD label had reading difficulties. Both studies indicated that most children who have reading problems experience difficulty with word-level skills. Most children served in special education programs who are identified as having LDs likely have WLRD as part of their disability (Lyon, 1995b).

Although dyslexia has always been reported to be more common in males than females, several studies indicate that the gender ratio among individuals with dyslexia is not different from the gender ratio within the population as a whole (DeFries & Gillis, 1991; Felton & Brown, 1991; Flynn & Rahbar, 1994; Shaywitz et al., 1990; Wood & Felton, 1994). Previous estimates indicating male preponderance tended to be based on clinic and school settings that were subject to referral bias. Boys are more likely to display externalizing behaviors that lead to referral, and the hyperactive–impulsive form of ADHD does appear to be more common in boys than girls (Barkley, 1997; Shaywitz et al., 1990).

Developmental Course

WLRD in particular and reading disabilities in general reflect persistent deficits rather than a developmental lag in linguistic and reading skills (Francis et al., 1996; Lyon, 1994b). Longitudinal studies show that of children classified as reading-disabled in the third grade, 74% remain thus classified in the ninth grade (Francis et al., 1996). Clearly these data reflect a pessimistic outcome for youngsters with LDs who have difficulties learning to read. However, at least three factors could be responsible for the lack of progress made by these youngsters. First, because most diagnostic criteria continue to require the use of a discrepancy between IQ and reading achievement in the eligibility process, many children are not identified until the third grade—the point at which their achievement has suffered enough to demonstrate the required discrepancy between the ostensible predictor (IQ) and reading skills. It is not coincidental that the largest increase in those eligible for special education in the LD category occurs in the 12- to 17-year age range. As Fletcher et al. (1998) have pointed out, initiating intervention after a child has failed for 2–3 years does not bode favorably for realistic gains in reading. Second, teaching interventions that are most efficacious for readers with LDs have not been implemented in most schools. Moreover, many of the children followed in the longitudinal studies described above were provided with several different types of interventions, without attention to how each intervention interacted with the next. Given this lack of systematic program planning and teaching, it is not surprising that only 20–25% of children made gains in reading. Unfortunately, those who did improve their reading ability were children with the least severe forms of reading disabilities (S. E. Shaywitz et al., 1992). Third, it is quite possible that the motivation to learn to read diminishes with time, given the extreme effort that many readers with LDs put into the learning process without success, resulting in protracted periods of failure. Recent studies clearly show relationships of early achievement in reading with subsequent behavioral difficulties (Kellam et al., 1996).

Core Processes

As could be expected, given the continuous and heterogeneous distribution of reading behaviors associated with reading ability and disabilities, both single-cause and multiple-cause theories have been advanced to represent the nature and etiologies of reading disorders. In the area of dyslexia, the phenotypic characteristics of the disorder are intimately interwoven with known and hypothesized causes of such characteristics. As such, this section is organized to review the most frequent types of reading deficits observed in children with dyslexia. Following this discussion, issues associated with single- versus multiple-cause models for these reading deficits are summarized.

The major academic deficits characterizing children with dyslexia are difficulties in decoding and the ability to read single words (Olson, Forsberg, Wise, & Rack, 1994; Perfetti, 1985; Shaywitz, 1996; Stanovich, 1986). These lead to a profound disturbance of reading ability that is the core of most forms of reading disabilities. Although this statement may appear at odds with those who argue that reading comprehension skills reflect the most salient abilities in reading development (Goodman, 1969, 1986; Smith, 1971), consider that comprehension is dependent upon one's ability to decode rapidly and recognize single words in an automatic and fluent manner. Stanovich (1994) places the substantial importance of word recognition vis-à-vis reading comprehension within the following perspective: "Reading for meaning [comprehension] is greatly hindered when children are having too much trouble with word recognition. When word recognition processes demand too much cognitive capacity, fewer cognitive resources are left to allocate to higher-level processes of text integration and comprehension" (p. 281).

The relatively greater importance of word recognition skills than of reading comprehension flies in the face of theories and models maintaining that the ability to use contextual information to predict upcoming words is the cornerstone of fluent reading (Goodman, 1969; Smith, 1971). However, work conducted by a number of investigators (see Rayner et al., 2002) has demonstrated that less skilled readers were more likely to depend upon text for word recognition; highly skilled readers did not rely on contextual information for decoding or single-word reading, since their word recognition processes were so rapid and automatic (Stanovich, 1994).

Given the converging evidence documenting the importance of word recognition, it is not surprising that the ability to read single words accurately and fluently has been the most frequently selected research target in the study of LDs in reading. Again, this is not to diminish the role of reading comprehension as an academic and cognitive skill to be taught and acquired. However, word recognition is not only a prerequisite behavior to comprehension; it is a more narrowly circumscribed behavior and is not related to numerous nonreading factors typically associated with comprehension (Wood et al., 1991). Therefore, it offers a more precise developmental variable for study. Many of the advances in reading research have resulted from the focus on definitions using word recognition, as opposed to simply lumping together children as having "LDs" or combining children with different bands of reading difficulties (see the sections on comprehension and fluency, below).

With the dependent variable thus identified, there continues to be some debate about the nonreading factor or factors (e.g., linguistic, perceptual, temporal processing speed) that account for deficits in single-word reading. Two different perspectives continue to exist. The first and more influential school of thought proposes that deficits in word recognition are primarily associated with, or caused by, one primary nonreading factor (i.e., phonological awareness, rapid temporal processing). The second school of thought is that deficits in the ability to read single words rapidly and automatically are referable to multiple factors, thus giving rise to hypothesized subtypes of reading disabilities. Any theory of dyslexia, however, must explain the core deficit, which is word decoding.

Single-Factor Models

Phonological Processing. The predominant single-factor model of dyslexia involves deficiencies in phonological processing, representing the phonological limitation hypothesis of investigators at the Haskins laboratories (Liberman, Shankweiler, & Liberman, 1989). "Phonological processing" refers to the use of phonological information, especially the sound structure of one's oral language, for processing written and oral information (Jorm & Share, 1983; Wagner & Torgesen, 1987; Wagner, Torgesen, Laughon, Simmons, & Rashotte, 1994). Speech sounds, or phonemes, are described by their phonetic properties, such as their manner or place of articulation, and their acoustic features or patterns of sound waves (Gerber, 1993).

English is an alphabetic language containing 44 phonemes. As in any alphabetic language, the unit characters (letters) that children learn to read and spell are keyed to the phonological structure of words (Liberman & Shankweiler, 1979;

Lukatela & Turvey, 1998). Thus a child's primary task in the early development of reading and spelling is to develop the realization that speech can be segmented into phonemes and that these phonemes represent printed forms (Blachman, 1991; Liberman, 1971; Lyon, 1995b). However, as Blachman (1997) has pointed out, this awareness that words can be divided into the smallest discernible segments of sound is a very difficult task for many children. The difficulty lies in large part in the fact that speech, unlike writing, does not consist of separate phonemes produced one after another "in a row over time" (Gleitman & Rosen, 1973, p. 460; see also Blachman, 1997). Instead, the sounds are "coarticulated" (overlapped with one another) to permit rapid communication of speech, rather than sound-by-sound pronunciation. This property of coarticulation—critical for speech, but possibly harmful to the beginning reader and speller—is explained by Liberman and Shankweiler (1991) as follows:

> The advantageous result of . . . coarticulation of speech sounds is that speech can proceed at a satisfactory pace—at a pace indeed at which it can be understood (Liberman, Cooper, Shankweiler, & Studdert-Kennedy, 1967). Can you imagine trying to understand speech if it were spelled out to you letter by painful letter? So coarticulation is certainly advantageous for the perception of speech. But a further result of coarticulation, and a much less advantageous one for the would-be reader, is that there is, inevitably, no neat correspondence between the underlying phonological structure and the sound that comes to the ears. Thus, though the word "bag," for example, has three phonological units, and correspondingly three letters in print, it has only one pulse of sound: The three elements of the underlying phonological structure—the three phonemes (/b/ /a/ /g/)—have been thoroughly overlapped (coarticulated) into the one beginning sound—"bag." . . . [Beginning readers] can understand, and properly take advantage of, the fact that the printed word *bag* has three letters, only if they are aware that the spoken word *"bag,"* with which they are already quite familiar, is divisible into three segments. They will probably not know that spontaneously, because as we have said, there is only one segment of sound, not three, and because the processes of speech perception that recover the phonological structure are automatic and quite unconscious. (pp. 5–6)

Thus the awareness of the phonological structure of the English language is the basis for the fluent recognition of known words necessary for basic reading, reading comprehension, spelling, and written expression (Shankweiler & Liberman, 1989; Rayner et al., 2002). When phonological awareness develops and the child understands the alphabetic principle, word recognition is mastered early in the reading process; the critical issues are then the automaticity of these processes and the development of comprehension ability, both of which develop along with accuracy, but have longer developmental trajectories. When the child does not understand the relationship of sound and print, word recognition will be delayed. The longer the child struggles to learn to read words, the more likely it is that a severe reading disability will emerge as the child cannot access print. Developing fluency and accessing comprehension abilities becomes increasingly difficult as the child loses exposure to sight words and the opportunity to access books. It is not surprising that at this point in time, the most common form of LD in reading involves word recognition ability.

There is substantial support for this relationship and its pivotal importance not only in learning to read, but also as a proximal cause of WLRD. Other causal factors identify difficulties experienced by children with reading difficulties, but are less adequate in explaining the word recognition problem (Fletcher, Foorman, Shaywitz, & Shaywitz, 1999).

Other Unitary Processes. There is a long history of identifying single factors in the etiology of dyslexia and other reading disabilities. This is clearly seen, for example, in the attempt to tie visual-perceptual difficulties to reading disabilities, a characteristic of much of the literature in the 1960s and 1970s (Vellutino, 1979). However, while it is common to observe the presence of difficulties with copying or matching geometric designs in comparisons of children who are disabled and nondisabled in reading, there is little evidence that the spatial processing problems per se are linked to reading disorders (Vellutino, Scanlon, & Fletcher, in press). At the same time, children with reading disabilities have problems that extend beyond the reading process. They are often observed to have comorbid difficulties involving math or attention, or other cognitive and motor difficulties that are frequently interpreted as clinically relevant in psychometric evaluations. This was clearly apparent in the older neuropsychological studies, which commonly focused on the emergence of a difference between groups as explanatory of the disorder (Doehring, 1978). Thus the history of behavioral research on children with reading disabilities is characterized by various attempts to compete and compare single-cause factors (Benton & Pearl, 1978). These studies invariably beg the question of how the presence of a particular factor in children with reading difficulties explains the reading problem; such research sometimes leads to convoluted theories in which the presumably causal factor is related to the reading process.

This same trend is apparent in more contemporary literature that attempts to relate sensory deficits in either the auditory or visual modality to dyslexia. In the visual area, there are studies using psychophysical methods involving visual persistence, contrast and flicker sensitivity, and the detection of motion thresholds; these studies are often interpreted to suggest a deficiency in the temporal processing of visual information (Stein, 2001). Such deficits are often related to specific difficulties in the magnocellular visual pathway. The magnocellular pathway is responsible for operations of the transient visual channel, which provides short, previsual responses to stimuli that are low in spatial frequency and move rapidly. In contrast, the parvocellular visual pathway is related to operations of the sustained visual channel, which provides a longer duration response to slow-moving stimuli that have high spatial frequency. In reading and other visual tasks, these two systems mutually inhibit one another. Various findings have suggested that individuals with reading difficulties have ineffective transient system inhibition that interferes with the saccadic suppression of visual information. This leads to persistence of retinal image, so that the words on a page may seem jumbled (Lovegrove, Martin, & Slaghuis, 1986; Stein, 2001).

This example illustrates some of the difficulties that arise in attempts to link these types of problems to the reading process. Although it is clear that individuals with reading disabilities differ from typically achieving individuals on measures involving the visual system, it is not clear how the magnocellular system can be involved in word recognition. The print itself is stationary, not moving. If words are jumbled when a person is scanning words, then the task would not seem to involve the perception of individual words, but groups of words as a person reads text (Iovino, Fletcher, Breitmeyer, & Foorman, 1999). The magnocellular system operates when a person is reading continuous text; the core problem in dyslexia involves the identification of words in isolation. Thus it is difficult to see how such a theory can explain the core reading problems associated with dyslexia.

More recent attempts to explain the visual processing difficulties observed in children with dyslexia relate these difficulties to the processing of the orthographic components of written language and assume that such deficits are not related to phonological decoding. Such explanations relate to the sometimes irregular relationship of the pronunciation of words and their representation in print. It is well established that the relationship of phonology and orthography in English is sometimes inconsistent, and that English spellings are commonly irregular (Rayner et al., 2002). Thus it is hypothesized that the visual system is related to the ability to immediately process words that cannot be sounded out automatically—a representation of the dual-route theory of reading. In this theory, words can be either accessed through a phonological route or recognized immediately through a visual route that bypasses the need for phonological processing (Castles & Coltheart, 1993). Talcott et al. (2000) found correlations between visual motion sensitivity and orthographic processing even when variance due to phonological processing and IQ was covaried from the relationship. However, this relationship was true for all children, regardless of the presence of a disability. In addition, there was no evidence that the relationship of orthographic processing to word recognition was stronger than the relationship of phonological processing. Eden, Stern, Wood, and Wood (1995) performed similar analyses in which they observed that measures of visual processing continued to contribute independently to prediction of reading skills after IQ and phonological processing were partialed out of the relationship. However, the amount of variance accounted for was relatively small, and the methods used capitalized on independence after the most highly correlated variables had been included. Therefore, the more recent visual processing hypotheses do not provide robust explanations for the core reading problems experienced by children with dyslexia; in this respect, they resemble any older hypotheses based on univariate comparisons of children with and without reading difficulties. Such differences between groups were easy to observe, but difficult to relate to the reading problem (Doehring, 1978; Satz & Fletcher, 1980).

Sensory hypotheses have also been developed in the auditory modality. The most prominent was developed by Tallal and colleagues (see Tallal, Miller, Jenkins, and Merzenich (1997). To summarize, in a long series of studies involving children with specific language impairment, differences between these children and normal youngsters were found in the ability to assess acoustic stimuli with spectral parameters that changed rapidly in intensity. Problems processing rapidly changing stimuli were observed for speech and nonspeech stimuli, leading Tallal and associates to hypothesize that language disabilities are caused by auditory processing problems involving their perception of rapidly changing stimuli. Tallal (1980) extended these findings to children with reading disabilities by using speech and nonspeech stimuli. She found that a subgroup of children with reading disabilities performed more poorly than nondisabled children on auditory perceptual tasks, and that performance was correlated with reading ability. However, the participants were obtained from a sample of children originally defined with oral language disorders, and the correlations may have been related to the complete inability of many children to read and thus the assignment of raw scores of 0 to these children. Nonetheless, Reed (1989) replicated the work of Tallal (1980), finding deficits on auditory stimuli that involved speech as well as nonspeech, whereas Mody, Studdert-Kennedy, and Brady (1997) did not replicate the findings for nonspeech stimuli.

Questions were raised about these studies because of the criteria used for defining the children as disabled, as well as the possibility that other factors could explain the differences between the groups, such as the high comorbidity of reading disabilities and ADHD. There were also concerns about the auditory stimuli. Two recent studies involved samples that controlled for the presence of ADHD and used well-established definitions of dyslexia. In a study by Waber et al. (2001), children with dyslexia and no ADHD were defined from a larger group of children originally referred for evaluation of learning impairments in a clinic setting. Waber et al. (2001) found a significant difference between children with good reading and dyslexia in their ability to discriminate speech and nonspeech stimuli, but across a variety of stimuli and not just those that showed rapid changes in their acoustic parameters. Breier, Fletcher, Foorman, and Gray (in press) used temporal-order judgment and discrimination tasks in children with dyslexia and no ADHD, dyslexia and ADHD, ADHD and no dyslexia, and typically achieving children with no ADHD. Children with dyslexia did not show a specific sensitivity to variations in interstimulus intervals. They also performed more poorly than children without dyslexia only on speech stimuli, but not on nonspeech stimuli. Phonological processing measures were consistently more closely related to speech than nonspeech stimuli. The results were independent of the presence of ADHD. Like Waber et al. (2001), Breier et al. (2002) concluded that children with dyslexia have difficulties with speech perception that correlate with reading and phonological processing ability, but little evidence for generalized auditory processing difficulties.

Altogether, these results do not provide compelling explanations of the core reading problem apparent in children with dyslexia. In this regard, they do not explain the word recognition difficulties in a parsimonious manner; nor is the weight of the evidence as strong as that associated with explanations based on phonological processing. It is absolutely true that dyslexia is more than a reading disability, and that children with dyslexia differ from normal children on a variety of dimensions. However, these differences do not explain the reading problem. They could be related to the nature of the underlying neurobiological problem that appears to be at the root of dyslexia, but the basis for these differences has yet to receive adequate exploration (Eden & Zeffiro, 1998).

Multiple-Factor Models

As we have noted above and in the first edition (Lyon, 1996b), LDs involve multiple domains, reflecting the fact that some children manifest reading deficits, whereas others have difficulties in oral language, written expression, and/or mathematics (Blashfield, 1993; Feagans, Short, & Meltzer, 1991; Fletcher, Francis, Rourke, Shaywitz, & Shaywitz, 1993; Fletcher & Morris, 1986; Hooper & Willis, 1989; Lyon & Risucci, 1989; Morris, 1993; Newby & Lyon, 1991; Rourke, 1985; Speece, 1993). Obviously comorbidities exist between and among these general conditions. Within specific LDs, such as dyslexia, it has also been hypothesized that a number of *subtypes* exist that can be identified on the basis of how their members perform on measures of cognitive–linguistic, perceptual, memory span, and achievement skills (Boder, 1973; Doehring & Hoshko, 1977; Fisk & Rourke, 1979; Lovett, 1984; Lyon, 1985a, 1985b, 1987; Lyon & Flynn, 1989, 1991; Lyon, Rietta, Watson, Porch, & Rhodes, 1981; Lyon, Stewart, & Freedman, 1982; Lyon & Watson, 1981; Mattis, French, & Rapin, 1975; Morris et al., 1998; Petrauskas & Rourke, 1979; Satz & Morris, 1981).

The argument for the existence of subtypes in the population with dyslexia has been based on the practical observation that even though children with dyslexia may appear very similar with respect to their reading deficits (i.e., word recognition deficits), they may differ significantly in the development of other skills that may be correlated with basic reading development (Lyon, 1985a). Thus, even within well-defined samples of children with dyslexia, there is large within-sample variance on some skills. This observation may explain, in part, why such children have been reported to differ from controls on so many variables related to reading (Doehring, 1978).

The literature on subtyping dyslexia and other reading disabilities is voluminous, comprising over 100 classification studies since 1963; the reader is referred to Hooper and Willis (1989), Newby and Lyon (1991), and the first edition of this chapter (Lyon, 1996b) for comprehensive reviews of this literature. For the purposes of the present chapter, two approaches to subtypes are reviewed: one that focuses on rational grouping of readers with LDs into subtypes on the basis of clinical observations and/or theories related to reading disabilities (Lovett, Ransby, & Barron, 1988; Wolf & Bowers, 1999; Wolf et al., 2001), and a second approach that exemplifies the use of empirical multivariate statistical methods to identify homogeneous subtypes of readers with LDs (Lyon, 1983, 1985a; Lyon et al., 1981; Morris et al., 1998).

Rational Subtyping Methods. As an example of a rational (clinical) approach to subtypes, Lovett (1984, 1987; Lovett, Steinbach, & Frijters, 2000) proposed two subtypes of reading disability, based on the hypothesis that word recognition develops in three successive phases. The three phases are related to response accuracy in identifying printed words, automatic recognition without the need to "sound out" words, followed by developmentally appropriate maximum speed as components of the reading process become consolidated in memory. Children who fail at the first phase are identified as "accuracy-disabled," and those who achieve age-appropriate word recognition but are markedly deficient in the second or third phase are termed "rate-disabled." The greatest strength of the Lovett subtype research program is its extensive external validation (Newby & Lyon, 1991). In a study of the two subtypes (rate-disabled vs. accuracy-disabled) and a normal sample matched on word recognition ability to the rate-disabled group, children in the accuracy-disabled group were deficient in a wide array of oral and written language areas external to the specific reading behaviors used to identify subtype members. On the other hand, the rate-disabled group's deficiencies were more restricted to deficient connected-text reading and spelling (Lovett, 1987). Reading comprehension was impaired on all measures for the accuracy-disabled group and was highly correlated with word recognition skill, but the rate-disabled group was impaired on only some comprehension measures. These additional subtype–treatment interaction studies (Lovett et al., 1988; Lovett, Ransby, Hardwick, & Johns, 1989; Lovett, Steinbach, & Frijters, 2000) found some differences between the accuracy- and rate-disabled groups on contextual reading, whereas word recognition improved for both groups.

Lovett's program is founded on explicit developmental reading theory, illustrates methodological robustness, and offers detailed, thoughtful alternative explanations for the complex external validation findings (Newby & Lyon, 1991). Important treatment outcome findings are muted somewhat by reading gains on standardized measures that did not move many children into the average, in spite of statistically significant results. There is little evidence of significant subtype–treatment interactions (Lyon & Flynn, 1989).

More recent research continues to emphasize the importance of this basic distinction between accuracy and rate. In the model developed by Wolf and associates (Wolf & Bowers, 1999; Wolf et al., 2001), the authors propose that although phonological processing contributes considerably to word recognition deficits, reading involves the ability to read both accurately and fluently. Children do demonstrate fluency deficits that are apparently independent of problems with phonological processing. When isolated deficits and fluency occur, the most reliable correlate occurs on tasks that require rapid naming of letters and digits. Thus Wolf and associates have postulated a "double-deficit model" of subtypes.

This model specifies essentially three subtypes: one characterized by deficits in both phonological processing and rapid naming; another with impairments only phonological processing; and a third with impairments only in rapid automatized naming. Wolf and associates have summarized evidence, largely rational but with reasonable approaches to validity, that supports this subtyping scheme. There are inherent methodological problems identified by Schatchneider, Carlson, Francis, Foorman, and Fletcher (2002) and Compton, DeFries, and Olson (2001) that involve difficulties in defining single- versus double-deficit typologies. When both phonological processing and rapid naming are impaired, a child is more severely impaired in both dimensions, which makes it difficult to match single- and double-deficit-impaired children. Thus children with double deficits tend to have more severe problems in either phonology or rapid naming as well as in reading, compared to children with a single deficit. An alternative is to use an empirical approach to subtyping to determine whether these subtypes emerge, which we address in the next section.

Empirical Subtyping Methods. There are numerous examples of empirical subtyping studies derived from achievement, neurocognitive, neurolinguistic, and combined classification models. Multiple models of LDs in reading have emerged through the application of multivariate statistical approaches. An integrated analysis of several prominent reading disability subtype systems that have been intensively investigated suggests some areas of convergence in the literature (Hooper & Willis, 1989). In particular, memory span, phonological, and orthographic processing in reading appear to be central in defining subtypes. Although a dichotomy of auditory–linguistic versus visual–spatial reading disability subtypes has been commonly proposed, this division has not been effectively validated (Newby & Lyon, 1991); nor is the evidence strong for any nonlinguistic variable as an explanation for the reading difficulties experienced by children with dyslexia.

In a series of studies employing multivariate cluster-analytic methods, Lyon and his colleagues (Lyon, 1983, 1985a, 1985b; Lyon et al., 1981, 1982; Lyon & Watson, 1981) identified six subtypes of older readers with LDs (11- to 12-year-old children) and five subtypes of younger readers with LDs (6- to 9-year-old children) on measures assessing linguistic skills, visual-perceptual skills, and memory span abilities. The theoretical viewpoint guiding this subtype research was based on Luria's (1966, 1973) observations that reading ability is a complex behavior effected by means of a complex functional system of cooperating zones of the cerebral cortex and subcortical structures. Within the context of this theoretical framework, it could be hypothesized that a deficit in any one or several zones of the functional system could impede the acquisition of fluent reading behavior. The identification of multiple subtypes within both age cohorts suggested the possibility that several different subtypes of reading disabilities exist, each characterized by different patterns of neuropsychological subskills relevant to reading acquisition.

We emphasize this example, as it attempted to identify subtype–treatment interactions, a research priority that is still infrequently addressed. Follow-up subtype–treatment interaction studies using both age samples (Lyon, 1985a, 1985b) only partially supported the independence of the subtypes with respect to response to treatment. It was found, however, that subtypes characterized at both age levels by significant deficits in blending sounds, rapid naming, and memory span did not respond to intervention methods employing synthetic phonics procedures. Rather, readers with this linguistic-deficit subtype first had to learn phonetically regular words by sight, and then learn the internal phonological structure, using the whole word as a meaningful semantic context. Again, this was true for both younger and older readers with the linguistic-deficit subtype.

In the past 10 years, the frequency of empirical subtyping studies has diminished. It is clear that many of these approaches to subtyping were largely atheoretical and simply involved the application of multivariate statistical algorithms to cognitive and academic variables. The resultant solutions were highly variable and often unreliable. Although there was some general replication across groups in terms of the types of clusters identified, the subtypes themselves were often difficult to relate to what is known about domain-specific reading disabilities or other LDs.

One recent empirical subtyping study provided support not only for the double-deficit model, but also for models that separate "specific" forms of reading disabilities from "garden variety" forms (Morris et al., 1998). This study differed from previous empirical approaches to subtyping, in that it was based on a model emphasizing the role of phonological processing in reading disabilities (Liberman et al., 1989; Stanovich, 1988). It also used other theories to select potential variables. Thus measures of rapid naming, short-term memory, vocabulary, and perceptual skills were included. From a methodological perspective, the sample was large and was selected on an a priori basis for a subtyping study (i.e., it was not just a sample of convenience). Multiple definitions were used to identify children. In addition to children defined with dyslexia, children with both dyslexia and math disabilities, children with isolated math disabilities, children with permutations involving ADHD, and typically achieving children were included. The application of the clustering algorithms was rigorous and followed guidelines ensuring both internal and external validity (Morris & Fletcher, 1988).

The nine resultant subtypes are portrayed in Figure 12.1. All profiles are depicted as z-scores relative to the sample mean. Here it is apparent that there are five subtypes with specific reading disabilities, two subtypes representing more pervasive impairments in language and reading, and two representing typically achieving groups of children. Six of the seven reading disability subtypes share, however, an impairment in phonological awareness skills. The five specific subtypes (see Figure 12.2) vary largely in rapid automatized naming and verbal short-term memory. We can see a large subtype in Figure 12.2 with impairments in phonological awareness, rapid naming, and verbal short-term memory. There are two subtypes with impairments in phonological awareness, and verbal short-term memory, varying in lexical and spatial skills; a subtype with phonological awareness and rapid naming difficulties; and a subtype without impairment in phonological awareness, but with deficits on any measure that required rapid processing, including rapid naming. This last subtype does not have a word recognition impairment, but has difficulties on measures of reading fluency and comprehension, consistent with Wolf's double-deficit model. The five specific subtypes can be differentiated from the "garden variety" subtypes on the basis of their vocabulary development. Children with specific subtypes of reading disabilities have vocabulary levels that are in the average range; children with more pervasive disturbances of reading and language have vocabulary levels that are in the low average range.

Altogether, these results are consistent with the phonological processing hypothesis advanced earlier in this chapter, as well as with Wolf's double-deficit model. The results are also consistent with Stanovich's (1988) model of phonological core variable differences. This model postulates that phonological processing is at the core of all WLRD. But reading disabilities are often more than just phonological processing problems. Children may have problems outside the phonological domain that do not contribute to the word recognition difficulties. This could be represented by impairments in vocabulary that would interfere with comprehension; more pervasive disturbances of language that would lead to a garden variety form of reading disability; or even fine motor and visual-perceptual problems that are demonstrably unrelated to dyslexia.

Neurobiological Factors

The hypothesis that LDs are "unexpected" stems in part from the belief that if children who experience low achievement due to such factors as economic disadvantage and inadequate instruction are excluded from the LD category, the cause in those who have low achievement not due to the exclusions must be intrinsic to the children. The history of research on LDs from the very beginning reflects this assumption and was significantly influenced by concepts like MBD. Although the emphasis on constitutional factors is only implicit in the federal definition of LDs through the subsuming of disorders represented by MBD and brain injury, it is explicit in other definitions. To illustrate, consider the NJCLD (1988) definition: "These disorders [LDs] are intrinsic to the individual, presumed to be due to central nervous system damage, and may occur across the life span" (p. 1). Similarly, the World Federation of Neurology definition explicitly indicates that dyslexia is "dependent upon fundamental cognitive disabilities, which are frequently of constitutional origin" (Critchley, 1970, p. 11).

As we have noted in our review of the history of LDs, the intrinsic nature of LDs was inferred from what was then known about the linguistic and behavioral characteristics of adults with documented brain injury. As the field progressed, definitions of LDs continued to attribute them to intrinsic (brain) rather than extrinsic (e.g., environmental, instructional) causes, even though there was no objective way to adequately assess

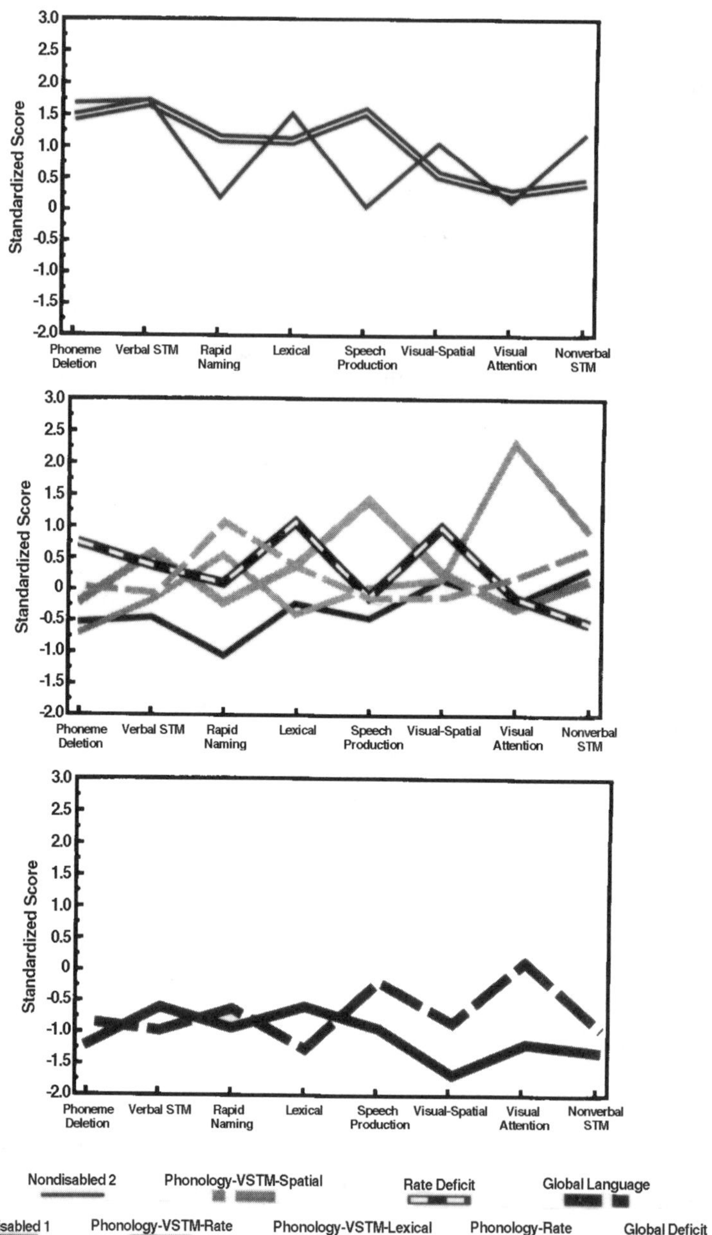

FIGURE 12.1. The *z*-scores for nine subtypes of children with reading disabilities, produced by cluster analysis of eight variables. The two subtypes in the upper panel represent typically achieving groups of children. The subtypes in the lower panel represent children with lower overall levels of functioning. The five subtypes in the middle panel represent children with relatively specific reading disabilities who show variable profile configurations. V, verbal; STM, short-term memory. Data from Morris et al. (1998).

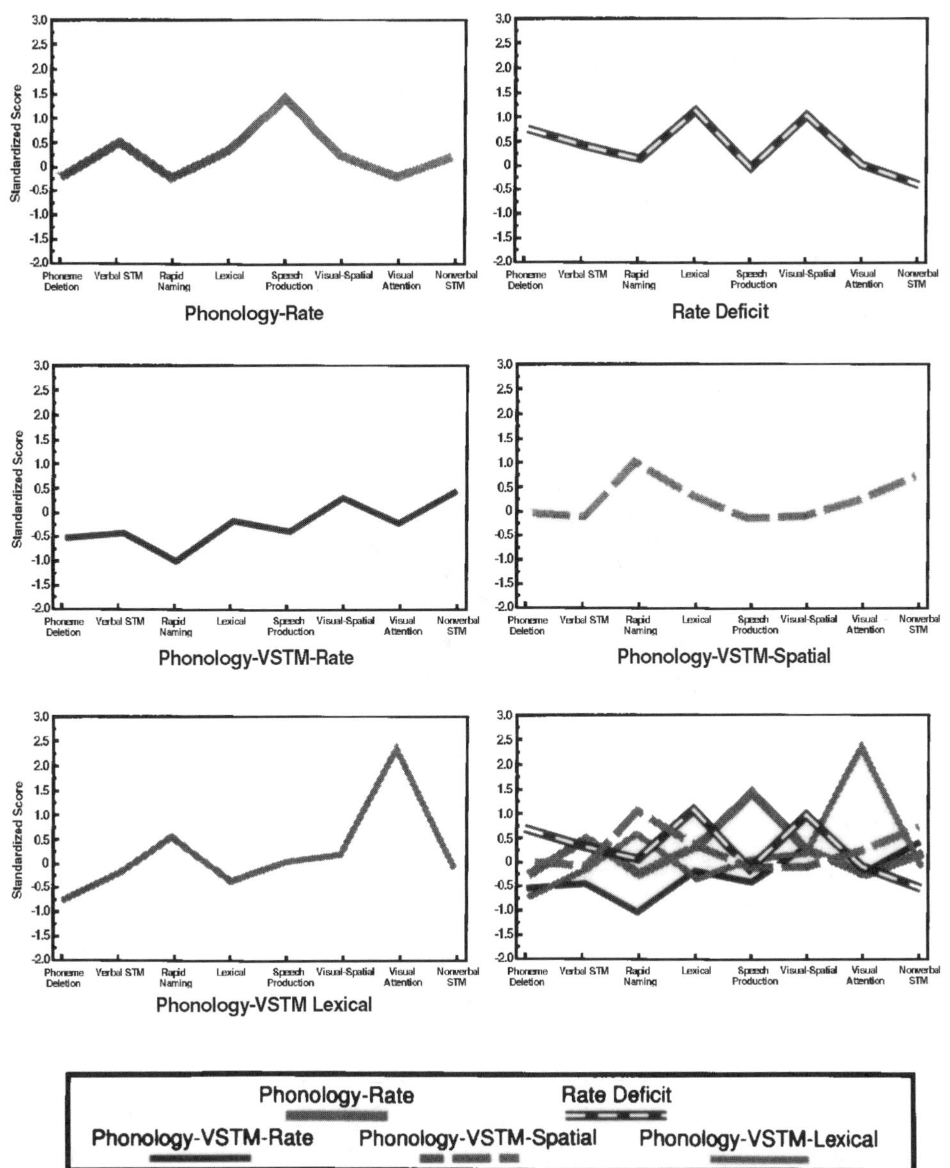

FIGURE 12.2. The z-scores for the five subtypes of children with specific reading disabilities, plotted separately for each subtype. V, verbal; STM, short-term memory. Data from Morris et al. (1998).

the presence of putative brain damage or dysfunction. And this problem was constantly dismissed as a matter that technology would eventually resolve! This conviction was reinforced by the common nonspecific association of indirect indices of neurological dysfunction with LDs, including perceptual–motor problems (i.e., difficulty copying geometric figures), paraclassical or "soft" neurological signs (e.g., gross motor clumsiness, fine motor incoordination), and anomalies on electrophysiological measures (Dykman et al., 1971; Taylor & Fletcher, 1983). Even at the time, the lack of specificity of these observations to either LDs or neurological integrity was widely acknowledged (Satz & Fletcher, 1980).

Over the past two decades, the quality of the evidence has improved. It is now possible to clearly support the hypothesis that LDs in general, and dyslexia in particular, have a locus in neurobiological factors. But the evidence also suggests that simplistic causal models in which neurobiological deficits produce a child with dyslexia are simplistic and do not take into account the complex interplay of the brain and environment in development. In this section, we review studies of (1) brain structure; (2) brain function; and (3) genetics. Most of these studies explicitly defined children as reading-disabled on the basis of word recognition and phonological processing abilities, so they tend to be specific to dyslexia. There is relatively little research on neurobiological factors involving LDs other than dyslexia.

Brain Structure. Research on brain structure involves either postmortem studies or the use of imaging techniques such as computed cerebral tomography (CT) and anatomical magnetic resonance imaging (aMRI). As CT did not prove particularly useful and is regarded as having poorer resolution than aMRI, we will not discuss CT. Reviews of this literature can be found in Hynd and Semrud-Clikeman (1989).

There are a few postmortem evaluations of the brain anatomy of adults with a history of dyslexia. Obviously these cases are rare, as dyslexia is not regarded as lethal. These studies, largely by a group led by Galaburda (1993), have involved a total of 10 brains accumulated over several years. The findings indicated that individuals with dyslexia are characterized by differences in the size of specific brain structures (e.g., planum temporale) and the presence of specific neuroanatomical anomalies (Filipek, 1996; Galaburda, 1993; Shaywitz et al., 2000).

Evaluations of cortical structures in adults with a history of reading problems as children have found that the planum temporale, a structure on the plane of the temporal lobe, is symmetrical in size in the left versus right hemisphere (Galaburda, Sherman, Rosen, Aboitiz, & Geschwind, 1985; Humphreys, Kaufmann, & Galaburda, 1990). In postmortem studies of adults who presumably did not have reading problems, this structure is often larger in the left hemisphere than the right hemisphere (Geschwind & Levitsky, 1968). Because this area of the left hemisphere supports language function, the absence of this anatomical difference has been viewed as partly the basis for language deficiencies that should lead to reading problems. In addition, microscopic examination of cortical architecture showed minor focal distortions called "ectopias." While also common in individuals with no history of dyslexia, these ectopias were more common than would be expected in individuals with a history of dyslexia. They were also more common in the left hemisphere. Finally, microscopic examinations of subcortical structures have also shown differences relative to normative expectations, particularly in the thalamus (Livingstone, Rosen, Drislane, & Galaburda, 1991). These structures of the thalamus are widely believed to be involved in visual processing.

Altogether, postmortem studies have found clear evidence of anomalies at both subcortical and cortical levels. However, these studies are limited because the reading characteristics, educational histories, and important factors that influence brain organization, such as handedness, are difficult to ascertain in a postmortem study. For example, it is not possible to correlate the size of the planum temporale or the frequency/location of ectopias with reading performance in a postmortem study, so it is difficult to establish the role of these findings in causing dyslexia.

Given the difficulties involved in ascertaining brains for postmortem evaluation, as well as the limitations of any postmortem study mentioned above, investigators have turned to aMRI for the evaluation of potential differences in brain structure. The use of aMRI is desirable because it is noninvasive and is safe for children. The aMRI data can also be quantitated, so that precise measurements of brain structure can be made. The findings can then be correlated with reading performance. Studies to date have examined a variety of structures (see Filipek, 1996). Given the interest generated by postmortem studies, these include the planum temporale and the temporal lobes. In addition, there have been some studies of the corpus callosum, which may reflect the fact that it is relatively easy to quantitate.

This research has yielded mixed results. Studies that compare the planum temporale in individuals with and without dyslexia report both symmetry (Hynd, Semrud-Clikeman, Lorys, Novey, & Eliopulos, 1990; Larson, Hoien, Lundberg, & Ödegaard, 1990) and even reversals in the expected patterns of asymmetry (Hynd et al., 1990) in the groups with dyslexia. However, other studies have not found an association between symmetry of the planum temporale in dyslexia (Rumsey et al., 1997; Schultz et al., 1994). Some studies report differences between dyslexic and normal individuals in temporal parietal brain regions (Duara et al., 1991; Kusch et al., 1993), but other studies do not find these differences (Hynd et al, 1990; Jernigan, Hesselink, Stowell, & Tallal, 1991). Finally, studies of the corpus callosum have also yielded mixed findings, with some studies reporting differences in the size (Duara et al., 1991; Hynd et al., 1995). But other studies have not found differences in corpus callosum measures (Larsen et al., 1990; Schultz et al., 1994).

More recent studies have continued to evaluate asymmetry in the planum region. An interesting study by Leonard et al. (1996) correlated reading performance and asymmetry of the temporal lobes; higher degrees of asymmetry favoring the left hemisphere were found to be associated with better reading performance, regardless of whether a child was disabled in reading. This finding implies lack of specificity to children with reading disabilities. However, Leonard et al. (2001) did not replicate this finding.

A recent study by Pennington et al. (1999) used extremely careful image acquisitions and elaborate morphometric analysis to measure multiple cortical and subcortical areas of the brain. These investigators found reductions bilaterally in the size of the insula and anterior superior cortex in individuals with dyslexia. In addition, the area of the brain posterior to the splenium of the corpus callosum—largely posterior temporal, parietal, and occipital regions—was larger in both the right and left hemispheres in individuals with dyslexia. These differences, however, were relatively small and occurred in a sample that had large differences between IQ scores of dyslexic and nondyslexic twin pairs, although the results were robust when age, gender, and IQ were controlled for.

The attempt to control for age, gender, and IQ (as well as handedness) in the Pennington et al. (1999) study is very important. Schultz et al. (1994) found statistically significant differences on multiple aMRI measures in children with dyslexia and age-matched controls, including the planum temporale and several left-hemisphere structures. However, when subject selection variables (especially gender and handedness) were controlled for statistically, these differences disappeared, and the only reliable finding was a reduction of the size of the left temporal lobe in individuals with dyslexia.

Altogether, there is some convergence indicating subtle differences in several brain structures between dyslexic and nonimpaired readers, especially in left-hemisphere regions supporting language. Comparisons across laboratories have been hampered by the use of different neuroimaging methods and data-analytic techniques, leading to difficulties replicating these findings (Filipek, 1996; Shaywitz et al., 2000). Many of these difficulties reflect the technical difficulties associated with aMRI quantitation, which requires manual drawing and a high degree of technical sophistication. These issues make analysis time-consuming (on the order of days for a single brain), inevitably leading to small samples and the types of methodological factors that have emerged.

New modalities for structural neuroimaging are on the horizon. In a recent study, Klingberg et al. (2000) used diffusion tensor imaging to evaluate the integrity of the cerebral white matter in areas known to support language in the left hemisphere. Comparisons of these measures in adults with and without a history of reading difficulties showed less development of white matter in those with a reading problem. These results suggested reduced myelination of these language-mediating areas. It will be interesting in the future to begin to combine these types of assessments with functional neuroimaging studies of the same person.

Brain Function. More recently, researchers have used different types of *functional* neuroimaging methods to measure brain activation in response to visual, linguistic, and reading tasks among individuals who read skillfully and individuals with dyslexia. Converging evidence from a range of functional imaging methods used in studies of both groups indicates that a network of brain areas is involved in the ability to recognize words accurately, and that adults and children with dyslexia manifest different patterns of activation in these areas when compared with skilled readers. These areas most consistently involve the basal temporal, temporoparietal, and inferior frontal regions, predominantly in the left hemisphere (Eden & Zeffiro, 1998; Shaywitz et al., 2000).

Functional neuroimaging in dyslexia is based on four different modalities that vary in their data acquisition and their spatial and temporal resolution (Papanicolaou, 1998): positron emission tomography (PET), fMRI, MSI, and magnetic resonance spectroscopy (MRS). We also mention measures involving electrophysiological methods in context, but do not mention them in detail, as their potential for brain mapping is less well developed than that of these other methods. All of these modalities attempt to measure changes in the brain that occur during cognitive processing, and then to construct maps that demonstrate where (and sometimes when) in the brain these changes occurred. For example, metabolic changes reflected by glucose utilization or shifts in blood flow from one part of the brain to another of the brain occur, depending on the mental operation and the parts of the brain that are involved in the operation. These changes can be recorded by PET or fMRI. Similarly, there are neurons that make connections in order to support a particular activity. When neurons make connections, there are changes in the properties of these neurons that alter brain electrical activity. This activity can be recorded by an electroencephalogram (EEG). There are also changes that occur in the magnetic fields surrounding these electrical sources when a person performs an activity. MSI measures these changes, providing information about what brain areas produce the magnetic signals. MRS measures changes in brain chemistry, such as lactate or glutamine, in response to some type of challenge (Hunter & Wang, 2001).

Regardless of the modality, the principles of functional imaging are relatively straightforward (Shaywitz et al., 2000). As a cognitive or motor task is performed, the changes in glucose metabolism (PET), blood flow (PET and fMRI), electrical activity (EEG), magnetic activity (MSI), or brain chemistry (MRS) are recorded. The changes in brain activation are recorded and superimposed on an MRI of the brain so that the areas of the brain responsible for the activity can be identified. Methods like fMRI, MSI, and MRS involve no radiation, are noninvasive, are safe, and can be used repeatedly even in children. Imaging with PET requires administration of a radioactive isotope to measure changes in blood flow and/or glucose utilization. Since the half-life of these isotopes is short, the time course of an experiment is limited. Children are not usually participants in PET studies unless they have a medical disorder and can directly benefit from the evaluation, as exposure to radioactive isotopes is involved. This exposure even limits the number of times that older individuals can participate in a PET study (Papanicolaou, 1998).

These modalities also vary in their spatial and temporal sensitivity. Metabolic techniques like PET and fMRI assess brain activity that occurs after the cognitive activity has occurred. They do not occur in real time. In fMRI, serial magnetic resonance images are acquired so rapidly that they can be used to capture the changes in blood flow associated with cognitive activity (Shaywitz et al., 2000). Thus spatial resolution with fMRI is excellent. Methods such as MSI (and EEG) occur in real time and provide considerable information on the time course of neural events. The spatial resolution of the brain maps themselves is poor, but this problem is handled by coregistering the MSI brain map on an aMRI scan. Evoked potential and EEG paradigms have excellent temporal resolution, but the spatial resolution is very poor even with coregistration, and these methods are not generally used for functional neuroimaging. MRS is devoted specifically to chemical shifts and is also dependent on coregistration with aMRI for spatial resection. The chemical shifts occur in real time, but require longer acquisitions to measure the shift (Hunter & Wang, 2001).

Previous research has used all four imaging modalities, and converging findings suggest that tasks requiring reading are associated with increased activation in a variety of areas, including the basal surface of the temporal lobe; the posterior portion of the superior and middle temporal gyri, extending into temporoparietal areas (supramarginal and angular gyri); and the inferior frontal lobe areas, primarily in the left hemisphere (Eden & Zeffiro, 1998; Rumsey et al., 1997; Shaywitz et al., 2000). There are inconsistencies among studies with respect to the engagement of a particular area (Poeppel, 1996). However, it is apparent that a network of areas are involved in word recognition, each of which may be activated to a different degree, depending upon specific task demands.

PET is an older technology, and studies of adults with good reading versus dyslexia were initially conducted using this modality. These studies found reductions in blood flow in the left temporoparietal area during performance of both reading and phonological processing tasks (Rumsey et al., 1992, 1997), but normal activation in the left inferior frontal areas among those with poor reading (Rumsey et al., 1994). In addition, the asymmetry of activity favoring the left hemisphere, which is usually observed in proficiently reading adults during reading tasks, was significantly reduced in adults with dyslexia (Gross-Glenn et al., 1991). Horwitz, Rumsey, and Donohue (1998) evaluated functional connectivity of the angular gyrus in adults at different levels of reading proficiency, and found that the activity in the left angular gyrus occurring during a phonological task was significantly correlated with other areas involved in reading in proficiently reading adults, but not in those with dyslexia. Horowitz et al. (1998) interpreted these data as suggesting a "functional disconnection" between these areas in people with dyslexia. Other studies have also shown evidence for right-hemisphere activation, which could be related to compensatory process or other nonlinguistic factors related to reading disability (see Grigorenko, 2001; Joseph, et al. 2001; Wood & Grigorenko, 2001)

Studies using fMRI have also found that lack of activation of the angular gyrus is commonly observed in adults with dyslexia. In an early fMRI study of adults, Shaywitz et al. (1998) found that adults who read well showed increased activation in temporoparietal areas (angular gyrus, Wernicke's area, and basal temporal areas) as demands for phonological analysis increased. Adults with dyslexia did not demonstrate this pattern, but showed more activation of anterior portions of the brain (inferior frontal gyrus (areas 44, 45). In addition, the dyslexic readers showed reversed (right greater than left) hemispheric asymmetries in activation in posterior temporal regions as compared to the group of nonimpaired readers—a finding that corresponds with previous reports of atypical patterns of hemispheric asymmetry in regional metabolism in persons with dyslexia (Rumsey et al., 1992). Pugh et al. (2000) also found evidence that the angular gyrus was poorly connected with other areas involving reading in adults with dyslexia. Studies of children using similar tasks have shown less activation of the inferior frontal area in those with dyslexia, but a similar pattern in more posterior regions of the brain (Shaywitz et al., 2002).

MSI studies of children have revealed highly reliable differences in activation patterns of children with dyslexia and typically achieving children. For these studies, activation maps were obtained while the children completed tasks in which they listened to or read real words, or read pseudowords in which the children had to decide whether the pseudowords rhymed (Simos, Breier, Fletcher, Bergman, & Papanicolaou, 2000; Simos, Breier, Fletcher, Foorman, et al., 2000). The two groups did not differ in activation patterns to the task in which they listened to words, showing patterns predominantly in the left hemisphere that would be expected for such a task. However, on both the word recognition tasks, striking differences in the activation patterns of the dyslexic and typically achieving groups (see Figure 12.3). In the typically achieving children, there was a characteristic pattern in which the occipital areas of the brain that support primary visual processing were initially activated (not shown in Figure 12.3). Then the ventral visual association cortices in both hemispheres were activated, followed by simultaneous activation of three areas in the *left* temporoparietal region (essentially the angular gyrus, Wernicke's area, and superior temporal gyrus). In the children with dyslexia, the same pattern and time course were apparent, but the temporoparietal areas of the *right* hemisphere were activated. On the whole, the findings are similar to those from the PET and fMRI studies, but the differences between the two groups are more strikingly lateralized.

Altogether, these findings suggest that in children with dyslexia, the functional connections between brain areas account for differences in brain activation, as opposed to specific or general dysfunction of any single brain area. A critical question is whether the patterns seen in these children are compensatory or reflect the failure of instruction to impact the brain in a manner necessary to form the neural networks that support word recognition. Thus the pattern may be similar to that seen in a young child who has not learned to read, and it may change by virtue of development, instruction, or even intervention. These studies may provide an example of how brain and environment interact in forming the neural networks supporting word recognition.

The relationship between neural imaging changes and response to an intervention has been evaluated in two recent studies (Richards et al., 2000; Simos et al., 2002). In the Richards et al. (2000) study, MRS was used to evaluate metabolic processes before and after a 3-week, 30-hour intervention focusing on phonological processing, word decoding, reading comprehension, and listening comprehension. Children received an MRS examination of the left anterior quadrant of the brain—known to be related to language processing—before and after the intervention. Prior to intervention, the MRS scans revealed a higher metabolic rate of lactate in this quadrant when children with dyslexia completed a task requiring them to decide whether words and nonwords rhymed. After the training program, lactate metabolism did not differentiate children

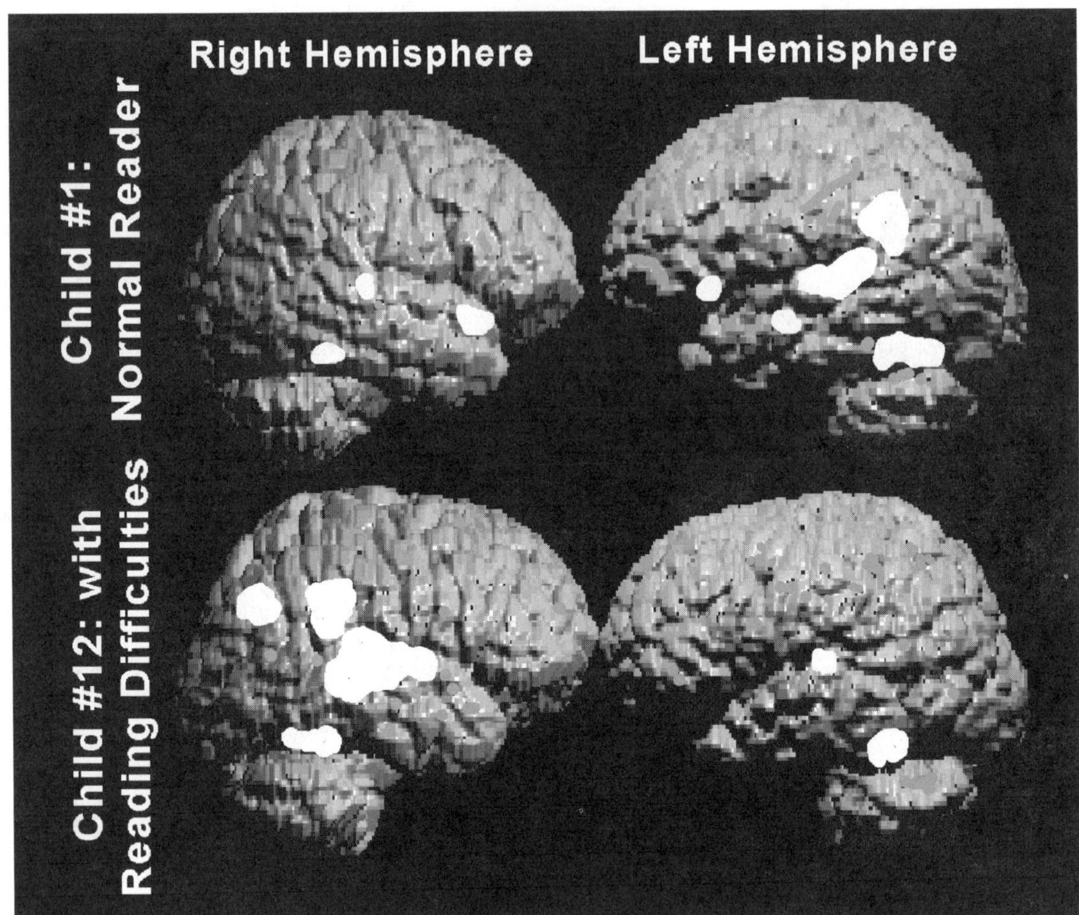

FIGURE 12.3. Three-dimensional brain activation maps scans from a child with dyslexia (lower set of images) and a proficiently reading child (top set of images) during pseudoword reading, based on MSI studies. Note the clustering of activity sources in left temporoparietal cortices in the proficient child, and in homotopic right-hemisphere areas in the child with dyslexia. Data from Simos, Breier, Fletcher, Foorman, et al. (2000).

with dyslexia from controls on the reading task. Although the investigators argued that the training program was responsible for the change in lactate metabolism, other reviewers (Gayan & Olson, 2001) have questioned the strength of these findings, largely focusing on the statistical analysis of the results.

In a second study, Simos, Fletcher, Bergman et al. (2002) employed MSI before and after children with severe dyslexia participated in an intense phonologically based intervention. These children ranged in age from 7 to 17 years and had very severe word recognition difficulties: Six of eight children read at the 3rd percentile or below, with the other two children reading at the 13th and 18th percentiles. The children received intervention for 2 hours a day, 5 days a week, over an 8-week period, for about 80 hours of intensive phonologically based instruction per child. Before intervention, the eight children with dyslexia uniformly displayed the aberrant pattern of activation in the right hemisphere that has been reliably identified with MSI. After intervention, the children's word-reading accuracy scores improved into the average range. In addition, in each case, there was significant activation of neural circuits in the left hemisphere commonly associated with proficient word-reading ability. There was also a tendency for reduction in right-hemisphere activity. Figure 12.4 provides a representative example of the changes before and after intervention. The changes were statistically

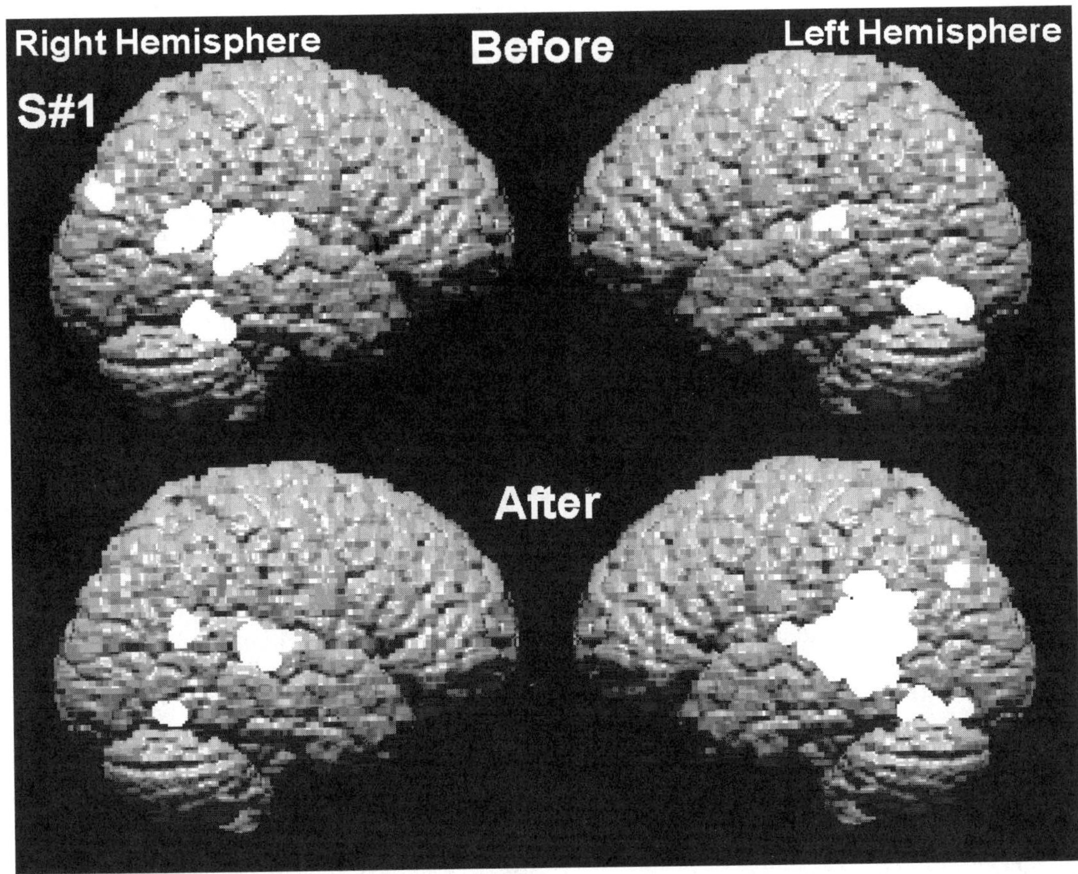

FIGURE 12.4. Activation maps from a child with dyslexia before and after an 8-week intense phonologically based intervention. The top set of images shows the typical brain activation map from MSI studies of dyslexia, with predominant activity in temporoparietal areas of the *right* hemisphere. In the lower set of images, there is a dramatic increase in *left* temporoparietal activation associated with the significant improvement in reading accuracy. Data from Simos et al. (2002).

significant, though the sample size was small. In addition, even with the improvement in word-reading accuracy, latency data from MSI continued to show delays in the evoked fields associated with the left-hemisphere response.

These studies are intriguing and do imply a far greater role for instruction in establishing the neural networks that support reading development. These findings received further support from Simos, Fletcher, Foorman et al. (2002), in which MSI was applied to children at the end of kindergarten who were identified as "at risk" for dyslexia, based on performance on screening tests of letter sounds and phonological awareness. These children demonstrated brain activation profiles that were quite similar to those identified in individuals with dyslexia as older children and adults. The children in this study are presently being followed after receiving an intensive intervention in grade 1 to determine whether there is additional normalization of their brain activation profiles. As this study also contains a comparison group of not-at-risk children, it will be possible to map neural changes that occur in association with learning to read in both at-risk and not-at-risk children. This study may provide additional evidence for the role of instruction in establishing the neural networks that support reading ability, and, when absent, reading disability.

Genetics. Genetic studies of reading ability stem from many years of observing that reading problems run in families. Reading problems clearly occur across family generations. The risk in the offspring of a parent with a reading disability is eight times higher than in the general population (Pennington, 1999). Yet studies of the heritability of dyslexia and other reading disabilities of reading disability show both genetic and environmental influences. These studies, reviewed by Pennington (1999), Olson et al. (1999), and Grigorenko (2001), show a long history of investigations at multiple levels. As Grigorenko (2001) has pointed out, three areas of research converge in demonstrating that dyslexia has a heritable component. These areas involve both twin and family studies of individuals in families with members who have dyslexia, along with linkage studies examining the role of specific genes that congregate within families that have significant heritability.

As reviewed by Grigorenko (2001) and Olson et al. (1999), 25–60% of the parents of children who have reading problems also display reading difficulties. The rate is higher in fathers (46%) than in mothers (33%). Children who have parents with reading difficulties are at much higher risk relative to the general population. The rates range from about 30% to 60%, depending on the method of ascertainment. If ascertainment depends on the parent's or school's identifying a child as dyslexic, the rate is closer to 30%. If the child and parent are actually evaluated by research instruments, the rate is significantly higher.

The limitation of family studies is that environments are also inherited. Twin studies can be used to address this issue by examining the concordance of dyslexia, as well as the heritability of reading achievement in general. As monozygotic twins have the same genotype, it would be expected that concordance rates would be much higher in monozygotic twins than in dizygotic twins, who share only 50% of the same genotype. However, monozygotic and dizygotic twins share the same environment. In general, concordance rates are quite high for monozygotic twins (almost always above 80%) relative to dizygotic twins (rarely above 50%). Therefore, differences in concordance presumably relate to the heritability.

Other approaches to twin studies of reading achievement also support the heritability of reading disabilities. These studies have employed statistical methods that help separate the variance in reading skills according to heritability and environmental factors (DeFries & Fulker, 1985), showing that 50–60% of the variance in reading achievement can be attributed to heritable factors. Studies of reading-related processes also show significant contributions of heritability. All of these studies also show that the environment exercises significant influence on reading skills, although the contribution of heritable factors is somewhat higher.

The final item of evidence comes from linkage studies that attempt to identify specific genes related to dyslexia. These studies tend to focus on families that have an unusually high number of members with dyslexia. The most significant finding involves an area on chromosome 6 that has been replicated in five different laboratories. There have also been findings implicating chromosome 15 (Smith, Pennington, Kimberling, & Ing, 1990; Grigorenko et al., 1997); these initial findings were not replicated, but subsequent studies have been more consistent in identifying an area of chromosome 15 in dyslexia. Potential markers have been identified on chromosomes 1 and 2. Though intriguing, these linkages have not been replicated (Grigorenko, 2001).

The genetic studies do provide strong evidence for the heritability of reading difficulties and help explain why reading problems have always been known to run in families. It is important to recognize that the evidence suggests that environmental factors are also important. It is likely that the tendencies of parents with dyslexia to read less frequently to their children and to have fewer books in the home contribute to the outcomes of parents and their children. In addition, the evidence does not show that the genetic influences are specific to individuals who read poorly; rather, the evidence suggests that what is inherited is a susceptibility to varying levels of proficiency in reading ability (Gilger & Kaplan, 2002). In many instances, reading disabilities may manifest themselves in the presence of specific interactions, or lack thereof, with the environment. The quality of reading instruction may be more critical when there is a family history of poor reading, which gives rise to limited environment–instructional interactions in the home (Olson et al., 1999; Pennington, 1999).

Summary: Dyslexia

It is possible to define the most common form of LD, dyslexia, using inclusionary criteria. These criteria focus on the relationship of word recognition and phonological processing. Differentiations are made relative to mental deficiency and to sensory disorders. No other exclusions seem essential, given the absence of evidence that word recognition problems vary according to putative causes. Moreover, although neurobiological explanations consistently identify differences in brain structure and brain function between children with dyslexia and typically achieving children, it is apparent that neurobiological and environmental factors interact to produce the phenotype associated with dyslexia.

Although the phonological processing hypothesis provides a robust explanation of the word-reading difficulties characteristic of dyslexia, it is also apparent that dyslexia is more than just a reading disability. Many children with dyslexia have problems in other areas, such as math and ADHD. Impairments in other components of the reading process, particularly fluency, are difficult to explain solely on the basis of phonological processing, although the failure to develop word recognition ability is the most parsimonious explanation of fluency and comprehension problems. There are explanations based on other factors that differentiate children with reading disabilities (not always well defined as dyslexia) and typically achieving children, but these hypotheses do not provide strong explanations of the core reading problem. This does not mean that dyslexia can be reduced just to a reading disorder, as the many individuals with dyslexia and comorbid conditions attest.

Perhaps the most exciting development in research, which is beyond the scope of this chapter, is the emerging data base on prevention and remediation of dyslexia, where positive results are emerging (Foorman & Torgesen, 2001; Lovett, Lacerenza, et al., 2000; Torgesen et al., 1999, 2001; Vellutino et al., 1996). Recent studies show that in many instances, dyslexia can be prevented through early identification and intervention (Foorman & Torgesen, 2001; Torgesen et al., 1999). In addition, other studies are beginning to show that remedial efforts have some efficacy with the word recognition component of dyslexia (Lovett, Lacerenza, 2000; Torgesen et al., 2001). In older children, the range of outcomes is rather narrow, but future research will probably broaden the outcomes to include the remediation of fluency and comprehension deficits. The importance of these latter processes will become clear as we turn to a discussion of readng disabilities involving reading comprehension and fluency.

Reading Comprehension Disability

Research on children with word recognition difficulties tends to (1) compare them with children who are typically achieving; and (2) not to consider impairments in other areas, such as fluency, comprehension, or even math and written expression. In many respects, this occurs because the findings of studies involving word recognition do not appear to vary because of other comorbidities, at least when the reading problem and its correlates are examined. But this is not the case in research on other forms of LDs, where inclusion of children with word recognition problems may obscure the results. Thus studies of children with specific problems in reading comprehension differ from studies of dyslexia because of the focus on comparisons of children with adequate word recognition accompanied by good reading comprehension skills, versus those who have good development of word recognition skills, but poor development of reading comprehension (Nation & Snowling, 1998; Oakhill, Yuill, & Parkin, 1986; Stothard & Hulme, 1996). This difference exists because if a study of reading comprehension contains a large number of children who decode words poorly (e.g., Perfetti, 1985; Shankweiler et al., 1999), the most likely cause of reading comprehension problems is the inability to decode. Proficient reading comprehension assumes fluent decoding.

There is good evidence that reading comprehension difficulties can occur in the absence of word recognition problems (Snow, 2002). The research base is much less developed than for disorders of word recognition, however. There is little work on neurobiological correlates or developmental course, though some studies of the latter are available. This section therefore does not address neurobiological correlates, although research on children with oral language disorders could potentially relate to this question (see Leonard et al., 2001).

Definitional Issues

Given the need to ensure adequacy of word recognition processes, defining children with reading comprehension problems is most difficult because of problems in measuring reading comprehension. There is always concern about how well reading comprehension tests measure processes specific to the comprehension of written language, as opposed to other language processes that must be in place in order for reading comprehension to take place. Measures of word recognition accuracy have a relatively transparent relationship between the content of the tests and performance requirements for word reading. However, standardized reading comprehension tests differ from everyday reading contexts along several potentially important dimensions, including passage length, immediate versus delayed recall, and learning and performance requirements (Pearson, 1998; Sternberg, 1991). The available assessments vary in what a child is asked to read (sentences, paragraphs, pages); in the response format (cloze, open-ended questions, multiple-choice, think-aloud); in memory demands (answering questions with and without the text available); and in the specific aspects of comprehension that are assessed (gist understanding, literal understanding, inferential comprehension). At this point in time, a single assessment may not be adequate, as it is difficult to determine the source of a child's comprehension difficulties based on a single measure.

Assessment is always an attempt to measure a latent construct (Fletcher et al., 1996). Any test is an imprecise measure of that construct. When a construct is multifaceted, as reading comprehension is, multiple assessments may be needed to adequately capture the underlying construct of interest. Reading comprehension tests, like other tests of complex cognitive functions, may also be limited both by a lack of ecological validity and by the absence of a model of the reading comprehension process that would guide test construction (Snow, 2002). As Lyon (1996b) noted in the first edition of this chapter, research in some LD domains has significant work to complete in the measurement area.

The role of IQ in defining the reading comprehension subgroup has also emerged differently from the way it has in dyslexia and other LDs. There are few studies that use IQ–achievement discrepancies to define groups of poor comprehenders. In fact, the discrepancy approach most often employed to define children with reading comprehension disability involves a discrepancy between scores on either word recognition or listening comprehension tests and scores on standardized tests of reading comprehension, without reference to IQ. One exception found that children with poor reading comprehension, but average intelligence and average word-reading skills, had difficulties in listening comprehension, working memory, and metacognitive aspects of comprehension (Cornoldi, DeBeni, & Pazzaglia, 1996). However, no comparison to children with "low achieverment" was made. Thus, the issue of IQ or IQ–achievement discrepancy has had little impact on research on reading comprehension disability.

Some studies of reading comprehension have used IQ as an outcome measure or covariate rather than as an inclusionary criterion for identifying disability. For example, children with specific reading comprehension difficulties show phonological skills and nonverbal intelligence similar to those of typically achieving children, but their Verbal IQ scores are lower (e.g., Stothard & Hulme, 1996). These findings suggest that more general verbal processing difficulties underlie the reading comprehension disability of children with good decoding but poor comprehension. As vocabulary and other lexical measures are related to both reading comprehension and Verbal IQ, the lower Verbal scores are hardly surprising (Fletcher et al., 1996). However, in a recent study of typically achieving readers, Verbal IQ was found to account for a small amount of the variability in reading comprehension skills (Badian, 1999; Oakhill, Cain, & Bryant, in press). After verbal intellectual skills were accounted for, significant variance in comprehension was predicted by text integration skills, metacognitive monitoring, and working memory. These relationships held over a 1-year follow-up. Cornoldi et al. (1996) found that these same skills best characterized their group of children with poor comprehension who had IQs that were discrepant from their reading comprehension achievement.

The simple assumption that the relation of intelligence and comprehension is represented by a path from higher verbal intelligence to reading comprehension is most likely incorrect. First, the relationship between reading comprehension and intelligence is probably bidirectional. Reading experience clearly facilitates growth of verbal intellectual skills (Stanovich, 1993). Second, measures of Verbal IQ assess vocabulary and verbal reasoning, and these are some of the same skills that are measured by tests of reading comprehension. A moderately strong relationship between verbal intelligence and reading comprehension is thus expected, but is uninformative.

Epidemiology and Developmental Course

Estimates of specific reading comprehension difficulties from epidemiological studies are not available. Sample-specific studies of children who have age-appropriate word recognition skills but poor reading comprehension range from 5% to 10%, depending on the exclusionary criteria used to define the groups (e.g., Cornoldi et al., 1996; Stothard & Hulme, 1996). These estimates have not been studied in relation to age, but it is likely that specific reading comprehension problems are more apparent in older children and emerge after the initial stage of learning to read. Shankweiler et al. (1999) were able to identify few second- and third-graders sampled for different types of LDs with good word recognition and poor comprehension skills. As with any definition of LDs, incidence varies depending on decisions about cutoff points on norm-referenced tests.

The developmental course of specific reading comprehension disability has not been studied. Recent studies in this area have addressed how poor comprehension early in a child's reading history may influence not only later reading comprehension, but also continued development of word-decoding skills. Although decoding and comprehension disabilities have been shown to be dissociable, children who are good at decoding but poor at comprehending may begin to fall behind in their decoding skills in the later school grades (Oakhill et al., in press) because of diminished experience with text. As they read less, and truncate their exposure to less common words (Cunningham & Stanovich, 1999), their sight word vocabularies do not keep pace with those of peers who have stronger comprehension abilities and read more frequently. Moreover, their poor ability to use semantic cues (a component of comprehension) to decode less frequent words may constrain higher levels of lexical development (Nation & Snowling, 1998).

Core Processes

Research on reading comprehension difficulties uses three major experimental designs in an attempt to identify core deficits underlying comprehension difficulties. One design compares age-matched children who are good at decoding but poor at comprehending with children who are good at both (chronological-age design). A second design compares children who are good at decoding/poor at comprehending with younger children matched for level of reading comprehension to the older disabled children (reading-level-match design). The third design attempts to train children in skills hypothesized to contribute to the reading comprehension deficit, to determine whether training actually improves reading comprehension.

The findings from the three methods are consistent. Children with good decoding/poor comprehending may have more basic deficits in vocabulary and understanding of syntax that impair reading comprehension (Stothard & Hulme, 1992, 1996). Other studies have shown that even when vocabulary and syntax are not deficient, deficits in reading comprehension still arise (Cain, Oakhill, & Bryant, 2000; Nation & Snowling, 1998) because of difficulties with inferencing and text integration, metacognitive skills related to comprehension, and working memory (Cornoldi et al., 1996; Oakhill et al., in press). In contrast, phonological skills, short-term memory, and verbatim recall of text are typically not deficient (Cain & Oakhill, 1999; Cataldo & Cornoldi, 1998; Nation, Adams, Bowyer-Crane, & Snowling, 1999; Oakhill, 1993; but see Stothard & Hulme, 1992).

Findings similar to those discussed for children with reading comprehension disability have been obtained in studies of children with brain injury. For example, Barnes and Dennis (1998, 2001) have evaluated the discourse and reading comprehension skills of children with spina bifida and hydrocephalus. These children are often characterized by intact word recognition skills, but deficient reading comprehension abilities. Barnes and Dennis have demonstrated that children with this form of brain injury have difficulty making inferences and assimilating nonliteral information from text. These difficulties with the reading domain parallel problems that the children have in comprehension of oral language, again attesting to the parallel relation of listening comprehension and reading comprehension.

It is well established that difficulties in listening comprehension parallel problems with reading comprehension (Shankweiler et al., 1999; Stothard & Hulme, 1996). Most studies comparing reading and listening comprehension in normative samples show high levels of overlap. Children cannot understand written language any better than they can understand oral language. It is possible that dissociations of listening and reading comprehension occur in some cases, so that reading comprehension is better than listening comprehension. This would seem most likely in older children and adults, but there is little research demonstrating these dissociations. Regardless, any language or cognitive difficulties that hinder oral language comprehension will also affect individuals' ability to read text or even to comprehend text read to them.

Summary: Reading Comprehension Disability

Although the comprehension-related deficits discussed above have been well documented and replicated across studies employing different procedures and criteria for group membership, there are questions concerning whether specific cognitive processes are primary causes or consequences of the comprehension deficits. Questions also remain about how to measure and define reading comprehension deficits, and debate ensues about the core cognitive processes that underlie reading comprehension disability (Snow, 2002; Stanovich, 1988). Nonetheless, studies of children with WLRDs, comprehension disability, or both (Connors & Olson, 1990; Oakhill, 1993); children with neurodevelopmental disorders such as hydrocephalus (Barnes & Dennis, 1998); and typically achieving children (Oakhill et al., in press) support a dissociation between these two components of reading. This work also shows that these two aspects of reading are associated with different cognitive deficits, suggesting that different forms of intervention will be necessary to remediate these two distinct forms of LDs.

Reading Fluency Disability

The question of whether there is a subgroup of reading disability characterized specifically by difficulties in reading fluency is controversial. As we have discussed above in the section on multiple-factor models, Wolf and Bowers (1999) and Lovett, Steinbach, & Fritters (2000) have argued for a "rate deficit" group that does not have problems in the phonological domain, but often has difficulties with comprehension because of a more general difficulty in rapidly processing information. The subtyping study of Morris et al. (1998) found evidence for a rate deficit subtype that was not phonologically impaired, but that showed difficulty on any task that required speeded processing. These tasks included measures including rapid automatized naming, visual attention, and rapid articulatory movements. As Wolf and Bowers hypothesized, this subtype also had difficulties with reading fluency and comprehension, but not word recognition. In this section, we review evidence on definitional issues, core processes, and interventions pertaining to reading fluency disability. There are few little data on epidemiology, developmental course, or neurobiological correlates that pertains specifically to this form of LD.

Definitional Issues

The critical question for a rate deficit subtype is similar to that identified for reading comprehension, which is whether processes associated with accuracy of word recognition can be differentiated from speed of either word decoding or text reading. Here there is ample evidence that these are dissociable processes and that fluency can also be differentiated from comprehension. However, all three processes are highly correlated, especially in younger children or in those who have reading difficulties. Fortunately, the measurement issue is not as daunting as for reading comprehension. Fluency essentially boils down to reading rate and is assessed by the amount of time needed to read single words, a list of words, short passages, or longer texts. These measures tend to be highly correlated, so assessing the construct is not difficult. Moreover, identifying individuals with rate deficits is no more difficult than identifying people with word recognition difficulties. It presently involves a decision about cutoff points on a dimension.

As we have discussed above, problems occur in the attempt to create groups of people who vary in their impairment in one but not the other area. For example, studies of the rate deficit hypothesis typically attempt to compare individuals who are weak in both accuracy and fluency with those who are weak in only one area. The problem is that accuracy and rate are moderately correlated. This means that on average, a group impaired in only one domain will tend to be less severely impaired than a group impaired in both domains. Moreover, it is possible that when impairment exists in both domains, the lower score in one domain leads to reduction in the other domain (Compton et al., 2001; Schatschneider et al., 2002).

This problem is enhanced when the assessment involves nonreading measures, such as phonological awareness and rapid naming. As the relationship of either domain to reading is nonlinear, increasingly poor reading ability makes the severity of reading difficulties greater in a person with two deficits than in a person with only a single deficit. These methodological issues make it difficult to compare reading disability subgroups if the expectation is that they are comparable in reading level. At the same time, the viability of reading rate (or rapid naming) as a construct that has independence from word recognition (or phonological processing) is well established.

Core Processes

The core process that has received the most attention in the rate deficit group involves rapid automatized naming. In reviewing research on rapid automatized naming, it should be noted that some investigators find evidence for deficiencies on any speeded process (e.g., Waber et al., 2001; Wolff, Michel, Ovrut, & Drake, 1990). However, this review focuses primarily on the evidence that relates rapid automatized naming to reading. There are essentially three lines of evidence supporting the relationship of naming speed as a separate contribution to reading difficulties. First, naming speed tasks, especially the ability to name letters rapidly, consistently contribute independently to variance in reading achievement beyond what can be attributed to phonological awareness ability. This finding is apparent not only in studies that attempt to predict longitudinal outcomes (Schatschneider et al., 2002; Wolf & Bowers, 1999), but also in studies that look at the relationship of different latent variables through confirmatory factor analysis (McBride-Chang & Manis, 1996; Wagner, Torgesen, & Rashotte, 1994). Second, there are subtyping studies that compare children who have deficits on both phonological awareness and rapid naming to children who have only a single deficit (Lovett, Steinbach, & Frijters, 2000; Wolf & Bowers, 1999). These studies show that children with "double deficits" have more severe reading difficulties than children who have only single deficits. However, these studies are subject to the methodological problems identified in the section on definitional issues. Finally, the cluster analysis study of Morris et al. (1998) found evidence for a subtype with impairment in both phonological awareness and naming speed, as well as subtypes with impairment in only phonological awareness or speed of processing. The subtype with double deficits was more impaired in reading than subtypes impaired in only one domain. Moreover, the subtype with rate impairment was not impaired in phonological awareness or the accuracy of word recognition—just in fluency and comprehension. At the same time, the rate deficit subtype occurred with low frequency, representing less than 10% of a large group of children with reading disabilities.

Despite this evidence, researchers argue about whether rapid naming contributes to reading achievement independently of its phonological component (Vellutino et al., in press). Obviously, any task that requires retrieving of information with an articulatory component has to involve phonological processing. As rapid naming tasks are moderately correlated with phonological awareness measures, this appears to be a reasonable conclusion. In this interpretation, naming speed is essentially a measure of how rapidly an individual can access phonologically based codes. The alternative view is that measures of naming speed involve nonphonological processes that are also related to reading (Wolf & Bowers, 1999; Wolf et al., 2001). In order to complete rapid naming tasks, it is apparent that a variety of cognitive processes may be involved. As reviewed above, rapid naming tests do contribute independently to reading outcomes, relative to contribution of phonological awareness tasks. However, the contributions are much higher if the outcome is a measure of fluency.

This latter finding begs the question of what rapid naming tests actually measure. It is significant that it is not naming speed per se that is most predictive. Although speed of naming colored objects is predictive of reading outcomes, it is not nearly as predictive as measures that involve the naming of letters or digits, and does not predict reading outcomes independently of the latter measures. Schatschneider et al. (2002) have suggested that the robust correlation of measures of letter naming with reading fluency measures later in development implies that rapid naming of letters is simply a rudimentary measure of reading speed. Although rapid naming may be independent of phonological awareness, it is not completely independent of reading per se, and thus is a primitive measure of reading fluency.

The final issue involves the apparent lack of specificity of rapid naming measures to reading difficulties. Waber et al. (2001) have demonstrated that unlike phonological awareness tasks, rapid naming measures do not differentiate children who have learning difficulties in other areas. For example, children with ADHD often have difficulties on measures of rapid automatized naming (Tannock, Martinussen, & Frijters, 2000). Based on these types of data, Waber et al. (2001) have argued that these difficulties reflect common brain-based problems with timing or rapid processing that occur across all forms of learning impairment.

Studies of children with brain injury provide evidence that the accuracy and speed of word recognition can and should be differentiated, but also contribute to concerns about the specificity of these difficulties to reading. Barnes, Dennis, and Wilkinson (1999) matched children with traumatic brain injury on their word-decoding accuracy. Comparisons of reading rate and naming speed showed that fluency was worse in children with traumatic brain injury, paralleling observations of non-brain-injured children with rate deficits (Waber et al., 2001; Wolf & Bowers, 1999). Moreover, fluency is related to reading comprehension scores in both populations (Barnes et al., 1999; Morris et al., 1998).

Although it is possible to differentiate accuracy and rate components on measures of phonological awareness and rapid naming, more research needs to be done on the presence of a subgroup specific to reading fluency. It is clear, however, that fluency must be considered independently of accuracy in evaluating the outcomes of reading intervention studies. Studies of older children show that accuracy may improve in children with severe reading difficulties without corresponding improvements in fluency (Torgesen et al., 2001).

Summary: Reading Fluency Disability

There is clear evidence for a dissociation of reading fluency deficits from those involving word recognition and comprehension. In addition, cognitive processes that focus on rapid naming and speed of processing appear related to fluency deficits. There are issues involved in how reading fluency deficits are defined, as well as issues concerning the specificity of rapid naming deficiencies to children with a reading disability. Regardless of these issues, intervention for fluency deficiencies is critically important, and research is rapidly accumulating on this issue. It is clear that many children who become accurate in word reading are still slow and labored when reading text. This interferes with comprehension, highlighting the critical importance of rate.

General Conclusions: Reading Disabilities

The preceding review of reading difficulties supports the hypothesis that at least three dissociable processes in reading may be differentially impaired in children with reading difficulties. The greatest amount of research is focused on children with word recognition deficits. This undoubtedly reflects the fact that this represents the most common form of LD in children and is a significant component of the LDs for 70–80% of all children identified with LDs in schools. Some criticize the focus on this form of LD as excessive (Kavale & Forness, 1998), but as long as it accounts for so many children, it must be the focus of considerable research.

Generally, this review of reading disabilities shows that current diagnostic approaches to LDs are not adequate and most likely hinder the ability of special education programs in schools to serve children. The approaches operate essentially as a "wait-to-fail" model, and children are commonly delayed in receiving services until they demonstrate serious reading problems. When an IQ–achievement discrepancy is used as an inclusionary criterion, this problem is greatly worsened. Alternative psychometric approaches to the identification of children with reading disabilities do not appear viable without rendering the current identification process more cumbersome. *It simply is not possible to shortcut the identification process without some attempt to operationalize the inadequate-instruction component of LD definitions, such as with response to intervention.* In this respect, it may be necessary to completely dismantle the current identification process in order to implement programs that research demonstrates are efficacious, and, in particular, to ensure that those children identified for special education services have had an opportunity to respond to high-quality instruction first (Donovan & Cross, 2002). Anything less than this is a disservice to individuals with LDs and will likely result in increasing numbers of older children requiring special education services—a trend already apparent in special education statistics (U.S. Department of Education, 1999). In many instances, these children are instructional casualties who simply did not receive the type of instruction that they needed early enough in their development.

Progress has also been made in terms of identifying the limitations of the focus on children with dyslexia. It is clear that there is another form of reading disability involving comprehension impairments, and most likely a third involving fluency difficulties. Methods for identifying these children need additional research, particularly from a measurement perspective, but this is emerging. In addition, there is little work on neurobiological correlates beyond those attributed to dyslexia.

MATHEMATICS DISORDERS

Definitional Issues

Deficits in math among individuals with LDs have been less extensively reported in the historical literature, though they have been noted for as long as reading difficulties have. In general, clinicians and researchers have paid less attention to children and adults with math difficulties, possibly because illiteracy has been considered to be more of a problem to society than math deficiency (Fleishner, 1994). Given this limited historical context, Keller and Sutton (1991) and Geary (1993) have argued for a research emphasis on the math abilities and performance of individuals with LDs.

Current definitions of LDs acknowledge that impairment in the ability to learn math should be considered as one of the major disorders subsumed within the category if certain inclusionary and exclusionary conditions are to be met. As noted earlier in this chapter, the federal definition of LDs refers to disabilities in mathematical calculations and concepts, whereas the NJCLD (1988) definition of LDs refers to significant difficulties in "math abilities." The DSM-IV (American Psychiatric Association, 1994) also refers to deficits in math via the term "mathematics disorder" and provides a number of criteria to be used in the diagnostic process. The ICD-10 (World Health Organization, 1992) provides research criteria for the identification of individuals with deficits in a highly specific domain termed "specific disorder of arithmetical skills." In this approach, the diagnosis of disorders of arithmetical skills is appropriate when such weaknesses occur against a background of normal reading and spelling development. All of these definitions of an LD in math, like definitions of LDs in reading and written expression, are based upon assumptions of normal or above-average ability to learn (as assessed by IQ measures), normal sensory function, adequate educational opportunity, and absence of developmental disorders and emotional disturbance. Like all other existing definitions of LDs except the definition of dyslexia provided by the International Dyslexia Research Committee (see Lyon, 1995b), the definitions are vague and remain difficult to operationalize. The limitations of these approaches have been documented in the section on IQ–achievement discrepancy and exclusions.

Because of this persistent vagueness and/or the parochial nature of the quality of extant definitions, no consistent standards have been established by which to judge the presence or absence of LDs in math. Adding to this dilemma is the fact that "LDs in math," "developmental arithmetic disorder," "math disabilities," and "specific math disabilities" are typically broad terms used for a variety of impairments in math skills. In addition, as Fleishner (1994) has pointed out, in some cases the term "math learning disability" has been used synonymously with the term "dyscalculia," to denote *specific* (as opposed to generalized) deficits in calculation or mathematical thinking. In these situations, there is often the assumption that oral language, reading, and writing are intact (e.g., see World Health Organization, 1992, and Strang & Rourke, 1985). However, math deficits are frequently associated with other LDs (Fuchs, Fuchs, & Prentice, in press; Fleishner, 1994; Rourke & Finlayson, 1978). It is clear that disorders of math calculations occur in isolation and, by definition, involve problems with concepts. Computational difficulty is a potential marker variable for some forms of LDs in math, though the underlying core processes may be different. Less clear is whether there is a separate disorder of math concepts that cannot be explained by difficulties with reading and language. Similarly, is a disability involving both reading and math a reading disability, a math disability, or a comorbid association? These issues are addressed below.

Epidemiology and Developmental Course

As Fleishner (1994) has pointed out, efforts to establish the prevalence of math LDs have produced similar estimates. Earlier studies by Badian and Ghublikian (1983), Kosc (1974), McKinney and Feagans (1984), and Norman and Zigmond (1980) all reported that approximately 6% of school-age children have some form of LD in math. More recent studies give estimates of 5–6% (Shalev, Auerbach, Manor, & Gross-Tsur, 2000) and 4.6% (Lewis, Hitch, & Walker, 1994). The latter study broke prevalence into those who only had arithmetic disability (1.3%) and those with both arithmetic and reading disabilities (2.3%). These estimates contrasted with 3.9% for specific reading disabilities. All the recent studies were European in origin, in which cutoff points tend to be more stringent (<5th percentile) than North American studies. Most studies have not found gender differences in math performance and achievement (Shalev et al., 2000; but see Lewis et al., 1994).

In terms of developmental course, there is little research, and none of it long-term. A 3-year longitudinal study (grades 4–7) by Shalev, Manor, Auerbach, and Gross-Tsur (1998) reported that 47% of those with math disabilities in grade 4 met criteria for such disabilities (arithmetic scores ≤ 5th percentile) in grade 7. As with reading problems, arithmetic difficulties tend to be persistent. Children with LDs in math can be identified early in schooling, and their difficulties tend to persist through adolescence (Cawley & Miller, 1989). Many of the children in these studies, however, also had reading difficulties. Little is known about the development of children with specific math disabilities.

Core Processes

The core processes that underlie disabilities in math have been studied for as long, but not as extensively, as those in reading disabilities. Much of the burgeoning research base focuses on children who have computational difficulties in math. This focus is not surprising, as the early neurological literature often described adults and children with "dyscalculia," based on their inability to perform simple arithmetic calculations either orally or on paper-and-pencil tasks. Older research tended to use neuropsychological models, which pioneered the focus on comparisons of children with disabilities in reading, in math, and in both that have become the preeminent paradigm in math disabilities research. This research, which is reviewed below in the section on subtypes, showed that children with impairments in both reading and math had pervasive problems with language and concept formation skills (Rourke, 1993). Children with impairments only in reading had problems restricted to the language domain, whereas children with impairments in math had difficulties with multiple aspects of nonverbal processing, including motor and somatosensory skills, problem-solving ability, and visual–spatial skills. This research tended to focus on the relationship the demands of math tasks for visual–spatial processing, but the relationship of visual–spatial skills to math has not been borne out (Geary, 1993; Rovet, Szekely, & Hockenberry, 1994).

A very recent development in the research on math disabilities has been the attempt to combine research strategies from the fields of cognitive development, mathematical cognition, and LDs (e.g., Geary, Hoard, & Hamson, 1999; Geary, Hamson, & Hoard, 2000; Jordan & Hanich, 2000). These studies follow children longitudinally and measure multiple competencies. These include development of early, informal arithmetic skills (such as counting and problem-solving strategies), arithmetic, and more formal indicators of mathematical competence (Geary et al., 1999, 2000; Ginsburg, Klein, & Starkey, 1998). Such studies attempt to relate cognitive marker skills or cognitive competencies that are purported to support the development of math to the acquisition of specific components of the math system, such as knowledge of counting principles (Geary et al., 1999). They also evaluate children with specific math disabilities and compare them to children who have both math and reading disabilities. In many ways, this new research strategy parallels earlier longitudinal studies of reading acquisition in typically developing children and in children with reading problems—the studies that proved critical to our understanding of reading disabilities at multiple levels. The current studies may lead to enhanced understanding of math skills and supporting cognitive competencies.

In discussing math disabilities, Geary (1993) has identified three classes of problems. The first involves difficulties in learning, representing, and retrieving math facts. These difficulties often manifested in terms of slow, inaccurate, or inconsistent computational problem-solving abilities. In some instances, such children tend to use counting methods because they do not appear to be able to retrieve a math fact. A second type of difficulty reflects problems with procedural aspects of math. This type of difficulty is manifested as problems with counting. Such children use developmentally immature strategies and algorithms that are incorrectly applied to solve computational problems. A third possible difficulty involves spatial representation and manipulation of numerical information. As this last type of difficulty has not held up in more recent research (Barnes et al., 2002; Geary et al., 2000; Rovet et al., 1994), it is not further discussed here. Suffice it to say that although many children with specific math disabilities appear to have difficulties with visual–spatial processing, efforts to link these difficulties specifically to math processes have yielded largely null results.

Difficulties in representing and retrieving math facts, and problems in learning and implementing procedures, do not appear to be orthogonal processes. In development, young children who experience math difficulties commonly experience problems with both math facts and procedural knowledge early in their schooling (Geary et al., 1999). However, in some children these difficulties seem persistent, whereas in other children the ability to represent and retrieve math facts begins to develop, but with subsequent difficulties in procedural knowledge. It is also apparent that difficulties with fact representation and retrieval are much more characteristic of individuals who have both a math disability and a comorbid reading disorder, whereas problems with procedures are more apparent in children who only experience a math disability and no reading problem. Thus Geary et al. (2000) found that in first grade, children with both math and reading disabilities had problems with counting and number comprehension tasks. Problems with number comprehension did not characterize children with a specific math disability, but these children had difficulties with counting knowledge in first and second grade. In addition, both types of children had more problems with counting procedures and retrieval of facts in first grade. The difference was that the difficulties with both types of errors persisted in children with comorbid reading and math disabilities, but the retrieval errors diminished in children who had a specific math disability. On tasks that were specifically designed to elicit retrieval errors, there was a clear tendency for children with comorbid reading and math disabilities to have more difficulties than children with only a math disability. Both these groups performed below the levels of children who had only a reading disability or no disability.

The core cognitive processes that appear to underlie these difficulties involve variations on working memory tasks (Bull & Johnston, 1997) and executive functions (Hooper, Swartz, Wakely, deKruif, & Montgomery, 2002). In a series of studies by Swanson and associates (Wilson & Swanson, 2001; Swanson & Sachse-Lee, 2001; Keeler & Swanson, 2001; see also Swanson & Siegel, 2001), the contributions of both verbal and visual–spatial working memory, executive processes that involve strategy knowledge, and the ability to use working memory efficiently have been studied in children with specific math disabilities and comorbid reading and math disabilities. Some studies have suggested that problems with visual–spatial working memory are more likely to characterize children with a specific math disability (Fletcher, 1985; Siegel & Ryan, 1989), whereas children with both reading and math disabilities have more pervasive language and verbal working memory difficulties. However, Keeler and Swanson (2001) found that math computational skills in individuals with a specific math disability were better predicted by verbal than by visual–spatial working memory. There was evidence for both domain-specific working memory difficulties, as well as problems with executive control that would lead to more pervasive problems with working memory. In contrast, Swanson and Sachse-Lee (2001) found that the domain-general system made a significant contribution to poor working memory in children with reading disabilities that was not directly related to their reading problems. Wilson and Swanson (2001) found that various measures of working memory that were both domain-general and domain-specific contributed to the ability to acquire strategies for math computations. As Geary et al. (2000) have pointed out, the relationship of working memory and math disabilities is complicated, and additional research is necessary to determine how these relationships relate to math disabilities in children with and without reading disabilities. Certainly, children who have both reading and math disabilities tend to have more severe problems in both areas than those who have problems in only one area (Fletcher et al., in press).

Other studies suggest that children who are impaired in both reading and math computations typically show more severe and pervasive disturbances of oral language than children who are only impaired in word recognition. Their difficulties reflect problems in learning, retaining, and retrieving math facts, which are essential to precise calculation; these lead to pervasive difficulties with math. Thus Jordan and Hanich (2000) found that children with both reading and mathematics difficulties showed problems in multiple domains of mathematical thinking.

Brain-injured children and those with other developmental disabilities commonly experience math problems (Shalev et al., 2000). Barnes et al. (2002) found that children with spina bifida or hydrocephalus who had good word recognition skills and poor math ability made more procedural errors than age-matched controls, but similar numbers of math fact retrieval and visual–spatial errors. Furthermore, their procedural errors were similar to those of younger children who were matched in math ability with these older brain-injured children. Thus children with hydrocephalus made errors in written computations that were developmentally immature for their age, but not different in kind from younger children with no math disability. These data are consistent with the hypothesis that children who are good at reading but poor at math can have a procedural deficit that involves the application of developmentally immature algorithms for solving written computations.

Subtypes of Math Disabilities

Children who manifest LDs in math are believed to display deficits in arithmetic calculation and/or math reasoning abilities. Historically, characteristics in math were described under the term "developmental dyscalculia," which refers to the failure to develop arithmetic competence (Novick & Arnold, 1988, p. 132). Classification of the characteristics of dyscalculia was first initiated by Kosc (1974), who identified the following six subtypes:

1. *Verbal dyscalculia*—an inability to name mathematical amounts, numbers, terms, symbols, and relationships.
2. *Practognostic dyscalculia*—an inability to enumerate, compare, and mathematically manipulate objects, either pictured or real.
3. *Lexical dyscalculia*—a disorder in reading mathematical symbols.
4. *Graphical dyscalculia*—a disability in writing mathematical symbols.
5. *Ideognostical dyscalculia*—a disorder in understanding mathematical concepts and in performing calculations mentally.
6. *Operational dyscalculia*—a disability in performing computational operations.

Kosc (1974) hypothesized that these math disability variants were functions of a congenital structural disorder of cortical regions of the brain involved in math abilities. To date, however, that has been no evidence to suggest either that these subtypes are distinct or that their deficiencies are associated with specific cortical regions. It is clear from Kosc's (1974) description of the characteristics of each type, that children diagnosed with LDs in math today would most likely manifest difficulties similar to those observed in ideognostical dyscalculia and/or operational dyscalculia.

Later attempts to characterize the population of children who manifest LDs in math contrasted children who varied in math and reading performance. For example, in a series of studies summarized by Rourke (1993), different patterns of performance on verbal–auditory and visual–spatial skills were identified in children who either: (1) had low achievement on all subtests of the Wide Range Achievement Test (WRAT); (2) had low achievement in reading and spelling, but not in arithmetic; and (3) had low achievement in arithmetic relative to reading and spelling. In the main, those children with low arithmetic performance relative to reading and spelling demonstrated high scores on auditory–verbal measures, with low scores on visual-perceptual and visual–spatial measures. These same patterns of performance were identified for children ranging from 7 to 14 years of age (Keller & Sutton, 1991).

Other studies of children with LDs, including those involving math computations, have described differences between groups of children with either specific reading or math disability and comorbid reading and math disabilities (e.g., Ackerman, Weir, Holloway, & Dykman, 1995; Fletcher, 1985; Morrison & Siegel, 1991; Rourke, 1993). The value of these distinctions is clearly established in many studies where children are defined as having word recognition difficulties, both word recognition and math computation difficulties, and only math computation difficulties. The latter children do not have problems with language of the sort experienced by children with WLRDs. They typically have difficulty with different forms of nonverbal processing and concept formation (Rourke, 1993). Although these studies reveal the importance of considering the specificity and comorbidity of LDs, they do not permit an analysis of the mechanisms by which the cognitive marker skills influence math learning. Furthermore, such subtyping studies were interested in the issue of LDs in math versus reading, rather than in understanding the basic math processes that contribute to scores on math achievement tests (Ginsburg et al., 1998).

Neurobiological Correlates

Studies of adults with brain lesions show that fairly specific math skills can be lost or preserved, depending on the pattern of brain injury (Dehaene

& Cohen, 1997). However, studies of either brain structure or brain function have not been carried out for children with LDs in math. Whether the development of math skills across different domains can be fractionated in ways apparent in studies of adults with brain injury is not clear. Also emerging are studies of the familial segregation and heritability of math disability, which are reviewed in this section.

Brain Structure and Function

A summary of lesional research on acalculia is beyond the scope of this chapter. However, these studies are interesting, in that they do suggest that distinct regions of the brain are involved in different arithmetic processes. These studies should be taken seriously, inasmuch as neuroimaging studies have found parallels between developmental and acquired reading disorders, with both implicating the angular gyrus as a critical structure in reading disabilities. To illustrate, Dehaene and Cohen (1997) described two patients with acalculia who experienced difficulties with calculations, but could read and write numbers. A patient with a left subcortical lesion, however, had a selective problem in retrieving verbal knowledge that extended to arithmetic tables. This patient had a subcortical lesion in the left hemisphere. In contrast, the second patient had difficulties with multiple tasks involving numerical knowledge. Although knowledge of rote arithmetical facts was reserved, the patient had difficulty subtracting and completing number by section tasks. The authors concluded that dissociable neural networks are involved in numerical knowledge. One involves the left hemisphere, which contributes to storage and retrieval of arithmetic facts. The second is a parietal network devoted to the ability to manipulate numerical quantities. These findings have been replicated in other studies (Chochon, Cohen, van de Moortele, & Dehaene, 1999).

Functional imaging studies using PET and fMRI have explored the representation of math in normal adults. These studies also show that the neural correlates of precise calculation and estimation are different (Dehaene, Spelke, Pinel, Stanescu, & Tsiukin, 1999). Precise calculation involves the inferior prefrontal cortex in the left hemisphere, as well as the left angular gyrus. These areas overlap substantially with those that mediate language functions. In contrast, estimation tasks showed bilateral activation in the inferior parietal lobes, which represent areas that overlap with spatial cognition. As many children with specific math disability have also been found to have spatial cognition difficulties, this overlap in neural representation of estimation and spatial cognition may help explain why the spatial processing difficulties do not seem to bear a strong relationship with math abilities in these children, but are often as profound as the math difficulties themselves. Any cognitive task that is sensitive to how these areas of the brain function will be deficient in children with a specific reading disability, but this does not mean that the cognitive deficits themselves are tightly linked.

Genetic Factors

As in reading disabilities, there is an emerging research base demonstrating heritable factors in math disabilities. It is clear that math disabilities are more common in certain families. Gross-Tsur, Manor, and Shalev (1996) found that 10% of children with a specific math disability had at least one other family member who complained of difficulties with math. Another 45% had another type of LD. Those with a family history of math disabilities were more likely to have persistent difficulties in math. Shalev et al. (2001) found that prevalence of math disabilities was quite high in mothers (66%), fathers (40%), and siblings (53%) of probands with math disabilities. Shalev et al. concluded that the prevalence of math disabilities was about 10 times higher in those with family members who had math disabilities than in the general population.

Heritability studies have focused on the comorbidity of reading and math disabilities, as well as specific math disabilities. In a twin study, Alarcon, DeFries, Light, and Pennington (1997) reported that 58% of monozygotic twins shared a math disability, compared to 39% of dizygotic twins. Knopik and DeFries (1999) found that genetic factors accounted for 83% of the shared variance between reading and math disabilities in a group of twins, compared to 58% of the shared variance in a controlled group. The contribution of shared environmental influences was quite small. Together, these figures suggest that genetic factors influence both reading and math disabilities. That there is substantial shared variance in heritability of reading and math disabilities is not surprising, in that 40–60% of individuals with a reading or math disability tend to have problems in both areas.

Summary: Math Disabilities

Altogether, there is burgeoning evidence for the existence of a group of children defined by difficulty in learning and retrieving math facts from memory, who tend to have problems with both reading and math. There is also evidence for the existence of a group of children who have difficulty learning math calculations because of procedural difficulties, but who do not have reading problems. Underlying these difficulties are cognitive processing problems involving working memory and executive functions that vary between the two groups, with the group that also has reading problems experiencing the language difficulties associated with reading disabilities. The language problems appear to disrupt math (Geary, 1993). There is little evidence for a separate subgroup with impairment in math concepts, but this possibility has not really been studied. In a sense, however, all children with disabilities in math probably have difficulty at some level with math concepts broadly conceived. The meaningfulness of this putative LD category—"math concepts disability"—is not clear. A better candidate would focus on difficulties with math problem solving, but whether these children are free of either reading problems or computational difficulties is not clear.

DISORDERS OF WRITTEN EXPRESSION

Disorders in the writing process have been discussed since the 1980s (Hooper et al., 1994). Well over a century ago, Ogle (1867) used the term "agraphia" to describe the relationship between aphasia and agraphia, although he noted that the two disorders were dissociable. In the first half of the 20th century, Goldstein (1948), Head (1926), and others applied clinical observation and case study methodology to explore the association and dissociation between written and oral expression. Wong (1991) has argued that deficits in written expression are clinically important, since they are frequently associated with reading disorders and/or are governed by similar metacognitive processes to include planning, self-monitoring, self-evaluation, and self-modification. Hooper et al. (1994) have reported that much of the research related to disorders of written expression and agraphia continues to employ case study methodology and, in the main, continues to rely on the study of individuals with acquired brain damage. More recent studies have used improved theoretical models and larger samples. However, studies of written expression have not followed the lead of math disabilities, and often do not separate children according to specific writing disabilities versus comorbidity with other LDs. This hampers definitional efforts. Altogether, as noted in the first edition's chapter, disorders of written expression have lagged behind the interests in reading and math disabilities.

Definitional Issues

A review of the available definitions for disorders of written expression reveals that the complexity and multidimensionality of these disorders continue to be ignored by formal characterizations or definitions. There are still no clear operational definitions of written language expression that address all components of the written language domain (see Berninger, 1994a and in press, for discussions of these issues). Emergent research on written language indicates that most, if not all, children with LDs have problems with at least one component of writing, whether it is handwriting, spelling, or written discourse (Hooper et al., 1994). No current definition identifies and defines these components in any objective or operational manner.

A number of authorities in this area have offered strategies to bolster definitions of disorders in written language (Graham, Harris, MacArthur, & Schwartz, 1991; Graham & Harris, 2000; Gregg, 1991). Spelling, handwriting, and more general aspects of formulating and producing written text are seen as somewhat separate components of a disorder of written language. But, other than descriptions of these processes and of children with disabilities in one or more of these areas, little work on definition and classification has been completed. Although it may be possible to identify children who have problems only in spelling and in handwriting as prototypes, children with problems only in "written expression" and in no other area appear difficult to identify. Given the complexity of the writing process and the fact that it is the last language domain to develop in children (Johnson & Myklebust, 1967; Hooper et al., 1994), it should not be surprising that deficits in written expression can co-occur with deficits in oral language, reading, and mathematics. However, as Berninger (1994a, in press) has pointed out, the relationship between these symbol systems is by no means invariant. For example, Abbott and Berninger (1993) found that written expression could not be explained just by oral expression; receptive written language ability always contributed uniquely to expressive written language ability. In addition, the widely held view that deficits in written expression invariably co-occur with reading disorders is not substantiated. More specifically, Berninger, Mizokowa, and Bragg (1991) and Berninger and Hart (1992, 1993) have demonstrated that reading and writing systems can be dissociated. Some children have reading problems but not writing problems, and other children have writing problems but not reading problems. But these patterns are infrequent, and most (but not all) children with writing deficits also manifest deficits in reading.

Despite continued difficulties in establishing exact criteria for disorders of written expression and in developing reliable and valid measures of the multiple processes involved in writing, research continues to focus on the characteristics of those who are good and poor at written expression. For instance, several investigators (Bereiter, 1980; Berninger, 1994a, 1994b; Hays & Flower, 1980; Hooper et al., 1994, in press) reported that individuals who write well are goal-directed; they understand the purpose of the writing assignment; they have a good knowledge of the topic prior to writing; they generate more ideas and use significant numbers of transitional ties; they produce a more cohesive text and flow of ideas; and they continuously monitor their written products for correctness of spelling and grammar.

On the other hand, Hooper et al. (1994) and others (De La Paz, Swanson, & Graham, 1998; Englert, 1990; Graham & Harris, 1987, 2000) report that writers with LDs demonstrate deficits in deploying strategies during production of written text and also have problems in actually generating text. When compared to "good" writers, writers with LDs produce shorter and less interesting essays, produce poorly organized text at the sentence and paragraph levels, and are less likely to review spelling, punctuation, grammar, or the body of their text to increase clarity (Hooper et al., 1994). But even here the description of children as "writers with LDs" is difficult, because most probably also have problems with oral language and reading development. A critical definitional issue relates to what is specific about disorders of written expression.

Epidemiology and Developmental Course

As Hooper et al. (1994) have pointed out, few epidemiological studies of disorders in written expression have been carried out. Likewise, the American Psychiatric Association (1994) explains that the prevalence rate for such disorders are difficult to establish, because "many studies focus on the prevalence of Learning Disorders in general without careful separation into specific disorders of reading, mathematics, or written expression. Disorder of Written Expression is rare when not associated with other Learning Disorders" (p. 52).

Basso, Taborelli, and Vignolo (1978) reported that acquired disorders of written expression occurred infrequently, at a rate of approximately 1 in every 250 subjects. However, given the high rate of developmental language disorders in the general population (8–15%) and the significantly high rate of disorders in basic reading skills (10–15% of the general population), one could predict that written language disorders affect at least 10% of the school-age population.

Berninger and Fuller (1992) reported that more boys than girls displayed written language deficits when level of achievement was used as the comparison variable, but there were no gender differences when IQ–achievement discrepancy criteria were used. Hooper et al. (1994) studied 30% of a middle school population that included an equal number of boys and girls and an equal number of white and nonwhite students. Of the children studied, approximately 34–47% fell more than one standard deviation below the mean on subtests of the Test of Written Language—Revised (Hammill & Larsen, 1988). Nonwhite students evidenced spontaneous writing problems at a ratio to white students of nearly 2:1, and boys showed a greater rate of impairment than girls, approximating a ratio of 1.5:1. Clearly, both the amount and accuracy of epidemiological data continue to be lacking, particularly in comparison to studies of oral language and reading.

Core Processes

Well over 30 years ago, Johnson and Myklebust (1967) presented a developmental model of language learning, which posited that the ability to write is dependent upon adequate development in listening, speaking, and reading. Hooper et al.

(1994) indicated that written expression and its disorders are multidimensional in nature. They conceptualized writing as a complex problem-solving process reflecting the writer's declarative knowledge, procedural knowledge, and conditional knowledge, all of which are subserved by a network of neuropsychological factors, personality factors, and other conditions (including teacher–student relationships, amount of writing instruction, and the teacher's knowledge of the writing process). Within this context, "declarative knowledge" refers to the specific writing and spelling subskills that the learner has acquired, whereas "procedural knowledge" refers to the learner's competence in using such knowledge while writing for meaning.

More recently, Berninger (in press) has differentiated the "transcription" component of writing from its "generational" component. The transcription component involves the production of letters and spelling, which are necessary to translate ideas into a written product. The generational component translates ideas into language representations that must be organized, stored, and then retrieved from memory. Over the past decade, progress has been made in research on both areas, although there has been more focus on the transcription than the generational component. This reflects in part the fact that transcription is specific to the writing process, whereas the generational component is applicable to many aspects of language and thought.

In a series of studies, Berninger and her associates (Berninger, 1994a, 1994b, in press; Berninger & Hart, 1993; Berninger et al., 1992) and Graham and colleagues (Graham, Weintraub, & Berninger, 2001; Graham, Harris, & Fink, 2000) have focused on the transcription component. They have reported that automaticity in the retrieval and production of alphabet letters, rapid coding of orthographic information, and speed of sequential finger movements are the best predictors of handwriting and composition skills. Automaticity predicts compositional fluency and quality. Fine motor skills also constrain handwriting, especially in the beginning stages of writing, which may be why sequential motor movement is related to letter production and legibility (Berninger, in press). Handwriting is more than a motor act, so that knowledge of orthography and planning ability also contributes to handwriting and spelling proficiency. Spelling abilities are predicted by orthographic phonological mappings and visual–motor integration (although see Lindamood, 1994, and Moats, 1994, for alternative predictions).

Berninger (in press) has suggested that neuropsychological, linguistic, and higher cognitive constraints may be recursive throughout the development of the writing process, but that each of these constraints may exert relatively more influence at different points in the developmental process (Hooper et al., 1994). This area needs more research. Hooper et al. (in press) have documented a role of executive functions in disorders of written expression. De La Paz et al. (1998) found that the difficulties experienced in revising written text by older (eighth-grade) students with writing problems were due in part to executive control issues. However, mechanical difficulties also contributed to these problems with revision. Obviously, the transcription and generation components must interact for an individual to produce high-quality written text.

Thus, although the research base is not large, it is clear that writing difficulties involve problems with handwriting, spelling, or the expression of ideas at the level of text. These problems have different correlates: spelling in conjunction with problems involving phonological analysis, knowledge of orthographic conventions specific to a child's language of instruction, and word recognition; handwriting in children with fine motor, motor planning, and working memory difficulties (with respect to the need for rapid retrieval of orthographic representations); and problems with executive functions and more pervasive oral language and reading difficulties (Berninger & Graham, 1998; Hooper et al., in press). Spelling and motor difficulties especially constrain the transcription component, whereas difficulties with executive functions and language constrain the generational component. The motor and executive function problems help explain why so many children with ADHD have disorders of written expression (Barkley, 1997).

In adults, writing difficulties often reflect an inability to spell that, even when remediated, is closely associated with difficulties in word recognition (Rourke, 1993). Even some children with specific math disabilities have difficulty with handwriting, often because they have impairments in their motor development. Their spelling errors, interestingly, are typically phonetically constrained, in contrast to those of children who have word recognition difficulties (Rourke, 1993). Once these two difficulties (spelling and motor skills) are taken into account, is there a subgroup of children whose difficulties are restricted to written expression? Here the classification research that is necessary to evaluate this hypothesis has not been completed, but there is some evidence for this possibility. In particular, some children have specific problems with handwriting and respond to preventative interventions (Graham, Harris, & Fink, 2000). Future research should target this possible subgroup in an effort to identify a prototype.

Multiple Etiologies

The multivariate nature of the developmental writing process suggests that disorders in written language can be referable to multiple etiologies, spanning biological, genetic, psychosocial, and environmental causes. Indeed, consider that in order to express thoughts in writing, one must formulate the idea; sequence relevant points in appropriate order; ensure that the written output is syntactically and grammatically correct; spell individual words correctly; and express the words, sentences, and passages in a legible manner via the graphomotor system.

Given this multidimensional nature of the writing process, multiple-cause models for deficits in writing are the rule. For example, Gregg (1991) reported that a variety of language-based deficits in phonology and word retrieval could impair several aspects of the writing task, as could deficits in visual–spatial skills and problems with executive functions (including organization, planning, and evaluating). Similarly, Roeltgen (1985) has proposed that deficits in linguistic, visual–spatial, and motor systems can interfere with the developmental writing process in distinct ways.

Neurobiological Correlates

There is little research on the neurobiological correlates of disorders of written expression. Studies of acquired disorders show that reading and writing can be fractionated, as in the example of "pure alexia," in which the patient loses reading ability but maintains the ability to write. Berninger (in press) has summarized a variety of findings from functional neuroimaging studies, showing that components involved in fine motor control and language generation can be related to areas of the frontal lobes and the cerebellum. These areas are well known to be involved in support of core processes that underlie writing, including motor control and planning, executive functions, and language. Barkley (1997) has used these findings to help explain why many children with ADHD have problems with writing.

There are few studies of heritability. Raskind, Hsu, Berninger, Thomson, and Wijsman (2000) found that spelling disorders, but not handwriting, aggregate in families. Other studies have found that spelling difficulties aggregate in families (Schulte-Korne, Deimel, Muller, Gutenbrunner, & Remschmidt, 1996). These findings are consistent with twin studies, which have found strong heritability of spelling abilities in twins that exceeded that found for reading abilities (Stevenson, Graham, Fredman, & McLoughlin, 1987). Nothen et al. (1999) reported a locus for spelling (and reading) on chromosome 15, which has also been reported for dyslexia (see Grigorenko, 2001). As reading and spelling abilities are highly correlated and represent a common factor that shares heritability (Marlow et al., 2001), it remains to be seen how these findings really differ from those reported above for spelling. Altogether, few specific neurobiological factors have been reported for disorders of written expression.

Summary: Disabilities of Written Expression

In contrast to our current understanding of oral language and reading disorders among children with LDs, less is known about the etiology, developmental course, prognosis, and treatment for disorders of written expression. The distinction of the motor and generational components is very important. Core processes have been identified, but these are shared with other disorders. Neurobiological research is only in its infancy. A key for the future is to attempt to identify subgroups of children with disorders of written expression that have some independence from other language-based disorders, with handwriting being the obvious example. But even here the comorbidity issue has not been adequately addressed, and the independence of ADHD and handwriting disorders is not established (Barkley, 1997).

CONCLUSIONS AND FUTURE DIRECTIONS

This chapter provides a review of the most recent research related to LDs in children. Within this context, the most productive research in LDs has been carried out in the language and reading areas, particularly in the study of the relationship between specific linguistic skills such as phonological processing and word recognition abilities. Research on this relationship in typically achieving populations versus those with LDs has led to an explosion of research on definition, core processes, neurobiological correlates, and intervention. Gaps continue to exist in our knowledge of math disabilities and disorders of written language. However, this gap is rapidly narrowing as the research base improves in these areas, as well as in areas involving reading comprehension and fluency.

A major advance that has occurred over the past decade in LD research has been the emphasis on conducting prospective, longitudinal studies to develop valid classification systems and definitions. This approach to classification and definition does not assume an a priori identification of children with LDs; rather, it requires the identification of large representative cohorts of preschool children who are followed for a period of several years. During this period, the children are administered a number of theoretically and conceptually grounded measures of cognitive, linguistic, academic, neurophysiological, and attentional skills at intervals of 6 months or 1 year. In studies of such unselected samples, problems associated with school-identified and clinic-referred samples can be reduced, and the emergence of abilities, disabilities, and comorbidities can be operationally defined and classified. Clearly with this type of methodology, substantial progress has been made in the classification and definition of LDs in reading. These findings should provide a stable context for additional prospective studies on various other LDs (written language, math) and allow better data to be gathered on their prevalence, developmental course, and response to various interventions.

Lyon (1996b) also noted in the first edition of this chapter that a promising development was the design and conduct of intervention studies for all types of LDs. Historically, little emphasis has been placed on understanding which specific types of interventions or combination of interventions are most efficacious for well-defined groups of children with LDs. This trend is changing, with major new treatment initiatives being sponsored by the National Institute of Child Health and Human Development (Lyon, 1995a) and the Office of Special Education Programs. The progress in reading is dramatic, for both remedial and preventative efforts. In the next few years, these efforts should expand to comprehension and fluency processes in reading, as well as to math and written expression (where research on intervention is just beginning to emerge).

While research flourishes, practice lags behind. This lag will make it difficult to implement what we know and to develop new research emphases in LD domains outside of reading. There are two obstacles. The first is reliance on concepts and definitions that had little research evidence to support them when they were adopted as policy. The second is the need to enhance personnel preparation to upgrade services for children in schools. The two are related and do not require separate discussion.

The resistance of practitioners and advocates to abandoning concepts that have no evidentiary basis is unfortunate. Two examples stand out. The first is the persistence of the federal definition of LDs. The second is the emphasis on the "unexpected" nature of LDs. As we have pointed out in this chapter, both concepts are outdated. First, the definition of LDs and the implementation of this definition in regulations are not lined up with the converging scientic evidence. The distance is rapidly increasing, as research continues and practice lags behind federal expenditure in this area of research. What educational legislation has a separate section devoted to research and its implementation through personnel preparation, demonstration grants, state improvement projects, and monitoring of process, other than Part D of IDEA? This area should be the easiest in which to implement research. In particular, there is little evidence that supports the IQ–achievement discrepancy model, and considerable evidence that it can harm children. It is not coincidental that the number of children in the 12- to 17-year age range is the fastest-growing in the LD category. As we have noted earlier, this reflects a "wait-to-fail" model that IDEA currently demands of special education with the focus on discrepancy and the fact that children must show lack of progress in order to qualify for services. Such an approach flies in the face of what research shows on prevention. The definition is not supported by research on the types of LDs. Little to no progress has been made at the regulatory level to make definitions of LDs inclusionary and not simply a set of vague exclusions. Most importantly, as our review of psychometric factors indicated, the definition must incorporate factors other than test scores. The obvious candidate is response to intervention. We stress this potential factor in the identification of LDs as we hypothesize that a significant number of children can be labeled as having LDs because of a lack of informed and adequate instruction. We also hypothesize that the reliance on a discrepancy model allows other students with LDs to go unrecognized—again, a circumstance that could be mitigated by identifying how children found to be at risk for failure through early screening respond to early intervention programs.

Misidentification of students with LDs is exacerbated due to the persistence of the notion that LDs are "unexpected." The research reviewed in this chapter clearly shows that LDs most certainly can be expected if children do not develop clearly specifiable cognitive competencies and are not adequately instructed. Conceptualizations of LDs need to abandon outmoded constructs like "discrepancy" and "unexpected," and to move toward inclusionary, intervention-oriented definitions.

It is time to move away from the advocacy that has been necessary to procure the recognition and services children with LDs need, and shift to an emphasis on the need to provide effective services to these children. Advocacy has helped these children enter schools with protections. It is now time to advocate for results through the rigorous scaling up and implementation of what we know from research. This will require enhanced preparation of personnel at all levels, but especially of the teachers who instruct all children in general and those in special education particularly. Addressing this latter issue is the key to results for children with LDs.

ACKNOWLEDGMENTS

The work of Jack M. Fletcher was supported in part by grants from the National Institute of Child Health and Human Development (No. P50 HD21888), the Center for Learning and Attention Disorders, and the National Science Foundation (No. NSF 9979968, Early Development of Reading Skills: A Cognitive Neuroscience Approach).

REFERENCES

Aaron, P. G. (1997). The impending demise of the discrepancy formula. *Review of Educational Research, 67*, 461–502.

Abbott, R. D., & Berninger, V. W. (1993). Structural equation modeling of relationships among developmental skills and writing skills in primary- and intermediate-grade writers. *Journal of Educational Psychology, 85*, 478–508.

Ackerman, P. T., Weir, N. L., Holloway, C. A., & Dykman, R. A. (1995). Adolescents earlier diagnosed as dyslexic show major IQ declines on the WISC-III. *Reading and Writing, 7*, 163–170.

Alarcon, M., DeFries, J. C., Light, J. C., & Pennington, B. F. (1997). A twin study of mathematics disability. *Journal of Learning Disabilities, 30*, 617–623.

American Psychiatric Association. (1980). *Diagnostic and statistical manual of mental disorders* (3rd ed.). Washington, DC: Author.

American Psychiatric Association. (1994). *Diagnostic and statistical manual of mental disorders* (4th ed.). Washington, DC: Author.

Badian, N. A. (1999). Reading disability defined as a discrepancy between listening and reading comprehension: A longitudinal study of stability, gender differences, and prevalence. *Journal of Learning Disabilities, 32*, 138–148.

Badian, N. A., & Ghublikian, M. (1983). The personal–social characteristics of children with poor mathematical computation skills. *Journal of Learning Disabilities, 16*, 154–157.

Barkley, R. A. (1997). *ADHD and the nature of self-control*. New York: Guilford Press.

Barkley, R.A. (1998). *Attention-deficit hyperactivity disorder: A handbook for diagnosis and treatment* (2nd ed.). New York: Guilford Press.

Barnes, M. A., & Dennis, M. (1998). Discourse after early-onset hydrocephalus: Core deficits in children of average intelligence. *Brain and Language, 61*, 309–334.

Barnes, M. A., & Dennis, M. (2001). Knowledge-based inferencing after childhood head injury. *Brain and Language, 76*, 253–265.

Barnes, M. A., Dennis, M., & Wilkinson, M. (1999). Reading after closed head injury in childhood: Effects on accuracy, fluency, and comprehension. *Developmental Neuropsychology, 15*, 1–24.

Barnes, M. A., Pengelly, S., Dennis, M., Wilkinson, M., Rogers, T., & Faulkner, H. (2002). Mathematics skills in good readers with hydrocephalus. *Journal of the International Neuropsychological Society, 8*, 72–82.

Basso, A., Taborelli, A., & Vignolo, L. A. (1978). Dissociated disorders of speaking and writing in aphasia. *Journal of Neurology, Neurosurgery and Psychiatry, 41*, 556–563.

Bastian, H. C. (1898). *Aphasia and other speech defects*. London: H. K. Lewis.

Bennett, D. E., & Clarizo, H. F. (1988). A comparison of methods for calculating a severe discrepancy. *Journal of School Psychology, 26*, 359–369.

Benton, R. L., & Pearl, D. (Eds.). (1978). *Dyslexia*. New York: Oxford University Press.

Bereiter, C. (1967). Some persisting dilemmas in the measurement of change. In C. W. Harris (Ed.), *Problems in the measurement of change* (pp. 3–20). Madison: University of Wisconsin Press.

Bereiter, C. (1980). Toward a developmental theory of writing. In L. W. Gregg & E. R. Steinberg (Eds.), *Cognitive processes in writing* (pp. 73–93). Hillsdale, NJ: Erlbaum.

Berninger, V. W. (1994a). Future directions for research on writing disabilities: Integrating endogenous and exogenous variables. In G. R. Lyon (Ed.), *Frames of reference for the assessment of learning disabilities: New views on measurement issues* (pp. 419–439). Baltimore: Brookes.

Berninger, V. W. (1994b). *Reading and writing acquisition: A developmental neuropsychological perspective*. Madison, WI: Brown & Benchmark.

Berninger, V. (in press). Understanding the graphic in developmental dysgraphia: A developmental neuropsychological perspective. In D. Dewey & D. Tupper (Eds.), *Developmental motor disorders: A neuropsychological perspective*. New York: Guilford Press.

Berninger, V. W., & Fuller, F. (1992). Gender differences in orthographic, verbal, and compositional fluency: Implications for assessing writing disabilities in primary grade children. *Journal of School Psychology, 30,* 363–382.

Berninger, V., & Graham, S. (1998). Language by hand: A synthesis of a decade of research in handwriting. *Handwriting Review, 12,* 11–25.

Berninger, V. W., & Hart, T. (1992). A developmental neuropsychological perspective for reading and writing acquisition. *Educational Psychologist, 27,* 415–434.

Berninger, V. W., & Hart, T. (1993). From research to clinical assessment of reading and writing disorders: The unit of analysis problem. In R. M. Joshi & C. K. Leong (Eds.), *Reading disabilities: Diagnosis and component processes* (pp. 33–61). Dordrecht, The Netherlands: Kluwer Academic.

Berninger, V. W., Mizokowa, D. T., & Bragg, R. (1991). Theory-based diagnosis and remediation of writing disabilities. *Journal of School Psychology, 29,* 57–79.

Berninger, V. W., Yates, C., Cartwright, A., Ruthberg, J., Remy, E., & Abbott, R. (1992). Lower-level developmental skills in beginning writing. *Reading and Writing: An Interdisciplinary Journal, 4,* 257–280.

Blachman, B. A. (1991). Getting ready to read. In J. F. Kavanagh (Ed.), *The language continuum: From infancy to literacy* (pp. 41–62). Parkton, MD: York Press.

Blachman, B. A. (Ed.). (1997). *Foundations of reading acquisition.* Mahwah, NJ: Erlbaum.

Blashfield, R. K. (1993). Models of classification as related to a taxonomy of learning disabilities. In G. R. Lyon, D. B. Gray, J. F. Kavanagh, & N. A. Krasnegor (Eds.), *Better understanding learning disabilities: New views from research and their implications for education and public policies* (pp. 17–26). Baltimore: Brookes.

Boder, E. (1973). Developmental dyslexia: A diagnostic approach based on three atypical reading–spelling patterns. *Developmental Medicine and Child Neurology, 15,* 663–687.

Breier, J. I., Fletcher, J. M., Foorman, B. R., & Gray, L. C. (2002). Perception of speech and nonspeech stimuli by children with and without reading disability and attention deficit hyperactivity disorder. *Journal of Experimental Child Psychology*, *82*, 226–250.

Broca, P. P. (1863). Localisation des fonctions cérébrales: Siège du langage articule. *Bulletin de la Société d'Anthropologie de Paris, 4,* 200–203.

Broca, P. P. (1865). Sur la siège du faculté de langage articule. *Bulletin de la Société d'Anthropologie de Paris, 6,* 377–393.

Bruck, M. (1985). The adult functioning of children with specific learning disabilities. In L. S. Sigel (Ed.), *Advances in applied developmental psychology* (Vol. 1, pp. 91–129). Norwood, NJ: Ablex.

Bruck, M. (1986). Social and emotional adjustments of learning disabled children: A review of the issues. In S. J. Ceci (Ed.), *Handbook of cognitive, social and neuropsychological aspects of learning disabilities* (pp. 361–380). Hillsdale, NJ: Erlbaum.

Bryan, T. H., Donahue, M., Pearl, T., & Sturm, C. (1981). Learning disabled conversational skills: The T.V. talk show. *Learning Disabilities Quarterly, 4,* 250–259.

Bull, R., & Johnston, R. S. (1997). Children's arithmetical difficulties: Contributions from processing speed, item identification, and short-term memory. *Journal of Experimental Child Psychology, 65,* 1–24.

Cain, K., & Oakhill, J. V. (1999). Inference making and its relation to comprehension failure in young children. *Reading and Writing: An Interdisciplinary Journal, 11,* 489–503.

Cain, K., Oakhill, J. V., & Bryant, P. (2000). Phonological skills and comprehension failures: A test of the phonological processing deficits hypothesis. *Reading and Writing, 13,* 31–56.

Casby, M. W. (1992). The cognitive hypothesis and its influence on speech–language services in schools. *Language, Speech, and Hearing Services in Schools, 23,* 198–202.

Castles, A., & Coltheart, M. (1993). Varieties of developmental dyslexia. *Cognition, 47,* 149–180.

Cataldo, M. G., & Cornoldi, C. (1998). Self-monitoring in poor and good reading comprehenders and their use of strategy. *British Journal of Developmental Psychology, 16,* 155–165.

Cawley, J. F., & Miller, J. H. (1989). Cross-sectional comparisons of the mathematical performance of children with learning disabilities: Are we on the right track toward comprehensive programming? *Journal of Learning Disabilities, 22,* 250–259.

Chochon, F., Cohen, L., van de Moortele, P. F., & Dehaene, S. (1999). Differential contributions of the left and right inferior parietal lobules to number processing. *Journal of Cognitive Neuroscience, 11,* 617–630.

Clairborne, J. H. (1906). Types of congenital symbol amblyopia. *Journal of the American Medical Association, 47,* 1813–1816.

Clements, S. D. (1966). *Minimal brain dysfunction in children* (NINDB Monograph No. 3). Washington, DC: U.S. Department of Health, Education and Welfare.

Cohen, J. (1983). The cost of dichotomization. *Applied Psychological Measurement*, *7*, 249–253.

Compton, D. L., DeFries, J. C., & Olson, R. K. (2001). Are RAN- and phonological awareness-deficits additive in children with reading disabilities? *Dyslexia, 3,* 125–149.

Connors, F. A., & Olson, R. K. (1990). Reading comprehension in dyslexic and normal readers: A component-skills analysis. In D. A. Balolta, G. B. Flores d'Arcais, & K. Rayner (Eds.), *Comprehension processes in reading* (pp. 557–579). Hillsdale, NJ: Erlbaum.

Cooley, E. J., & Ayers, R. R. (1988). Self-concept and success–failure attributions of nonhandicapped students and students with learning disabilities. *Journal of Learning Disabilities, 21,* 174–178.

Cornoldi, C., DeBeni, R., & Pazzaglia, F. (1996). Profiles of reading comprehension difficulties: An analysis of single cases. In C. Cornoldi & J. Oakhill (Eds.), *Reading comprehension difficulties: Processes and intervention* (pp. 113–136). Mahwah, N.J.: Erlbaum.

Critchley, M. (1970). *The dyslexic child.* Springfield, IL: Thomas.

Cunningham, A. E., & Slavonic, K. E. (1998). What reading does for the mind. *American Educator, 4,* 8–15.

Cruickshank, W. M., Bentzen, F. A., Ratzburg, F. H., & Tannenhauser, M. T. (1961). *A teaching method for brain-injured and hyperactive children.* Syracuse, NY: Syracuse University Press.

Cruickshank, W. M., Bice, H. V., & Wallen, N. E. (1957). *Perception and cerebral palsy.* Syracuse, NY: Syracuse University Press.

Cunningham, A. E., & Stanovich, K. E. (1999). What reading does for the mind. *American Educator, 4,* 8–15.

DeFries, J. C., & Fulker, D. W. (1985). Multiple regression analysis of twin data. *Behavior Genetics, 15,* 467–478.

DeFries, J. C., & Gillis, J. J. (1991). Etiology of reading deficits in learning disabilities: Quantitative genetic analyses. In J. E. Obrzut & G. W. Hynd (Eds.), *Neuropsychological foundations of learning disabilities: A handbook of issues, methods, and practice* (pp. 29–48). San Diego, CA: Academic Press.

Dehaene, S., & Cohen, L. (1997). Cerebral pathways for calculation: Double dissociation between rote verbal and quantitative knowledge of arithmetic. *Cortex, 33,* 219–250.

Dehaene, S., Spelke, E., Pinel, P., Stanescu, R., & Tsiukin, S. (1999). Sources of mathematical thinking: Behavioral and brain-injury evidence. *Science, 284,* 970–974.

de Hirsch, K., Jansky, J., & Langsford, W. (1965). *Predicting reading failure.* New York: Harper & Row.

De La Paz, S., Swanson, P. M., & Graham, S. (1998). The contribution of executive control to the revising by students with writing and learning difficulties. *Journal of Educational Psychology, 90,* 448–460.

Dobbins, D. A. (1988). Yule's "hump" revisited. *British Journal of Educational Psychology, 58,* 338–344.

Doehring, D. G. (1978). The tangled web of behavioral research on developmental dyslexia. In A. L. Benton & D. Pearl (Eds.), *Dyslexia* (pp. 123–137). New York: Oxford University Press.

Doehring, D. G., & Hoshko, I. M. (1977). Classification of reading problems by the Q-technique of factor analysis. *Cortex, 13,* 281–294.

Donovan, M. S., & Cross, C. T. (2002). *Minority students in special and gifted education.* Washington, DC: National Academy Press.

Doris, J. L. (1993). Defining learning disabilities: A history of the search for consensus. In G. R. Lyon, D. B Gray, J. F. Kavanagh, & N. A. Krasnegor (Eds.), *Better understanding learning disabilities: New views from research and their implications for education and public policies* (pp. 97–116). Baltimore: Brookes.

Duara, R., Kuslch, A., Gross-Glenn, K., Barker, W., Jallad, B., Pascal, S., Loewenstein, d.A., Sheldon, J., Rabin, M., Levin, B., & Lubs, H. (1991). Neuroanatomic differences between dyslexic and normal readers on magnetic resonance imaging scans. *Archives of Neurology, 48,* 410–416.

Dykman, R. A., Ackerman, P. T., Clements, S. D., & Peters, J. E. (1971). Specific learning disabilities: An attentional deficit syndrome. In H.R. Myklebust (Ed.), *Progress in learning* (Vol. 2, pp. 56–93). New York: Grune & Stratton.

Eden, G. F., Stern, J. F., Wood, M. H., & Wood, F. B. (1995). Verbal and visual problems in dyslexia. *Journal of Learning Disabilities, 28,* 282–290.

Eden, G. F., & Zeffiro, T. A. (1998). Neural systems affected in developmental dyslexia revealed by functional neuroimaging. *Neuron, 21,* 279–282.

Englert, C. S. (1990). Unraveling the mysteries of writing through strategy instruction. In T. E. Scruggs & B. Y. L. Wong (Eds.), *Intervention research in learning disabilities* (pp. 220–262). New York: Springer-Verlag.

Feagans, L., Short, E., & Meltzer, L. (1991). *Subtypes of learning disabilities.* Hillsdale, NJ: Erlbaum.

Felton, R. H., & Brown, I. S. (1991). Neuropsychological prediction of reading disabilities. In J. E. Obrzut & G. W. Hynd (Eds.), *Neuropsychological foundations of learning disabilities: A handbook of issues, methods, and practice* (pp. 387–410). New York: Academic Press.

Filipek, P. (1996). Structural variations in measures in the developmental disorders. In R. Thatcher, G. Lyon, J. Rumsey, & N. Krasnegor (Eds.), *Developmental neuroimaging: Mapping the development of brain and behavior* (pp. 169–186). San Diego, CA: Academic Press.

Fisk, J. L., & Rourke, B. P. (1979). Identification of subtypes of learning disabled children at three age levels: A neuropsychological multivariate approach. *Journal of Clinical Neuropsychology, 1,* 289–310.

Fleishner, J. E. (1994). Diagnosis and assessment of mathematics learning disabilities. In G. R. Lyon (Ed.), *Frames of reference for the assessment of learning disabilities: New views on measurement issues* (pp. 441–458). Baltimore: Brookes.

Fletcher, J. M. (1985). Memory for verbal and nonverbal stimuli in learning disability subgroups: Analysis by selective reminding. *Journal of Experimental Child Psychology, 40,* 244–259.

Fletcher, J. M., & Morris, R. (1986). Classification of disabled learners: Beyond exclusionary definitions. In S. J. Cici (Ed.), *Handbook of cognitive, social, and neuropsychological aspects of learning disabilities* (pp. 55–80). Hillsdale, NJ: Erlbaum.

Fletcher, J. M., Foorman, B. R., Boudousquie, A. B., Barnes, M. A., Schatschneider, C., & Francis, D. J. (2002). Assessment of reading and learning disabilities: A research-based, intervention-oriented approach. *Journal of School Psychology, 40,* 27–63.

Fletcher, J. M., Foorman, B. R., Shaywitz, S. E., & Shaywitz, B. A. (1999). Conceptual and methodological issues in dyslexia research: A lesson for developmental disorders. In H. Tager-Flusberg (Ed.), *Neurodevelopmental disorders* (pp. 271–306). Cambridge, MA: MIT Press.

Fletcher, J. M., Francis, D. J., Rourke, B. P., Shaywitz, S. E., & Shaywitz, B. A. (1993). Classification of learning disabilities: Relationships with other childhood disorders. In G. R. Lyon, D. B. Gray, J. F. Kavanagh, & N. A. Krasnegor (Eds.), *Better understanding learning disabilities: New views from research and their implications for education and public policies* (pp. 27–56). Baltimore: Brookes.

Fletcher, J. M., Francis, D. J., Shaywitz, S. E., Lyon, G. R., Foorman, B. R., Stuebing, K. K., & Shaywitz, B. A. (1998). Intelligent testing and the discrepancy model for children with learning disabilities. *Learning Disabilities Research and Practice, 13,* 186–203.

Fletcher, J. M., Francis, D. J., Stuebing, K. K., Shaywitz, B. A., Shaywitz, S. E., Shankweiler, D. P., Katz, L., & Morris, R. (1996). Conceptual and methodological issues in construct definition. In G.R. Lyon and N.A. Krasnegor (Eds.), *Attention, memory, and executive functions* (pp. 17–42). Baltimore: Brookes.

Fletcher, J. M., Shaywitz, S. E., & Shaywitz, B. A. (1999). Comorbidity of learning and attention disorders: Separate but equal. *Pediatric Clinics of North America, 46,* 885–897.

Fletcher, J. M., Shaywitz, S. E., Shankweiler, D. P., Katz, L., Liberman, I. Y., Stuebing, K. K., Francis, D. J., Fowler, A., & Shaywitz, B. A. (1994). Cognitive profiles of reading disability: Comparisons of discrepancy and low achievement definitions. *Journal of Educational Psychology, 86,* 1–18.

Fletcher, J. M., Lyon, G. R., Barnes, M., Stuebing, K. K., Francis, D. J., Olson, R. K., Shaywitz, S. E., & Shaywitz, B. A. (in press). Classification of learning disabilities: An evidenced-based evaluation. In R. Bradley, L. Danielson, & D. Hallahan (Eds.), *Identification of learning disabilities: Research to practice*. Mahwal, NJ: Lawrence Erlbaum.

Flowers, L., Meyer, M., Lovato, J., Wood, F., & Felton, R. (2001). Does third grade discrepancy status predict the course of reading development? *Annals of Dyslexia, 51*, 49–71.

Flynn, J. M., & Rahbar, M. H. (1994). Prevalence of reading failure in boys compared with girls. *Psychology in the Schools, 31*, 66–70.

Foorman, B. R., & Torgesen, J. (2001). Critical elements of classroom and small-group instruction promote reading success in all children. *Learning Disabilities Research and Practice, 16,* 203–212.

Foorman, B. R., Francis, D. J., Fletcher, J. M., Schatschneider, C., & Mehta, P. (1998). The role of instruction in learning to read: Preventing reading failure in at-risk-children. *Journal of Educational Psychology, 90,* 37–55.

Foorman, B. R., Francis, D. J., Winikates, D., Mehta, P., Schatschneider, C., & Fletcher, J. (1997). Early interventions for children with reading disabilities. *Scientific Studies of Reading, 1,* 255–276.

Francis, D. J., Fletcher, J. M., Stuebing, K. K., Lyon, G. R., Shaywitz, S. A., & Shaywitz, B. A. (2002). *Psychometric approaches to the identification of learning disabilities. Test scores are not sufficient*. Manuscript under review.

Francis, D. J., Shaywitz, S. E., Stuebing, K. K., Shaywitz, B. A., & Fletcher, J. M. (1996). Developmental lag versus deficit models of reading disability: A longitudinal, individual growth curves analysis. *Journal of Educational Psychology, 88,* 3–17.

Fuchs, D., Fuchs, L. S., Thompson, A., Al Otaiba, S., Yen, L., Yang, N. Y., Braun, M., & O'Connor, R. E. (2001). Is reading important in reading-readiness programs?: A randomized field trial with teachers as field implementers. *Journal of Educational Psychology, 93,* 251–267.

Fuchs, L. S., & Fuchs, D. (1998). Treatment validity: A unifying concept for reconceptualizing identification of learning disabilities. *Learning Disabilities Research and Practice, 13,* 204–219.

Fuchs, L. S., Fuchs, D., & Prentice, K. (in press). Responsiveness to mathematical problem solving instruction among students with and without comorbid reading disability. *Journal of Educational Psychology.*

Galaburda, A. M. (1993). The planum temporale. *Archives of Neurology, 50,* 457.

Galaburda, A. M., Sherman, G. P., Rosen, G. D., Aboitiz, F., & Geschwind, N. (1985). Developmental dyslexia: Four consecutive patients with cortical anomalies. *Annals of Neurology, 18,* 222–233.

Gayan, J., & Olson, R. K. (2001). Genetic and environmental influences on orthographic and phonological skills in children with reading disabilities. *Developmental Neuropsychology, 20,* 483–507.

Geary, D. C. (1993). Mathematical disabilities: Cognitive, neuropsychological, and genetic components. *Psychological Bulletin, 114,* 345–362.

Geary, D. C., Hamson, C. O., & Hoard, M. K. (2000). Numerical and arithmetical cognition: A longitudinal study of process and concept deficits in children with learning disability. *Journal of Experimental Child Psychology, 77,* 236–263.

Geary, D. C., Hoard, M. K., & Hamson, C. O. (1999). Numerical and arithmetical cognition: Patterns of functions and deficits in children at risk for a mathematical disability. *Journal of Experimental Child Psychology, 74,* 213–239.

Gerber, A. (1993). *Language-related learning disabilities: Their nature and treatment.* Baltimore: Brookes.

Geschwind, N., & Levitsky, W. (1968). Human brain: Left-right asymmetries in temporal speech region. *Science, 161,* 186–187.

Gilger, J. W. (2000). Contributions and promise of human behavioral genetics. *Human Biology, 72,* 229–255.

Gilger, J. W., & Kaplan, B. J. (2002). Atypical brain development: A conceptual framework for understanding develop-mental learning disabilities. *Developmental Neuro-psychology.*

Ginsburg, H. P., Klein, A., & Starkey, P. (1998). The development of children's mathematical thinking: Connecting research with practice. In W. Damon (Series Ed.), & I. E. Siegel & K. A. Renninger (Vol. Eds.), *Handbook of child psychology: Vol. 4. Child psychology in practice* (5th ed., pp. 401–476). New York: Wiley.

Gleitman, L. R., & Rosen, P. (1973). Teaching reading by use of a syllabary. *Reading Research Quarterly, 8,* 447–483.

Goldstein, K. (1948). *Language and language disorders.* New York: Grune & Stratton.

Goodman, K. S. (1969). Words and morphemes in reading. In K. S. Goodman & J. Fleming (Eds.), *Psycholinguistics and the teaching of reading* (pp. 3–36). Newark, DE: International Reading Association.

Goodman, K. S. (1986). *What's whole about whole language?* Portsmouth, NH: Heinemann.

Graham, S., & Harris, K. R. (1987). Improving composition skills of inefficient learners with self-instructional strategy training. *Topics in Language Disorders, 7,* 67–77.

Graham, S., & Harris, K. R. (2000). Helping children who experience reading difficulties: Prevention and intervention. In L. Baker, M. J. Dreher, & J. T. Guthrie (Eds.), *Engaging young readers: Promoting achievement and motivation* (pp. 43–67). New York: Guilford Press.

Graham, S., Harris, K. R., & Fink, B. (2000). Is handwriting causally related to learning to write?: Treatment of handwriting problems in beginning writers. *Journal of Educational Psychology, 92,* 620–633.

Graham, S., Harris, K., MacArthur, C., & Schwartz, S. (1991). Writing and writing instruction with students with learning disabilities: A review of a program of research. *Learning Disability Quarterly, 14,* 89–114.

Graham, S., Weintraub, N., & Berhinger, V. (2001). Which manuscript letters do primary grade children write legibly? *Journal of Educational Psychology, 93,* 488–497.

Gregg, N. (1991). Disorders of written expression. In A. Bain, L. Bailet, & L. Moats (Eds.), *Written language disorders: Theory into practice* (pp. 65–97). Austin, TX: Pro-Ed.

Gresham, F. M. (in press). Response to treatment. In R. Bradley, L. Danielson, & D. Hallahan (Eds.), *Identification of learning disabilities: Research to practice*. Mahwah, NJ: Erlbaum.

Grigorenko, E. L. (2001). Developmental dyslexia: An update on genes, brains, and environments. *Journal of Child Psychology and Psychiatry, 42,* 91–125.

Grigorenko, E. L., Wood, F. B., Meyer, M. S., Hart, L. A., Speed, W. C., Shuster, A., & Pauls, D. L. (1997). Susceptibility loci for distinct components of developmental dyslexia on chromosome 6 and 15. *American Journal of Human Genetics, 60,* 27–39.

Gross-Glenn, K., Duara, R., Barker, W. W., Loewenstein, D., Chang, J. Y., Yoshii, F., Apicella, A. M., Pascal, S.,

Boothe, T., Sevush, S., Jallad, B. J., Novoa, L., & Lubs, H. A. (1991). Positron emission tomographic studies during serial word-reading by normal and dyslexic adults. *Journal of Clinical and Experimental Neuropsychology, 13,* 531–544.

Gross-Tsur, V., Manor, O., & Shalev, R. S. (1996). Developmental dyscalculia: Prevalence and demographic features. *Developmental Medicine and Child Neurology, 38,* 25–33.

Hallahan, D. P., & Cruickshank, W. M. (1973). *Psychoeducational foundations of learning disabilities.* Englewood Cliffs, NJ: Prentice-Hall.

Hammill, D. D. (1993). A brief look at the learning disabilities movement in the United States. *Journal of Learning Disabilities, 26,* 295–310.

Hammill, D. D., & Larsen, S. (1988). *Test of Written Language—Revised.* Austin, TX: Pro-Ed.

Hammill, D. D., Leigh, J., McNutt, G., & Larsen, S. (1981). A new definition of learning disabilities. *Journal of Learning Disabilities, 4,* 336–342.

Hart, B., & Risley, T. R. (1995). *Meaningful differences in the everyday experience of young American children.* Baltimore: Brookes.

Hatcher, P., & Hulme, C. (1999). Phonemes, rhymes, and intelligence as predictors of children's responsiveness to remedial reading instruction. *Journal of Experimental Child Psychology, 72,* 130–153.

Hays, J. R., & Flower, L. S. (1980). Identifying the organization of the writing process. In L. W. Gregg & E. R. Steinberg (Eds.), *Cognitive processes in writing* (pp. 3–30). Hillsdale, NJ: Erlbaum.

Head, H. (1926). *Aphasia and kindred disorders of speech.* London: Cambridge University Press.

Hinshelwood, J. (1895). Word-blindness and visual memory. *Lancet, ii,* 1564–1570.

Hinshelwood, J. (1900). Congenital word-blindness. *Lancet, i,* 1506–1508.

Hinshelwood, J. (1917). *Congenital word-blindness.* London: H. K. Lewis.

Hooper, S. R., Montgomery, J., Swartz, C., Reed, M., Sandler, A., Levine, M., & Watson, T. (1994). Measurement of written language expression. In G. R. Lyon (Ed.), *Frames of reference for the assessment of learning disabilities: New views on measurement issues* (pp. 375–418). Baltimore: Brookes.

Hooper, S. R., Swartz, C., Wakely, M., deKruif, R., & Montgomery, J. (2002). Executive functions in elementary school children with and without problems in written expression. *Journal of Learning Disabilities, 35,* 59–68.

Hooper, S. R., & Willis, W. G. (1989). *Learning disability subtyping: Neuropsychological foundations, conceptual models, and issues in clinical differentiation.* New York: Springer-Verlag.

Horwitz, B., Rumsey, J. M., & Donohue, B. C. (1998). Functional connectivity of the angular gyrus in normal reading and dyslexia. *Proceedings of the National Academy of Sciences USA, 95,* 8939–8944.

Hoskyn, M., & Swanson, H. L (2000). Cognitive processing of low achievers and children with reading disabilities: A selective meta-analytic review of the published literature. *School Psychology Review, 29,* 102–119.

Humphreys, P., Kaufmann, W. E., & Galaburda, A. M. (1990). Developmental dyslexia in women: Neuropathological findings in three patients. *Annals of Neurology, 28,* 727–738.

Hunter, J. V., & Wang, Z. J. (2001). MR spectroscopy in pediatric neuroradiology. *MRI Clinics of North America, 9,* 165–189.

Hynd, G. W., Hall, J., Novey, E. S., Etiopulos, D., Black, K., Gonzales, J. J., Edmonds, J. E., Riccio, C., & Cohen, M.. (1995). Dyslexia and corpus callosum morphology. *Archives of Neurology, 52,* 32–38.

Hynd, G. W., & Semrud-Clikeman, M. (1989). Dyslexia and brain morphology. *Psychological Bulletin, 106,* 447–482.

Hynd, G. W., Semrud-Clikeman, M., Lorys, A. R., Novey, E. S., & Eliopulos, D. (1990). Brain morphology in developmental dyslexia and attention deficit disorder/hyperactivity. *Archives of Neurology, 47,* 919–926.

Hynd, G. W., & Willis, W. G. (1988). *Pediatric neuropsychology.* Orlando, FL: Grune & Stratton.

Iovino, I., Fletcher, J. M., Breitmeyer, B. G., & Foorman, B. R. (1999). Colored overlays for visual perceptual deficits in children with reading disability and attention deficit/hyperactivity disorder: Are they differentially effective? *Journal of Clinical and Experimental Neurospychology, 20,* 791–806.

Jackson, E. (1906). Developmental alexia. *American Journal of Medical Science, 131,* 843–849.

Jernigan, T. L., Hesselink, J. R., Stowell, E., & Tallal, P. (1991). Cerebral structure on magnetic resonance imaging in language- and learning-impaired children. *Archives of Neurology, 48,* 539–545.

Johnson, D. J., & Blalock, J. (Eds.). (1987). *Adults with learning disabilities.* Orlando, FL: Grune & Stratton.

Johnson, D. J., & Myklebust, H. (1967). *Learning disabilities: Educational principles and practices.* New York: Grune & Stratton.

Jordan, N. C., & Hanich, L. B. (2000). Mathematical thinking in second-grade children with different forms of LD. *Journal of Learning Disabilities, 33,* 567–578.

Jorm, A. F., & Share, D. L. (1983). Phonological reading and acquisition. *Applied Psycholinguistics, 4,* 103–147.

Jorm, A. F., Share, D. L., Matthews, M., & Matthews, R. (1986). Cognitive factors at school entry predictive of specific reading retardation and general reading backwardness: A research note. *Journal of Child Psychology and Psychiatry, 27,* 45–54.

Joseph, J., Noble, K., & Eden, G. (2001). The neurobiological basis of reading. *Journal of Learning Disabilities, 34, 566–579.*

Kavale, K. A. (1988). Learning disability and cultural disadvantage: The case for a relationship. *Learning Disability Quarterly, 11,* 195–210.

Kavale, K. A., & Forness, S. (1985). *The science of learning disabilities.* Boston: College-Hill Press.

Kavale, K. A., & Forness, S. R. (1996). Social skill deficits and learning disabilities: A meta-analysis. *Journal of Learning Disabilities, 29,* 226–237.

Kavale, K. A., & Forness, S. R. (1988). The politics of learning disabilities. *Learning Disability Quarterly, 21,* 245–273.

Kavale, K. A., & Forness, S. R. (2000). What definitions of learning disability say and don't say: A critical analysis. *Journal of Learning Disabilities, 33,* 239–256.

Kavale, K. A., & Nye, C. (1981). Identification criteria for learning disabilities: A survey of the research literature. *Learning Disability Quarterly, 4,* 383–388.

Kavale, K. A., & Reese, L. (1992). The character of learning disabilities: An Iowa profile. *Learning Disability Quarterly, 15,* 74–94.

Kavanagh, J. F., & Truss, T. J. (Eds.). (1988). *Learning disabilities: Proceedings of the national conference.* Parkton, MD: York Press.

Keeler, M. L., & Swanson, H. L. (2001). Does strategy knowledge influence working memory in children with mathematical disabilities? *Journal of Learning Disabilities, 34*, 418–434.

Kellam, S. G., Rebok, G. W., Mayer, L. S., Ialongo, N., & Kalodner, C. R. (1994). Depressive symptoms over first grade and their response to a developmental epidemiologically based preventive trial aimed at improving achievement. *Development and Psychopathology*, *6*, 463–481.

Keller, C. E., & Sutton, J. P. (1991). Specific mathematics disorders In J. E. Obrzut & G. W. Hynd (Eds.), *Neuropsychological foundations of learning disabilities: A handbook of issues, methods, and practice* (pp. 549–572). New York: Academic Press.

Keogh, B. K. (1993). Linking purpose and practice: Social/political and developmental perspectives on classification. In G. R. Lyon, D. B. Gray, J. F. Kavanagh, & N. A. Krasnegor (Eds.), *Better understanding learning disabilities: New views from research and their implications for education and public policies* (pp. 311–324). Baltimore: Brookes.

Kirk, S. A. (1963). Behavioral diagnosis and remediation of learning disabilities. *Conference Exploring Problems of the Perceptually Handicapped Child, 1,* 1–23.

Klingberg, T., Hedehus, M., Temple, E., Salz, T., Gabrieli, J. D., Moseley, M. E., & Poldrack, R. A. (2000). Microstructure of temporo-parietal white matter as a basis for reading ability: Evidence from diffusion tensor magnetic resonance imaging. *Neuron, 25,* 493–500.

Knopik, V. S., & DeFries, J. C. (1999). Etiology of covariation between reading and mathematics performance: A twin study. *Twin Research, 2,* 226–234.

Kosc, L. (1974). Developmental dyscalculia. *Journal of Learning Disabilities, 7,* 164–177.

Kusch, A., Gross-Glenn, K., Jallad, B., Lubs, H., Rabin, M., Feldman, E., & Duara, R. (1993). Temporal lobe surface area measurements on MRI in normal and dyslexic readers. *Neuropsychologia, 31,* 811–821.

Kussmaul, A. (1877). Disturbance of speech. *Cyclopedia of Practical Medicine, 14,* 581–875.

Larsen, J. P., Hoien, T., Lundberg, I., & Ödegaard, H. (1990). MRI evaluation of the size and symmetry of the planum temporale in adolescents with developmental dyslexia. *Brain and Language, 39,* 289–301.

Leonard, C. M., Eckert, M. A., Lombardino, L. J., Oakland, T., Franzier, J., Mohr, C. M., King, W. M., & Freeman, A. (2001). Anatomical risk factors for phonological dyslexia. *Cerebral Cortex, 11,* 148–157.

Leonard, C. M., Lombardino, L. J., Mercado, L. R., Browd, S. R., Breier, J. I., & Agee, O. F. (1996). Cerebral asymmetry and cognitive development in children: A magnetic resonance imaging study. *Psychological Science, 7,* 89–95.

Lerner, J. (1989). Educational intervention in learning disabilities. *Journal of the American Academy of Child and Adolescent Psychiatry*, *28*, 326–331.

Lewis, C., Hitch, G. J., & Walker, P. (1994). The prevalence of specific arithmetic difficulties and specific reading difficulties in 9- to 10-year-old boys and girls. *Journal of Child Psychology Psychiatry, 35,* 283–292.

Liberman, A. M., Cooper, F. S., Shankweiler, D., & Studdert-Kennedy, M. (1967). Perception of the speech code. *Psychological Review, 74,* 431–461.

Liberman, I. Y. (1971). Basic research in speech and lateralization of language. *Bulletin of the Orton Society, 21,* 72–87.

Liberman, I. Y., & Shankweiler, D. (1979). Speech, the alphabet, and teaching to read. In L. B. Resnick & P. A. Weaver (Eds.), *Theory and practice in early reading* (Vol. 2, pp. 109–134). Hillsdale, NJ: Erlbaum.

Liberman, I. Y., & Shankweiler, D. (1991). Phonology and beginning reading: A tutorial. In L. Rieben & C. A. Perfetti (Eds.), *Learning to read: Basic research and its implications* (pp. 46–73). Hillsdale, NJ: Erlbaum.

Liberman, I. Y., Shankweiler, D., & Liberman, A. (1989). The alphabetic principle and learning to read. In D. Shankweiler & I. Y. Liberman (Eds.), *Phonology and reading disability: Solving the reading puzzle* (pp. 1–34). Ann Arbor: University of Michigan Press.

Lindamood, P. C. (1994). Issues in researching the link between phonological awareness, learning disabilities, and spelling. In G. R. Lyon (Ed.), *Frames of reference for the assessment of learning disabilities: New views on measurement issues* (pp. 351–374). Baltimore: Brookes.

Livingstone, M. S., Rosen, G. D., Drislane, F. W., & Galaburda, A. M. (1991). Physiological and anatomical evidence for a magnocellular defect in developmental dyslexia. *Proceedings of the National Academy of Sciences USA, 88,* 7943–7947.

Lovegrove, W., Martin, F., & Slaghuis, W. (1986). A theoretical and experimental case for a visual deficit in specific reading disability. *Cognitive Neuropsychology, 3,* 225–267.

Lovett, M. W. (1984). A developmental perspective on reading dysfunction: Accuracy and rate criteria in the subtyping of dyslexic children. *Brain and Language, 22,* 67–91.

Lovett, M. W. (1987). A developmental approach to reading disability: Accuracy and speed criteria of normal and deficient reading skill. *Child Development, 58,* 234–260.

Lovett, M. W., Lacerenza, L., Borden, S. L., Frijters, J. C., Steinbach, K. A.,, & DePalma, M. (2000). Components of effective remediation for developmental reading disabilities: Combining phonological and strategy-based instruction to improve outcomes. *Journal of Educational Psychology, 92,* 263–283.

Lovett, M. W., Ransby, M. J., & Barron, R. W. (1988). Treatment, subtype, and word type effects in dyslexic children's response to remediation. *Brain and Language, 34,* 328–349.

Lovett, M. W., Ransby, M. J., Hardwick, N., & Johns, M. S. (1989). Can dyslexia be treated?: Treatment-specific and generalized treatment effects in dyslexic children's response to remediation. *Brain and Language, 37,* 90–121.

Lovett, M. W., Steinbach, K. A., & Frijters, J. C. (2000). Remediating the core deficits of reading disability: A double-deficit perspective. *Journal of Learning Disabilities, 33,* 334–358.

Lukatela, G., & Turvey, M. T. (1998). Reading in two alphabets. *American Psychologist, 53,* 1057–1072.

Luria, A. R. (1966). *Higher cortical functions in man.* New York: Basic Books.

Luria, A. R. (1973). *The working brain.* New York: Basic Books.

Lyon, G. R. (1983). Learning-disabled readers: Identification of subgroups. In H. R. Myklebust (Ed.), *Progress in learning disabilities* (Vol. 5, pp. 103–134). New York: Grune & Stratton.

Lyon, G. R. (1985a). Educational validation studies of learning disability subtypes. In B. P. Rourke (Ed.), *Neuropsychology of learning disabilities: Essentials of subtype analysis* (pp. 228–256). New York: Guilford Press.

Lyon, G. R. (1985b). Identification and remediation of learning disability subtypes: Preliminary findings. *Learning Disability Focus, 1,* 21–35.
Lyon, G. R. (1987). Learning disabilities research: False starts and broken promises. In S. Vaughn & C. Bos (Eds.), *Research in learning disabilities: Issues and future directions* (pp. 69–85). Boston: College-Hill Press.
Lyon, G. R. (Ed.). (1994a). *Frames of reference for the assessment of learning disabilities: New views on measurement issues.* Baltimore: Brookes.
Lyon, G. R. (1994b). Critical issues in the measurement of learning disabilities. In G. R. Lyon (Ed.), *Frames of reference for the assessment of learning disabilities: New views on measurement issues* (pp. 3–13). Baltimore: Brookes.
Lyon, G. R. (1995a). Research initiatives and discoveries in learning disabilities. *Journal of Child Neurology, 10,* 120–126.
Lyon, G. R. (1995b). Toward a definition of dyslexia. *Annals of Dyslexia, 45,* 3–27.
Lyon, G. R. (1996a). The future of children: Special education for students with disabilities. *Learning Disabilities, 6,* 54–76.
Lyon, G. R. (1996b). Learning disabilities. In E. J. Mash & R. A. Barkley (Eds.), *Child psychopathology* (pp. 390–435). New York: Guilford Press.
Lyon, G. R., Fletcher, J. M., Shaywitz, S. E., Shaywitz, B. A., Torgesen, J. K., Wood, F. B., Schulte, A., & Olson, R. (2001). Rethinking learning disabilities. In C. E. Finn, Jr., R. A. J. Rotherham, & C. R. Hokanson, Jr. (Eds.), *Rethinking special education for a new century* (pp. 259–287). Washington, DC: Thomas B. Fordham Foundation and Progressive Policy Institute.
Lyon, G. R., & Flynn, J. M. (1989). Educational validation studies with subtypes of learning disabled readers. In B. P. Rourke (Ed.), *Neuropsychological validation of learning disability subtypes* (pp. 243–242). New York: Guilford Press.
Lyon, G. R., & Flynn, J. M. (1991). Assessing subtypes of learning disabilities. In H. L. Swanson (Ed.), *Handbook on the assessment of learning disabilities: Theory, research, and practice* (pp. 59–74). Austin, TX: Pro-Ed.
Lyon, G. R., Gray, D. B., Kavanagh, J. F., & Krasnegor, N. A. (Eds.). (1993). *Better understanding learning disabilities: New views from research and their implications for education and public policies.* Baltimore: Brookes.
Lyon, G. R., & Moats, L. C. (1993). An examination of research in learning disabilities: Past practices and future directions. In G. R. Lyon, D. B. Gray, J. F. Kavanagh, & N. A. Krasnegor (Eds.), *Better understanding learning disabilities: New views from research and their implications for education and public policies* (pp. 1–14). Baltimore: Brookes.
Lyon, G. R., Rietta, S., Watson, B., Porch, B., & Rhodes, J. (1981). Selected linguistic and perceptual abilities of empirically derived subgroups of learning disabled readers. *Journal of School Psychology, 19,* 152–166.
Lyon, G. R., & Risucci, D. (1989). Classification of learning disabilities. In K. A. Kavale (Ed.), *Learning disabilities: State of the art and practice* (pp. 40–70). Boston: College-Hill Press.
Lyon, G. R., Stewart, N., & Freedman, D. (1982). Neuropsychological characteristics of empirically derived subgroups of learning disabled readers. *Journal of Clinical Neuropsychology, 4,* 343–365.
Lyon, G. R., & Watson, B. (1981). Empirically derived subgroups of learning disabled readers: Diagnostic characteristics. *Journal of Learning Disabilities, 14,* 256–261.
MacMillan, D. L., & Siperstein, G. N. (2002). *Learning disabilities as operationally defined by schools.* Washington, DC: U. S. Department of Education.
Mann, L. (1979). *On the trail of process.* New York: Grune & Stratton.
Marlow, A. J., Fisher, S. E., Richardson, A. J., Talcott, J. B., Monaco, A. P., Stein, J. F., & Cardon, L. R. (2001). Investigation of quantitative measures related to reading disability in a large sample of sib-pairs from the UK. *Behavior Genetics, 31*(2), 219–230.
Martin, E. W. (1993). Learning disabilities and public policy: Myths and outcomes. In G. R. Lyon, D. B. Gray, J. F. Kavanagh, & N. A. Krasnegor (Eds.), *Better understanding learning disabilities: New views from research and their implications for education and public policies* (pp. 27–56). Baltimore: Brookes.
Mathes, P. G., Howard, J. K, Allen, S., & Fuchs, D. (1998). Peer-assisted learning strategies for first-grade readers: Making early reading instruction responsive to the needs of diverse learners. *Reading Research Quarterly, 33,* 62–94.
Mattis, S., French, J. H., & Rapin, I. (1975). Dyslexia in children and adults: Three independent neuropsychological syndromes. *Developmental Medicine and Child Neurology, 17,* 150–163.
McBride-Chang, C., & Manis, F. R. (1996). Structural invariance in the associations of naming speed, phonological awareness, and verbal reasoning in good and poor readers: A test of the double deficit hypothesis. *Reading and Writing, 8,* 323–339.
McKinney, J. D., & Feagans, L. (1984). Academic and behavioral characteristics: Longitudinal studies of learning disabled children and average achievers. *Learning Disability Quarterly, 7,* 251–265.
Miles, T. R., & Haslum, M. N. (1986). Dyslexia: Anomaly or normal variation. *Annals of Dyslexia, 36,* 103–117.
Moats, L. C. (1994). The missing foundation in teacher education: Knowledge of the structure of spoken and written language. *Annals of Dyslexia, 44,* 81–102.
Moats, L. C., & Lyon, G. R. (1993). Learning disabilities in the United States: Advocacy, science, and the future of the field. *Journal of Learning Disabilities, 26,* 282–294.
Mody, M., Studdert-Kennedy, M., & Brady, S. (1997). Speech perception deficits in poor readers: Auditory processing or phonological coding? *Journal of Experimental Child Psychology, 64,* 199–231.
Morgan, W. P. (1896). A case of congenital word blindness. *British Medical Journal, ii,* 1378.
Morris, R. D. (1993). Issues in empirical versus clinical identification of learning disabilities. In G. R. Lyon, D. B. Gray, J. F. Kavanagh, & N. A. Krasnegor (Eds.), *Better understanding learning disabilities: New views from research and their implications for education and public policies* (pp. 73–94). Baltimore: Brookes.
Morris, R. D. (in press). The sociopolitical process of classification: Making the implicit explicit in learning disabilities. In R. Bradley, L. Danielson, & D. Hallahan (Eds.), *Identification of learning disabilities: Research to practice.* Washington, DC: U.S. Department of Education.
Morris, R. D., & Fletcher, J. M. (1988). Classification in neuropsychology: A theoretical framework and research paradigm. *Journal of Clinical and Experimental Neuropsychology, 10,* 640–658.
Morris, R. D., Stuebing, K. K., Fletcher, J. M., Shaywitz, S. E., Lyon, G. R., Shankweiler, D. P., Katz, L., Francis,

D. J., & Shaywitz, B. A. (1998). Subtypes of reading disability: Variability around a phonological core. *Journal of Educational Psychology, 90*, 347–373.

Morrison, S. R., & Siegel, L. S. (1991). Learning disabilities: A critical review of definitional and assessment issues. In J. E. Obrzut & G. W. Hynd (Eds.), *Neuropsychological foundations of learning disabilities: A handbook of issues, methods, and practice* (pp. 79–98). New York: Academic Press.

Myers, P., & Hammill, D. D. (1990). *Learning disabilities.* Austin, TX: Pro-Ed.

Nation, K., Adams, J. W., Bowyer-Crane, A., & Snowling, M. J. (1999). Working memory deficits in poor comprehenders reflect underlying language impairments. *Journal of Experimental Child Psychology, 73*, 139–158.

Nation, K., & Snowling, M. J. (1998). Semantic processing and the development of word-recognition skills: Evidence from children with reading comprehension difficulties. *Journal of Memory and Language, 37*, 85–101.

National Joint Committee on Learning Disabilities (NJCLD). (1988, April). [Letter from NJCLD to member organizations]. Austin, TX: Author.

National Reading Panel. (2000). *Teaching children to read: An evidence-based assessment of the scientific research literature on reading and its implications for reading instruction.* Washington, DC: National Institute of Child Health and Human Development.

Newby, R. F., & Lyon, G. R. (1991). Neuropsychological subtypes of learning disabilities. In J. E. Obrzut & G. W. Hynd (Eds.), *Neuropsychological foundations of learning disabilities: A handbook of issues, methods, and practice* (pp. 355–385). New York: Academic Press.

Norman, C. A., & Zigmond, N. (1980). Characteristics of children labeled and served as learning disabled in school systems affiliated with Child Service Demonstration Centers. *Journal of Learning Disabilities, 13*, 542–547.

Nothen, M. M., Schulte-Korne, G., Grimm, T., Cichon, S., Vogt, I. R., Muller-Myhsok, B., Propping, P., & Remschmidt, H. (1999). Genetic linkage analysis with dyslexia: Evidence for linkage of spelling disability to chromosome 15. *European Child and Adolescent Psychiatry, 3*, 56–59.

Novick, B. Z., & Arnold, M. M. (1988). *Fundamentals of clinical child neuropsychology.* Philadelphia: Grune & Stratton.

Oakhill, J. (1993). Children's difficulties in reading comprehension. *Educational Psychology Review, 5*, 1–15.

Oakhill, J. V., Cain, K., & Bryant, P. E. (in press). The dissociation of single-word and text comprehension: Evidence from component skills. *Language and Cognitive Processes.*

Oakill, J., & Yuill, N. (1996). Higher order factors in comprehension disability: Processes and remediation. In C. Cornoldi & J. Oakhill (Eds.), *Reading comprehension difficulties: Processes and interventions* (pp. 69–92). Mahwah, NJ: Erlbaum.

Oakhill, J. V., Yuill, N., & Parkin, A. (1996). On the nature of the difference between skilled and less-skilled comprehenders, *Journal of Research in Reading, 9*, 80–91.

Ogle, J. W. (1867). Aphasia and agraphia. *Report of the Medical Research Council of Saint George's Hospital, 2*, 83–122.

Olson, R. K., Forsberg, H., Gayan, J., & DeFries, J. C. (1999). A behavioral-genetic analysis of reading disabilities and component processes. In R. M. Klein & P. A. McMullen (Eds.), *Converging methods for understanding reading and dyslexia* (pp. 133–153). Cambridge, MA: MIT Press.

Olson, R. K., Forsberg, H., Wise, B., & Rack, J. (1994). Measurement of word recognition, orthographic, and phonological skills. In G. R. Lyon (Ed.), *Frames of reference for the assessment of learning disabilities* (pp. 243–278). Baltimore: Brookes.

Orton, S. (1928). Specific reading disability—strephosymbolia. *Journal of the American Medical Association, 90*, 1095–1099.

Orton, S. (1937). *Reading, writing and speech problems in children: A presentation of certain types of disorders in the development of the language faculty.* New York: Norton.

Papanicolaou, A. C. (1998). *Fundamentals of functional brain imaging.* Lisse, The Netherlands: Swets & Zeitlinger.

Paris, S., & Ika, E. R. (1989). Strategies for comprehending text and coping with reading disabilities. *Learning Disabilities Quarterly, 12*, 32–42.

Pearson, P. D. (1998). Standards and assessment: Tools for crafting effective instruction? In F. Lehr & J. Osborn (Eds.), *Literacy for all: Issues in teaching and learning* (pp. 264–288). New York: Guilford Press.

Pennington, B. F. (1999). Dyslexia as a neurodevelopmental disorder. In H. Tager-Flusberg (Ed.), *Neurodevelopmental disorders* (pp. 307–330). Cambridge, MA: MIT Press.

Pennington, B. F., Filipek, P. A., Churchwell, J., Kennedy, D. N., Lefley, D., Simon, J. H., Filley, C. M., Galaburda, A., Alarcon, M., & DeFries, J. C. (1999). Brain morphometry in reading-disabled twins. *Neurology, 53*, 723–729.

Pennington, B. F., Gilger, J. W., Olson, R. K., & DeFries, J. C. (1992). The external validity of age- versus IQ-discrepancy definitions of reading disability: Lessons from a twin study. *Journal of Learning Disability, 25*, 562–573.

Perfetti, C. A. (1985). *Reading ability.* New York: Oxford University Press.

Peters, J. E., Davis, J. J., Goolshy, C. M., & Clements, S. D. (1973). *Physicians' handbook: Screening for MBD.* New York: CIBA Medical Horizons.

Petrauskas, R., & Rourke, B. P. (1979). Identification of subgroups of retarded readers: A neuropsychological multivariate approach. *Journal of Clinical Neuropsychology, 1*, 17–37.

Poeppel, D. (1996). A critical review of PET studies of phonological processing. *Brain and Language, 55*, 317–351.

Pugh, K. R., Mencl, W. E., Shaywitz, B. A., Shaywitz, S. E., Fulbright, R. K., Constable, R. T., Skudlarski, P., Marchione, K. E., Jenner, A. R., Fletcher, J. M., Liberman, A. M., Shankweiler, D. P., Katz, L., Lacadie, C., & Gore, J. C. (2000). The angular gyrus in developmental dyslexia: Task-specific differences in functional connectivity within posterior cortex. *Psychological Science, 11*, 51–56.

Raskind, W. H., Hsu, L., Berninger, V. W., Thomson, J. B, & Wijsman, E. M. (2000). Familial aggregation of dyslexia phenotypes. *Behavior Genetics, 30*(5), 385–396.

Rayner, K., Foorman, B. R., Perfetti, C. A., Pesetsky, D., & Seidenberg, M. S. (2002). How psychological science informs the teaching of reading. *Psychological Science in the Public Interest, 2*, 31–74.

Reed, M. A. (1989). Speech perception and the discrimination of brief auditory cues in reading disabled children. *Journal of Experimental Child Psychology, 48*, 270–292.

Reynolds, C. (1984–1985). Critical measurement issues in learning disabilities. *Journal of Special Education, 18*, 451–476.

Richards, T. L., Cornia, D., Serafini, S., Steury, K., Echelard, D. R., Dager, S. R., Marro, K., Abbott, R. D., Maravilla, K. R., & Berninger, V. W. (2000). The effects of a phonologically driven treatment for dyslexia on lactate levels as measured by proton MRSI. *American Journal of Neuroradiology, 21,* 916–922.

Rodgers, B. (1983). The identification and prevalence of specific reading retardation. *British Journal of Educational Psychology, 53,* 369–373.

Roeltgen, D. (1985). Agraphia. In K. M. Heilman & E. Valenstein (Eds.), *Clinical neuropsychology* (pp. 75–96). New York: Oxford University Press.

Rogosa, D. (1995). Myths and methods: "Myths about longitudinal research" (plus supplemental questions. In J. M. Gottman (Ed.), *The analysis of change* (pp. 3–66). Mahwah, NJ: Erlbaum.

Rourke, B. P. (Ed.). (1985). *Neuropsychology of learning disabilities: Essentials of subtype analysis.* New York: Guilford Press.

Rourke, B. P. (1989). *Nonverbal learning disabilities: The syndrome and the model.* New York: Guilford Press.

Rourke, B. P. (1993). Arithmetic disabilities specific and otherwise: A neuropsychological perspective. *Journal of Learning Disabilities, 26,* 214–226.

Rourke, B. P., & Finlayson, M. A. J. (1978). Neuropsychological significance of variations in patterns of academic performance: Verbal and visual–spatial abilities. *Journal of Pediatric Psychology, 3,* 62–66.

Rovet, J., Szekely, C., & Hockenberry, M. N. (1994). Specific arithmetic calculation deficits in children with Turner syndrome. *Journal of Clinical Experiemental Neuropsychology, 16,* 820–839.

Rumsey, J. M., Andreason, P., Zametkin, A. J., Aquino, T., King, A., Hamburger, S., Pileus, A., Rapport, J., & Cohen, R. (1992). Failure to activate the left temporoparietal cortex in dyslexia: An oxygen 15 positron emission tomographic study. *Archives of Neurology, 49,* 527–534.

Rumsey, J. M., Nace, K., Donohue, B., Wise, D., Maisog, J. M., & Andreason, P. (1997). A positron emission tomographic study of impaired word recognition and phonological processing in dyslexic men. *Archives of Neurology, 54,* 562–573.

Rumsey, J. M., Zametkin, A. J., Andreason, P., Hanchan, A. P., Hamburger, S. D., Aquino, T., King, C., Pikus, A., & Cohen, R. M. (1994). Normal activation of frontotemporal language cortex in dyslexia, as measured with oxygen 15 positron emission tomography. *Archives of. Neurology, 51,* 27–38.

Rutter, M. (1982). Syndromes attributed to "minimal brain dysfunction" in childhood. *American Journal of Psychiatry, 139,* 21–33.

Rutter, M., & Yule, W. (1975). The concept of specific reading retardation. *Journal of Child Psychology and Psychiatry, 16,* 181–197.

Sattler, J. M. (1993). *Assessment of children's intelligence and special abilities.* Boston: Allyn & Bacon.

Satz, P., Buka, S., Lipsitt, L., & Seidman, L. (1998). The long-term prognosis of learning disabled children: A review of studies (1954–1993). In B. K. Shapiro, P. J. Accardo, & A. J. Capute (Eds.), *Specific reading disability: A view of the spectrum* (pp. 223–250). Parkton, MD: York Press

Satz, P., & Fletcher, J. M. (1980). Minimal brain dysfunctions: An appraisal of research concepts and methods. In H. Rie & E. Rie (Eds.) *Handbook of minimal brain dysfunctions: A critical view* (pp. 669–715). New York: Wiley–Interscience.

Satz, P., & Morris, R. (1981). Learning disability subtypes: A review. In F. J. Pirozzolo & M. C. Wittrock (Eds.), *Neuropsychological and cognitive processes in reading* (pp. 109–141). New York: Academic Press.

Schatschneider, C., Carlson, C. D., Francis, D. J., Foorman, B. R., & Fletcher, J. M. (2002). Relationships of rapid automatized naming and phonological awareness in early reading development: Implications for the double deficit hypothesis. *Journal of Learning Disabilities, 35,* 245–256.

Schulte-Korne, G., Deimel, W., Muller, K., Gutenbrunner, C., & Remschmidt, H. (1996). Familial aggregation of spelling disability. *Journal of Child Psychology and Psychiatry, 37*(7), 817–822.

Schultz, R. T., Cho, N. K., Staib, L. H., Kier, L. E., Fletcher, J. M., Shaywitz, S. E., Shankweiler, D. P., Katz, L., Gore, J. C., Duncan, J. S., & Shaywitz, B. A. (1994). Brain morphology in normal and dyslexic children: The influence of sex and age. *Annals of Neurology, 35,* 732–742.

Senf, G. M. (1981). Issues surrounding the diagnosis of learning disabilities: Child handicap versus failure of the child–school interaction. In T. R. Kratochwill (Ed.), *Advances in school psychology* (Vol. 1, pp. 126–142). Hillsdale, NJ: Erlbaum.

Senf, G. M. (1986). LD research in sociological and scientific perspective. In J. K. Torgesen & B. Y. Wong (Eds.), *Psychological and educational perspectives on learning disabilities* (pp. 27–53). New York: Academic Press.

Senf, G. M. (1987). Learning disabilities as sociological sponge: Wiping up life's spills. In S. Vaughn & C. Bos (Eds.), *Research in learning disabilities: Issues and future directions* (pp. 87–101). Boston: Little, Brown.

Shalev, R. S., Auerbach, J., Manor, O., & Gross-Tsur, V. (2000). Developmental dyscalculia: prevalence and prognosis. *European Child and Adolescent Psychiatry, 9,* 58–64.

Shalev, R. S., & Gross-Tsur, V. (2001). Developmental dyscalculia. *Pediatric Neurology, 24,* 337–342.

Shalev, R. S., Manor, O., Auerbach, J., & Gross-Tsur, V. (1998). Persistence of developmental dyscalculia: what couts? Results from a 3-year prospective follow-up study. *Journal of Pediatrics, 133,* 358–362.

Shalev, R. S., Manor, O., Kerem, B., Ayali, M., Badichi, N., Friedlander, Y., & Gross-Tsur, V. (2001). Developmental dyscalculia is a familial learning disability. *Journal of Learning Disabilities, 34,* 59–65.

Shankweiler, D., & Liberman, I. Y. (Eds.). (1989). *Phonology and reading disability: Solving the reading puzzle.* Ann Arbor: University of Michigan Press.

Shankweiler, D., Lundquist, E., Katz, L., Stuebing, K, Fletcher, J., Brady, S., Fowler, A., Dreyer, L., Marchoine, K., Shaywitz, S., & Shaywitz, B. (1999). Comprehension and decoding: Patterns of association in children with reading difficulties. *Scientific Studies of Reading, 3,* 69–94.

Share, D. J., Jorm, A. F., MacLean, R., & Matthews, R. (1984). Sources of individual differences in reading achievement. *Journal of Educational Psychology, 76,* 466–477.

Share, D. L., McGee, R., & Silva, P. D. (1989). I.Q. and reading progress: A test of the capacity notion of I.Q. *Journal of the American Academy of Child and Adolescent Psychiatry, 28,* 97–100.

Shaywitz, B. A., Shaywitz, S. E., Pugh, K. R., Mencl, W. E., Fulbright, R. K., Constable, R. T., Skudlarski, P., Jenner, A., Fletcher, J. M., Marchione, K. E., Shankweiler, D., Katz, L., Lacadie, C., & Gore, J. C. (2002). Disruption of the neural circuitry for reading in children with developmental dyslexia. *Biological Psychiatry,* 52, 101–110.

Shaywitz, S. E. (1996). Dyslexia. *Scientific American, 275,* 98–104.

Shaywitz, S. E., Escobar, M. D., Shaywitz, B. A., Fletcher, J. M., & Makuch, R. (1992). Evidence that dyslexia may represent the lower tail of a normal distribution of reading ability. *New England Journal of Medicine, 326,* 145–150.

Shaywitz, S. E., Fletcher, J. M., & Shaywitz, B. A. (1994). Issues in the definition and classification of attention deficit disorder. *Topics in Language Disorders, 14,* 1–25.

Shaywitz, S. E., Fletcher, J. M., Holahan, J. M., Shneider, A. E., Marchione, K. E., Stuebing, K. K., Francis, D. J., & Shaywitz, B. A. (1999). Persistence of dyslexia: The Connecticut Longitudinal Study at adolescence. *Pediatrics, 104,* 1351–1359.

Shaywitz, S. E., Pugh, K. R., Jenner, A. R., Fulbright, R. K., Fletcher, J. M., Gore, J. C., & Shaywitz, B. A. (2000). The neurobiology of reading and reading disability (dyslexia). In M. L. Kamil, P. B. Mosenthal, P. D. Pearson, & R. Barr (Eds.), *Handbook of reading research* (Vol. 3, pp. 229–249). Mahwah, NJ: Erlbaum.

Shaywitz, S. E., Shaywitz, B. A., Fletcher, J. M., & Escobar, M. D. (1990). Prevalence of reading disability in boys and girls: Results of the Connecticut Longitudinal Study. *Journal of the American Medical Association, 264,* 998–1002.

Shaywitz, S. E., Shaywitz, B. A., Pugh, K. R., Fulbright, R. K., Constable, R. T., Mencl, W. E., Shankweiler, D. P., Liberman, A. M., Skudlarski, P., Fletcher, J. M., Katz, L., Marchione, K. E., Lacadie, C., Gatenby, C., & Gore, J. C. (1998). Functional disruption in the organization of the brain for reading in dyslexia. *Proceedings of the National Academy of Sciences USA, 95,* 2636–2641.

Shaywitz, S. E., Shaywitz, B. A., Schnell, C., & Towle, V. R. (1988). Concurrent and predictive validity of the Yale Children's Inventory: An instrument to assess children with attentional deficits and learning disabilities. *Pediatrics, 81,* 562–571.

Shelton, T. L., & Barkley, R. A. (1994). Critical issues in the assessment of attention deficit disorders in children. *Topics in Language Disorders, 14,* 26–41.

Siegel, L. S. (1992). An evaluation of the discrepancy definition of dyslexia. *Journal of Learning Disabilities, 25,* 618–629.

Siegel, L. S., & Ryan, E. B. (1989). The development of working memory in normally achieving and subtypes of learning disabled. *Child Development, 60,* 973–980.

Silva, P. A., McGee, R., & Williams, S. (1985). Some characteristics of 9-year-old boys with general reading backwardness or specific reading retardation. *Journal of Child Psychology and Psychiatry, 26,* 407–421.

Simos, P. G., Breier, J. I., Fletcher, J. M., Bergman, E., & Papanicolaou, A. C. (2000). Cerebral mechanisms involved in word reading in dyslexia children: A magnetic source imaging approach. *Cerebral Cortex, 10,* 809–816.

Simos, P. G., Breier, J. I., Fletcher, J. M., Foorman, B. R., Bergman, E., Fishbeck, K., & Papanicolau, A. C. (2000). Brain activation profiles in dyslexic children during nonword reading: A magnetic source imaging study. *Neuroscience Reports, 290,* 61–65.

Simos, P. G., Fletcher, J. M., Bergman, E., Breier, J. I., Foorman, B. R., Castillo, E. M., Fitzgerald, M., & Papanicolaou, A. C. (2002). Dyslexia-specific brain activation profile becomes normal following successful remedial training. *Neurology, 58,* 1–10.

Simos, P. G., Fletcher, J. M., Foorman, B. R., Francis, D. J., Castillo, E. M., Davis, R. N., Fitzgerald, M., Mathes, P. G., Denton, C., & Papanicolaou, A. C. (2002). Brain activation profiles during the early stages of reading acquisition. *Journal of Child Neurology, 17,* 159–163.

Simos, P. G., Papanicolaou, A. C., Breier, J. I., Fletcher, J. M., Wheless, J. W., Maggio, W. W., Gormley, W., Constantinou, J. E. C., & Kramer, L. (2000). Insights into brain function and neural plasticity using magnetic source imaging. *Journal of Clinical Neurophysiology, 17,* 143–162.

Smith, F. (1971). *Understanding reading: A psycholinguistic analysis of reading and learning to read.* New York: Holt, Rinehart & Winston.

Smith, S. D., Pennington, B. F., Kimberling, W. J., & Ing., P. S. (1990). Familial dyslexia: Use of genetic linkage data to define subtypes. *Journal of the American Academy of Child and Adolescent Psychiatry, 29,* 338–348.

Snow, C. (2002). *Reading for understanding.* Santa Monica, CA: Rand.

Snow, C., Burns, M. S., & Griffin, P. (Eds.). (1998). *Preventing reading difficulties in young children.* Washington, DC: National Academy Press.

Snowling, M. J., Bishop, D. V. M., & Stothard, S. E. (2000). Is preschool language impairment a risk factor for dyslexia in adolescence? *Journal of Child Psychology and Psychiatry, 41,* 587–600.

Speece, D. L. (1993). Broadening the scope of classification research. In G. R. Lyon, D. B. Gray, J. F. Kavanagh, & N. A. Krasnegor (Eds.), *Better understanding learning disabilities: New views from research and their implications for education and public policies* (pp. 57–72). Baltimore: Brookes.

Speece, D. L., & Case, L. P. (2001). Classification in context: An alternative approach to identifying early reading disability. *Journal of Educational Psychology, 93,* 735–749.

Spreen, O. (1989). Learning disability, neurology, and long-term outcome: Some implications for the individual and for society. *Journal of Clinical and Experimental Neuropsychology, 11,* 389–408.

Stanovich, K. E. (1986). Matthew effects in reading: Some consequences of individuals differences in the acquisition of literacy. *Reading Research Quarterly, 21,* 360–407.

Stanovich, K. E. (1988). Explaining the differences between the dyslexic and the garden-variety poor reader: The phonological–core variable difference model. *Journal of Learning Disabilities, 21,* 590–604.

Stanovich, K. E. (1991). Word recognition: Changing perspectives. In M. L. Kamil, P. Mosenthal, & P. D. Pearson (Eds.), *Handbook of reading research* (Vol. 2, pp. 418–452). New York: Longman.

Stanovich, K. E. (1993). The construct validity of discrepancy definitions of reading disability. In G. R. Lyon, D. B. Gray, J. F. Kavanagh, & N. A. Krasnegor (Eds.), *Better understanding learning disabilities: New views on research and their implications for education and public policies* (pp. 273–307). Baltimore: Brookes.

Stanovich, K. E. (1994). Romance and reality. *The Reading Teacher, 47,* 280–291.

Stanovich, K. E., & Siegel, L. S. (1994). Phenotypic performance profile of children with reading disabilities: A regression-based test of the phonological–core variable–difference model. *Journal of Educational Psychology, 86,* 24–53.

Stephenson, S. (1905). Six cases of congenital word blindness affecting three generations of one family. *Opthalmoscope, 5,* 482–484.

Stein, J. (2001). The sensory basis of reading problems. *Developmental Neuropsychology, 20,* 509–534.

Sternberg, R. J. (1991). Are we reading too much into reading comprehension tests? *Journal of Reading, 34,* 540–545.

Sternberg, R. J., & Grigorenko, E. L. (2002). Difference scores in the identification of children with learning disabilities: It's time to use a different method. *Journal of School Psychology, 40,* 65–84.

Stevenson, J., Graham, P., Fredman, G., & McLoughlin, V. (1987). A twin study of genetic influences on reading and spelling ability and disability. *Journal of Child Psychology and Psychiatry, 28*(2), 229–247.

Stothard, S. E., & Hulme, C. (1992). Reading comprehension difficulties in children: the role of language comprehension and working memory skills. *Reading and Writing, 4,* 245–256.

Stothard, S. E., & Hulme, C. (1996). A comparison of reading comprehension and decoding difficulties in children. In C. Cornoldi & J. Oakhill (Eds.), *Reading comprehension difficulties: Processes and intervention* (pp. 93–112). Mahwah, NJ: Erlbaum.

Strang, J. D., & Rourke, B. P. (1985). Arithmetic disability subtypes: The neuropsychological significance of specific arithmetic impairment in childhood. In B. P. Rourke (Ed.), *Neuropsychology of learning disabilities: Essentials of subtype analysis.* (pp. 167–186). New York: Guilford Press.

Strauss, A. A., & Lehtinen, L. E. (1947). *Psychopathology and education of the brain-injured child: Vol. 2. Progress in theory and clinic.* New York: Grune & Stratton.

Strauss, A. A., & Werner, H. (1943). Comparative psychopathology of the brain-injured child and the traumatic brain-injured adult. *American Journal of Psychiatry, 19,* 835–838.

Stuebing, K. K., Fletcher, J. M., LeDoux, J. M., Lyon, G. R., Shaywitz, S. E., & Shaywitz, B. A. (2002). Validity of IQ-discrepancy classifications of reading disabilities: A meta-analysis. *American Educational Research Journal, 39,* 465–518.

Swanson, H. L. (1999). Reading research for students with LD: A meta-analysis of intervention outcomes. *Journal of Learning Disabilities, 32,* 504–532.

Swanson, H. L., & Sachse-Lee, C. (2001). A subgroup analysis of working memory in children with reading disabilities: Domain-general or domain-specific deficiency? *Journal of Learning Disabilities, 34,* 249–263.

Swanson, H. L., & Siegel, L. (2001). Learning disabilities as a working memory deficit. *Issues in Education, 7,* 1–48.

Tager-Flusberg, H., & Cooper, J. (1999). Present and future possibilities for defining a phenotype for specific language impairment. *Journal of Speech, Language, and Hearing Research, 42,* 1275–1278.

Talcott, J. B., Witton, C., McClean, M., Hansen, P. C., Rees, A., Green, G. G. R., & Stein, J. F. (2000). Visual and auditory transient sensitivity determines word decoding skills. *Proceedings of the Natural Academy of Sciences, USA, 97,* 2952–2958.

Tallal, P. (1980). Auditory temporal perception, phonics, and reading disabilities in children. *Brain and Language, 9,* 182–198.

Tallal, P. (1988). Developmental language disorders. In J. F. Kavanagh & T. Truss (Eds.), *Learning disabilities: Proceedings of the national conference* (pp. 181–272). Parkton, MD: York Press.

Tallal, P., Miller, S., Jenkins, W. M., & Merzenich, M. M. (1997). The role of temporal processing in developmental language-based learning disorders: Research and clinical implications. In B. A. Blachman (Ed.), *Foundations of reading acquisition and dyslexia: Implications for early intervention* (pp. 49–66). Mahwah, NJ: Erlbaum.

Tannock, R., Martinussen, R., & Frijters, J. (2000). Naming speed performance and stimulant effects indicate effortful, semantic processing deficits in attention-deficit/hyperactivity disorder. *Journal of Abnormal Child Psychology, 28,* 237–252.

Taylor, H. G., & Fletcher, J. M. (1983). Biological foundations of specific developmental disorders: Methods, findings, and future directions. *Journal of Child Clinical Psychology, 12,* 46–65.

Tomblin, J. B., & Zhang, X. (1999). Language patterns and etiology in children with specific language impairment. In H. Tager-Flusberg (Ed.), *Neurodevelopmental disorders* (pp. 361–382). Cambridge, MA: MIT Press.

Torgesen, J. K. (1991). Learning disabilities: Historical and conceptual issues. In B. Y. L. Wong (Ed.), *Learning about learning disabilities* (pp. 3–39). New York: Academic Press.

Torgesen, J. K. (2000). Individual responses in response to early interventions in reading: The lingering problem of treatment resisters. *Learning Disabilities Research and Practice, 15,* 55–64.

Torgesen, J. K., Alexander, A. W., Wagner, R. K., Rashotte, C. A., Voeller, K. K. S., & Conway, T. (2001). Intensive remedial instruction for children with severe reading disabilities: Immediate and long-term outcomes from two instructional approaches. *Journal of Learning Disabilities, 34,* 33–58.

Torgesen, J. K., & Wagner, R. K. (1998). Alternative diagnostic approaches for specific developmental reading disabilities. *Learning Disabilities Research and Practice, 13,* 220–232.

Torgesen, J. K., Wagner, R. K., Rashotte, C. A., Rose, E., Lindamood, P., Conway, J., & Garvan, C. (1999). Preventing reading failure in young children with phonological processing disabilities: Group and individual responses to instruction. *Journal of Educational Psychology, 91,* 579–594.

U.S. Department of Education. (1999). 34 CFR Parts 300 and 303: Assistance to the states for the education of children with disabilities and the early intervention program for infants and toddlers with disabilities. Final regulations. *Federal Register, 64*(48), 12406–12672.

U.S. Office of Education. (1968). *First annual report of the National Advisory Committee on Handicapped Children.* Washington, DC: U.S. Department of Health, Education and Welfare.

U.S. Office of Education. (1977). Assistance to states for education for handicapped children: Procedures for evaluating specific learning disabilities. *Federal Register, 42,* G1082–G1085.

van der Wissell, A., & Zegers, F. E. (1985). Reading retardation revisited. *British Journal of Developmental Psychology, 3,* 3–9.

Vaughn, S. R., Linan-Thompson, S., & Hickman-Davis, P. (2002). *Response to treatment as a means of identifying students with reading/learning disabilities.* Manuscript submitted for publication.

Vellutino, F. R. (1979). *Dyslexia: Theory and research.* Cambridge, Mass.: The M.I.T. Press.

Vellutino, F. R. (2001). Further analysis of the relationship between reading achievement and intelligence: Response to Naglieri. *Journal of Learning Disabilities, 34,* 306–310.

Vellutino, F. R., Scanlon, D., & Fletcher, J. M. (in press). Research in the study of specific reading disability (dyslexia): What have we learned in the past four decades? *British Journal of Psychology*.

Vellutino, F. R., Scanlon, D. M., & Lyon, G. R. (2000). Differentiating between difficult-to-remediate and readily remediated poor readers: More evidence against the IQ–achievement discrepancy definition for reading disability. *Journal of Learning Disabilities, 33,* 223–238.

Vellutino, F. R., Scanlon, D. M., Sipay, E. R., Small, S. G., Pratt, A., Chen, R., & Denckla, M. B. (1996). Cognitive profiles of difficult-to-remediate and readily remedeated poor readers: Early intervention as a vehicle for distinguishing between cognitive and experimental deficits as basic causes of specific reading disability. *Journal of Educational Psychology, 88,* 601–638.

Waber, D. P., Weiler, M. D., Wolff, P. H., Bellinger, D., Marcus, D. J., Ariel, R., Forbes, P., & Wypij, D. (2001). Processing of rapid auditory stimuli in school-age children referred for evaluation of learning disorders. *Child Development, 72,* 37–49.

Wadsworth, S. J., Olson, R. K., Pennington, B. F., & DeFries, J. C. (2000). Differential genetic etiology of reading disability as a function of IQ. *Journal of Learning Disabilities, 33,* 192–199.

Wagner, R. K., & Torgesen, J. K. (1987). The nature of phonological processing and its causal role in the acquisition of reading skills. *Psychological Bulletin, 101,* 192–212.

Wagner, R. K., Torgesen, J. K., Laughon, P., Simmons, K., & Rashotte, C. A. (1993). Development of young readers' phonological processing abilities. *Journal of Educational Psychology, 85,* 83–103.

Wagner, R. K., Torgesen, J. K., & Rashotte, C. A. (1994). The development of reading-related phonological processing abilities: New evidence of bi-directional causality from a latent variable longitudinal study. *Developmental Psychology, 30,* 73–87.

Wernicke, C. (1894). *Grundriss der Psychiatrie: Psychophysiologische Eindeitung*. Wiesbaden, Germany.

Wiederholt, J. L. (1974). Historical perspectives on the education of the learning disabled. In L. Mann & D. A. Sabatino (Eds.), *The second review of special education* (pp. 103–152). Austin TX: Pro-Ed.

Willcutt, E. G., & Pennington, B. F. (2000). Psychiatric comorbidity in children and adolescents with reading disability. *Journal of Child Psychology and Psychiatry, 41,* 1039–1048.

Wilson, K. M., & Swanson, H. L. (2001). Are mathematics disabilities due to a domain-general or a domain-specific working memory deficit? *Journal of Learning Disabilities, 34,* 237–248.

Wise, B. W., Ring, J., & Olson, R. K. (2000). Individual differences in gains from computer-assisted remedial reading. *Journal of Experimental Child Psychology, 77,* 197–235.

Wolf, M., & Bowers, P. G. (1999). The double deficit hypothesis for the developmental dyslexias. *Journal of Educational Psychology, 91,* 415–438.

Wolf, M., Bowers, P. G., & Biddle, K. (2001). Naming-speed processes, timing, and reading: A conceptual review. *Journal of Learning Disabilities, 33,* 387–407.

Wolff, P. H., Michel, G. F., Ovrut, M., & Drake, C. (1990). Rate and timing precision of motor coordination in developmental dyslexia. *Developmental Psychology, 26,* 349–359.

Wong, B. Y. L. (1991). *Learning about learning disabilities.* New York: Academic Press.

Wood, F. B., & Felton, R. H. (1994). Separate linguistic and attentional factors in the development of reading. *Topics in Language Disorders, 14,* 42–57.

Wood, F. B, Felton, R. H., Flowers, L., & Naylor, C. (1991). Neurobehavioral definition of dyslexia. In D. D. Duane & D. B. Gray (Eds.), *The reading brain: The biological basis of dyslexia* (pp. 1–26). Parkton, MD: York Press.

Wood, F. B., & Grigorenko, E. L. (2001). Emerging issues in the genetics of dyslexia: A methodological preview. *Journal of Learning Disabilities, 34,* 503–512.

World Health Organization. (1992). *The ICD-10 classification of mental and behavioral disorders: Clinical descriptions and diagnostic guidelines.* Geneva: Author.

Wristers, K. J., Francis, D. J., Foorman, B. R., Fletcher, J. M., & Swank, P. R. (2002). Growth in precursor reading skills: Do low-achieving and IQ-discrepant readers develop differently? *Learning Disability Research and Practice, 17,* 19–34.

Ysseldyke, J. E., & Algozzine, B. (1983). LD or not LD?: That's not the question. *Journal of Learning Disabilities, 16,* 29–31.

Zigmond, N. (1993). Learning disabilities from an educational perspective. In G. R. Lyon, D. B. Gray, J. F. Kavanagh, & N. A. Krasnegor (Eds.), *Better understanding learning disabilities: New views from research and their implications for education and public policies* (pp. 27–56). Baltimore: Brookes.

V

INFANTS AND CHILDREN AT RISK FOR DISORDER

CHAPTER THIRTEEN

Disorder and Risk for Disorder during Infancy and Toddlerhood

Karlen Lyons-Ruth
Charles H. Zeanah
Diane Benoit

Sameroff (1992) has noted that the study of behavior in context was the most significant advance in developmental research in the latter part of the 20th century. This is no surprise to those who study, observe, or treat infants and young children; all of these professionals must be impressed again and again with the extraordinary importance of context for infant development. Increasingly, the infant's relationship with the primary caregiver has been considered the most important context in which to consider infant development and psychopathology (Crockenberg & Leerkes, 2000; Zeanah, Larrieu, Valliere, & Heller, 2000).

Nevertheless, this observation also underscores a major challenge of attempting to conceptualize disorders of infancy. A series of questions challenges our efforts to define these disorders. Can infants be diagnosed as having within-the-person psychiatric disorders or are their symptoms relationship-specific? To what degree should the caregiving contexts of infants' development be considered an integral part of a relationship disorder, as opposed to an associated feature of individual disordered behavior? Are disturbed behaviors in infants indicative of disorder per se, or do they merely indicate risk for subsequent disorder? To what degree are we to take into account here-and-now suffering, or must we also demonstrate links between infant developmental disturbances and subsequent disorders? How we answer these questions may lead us in different directions.

There are, in fact, two major and quite different traditions in infant mental health regarding how to conceptualize psychiatric disturbances in young children. These approaches make different assumptions about disturbances, and seem likely to direct efforts at intervention differently as well.

One tradition (which has dominated research in developmental psychology and developmental psychopathology) suggests that infants may be considered as having a number of specific risk factors increasing, and/or protective factors decreasing, the probability that they will develop a given disorder in later childhood. These risk and protective factors may be biological (intrinsic), social (contextual), or both. Much of contemporary research has been devoted to detecting early "markers" of subsequent disorder, with the aim of delineating developmental pathways or trajectories of at-risk infants.

Another tradition (which has more clinical than empirical roots) suggests that infants may have formal psychiatric disorders, even in the first 3 years of life. Research in support of this tradition is only beginning to appear, and there is much work to be done to test some of the assertions that have been made. Nonetheless, this approach to disorders of infancy appears to have widespread support (Minde, 1995; Zeanah, 1993; Zero to Three/National Center for Clinical Infant Programs, 1994).

The plan for this chapter is first to consider some of the conceptual controversies regarding relational versus individual approaches to diagnostic classification issues, which emerge with particular clarity in the study of disorders of infancy. Current competing approaches to diagnosis in infancy are discussed. Research relevant to the definitions and correlates of the various particular "disorders" of infancy is then reviewed—including research on common clinical problems not yet represented in the fourth edition of the *Diagnostic and Statistical Manual of Mental Disorders* (DSM-IV; American Psychiatric Association [APA], 1994), such as colic or regulatory disorders. In the final section, longitudinal developmental research exploring both infant behavioral constellations and family characteristics that may constitute risk factors, precursors, or prodromal forms of later childhood disorders is selectively reviewed. Three particularly active areas of current research are considered: studies of the intergenerational transmission of patterns of relational behavior; research exploring the context and correlates of disorganized/disoriented infant attachment behaviors; and recent studies of early predictors of later psychiatric symptomatology, including aggressive behavior disorders, anxiety disorders, and depressive and dissociative symptoms.

DIAGNOSTIC CLASSIFICATION IN INFANCY

The clinical tradition of examining disorders of infancy requires us to consider some of the special challenges of diagnostic classification relevant to this age group. Emde, Bingham, and Harmon (1993) have suggested that these challenges include the multidisciplinary nature of infant mental health, the developmental perspective inherent in infant mental health, the multigenerational focus of problems, and the prevention orientation of the field. These features complicate the diagnostic process in infancy, but the failure to include such features may also be responsible in part for the widespread dissatisfaction among clinicians with the approach to disorders of infancy taken by standard nosologies (Zeanah, 1993).

DSM-IV and Disorders of Infancy

The disorders of infancy and early childhood described in DSM-IV (APA, 1994; see Table 13.1) are limited in both number and scope, and with few exceptions, they use the same criteria for children under 3 years of age that they use for children older than 3 years. Thus they fail to take into account possible developmental differences in symptom picture, the implications of rapid developmental change over the first 3 years of life, and the likelihood of symptoms or syndromes specific to this developmental period.

The Zero to Three Scheme and Disorders of Infancy

In response to these issues, a task force from the Zero to Three/National Center for Clinical Infant Programs proposed a more detailed classificatory scheme for disorders apparent in the first 3 years of life. Chaired initially by Stanley Greenspan, and later by Serena Wieder, this group included a number of influential figures in infant mental health who met regularly to formulate approaches to the problem. This effort resulted in the publication of a manual (Zero to Three, 1994) delineating criteria intended to capture the clinical phenomenology of disorders of infancy (see Table 13.2). This scheme—referred to in brief as the *Diagnostic Classification: 0–3* (DC:0–3)—describes seven specific types of disorders believed to occur in infants and young children and provides criteria for diagnosing them. In addition, it adopts a multiaxial approach to diagnosis similar to that of the DSM (APA, 1980, 1987, 1994), although its axes are somewhat different. The DC:0–3 Axis I includes the disorders listed in the first part of Table 13.2.

The DC:0–3 Axis II comprises a classification of relationship disorders—that is, a relationship with a caregiver that is so disturbed as to constitute a disorder. Nevertheless, the relationship disorder is believed to exist between the caregiver and infant rather than within the infant. Types of disordered relationships defined include "overinvolved," "underinvolved," "anxious/tense," "angry/hostile," "abusive," and "mixed." In this

TABLE 13.1. Psychiatric Disorders and Conditions of the First 3 Years: DSM-IV, Axis I

Feeding and eating disorders of infancy or early childhood
- Pica
- Rumination disorder
- Feeding disorder of infancy or early childhood

Reactive attachment disorder of infancy or early childhood

Pervasive developmental disorders
- Autistic disorder
- Rett's disorder
- Childhood disintegrative disorder (after age 2)

Problems related to abuse or neglect
- Physical abuse of child
- Sexual abuse of child
- Neglect of child

Relational problems
- Parent–child relational problem

Note. Axis I diagnostic categories particularly relevant to infants and toddlers appearing in American Psychiatric Association (1994).

TABLE 13.2. Diagnostic Classification: 0–3 (DC:0–3)

Axis I: Primary diagnosis
- Disorders of relating and communicating
  - Multisystem developmental disorder
- Regulatory disorders
- Eating behavior disorder
- Sleep behavior disorder
- Traumatic stress disorder
- Disorders of affect
  - Anxiety disorders
  - Mood disorders
  - Mixed disorder of emotional expressiveness
  - Gender identity disorder
  - Reactive attachment disorder
- Adjustment disorder

Axis II: Relationship disorder classification
- Overinvolved
- Underinvolved
- Anxious/tense
- Angry/hostile
- Abusive
- Mixed

Axis III: Other medical and developmental conditions

Axis IV: Psychosocial stressors

Axis V: Functional emotional developmental level

Note. Diagnostic system presented in Zero to Three/National Center for Clinical Infant Programs (1994).

classificatory system, a relationship disorder may occur with or without an Axis I disorder, and vice versa.

The DC:0–3 Axes III and IV are quite similar to their DSM-IV counterparts. Axis III includes physical, neurological, or developmental problems not considered elsewhere. These may or may not be related to the Axis I or Axis II diagnoses. Axis IV comprises a rating of psychosocial stressors. Axis V is used to describe the infant's functional emotional level. A Parent–Infant Relationship Global Assessment Scale (PIRGAS) is also included in an appendix for the purpose of rating the level of relationship adaptation or disturbance. Ratings range from "well adapted" through "perturbed," "disturbed," and "disordered" to "frankly dangerous." Only if the relationship is determined to be disordered or dangerously impaired on this scale does an Axis II classification apply.

Although widely adopted by clinicians, the DC:0–3 nosology has not been well studied. Eight years after its publication, there are only a handful of studies examining the reliability and validity of its criteria. This is disappointing, indeed, as a major hope for the system was to stimulate research. A significant problem is that although some disorders are described clearly with well-delineated decision rules (e.g., traumatic stress disorder), others are vaguely defined (e.g., reactive attachment disorder [RAD]) or unclear with regard to how many criteria are needed to make a diagnosis (e.g., regulatory disorders). This has led to calls for a new research agenda to focus on disorders of early childhood (Leckman, 2000). The American Academy of Child and Adolescent Psychiatry has provided preliminary support for an effort to develop "research diagnostic criteria" for disorders of early childhood (ages 2–5 years), in order to advance research and enhance clinical practice. It remains to be seen whether this will prove more stimulating to investigators concerned about the validity of early childhood disorders.

Other Diagnostic Issues

With both the DSM-IV and DC:0–3 diagnostic systems, there is an implicit acceptance of the traditional biomedical model of a categorical typology of disorders. Nevertheless, we might reasonably ask whether a continuous or dimensional approach to psychopathology during infancy may have important advantages over a categorical or disorder approach, as some have suggested (Rutter, 1994). Some have advocated a continuous approach to diagnosis with older children as well, although there is considerable controversy about this (Quay, 1986). RAD is an example of a disorder in which both approaches are being explored in young children (Zeanah & Boris, 2000).

Another issue to be considered is whether disorders of infancy are better conceptualized as within individuals or as between infants and their primary caregivers. Sameroff and Emde (1989) have suggested that with a few notable exceptions, such as autistic spectrum disorders, most disorders of early infancy are relationship disorders rather than individual disorders. Anchoring their approach in disturbances in the infant–caregiver relationship, and particularly in the caregiver's regulatory function for the infant, they have defined different levels of disturbance (relationship perturbations, disturbances, and disorders) and provided some preliminary ideas about diagnosis (Anders, 1989). The Zero to Three task force members have made two efforts to incorporate an approach to relationship difficulties. First, they have included an axis of relationship disorders (Axis II) in DC:0–3, although the types of disordered relationships described in the DC:0–3 system are quite different from those proposed by Sameroff and Emde (1989). An infant may be diagnosed as having an Axis I disorder or an Axis II disorder or both in this system. Second, they have included the PIRGAS, a continuous scale of relationship adaptation, which was developed specifically from Sameroff and Emde's (1989) proposed continuum of relationship difficulties. Nevertheless, data about the reliability and validity of the PIRGAS are still preliminary. An important question is whether it is possible or desirable to accommodate such divergent views about the nature of developmental disturbances in the same classificatory system.

In summary, the extant systems of classifying disorders of infancy are preliminary (in the case of DC:0–3) or underdeveloped (in the case of DSM-IV). An attempt to validate the classification systems and the specific criteria included for various disorders is a necessary next step. For the discussion that follows, we have selected for review common problems seen by infant mental health clinicians. We begin with problems commonly believed to be more biologically rooted, such as regulatory disorders and colic, and conclude with disorders believed to be more experientially rooted, such as posttraumatic stress disorder (PTSD) and RAD. Between these two poles of the spectrum are disorders believed to have more variable or mixed contributions from individual differences in central nervous system functioning and psychological experiences. Throughout the discussion we emphasize the ongoing importance of contextual factors, and especially the primary caregiving relationship, for the expression and experience of disorders throughout this spectrum.

DISORDERS OF INFANCY AND TODDLERHOOD

Regulatory Disorders

As just discussed, several common problems encountered during infancy are not included in DSM-IV. However, given the frequency of presentation of these problems and the controversies surrounding infant diagnosis, they are reviewed here.

Description of the Disorders

Regulatory disorders are characterized by "difficulties in regulating physiological, sensory, attentional, and motor or affective processes, and in organizing a calm, alert, or affectively positive state" (Greenspan & Wieder, 1993, p. 282). Clinically, infants with regulatory disorders are behaviorally (or temperamentally) difficult. They may present with an inability to regulate sleep–wake cycles, mood, and self-soothing, or with such difficulties as irritability, feeding problems, hypersensitivities to stimulation, and a lack of cuddliness. (Colic, another symptom that many regard as a disorder in its own right, is discussed separately below.) Most of these difficulties are believed to reflect, or be associated with, problems in sensory, sensory–motor, or processing capacities; these may include impaired reactivity to auditory, visual, tactile, gustatory, vestibular, or olfactory stimulation, temperature, motor tone, motor planning skills, fine motor skills, and capacity to discriminate or integrate auditory–verbal or visual–spatial stimuli. "Sensory integration" is a central concept of regulation and regulatory disorders. The theory of sensory integration strongly emphasizes the importance of vestibular, proprioceptive, and tactile stimulation and processing capacity to development and behavior; describes hierarchical levels of brain function and sequential stages in neurological development; and views sensory integration as requisite to all perceptual–motor activities and all "higher-level" activities. Several instruments have been developed to assess children's sensory integration, but these are often intended for children older than 3 years old (described in Barton & Robins, 2000, and Hoehn & Baumeister, 1994). Most of the research on sensory integration and sensory integration therapy (which was first developed for use with children with cerebral palsy, was then used with children with mental retardation and learning disabilities, is costly, and typically requires more than 1 year) has likewise been conducted on children over age 3. Critical reviews of the literature (Hoehn & Baumeister, 1994; Polatajko, Kaplan, & Wilson, 1992) and a recent meta-analysis (Vargas & Camilli, 1998) raise serious questions about the validity of the concept of sensory integration, as well as the efficacy of sensory integration therapy (showing a weighted average effect size of .03, not significantly different from zero).

Diagnostic Considerations

Although regulatory disorders are not included in the diagnostic nomenclature of DSM-IV, Greenspan and Wieder (1993) have described six types of regulatory disorders, each including specific diagnostic criteria: Type I (hypersensitive type), Type II (underreactive type), Type III (active/aggressive type), Type IV (mixed type), Type V (sleeping difficulties), and Type VI (eating difficulties). They suggest that regulatory disorders may affect one or more areas of development and may range in severity from mild to severe. In the most severe regulatory disorders, physiological or state repertoires are affected. For example, infants may have irregular breathing, startles, gagging, and so forth. In the mildest regulatory disorders, infants may exhibit sleep, eating, or elimination problems. Between these two extremes of severity, other difficulties may be found in the area of (1) gross and fine motor activity (e.g., abnormal tonus or posture, jerky or limp movements, poor motor planning); (2) attentional organization (e.g., driven or perseverating on small details); or (3) affective organization (including predominant affective tone, range, and modulation of affective experiences).

Regulatory disorders are diagnosed only in infants older than 6 months, because transient difficulties with self-regulation (e.g., sleep problems) are common in young infants and resolve spontaneously by 5–6 months of age (DeGangi, Craft, & Castellan, 1991). Furthermore, in order for a diagnosis of a regulatory disorder to be made, both behavioral and constitutional maturational elements must be present, and the difficulties in sensory, sensory–motor, or processing capacities must affect daily adaptation and relationships (DeGangi, Craft, & Castellan, 1991; Greenspan & Wieder, 1993). There are no data regarding the reliability and validity of regulatory disorders. Although the concept of regulatory disorders has been helpful clinically, the subtypes remain confusing and ambiguous (Barton & Robins, 2000). Moreover, of the children who experience some of the symptoms described for regulatory disorders, there are no guidelines regarding who may suffer from regulatory "difficulties" and not a regulatory "disorder."

Developmental Course and Prognosis

There are no documented adult equivalents of regulatory disorders. To date, only one study (DeGangi, Porges, Sickel, & Greenspan, 1993) has examined the natural history and prognosis of regulatory disorders. In this follow-up study, 9 out of 11 infants with a regulatory disorder diagnosed at ages 8–10 months (and 13 out of 24 controls) were followed for 4 years. Findings from this study showed that 8 of the 9 regulatory-disordered infants had developmental, sensory–motor, and/or emotional and behavioral problems at 4 years of age. In addition, there were significant group differences on measures of cognitive abilities, attention span and activity level, emotional maturity, motor maturity, and tactile sensitivity between those preschoolers without and those with regulatory disorders (in the expected direction). The authors concluded that if left untreated, regulatory disorders and the associated behavioral difficulties may persist.

Epidemiology

The incidence and prevalence rates of regulatory disorders have not yet been established. However, regulatory disorders are believed to be rare, and there may be an overrepresentation of male subjects (DeGangi, Craft, Castellan, 1991). No information is yet available on either socioeconomic or cultural variations of regulatory disorders.

Etiology

Although the etiology of regulatory disorders is unclear, dysfunctions in the autonomic nervous system have been hypothesized; however, such dysfunctions may be physiological correlates of these disorders rather than etiological factors. In support of this hypothesis, DeGangi, DiPietro, Greenspan, and Porges (1991) found that some physiological responses relating to vagal tone (heart period and cardiac vagal tone) differentiated 8- to 11-month-old infants with regulatory disorders (n = 11) from infants without regulatory disorders (n = 24). Specifically, the infants with regulatory disorders tended to have higher baseline vagal tone and showed inconsistent vagal reactivity (i.e., heterogeneous response to sensory and cognitive tasks). These findings suggest that infants with regulatory disorders may have autonomic (parasympathetic) hyperirritability caused by defective central neural programs and mediated via neurotransmitters through the vagus nerve (DeGangi, DiPietro, et al., 1991; Porges, 1991).

In a study to identify early physiological correlates of regulatory disorders, Zeskind, Marshall, and Goff (1996) studied the autonomic regulation of newborn infants found to be normal and healthy by routine physical and neurological examinations. They measured the children's cry threshold, as characteristics of the cries of a newborn infant, such as threshold and sound, are sensitive to individual differences in the functional integrity of the infant's developing parasympathetic and sympathetic nervous system. In addition, Zeskind et al. (1996) completed a spectrum analysis of heart rate and made observations of the infants' behavior (e.g., cry reactivity, behavioral state, behavioral startles). Thirty-seven infants had a typical cry threshold (i.e., they required one rubber band snap to the sole of the foot to elicit crying), and 17 infants had a high cry threshold (i.e., they required three or more rubber band snaps to the sole of the foot to elicit crying; high cry threshold has been described as reflecting nervous system dysfunction). Behaviors long described as characteristic of difficult temperament differentiated infants in the study (such behaviors include less biobehavioral rhythmicity, and variations in self-regulation and in the threshold, latency, and duration of infant reactivity and heart rate variability). Results provided evidence that infants with a high cry threshold showed a wide range of biobehavioral measures previously described as reflecting the homeostasis properties and regulation of an infant's autonomic nervous systems. The study did not follow the children beyond the neonatal period and did not examine whether the infants with high cry threshold developed regulatory disorders. No genetic etiological contributor has yet been hypothesized for these disorders.

DeGangi (1991) examined possible environmental factors, especially caregiving environment, that might contribute to regulatory disorders. Her group found that, compared to mothers of infants without regulatory disorders, mothers of infants with regulatory disorders showed less contingent responses, less physical proximity, and more flat affect during play interactions. Parents of infants with regulatory disorders also have more negative perceptions of their infants than do parents of infants without regulatory disorders (DeGangi et al., 1993). Although findings from these studies do not point directly to an environmental etiology for regulatory disorders, they suggest that the quality of the caregiving environment may contribute to the improvement or perpetuation of some regulatory disorders.

Future Directions

To date, a few case vignettes of children affected by regulatory disorders have been described (Barton & Robins, 2000; Benoit, 2000b; Maldonado-Duran & Sauceda-Garcia, 1996). More research is necessary to validate this diagnostic grouping; to determine the disorders' prevalence, physiological correlates, developmental course, and prognosis; and to examine the relative contributions of both the autonomic nervous system and the caregiving environment to regulatory disorders. The relationship between sleeping and feeding disorders and regulatory disorders should be explored as well. Finally, future research should examine prevention and treatment issues.

Colic

Although colic is not a DSM-IV diagnosis, it is a common problem during infancy. Because colic is often viewed as a form of excessive crying, it is useful to review normal patterns of crying during infancy. In his landmark study of 80 mothers who kept detailed diaries of their infants' daily patterns of crying for 3 months, Brazelton (1962) found that in normal, healthy infants, the duration of crying increases progressively from birth to 6 weeks of age. By 6 weeks old, normal infants reach a peak of crying, with approximately 2 hours and 45 minutes of crying per day. By 12 weeks old, the average duration of crying decreases to approximately 1 hour per day. Brazelton also found that normal crying patterns tend to cluster around the evening hours, beginning at 3 weeks, peaking at 6 weeks, and gradually disappearing by 12 weeks. Barr, Kramer, Pless, Boisjoly, and Leduc (1989), found that the amount of crying over 24 hours or by period of day was not affected by method of feeding (breast vs. bottle).

Description of the Disorder

Lester, Boukydis, Garcia-Coll, and Hole (1990) described the physical and behavioral signs of colic as including facial grimacing, flexed elbows, clenched fists, drawn up or stiff and extended knees, tense and distended abdomen, tightly closed or widely opened eyes, arched back, red face, cold feet, brief breath-holding episodes, increased bowel sounds, and gas. Associated features of colic include spasms in the gastrointestinal tract. These spasms are believed to be secondary to the colic rather than causing the colic (Lester et al., 1990). Infants with colic are more likely to have or develop difficult temperament than noncolicky infants even after the colic has ended (Lester et al., 1990). Sleep problems have been found in infants with colic (Stahlberg & Savilahti, 1986; Weissbluth, 1987). In fact, Weissbluth (1987) suggests that colic reflects a disturbance of the sleep–wake control mechanisms, suggesting an underlying autonomic imbalance and providing some support for Greenspan and Wieder's (1993) view that colic may represent one manifestation of a child's difficulty in self-regulation.

Diagnostic Considerations

Several attempts have been made to provide empirical definitions for normal crying, excessive crying, and colic in infancy (Barr, Rotman, Yaremko, Leduc, & Francoeur, 1992; Lester et al., 1990; Wessel, Cobb, Jackson, Harris, & Detwilet, 1954). Many clinicians and researchers use "colic" and "excessive crying" interchangeably, or view colic as an extreme form of the normal crying activity in infants (Barr, 1990; Brazelton, 1990). Wessel et al. (1954) have provided the most widely used definition of colic (also known as the "rule of 3"), in which colic is defined as crying or fussing (paroxysmal onset) occurring for more than 3 hours per day, 3 days per week, and for 3 weeks in otherwise healthy infants during the first 3–4 months of life. Lester et al. (1990) empirically define colic as a syndrome consisting of four major characteristics: (1) paroxysmal onset; (2) distinctive, high-pitched pain cry; (3) physical signs associated with hypertonia (described above); and (4) inconsolability.

Barr et al. (1992) found that infants with colic in one sample could be classified into two groups, based on their symptomatology: (1) those with "Wessel colic," for whom mothers reported the symptomatology originally described by Wessel et al. (1954); and (2) those with "non-Wessel colic," for whom mothers reported crying and fussing periods on fewer than 3 days per week. Barr and his colleagues reported that "maternal measures of total daily crying/fussing duration, crying/fussing bout length, and infant temperament and objective analyses of facial activity showed a consistent pattern of differences in which Wessel's colic infants differed from both non-Wessel's colic and control infants, who in turn did not differ from each other" (1992, p. 14). Mothers of infants in both groups characterized their infants' cries following feeds as being more "sick-sounding."

Developmental Course and Prognosis

Several studies have examined prospectively the outcome of children who had colic during infancy and provide contradictory evidence with respect to the long-term consequences of colic. In a survey 1 year after infants had colic, Räihä, Lehtonen, Korhonen, and Korvenranta (1996) studied 49 families of infants with colic (classified as severe colic in 32 cases and moderate colic in 17 cases) and 49 controls. Findings showed that the overall "atmosphere" in the families had improved, compared to the period when the infants were colicky. However, families in the group with severe colic had more difficulties in communication, more unresolved conflicts, more dissatisfaction, and a greater lack of empathy than the control families. Families of children who had had moderate colic coped nearly as well as the controls. Three years after the same infants were diagnosed with colic, Räihä, Lehtonen, Korhonen, and Korvenranta (1997) found that the same families of infants who had had moderately to severely colicky infants did not differ significantly from control families with respect to family characteristics. No objective assessment of family functioning was completed; only self-report inventories were completed by subjects (usually one family member). Furthermore, different tools were used at the 1-year and 3-year follow-up periods, making comparisons between time periods difficult.

In a Finnish follow-up study 3 years after colic, Rautava, Lehtonen, Helenius, and Sillanpää (1995) examined 338 infants with colic and 866 infants without colic, using the Achenbach Child Behavior Checklist; the Denver Developmental Screening Test; and questionnaires completed by mothers, fathers, and nurses regarding interactions within the family, parents' satisfaction with daily life, child caring, and child behavior and development. Results showed that families of children who had been colicky during infancy were experiencing more distress 3 years later.

Canivet, Jakobsson, and Hagander (2000) found that 4 years after infants had colic (according to Wessel's criteria and modifications of these criteria), they and their families did not differ from control children without colic and their families on measures of behavior, sleeping habits, number of hospital stays, weight and height, "family climate," parental education, and parental socioeconomic status (SES). Children who had a history of colic during infancy differed from those who did not with respect to temperamental characteristics as reported by their parents: The formerly colicky children displayed more negative emotions, including more temper tantrums. These children also differed from those with no history of colic in regard to their mealtime behavior: Compared to controls, the formerly colicky children displayed more negative moods during meals, were less likely to enjoy meals and to like eating, and refused certain foods more often. More formerly colicky children than controls also reported psychosomatic complaints, specifically stomachaches.

Lehtonen, Korhonen, and Korvenranta (1994) compared 59 colicky infants and 58 controls with respect to their mothers' perceptions of temperament and sleeping patterns. Results showed that at age 3 months, the infants with colic were described by their mothers as more intense in their reactions, less persistent, more distractible, and more negative in their moods, compared to matched counterparts. At 12 months old, infants who had a history of colic and those who did not were rated similarly overall by their mothers on a temperament questionnaire, although infants with a history of colic were described by their mothers during interviews as more active and less persistent, and as more difficult than average in 23% of cases, compared to 5% of controls. No difference was found between the two groups with respect to their sleeping patterns at 8 and 12 months.

Some researchers have found an association between the amount of crying at 6–8 weeks old and family disruption 3 years later, but early crying had little impact on a child's later behavior (Elliott, Pederson, & Mogan, 1997). No mortality associated with colic has been documented. Colic continues to be perceived by clinicians as a transitory phenomenon that spontaneously improves after the first 4–6 months of life. There is no known adult equivalent of the disorder.

Epidemiology

Because of the absence of universally accepted definitions of excessive crying and colic, incidence and prevalence estimates vary greatly. Such estimates, ranging from 3% to 40% (Brazelton, 1990; Canivet et al., 2000; Lehtonen & Korvenranta, 1995; Lester et al., 1990), may actually magnify the "true" incidence and prevalence rates of colic, as they probably reflect the incidence and prevalence rates for both excessive crying and colic.

The incidence rates of colic are similar for full-term and age-corrected preterm infants. Controlled studies have shown that there is no difference in the prevalence of colic between infants who are breast-fed and infants who are bottle-fed (Forsyth, McCarthy, & Leventhal, 1985; Illingworth, 1954; Paradise, 1966; Stahlberg, 1984). There are no documented sex differences or socioeconomic factors, although some cultural variations in crying have been documented (e.g., Barr, 1990).

Etiology

Little is known about the etiology and pathophysiology of colic. Several potential causes of colic have been studied, but findings from these studies remain inconclusive. A distinction between "intrinsic" (or biological) and "extrinsic" (or environmental) causes of colic has been made (Illingworth, 1985).

Suspected intrinsic causes or risk factors for colic include food allergy (particularly to cow's milk protein), hypertonia secondary to gastrointestinal contractions, immaturity of the gastrointestinal tract, and progesterone deficiency. Suspected extrinsic causes of colic include maternal anxiety, personality factors, inappropriate handling, the mother–infant relationship, tobacco smoking, maternal diet, and inadequate feeding (Garrison & Christakis, 2000; see Lester et al., 1990, for a review; see Lucassen et al., 1998, for a review of the effects of various interventions from 27 controlled trials; see also Lust, Brown, & Thomas, 1996; Reijneveld, Brugman, & Hirasing, 2000). For example, mothers of infants with excessive crying have been described as depressed, exhausted, and angry, and as providing fewer positive responses to their infants than controls. Some researchers showed differences between measures of maternal feelings and causal attribution of infant crying between mothers of colicky infants and mothers of infants without colic (Pauli-Pott, Becker, Mertesacker, & Beckmann, 2000). In a longitudinal study of 40 infant–mother pairs (20 with "irritable" infants who had colic and 20 controls), Keefe, Kotzer, Froese-Fretz, and Curtin (1996) found significant differences between the two groups: The irritable infants showed more crying, more intense crying, more disruption in sleep–wake cycles, and less synchrony in mother–infant interactions. On the Nursing Child Assessment Feeding Scale, mothers of irritable infants showed fewer social and emotional growth-fostering behaviors, and scored lower overall on the feeding observation; irritable infants were less responsive to their mothers and scored significantly lower on the subtotal of infant items than the nonirritable infants. However, when the feeding observation was repeated at 16 weeks of age, no significant differences in interactive behaviors were noted for the mothers or infants in either group. Because of inconclusive evidence from research on etiology and pathophysiology, some researchers and clinicians view colic as the final common pathway between various intrinsic and extrinsic factors. The direction of effects has not been clarified.

Lester and his colleagues (Lester & Boukydis, 1991; Lester et al., 1990) argue that colic may be caused by an imbalance in the autonomic (interplay between the sympathetic and parasympathetic) nervous system. They base their argument in part on their findings about the specific acoustic characteristics of the cry of infants with colic. Indeed, they argue that the vagal complex (cranial nerves IX to XII) and the phrenic and thoracic nerves control the acoustic characteristics of the cry, in addition to influencing some of the muscles of the larynx (Lester, 1987; Lester & Boukydis, 1991). Some infants may experience sympathetic dominance, which triggers the sudden onset of crying, the high-pitched pain cry, and the hypertonia characteristic of colic. Lester et al. (1990) argue that infants with colic have lower thresholds of reactivity, which can be traced to the hypothalamic–limbic circuits that initiate the cry (Lester & Boukydis, 1991) and which result in higher levels of motor arousal to stimulation (hypertonia). Lester and his colleagues argue that because of the diminished parasympathetic inhibition, an infant with colic lacks regulatory capacities for self-soothing, cannot be soothed by the caregiver, and is thus difficult to console.

Prudhomme White, Gunnar, Larson, Donzella, and Barr (2000) have provided evidence that colic may be associated with a disruption or delay in the establishment of the circadian rhythm in activity of the hypothalamic–pituitary–adrenocortical (HPA) axis and associated sleep–wake activity. They found no evidence of greater responsivity in the physiological substrate of difficult temperament for colicky infants and provided evidence of similarity in temperament once colic was resolved. Compared with controls, infants with colic displayed a blunted rhythm in cortisol production at home and slept about 2 hours less than controls. Nighttime sleep was statistically different between the groups when fussing and crying were controlled for statistically.

Lester et al. (1990) also found that the cry characteristics of infants with colic differed from those of infants without colic. They studied a group of 16 full-term and preterm infants between the ages of 1 and 4 months who met the criteria for excessive crying (which they defined as crying for at least 3 hours per day, 3 days per week, for 3 weeks) and colic (as defined by paroxysmal or sudden onset of cry; distinctive, high-pitched pain cry; physical signs associated with hypertonia; and inconsolability). The acoustic characteristics of the cries of the 16 infants with colic were compared to those of a group of infants without colic, matched for age, prematurity, medical illness, and SES. Findings showed that the cries of the infants with colic had a 25% higher pitch, a 30% greater pitch variability, and more than twice the turbulence or disphonation than the cries of the control infants. In that study, mothers of infants with colic rated the cries of their infants as more urgent, more piercing, more grating, and more arousing than did mothers in the control group. Fuller, Keefe, and Curtin (1994) also found that compared to the cries of 11 nonirritable infants, the cries of 11 irritable infants were higher in jitter, shimmer, proportion of noise, and tenseness. However, St. James-Roberts (1999) found no evidence that crying in colicky infants from a community sample had distinct acoustic features.

In an attempt to examine the social origins of colic, Crowcroft and Strachan (1997) used a questionnaire administered by health visitors on 76,747 infants born in Sheffield, England, between August 1, 1975 and May 31, 1988, when infants were 1 month old. Results showed that the odds of reporting colic were increased by breast feeding, increased parental age, lower parity, increased parental age at leaving full-time education, and more affluent home and districts of residence. The authors reported that in a logistic regression analysis, maternal age, parity, and socioeconomic factors remained the most important risk factors for infantile colic, and the effect of breast feeding was attenuated. Dietary factors contributed little to the reporting of colic.

Future Directions

The absence of a standard definition and accepted diagnostic criteria for colic has hampered research on colic, including its etiology, pathophysiology, and management (Lester et al., 1990). As a first step, Lester et al. (1990) recommend differentiating colic from excessive crying. Other areas in need of research include the contribution of parental characteristics, including quality of caregiving, to the onset and/or perpetuation of colic.

Failure to Thrive

Description of the Disorder

Although there is no universally accepted definition of failure to thrive (FTT), FTT is an Axis I diagnosis in DSM-IV under the name "feeding disorder of infancy or early childhood" (see Table 13.3). Considerable heterogeneity exists with respect to characteristics of infants with FTT, their caregivers, and their family and social circumstances (see Benoit, 1993a, 1993b, 2000a, for reviews).

Infants with FTT. Because of their state of malnutrition, infants with FTT often look cachectic, are prone to recurrent infections, and show a decreased ability to recover from them. They are often developmentally delayed and may exhibit unusual postures. Infants with FTT may look depressed, withdrawn, sad, apathetic, wary or hypervigilant, irritable, and angry. A retrospective population-based survey of 97 infants with FTT, identified by population screening at a median age of 15.1 months and compared to a control group of 28 infants without FTT who had similar levels of deprivation, showed that the parents of infants with FTT reported an early history of feeding problems more often than the parents of infants in the control group. Despite the problems associated with retrospective accounts of earlier problems, the findings identify early feeding problems as a potential risk factor for the development of FTT (Wright & Birks, 2000). In a prospective study of 35 neonates with a median gestational age at birth of 34 weeks admitted to a neonatal intensive care unit for a minimum of 5 days, Hawdon, Beauregard, Slattery, and Kennedy (2000) examined risk factors for later feeding problems. At 36–40 weeks postmenstrual age, a feeding assessment was done using the Neonatal Oral Motor Assessment Scale, and each infant's feeding pattern was categorized as normal (n = 21), disorganized (immature; n = 12), and dysfunctional (abnormal; n = 2). A high incidence (14 of 35, or 40%) of infants had disorganized or dysfunctional feeding patterns. Compared to infants with normal feeding patterns at the original feeding assessment, these infants were six times were likely to have problems with vomiting and three times more likely to cough when offered solids at 6 months old. By 12 months of age, infants who had had disorganized and dysfunctional early feeding patterns were nine times more likely to cough

TABLE 13.3. DSM-IV Diagnostic Criteria for Feeding Disorder of Infancy or Early Childhood

A. Feeding disturbance as manifested by persistent failure to eat adequately with significant failure to gain weight or significant loss of weight over at least 1 month.

B. The disturbance is not due to an associated gastrointestinal or other general medical condition (e.g., esophageal reflux).

C. The disturbance is not better accounted for by another mental disorder (e.g., Rumination Disorder) or by lack of available food.

D. The onset is before age 6 years.

Note. From American Psychiatric Association (1994, pp. 99–100).

with meals and four times less like to tolerate lumpy textures. Hawdon et al. (2000) suggest that these feeding problems might contribute to failure to thrive and psychosocial distress in some of these infants and their families.

Caregivers of Infants with FTT. Mothers of infants with FTT have been described (in both controlled and noncontrolled studies) as exhibiting a wide variety of clinical problems, such as affective disorders, substance abuse, and personality disorders (e.g., Crittenden, 1987; Polan et al., 1991). However, conflicting findings continue to surround this area of research (see Benoit, 1993a, 1993b, 2000a, for reviews). In their controlled study of maternal attachment characteristics, Benoit and colleagues (Benoit, Zeanah, & Barton, 1989; Coolbear & Benoit, 1999) found that mothers of infants with FTT were more likely than their matched counterparts to be classified as insecure with respect to attachment (on the Adult Attachment Interview [AAI]; George, Kaplan, & Main, 1985). These findings suggest that mothers of infants with FTT are either more passive, confused, and intensely angry than their matched counterparts when discussing past and current attachment relationships, or else they dismiss attachment relationships as unimportant and noninfluential. Such patterns of responses are usually characterized by insensitive caregiving (van IJzendoorn, 1995). Polan and Ward (1994) demonstrated that types of maternal touch that may promote growth or facilitate feeding are reduced in FTT, due (in extreme cases) to maternal and child touch aversion. Black, Hutcheson, Dubowitz, and Berenson-Howard (1994) showed that parents of children with nonorganic FTT were less nurturing and more neglecting than parents of control children. However, findings from these studies do not elucidate the direction of effects.

Family, Caregiving, and Social Characteristics of Infants with FTT. Several controlled (Chatoor, Ganiban, Colin, Plummer, & Harmon, 1998; Crittenden, 1987; Valenzuela, 1990) and noncontrolled (Drotar et al., 1985; Gordon & Jameson, 1979) studies have documented increased rates of insecure attachment between infants with FTT and their mothers. Furthermore, Chatoor (1989) reported that compared to matched controls, infants with FTT interacted with their mothers in ways characterized by more conflict, less dyadic reciprocity, more struggle for control, and more negative affect (e.g., anger, sadness, frustration). In fact, mothers of infants with FTT used more rough, abrupt, and controlling interactions, fewer positive vocalizations, and more criticism or threats when interacting with their infants, and were generally less responsive and more intrusive than the control mothers (Chatoor, Egan, Getson, Menvielle, & O'Donnell, 1987; Berkowitz & Senter, 1987; Finlon et al., 1985). These findings identify an association between FTT and the quality of mothers' interactions with their infants with FTT, but not a direction of effect.

To date, most studies on FTT have reported that infants with FTT generally have a late birth order in a two-parent family (Benoit et al., 1989; Crittenden, 1987), with three to four children close in age (Benoit et al., 1989). Controlled studies have documented various family and marital/couple problems (Benoit et al., 1989; Crittenden, 1987) including inadequate housing, frequent moves, poverty, unemployment, substance abuse, violence, social isolation, and child maltreatment (Benoit, 2000a).

Diagnostic Considerations

Several attempts at classification (e.g., DSM-IV [APA, 1994]; the *International Classification of Diseases*, 10th revision [ICD-10; World Health Organization, 1993]; Chatoor, Dickson, Schaefer, & Egan, 1985; Dahl & Sundelin, 1986; Gremse, Lytle, Sacks, & Balistreri, 1998; Woolston, 1985) have failed to use operationalized diagnostic criteria to cover the spectrum of feeding disorders and FTT or to distinguish between other feeding disorders and FTT. Despite these problems, a common definition of FTT includes weight below the 5th percentile for age on standardized growth charts and/or deceleration in the rate of weight gain from birth to the present of at least two standard deviations on standard growth charts.

Developmental Course and Prognosis

Several factors are associated with the outcome and prognosis of FTT. Children with a previous history of FTT are shorter and gain less weight over time (Boddy, Skuse, & Andrews, 2000; Reif, Beler, Villa, & Spirer, 1995). Findings from controlled studies show conflicting results regarding whether FTT is associated with learning problems, lower intelligence, or developmental delay (Corbett, Drewett, & Wright, 1996; Drewett, Corbett, & Wright, 1999; Puckering et al., 1995; Reif et al., 1995). The degree of growth retardation and duration of follow-up have no significant effect on the outcome in these studies. Good indicators of catching up capabilities in terms of weight and height include birthweight, maternal height, SES, and (to a lesser extent) paternal parameters. Children with a history of FTT who caught up faster had better school performances and were from families with higher SES.

Mackner, Starr, and Black (1997) demonstrated that the cognitive performance of children with both FTT and neglect was significantly below that of children with neglect only, children with FTT only, and controls with neither FTT nor neglect; this finding suggests a cumulative effect of neglect and FTT on cognitive functioning. Kerr, Black, and Krishnakumar (2000) found that children with a history of both FTT and maltreatment had more behavior problems and worse cognitive performance and school functioning than children with neither risk factor. Children with only one risk factor (either FTT or maltreatment) achieved intermediate scores. In a prospective, controlled study of family environments of children who had been hospitalized with FTT, Drotar, Pallotta, and Eckerle (1994) found that the quality of family relationships at the point of diagnosis did not predict family relationships, residence, or constellation changes on average 3.5 years later. However, mothers of children who had been hospitalized for FTT reported less adaptive relationships within the family than controls. Again, findings from these various studies do not help to elucidate the direction of effects.

Epidemiology

In the United States, FTT is estimated to affect from 1% to 5% of infants admitted to hospitals, 10% of those living below the poverty level in rural and urban areas, 20% of infants born prematurely, and up to 30% of infants seen in inner-city emergency room and ambulatory care settings (Casey et al., 1994, Frank & Ziesel, 1988; Powell, Low, & Speers, 1987). Male and female infants are equally affected. In Britain, 1.8% of infants in the community and 3.3% of those born full-term and of appropriate weight for gestational age are affected (Skuse, Gill, Reilly, Wolke & Lynch, 1995; Skuse, Wolke,, & Reilly, 1992). In Israel, 3.9% of full-term infants in the community develop FTT (Wilensky et al., 1996). By definition, all infants with FTT share a serious underlying medical ("organic") problem: malnutrition. Only 16–30% of children with FTT have organic problems (in addition to malnutrition) severe enough to explain their growth failure, however (Berwick, Levy, & Kleinerman, 1982).

Etiology

Many etiological factors have been suggested and reflect the apparent heterogeneity of FTT. The common denominator in all cases of FTT is that the infants are not receiving an adequate amount of calories to meet nutritional and caloric needs. There are many possible reasons why an infant with FTT is not receiving an adequate number of calories. Such reasons may, of course, include various underlying medical problems that increase the caloric/nutritional needs of the child (e.g., some hypermetabolic states, malabsorption). No genetic contributor per se has been identified as causing FTT or feeding disorders. However, some genetic disorders (e.g., inborn errors of metabolism, cystic fibrosis) have been associated with FTT. Importantly, not all children with genetic or metabolic disorders have FTT. Other possible etiological factors may include a disordered caregiver–infant relationship, various forms of infant maltreatment, and various family problems (see Benoit, 1993a, 1993b, 2000a, for reviews).

Despite warnings that the traditional use of "organic" versus "nonorganic" (or environmental) as an etiological dichotomy is misleading, it is still widely used in clinical settings. A "mixed" etiology (i.e., both organic and nonorganic factors are simultaneously present and likely to be contributing to the onset and/or perpetuation of FTT) can be found in 15–35% of infants with FTT (Singer, 1986). As stated earlier, only 16–30% of children with FTT have organic diseases severe enough to explain their growth failure. There has been a recent impetus to examine simultaneously both organic and nonorganic contributors to FTT (Casey, 1988).

Future Directions

The lack of a universally accepted definition of FTT, as well as of a validated classification system, continues to hamper research in this area. Research in the field is characterized by inconsistencies in diagnostic criteria and paucity of treatment data (Benoit, 1993a, 2000a). Much of the research fails to address the direction of effects. Future research should address the shortcomings of prior research.

Other Feeding Disorders

Description of the Disorders

Rumination Disorder. As seen in Table 13.4, rumination disorder (see Benoit, 1993a, 2000a, for reviews) consists of repeated voluntary regurgitation of food, followed by rechewing and reswallowing the food in a state of relaxation, self-absorption, and pleasure. The age of onset is usually between 3 and 12 months of age. The condition is usually self-limited. Complications of rumination disorder may include malnutrition/FTT, dehydration, gastric problems, and a 25% mortality rate. Boys are affected five times more often than girls. Rumination disorder is rare. Two types of rumination disorder have been described: (1) psychogenic (with a younger age of onset and associated significant disturbances or inadequacies in the caregiving environment); and (2) self-stimulation (with a later age of onset and associated mental retardation in the affected child).

Pica. Pica (see Benoit, 1993a, 2000a, for reviews) is the repeated ingestion of nonnutritive substances such as clay, dirt, sand, stones, pebbles, hair, feces, and many other substances, as shown in Table 13.5. The ingestion of nonnutritive substances must have been occurring for at least 1 month in order for a diagnosis of pica to be made. Pica usually appears during the second year of life and often remits spontaneously during early childhood. Children with mental retardation and autism are affected more frequently than children without these problems. Possible "physical" etiological factors have been identified, such as deficiencies in iron, calcium, and zinc. Other possible etiological or associated factors include poverty, child maltreatment, parental psychopathology, lack of stimulation, and family disorganization.

Posttraumatic Feeding Disorder. Posttraumatic feeding disorder (PTFD) was first described by Chatoor, Conley, and Dickson (1988) in children of latency age. PTFD is said to occur when an infant or child exhibits food refusal after one or more traumatic events to the oropharynx or esophagus (e.g., choking, reflux, forced feeding) that trigger intense distress, are associated with anticipatory anxiety (e.g., crying at the sight of food), and result in resistance to feeding (with increasing distress when force-fed). The incidence and prevalence rates pf PTFD are unknown, but it is believed to be on the increase because of advances in medical technology that now contribute to the survival of infants with complex medical problems, whose survival is often contingent upon prolonged periods of tube feeding. Several reports suggest that infants who are tube-fed are at risk for developing severe feeding difficulties (e.g., extreme food selectivity, conditioned avoidance, or "food phobia") when oral feedings are

TABLE 13.4. DSM-IV Diagnostic Criteria for Rumination Disorder

A. Repeated regurgitation and rechewing of food for a period of at least 1 month following a period of normal functioning

B. The behavior is not due to an associated gastrointestinal or other general medical condition (e.g., esophageal reflux).

C. The behavior does not occur exclusively during the course of Anorexia Nervosa or Bulimia Nervosa. If the symptoms occur exclusively during the course of Mental Retardation or a Pervasive Developmental Disorder, they are sufficiently severe to warrant independent clinical attention.

Note. From American Psychiatric Association (1994, p. 98).

TABLE 13.5. DSM-IV Diagnostic Criteria for Pica

A. Persistent eating of nonnutritive substances for a period of at least 1 month.

B. The eating of nonnutritive substances is inappropriate to the developmental level.

C. The eating behavior is not part of a culturally sanctioned practice.

D. If eating behavior occurs exclusively during the course of another mental disorder (e.g., Mental Retardation, Pervasive Developmental Disorder, Schizophrenia), it is sufficiently severe to warrant independent clinical attention.

Note. From American Psychiatric Association (1994, p. 96).

introduced (Blackman & Nelson, 1985, 1987; Geertsma, Hyams, Pelletier, & Reiter, 1985; Levy, Winters, & Heird, 1980; Linscheid, Tarnowski, Rasnake, & Brams, 1987; Palmer, Thompson, & Linscheid, 1975). The traumatic oral experiences related to medical treatment (e.g., suctioning, repeated insertion of nasogastric or endotracheal tubes) that many of these children experience, or episodes of choking and gagging on food or medicine, may lead to pervasive problems with refusal of solids and fluids. Because many of these infants are tube-fed, they may not suffer from FTT even though they often have a severe feeding disorder. And because of the traumatic nature of their earlier oral experiences, these children have been described as suffering from a "posttraumatic" disorder (Chatoor et al., 1988).

Chatoor, Ganiban, Harrison, and Hirsch (2001) compared children with PTFD and children with "infantile anorexia" (FTT) and found that both groups of children showed more problematic feeding interactions than did children in a control group. The children with PTFD exhibited more resistance during feeding interactions than did the other two groups, particularly resistance to swallowing food. The authors concluded that infants' medical and feeding histories, as well as observations of feeding, are important to making the diagnosis of PTFD and differentiating it from other feeding disorders.

Diagnostic Considerations

The field of feeding disorders in infancy and early childhood is plagued with the same kinds of definitional, diagnostic, and classification problems described in the section on FTT. Various groups of researchers have attempted to classify feeding disorders in children, but there is no consensus (Burklow, Phelps, Schultz, McConnell, & Rudolph, 1998; Chatoor et al., 1988).

Whelan and Cooper (2000) found that compared with mothers of control children and mothers of children with a non-feeding-related form of disturbance, mothers of 4-year-old children with feeding problems had no raised rates of mood disorders (either current or past), but they had a markedly raised rate of both current and past DSM-IV eating disorders. The odds ratio of a maternal eating disorder for the children with feeding problems was 11: 1. Research is needed to document the frequency of association between FTT and other feeding disorders.

Developmental Course and Prognosis

In a survey of predominantly non-Hispanic, European American parents in five Chicago-area pediatric offices, Reau, Senturia, Lebailly, and Christoffel (1996) compared the range of feeding times for infants (3–12 months old; $n = 130$) and toddlers (13–27 months old; $n = 151$.). Results showed that feeding time distribution did not differ by age and had a mean duration of 15.9 to 22.5 minutes. In their survey, Reau et al. (1996) found that the most common problematic feeding behavior was "not always hungry at mealtime"—a complaint reported by 33% of parents of infants and 54% of parents of toddlers. These authors demonstrated that toddlers who were picky eaters ate more slowly (means of 23.3 minutes vs. 19.7 minutes; $p < .04$). The children who had feeding problems at both 6 and 12 months ate most slowly (mean = 37.5 minutes; $p = .05$). Reau et al. (1996) concluded that infants and toddlers who take more than 30 minutes to feed are slow eaters. In addition, although reports of behavioral feeding problems are common in toddlers, only picky eating was associated with lengthened feeding time. Reau and her colleagues reported that their findings were in line with findings from another survey in two inner-city Hispanic community clinics (Uribe & Senturia, 1994). This study was a retrospective self-report, suggesting that perhaps parents of toddlers with current behavioral feeding problems may be more likely to recall past problematic behaviors. Marchi and Cohen (1990) followed a sample of over 800 children over a 10-year period (from early–middle childhood to late childhood–adolescence). They found that feeding problems in young children were stable over time. Maladaptive eating behavior and pica in early childhood were significant risk factors for bulimia nervosa in 9- to 18-year-old children and young adolescents, whereas picky eating and "digestive problems" were risk factors for later anorexia nervosa. Findings from this study suggest that eating problems in infancy and early childhood may persist into later childhood and adolescence. More research is needed to determine whether eating problems in infancy and early childhood are also risk factors for eating disorders in adulthood.

Epidemiology

Feeding disorders are believed to affect from 6% to 35% of young children (Jenkins, Bax, & Hart, 1980; Palmer & Horn, 1978; Richman, 1981).

However, because the terms "FTT" and "feeding disorder" have often been used interchangeably in the literature, and because there is no universally accepted definition of either term, it is impossible to determine the accurate incidence or prevalence rates of particular types of disorders.

Future Directions

As with other problems of infancy and early childhood, the lack of a standard definition and accepted diagnostic criteria for feeding disorders, in addition to the lack of distinction between FTT and other feeding disorders, have hampered research on infant feeding disorders. Possible factors contributing to the onset and/or perpetuation of feeding disorders (e.g., parental characteristics; quality of the caregiving environment and of the parent–infant relationship) should also be systematically examined. Future research should address issues of definition, etiology, pathophysiology, prevention, and treatment. In her review of the literature on treatments for severe feeding problems in children (some of which have been used with toddlers), Kerwin (1999) notes that contingency management treatments including both positive reinforcement of appropriate feeding responses (e.g., accepting rather than removing the spoon during food refusal training and swallow induction) and ignoring or guiding of inappropriate responses are effective interventions. Future research should address the questions of for whom, when, and why empirically supported treatments of feeding problems are appropriate.

Sleep Disorders

Description of the Disorders

Sleep problems represent one of the most common pediatric problems during the first 3 years of life. As Sadeh and Anders (1993) and Anders, Goodlin-Jones, and Sadeh (2000) argue, familiarity with normal sleep states, diurnal organization (sleep–wake cycle), and ultradian organization (the cycle of rapid-eye-movement [REM] and non-rapid-eye-movement [NREM] sleep) is useful to understand sleep disorders occurring during infancy and early childhood (see Anders, 1975; Anders, Carskadon, & Dement, 1980; and Anders et al., 2000, for reviews). The most common sleep disturbances in infants include difficulties in falling asleep, night waking, or both, which are considered "dyssomnias." The most common sleep problems in preschool and school-age children are "parasomnias" (or disturbances of NREM sleep) and include nightmares, night terrors, sleepwalking, sleep talking, and certain types of enuresis (see Anders et al., 1980, for a review). We confine our discussion in the remainder of this section to dyssomnias.

Diagnostic Considerations

Three classifications of sleep disorders in infancy and early childhood exist. They include the *International Classification of Sleep Disorders: Diagnostic and Coding Manual* (ICSD:DCM; American Sleep Disorders Association, 1990), DSM-IV (APA, 1994), and DC:0–3 (Zero to Three, 1994). For an excellent comparison among the three classification systems, and a new, alternative classification based on research findings and clinically relevant symptomatology, see Anders et al. (2000). DSM-IV criteria for primary insomnia, the most common dyssomnia diagnosis in infants, are shown in Table 13.6.

Developmental Course and Prognosis

Reports suggest that about 14% of 3-year-olds and about 8% of 4-year-olds have sleep problems (Jenkins et al., 1980; Richman, 1981; Richman, Stevenson, & Graham, 1982). As pointed out by Anders et al. (2000), nearly half of infants with sleep problems continue to have sleep problems in later years, suggesting that the myth about children outgrowing their sleep problems is refuted by research findings. However, the only longitudinal study of sleep disorder reported that 30% of full-term night wakers at 5 months were also night wakers at 20 months, but that only 17% remained night wakers at 56 months. More longitudinal data are needed to examine the developmental course of sleep disorders from infancy into adulthood.

Epidemiology

It is estimated that from 15% to 30% of infants and toddlers have sleep problems, including resisting going to bed and/or settling down to sleep or night waking (Lozoff, Wolf, & Davis, 1985; Richman, 1981). No gender differences have been identified with respect to night waking (Paret, 1983). No known socioeconomic factors are associated with sleep problems in infancy and

TABLE 13.6. DSM-IV Diagnostic Criteria for Primary Insomnia

A. The predominant complaint is difficulty initiating or maintaining sleep, or nonrestorative sleep, for at least 1 month.

B. The sleep disturbance (or associated daytime fatigue) causes clinically significant distress or impairment in social, occupational, or other important areas of functioning.

C. The sleep disturbance does not occur exclusively during the course of Narcolepsy, Breathing-Related Sleep Disorder, Circadian Rhythm Sleep Disorder, or a Parasomnia.

D. The disturbance does not occur exclusively during the course of another mental disorder (e.g., Major Depressive Disorder, Generalized Anxiety Disorder, a delirium).

E. The disturbance is not due to the direct physiological effects of a substance (e.g., a drug of abuse, a medication) or a general medical condition.

Note. From American Psychiatric Association (1994, p. 557).

early childhood. However, an association between breast feeding and sleep problems in infancy has been reported (Carey, 1974; Paret, 1983). There are cultural variations and individual family differences in sleeping habits and routines (e.g., some families and cultures have adults and children sleep in close proximity, whereas others isolate children from adults during sleep).

Etiology

Transient sleep difficulties may be associated with physical illness (e.g., ear infection, cold) or pain from teething during the first 2 years of life. Stress, maturational factors, and temperament have repeatedly been related to sleep state organization. Other factors such as allergies, cosleeping, nutritional factors, colic, and states of physical discomfort, may also be contributing, but findings are contradictory (see Anders et al., 2000, for a review). As discussed earlier, some clinicians and researchers view sleep disorders as a manifestation of an underlying regulatory disorder (Greenspan & Wieder, 1993). No genetic determinant of sleep problems has been identified.

Environmental factors (e.g., parental conflict, maternal psychopathology, family stress, parent–child relationship disturbances) have been identified as contributing to the onset and/or perpetuation of sleep problems in infancy and toddlerhood (e.g., Benoit, Zeanah, Boucher, & Minde, 1992; Bernal, 1973; Paret, 1983). One of the most consistent research findings is the association between sleep problems and parent–child interactions at bedtime. In addition, Benoit et al. (1992) found that, compared to their matched counterparts ($n = 21$), mothers of toddlers with sleep problems ($n = 20$) were rated on the AAI as significantly more insecure with respect to attachment than mothers of toddlers without sleep problems. These findings suggest that some mothers of toddlers with severe sleep problems are more insensitive in reading their toddlers' cues and signals of distress and in responding to them. The types of insensitivity associated with maternal insecurity in the attachment literature include rejection and inconsistency.

Future Directions

Future research might examine factors within the sleep-disordered infant and the caregiving environment that might contribute to the onset and perpetuation of sleep problems. Research on prevention and outcome of sleep problems during infancy is also necessary.

Posttraumatic Stress Disorder

Description of the Disorder

PTSD includes symptom clusters of reexperiencing the traumatic event, avoidance of reminders, numbing of responsiveness, and increased arousal as central features (APA, 1994; Fletcher, Chapter 7, this volume). These types of symptoms have been noted in both children (Pynoos, 1990; Terr, 1990) and adults (Davidson & Fairbank, 1993), but some have questioned whether criteria developed to describe a disorder in adults can be effectively applied to young children even if the disorder occurs in them (Zeanah, 1994). Notable in this regard is that the field tests of DSM-IV criteria for PTSD were conducted exclusively with adults.

Diagnostic Considerations

Drell, Siegel, and Gaensbauer (1993), based on a thorough review of the salient developmental literature, concluded that infants are capable of remembering events, including traumatic ones, from the first few months of life. Furthermore, they asserted that PTSD can and does occur in the first few years of life. Nevertheless, until the past few years, it was not clear whether traumatized infants actually met criteria for PTSD.

Scheeringa, Zeanah, Drell, and Larrieu (1995) evaluated the usefulness of DSM-IV criteria for diagnosing PTSD in children less than 48 months old. The investigators identified 20 cases of traumatized young children who had experienced a severe trauma (e.g., an attack by an animal, abuse, or witnessing the murder of a parent) and had been evaluated by a mental health professional prior to age 48 months. The results of this study were provocative. Despite the fact that most of the traumatized infants had signs and symptoms similar to what has been described in older children and adults, none of the infants met criteria sufficient for a diagnosis of PTSD. A number of the criteria were noted to be developmentally inappropriate, because they required cognitive and communicative skills not yet available to infants.

Scheeringa et al. (1995) then developed an alternative set of criteria based upon DSM-IV criteria and clinical experiences with traumatized infants and tested this set with a second sample. The new criteria were developed to be more behaviorally anchored and developmentally appropriate for young children. When DSM-IV criteria were used, only one severely traumatized infant could be diagnosed with PTSD. When the alternative criteria were used, 8 of the 12 traumatized infants met criteria for PTSD. In addition, interrater reliabilities among four untrained raters were unacceptably low for DSM-IV criteria (mean kappa for all items = .50) but much better for the alternative criteria (mean kappa for all items = .67). Because each of the cases involved a young child who had experienced a severe trauma, the investigators concluded that PTSD occurs in infancy, but that the DSM-IV criteria require modification because of important developmental differences.

Two subsequent studies with traumatized young children have replicated and extended these findings. Both studies replicated the finding that the alternative criteria were more sensitive to detecting disorders in traumatized young children than DSM-IV criteria. The first study also demonstrated procedural, criterion, and discriminant validity of PTSD in early childhood, using a combination of a structured interview of mothers and direct observations of child play with an examiner and interaction with mothers (Scheeringa, Peebles, Cook, & Zeanah, 2001). Interestingly, only 12% of the signs of PTSD identified were derived from clinician observation, while 88% were derived from maternal report. A second study demonstrated that comorbidity is common in traumatized young children and that most of the comorbid disorders appear after the onset of the traumatic event (Scheeringa, Zeanah, Myers, & Putnam, 2002).

Developmental Course and Prognosis

Physically and sexually abused young children have been noted to develop posttraumatic symptoms, although in many of these cases the trauma may not have been a single, discrete event but rather a series of traumatic events or even an enduring circumstance. In examining the effects of acute versus chronic traumas, Scheeringa and Zeanah (1995) found that infants who had suffered acute traumas were more severely affected overall and had more symptoms of reexperiencing the traumatic event than infants who had experienced chronic traumas. This should not suggest that acute traumas are more injurious than chronic traumas but only that the symptom picture differs in the two instances. Some have suggested, for example, that the effects of chronic traumas may be more apparent in long-term effects on personality or other developmental domains than in acute symptomatology (Zero to Three, 1994).

Another important consideration consists of age at the time of the trauma and its effects on traumatic memories. Terr (1988) has suggested, based on her clinical experiences, that infants experiencing traumas occurring prior to 28 months are less likely to have "full verbal recollection" (p. 103) than older infants. Nevertheless, other case reports strongly suggest that verbal recollection may be available at least from the latter part of the second year of life (Sugar, 1992). From a developmental perspective, a change might be expected after 18 months, given the well-known qualitative advance in symbolic representation that occurs about this time (Kagan, 1981). With this in mind, Scheeringa and Zeanah (1995) found that infants over 18 months of age were likely to have significantly more reexperiencing symptoms than infants under 18 months. This finding makes sense, given that reexperiencing symptoms probably require fairly developed capacities for symbolic functioning. Nevertheless, it is also clear that some infants under 18 months of age are capable of later representing the catastrophic traumatic events symbolically in vivid detail (see Gaensbauer, Chatoor, Drell, Siegel, & Zeanah, 1995). How implicit traumatic memories become transformed later into explicit memories remains to be demonstrated.

Increasingly, questions have been raised about the harmful effects on children of witnessing traumatic events rather than experiencing them directly (Osofsky, 1995; Zeanah & Scheeringa, 1997). Here, of course, cognitive immaturity may serve a protective function for infants in the first year of life, who have a limited ability to understand and to anticipate threat, danger, and even loss. By the second and third years, however, one might expect increased vulnerability to the witnessing of violence. Scheeringa and Zeanah (1995) found that infants who had witnessed violent traumas rather than experienced them directly were likely to exhibit more symptoms of hyperarousal. Also, they found that infants whose caregivers were threatened in the traumatic events were significantly more symptomatic than infants whose caregivers were not threatened.

Data about the long-term adaptation of traumatized young children are quite limited. Nevertheless, Terr (1990) has suggested that effects are likely to be far-reaching, and some case reports provide support for that assertion (Pruett, 1979; Terr, 1990). Factors that may be related to outcome, including gender, age at exposure, comprehension of danger, premorbid functioning, and available support, should be addressed in future research. Most clinicians seem to agree that the nature of supports available in the posttraumatic environment is likely to be crucial for facilitating adaptation (Pruett, 1979; Zeanah & Burk, 1984; Drell et al., 1993; Pynoos & Eth, 1985).

Future Directions

An important area for future exploration concerns the neurobiology of trauma in young children. There is a large and ever-growing literature on the neurobiology of trauma in adults and older children. Our knowledge of the importance of brain development in the first few years of life (Nelson & Bosquet, 2000) and speculation about the putative effects of trauma not just on brain functioning, but also on brain structure (Perry, 1997), all make this an important area.

Another important area for future research concerns the relationship context of trauma in early childhood. Scheeringa and Zeanah (1995) found that the single best predictor of severity of posttraumatic symptomatology in young children was whether or not their caregivers had been threatened by the traumatic events. This was a stronger predictor even than whether or not the young children were injured during the traumatic events. The investigators advanced two possible reasons for this finding. First, in a direct effect, young children might appreciate the threat to themselves posed by a threat to their primary caregivers, leading to an intensification of their own symptoms. Second, in an indirect effect, a caregiver may be traumatized by the same event that traumatizes a child. This may result in the caregiver's being less able to respond empathically to the child, leading to an intensification of the child's posttraumatic symptoms. Either way, it is clear that the parent–child relationship is importantly related to the child's symptomatology.

Scheeringa and Zeanah (2001a) have recently reviewed the literature on the relationship context of trauma in early childhood and described ways in which the parent–child relationship mediates or moderates the effects of trauma on young children. They have proposed "relational PTSD" as the co-occurrence of PTSD in parent and young child, in which the symptomatology of each partner exacerbates and complicates that of the other. They describe several patterns of relational PTSD, including a "withdrawn/ unresponsive/unavailable" pattern, an "overprotective/constricting" pattern, and a "reenacting/endangering/ frightening" pattern. At this point, empirical validation of these patterns will be an important next step in clarifying the role of the parent–child relationship in cases of traumatized young children. These findings are likely to have important implications for treatment of such children and their parents.

Reactive Attachment Disorder

Description of the Disorder

Despite concerns about clinical disorders of attachment in the scientific literature dating back to the beginning of the 20th century, RAD first appeared in official psychiatric nomenclatures only in 1980, with the publication of DSM-III (APA, 1980). Criteria describing this disorder were revised substantially in DSM-III-R (APA, 1987), but only minor changes were made subsequently in DSM-IV (APA, 1994). Although controversies abound about the specific characteristics of RAD and more recently proposed attachment disorders, there is a general consensus that they describe symptom pictures unaccounted for by other disorders (Rutter, 1994; Volkmar, 1997; Zeanah & Emde, 1994).

There are two distinct types of RAD outlined in DSM-IV: an inhibited and a disinhibited type (see Table 13.7). In the first type, inhibited, unresponsive, and/or hypervigilant social responses are characteristic. In the second type, the infant exhibits indiscriminate oversociability, a failure to show selective attachments, a relative lack of selectivity in the persons from whom comfort is sought, and poorly modulated social interactions with unfamiliar persons across a range of social situations.

Curiously, despite hundreds of studies of attachment in developmental research in the past 20 years, there were no studies of RAD until quite recently. The DSM-IV criteria for RAD were derived from studies of the social behaviors of maltreated children and studies of institutionalized children (see Zeanah & Emde, 1994, for a review). Tizard and Rees (1975), for example, studied children institutionalized from birth. Of 26 children in that study who remained in the institution for the first 4 years of life, 8 were noted to be emotionally withdrawn and socially bizarre, as they were largely unresponsive to anyone. Another 10 of the 26 institutionalized children had superficial attachments to staff members, with attention seeking, clinginess, and overfriendly behavior with strangers.

When the first edition of this volume was published, there had been no studies addressing the reliability or validity of RAD. In the past few years, eight empirical papers have been published on this topic, several others have been presented at scientific meetings, and even more longitudinal studies are underway. These studies include at least eight different samples of children from six countries, suggesting that the research base of this disorder is beginning to grow.

Diagnostic Considerations

The first study that examined the criteria for RAD was a retrospective review of 48 consecutive clinic-referred children less than 3 years of age (Boris, Zeanah, Larrieu, Scheeringa, & Heller, 1998). Perhaps because 79% of the children in that study were referred to the clinic by child protective services, 42% met criteria for an attachment disorder (though not necessarily RAD as defined by DSM-IV). Ratings of alternative criteria for the emotionally withdrawn/inhibited and indiscriminately social patterns had higher levels of interrater reliability than did the DSM-IV criteria. Finally, children who met criteria for attachment disorders had significantly more impairments in the parent–child relationship than children who did not meet criteria for such disorders.

Studies of children from institutions in Romania have also contributed to this literature. The two patterns of RAD described in DSM-IV (APA, 1994) have been noted in children adopted from Romanian institutions, although the disinhibited/indiscriminate pattern appears to be far more common than the inhibited/emotionally withdrawn pattern, at least in follow-up studies months to years after adoption (O'Connor, in press; Zeanah, 2000). In contrast, children demonstrating signs of the emotionally withdrawn/inhibited pattern of RAD were readily apparent in the only study of currently institutionalized children in Romania (Smyke, Dumitrescu, & Zeanah, in press). This seeming discrepancy probably reflects the tendency of children with the emotionally withdrawn/inhibited pattern of RAD to recover when placed in more favorable environments. This same tendency for emotionally withdrawn/inhibited RAD to resolve in maltreated children soon after placement in foster care has been noted anecdotally (Hinshaw-Fuselier, Boris, & Zeanah, 1999; Zeanah & Boris, 2000; Zeanah, Mammen, & Lieberman, 1993). An important remaining question is about the degree of their recovery. Atypical features of attachment in variants of the Strange Situation (Ainsworth, Blehar, Waters, & Wall, 1978) are common in adopted, formerly institutionalized children (Chisholm, 1998; Marvin & O'Connor, 1999; Marcovitch et al., 1997).

The major finding to emerge from contemporary research on formerly institutionalized children is that indiscriminate sociability is linked to lack of a discriminated attachment figure in children in institutions, but it persists long after these children have developed attachment figures in the more favorable caregiving environment of the adoptive home. That is, the recovery paths of indiscriminate sociability and attachment appear to diverge (Chisholm, 1998; Chisholm, Carter, Ames, & Morison, 1995; O'Connor, Bredenkamp, & Rutter, 1999; O'Connor & Rutter, 2000).

TABLE 13.7. DSM-IV Diagnostic Criteria for Reactive Attachment Disorder of Infancy or Early Childhood

A. Markedly disturbed and developmentally inappropriate social relatedness in most contexts, beginning before age 5 years, as evidenced by either (1) or (2).

(1) persistent failure to initiate or respond in a developmentally appropriate fashion to most social interactions, as manifest by excessively inhibited, hypervigilant, or highly ambivalent and contradictory responses (e.g., the child may respond to caregivers with a mixture of approach, avoidance, and resistance to comforting, or may exhibit frozen watchfulness)
(2) diffuse attachments as manifest by indiscriminate sociability with marked inability to exhibit appropriate selective attachments (e.g., excessive familiarity with relative strangers or lack of selectivity in choice of attachment figures)

B. The disturbance in Criterion A is not accounted for solely by developmental delay (as in Mental Retardation) and does not meet criteria for a Pervasive Developmental Disorder.

C. Pathogenic care as evidenced by at least one of the following.

(1) persistent disregard of the child's basic emotional needs for comfort, stimulation, and affection
(2) persistent disregard of the child's basic physical needs
(3) repeated changes of primary caregiver that prevent formation of stable attachments (e.g., frequent changes in foster care)

D. There is a presumption that the care in Criterion C is responsible for the disturbed behavior in Criterion A (e.g., the disturbances in Criterion A began following the pathogenic care in Criterion C).

Specify type:
Inhibited Type: if Criterion A1 predominates in the clinical presentation
Disinhibited Type: if Criterion A2 predominates in the clinical presentation

Note. From American Psychiatric Association (1994, p. 118). Copyright 1994 by the American Psychiatric Association. Reprinted by permission.

In addition, a recent study has documented that signs of indiscriminate RAD may be demonstrated in young children in institutions, whether or not they have a preferred attachment figure and whether or not they have signs of emotionally withdrawn/inhibited RAD (Smyke et al., in press; Zeanah, Smyke, & Dumitrescu, 2002). Similar findings have been demonstrated in a retrospective study of maltreated toddlers in foster care (Zeanah, Smyke, Boris, & Scheeringa, 2001). Several different explanations have been advanced to account for these findings. O'Connor (in press), for example, has suggested that recovery of attachment in children who have experienced extreme deprivation is incomplete; therefore, measures of secure attachment in children with high levels of indiscriminate behavior are flawed. Chisholm and colleagues (Ames & Chisholm, 2001; Chisholm, 1998), on the other hand, have emphasized the adaptive value of indiscriminate "friendliness" and suggested that it may not reflect disordered attachment at all. Instead, they have argued that indiscriminate behavior is learned and persists because it remains adaptive. Zeanah and colleagues (Zeanah, 2000; Zeanah & Smyke, in press) have posited a lasting breakdown in the regulation of attachment and affiliative behavior (which ordinarily occurs in the second half of the first year of life) as an explanation for the divergence of attachment and indiscriminate behavior. Indiscriminate sociability, in this model, represents the failure in selective inhibition of affiliative behavior by the onset of focused attachment behaviors at 7–9 months of age.

Developmental research has demonstrated clearly that attachment, whether disordered or not, may be expressed differentially in different relationships. It is possible to define a disorder within an individual even if its expression is not cross-contextual. Some efforts have been made to develop criteria compatible with the findings of developmental attachment research (Lieberman & Zeanah, 1995; Zeanah et al., 2000) that include seriously disturbed attachment relationships as disorders. Specific types of such disorders include relationship-specific patterns of self-endangering, vigilant/hypercompliant behavior, and role-reversed behavior, as well as disrupted attachment disorder (unresolved grief following loss of attachment figure). Although validity data remain limited about these patterns, each has been identified in one retrospective study (Boris et al., 1998) and one prospective study (Boris et al., 2000). The reliability data about attachment disorder with role reversal have been unacceptably low, however (Boris et al., 1998, 2000).

Disrupted attachment disorder, as just noted, describes the grief responses of young children who lose their major attachment figure. These reactions were originally noted by Robertson and Robertson (1989) in their work with children separated from their parents. Because of the central importance of the attachment figure in the first 3 years of life, the loss of an attachment figure at this time may be qualitatively different than if the loss occurs at other points in the life cycle. Indeed, there is evidence that loss before age 5 years places a child at increased risk for subsequent psychopathology (Brown, Harris, & Bifulco, 1986). Nevertheless, validity data about this proposed disorder are lacking.

Developmental Course and Prognosis

There are no direct data available about the course of RAD or other disorders of attachment. Nevertheless, data about the consequences of insecure attachment in infancy and about children raised in institutions converge to suggest that attachment difficulties in infancy are likely to be related to a number of subsequent problems. These include relatively profound effects in the areas of social competence, peer relations, and family relations, but fewer effects on behavior problems and cognition (Zeanah & Emde, 1994; Boris & Zeanah, 1999). Thus it is clear that the quality of early attachment relationships is important to subsequent adaptation (see also the following section), and that significant disruptions in an infant's access to a relatively small number of emotionally available caregivers in the first few years of life appear to be associated with serious deviation in social relationships.

Still, it is unclear what happens to children experiencing clinical disorders of attachment in infancy at later points in development. Research on the sequelae of disorganized/disoriented attachments in infancy discussed later in this chapter (see "Infant Attachment and Later Psychiatric Symptomatology") points to aggressive behavior disorders and dissociative symptoms, as well as overall psychopathology, as disorders that are related to early attachment problems.

Future Directions

Advances in the study of disordered attachment have been notable since the first edition of this volume appeared. In fact, virtually all we know about these disorders comes from studies conducted in the past 5 years. Preliminary validity data have supported the two types of RAD described in DSM-IV (APA, 1994) and ICD-10 (WHO, 1993). Nevertheless, the independence of these two types is in question, as accumulating evidence suggests that mixed patterns exist (Zeanah et al., in press; Zeanah et al., 2001) and that indiscriminate sociability occurs in children who become attached following adoption from institutions (Chisholm, 1998; Marvin & O'Connor, 1999). Other forms of disordered attachment may also exist, although validity data about these other types is more limited. Importantly, no studies of discriminant validity have been reported to date. In addition, the relationship between insecure (especially disorganized) attachment and attachment disorders needs to be clarified.

It is already clear that thinking about attachment disorders can be greatly enhanced by drawing on the rich body of longitudinal data available from developmental attachment research (van IJzendoorn & Bakersman-Kranenburg, in press; Zeanah, 1996; Zeanah & Emde, 1994). It seems likely that such an integration will be useful to both clinicians and to investigators. The remainder of the chapter reviews recent prospective longitudinal work on the intergenerational family context of risk for disorder, with a particular emphasis on new findings in the attachment literature.

LONGITUDINAL RESEARCH ON FAMILY CONTEXT AND INFANTS' RISK FOR LATER DISORDERS

Introduction to the Research

The Child in the Family Context

Because of the unique location of infancy at the beginning of the developmental process, infant clinicians and researchers have a special charge to maintain an orientation toward prevention of mental disorder as well as treatment of existing conditions. As longitudinal research increasingly makes clear, family factors that substantially increase the risk of a child's "suffering death, pain, disability, or an important loss of freedom" (APA, 1994, p. xxi) associated with mental disorder are beginning to be traced back to the infancy or prebirth periods, before the child him- or herself may be symptomatic. Because of the rapidity of developmental changes characteristic of the early years, family factors may also be more stable predictors of later child status than particular infant symptoms, although this remains an important question for research.

Child factors are also important correlates of a wide range of psychiatric disorders, as documented by chapters in the current volume. Child factors correlated with or predictive of disorder have included inhibited temperament, specific genetic markers, and nonspecific genetic contributions identified by behavioral genetic studies. Family factors may also be shaped by genetic inheritance. The relatively recent application of sophisticated longitudinal research methods to the study of child psychopathology now offers the potential to delineate predictable relations in how family genetic and environmental influences and child factors interact and produce identifiable developmental trajectories over time.

The Importance of High-Risk Longitudinal Studies

Because of the dramatic cognitive and behavioral reorganizations that take place during the first 4 years of life, early behavioral maladaptation at either the child or family level may have little surface similarity to forms of individual or family psychopathology exhibited later in development. Because of this phenotypic discontinuity over developmental epochs, particular early behaviors or family relational patterns may not initially be recognized as important precursors, prodromes, or disorders of infancy. Therefore, prospective longitudinal studies from the early years of life are a particularly powerful methodology for exploring whether there are identifiable environmental or biological markers, risk conditions, or early precursor forms of child behavior that contribute to the development of a deviant trajectory over time. For example, certain forms of child caregiving toward the parent or odd behaviors in the presence of the parent, such as those being described in current attachment studies, may only gain significance as indicators of infant disorder if they are shown to be systematically related to later serious psychopathology. Thus studies of infant diagnostic groupings need to proceed in concert with more broadly based community studies of high-risk groups if the full range of early signs of disorder is to be identified.

The Role of Early Relationships

The past two decades of infancy research have also been distinctive in maintaining a concentrated focus on how to conceptualize and assess parent–infant relationships at both a behavioral and a representational level. A focus on understanding the role and patterning of relationships is critical to a complete understanding of early biobehavioral development and its relation to later emotional disorder (Lyons-Ruth, 1995). However, the study of family relationships has been relatively neglected in recent psychopathology research because of the methodological and conceptual challenges inherent in directly observing relational behavior. This lack needs to be redressed in light of recent animal studies indicating that parental nurturing behaviors are critical to setting up enduring parameters of the infant's neuroanatomy and neurochemistry (see below).

Although there has been a relative dearth of systematic research on diagnostically defined disorders of infancy, a sophisticated research literature exists delineating family contextual features evident before or during infancy that are associated with infant or child maladaptation. In this section, three particularly active areas of infant-oriented longitudinal work relevant to exploring the developmental trajectories leading to childhood psychopathology are reviewed: research on intergenerational transmission of relational behavior; research on the context and correlates of disorganized/disoriented infant attachment behaviors; and research on early predictors of later psychiatric symptomatology.

Intergenerational Transmission of Relational Behavior

Researchers from various traditions have been demonstrating that the caregiving patterns established in relation to the infant not only have a degree of stability over time, but have roots in the adaptation of the parent *prior* to the birth of the child. One clear implication of this literature is that parental developmental history and psychological structure, as well as parental genetic transmission, make contributions to the shaping of the child's relational behavior and biology; thus these factors need to be understood in their own right if the complex interplay between parent and child contributions to deviant pathways is to be understood.

Caregiving Received in Parents' Childhoods and Subsequent Parenting

A number of earlier studies have documented univariate prediction from single prenatal variables (e.g., unplanned pregnancy) to aspects of subsequent parenting and have found associations between a parent's childhood experiences (e.g., abuse) and aspects of later parental and marital/couple relationships (for a review, see Belsky & Pensky, 1988). However, other infancy work has been more sophisticated in using multimethod, prospective longitudinal designs and searching for mediating processes that might explain how prenatal adaptation and/or a parent's childhood experiences influence the early parent–child relationship. For example, Heinecke, Diskin, Ramsey-Klee, and Oates (1986) followed 46 families from midpregnancy until an infant was 2 years of age and found that the child's modulation of aggression at age 2 years was predicted by a path model that included both direct and indirect effects of three of the four prebirth parental variables assessed. The three variables that influenced child aggression directly were prebirth husband–wife adaptation, maternal competence, and maternal Minnesota Multiphasic Personality Inventory warmth scores. In contrast, maternal prebirth IQ scores did not contribute to the prediction of child aggression modulation, but did predict 2-year-old attention and verbal expressiveness. A mother's prebirth characteristics (such as maternal adaptation, competence, and warmth) also contributed to the child's aggression modulation indirectly, because prebirth characteristics were in turn related to the mother's higher responsiveness to infant needs at 1, 3, 6, 12, and 24 months of age, with responsiveness in turn related to decreased infant fretting over the first 2 years of life and decreased aggression at age 2 years.

In a second study, Cox et al. (1985) found that prebirth maternal characteristics predicted 41% of the variance in positive quality of mother–infant interaction at 3 months of age. In this study as well, the maternal prebirth assessments included measures of prenatal marital competence (assessed both through interview and observational measures) and individual psychological health based on 10 standardized measures. In addition, this study included a measure of the quality of parenting received in a parent's family of origin. Unexpectedly, the family-of-origin reports were much stronger predictors of mothers' parenting than were the marital and psychological health variables, and the latter variables accounted for no further variance after family-of-origin variables were entered. The mothers' reports of their own parents' hostility and intrusiveness were particularly strong predictors of their own parenting.

The power of family-of-origin interview assessments has been replicated in other multivariate studies. Belsky, Hertzog, and Rovine (1986) gathered data on the contributions of prebirth maternal personality and marital adjustment, quality of care in family of origin, maternal social network contact assessed at 3 and 9 months, and infant temperament assessed at 3 and 9 months. They evaluated how well this set of measures predicted a composite measure of mother–infant interaction observed in the home when an infant was 1, 3, and 9 months old. The authors had expected to find that effects of mother's family history on her parenting would be mediated through current personality variables, and such a mediated path did occur. However, as Belsky et al. (1986) noted, "The most important contradiction [to the hypothesized model] . . . involved the direct and unmediated effect of developmental history on maternal interaction with the infant" (p. 188). The variance accounted for by the direct effect of the mother's family history outweighed the mediated effects, and the family-of-origin assessment made the greatest overall contribution of any variable to the prediction of parenting.

Lyons-Ruth and colleagues (Lyons-Ruth, Zoll, Connell, & Grunebaum, 1989; Lyons-Ruth, 1992), studying an impoverished, socially at-risk sample, predicted that influences of family history on parenting would be mediated through influences on the mother's current depressive symptoms, marital status, number of children, and age of first childbearing. Again, these mediated effects of childhood history were overshadowed by the large direct effects of the mother's childhood experiences on her own behavior toward her child, with the childhood experience measure accounting for more overall variance in parenting (27%) than all other risk factors. In response to these accumulated findings, Lyons-Ruth (1992) concluded that implicit representations of strategies of interaction in intimate relationships may be developed in early family relationships and reaccessed directly as parents establish relationships with their infants.

The most impressive demonstration of intergenerational continuity in parenting has come from Elder and colleagues' longitudinal study using the Berkeley Guidance Study Archives (Elder, Caspi, & Downey, 1986). Although not focused on infancy per se, this longitudinal study, begun in 1928, has included four generations—encompassing grandparents, parents, children, and grandchildren—so that measures of childhood experience were obtained *prospectively*, rather than by retrospective report as in the studies above. They found that personality measures, marital conflict, and parenting styles tended to be correlated within families across generations, and these correlated parental qualities were in turn related to child behavior. Parents who displayed conflicted, unstable personalities also experienced marital tension and displayed irritable, explosive behavior toward their children. Their children in turn displayed irritable, explosive behavior in both childhood and adulthood. However, if unstable personality and marital conflict did not find expression in punitive parental behavior toward children, intergenerational transmission did not occur.

These intergenerational continuities are undoubtedly complex products of learned relational behavior and of both genetic and environmental effects on physiological functioning (see below). The next generation of research on intergenerational continuity and discontinuity needs to incorporate experimental manipulations (such as randomized interventions), in concert with genetic analyses, close observation of early interactions, and assessments of parent and infant physiological responses, in order to begin to tease apart these correlated etiological factors.

Parental Attachment Strategies and Subsequent Infant Attachment Strategies

Recent research guided by attachment theory is also underscoring the power of assessments that explore parents' childhood experiences by demonstrating the strong associations between prenatal scores on the Adult Attachment Interview (AAI; George et al., 1985) and infant attachment behavior assessed at 1 year of age (see below). The AAI was developed to explore the implicit mental representations or "internal working models" that parents have formed of their own early attachment-related experiences. The scoring of the AAI has been revolutionary, however, in enabling investigators to go beyond a focus on the objective content of early experience and beyond a reliance on the adult's conscious reporting to a focus on the underlying forms of discourse and cognition through which those experiences are presented (for the latest version of the scoring manual, see Main & Goldwyn, 1998). A summary description of the interview and its coding procedures can be found in van IJzendoorn and Bakermans-Kranenburg (1996).

In several prospective studies, parental attachment classification assessed before the birth of the first child was found to predict the infant's attachment classification 1 year later, with 70% agreement between three-category maternal and infant classification systems. In a meta-analysis of 18 studies, including both prospective and concurrent designs, van IJzendoorn (1995) confirmed a 75% correspondence rate between secure versus insecure mother and child attachment classifications, with an overall effect size of .47 (see next section for descriptions of secure and insecure attachment patterns). Prediction from fathers to infants was somewhat lower (Fonagy, Steele, & Steele, 1991; Radojevic, 1992; Steele & Steele, 1994; Suess, Grossmann, & Sroufe, 1992).

van IJzendoorn (1995) also evaluated the relationship between parental AAI classification and parental sensitive responsiveness toward the infant, because sensitive parental behavior is hypothesized to mediate the relationship between parent and infant attachment classifications. For 10 studies, the effect size was .34 in the expected direction. As van IJzendoorn points out, this effect size indicates that parental interactive behavior (as currently assessed) is not accounting for all the correspondence between parent and infant attachment classification, so that other factors such as genetic resemblance may also play a role in the obtained correspondences. With recent advances in noninvasive DNA sampling and linkage analysis, studies evaluating the relative contributions of genetic and environmental factors to intergenerational transmission of attachment patterns will occur over the next decade.

In five available studies (n = 148), mothers of young children with psychiatric problems (sleep disorders, FTT, conduct problems) displayed a highly deviant distribution of attachment classifications, with only 14% of parents in the secure group. This distribution is similar to that of adults with psychiatric diagnoses themselves, among whom 12% were classified as "autonomous" on the AAI (van IJzendoorn & Bakermans-Kranenburg, 1996). The extent of the deviation in attachment classifications among parents of clinic-referred children is striking, given the outpatient nature of the samples.

The possibility that a child's problem behavior negatively influenced the coherence of a parent's discourse concerning his or her own earlier attachment experiences seems unlikely. For example, earlier meta-analytic findings have shown that serious infant medical problems during the first year (congenital heart problems, extreme prematurity, cystic fibrosis, retardation) did *not* result in lowered proportions of secure infant attachment classifications. In contrast, serious parental psychiatric problems substantially altered the proportion of secure infant classifications (van IJzendoorn, Goldberg, Kroonenberg, & Frenkel, 1992). Thus most parents may be able to compensate even for severe deviations in infants' behavior and development, although infants are not similarly able to compensate for parental disturbance.

Work documenting conditions of *discontinuity* from childhood experience to later parenting is also beginning to emerge, with several studies indicating that a supportive marriage may buffer women from the detrimental effects of difficult childhood experiences (Belsky, Youngblade, & Pensky, 1989; Quinton, Rutter, & Liddle, 1984). Why some women can make such supportive matches and others do not remains a question for investigation, however. Recent studies suggest that a positive relationship with another adult in childhood and/or a positive therapeutic relationship in adulthood may alter the process of intergenerational transmission (Egeland, Jacobvitz, & Sroufe, 1988). Other studies point to a role for positive peer relationships in childhood (Lyons-Ruth, 1992; Quinton, Pickles, Maughan, & Rutter, 1993) and for physical attractiveness (Belsky et al., 1989; Elder, Van Nguyen, & Caspi, 1985) in leading to more positive parenting behavior by adults with difficult childhoods. Studies of adult patterns of attachment are also pointing to sizable subgroups of parents who exhibit secure adult patterns of attachment despite difficult or traumatic childhood relationships (Grossmann, Fremmer-Bombik, Rudolph, & Grossmann, 1988; Jacobvitz, Goldetsky, & Hazen, 1993). A reliable body of work on processes related to changes in adult attachment patterns has not yet emerged, however.

Parental Caregiving Behavior and Subsequent Infant Neurophysiology: Animal Models

The continuity being demonstrated in patterns of relational behavior across generations is undoubtedly influenced by genetic factors, including complex interactions between genetic and behavioral processes. However, recent neuroscience research using randomized rearing conditions with both rats and rhesus macaques has confirmed the independent contribution of parental nurturance to offspring physiology as well as the enduring nature of those developmental effects. These studies are demonstrating that both infant neurotransmitter systems and the infant stress response system mediated by the HPA axis are open systems at birth that depend on the patterning of caregiver behavior to set enduring parameters of their functioning across the life span. Therefore, the early caregiving environment may be foundational at a physiological level in setting up relatively irreversible patterns of neurotransmitter activity and levels of HPA axis responsivity to stress or threat. For example, when caregiving behavior is impaired among macaque mothers due to uncertainty about the ease of obtaining food, macaque infants develop enduring fearful behaviors and elevated levels of corticotropin-releasing factor, which do not wane after a predictable food supply is reestablished (Coplan et al., 1996; Nemeroff, 1996).

Similarly, using a randomized cross-fostering design with newborn rat pups, Meaney and colleagues (Francis, Diorio, Liu, & Meaney, 1999; Liu et al., 2000) have demonstrated that both a pup's physiological stress responses mediated by the HPA axis and the degree of synaptogenesis in the hippocampus were related to the degree of nurturing received from the mother. More important, if pups genetically related to nonnurturing mothers were fostered to nurturing mothers, their own HPA axis and hippocampal development were similar to those of the pups of nurturing mothers. They in turn exhibited enhanced nurturing toward their own offspring, and their own enhanced HPA axis functioning and hippocampal development were transmitted intergenerationally, independent of genetic influence. A number of researchers are now exploring whether experiences of problematic caregiving in human infancy may also be related to enduring alterations in HPA axis or neurotransmitter function (e.g., Kaufman et al., 1997; Ito et al., 1993; Rogeness & McClure, 1996).

Other well-controlled research indicates that genetic diathesis and rearing conditions interact, often in unexpected ways, to produce complex social behavior and psychopathology (Cutrona et al., 1994; Cadoret, Yates, Troughton, Woodworth, & Stewart, 1995; Cadoret et al., 1996; Tienari et al., 1987; Arcus, Gardner, & Anderson, 1992; Suomi, 1987; Suomi & Champeaux, 1992). Given the lack of power of current behavioral genetic designs in human populations to assess gene–environment interactions reliably (e.g., Wahlsten, 1991), we will need to continue to treat family interactive behavior as a complex product of both inherited and acquired tendencies. Studies of the intergenerational transmission of relational patterns indicate that finely meshed, complementary patterns of parent and infant behavior, accompanied by detailed "internal models" of relationships, operate as an influential interface in this transmission process.

Disorganized/Disoriented Attachment Patterns and Infant Risk

These findings on the intergenerational transmission of relational patterns have increased interest in understanding how an infant organizes patterns of relational behavior within particular caregiving contexts. One influential research tradition now exploring the interface between normal and disturbed behavior in infancy is that of attachment studies. This literature began by exploring the organization of infant attachment behavior in normal samples, but it has more recently begun to document the occurrence of disorganized/disoriented forms of infant behavior in disturbed family contexts. The emerging data on the context and correlates of disorganized/disoriented infant behavior are creating interest in these behaviors as possible symptoms of current disorder or as precursors or risk factors for later clinical disorders. In this section, we review what is known about the infant context of disorganized/disoriented attachment behaviors; in the section that follows, we link this literature to longitudinal studies of the psychiatric sequelae of those infant behaviors.

The Attachment Behavioral System

As defined initially by John Bowlby (1969), the attachment behavioral system includes those infant behaviors that are activated by stress and that have as a goal the reinstating of a sense of security, usually best achieved in infancy by close physical contact with or proximity to a familiar caregiver. The attachment system can be thought of as the psychological version of the immune system, in that the attachment system is the preadapted behavioral system for combating and reducing stress or fearful arousal, just as the immune system is the biological system for combating physical disease. Under normal conditions, an adequately functioning attachment relationship will serve to buffer the infant (and adult) against extreme levels of fearful arousal.

Although the attachment system is viewed as only a single, circumscribed motivational system among other systems, it is also regarded as preemptive when aroused, since it mobilizes responses to fear or threat. In that sense, the quality of regulation of fearful affect is foundational to the developing child's freedom to turn attention away from issues of threat toward other developmental achievements, such as exploration, learning, and play. Because the attachment behavioral system is a system activated by experienced stress, attachment behaviors may not be evident in familiar, low-stress environments. Therefore, the assessment paradigm of choice has involved two brief separations in an unfamiliar setting (termed the "Strange Situation" assessment) (Ainsworth et al., 1978).

From 1970 to 1985, investigators focused on replicating and extending the original discovery of Ainsworth et al. (1978) that three organized patterns of infant behavior toward the caregiver were identifiable at 1 year of age in response to mild stress. These behavioral profiles were termed "secure," "avoidant," and "ambivalent" attachment patterns, and their characteristics are summarized in Table 13.8. Main (1990) describes secure infants as maintaining a stance, or strategy, of open communication of both positive and negative affect. Infants in the ambivalent group are viewed as maintaining a strategy of heightening signals of anger and distress, with the goal of eliciting a response from a less responsive caregiver. Main (1990) characterizes the underlying organized strategy of avoidant infants as one of restricting the communication of anger and distress by displacing attention onto the inanimate environment, away from cues that might intensify the desire to seek comfort from a parent who rejects attachment behavior. Secure, avoidant, and ambivalent patterns of infant behavior were empirically related to both current and prior differences in maternal caregiving behavior observed at home, with mothers of infants classified as secure rated as more sensitive and responsive than mothers of infants in the other two groups (Ainsworth et al., 1978). A series of subsequent studies demonstrated that infants displaying secure patterns of attachment behavior also exhibited more positive social behaviors toward both parents and peers throughout the preschool years (for reviews, see Cassidy & Shaver, 1999).

Four sources of evidence indicate that infant attachment patterns are not primarily dispositional traits, but have their origins in patterns of relationship developed with a particular caregiver:

1. The attachment strategy shown with one parent is not strongly associated with the attachment pattern shown to the other parent (Fox, Kimmerly, & Schafer, 1991; Grossmann, Grossmann, Huber, & Wartner, 1981; Main & Weston, 1981).
2. In 70% of cases, the infant attachment strategy shown to the primary caregiver is predictable from the caregiver's state of mind with regard to attachment issues assessed prior to the birth of the infant, as noted earlier.
3. The attachment strategy displayed toward the primary caregiver is more predictive of later social adaptation than are strategies shown toward other caregivers (Main, Kaplan, & Cassidy, 1985; Main & Weston, 1981; Suess et al., 1992), even when the primary caregiver is not biologically related (Oppenheim, Sagi, & Lamb, 1988).
4. Various measures of infant temperament have predicted distress to separation, but have not predicted whether the distressed or nondistressed behavior pattern is classified as secure or insecure (Belsky & Rovine, 1987; Kochanska, 1998; Vaughn, Lefever, Seifer, & Barglow, 1989).

Other scattered relationships between temperament and aspects of attachment behavior have appeared in the literature, but have not yielded a replicated and clearly interpretable body of data (Bates, Maslin, & Frankel, 1985; Calkins & Fox, 1992; Crockenberg, 1981; Crockenberg & McCluskey, 1986; Grossmann, Grossmann, Spangler, Suess, & Unzner, 1985; Miyake, Chen, & Campos, 1985).

Disorganized/Disoriented Attachment Behavior

From 1985 to the present, as attachment researchers increasingly began to study high-risk families and clinical samples, it became apparent that the behaviors of some infants did not fit any of the three behavioral patterns common among low-risk cohorts. Main and Solomon (1990) then developed coding criteria for a fourth infant attachment category, labeled "disorganized/disoriented" attachment behavior. Disorganized/

TABLE 13.8. Organized Patterns of Attachment Behavior during Infancy

Secure strategy	Avoidant strategy	Ambivalent strategy
Open communication of affect	Restricted communication of affect	Heightened communication of affect
May or may not be distressed at separation	Little display of distress	Heightened distress
Positive greeting or contact seeking	Avoidance of contact	Anger and contact seeking combined
Soothing effective if distressed	Displacement of attention	Failure of soothing
Few avoidant or ambivalent behaviors	Displacement of anger	Possible heightened passivity/helplessness
Low cortisol secretion	Possible higher cortisol secretion	(No cortisol data)
55% incidence	23% incidence	8% incidence
Organized strategy	Organized strategy	Organized strategy

disoriented infant attachment behaviors are now gaining empirical support as precursors or prodromal forms of various child and adult psychiatric symptoms (see below). The term "disorganized/disoriented" refers to the apparent lack of a consistent strategy for organizing responses to the need for comfort and security when the individual is under stress. The term does *not* refer to mental disorganization or to behavioral disorganization more generally, although other infant correlates of disorganized attachment behavior are only beginning to be explored. Approximately 15% of infants in two-parent, middle-class families display disorganized/disoriented attachment behavior. The incidence of such behavior increases under attachment-relevant family risk conditions such as child maltreatment, maternal alcohol consumption, maternal depression, adolescent parenthood, or multiproblem family status, with estimates ranging from 24% among infants of middle-income depressed parents to a high of 82% among low-SES maltreated infants (see van Ijzendoorn, Schuengel, & Bakermans-Kranenburg, 1999, for a meta-analytic review).

Infants who show disorganized/disoriented behavior do not consistently manage distress and approach tendencies by avoidance and displacement, as in the avoidant attachment pattern; nor do they consistently voice their distress at separation and actively seek contact when their mothers return, as usually occurs in the secure or ambivalent patterns. The particular forms and combinations of disorganized/disoriented behaviors tend to be fairly idiosyncratic from child to child, but they include apprehensive, helpless, or depressed behaviors; unexpected alternations of approach and avoidance toward the attachment figure; or other conflict behaviors, such as prolonged freezing or stilling, or slowed "underwater" movements. Table 13.9 summarizes these behaviors (see Main & Solomon, 1990, for a full description of the coding system). Often the outlines of a "best-fitting" or "forced" secure, avoidant, or ambivalent strategy can also be discerned in the context of an infant's disorganized/disoriented attachment behavior. Therefore, all such infants are also assigned a secondary organized strategy, yielding final classifications as "disorganized–secure," "disorganized–avoidant," or "disorganized–ambivalent." Given the array of odd or contradictory behaviors contributing to the disorganized/disoriented category, further work is needed to identify distinct subgroups that might share a particular etiology and/or a subsequent developmental pathway. It is not yet clear whether the "forced" or secondary classifications now assigned are the most empirically useful subgroupings.

Physiological Correlates

In support of the view that infant disorganized/disoriented attachment behavior constitutes the least adaptive behavior pattern, Spangler and Grossmann (1993) demonstrated that infants with this pattern exhibited significantly greater heart rate elevation during the Strange Situation assessment than secure or avoidant infants did (ambivalent infants were not studied), even though overt distress was similar among disorganized and secure infants. In addition, cortisol levels assessed 30 minutes after the assessment remained significantly elevated among infants with disorganized strategies compared to infants with secure strategies, whereas cortisol levels of avoidant infants were intermediate in value (see also Hertsgaard, Gunnar, Erickson, & Nachmias, 1995). Spangler and Grossmann (1993) interpret these data as consistent with animal data indicating that the adrenocortical system is only activated when adequate behavioral strategies cannot be applied.

Cognitive Correlates

Lyons-Ruth, Repacholi, McLeod, and Silva (1991) reported that disorganized/disoriented infant attachment behavior accounted for variance in infant mental development scores at 18 months, independent of variance related to maternal behavior and maternal IQ. Infant physical development quotients were not lowered, producing a pattern of "mental lag" or disparity between mental and performance scores, which occurred almost exclusively among a subset of disorganized infants. This link between disorganized attachment strategies and less effective cognitive functioning has also been demonstrated in an Icelandic cohort followed from ages 7 to 17 years (Jacobsen, Edelstein, & Hoffman, 1994). In addition, a strong relation has been demonstrated between elevated cortisol levels and decreased mental development scores among infants in Romanian orphanages (Carlson & Earls, 1997). Given the well-established link between chronically elevated cortisol levels and structural changes in the hippocampus, further work is needed on the interrelations among disorganiza-

TABLE 13.9. Indices of Disorganization/Disorientation in Presence of Parent

1. Sequential display of contradictory behavior patterns, such as strong attachment behavior followed by avoidance or disorientation.
2. Simultaneous display of contradictory behavior patterns, such as strong avoidance with strong contact seeking, distress, or anger.
3. Undirected, misdirected, incomplete, and interrupted movements and expressions.
4. Stereotypies, asymmetrical movements, mistimed movements, and anomalous postures.
5. Freezing, stilling, or "slow-motion" movements and expressions.
6. Direct indices of apprehension regarding the parent.
7. Direct indices of disorganization or disorientation in presence of parent, such as disoriented wandering, confused or dazed expressions, or multiple, rapid changes of affect.

Note. See Main and Solomon (1990) for complete descriptions.

tion of attachment strategies, HPA activity, and cognitive development (Liu et al., 2000).

Developmental Reorganization

As disorganized/disoriented infants and toddlers make the transition into the preschool years, a developmental reorganization occurs for many of these children, with the signs of conflict, apprehension, or helplessness characteristic of disorganized attachment strategies in infancy becoming augmented or replaced by various forms of controlling behaviors toward the parent, including caregiving behavior or punitive behavior (Main et al., 1985; Wartner, Grossmann, Fremmer-Bombik, & Suess, 1994). Solomon, George, and De Jong (1995) have also reported differences in the fantasy play behavior of caregiving and punitive children. Caregiving children tended to inhibit their fantasy play, while punitive children exhibited more chaotic play scenarios, with themes of unresolved danger and blocked assess to care and safety. In other work, similar deviations in the organization and thematic content of fantasy play have been related to clinical problems at age 5 (Oppenheim, Emde, & Warren, 1996). Additional longitudinal studies investigating this shift in behavioral organization are needed, however, particularly among high-risk or clinically referred infants. For example, Cicchetti and Barnett (1991) found that the disorganized behaviors seen in infancy were still more prominent than controlling patterns among maltreated children from 30 to 48 months of age.

Parental Correlates

During the AAI, parents of infants exhibiting disorganized/disoriented attachment behavior have been found to display lapses of monitoring of reasoning or discourse in discussing childhood experiences of loss or trauma (see van IJzendoorn, 1995), leading Main and Goldwyn (1998) to classify them as "unresolved" with respect to those experiences. van IJzendoorn (1995), in his meta-analysis, reports an overall association of .31 between a mother's unresolved AAI classification and an infant's disorganized attachment behavior. However, the relationship between a parent's unresolved status on the AAI and disorganized infant attachment status has been explored primarily in nonclinical samples. Recent studies indicate that AAI protocols of adults in clinical samples are often placed in rare and less well-described AAI coding categories (e.g., "cannot classify" or "overwhelmed by trauma"), in addition to or in place of categorization in the unresolved group (Holtzworth-Munroe, Stuart, & Hutchinson, 1997; Lyons-Ruth, Melnick, & Yellin, 2001; Patrick, Hobson, Castle, Howard, Maughn, & 1994). The infant behaviors correlated with these forms of maternal or paternal attachment organization have not been identified. Therefore, further description is needed of parental states of mind regarding attachment in clinical cohorts and their relationship to infant behavior.

Results from a number of studies using parental behavior measures have indicated that, as a group, mothers of disorganized infants demonstrate the least optimal interactive behaviors with their children. In addition, all of the more distal correlates of disorganized or controlling behaviors, such as parental unresolved attachment classifications or parental psychosocial risk factors, point to a contribution of parent–infant interaction to the genesis of infant disorganization (see Lyons-Ruth & Jacobvitz, 1999; van IJzendoorn et al., 1999). However, it appears that parental behaviors other than those captured by Ainsworth et al.'s (1978) sensitivity scale must be investigated, since studies using that scale in particular have generated only a small association, albeit a reliable one, between parental behavior and infant disorganization (van IJzendoorn et al., 1999).

Main and Hesse (1990) have hypothesized that disorganization of infant attachment strategies results from parental unresolved fear, which is then transmitted through behavior that is either frightened or frightening to the infant. Studies directly exploring the contribution of frightened/frightening caregiving to infant disorganization are slowly beginning to accumulate. Lyons-Ruth, Bronfman, and Parsons (1999) explored a broader fear-related hypothesis that differs from the Main and Hesse (1990) hypothesis slightly in viewing infant fearful arousal as stemming from an absence of adequate parental regulatory responses, rather than from parental frightened or frightening behaviors per se. In this view, parental withdrawing behaviors or role-confused behaviors that leave the infant without adequate parental regulation of fearful affect should also be disorganizing, whether or not the parent's own behaviors are directly frightened or frightening to the infant.

Lyons-Ruth, Bronfman, and Parsons (1999) used the Atypical Maternal Behavior Inventory in Assessment and Classification (the AMBIANCE), which indexed the frequency of maternal withdrawing, negative/intrusive, role-confused, disoriented, and contradictory behaviors in response to infant cues, as well as the frightened/frightening behaviors included on the Main and Hesse (1992) coding inventory. As predicted, the frequency of atypical caregiving behaviors was significantly related to an infant's display of disorganized attachment behaviors. Maternal atypical behavior in the lab was also associated with increased infant distress at home.

When examined separately, the maternal frightened/frightening behaviors from the Main and Hesse (1992) protocol also significantly discriminated mothers with disorganized infants. However the frightened/frightening behaviors identified by Main and Hesse constituted only 17% of the atypical behaviors coded, and the remaining atypical behaviors continued to distinguish mothers of disorganized infants after all frightened/frightening behaviors were removed. This suggests that both maternal frightened/frightening behavior and infant disorganization occur in a broader context of disregulated and atypical communication between mother and infant.

Recent studies using the AMBIANCE coding scales have replicated the links between maternal atypical behavior and both infant disorganization and maternal unresolved status on the AAI across a wide range of SES groups (Benoit, Blokland, & Madigan, 2001; Lyons-Ruth et al., 2001; Grienenberger & Kelly, 2001; Madigan, 2002). Both Schuengel, Bakermans-Kranenburg, and van IJzendoorn (1999) and Jacobvitz, Hazen, and Riggs (1997) have also documented the link between frightened/frightening behavior and infant disorganization.

Genetic Correlates

A recent report has also documented a genetic contribution to infant disorganization, manifested in an association between disorganized/disoriented attachment and a particular polymorphism (7-repeat allele) on the dopamine D4 receptor gene. In a low-risk Hungarian sample, the risk for disorganized attachment was increased fourfold among infants carrying the 7-repeat allele (Lakatos et al., 2000). Further work is needed to replicate this effect in other samples. In addition, work is needed to assess whether maternal atypical behaviors have a similar genetic loading, and whether atypical caregiving behavior acts to mediate or potentiate the genetic link between the dopamine D4 receptor allele and infant behavior.

In summary, disorganized/disoriented infant attachment behaviors are emerging as potential indices of a relational disorder of infancy, since they are often characterized by signs of conflict and dysphoria, by increased infant distress, and by increased physiological markers of unmodulated infant stress. As currently described, however, these behaviors are subtle, need considerable training to identify reliably, and include a wide range of infant presentations. The diversity of behavioral presentations also raises the possibility that a number of subgroups may exist within the overall category, with different implications for current disorder or later prognosis. However, the established reliability and concurrent validity of these infant behaviors mandate continued research to distill the most powerfully predictive and clinically usable indicators of disorganized/disoriented attachment status and integrate them into current diagnostic thinking. New data on the longitudinal prediction of psychiatric symptomatology from early assessments of disorganized attachment status and family context, which are reviewed next, further underscore this conclusion.

Infant Attachment and Later Psychiatric Symptomatology

Aggressive Behavior Disorders

The research literatures on conduct disorder and antisocial personality disorder have long pointed to the early onset of aggressive behavior disorders among a substantial subgroup of cases identified in adolescence or adulthood (e.g., Hinshaw & Lee, Chapter 3, this volume). Recent work is now beginning to identify predictors of childhood aggressive disorders evident during the first 3 years of life (see Lyons-Ruth, 1996, for a review).

The literature on childhood correlates of conduct disorder indicates that, compared to families of children with attention-deficit/hyperactivity disorder, families of children with conduct disorder have particularly elevated scores on measures of family adversity (Blanz, Schmidt, & Esser, 1991); these families also have higher rates of diagnosable disorder, including antisocial personality disorder, major depression, and substance abuse (Biederman, Munir, & Knee, 1987; Lahey, Russo, Walker, & Piacentini, 1989). Even more well documented is the relationship between harsh and ineffective parental discipline and aggressive behavior problems—a relationship now documented as early as 2 and 3 years of age (e.g., Campbell, 1991). Patterson and Bank (1989) have shown that parental dispositions placing a family at risk for initiation of coercive cycles of interaction include parental lack of social skills, parental antisocial traits (self-reported aggression and motor vehicle violations), and parent-reported child difficult temperament. These variables are substantially correlated and predict variance primarily among single-parent families.

Work by Dodge and others has further established that both aggressive boys and their mothers tend to attribute hostile intentions to others in ambiguous situations, with mothers of aggressive children attributing child misbehavior more to negative personality dimensions and endorsing more forceful disciplinary responses, and children of mothers who make hostile attributions displaying more aggression (Dix & Lochman, 1990; Dodge, Pettit, McClaskey, & Brown, 1986; Pettit, Dodge, & Brown, 1988). Another robust finding has been the documentation of a Verbal IQ deficit of about 8 points, or half a standard deviation, among children with conduct disorder, compared both to nondeviant peers and to the children's own Performance IQ scores (see Moffitt, 1993).

Infant research is now indicating that all these correlates of disorder may be evident and predictive of later aggression during the first 18 months of life, before the onset of coercive cycles of interaction. Egeland, Pianta, and O'Brien (1993), studying a large low-income cohort before the discovery of the disorganized form of infant attachment behavior, demonstrated that maternal intrusive control, observed when children were 6 months old, predicted insecure infant attachment behavior at 12 months of age; negative, noncompliant, and hyperactive behavior at age 3½ years; and elevated teacher ratings of both internalizing and externalizing problems in first grade. When assessed in infancy, intrusive mothers reported more anxiety and suspiciousness, displayed less appreciation of the need for reciprocity with the child, and were unlikely to be living with a partner. In a later follow-up, both insecure attachment in infancy and maternal hostility at age 3½ years predicted first- through third-grade teacher-rated aggression.

Lyons-Ruth, Alpern, and Repacholi (1993), following a cohort of 64 low-income families from infancy, found that maternal psychosocial problems (particularly chronic depressive symptoms) and disorganized/disoriented infant attachment behavior made additive contributions to the prediction of child hostile/aggressive behavior in kindergarten. If the mothers had psychosocial problems *and* the attachment relationships were disorganized, a majority of infants (56%) exhibited highly hostile behavior in kindergarten, compared to 5% of low-income children with neither risk factor. The predictive effect of maternal psychosocial problems was mediated through the increased hostile/intrusive behavior shown by such mothers in interaction with their infants at home at 18 months of age. A number of other studies in both low- and middle-income samples have now confirmed this link between disorganized attachment and preschool behavior problems (van IJzendoorn et al., 1999).

At school age in the same cohort, Lyons-Ruth, Easterbrooks, and Cibelli (1997) found that a deviant level of externalizing behavior at age 7 was correctly predicted in 87% of cases from the infancy assessments. Disorganized attachment behavior in infancy predicted externalizing behavior at age 7, but only if a child had also displayed lowered mental development scores in infancy. In forward predictions, 50% of the disorganized/low-mental-development infants displayed deviant levels of externalizing symptoms at age 7 years, compared to 5% of other infants. In backward predictions, 83% of deviant children were in the disorganized/low-mental-development group at 18 months of age compared, to only 13% of nondeviant children. Mothers of deviant children had slightly *higher* Verbal IQ scores than mothers of nondeviant children. Fifty percent of disorganized infants were later rated by teachers as showing very poor adaptation to the school environment, compared to 20% of children whose infant attachment strategies were organized.

A similar pattern of findings has also emerged in two cross-sectional studies of 4- to 5-year-old clinic-referred children, one of which used DSM-III-R criteria for defining oppositional defiant disorder (Greenberg, Speltz, DeKlyen, & Endriga, 1991; Speltz, Greenberg, & DeKlyen, 1990). In both studies, oppositional children were significantly more likely to display insecure attachment patterns, with a majority of such children (67% and 58% in each study, respectively) exhibiting disorganized attachment behaviors of the controlling type.

This body of infant studies considerably broadens and deepens our view of the developmental pathways leading to conduct problems. This literature identifies many of the same correlates of child aggression evident in the literature on school-age children, such as poor parental social skills, intrusive and rejecting parental behavior, and child verbal deficits. However, this literature also indicates that a child's coercive behavior is likely to be preceded by serious disturbances in the security of the attachment relationship in infancy. In addition, the literature suggests substantial phenotypic discontinuity in the presentation of to-be-aggressive children from infancy to school age, with the disorganization in infancy characterized by indicators of conflict, apprehension, helplessness, and distress rather than by coercive behavior per se. Attachment theory would interpret these behaviors as responses to dysfunctions in the infant's primary attachment relationships, which leave the infant unable to develop an organized relational strategy for regulating arousal.

Dissociative Symptoms, Depressive Symptoms, Anxiety Disorders, and Overall Psychopathology

As noted just above, a number of studies have found that disorganized attachment strategies (or disorganized strategies that later become controlling) predicted elevations in both internalizing and externalizing behavior problems as rated by teachers in middle childhood. This is not surprising, since depressive and anxiety symptoms are elevated among many youths with conduct disorder (see Hinshaw & Lee, Chapter 3, this volume).

What is less clear is whether disorganized/disoriented attachment primarily predicts internalizing symptoms that are comorbid with externalizing disorders, or whether purely internalizing disorders are also related to early attachment disorganization. Lyons-Ruth et al. (1997) reported that purely internalizing symptoms were predicted by early organized avoidant attachments, while comorbid internalizing and externalizing symptoms were predicted by attachment behaviors that were both avoidant and disorganized. Hubbs-Tait, Osofsky, Hann, and Culp (1994) and Goldberg, Gotowiec, and Simmons (1995) also found that internalizing symptoms were more strongly related to avoidant attachment behavior. Additional studies are needed that differentiate between comorbid and non-comorbid internalizing symptoms.

Dissociative symptomatology is one type of internalizing symptom that has been related to early disorganized/disoriented attachment strategies both theoretically and empirically. Liotti (1992) has pointed out the phenotypic similarity between the contradictory and unintegrated quality of disorganized behaviors in infancy and the contradictory and unintegrated nature of dissociated mental states in adulthood, and has speculated that disorganized behaviors represent a developmental anlagen or precursor state for later dissociative symptoms. Ogawa, Sroufe, Weinfeld, Carlson, and Egeland (1997) tested this hypothesis in a study from infancy to adolescence of 126 children from low-income families. From a wide array of potential predictors from infancy, preschool, and middle childhood, the best predictors of symptoms on the Dissociative Experiences Scale at age 19 were disorganized attachment at 12–18 months and mother's psychological unavailability from 0 to 24 months. The variance in dissociative symptoms related to sexual or physical abuse was not uniquely predictive once the quality of the early caregiving relationship was accounted for.

Disorganized attachment also predicted teacher-rated items on the Child Behavior Checklist—Teacher Report Form that indexed dissociation-like phenomena in elementary school and high school. Only during elementary school did the occurrence of physical abuse add to the variance in symptoms accounted for by early attachment. Using data from the same sample, Carlson (1998) also found that early disorganization predicted overall psychopathology at age 17½ assessed on the Schedule for Affective Disorders and Schizophrenia for School-Age Children.

The most surprising aspect of both these findings is that the prediction from infancy to adolescence was direct and unmediated by a number of other well-chosen variables. These intervening variables, such as incidence of abuse or childhood behavior problems, would be expected to "carry forward" or mediate the variance in adaptation initially associated with infant disorganization. Instead, the early caregiving relationship appears to create a broader vulnerability to late adolescent psychiatric symptoms than can be captured by our current assessments of preschool and school-age symptoms and risk factors.

Two other papers from the same study sample have explored infancy, preschool, and school-age predictors of adolescent depressive or anxiety disorders, although for unclear reasons disorganized/disoriented attachment status was not included as a variable for analysis in either study. In relation to depressive symptoms, Duggal, Carlson, Sroufe, and Egeland (2001) examined only maternal contributors to both childhood (first through third grades) and adolescent (16–17½ years) depression among 168 families. Predictors examined included maternal depressive symptoms (7 years), early maternal stress (12–64 months), later maternal stress (6–17 years), support for parenting (12–64 months), early maternal supportive care to child (12–42 months), later maternal supportive care (13 years), and maternal abuse of child (0–64 months). Significant associations were found between all variables and depressive symptoms in childhood, but only the extent of maternal abuse and the degree of early maternal stress made unique contributions in a multiple-regression analysis. In contrast, depression in adolescence across gender was related most strongly to lack of supportive early care. This was particularly true of boys, whereas for girls the primary predictor was maternal depressive symptoms at age 7. Other variables did not add to the variance accounted for by these two predictors. The only predictor of *adolescent-onset* depressive symptoms, as compared to depressive symptoms that began earlier in life, was mother's depressive symptoms at age 7.

Warren, Huston, Egeland, and Sroufe (1997) assessed whether variables coded during the first year of life were related to anxiety disorders at 17½ years in the same sample. The factors examined included nurse-rated and examiner-rated neonatal temperament, maternal trait anxiety, and anxious/resistant (i.e., ambivalent) attachment as assessed at 12 months of age. The 18-month attachment assessment was not entered into this analysis. Only ambivalent attachment and Neonatal Behavior Assessment Scale range-of-state scores accounted for unique portions of variance in adolescent anxiety. However, the relation between range-of-state scores and adolescent anxiety was in the opposite direction to prediction, leading the investigators to speculate to that it was a chance finding. Ambivalent attachment accounted for only 4% of the variance, however. Other variables related to quality of maternal care (including disorganized/disorganized attachment and the other above- mentioned predictors of depressive and dissociative symptoms) were not examined, so it remains unclear whether ambivalent attachment indexes a unique aspect of the early parent-child relationship.

Other work examining the concept of "behavioral inhibition," using Kagan, Reznick, Clarke, Snidman, and Garcia-Coll's (1984) criteria, has shown a relation between behavioral inhibition at 21 months of age and anxiety disorders in childhood, as well as between parental anxiety disorder and offspring behavioral inhibition at 2 to 7 years of age (Biederman et al., 1993; Kagan, Snidman, Zentner, & Peterson, 1999). However, complex transactional effects seem to categorize the relations between caregiving and behavioral inhibition. In other work from Kagan's lab, Arcus et al. (1992) found that maternal directive caregiving style interacted with infant temperament, reducing the tendency for infants with "high-reactive" temperament at 4 months to become behaviorally inhibited by 14 months.

Complex transactional effects also seem to characterize the relations between attachment security and behavioral inhibition. Calkins and Fox (1992), examining 33 measures of temperament across the first year, found that only 1 of the 33 measures predicted ambivalent attachment at 14 months, but that attachment at 14 months predicted behavioral inhibition at 24 months. Kochanska (1998) found that behavioral inhibition did not predict whether an infant was classified as secure or insecure, but did predict type of insecurity (inhibited insecure children were classified as ambivalent rather than avoidant).

In one of the few studies that has examined security of attachment among mothers with anxiety disorders and their young children aged 18–59 months, Manassis, Bradley, Goldberg, Hood, and Swinson (1994) found that 78% of these mothers were classified "unresolved with respect to loss or trauma," and that 65% of the children of these mothers (n = 20) were classified as disorganized in their attachment strategies. Behavioral inhibition was also assessed, and 65% of offspring were classified as behaviorally inhibited (Manassis, Bradley, Goldberg, Hood, & Swinson, 1995). There was no statistical relation between behavioral inhibition and insecure attachment, with three of the four secure children classed as inhibited. On parent-reported symptom scales, inhibited children displayed more somatic symptoms, while insecure children displayed more internalizing symptoms, social withdrawal, depressive symptoms, somatic problems, and destructive behaviors. Of the three children with DSM-III-R anxiety disorders, all were insecurely attached, but only one was behaviorally inhibited. In sum, studies to date indicate that both infant temperament and the quality of early caregiving and attachment contribute to the development of anxiety disorders, but there is disagreement across studies as to how the two classes of variables relate to one another.

CONCLUDING COMMENTS

The body of infant research reviewed here has implications for our conception of childhood disorder more generally. First, this literature points up the need for a longitudinal–developmental conception of childhood psychopathology, since both internalizing and externalizing symptoms appear to be more strongly related to early precursors or risk factors than previously thought. Second, this literature converges with the broader clinical literature in pointing to the importance of the biological and social regulation available in the family context as one mediator of childhood psychopathology. Longitudinal research from infancy has constituted particularly fertile ground for the development of sophisticated theoretical and research approaches to the assessment of relational processes between parents and children, including both the biological concomitants and the representational processes associated with patterns of family interaction. As noted earlier, case–control studies of such infant disorders as feeding, sleep, and regulatory disorders have implicated both current parent–child interactional problems and problematic parental attachment histories as correlates of child disorders. This literature presses us to extend more sophisticated relational assessments to the study of psychopathology, including a more comprehensive view of parental affect and behavior toward the child, increased information about parental relationship histories and implicit representational models for guiding caregiving behavior, and increased study of the intergenerational transmission of particular patterns of relating. These relational methods in turn need to be integrated into genetic and intervention designs with the potential to evaluate causal influences.

Finally, the infancy literature (as well as the larger developmental and clinical research literatures) is pressing us to reexamine our tradition of individually oriented diagnostic criteria and assessment practices, and to move toward more systematic assessment of family context and relational behavior. Current diagnostic criteria are inconsistent in emphasizing relational behavior as intrinsic to some disorders (e.g., externalizing disorders and character disorders) but not others (e.g., most internalizing disorders). Infant research is urging us toward a more systematic and developmental view of implicit representation, affect, stress responsivity, and relational behavior as inextricably linked expressions of interpersonal relational systems with potentially intergenerational trajectories. These accumulated insights into family relational systems will need to be integrated with work in genetic analysis, child temperament, and psychophysiology to clarify how genetic diathesis and temperamental or regulatory qualities of the individual interact with the quality of biopsychological regulation provided in the family system to produce developmental trajectories culminating in psychological disorders.

ACKNOWLEDGMENTS

During the writing of this chapter, Karlen Lyons-Ruth was supported in part by National Institute of Mental Health Grant No. R01 MH62030. Charles H. Zeanah's work described in this chapter was supported in part by the MacArthur Foundation Research Network, "Early Experience and Brain Development."

REFERENCES

Ainsworth, M. D. S., Blehar, M. C., Waters, E., & Wall, S. (1978). *Patterns of attachment: A psychological study of the Strange Situation*. Hillsdale, NJ: Erlbaum.

American Psychiatric Association (APA). (1980). *Diagnostic and statistical manual of mental disorders* (3rd ed.). Washington, DC: Author.

American Psychiatric Association (APA). (1987). *Diagnostic and statistical manual of mental disorders* (3rd ed., rev.). Washington, DC: Author.

American Psychiatric Association (APA). (1994). *Diagnostic and statistical manual of mental disorders*, (4th ed.). Washington, DC: Author.

American Sleep Disorders Association. (1990). *The international classification of sleep disorders: Diagnostic and coding manual (ICSD:DCM)*. Kansas City, KS: Allen Press.

Ames, E., & Chisholm, K. (2001). Social and emotional development in children adopted from institutions. In D. B. Bailey, J. T. Bruer, F. J. Symons, J. W. Lichtman (Eds.), *Critical thinking about critical periods* (pp. 129–148), Baltimore: Brookes.

Anders, T. F. (1975). Maturation of sleep patterns in the newborn infant. *Advances in Sleep Research*, *2*, 43–66.

Anders, T. F. (1989). Clinical syndromes, relationship disturbances and their assessment. In A. J. Sameroff & R. N. Emde (Eds.), *Relationship disturbances in early childhood* (pp. 125–144). New York: Basic Books.

Anders, T. F., Carskadon, M. A., & Dement, W. C. (1980). Sleep and sleepiness in children and adolescents. *Pediatric Clinics of North America*, *27*, 29–43.

Anders, T., Goodlin-Jones, B., & Sadeh, A. (2000). Sleep disorders. In C.H. Zeanah (Ed.), *Handbook of infant mental health* (2nd ed., pp. 326–338). New York: Guilford Press.

Arcus, D., Gardner, S., & Anderson, C. (1992, May). Infant reactivity, maternal style, and the development of inhibited and uninhibited behavioral profiles. In D. Arcus (Chair), *Temperament and environment*. Symposium conducted at the biennial meeting of the International Society for Infant Studies, Miami, FL.

Barr, R. G. (1990). The "colic" enigma: Prolonged episodes of a normal predisposition to cry. *Infant Mental Health Journal*, *11*, 340–348.

Barr, R. G., Kramer, M. S., Pless, I. B., Boisjoly, C., & Leduc, D. (1989). Feeding and temperament as determinants of early infant cry/fuss behavior. *Pediatrics*, *84*, 514–521.

Barr, R. G., Rotman, A., Yaremko, J., Leduc, D., & Francoeur, T. E. (1992). The crying of infants with colic: A controlled empirical description. *Pediatrics*, *90*, 14–21.

Barton, M. L., & Robins, D. (2000). Regulatory disorders. In C. H. Zeanah (Ed.), *Handbook of infant mental health* (2nd ed. pp. 311–325). New York: Guilford Press.

Bates, J. E., Maslin, C. A., & Frankel, K. A. (1985). Attachment security, mother–child interaction, and temperament as predictors of behavior-problem ratings at age three years. In I. Bretherton & E. Waters (Eds.), Growing points of attachment theory and research. *Monographs of the Society for Research in Child Development*, *50*(1–2, Serial No. 209), 167–193.

Belsky, J., & Pensky, E. (1988). Developmental history, personality, and family relationships: Toward an emergent family system. In R. A. Hinde & J. Stevenson-Hinde (Eds.), *Relationships within families: Mutual influences* (pp. 193–217). New York: Oxford University Press.

Belsky, J., & Rovine, M. (1987). Temperament and attachment security in the Strange Situation: An empirical rapprochement. *Child Development*, *58*, 787–795.

Belsky, J., Hertzog, C., & Rovine, M. (1986). Causal analyses of multiple determinants of parenting: Empirical and methodological advances. In M. Lamb, A. Brown, & B. Rogoff (Eds.), *Advances in developmental psychology* (Vol. 4, pp. 153–202). Hillsdale, NJ: Erlbaum.

Belsky, J., Youngblade, L., & Pensky, E. (1989). Childrearing history, marital quality, and maternal affect: Intergenerational transmission in a low-risk sample. *Developmental Psychopathology*, *1*, 291–304.

Benoit, D. (1993a). Failure to thrive and feeding disorders. In C. H. Zeanah (Ed.), *Handbook of infant mental health* (pp. 317–331). New York: Guilford Press.

Benoit, D. (1993b). Phenomenology and treatment of failure to thrive. *Child and Adolescent Psychiatric Clinics of North America*, *2*, 61–73.

Benoit, D. (2000a). Feeding disorders, failure to thrive, and obesity. In C. H. Zeanah (Ed.), *Handbook of infant mental health* (2nd ed., pp. 339–352). New York: Guilford Press.

Benoit, D. (2000b). Regulation and its disorders. In C. Violato, E. Oddone-Paolucci, & M. Genuis (Eds.), *The changing family and child development* (pp. 149–161). Aldershot, England: Ashgate.

Benoit, D., Blokland, K., & Madigan, S. (2001). Maternal representations of their child and attachment during pregnancy: Association with maternal postnatal disrupted behavior. In O. Mayseless & M. Scharf (Chairs), *Mothers' parenting representations, their own, and their children's functioning and adaptation*. Symposium conducted at the biennial meeting of the Society for Research in Child Development, Minneapolis, MN.

Benoit, D., Zeanah, C. H., & Barton, L. M. (1989). Maternal attachment disturbances in failure to thrive. *Infant Mental Health Journal*, *10*, 185–202.

Benoit, D., Zeanah, C. H., Boucher, C., & Minde, K. K. (1992). Sleep disorders in early childhood: Association with insecure maternal attachment. *Journal of the American Academy of Child and Adolescent Psychiatry*, *31*, 86–93.

Berkowitz, C. D., & Senter, S. A. (1987). Characteristics of mother–infant interactions in nonorganic failure to thrive. *Journal of Family Practice*, *25*, 377–381.

Bernal, J. (1973). Night waking in infants during the first 14 months. *Developmental Medicine and Child Neurology*, *14*, 362–372.

Berwick, D. M., Levy, J. C., & Kleinerman, R. (1982). Failure to thrive: Diagnostic yield of hospitalization. *Archives of Disease in Childhood*, *57*, 347–351.

Biederman, J., Munir, K., & Knee, D. (1987). Conduct and oppositional disorder in clinically referred children with attention deficit disorder: A controlled family study. *Journal of the American Academy of Child and Adolescent Psychiatry*, *26*, 724–727.

Biederman, J., Rosenbaum, J. F., Bolduc-Murphy, E. A., Farone, S. V., Chaloff, J., Hirshfeld, D. R., & Kagan, J. (1993). A 3-year follow-up of children with and without behavioral inhibition. *Journal of the American Academy of Child and Adolescent Psychiatry*, *32*, 814–821.

Black, M.M., Hutcheson, J., Dubowitz, H., & Berenson-Howard, J. (1994). Parenting style and developmental status among children with nonorganic failure to thrive. *Journal of Pediatric Psychology*, *19*, 689–707.

Blackman, J. A., & Nelson, C. L. A. (1985). Reinstituting oral feedings in children fed by gastrostomy tube. *Clinical Pediatrics*, *24*, 434–438.

Blackman, J. A., & Nelson, C. L. A. (1987). Rapid introduction of oral feedings to tube-fed patients. *Journal of Developmental and Behavioral Pediatrics*, *8*(2), 63–67.

Blanz, B., Schmidt, M. H., & Esser, G. (1991). Familial adversities and child psychiatric disorder. *Journal of Child Psychology and Psychiatry*, *32*, 939–950.

Boddy, J., Skuse, D., & Andrews, B. (2000). The developmental sequelae of nonorganic failure to thrive. *Journal of Child Psychology and Psychiatry*, *41*, 1003–1014.

Boris, N. W., Hinshaw-Fuselier, S., Heller, S. S., Smyke, A. T. S., Scheeringa, M., & Zeanah, C. H. (2000, July). *Attachment disorders: diagnostic challenges*. Paper presented at the Sixth International Congress of the World Association for Infant Mental Health, Montreal, Canada.

Boris, N. W., & Zeanah, C. H. (1999). Disturbances and disorders of attachment in infancy: An overview. *Infant Mental Health Journal*, *20*, 1–9.

Boris, N., W., Zeanah, C. H., Larrieu, J., Scheeringa, M., & Heller, S. (1998). Attachment disorders in infancy and early childhood: A preliminary study of diagnostic criteria. *American Journal of Psychiatry*, *155*, 295–297.

Bowlby, J. (1969). *Attachment and loss: Vol. 1. Attachment.* New York: Basic Books.

Brazelton, T. B. (1962). Crying in infancy. *Pediatrics*, *29*, 579–588.

Brazelton, T. B. (1990). Crying and colic. *Infant Mental Health Journal*, *11*, 349–356.

Brown, G. W., Harris, T. O., & Bifulco, A. (1986). Long-term effects of early loss of a parent. In M. Rutter, C. E. Izard, & P. B. Read (Eds.), *Depression in young people* (pp. 251–296). New York: Guilford Press.

Burklow, K. A., Phelps, A. N., Schultz, J. R., McConnell, K., & Rudolph, C. (1998). Classifying complex pediatric feeding disorders. *Journal of Pediatric Gastroenterology and Nutrition*, *27*, 143–147.

Cadoret, R. J., Winokur, G., Langbehn, D., Troughton, E., Yates, W. R., & Stewart, M. A. (1996). Depression spectrum disease: I. The role of gene–environment interaction. *American Journal of Psychiatry*, *153*, 892–899.

Cadoret, R. J., Yates, W. R., Troughton, E., Woodworth, G., & Stewart, M. A. (1995). Genetic–environmental interaction and the genesis of aggressivity and conduct disorders. *Archives of General Psychiatry*, *52*, 916–924.

Calkins, S., & Fox, N. (1992). The relations among infant temperament, security of attachment, and behavioral inhibition at twenty-four months. *Child Development*, *63*, 1456–1472.

Campbell, S. B. (1991). Longitudinal studies of active and aggressive preschoolers: Individual differences in early behavior and in outcome. In D. Cicchetti & S. L. Toth (Eds.), *Rochester Symposium on Developmental Psychopathology: Vol. 2. Internalizing and externalizing expression of dysfunction* (pp. 57–89). Hillsdale, NJ: Erlbaum.

Canivet, C., Jakobsson, I., & Hagander, B. (2000). Infantile colic: Follow-up at four years of age. Still more "emotional." *Acta Paediatrica*, *89*, 13–17.

Carey, W. B. (1974). Night waking and temperament in infancy. *Journal of Pediatrics*, *84*, 756–758.

Carlson, E. A. (1998). A prospective longitudinal study of disorganized/disoriented attachment. *Child Development*, *69*, 1970–1979.

Carlson, M., & Earls, F. (1997). Psychological and neuroendocrinological sequelae of early social deprivation in institutionalized children in Romania. *Annals of the New York Academy of Sciences*, *807*, 419–428.

Casey, P. H. (1988). Failure-to-thrive: Transitional perspective. *Journal of Developmental and Behavioral Pediatrics*, *8*, 37–38.

Casey, P. H., Kelleher, K. J., Bradley, R. H., Kellogg, K. W., Kirby, R. S., & Whiteside, L. (1994). A multifaceted intervention for infants with failure to thrive. *Archives of Pediatrics and Adolescent Medicine*, *148*, 1071–1077.

Cassidy, J., & Shaver, P. R. (Eds.). (1999). *Handbook of attachment: Theory, research, and clinical implications.* New York: Guilford Press.

Chatoor, I. (1989). Infantile anorexia nervosa: A developmental disorder of separation and individuation. *Journal of the American Academy of Psychoanalysis*, *17*(1), 43–64.

Chatoor, I., Conley, C., & Dickson, L. (1988). Food refusal after an incident of choking: A posttraumatic eating disorder. *Journal of the American Academy of Child and Adolescent Psychiatry*, *27*, 105–110.

Chatoor, I., Dickson, L., Schaefer, S., & Egan, J. (1985). A developmental classification of feeding disorders associated with failure to thrive: Diagnosis and treatment. In D. Drotar (Ed.), *New directions in failure to thrive: Implications for research and practice* (pp. 235–258). New York: Plenum Press.

Chatoor, I., Egan, J., Getson, P., Menvielle, E., & O'Donnell, R. (1987). Mother–infant interactions in infantile anorexia nervosa. *Journal of the American Academy of Child and Adolescent Psychiatry*, *27*(5), 535–540.

Chatoor, I., Ganiban, J., Colin, V., Plummer, N., & Harmon, R. J. (1998). Attachment and feeding problems: A reexamination of nonorganic failure to thrive and attachment security. *Journal of the American Academy of Child and Adolescent Psychiatry*, *37*, 1217–1224.

Chatoor, I., Ganiban, J., Harrison, J., & Hirsch, R. (2001). Observation of feeding in the diagnosis of posttraumatic feeding disorder in infancy. *Journal of the American Academy of Child and Adolescent Psychiatry*, *40*, 595–602.

Chisholm, K. (1998). A three year follow-up of attachment and indiscriminate friendliness in children adopted from Romanian orphanages. *Child Development*, *69*, 1092–1106.

Chisholm, K., Carter, M. C., Ames, E. W., & Morison, S. J. (1995). Attachment security and indiscriminantly friendly behavior in children adopted from Romanian orphanages. *Development and Psychopathology*, *7*, 283–294.

Cicchetti, D., & Barnett, D. (1991). Attachment organization in maltreated preschoolers. *Development and Psychopathology*, *3*, 397–411.

Coolbear, J., & Benoit, D. (1999). Failure to thrive: Risk for clinical disturbance of attachment? *Infant Mental Health Journal*, *20*, 87–104.

Coplan, J., Andrews, M., Rosenblum, L., Owens, M., Friedman, S., Gorman, J., & Nemeroff, C. (1996). Persistent elevations of cerebrospinal fluid concentrations of corticotropin-releasing factor in adult nonhuman primates exposed to early-life stressors: Implications for the pathophysiology of mood and anxiety disorders. *Proceedings of the National Academy of Sciences USA*, *93*, 1619–1623.

Corbett, S. S., Drewett, R. F., & Wright, C. M. (1996). Does a fall down a centile chart matter?: The growth and developmental sequelae of mild failure to thrive. *Acta Paediatrica*, *85*, 1278–1283.

Cox, M. J., Owen, M. T., Lewis, J. M., Riedel, C., Scalf-McIver, L., & Suster, A. (1985). Intergenerational influences on the parent–infant relationship in the transition to parenthood. *Journal of Family Issues*, *6*, 543–564.

Crittenden, P. M. (1987). Non-organic failure to thrive: Deprivation or distortion? *Infant Mental Health Journal*, *8*, 51–64.

Crockenberg, S. B. (1981). Infant irritability, mother responsiveness, and social support influences on the security of infant–mother attachment. *Child Development*, *52*, 857–865.

Crockenberg, S. B., & Leerkes, E. (2000). Infant social and emotional development in family context. In C. H. Zeanah (Ed.), *Handbook of infant mental health* (2nd ed., pp. 60–90). New York: Guilford Press.

Crockenberg, S. B., & McCluskey, K. (1986). Change in maternal behavior during the baby's first year of life. *Child Development*, *57*, 746–753.

Crowcroft, N. S., & Strachan, D. P. (1997) The social origins of infantile colic: Questionnaire study covering 76,747 infants. *British Medical Journal*, *314*, 1325–1328.

Cutrona, C. E., Cadoret, R. J., Suhr, J. A., Richards, C. C., Troughton, E., Schutte, K., & Woodworth, G. (1994). Interpersonal variables in the prediction of alcoholism among adoptees: Evidence for gene–environment interactions. *Comprehensive Psychiatry*, *35*(3), 171–179.

Dahl, M., & Sundelin, C. (1986). Early feeding problems in an affluent society: I. Categories and clinical signs. *Acta Paediatrica Scandinavica*, *75*, 370–379.

Davidson, J. R., & Fairbank, J. A. (1993). The epidemiology of posttraumatic stress disorder. In J. R. Davidson & E. B. Foa (Eds.), *Posttraumatic stress disorder: DSM-IV and beyond* (pp. 147–169). Washington, DC: American Psychiatric Press.

DeGangi, G. A. (1991). Assessment of sensory, emotional, and attentional problems in regulatory disordered infants: Part 1. *Infants and Young Children*, *3*, 1–8.

DeGangi, G. A., Craft, P., & Castellan, J. (1991). Treatment of sensory, emotional, and attentional problems in regulatory disordered infants: Part 2. *Infants and Young Children*, *3*, 9–19.

DeGangi, G. A., DiPietro, J. A., Greenspan, S. I., & Porges, S. W. (1991). Psychophysiological characteristics of the regulatory disordered infant. *Infant Behavior and Development*, *14*, 37–50.

DeGangi, G. A., Porges, S. W., Sickel, R. Z., & Greenspan, S. I. (1993). Four-year follow-up of a sample of regulatory disordered infants. *Infant Mental Health Journal*, *14*, 330–343.

Dix, T. H., & Lochman, J. E. (1990). Social cognition and negative reactions to children: A comparison of mothers of aggressive and nonaggressive boys. *Journal of Social and Clinical Psychology*, *9*, 418–438.

Dodge, K. A., Pettit, G. S., McClaskey, C. L., & Brown, M. M. (1986). Social competence in children. *Monographs of the Society for Research in Child Development*, *51*(2, Serial No. 213).

Drell, M. J., Siegel, C. H., & Gaensbauer, T. J. (1993). Posttraumatic stress disorder. In C. H. Zeanah (Ed.), *Handbook of infant mental health* (pp. 291–304). New York: Guilford Press.

Drewett, R. F., Corbett, S. S., & Wright, C. M. (1999). Cognitive and educational attainments at school age of children who failed to thrive in infancy: A population-based study. *Journal of Child Psychology and Psychiatry*, *40*, 551–561.

Drotar, D., Malone, C. A., Devost, L., Brickell, C., Mantz-Clumpner, L., Negray, J., Wallace, M., Waychik, J., Wyatt, B., Eckerle, D., Bush, L., Finlon, M. A., ElAmin, D., Nowak, M., Satola, J., & Pallotta, J. (1985). Early preventive interventions in failure to thrive: Methods and early outcome. In D. Drotar (Ed.), *New directions in failure to thrive: Implications for research and practice* (pp. 119–138). New York: Plenum Press.

Drotar, D., Pallotta, J., & Eckerle, D. (1994). A prospective study of family environments of children hospitalized for nonorganic failure to thrive. *Journal of Developmental and Behavioral Pediatrics*, *15*, 78–85.

Duggal, S., Carlson, L., Sroufe, A., & Egeland, B. (2001). Depressive symptomatology in childhood and adolescence. *Development and Psychopathology*, *13*, 143–164.

Egeland, B., Jacobvitz, D., & Sroufe, L. A. (1988). Breaking the cycle of abuse. *Child Development*, *59*, 1080–1088.

Egeland, B., Pianta, R., & O'Brien, M. A. (1993). Maternal intrusiveness in infancy and child maladaptation in early school years. *Development and Psychopathology*, *5*, 359–370.

Elder, G., Caspi, A., & Downey, G. (1986). Problem behavior and family relationships: Life course and intergenerational themes. In A. Sorensen, F. Weinert, & L. Sherrod (Eds.), *Human development: Interdisciplinary perspectives* (pp. 293–340). Hillsdale, NJ: Erlbaum.

Elder, G., Van Nguyen, T., & Caspi, A. (1985). Linking family hardships to children's lives. *Child Development*, *56*, 361–375.

Elliott, M. R., Pederson, E. L., & Mogan, J. (1997). Early infant crying: Child and family follow-up at three years. *Canadian Journal of Nursing Research*, *29*, 47–67.

Emde, R. N., Bingham, R. D., & Harmon, R. J. (1993). Classification and the diagnostic process in infancy. In C. H. Zeanah (Ed.), *Handbook of infant mental health* (pp. 225–235). New York: Guilford Press.

Finlon, M. A., Drotar, D., Satola, J., Pallotta, J., Wyatt, B., & El-Amin, D. (1985). Home observation of parent–child transaction in failure to thrive. In D. Drotar (Ed.), *New directions in failure to thrive: Implications for research and practice* (pp. 177–190). New York: Plenum Press.

Fonagy, P., Steele, H., & Steele, M. (1991). Maternal representations of attachment during pregnancy predict the organization of infant–mother attachment at one year of age. *Child Development*, *62*, 891–905.

Forsyth, B. W. C., McCarthy, P. L., & Leventhal, J. M. (1985). Problems of early infancy, formula changes, and mothers' beliefs about their infants. *Journal of Pediatrics*, *106*, 1012–1017.

Fox, N. A., Kimmerly, N. L., & Schafer, W. D. (1991). Attachment to mother/attachment to father: A meta-analysis with emphasis on the role of temperament. *Child Development*, *62*, 210–225.

Francis, D., Diorio, J., Liu, D., & Meaney, M. (1999). Non genomic transmission across generations of maternal behavior and stress responses in the rat. *Science*, *286*, 1155–1158.

Frank, D. A., & Ziesel, S. H. (1988). Failure to thrive. *Pediatric Clinics of North America*, *35*(6), 1187–1206.

Fuller, B. F., Keefe, M. R., & Curtin, M. (1994). Acoustic analysis of cries from "normal" and "irritable" infants. *Western Journal of Nursing Research*, *16*, 243–253.

Gaensbauer, T. J., Chatoor, I., Drell, M., Siegel, D., & Zeanah, C. H. (1995). Traumatic loss in a one-year-old girl. *Journal of the American Academy of Child and Adolescent Psychiatry*, *34*, 94–102.

Garrison, M. M., & Christakis, D. A. (2000). Early childhood: Colic, child development, and poisoning prevention. A systematic review for treatments of infant colic. *Pediatrics*, *106*, 184–190.

Geertsma, M. A., Hyams, J. S., Pelletier, J. M., & Reiter, S. (1985). Feeding resistance after parental hyperalimentation. *American Journal of Diseases of Children*, *139*, 255–256.

George, C., Kaplan, N., & Main, M. (1985). *Adult Attachment Interview*. Unpublished manuscript, University of California, Berkeley.

Goldberg, S., Gotowiec, A., & Simmons, R. J. (1995). Infant–mother attachment and behavior problems in healthy and chronically ill preschoolers. *Development and Psychopathology*, *7*, 267–282.

Gordon, A. H., & Jameson, J. C. (1979). Infant–mother attachment in patients with nonorganic failure to thrive syndrome. *Journal of the American Academy of Child Psychiatry*, *18*, 251–259.

Greenberg, M. T., Speltz, M. L., DeKlyen, M., & Endriga, M. C. (1991). Attachment security in preschoolers with and without externalizing problems: A replication. *Development and Psychopathology*, *3*, 413–430.

Greenspan, S. I., & Wieder, S. (1993). Regulatory disorders. In C. H. Zeanah (Ed.), *Handbook of infant mental health* (pp. 280–290). New York: Guilford Press.

Gremse, D. A., Lytle, J. M., Sacks, A. I., & Balistreri, W. F. (1998). Characterization of failure to imbibe in infants. *Clinical Pediatrics*, *37*, 305–310.

Grienenberger, J., & Kelly, K. (2001). Maternal reflective functioning and caregiving: Links between mental states and observed behavior in the intergenerational transmission. In A. Slade (Chair), *Maternal reflective functioning in relation to the child: Attachment, caregiving, and disrupted relationships*. Symposium conducted at the biennial meeting of the Society for Research in Child Development, Minneapolis, MN.

Grossmann, K., Fremmer-Bombik, E., Rudolph, J., & Grossmann, K. (1988). Maternal attachment representations as related to patterns of infant–mother attachment and maternal care during the first year. In R. Hinde & J. Stevenson-Hinde (Eds.), *Relationships within families: Maternal influences* (pp. 241–260). Oxford: Oxford University Press.

Grossmann, K. E., Grossmann, K., Huber, F., & Wartner, U. (1981). German children's behaviour towards their mothers at 12 months and their fathers at 18 months in Ainsworth's Strange Situation. *International Journal of Behavioral Development*, *4*, 157–181.

Grossmann, K., Grossmann, K. E., Spangler, G., Suess, G., & Unzner, L. (1985). Maternal sensitivity and newborns' orientation responses as related to quality of attachment in northern Germany. In I. Bretherton & E. Waters (Eds.), Growing points of attachment theory and research. *Monographs of the Society for Research in Child Development*, *50*(1–2, Serial No. 209), 233–256.

Hawdon, J. M., Beauregard, N., Slattery, J., & Kennedy, G. (2000). Identification of neonates at risk of developing feeding problems in infancy. *Developmental Medicine and Child Neurology*, *42*, 235–239.

Heinecke, C. M., Diskin, S. D., Ramsey-Klee, D. M., & Oates, D. S. (1986). Pre- and postbirth antecedents of 2-year-old attention, capacity for relationships, and verbal expressiveness. *Developmental Psychology*, *22*, 777–787.

Hertsgaard, L., Gunnar, M., Erickson, M., & Nachmias, M. (1995). Adrenocortical response to the Strange Situation in infants with disorganized/disoriented attachment relationships. *Child Development*, *66*, 1100–1106.

Hinshaw-Fuselier, S., Boris, N., & Zeanah, C. H. (1999). Reactive attachment disorder in maltreated twins. *Infant Mental Health Journal*, *20*, 42–59.

Hoehn, T. P., & Baumeister, A. A. (1994). A critique of the application of sensory integration therapy to children with learning disabilities. *Journal of Learning Disabilities*, *27*, 338–350.

Holtzworth-Munroe, A., Stuart, G. L., & Hutchinson, G. (1997). Violent vs. nonviolent husbands: Differences in attachment patterns, dependency, and jealousy. *Journal of Family Psychology*, *11*, 314–331.

Hubbs-Tait, L., Osofsky, J., Hann, D., & Culp, A. (1994). Predicting behavior problems and social competence in children of adolescent mothers. *Family Relations*, *43*, 439–446.

Illingworth, R. S. (1954). "Three months' colic." *Archives of Disease in Childhood*, *29*, 165–174.

Illingworth, R. S. (1985). Infantile colic revisited. *Archives of Disease in Childhood*, *60*, 981–985.

Ito, Y., Teicher, M. H., Glod, C. A., Harper, D., Magnus, E., & Gelbard, H. (1993). Increased prevalence of electrophysiological abnormalities in children with psychological, physical, and sexual abuse. *Journal of Neuropsychiatry and Clinical Neurosciences*, *5*(4), 401–408.

Jacobsen, T., Edelstein, W., & Hoffman, V. (1994). A longitudinal study of the relation between representations of attachment in childhood and cognitive functioning in childhood and adolescence. *Developmental Psychology*, *30*, 112–124.

Jacobvitz, D., Goldetsky, G., & Hazen, N. (1993, March). Romantic and caregiving relationships in "earned-secure" adults. In P. Costanzo (Chair), *Mental representations of relationships: Intergenerational and temporal continuity?* Symposium conducted at the biennial meeting of the Society for Research in Child Development, New Orleans, LA.

Jacobvitz, D., Hazen, N., & Riggs, S. (1997, April). *Disorganized mental processes in mothers, frightened/frightening caregiving, and disoriented/disorganized behavior in infancy*. Paper presented at the biennial meeting of the Society for Research in Child Development, Washington, DC.

Jenkins, S., Bax, M., & Hart, H. (1980). Behavior problems in pre-school children. *Journal of Child Psychology and Psychiatry*, *21*, 5–17.

Kagan, J. (1981). *The second year: The emergence of self-awareness.* Cambridge, MA: Harvard University Press.

Kagan, J., Reznick, J. S., Clarke, C., Snidman, N., & Garcia-Coll, C. (1984). Behavioral inhibition to the unfamiliar. *Child Development*. 55, 2212–2225.

Kagan, J., Snidman, N., Zentner, M., & Peterson, E. (1999). Infant temperament and anxious symptoms in school age children. *Development and Psychopathology*, 11, 209–224.

Kaufman, J., Birmaher, B., Perel, J., Dahl, R. D., Moreci, P., Nelson, B., Wells, W., & Ryan, N. D. (1997). The corticotropin-releasing hormone challenge in depressed abused, depressed nonabused, and normal control children. *Biological Psychiatry*, *42*, 669–679.

Keefe, M. R., Kotzer, A. M., Froese-Fretz, A., & Curtin M. (1996). A longitudinal comparison of irritable and non-irritable infants. *Nursing Research*, *45*, 4–9.

Kerr, M. A., Black, M. M., & Krishnakumar, A. (2000). Failure-to-thrive, maltreatment and the behavior and development of 6–year-old children from low-income, urban families: A cumulative risk model. *Child Abuse and Neglect*, *24*, 587–598.

Kerwin, M. E. (1999). Empirically supported treatments in pediatric psychology: Severe feeding problems. *Journal of Pediatric Psychology*, *24*, 193–214.

Kochanska, G. (1998). Mother–child relationship, child fearfulness, and emerging attachment: A short-term longitudinal study. *Developmental Psychology*, *34*(3), 480–490.

Lakatos, K., Toth, I., Nemoda, Z., Ney, K., Sasvari-Szekely, M., & Gervai, J. (2000). Dopamine D4 receptor (DRD4) gene polymorphism as associated with attachment disorganization in infants. *Molecular Psychiatry*, *5*, 633–637.

Lahey, B. B., Russo, M. F., Walker, J. L., & Piacentini, J. C. (1989). Personality characteristics of the mothers of children with disruptive behavior disorders. *Journal of Consulting and Clinical Psychology*, *57*, 512–515.

Leckman, J. (2000, October). *A research agenda for preschool psychopathology*. Paper presented at the Research Forum of the annual meeting of the American Academy of Child and Adolescent Psychiatry, New York.

Lehtonen, L., & Korvenranta, H. (1995). Infantile colic: Seasonal incidence and crying profiles. *Archives of Pediatrics and Adolescent Medicine*, *149*, 533–536.

Lehtonen, L., Korhonen, T., & Korvenranta, H. (1994). Temperament and sleeping patterns in colicky infants during the first year of life. *Journal of Developmental and Behavioral Pediatrics*, *15*, 416–420.

Lester, B. M. (1987). Prediction of developmental outcome from acoustic cry analysis in term and preterm infants. *Pediatrics*, *80*, 529–534.

Lester, B. M., & Boukydis, C. F. Z. (1991). No language but a cry. In H. Papousek (Ed.), *Origin and development of non-verbal communication.* New York: Cambridge University Press.

Lester, B. M., Boukydis, C. F. Z., Garcia-Coll, C. T., & Hole, W. T. (1990). Colic for developmentalists. *Infant Mental Health Journal*, *11*, 321–333.

Levy, J. S., Winters, R. W., & Heird, W. (1980). Total parenteral nutrition in pediatric patients. *Pediatrics*, *2*, 99–106.

Lieberman, A. F., & Zeanah, C. H. (1995). Disorders of attachment in infancy. *Child and Adolescent Psychiatric Clinics of North America*, *4*, pp. 571–588.

Linscheid, T. R., Tarnowski, K. J., Rasnake, L. K., & Brams, J. S. (1987). Behavioral treatment of food refusal in a child with short-gut syndrome. *Journal of Pediatric Psychology*, *12*(5), 451–459.

Liotti, G. (1992). Disorganized/disoriented attachment in the etiology of the dissociative disorders. *Dissociation*, *4*, 196–204.

Liu, D., Diorio, J., Day, J. C., Francis, D. D., & Meaney, M. J. (2000). Maternal care, hippocampal synaptogenesis and cognitive development in rats. *Nature Neuroscience*, *8*, 799–806.

Lozoff, B., Wolf, A. W., & Davis, N. S. (1985). Sleep problems seen in pediatric practice. *Pediatrics*, *75*, 477–483.

Lucassen, P. L. B. J., Assendelft, W. J. J., Gubbels, J. W., van Eijk, J. T. M., van Geldrop, W. J., & Knuistingh Neven, A. (1998). Effectiveness of treatments for infantile colic: Systematic review. *British Medical Journal*, *316*, 1563–1569.

Lust, K. D., Brown, J. E., & Thomas, W. (1996). Maternal intake of cruciferous vegetables and other food and colic symptoms in exclusively breast-fed infants. *Journal of the American Dietetic Association*, *96*, 47–48.

Lyons-Ruth, K. (1992). Maternal depressive symptoms, disorganized infant–mother attachment relationships and hostile–aggressive behavior in the preschool classroom: A prospective longitudinal view from infancy to age five. In D. Cicchetti & S. Toth (Eds.), *Rochester Symposium on Developmental Psychopathology: Vol. 4. A developmental approach to affective disorders* (pp. 131–171). Rochester, NY: University of Rochester Press.

Lyons-Ruth, K. (1995). Broadening our conceptual frameworks: Can we reintroduce relational strategies and implicit representational systems to the study of psychopathology? *Developmental Psychology*, *31*, 432–436.

Lyons-Ruth, K. (1996). Attachment relationships among children with aggressive behavior problems: The role of disorganized early attachment patterns. *Journal of Consulting and Clinical Psychology*, *64*, 64–73.

Lyons-Ruth, K., Alpern, L., & Repacholi, B. (1993). Disorganized infant attachment classification and maternal psychosocial problems as predictors of hostile–aggressive behavior in the preschool classroom. *Child Development*, *64*, 572–585.

Lyons-Ruth, K., Bronfman, E., & Parsons, E. (1999). Maternal disrupted affective communication, maternal frightened or frightening behavior, and disorganized infant attachment strategies. In J. Vondra & D. Barnett (Eds.), Atypical patterns of infant attachment: Theory, research and current directions. *Monographs of the Society for Research in Child Development*, *64*(3)(Serial No. 258), 67–96.

Lyons-Ruth, K., Easterbrooks, M A., & Cibelli, C. D. (1997). Infant attachment strategies, infant mental lag, and maternal depressive symptoms: Predictors of internalizing and externalizing problems at age 7. *Developmental Psychology*, *33*(4), 681–692.

Lyons-Ruth, K., & Jacobvitz, D. (1999). Attachment disorganization: Unresolved loss, relational violence, and lapses in behavioral and attentional strategies. In J. Cassidy & P. Shaver (Eds.), *Handbook of attachment: Theory, research, and clinical implications* (pp. 520–554). New York: Guilford Press.

Lyons-Ruth, K., Melnick, S., & Yellin, C. (2001). Autonomous AAI's in clinical samples: Using thick data to unravel relations among caregiving, child attachment, and mothers' AAI's. In J. Crowell & J. Allen (Chairs), *Forks in the road: Using "thick" data to understand lawful discontinuities in attachment and adaptation across the lifespan*. Symposium conducted at the biennial meeting of the Society for Research in Child Development, Minneapolis, MN.

Lyons-Ruth, K., Repacholi, B., McLeod, S., & Silva, E. (1991). Disorganized attachment behavior in infancy: Short-term stability, maternal and infant correlates, and risk-related subtypes. *Development and Psychopathology*, *3*, 377–396.

Lyons-Ruth, K., Zoll, D., Connell, D., & Grunebaum, H. (1989). Family deviance and family disruption in childhood: Associations with maternal behavior and infant maltreatment during the first two years of life. *Development and Psychopathology*, *1*, 219–236.

Mackner, L. M., Starr, R. H., & Black, M. M. (1997). The cumulative effect of neglect and failure to thrive on cognitive functioning. *Child Abuse and Neglect*, *7*, 691–700.

Madigan, S. (2002). *Anomalous mother–infant interaction, unresolved states of mind, and disorganized attachment relationships*. Unpublished master's thesis, University of Western Ontario, London, Ontario, Canada.

Main, M. (1990). Cross-cultural studies of attachment organization: Recent studies, changing methodologies, and the concept of conditional strategies. *Human Development*, *33*, 48–61.

Main, M., & Goldwyn, R. (1998). *Adult attachment scoring and classification systems*. Unpublished classification manual, University of California, Berkeley.

Main, M., & Hesse, E. (1990). Parents' unresolved traumatic experiences are related to infant disorganized attachment status: Is frightened and/or frightening parental behavior the linking mechanism? In M. Greenberg, D. Cicchetti, & E. M. Cummings (Eds.), *Attachment in the preschool years: Theory, research and intervention* (pp. 161–184). Chicago: University of Chicago Press.

Main, M., & Hesse, E. (1992). *Frightening/frightened, dissociated, or disorganized behavior on the part of the parent: A coding system for parent–infant interactions* (4th ed.). Unpublished manuscript, University of California, Berkeley.

Main, M., Kaplan, H., & Cassidy, J. (1985). Security in infancy, childhood and adulthood: A move to the level of representation. In I. Bretherton & E. Waters (Eds.), Growing points of attachment theory and research. *Monographs of the Society for Research in Child Development*, *50*(1–2, Serial no. 209), 66–104.

Main, M., & Solomon, J. (1990). Procedures for identifying infants as disorganized/disoriented during the Ainsworth Strange Situation. In M. Greenberg, D. Cicchetti, & E. M. Cummings (Eds.), *Attachment in the preschool years: Theory, research and intervention* (pp. 121–160). Chicago: University of Chicago Press.

Main, M., & Weston, D. R. (1981). The quality of the toddler's relationship to mother and to father: Related to conflict behavior and the readiness to establish new relationships. *Child Development*, *52*, 932–940.

Maldonado-Duran, M., & Sauceda-Garcia, J. (1996). Excessive crying in infants with regulatory disorders. *Bulletin of the Menninger Clinic*, *60*(1), 62–78.

Manassis, K., Bradley, S., Goldberg, S., Hood, J., & Swinson, R. P. (1994). Attachment in mothers with anxiety disorders and their children. *Journal of the American Academy of Child and Adolescent Psychiatry*, *33*(8), 1106–1113.

Manassis, K., Bradley, S., Goldberg, S., Hood, J., & Swinson, R. P. (1995). Behavioural inhibition, attachment and anxiety in children of mother with anxiety disorders. *Canadian Journal of Psychiatry*, *40*(2), 87–92.

Marchi, M., & Cohen, P. (1990). Early childhood eating behaviors and adolescent eating disorder. *Journal of the American Academy of Child and Adolescent Psychiatry*, *29*, 112–117.

Marcovitch, S., Goldberg, S., Gold, A., Washington, J., Wasson, C., Krekewich, K., & Handley-Derry, M. (1997). Determinants of behavioural problems in Romanian children adopted in Ontario. *International Journal of Behavioural Development*, *20*, 17–31.

Marvin, R., & O'Connor, T. (1999). *The formation of parent–child attachment following privation*. Paper presented at the biennial meeting of the Society for Research in Child Development, Albuquerque, NM.

Minde, K. K. (Ed.). (1995). Infant psychiatry. *Child and Adolescent Psychiatric Clinics of North America*, *4*.

Miyake, K., Chen, S., & Campos, J. (1985). Infant temperament, mother's mode of interaction, and attachment in Japan: An interim report. In I. Bretherton & E. Waters (Eds.), Growing points of attachment theory and research. *Monographs of the Society for Research in Child Development*, *50*(1–2, Serial No. 209), 276–297.

Moffitt, T. E. (1993). Adolescence-limited and life-course-persistent antisocial behavior: A developmental taxonomy. *Psychological Review*, *100*(4), 674–701.

Nelson, C. A., & Bosquet, M. (2000). Neurobiology of fetal and infant development: Implications for infant mental health. In C. H. Zeanah (Ed.), *Handbook of infant mental health* (2nd ed., pp. 37–59). New York: Guilford Press.

Nemeroff, C. (1996). The corticotropin-releasing factor (CRF) hypothesis of depression: New findings and new directions. *Molecular Psychiatry*, *1*, 336–342.

O'Connor, T. (in press). Attachment disorders of infancy and childhood. In M. Rutter & E. Taylor (Eds.), *Child and adolescent psychiatry: Modern approaches* (4th ed.). Oxford: Blackwell.

O'Connor, T., Bredenkamp, D., & Rutter, M. (1999). Attachment disturbances and disorders in children exposed to early severe deprivation. *Infant Mental Health Journal*, *20*, 10–29.

O'Connor, T., & Rutter, M. (2000). Attachment behavior disorder following severe early deprivation: Extension and longitudinal follow-up. *Journal of the American Academy of Child and Adolescent Psychiatry*, *39*, 703–712.

Ogawa, J. R., Sroufe, L., Weinfield, N. S., Carlson, E. A., & Egeland, B. (1997). Development and the fragmented self: Longitudinal study of dissociative symptomatology in a nonclinical sample. *Development and Psychopathology*, *9*, 855–879.

Oppenheim, D., Emde, R., & Warren, S. L. (1996). Can emotions and themes in children's play predict behavior problems? *Journal of the American Academy of Child and Adolescent Psychiatry*, *35*(10), 1331–1337.

Oppenheim, D., Sagi, A., & Lamb, M. (1988). Infant–adult attachments on the kibbutz and their relation to socioemotional development four years later. *Developmental Psychology*, *24*, 427–433.

Osofsky, J. D. (1995). The effects of exposure to violence on young children. *American Psychologist*, *50*, 782–788.

Palmer, S., & Horn, S. (1978). Feeding problems in children. In S. Palmer & S. Ekvall (Eds.), *Pediatric nutrition in developmental disorders* (pp. 107–129). Springfield, IL: Thomas.

Palmer, S., Thompson, R. J., & Linscheid, T. R. (1975). Applied behavior analysis in the treatment of childhood feeding disorders. *Developmental Medicine and Child Neurology, 17,* 333–339.

Paradise, J. L. (1966). Maternal and other factors in the etiology of infant colic. *Journal of the American Medical Association, 197,* 191–199.

Paret, I. (1983). Night waking and its relation to mother–infant interaction in nine-month-old infants. In J. D. Call & E. Galenson (Eds.), *Frontiers of infant psychiatry* (Vol. 1, pp. 171–177). New York: Basic Books.

Patrick, M., Hobson, R. P., Castle, D., Howard, R., & Maughn, B. (1994). Personality disorder and the mental representation of early social experience. *Development and Psychopathology, 6,* 375–388.

Patterson, G. R., & Bank, L. (1989). Some amplifying mechanisms for pathologic processes in families. In M. R. Gunnar & E. Thelen (Eds.), *The Minnesota Symposia on Child Psychology: Vol. 22. Systems and development* (pp. 16–20). Hillsdale, NJ: Erlbaum.

Pauli-Pott, U., Becker, K., Mertesacker, T., & Beckmann, D. (2000). Infants with "Colic"—Mothers' perspectives on the crying problem. *Journal of Psychosomatic Research, 48*(2), 125–132.

Perry, B. (1997). Incubated in terror: Neurodevelopmental factors in the "cycle of violence." In J. D. Osofsky (Ed.), *Children in a violent society* (pp. 124–149). New York, Guilford Press.

Pettit, G. S., Dodge, K. A., & Brown, M. M. (1988). Early family experience, social problem solving patterns and children's social competence. *Child Development, 59,* 107–120.

Polan, H. J., Leon, A., Kaplan, M. D., Kessler, D. B., Stern, D. N., & Ward, M. J. (1991). Disturbances of affect expression in failure to thrive. *Journal of the American Academy of Child and Adolescent Psychiatry, 30,* 897–903.

Polan, H. J., & Ward, M. J. (1994). Role of the mother's touch in failure to thrive: A preliminary investigation. *Journal of the American Academy of Child and Adolescent Psychiatry, 33,* 1098–1105.

Polatajko, H. J., Kaplan, B., & Wilson, B. (1992). Sensory integration treatment for children with learning disabilities: Its status 20 years later. *Occupational Therapy Journal of Research, 12,* 323–341.

Porges, S. W. (1991). Vagal tone: A mediator of affect. In J. A. Garber & K. A. Dodge (Eds.), *The development of affect regulation and dysregulation.* New York: Cambridge University Press.

Powell, G. F., Low, J. F., & Speers, M. A. (1987). Behavior as a diagnostic aid in failure to thrive. *Journal of Developmental and Behavioral Pediatrics, 8,* 18–24.

Prudhomme White, B., Gunnar, M. R., Larson, M. C., Donzella, B., & Barr, R. G. (2000). Behavioral and physiological responsivity, sleep, and patterns of daily cortisol production in infants with and without colic. *Child Development, 71,* 862–877.

Pruett, K. D. (1979). Home treatment for two infants who witnessed their mother's murder. *Journal of the American Academy of Child Psychiatry, 18,* 647–657.

Puckering, C., Pickels, A., Skuse, D., Heptinstall, E., Dowdney, L., & Zur-Szpiro, S. (1995). Mother–child interaction and the cognitive and behavioural development of four-year-old children with poor growth. *Journal of Child Psychology and Psychiatry, 36,* 573–595.

Pynoos, R. S. (1990). Post-traumatic stress disorder in children and adolescents. In B. Garfinkel, G. Carlson, & E. Weller (Eds.), *Psychiatric disorders in children and adolescents* (pp. 48–63). Philadelphia: Saunders.

Pynoos, R. S., & Eth, S. (1985). Children traumatized by witnessing acts of personal violence: Homicide, rape or suicide behavior. In S. Eth & R. S. Pynoos (Eds.), *Posttraumatic stress disorder in children* (pp. 17–44). Washington, DC: American Psychiatric Association.

Quay, H. C. (1986). Classification. In H. C. Quay & J. S. Werry (Eds.), *Psychopathological disorders of childhood* (pp. 1–34). New York: Wiley.

Quinton, D., Pickles, A., Maughan, B., & Rutter, M. (1993). Partners, peers, and pathways: Assortative pairing and continuities in conduct disorder. *Development and Psychopathology, 5*(4), 763–783.

Quinton, D., Rutter, M., & Liddle, C. (1984). Institutional rearing, parenting difficulties, and marital support. *Psychological Medicine, 14,* 107–124.

Radojevic, M. (1992, July). *Predicting quality of infant attachment to father at 15 months from pre-natal paternal representations of attachment*: An Australian contribution. Paper presented at the 25th International Congress of Psychology, Brussels.

Räihä, H., Lehtonen, L., Korhonen, T., & Korvenranta, H. (1996). Family life 1 year after infantile colic. *Archives of Pediatrics and Adolescent Medicine, 150,* 1032–1036.

Räihä, H., Lehtonen, L., Korhonen, T., & Korvenranta, H. (1997). Family functioning 3 years after infantile colic. *Journal of Developmental and Behavioral Pediatrics, 18,* 290–294.

Rautava, P., Lehtonen, L., Helenius, H., & Sillanpää, M. (1995). Infantile colic: Child and family three years later. *Pediatrics,* 96, 43–47.

Reau, N. R., Senturia, Y. D., Lebailly, S. A., & Christoffel, K. K. (1996). Infant and toddler feeding patterns and problems: Normative data and new directions. *Journal of Developmental and Behavioral Pediatrics, 17,* 149–153.

Reif, S., Beler, B., Villa, Y., & Spirer, Z. (1995). Long-term follow-up and outcome of infants with non-organic failure to thrive. *Israel Journal of Medical Science, 31*(8), 483–489.

Reijneveld, S. A., Brugman, E., & Hirasing, R. A. (2000). Infantile colic: maternal smoking as potential risk factor. *Archives of Disease in Childhood, 83,* 302–303.

Richman, N. (1981). A community survey of the characteristics of the 1–2-year-olds with sleep disruptions. *Journal of the American Academy of Child Psychiatry, 20,* 281–291.

Richman, N., Stevenson, J., & Graham, P. J. (1982). *Preschool to school: A behavioral study.* New York: Academic Press.

Robertson, J., & Robertson, J. (1989). *Separation and the very young.* London: Free Association Books.

Rogeness, G.A., & McClure, E.B. (1996). Development and neurotransmitter–environmental interactions. *Development and Psychopathology, 8,* 183–199.

Rutter, M. (1994, July). *Clinical implications of attachment concepts: Retrospect and prospect.* Paper presented as the Bowlby Memorial Lecture at the 13th International Congress, International Association of Child and Adolescent Psychiatry and Allied Professions, San Francisco.

Sadeh, A., & Anders, T. F. (1993). Sleep disorders. In C. H. Zeanah (Ed.), *Handbook of infant mental health* (pp. 305–316). New York: Guilford Press.

Sameroff, A. (1992). Systems, development and early intervention: A commentary. In J. Shonkoff, P. Hauser-Cram,

M. W. Krauss, & C. C. Upshur (Eds.), Development of infants with disabilities and their families. *Monographs of the Society for Research in Child Development*, 57(6, Serial No. 230), 154–163.

Sameroff, A., & Emde, R. N. (1989). *Relationship disturbances in early childhood.* New York: Basic Books.

Scheeringa, M., Peebles, C., Cook, C., & Zeanah, C. H. (2001). Towards establishing the procedural, criterion, and discriminant validity of PTSD in early childhood. *Journal of the American Academy of Child and Adolescent Psychiatry*, *40*, 52–60.

Scheeringa, M., & Zeanah, C. H. (1995). Symptom expression and trauma variables in children under 48 months of age. *Infant Mental Health Journal*, *16*, 259–270.

Scheeringa, M., & Zeanah, C. H. (2001). A relationship perspective on PTSD in infancy. *Journal of Traumatic Stress*, *14*, 799–815.

Scheeringa, M., Zeanah, C. H., Drell, M., & Larrieu, J. (1995). Two approaches to the diagnosis of post-traumatic stress disorder in infancy and early childhood. *Journal of the American Academy of Child and Adolescent Psychiatry*, *34*, 191–200.

Scheeringa, M., Zeanah, C. H., Myers, L., & Putnam, F. (2002). *Comorbidity of traumatized preschool children with and without PTSD.* Manuscript submitted for publication.

Schuengel, C., Bakermans-Kranenburg, M., & van IJzendoorn, M. (1999). Frightening maternal behavior linking unresolved loss and disorganized infant attachment. *Journal of Consulting and Clinical Psychology*, *67*, 54–63.

Singer, L. (1986). Long-term hospitalization of failure-to-thrive infants: Developmental outcome at three years. *Child Abuse and Neglect*, *10*, 479–486.

Skuse, D. H., Gill, D., Reilly, S., Wolke, D. & Lynch, M. A. (1995). Failure to thrive and the risk of child abuse: A prospective population survey. *Journal of Medical Screening*, *2*, 145–149.

Skuse, D. H., Wolke, D. & Reilly, S. (1992). Failure to thrive: Clinical and developmental aspects. In H. Remschmidt & M. H. Schmidt (Eds.), *Developmental psychopathology* (pp. 46–71). Lewiston, NY: Hogrefe & Huber.

Smyke, A. T., Dumitrescu, A., & Zeanah, C. H. (2002). Disturbances of attachment in Romanian children: I. The continuum of caretaking casualty. *Journal of the American Academy of Child and Adolescent Psychiatry*, *41*, 972–982.

Solomon, J., George, C., & De Jong, A. (1995). Children classified as controlling at age six: Evidence of disorganized representational strategies and aggression at home and at school. *Development and Psychopathology*, *7*, 447–463.

Spangler, G., & Grossmann, K.E. (1993). Biobehavioral organization in securely and insecurely attached infants. *Child Development*, *64*, 1439–1450.

Speltz, M. L., Greenberg, M. T., & DeKlyen, M. (1990). Attachment in preschoolers with disruptive behavior: A comparison of clinic-referred and nonproblem children. *Development and Psychopathology*, *2*, 31–46.

St. James-Roberts, I. (1999). What is distinct about infants' "colic" cries? *Archives of Disease in Childhood*, *80*, 56–62.

Stahlberg, M. R. (1984). Infantile colic: Occurrence and risk factors. *European Journal of Pediatrics*, *143*, 108–111.

Stahlberg, M. R., & Savilahti, E. (1986). Infantile colic and feeding. *Archives of Disease in Childhood*, *61*, 1232–1233.

Steele, H., & Steele, M. (1994). Intergenerational patterns of attachment. In K. Bartholomew & D. Perlman (Eds.),. *Advances in personal relationships: Vol. 5. Attachment processes during adulthood* (pp. 93–120). London: Jessica Kingsley.

Suess, G. J., Grossmann, K. E., & Sroufe, L. A. (1992). Effects of infant attachment to mother and father on quality of adaptation to preschool: From dyadic to individual organization of self. *International Journal of Behavioural Development*, *15*, 43–65.

Sugar, M. (1992). Toddlers' traumatic memories. *Infant Mental Health Journal*, *13*, 245–251.

Suomi, S. J. (1987). Genetic and maternal contributions to individual differences in rhesus monkey biobehavioral development. In N. Krasnegor (Ed.), *Perinatal development: A psychological perspective* (pp. 397–419). New York: Academic Press.

Suomi, S. J., & Champeaux, M. (1992, May). Genetic and environmental influences on rhesus monkey biobehavioral development: A cross-fostering study. In D. Arcus (Chair), *Temperament and environment.* Symposium conducted at the Biennial Meeting of the International Society for Infant Studies, Miami, FL.

Terr, L. C. (1988). What happens to early memories of trauma?: A study of twenty children under age five at the time of documented traumatic events. *Journal of the American Academy of Child and Adolescent Psychiatry*, *27*, 96–104.

Terr, L. C. (1990). *Too scared to cry.* New York: Harper & Row.

Tienari, P., Sorri, A., Lahti, I., Naarala, M., Wahlberg, K.-E., Moring, J., Pohjola, J., & Wynne, L. (1987). Genetic and psychosocial factors in schizophrenia: The Finnish Adoptive Family Study. *Schizophrenia Bulletin*, 13, 477–484.

Tizard, B., & Rees, J. (1975). The effect of early institutional rearing on the behaviour problems and affectional relationships of four-year-old children. *Journal of Child Psychology and Psychiatry*, *16*, 61–73.

Uribe, V., & Senturia, Y. D. (1994). The PPRG: Hispanic infant and toddler feeding study. *Clinical Research*, *42*, 379.

Valenzuela, M. (1990). Attachment in chronically underweight young children. *Child Development*, *61*, 1984–1996.

van IJzendoorn, M. (1995). Adult attachment representations, parental responsiveness, and infant attachment: A meta-analysis on the predictive validity of the Adult Attachment Interview. *Psychological Bulletin*, *117*, 387–403.

van IJzendoorn, M., & Bakermans-Kranenburg, M. J. (1996). Attachment representations in mothers, fathers, adolescents, and clinical groups: A meta-analytic search for normative data. *Journal of Consulting and Clinical Psychology*, *64*, 8–21.

van IJzendoorn, M., & Bakermans-Kranenburg, M. (in press). Disorganized attachment and the dysregulation of negative emotions. *Johnson & Johnson Pediatric Roundtable.*

van IJzendoorn, M. H., Goldberg, S., Kroonenberg, P. M., & Frenkel, O. J. (1992). The relative effects of maternal and child problems on the quality of attachment: A meta-analysis of attachment in clinical samples. *Child Development*, *63*, 840–858.

van IJzendoorn, M. H., Schuengel, C., & Bakermans-Kranenburg, M. K. (1999). Disorganized attachment in early childhood: Meta-analysis of precursors, concomitants and sequelae. *Development and Psychopathology*, *11*, 225–249.

Vargas, S., & Camilli, G. (1998). A meta-analysis of research on sensory integration treatment. *American Journal of Occupational Therapy*, *53*, 189–198.

Vaughn, B. E., Lefever, G. B., Seifer, R., & Barglow, P. (1989). Attachment behavior, attachment security, and temperament during infancy. *Child Development*, *60*, 728–737.

Volkmar, F. (1997). Reactive attachment disorders: Issues for DSM-IV. In A. Frances (Ed.), *DSM-IV source book* (pp. 255–263). Washington, DC: American Psychiatric Association.

Wahlsten, D. (1991). Insensitivity of the analysis of variance to heredity–environment interaction. *Behavioral and Brain Sciences*, *13*, 109–161.

Warren, S., Huston, L., Egeland, B., & Sroufe, A. L. (1997). Child and adolescent anxiety disorders and early attachment. *Journal of the American Academy of Child and Adolescent Psychiatry*, *36*(5), 637–644.

Wartner, U. G., Grossmann, K., Fremmer-Bombik, E., & Suess, G. (1994). Attachment patterns at age six in south Germany: Predictability from infancy and implications for preschool behavior. *Child Development*, *65*, 1014–1027.

Weissbluth, M. (1987). Sleep and the colicky infant. In C. Guilleminault (Ed.), *Sleep and its disorders in children* (pp. 129–140). New York: Raven Press.

Wessel, M. A., Cobb, J. C., Jackson, E. B., Harris, G. S., & Detwilet, A. C. (1954). Paroxysmal fussing in infancy, sometimes called "colic." *Pediatrics*, *14*, 421–434.

Whelan, E., & Cooper, P. J. (2000). The association between childhood feeding problems and maternal eating disorder: A community study. *Psychological Medicine*, *30*, 69–77.

Wilensky, D. S., Ginsberg, G., Altman, M., Tulchinsky, T. H., Ben Yishay, F., & Atterbach, J. (1996). A community based study of failure to thrive in Israel. *Archives of Disease in Childhood*, *75*, 145–148.

Woolston, J. L. (1985). The current challenge in failure to thrive syndrome research. In D. Drotar (Ed.), *New directions in failure to thrive: Implications for research and practice* (pp. 225–235). New York: Plenum Press.

World Health Organization. (1993). *The ICD-10 classification of mental and behavioural disorders: Clinical description and diagnostic guidelines*. Geneva: Author.

Wright, C., & Birks, E. (2000). Risk factors for failure to thrive: A population-based survey. *Child Care, Health and Development*, *26*, 5–16

Zeanah, C. H. (Ed.). (1993). *Handbook of infant mental health*. New York: Guilford Press.

Zeanah, C. H. (1994). Assessment and treatment of infants exposed to violence. In J. Osofsky & E. Fenichel (Eds.), *Hurt, healing and hope* (pp. 29–37). Washington, DC: Zero to Three/National Center for Clinical Infant Programs.

Zeanah, C. H. (1996). Beyond insecurity: A reconceptualization of attachment disorders of infancy. *Journal of Consulting and Clinical Psychology*, *64*, 42–52.

Zeanah, C. H. (2000). Disturbances of attachment in young children adopted from institutions. *Journal of Developmental and Behavioral Pediatrics*, *21*, 230–236.

Zeanah, C. H., & Boris, N. W. (2000). Disturbances and disorders of attachment in early childhood. In C. H. Zeanah (Ed.), *Handbook of infant mental health* (2nd ed., pp. 353–368). New York: Guilford Press.

Zeanah, C. H., Boris, N. W., Bakshi, S., & Lieberman, A. (2000). Disorders of attachment. In J. Osofsky & H. Fitzgerald (Eds.), *WAIMH handbook of infant mental health* (pp. 92–122). New York: Wiley.

Zeanah, C. H., Boris, N., & Lieberman, A. (2000). Attachment disorders of infancy. In A. Sameroff, M. Lewis, & S. M. Miller (Eds.), *Handbook of developmental psychopathology* (2nd ed., pp. 293–307). New York: Kluwer Academic/Plenum.

Zeanah, C. H., Boris, N. W., O'Connor, T., & Smyke, A. T. (2000, July). *Three studies of reactive attachment disorder*. Paper presented at the 7th World Congress of the World Association for Infant Mental Health, Montreal.

Zeanah, C. H., & Emde, R. N. (1994). Attachment disorders in infancy. In M. Rutter, L. Hersov, & E. Taylor (Eds.), *Child and adolescent psychiatry: Modern approaches* (3rd ed., pp. 490–504). Oxford: Blackwell.

Zeanah, C. H., Larrieu, J. A., Valliere, J., & Heller, S. S. (2000). Infant–parent relationship assessment. In C. H. Zeanah (Ed.), *Handbook of infant mental health* (2nd ed., pp. 222–235). New York: Guilford Press.

Zeanah, C. H., Mammen, O., & Lieberman, A. (1993). Disorders of attachment. In C. H. Zeanah (Ed.), *Handbook of infant mental health* (pp. 332–349). New York: Guilford Press.

Zeanah, C. H., & Scheeringa, M. (1997). The experience and effects of violence in infancy. In J. D. Osofsky (Ed.), *Children in a violent society* (pp. 97–123). New York: Guilford Press.

Zeanah, C. H., & Smyke, A. T. (2002). Clinical disorders of attachment in young children: consensus and controversies. In B. Zuckerman, A. F. Lieberman, & N. A. Fox (Eds.), *Emotion regulation and developmental health: Infancy and early childhood* (pp. 139–152). Johnson and Johnson Pediatric Institute.

Zeanah, C. H., Smyke, A. T., Boris, M., & Scheeringa, M. (2001, April). *Disorders of attachment in abused/neglected toddlers*. Paper presented at the biennial meeting of the Society for Research in Child Development, Minneapolis, MN.

Zeanah, C. H., Smyke, A. T., & Dumitrescu, A. (2002). Disturbances of attachment in Romanian children: II. Indiscriminate behavior and institutional care. *Journal of the American Academy of Child and Adolescent Psychiatry*, *41*, 983–989.

Zero to Three/National Center for Clinical Infant Programs. (1994). *Diagnostic classification of mental health and developmental disorders of infancy and early childhood (Diagnostic Classification: 0–3)*. Washington, DC: Author.

Zeskind, P. S., Marshall, T. R., & Goff, D. M. (1996). Cry threshold predicts regulatory disorder in newborn infants. *Journal of Pediatric Psychology*, *21*, 803–819.

CHAPTER FOURTEEN

Child Maltreatment

Christine Wekerle
David A. Wolfe

When you are a child of abuse and no one listens to you and no one confirms that you are being abused, you feel like you are insane.
—HECHE (2001, p. 223)

Child maltreatment is a tragedy of human error and human circumstances. At its most basic level, child maltreatment denotes parenting failure—a failure to protect a child from harm, and a failure to provide the positive aspects of a parent–child relationship that can foster development. The responsibility for this failure is shared not only by the individual parents for not adequately providing for their child, but also by society, for not adequately providing the parents with supports and safety nets. About 3 million reports of child maltreatment are made to child protective services (CPS) each year (U.S. Department of Health and Human Services [DHHS], 2001), confirming that such acts represent a major and urgent public health concern. With this conern comes a keener sense of responsibility for research-based assessment, prevention, and treatment efforts directed toward the child and family.

Most maltreating parents do not have psychotic or other serious mental illness, and some show no apparent psychological or personality dysfunction (Francis, Hughes, & Hitz, 1992; Wolfe, 1999). However, many have problems in related areas of depression, anxiety (including posttraumatic stress disorder [PTSD]), domestic violence, substance abuse and dependence (alcohol, other drugs, or multiple substances), personality disturbances, social isolation, and poverty, with several of these problems overlapping in both community and clinical samples (see Wekerle & Wall, 2002a, 2002b). For instance, first-degree relatives of depressed, abused children have a ninefold greater likelihood of lifetime depression than controls (Kaufman et al., 1998). Although some of the co-occurring disorders are treatable, appropriate treatment is often lacking due to numerous obstacles. Even if maltreatment is detected by formal systems, the focus of professional attention is on child protection and risk assessment, with fewer resources available for treating adult disorders or circumstances. This narrow response may fail to protect against further abuse by overlooking significant risk factors, such as substance misuse or parental disorders (English, Marshall, Brummel, & Orme, 1999).

Although child characteristics may play a factor in parental abuse (Wolfe, 1999), a child is never responsible for being abused (deYoung & Lowry, 1992). Child abuse is an adult act, and without this adult behavior the child would have fewer developmental problems and disorders. Moreover, maltreatment-induced psychopathology in childhood is preventable. Given its association with health risk behaviors, medical illness, and greater rates of psychiatric and medical services needs, child maltreatment may be the single most preventable and intervenable contributor to child and adult mental illness (DeBellis, 2001). Once a child has been maltreated, there may a long and winding road ahead to support a transition from victim to survivor, and from surviving to living.

Despite difficulties, most childhood victims achieve a level of successful adaptation in one or more life domains, as is suggested by the developing literature on resilience (e.g., Heller, Larrieu, D'Imperio, & Boris, 1999; Kaufman, Cooke, Arny, Jones, & Pittinsky, 1994; Luthar, Cicchetti, & Becker, 2000). For example, in a prospective study, only 22% of maltreated children were resilient in adulthood, defined as having no period of homelessness, consistent employment, and no juvenile or adult arrests (McGloin & Widom, 2001); this represented a significant difference from matched controls. Mechanisms of resilience are beginning to attract the interest of researchers and clinicians, in addition to psychopathology and other negative sequelae of maltreatment discussed herein.

Children's dependency sets the stage for their greater vulnerability to a wide range of damaging experiences, including maltreatment (Finkelhor & Dziuba-Leatherman, 1994). Child maltreatment is typically categorized into neglect, physical abuse, psychological/emotional abuse, and sexual abuse. Although neglect is the most prevalent and chronic form of maltreatment (Sedlak & Broadhurst, 1996; Trocme & Wolfe, 2001), it remains the least understood (Hildyard & Wolfe, 2002). Psychological abuse is also of concern, due to its co-occurrence with most other forms of maltreatment and its assumed contribution to maladjustment (Claussen & Crittenden, 1991; McGee & Wolfe, 1991; National Research Council, 1993). Because these types of child maltreatment usually co-occur to some degree, research studies typically focus on the common developmental issues shared by all forms, noting differences by abuse characteristics (type, severity, age of onset, etc.) where appropriate.

Importantly, child maltreatment occurs in a relational context and may be viewed as a "relational psychopathology" resulting from a poor fit of the parent, child, and environment (Cicchetti & Olsen, 1990). Insecure child attachment to the parent and poor parental bonding may set the stage for maltreatment by fostering role reversal, rejection, fear of closeness, low emotional investment, and unresolved conflict (Alexander, 1992, 1993). This relational context provides significant emotional weight to the abuse experience. The co-occurrence of violence and other forms of child maltreatment (e.g., physical injury during sexual abuse) creates a situation of trauma within a relational context (Herman, 1992; Terr, 1991). Thus a posttraumatic stress response is one important conceptualization of how child maltreatment affects the individual's developmental course, as discussed later in this chapter.

This chapter is oriented toward the importance of the parent–child relational context and the developmental traumatology model of child maltreatment. First, we present the historical context, definitions, and epidemiology of maltreatment. Next, each type of child maltreatment is discussed in terms of its influence on domains in child development development (physical, cognitive, socioemotional). Salient themes that cut across maltreatment types (e.g., dissociation, self-blame) are then presented, along with relevant empirical findings. Theoretical perspectives, including a greater discussion of developmental traumatology theory (e.g., DeBellis & Putnam, 1994; DeBellis, 2001) and PTSD (American Psychiatric Association, 2000), are highlighted. Finally, etiology and future directions are presented.

HISTORICAL CONTEXT

Maltreatment of children rarely raised concern prior to the middle of the 20th century, because societies viewed harsh forms of discipline and corporal punishment as inconsequential and as a parent's right and responsibility. Abusive acts have, in all likelihood, been commonplace throughout history (Radbill, 1968). Children who saw violence between their parents remained silent witnesses, as wives were considered the property of their husbands, and violence against them and their children was accepted. For centuries, maltreatment continued undaunted by any countermovement to seek more humane treatment for children. The medical establishment created momentum with clinical descriptions of the "battered child syndrome" in the early 1960s (Kempe, Silverman, Steele, Droegenmueller, & Silver, 1962), providing impetus for the drafting of model child abuse legislation and mandatory reporting laws. Such laws required, for the first time, that all adults who come into contact with children as part of their professional responsibilities (e.g., teachers, doctors, school bus drivers) must report any suspicion of child abuse to official child protection authorities or police. The "child protection movement," which began in the 1930s and 1940s primarily in response to the need for alternative care for orphans and unwanted children, responded to growing public awareness to seek alternative care for children deemed to be at risk of harm. Not until the passage of the first Child Abuse and Neglect Treatment Act in 1974, however, were funds earmarked for research on its causes and effects. Fortunately, counterefforts to value the rights and needs of children, and to recognize their exploitation and abuse, began to take root during the latter part of the 20th century in many developed countries, spurred by the Convention on the Rights of the Child (United Nations General Assembly, 1989).

Although still in its infancy, the growing recognition of child maltreatment has brought worldwide interest to document and reduce its incidence. Today, 32 countries have an official government policy regarding child abuse and neglect, and about one-third of the world's population is included in countries that conduct an annual count of child abuse and neglect cases (Bross, Miyoshi, Miyoshi, & Krugman, 2000). Such efforts provide the critical first steps to identifying the scope of the problem, and justify the implementation of important societal, community, and cultural changes to combat child abuse.

DEFINITION OF CHILD MALTREATMENT

"Child maltreatment" is a generic term referring to four primary acts: physical abuse, emotional abuse, sexual abuse, and neglect. Determining when a parental act represents maltreatment is complicated by many factors. These include sociodemographic factors related to safety (e.g., quality of the home environment in the context of poverty and community violence) and risk (e.g., parental substance misuse and how it affects parenting), physical or medical evidence of injury severity, and systemic factors (e.g., caseworker caseload, degree of family monitoring) (Cicchetti & Manly, 2001; Emery & Laumann-Billings, 1998; McGee & Wolfe, 1991). A World Health Organization (WHO, 1999) report defines "child abuse" as that which "constitutes all forms of physical and/or emotional ill-treatment, sexual abuse, neglect or negligent treatment or commercial or other exploitation, resulting in actual or potential harm to the child's health, survival, development or dignity in the context of a relationship of responsibility, trust or power" (p. 15). The United Nations Children's Fund (UNICEF, 2000) considers maltreated children to be persons under age 18 who suffer occasional or habitual acts of physical, sexual, or emotional violence, be it in the family group or in social institutions. A common element of all definitions is that maltreatment includes not only acts of aggression and exploitation, but also acts of omission (such as abandonment or failure to provide), and highlights the context as a power-abusive relationship. The following definitions of maltreatment are based on a consensus meeting by WHO (1999, pp. 15–16).

Physical Abuse

WHO defines "physical abuse" of a child as acts that result in actual or potential physical harm, stemming from an interaction (or lack of an interaction) that is reasonably within the control of a parent or person in a position of responsibility, power, or trust. There may be single or repeated incidents. Some of the more prominent, acute physical signs for children who have been physically abused include external signs of physical injury, such as bruises, lacerations, scars, abrasions, burns, sprains, and broken bones. Internal injuries may be present, such as head injury (intracerebral and occular hemorrage from violent shaking [so-called "shaken baby syndrome"] or contact with a hard object), and intra-abdominal injuries (e.g., ruptured liver or spleen). Other physical indications may arise from harsh physical blows, such as missing teeth.

Female genital mutilation (FGM) is included in the WHO discussion of physical abuse. Although it is a deeply rooted traditional practice with cultural acceptance in African countries and a few countries in the Middle East and Asia, it becomes a child protection issue for communities of immigrants from these countries in the Western world. The percentages of women of reproductive age who have been genitally cut range from 18% to 98%, with wide variations across countries. This translates into over 130 million girls and women who have undergone some form of FGM, with 2 million girls being at risk each year. FGM has serious health consequences (infection, insufficient opening for intercourse and childbirth, etc.), especially in its more severe forms. Its detection, however, is a challenge, as a girl may be sent back to the country of origin for the procedure, or it is performed within a protective subculture (Barstow, 1999).

Emotional Abuse

WHO defines "emotional abuse" as the failure to provide a developmentally appropriate, supportive environment, including the availability of a primary attachment figure, so that a child can establish a stable and full range of emotional and social competencies commensurate with his or her personal potential, and in the context of the society in which the child lives. There may also be acts toward the child that cause or have a high probability of causing harm to the child's health or physical, mental, spiritual, moral, or social development. These acts must be reasonably within the control of a parent or person in a position of responsibility, power, or trust. Acts include restriction of movement (e.g., tying, confinement), as well as patterns of belittling, denigrating, scapegoating, threatening, scaring, discriminating, ridiculing, or other nonphysical forms of hostile or rejecting treatment.

Some countries, such as the United States and Canada, include children's exposure to domestic violence as a form of emotional abuse or neglect (Trocme & Wolfe, 2001). This is in recognition that it is emotionally harming to a child to witness injury to a loved parent with whom the child identifies and on whom he or she relies for care. Furthermore, research shows that witnessing has a pronounced effect on children's adjustment (for reviews, see Carlson, 2000; Mohr, Lutz, Fantuzzo, & Perry, 2000), and that domestic violence often overlaps with physical abuse of the child (Appel & Holden, 1998). For example, one study showed that in the most recent domestic violent episode, mothers received 70% of injuries and children received 12% (Graham-Bermann, 2000). Despite considerable agreement that emotional abuse is harmful and widespread, efforts to document the incidence have not as yet overcome the difficult challenges posed by this broad definition.

Neglect

WHO (1999) describes "neglect" as the failure to provide for a child in all spheres: physical and mental health, education, nutrition, shelter, and safe living conditions, in the context of resources reasonably available to the family or caretakers. The neglect causes or has a high probability of causing harm to the child's health or physical, mental, spiritual, moral, or social development. This includes the failure to properly supervise and protect the child from physical harm and to provide the emotional security of being cared for. Although exploitation is discussed as a separate category, it clearly constitutes neglect in terms of failing to allow a childhood and exluding normative child activities (e.g., play, education, proper nutrition, and safety). WHO describes exploitation of a child as the use of the child in work or other activities for the benefit of others. This includes (but is not limited to) child labor and child prostitution, the latter being considered sexual abuse as well. Countless children worldwide are pressed into dangerous work for long hours, putting them at risk for death. According to estimates from the International Labour Organization (ILO, 2001), there are close to 15 million child workers under the age of 15 in Latin America and the Caribbean, and 250 million worldwide. The ILO estimates that well over half of all working children in the world are girls.

Sexual Abuse

WHO (1999) defines "sexual abuse" as the involvement of a child or youth in sexual activity (1) that the young person does not fully comprehend, (2) that he or she is unable to give informed consent to, (3) that he or she is not developmentally prepared for and cannot give consent to, or (4) that violates the laws or social taboos of society. The perpetrator is an adult or another child who by development or age (typically considered 5 or more years older) is in a relationship of responsibility, trust, or power, and the sexual activity is intended to gratify or satisfy the needs of the perpetrator. This may include (but is not limited to) the inducement or coercion of a child to engage in any unlawful sexual activity (e.g., fondling, exposure, intercourse), child prostitution, and the use of children in pornography.

EPIDEMIOLOGY

Population-based studies (i.e., those that rely on adult self-report rather than officially reported cases) estimate that approximately 10% (Straus & Gelles, 1986) to 25% (MacMillan et al., 1997) of all adults were physically abused at some point during their childhood. Whereas most acts of physical abuse involve bruises and cuts, WHO (1999) estimates that as many as 1 in 5,000 to 1 in 10,000 children under the age of 5 die each year from physical violence. With regard to sexual abuse, international studies conducted in 19 countries—including, for example, South Africa, Sweden, and the Dominican Republic—have reported prevalence rates ranging from 7% to 34%

among girls, and from 3% to 29% among boys. Estimates for African, Middle Eastern, or Far Eastern countries, however, are not currently available (for a recent discussion of the realities of sexual abuse disclosure in the Arab world, see Shalhoub-Kevorkian, 1999). An especially pernicious form of abuse is child prostitution, affecting an estimated 1 million children annually worldwide. As many as 10 million children may be forced to engage in child prostitution, the sex industry, sex tourism, and pornography, although accurate statistics are not available (WHO, 1999). A UNICEF-supported study by the 1996 World Conference against Sexual Exploitation of Children revealed that 47% of sexually exploited girls in Central American countries were abused and raped in their homes. Almost half of them had begun commercial sexual activity between the age of 9 and 13, and the majority had used drugs to sustain such exploitation (UNICEF, 2000).

In the United States, the rate of reported child abuse and neglect is declining from a peak in 1993, but the numbers remain epidemic ("Bruised and Abused," 2001). Based on the states' responses to the 1999 National Child Abuse and Neglect Reporting System (NCANDS), 2,974,000 referrals were received to CPS, of which 39.6% were "screened out" and not referred for further investigation or assessment (U.S. DHHS, 2001). Fewer than one-third (29.2%) resulted in a disposition of either substantiated or indicated child maltreatment, where the weight of the evidence (e.g., physical evidence, perpetrator admission etc.) either confirmed or suggested high probability of maltreatment. Thus in 1999 there were 826,000 maltreated children nationwide, for a rate of 11.8 per 1,000 children. The breakdown across type of maltreatment was as follows: 58.4% neglect; 21.3% physical abuse; 11.3% sexual abuse; 35.9% other, including psychological maltreatment (rate of 0.9/1,000), abandonment, congenital drug addiction, and so forth. In addition, 35.9% were reported for more than one type. The child maltreatment fatality rate has remained fairly stable over the years. The mortality rate is 1.62 deaths per 100,000 children in the general population, largely accounted for by children age 1 year or younger (42.6%) suffering from neglect. A small percentage of these fatal cases (12.5%) had CPS involvement in the 5 years prior to the children's death (U.S. DHHS, 2001).

Although over half of reports to CPS were received from professionals (e.g., 15% education personnel, 8.5% medical personnel), there remains a salient role for reporting by community and family members (45.3%). This distribution of reporters is noted as having remained stable for several years. Most states have time standards for initiating an investigation. The average time lapse was 63.8 hours, indicating a reasonable if not rapid response to initial calls, when it is considered that the average annual caseload of CPS workers is 72 investigations. In some states, high-priority reports require an immediate response within 24 hours (U.S. DHHS, 2001).

Child maltreatment cuts across all lines of gender, national origin, language, religion, age, ethnicity, disability, and sexual orientation. Based on 1999 official reports, maltreated children are most often infants and toddlers (i.e., for those 0 to 3 years old, the rate is 13.9/1,000 same-age children in the population). Recurrence of maltreatment reports are also most evident for younger children, with the highest likelihood attached to neglect, followed by physical abuse, then sexual abuse (Fluke, Yuan, & Edwards, 1999). The rate of physical abuse for boys was highest in the 4- to 7-year-old and 8- to 11-year-old ranges. For girls, the peak for physical abuse was in the 12- to 15-year-old range. Otherwise, maltreatment types are similar for males and females. One clear exception is sexual abuse (female-to-male ratio of 1.6:0.4). Overall, however, female parents were identified as the perpetrators of neglect and physical abuse for the highest percentage of children (U.S. DHHS, 2001). Although males are the dominant perpetrators in sexual abuse, the most common perpetrator pattern for maltreatment in general is a female parent acting alone who is typically younger than 30 years of age. A notable difference is in the fatality rate, where the majority of maltreatment deaths were *less frequently* perpetrated by a parent acting alone (57.8%).

Rates by ethnicity ranged from a low of 4.4 Asians/Pacific Islanders per 1,000 children of the same race in the population to a high of 25.2 African Americans per 1,000 (for American Indians/Alaska Natives, the rate was 20.1/1,000). Morton (1999) discusses this "colorization" of the child welfare system, advancing the view that CPS has a more pervasive and invasive impact on African American families than any other ethnic group. Morton notes, for example, that in 1995, African American children constituted 15% of the U.S. child population, but represented 41% of the child welfare population, 49% of children in foster and group care, and 40% of maltreatment-related fatalities. Traditionally, this has been considered a reflection of the effect of poverty. Families with annual incomes under $15,000 have a 26.5 times higher maltreatment incidence rate. Also, the link between female-headed households (52% of African American children live with their mothers only) has been advanced as a contributing factor. Other considerations remain, including a bias preceding system entry, at the reporting or decision-to-investigate stage. Hispanic and Asian/Pacific Islander children are underrepresented, while African American and Native American children are overrepresented. Another possibility is less effective service delivery or intervention effectiveness, given the issue of culture competence. For instance, Garland et al. (2000) found that even after controls for age, gender, and total behavior problems, African American and Hispanic American children in foster care received fewer mental health services than their European American counterparts. When care was received, the frequency of outpatient visits was predicted by race and ethnic background. Cultural competency in the child welfare system merits further consideration.

COST OF CHILD MALTREATMENT

Prevent Child Abuse America released a report in 2001 (cited in Levine, 2001) estimating the cost of maltreatment, using data sources such as involvement in the mental health care and juvenile justice systems, lost workplace productivity, and so on. This report estimated that child abuse costs the United States over $94 billion every year or $258 million a day, with such major expenditures as the child welfare system ($39.5 million), hospitalization ($17 million), juvenile delinquency ($24 million), and adult criminality ($152 million), for example. A further illustration of the cost of maltreatment versus prevention was provided by the state of Michigan (Caldwell, 1992). Summing across all the child-maltreatment-related costs yielded an astounding estimate of $823 million during 1 year in Michigan, when the long- and short-term consequences of inadequate prenatal care and child abuse were taken into consideration. In contrast, if a comprehensive parent education program had been offered to every family having its first baby in the state of Michigan, the cost would have been $28.67 million, and a comprehensive home-visiting program provided to these same families would have cost $57.59 million. These figures persuasively argue for prevention as a fiscally responsible approach. We now turn our attention to describing the specific types of child maltreatment.

THE PHYSICALLY ABUSED CHILD

Physical victimization can take many forms, including acts experienced by the majority of children (e.g., physical punishment, sibling violence, peer assault), as well as acts experienced by a significant minority, such as physical abuse (Finkelhor & Dziuba-Leatherman, 1994). Physical abuse involves both minor and more severe injuries to the child, as well as a relatively rare form called "Munchausen by proxy syndrome" (MBPS). MBPS involves intentionally injuring the child (e.g., inducing vomiting) in order to present the child for medical investigation and treatment for some fictitious or unknown medical condition (Schreier & Libow, 1993). Although most physical abuse incidents occur in the context of discipline and child management (see Trocme & Wolfe, 2001), such acts as scalding, burning, and MBPS appear more sadistic, given their purposeful and sequential nature. There would seem to be a clear intent to hurt the child.

Cognitive Development

In the case of shaken baby syndrome, an infant or toddler is shaken back and forth. Surviving children often have significant neurological and visual impairment, and death occurs in about a third of such cases (Kivlin, Simons, Lazoritz, & Ruttum, 2000; McCabe & Donahue, 2000). Children who are otherwise physically abused appear to have delayed social-cognitive and academic/intellectual development, in comparison to their age-mates. Physically abused children presenting to a psychiatric facility have been found to exhibit more mild neurological impairments, and more serious and minor physical injuries, than their nonabused counterparts (Kolko, Moser, & Weldy, 1990; for a review, see Kolko, 2002). Social-cognitive development (i.e., the child's emerging view of the world and development of moral reasoning) is fostered by healthy parental guidance and control. It stands to reason, therefore, that because abused children have been raised in an atmosphere of power assertion and external control, their level of moral reasoning would be significantly below their nonabused peers. Typically, abusive parents fail to invoke in their children concern for the welfare of others, especially in a manner that the children will internalize and imitate.

Smetana, Kelly, and Twentyman (1984) considered preschoolers' judgments regarding the dimensions of seriousness, deserved punishment, rule contingency (the permissibility of actions in the absence of rules), and generalizability of familiar moral and conventional nursery school transgressions (e.g., pictures depicting physical harm, psychological distress, and resource distribution). Physically abused children considered transgressions entailing psychological distress to be more universally wrong for others (but not for themselves), whereas neglected children considered the unfair distribution of resources to be more universally wrong for themselves (but not for others). These findings are consistent with the type of maltreatment experienced by each of these two groups of children. It appears that abused children, as a function of their physical and psychological maltreatment, may have a heightened sensitivity to the intrinsic wrongness of such offenses. Subsequent work found that maltreated children did not differ from nonmaltreated children in cognitive judgments of "right" versus "wrong," but differed in their affective responses (Smetana, Daddis, et al., 1999; Smetana, Toth, et al., 1999).

Academic performance and language development are also delayed among physically abused children, including lower IQ and achievement (e.g., Appelbaum, 1977; Barahal, Waterman, & Martin, 1981; Erickson, Egeland, & Pianta, 1989; Hoffman-Plotkin & Twentyman, 1984; Salzinger, Kaplan, Pelcovitz, Samit, & Krieger, 1984). Among adolescents with a history of physical abuse, expressive and receptive language deficits have been noted (McFadyen & Kitson, 1996). In research using event history analysis, an intensification of academic risk has been noted in adolescence (after age 14), when maltreated children are at increased risk for absenteeism and decline in grade point average (Leiter & Johnsen, 1997). Cognitive deficits may be due to the limited stimulation received in the home from parents who are overly concerned with a child's behavioral appearance and obedience—impairing the child's freedom to explore, attempt new challenges, learn cooperatively with others, and engage in a variety of cognitive and social stimuli.

Behavioral Development

The most notable behavioral signs associated with physical abuse are heightened aggression and hostility toward others (especially authority figures), and angry oubursts, sometimes to minor provocation (for reviews, see Kolko, 1992, 2002). Pelcovitz, Kaplan, DeRosa, Mandel, and Salzinger (2000) found that physically abused teens had higher rates of conduct and oppositional defiant disorders than nonabused youths recruited from a social services department (64% of youths with physical abuse histories also had exposure to domestic violence). Physical abuse during the preschool period, especially as it overlaps with emotional maltreatment, predicts externalizing behavior problems (Manly, Kim, Rogosch, & Cicchetti, 2001). Physically abused children are more disliked and less popular than their nonabused peers (Salzinger, Feldman, Hammer, & Rosario, 1993). This relationship is mediated by the children's aggressive versus prosocial behavior toward others (Salzinger, Feldman, Ng-Mak, Mojica, & Stockhammer, 2001). With close friends, maltreated children exhibit less intimacy, more conflict, and more negative affect than their nonabused counterparts (Parker & Herrera, 1996). These peer difficulties remain even when poverty and negative life events are taken into account (Okun, Parker, & Levendosky, 1994). In addition, physically abused children may form a hostile attributional bias toward peers (i.e., they automatically presume that a peer means harm), which facilitates an aggressive response. For example, Brown and Kolko (1999) found that self-oriented attributions (e.g., self-blame) were associated with internalizing symptoms, and other-oriented attributions (e.g., seeing the world as dangerous) tended to be linked to externalizing symptoms. The relationship between physical abuse and aggression may be mediated by impairments in acquired social knowledge, where learning is hampered by the abusive context (Shirk, 1988), especially in social problem-solving skills (Rogosch, Cicchetti, & Aber, 1995).

Another behavioral pattern among younger physically abused children has been labeled "compulsive compliance" (Crittenden & DiLalla, 1988). This term refers to a child's ready and quick compliance to significant adults, which occurs in the context of the child's general state of vigilance or watchfulness for adult cues. A child's compulsively compliant behavior may be accompanied by masked facial expressions (e.g., false positive affect, suppressed fear or anger), ambiguous affect, nonverbal–verbal incongruence, and rote verbal responses. Such behavior seems to emerge in pace with the child's abstraction abilities, at about 12 months of age, concurring with the child's ability to form a stable mental representation of the caregiver. It has been suggested that abused infants learn to inhibit behaviors that have been associated with maternal anger (e.g., requests for attention, protests against intrusions), and that in toddlerhood, such children may actively behave in a manner designed to please their mothers. This early pattern may lead to inflexible strategies of behavior, with the consequence of reduced reciprocity in interactions (Crittenden, 1992; see also Crittenden & Claussen, 2002).

Socioemotional Development

The above-described behavioral symptoms of aggression and excessive compliance can be understood in terms of the nature of the caregiver–child interaction that provides a basis for the child's formation of an interpersonal style (Sroufe & Fleeson, 1986). The primary attachment relationship has been theoretically linked to the intergenerational transmission of abuse (e.g., Kaufman & Zigler, 1989), the failure of maltreated children to form harmonious relationships with others (Erickson, Sroufe, & Egeland, 1985), and their vulnerability to additional developmental failures that rely to some extent on early attachment success (Aber & Allen, 1987). Attachment research shows that the vast majority of maltreated infants form insecure attachments with their caregivers (from 70% to 100% across studies; Cicchetti, Toth, & Bush, 1988). This suggests that such a child lacks confidence in the mother as an available and responsive provider, and that the mother has difficulty in providing sensitive, nurturant, and responsive care. Of note is a greater likelihood of a disorganized/disoriented attachment, where no clear attachment strategy is utilized; rather, a mixture of approach, avoidance, and atypical (e.g., freezing) behavioral responses is deployed by the child (Barnett, Ganiban, & Cicchetti, 1999). Although these reactions may be adaptive in the short term, it is suggested that such nonoptimal attachment may be most significant in terms of influencing a child's relationship formation with peers, future partners, and future offspring (Cicchetti, Toth, & Maughan, 2000).

As abused children enter school, their development of relationships with both peers and adults is challenged. At this time, their manifestations of sensitivity to others' emotions and problems in their early prosocial behavior development become paramount. Because a positive bond or relationship between parent and child is an important learning context, abused children would be expected to show problems in the affective domain. Physically abused children have a higher incidence of depressive symptoms and diagnoses than either nonabused controls or neglected children do (Kolko, 2002). For example, Toth, Manly, and Cicchetti (1992) compared physically abused, neglected, and nonmaltreated children, using several measures of depression and social adjustment. After the researchers controlled for age and cognitive functioning, the physically abused group differed significantly from both the neglected and nonmaltreated samples, which did not differ from each other. Abused children do tend to isolate themselves, to respond aggressively under a range of circumstances, and to respond with anger and aversion to the distress of others (Main & George, 1985). Pelcovitz et al. (2000) found that adolescents who were physically abused and witnessed domestic violence were at greater risk for major depression, separation anxiety disorder, and PTSD than were their nonabused counterparts. Pollak, Cicchetti, Hornung, and Reed (2000) found that physically abused children had difficulties recognizing emotions such as sadness and disgust, although their accuracy in recognizing anger did not differ from nonmaltreated controls. These authors conclude that physically abusive environments appear to compromise the ability to recognize and differentiate some emotions, while concurrently heightening the awareness of others (e.g., anger), perhaps due to an overabundance of hostile emotional cues and a familial context of limited affective range.

Munchausen by Proxy Syndrome

MBPS varies widely in terms of symptom presentation (Schreier & Libow, 1993). Clues to the problem are usually a pattern of unexpected symptoms in the child, and chronic and varied child illness behaviors. Gastrointestinal symptoms and seizures tend to dominate the MBPS picture. Infants and preverbal children seem to be at greatest risk, because intrusive, active induction of illness is most likely (e.g., active suffocation, diarrhea, vomiting, seizures). Older children tend to present with falsified reports or simulated symptoms (e.g., misrepresentation of medical history, contamination of laboratory specimens). Adolescents may become involved with validating their parents' fabrications or even in directly harming themselves.

MBPS is typically perpetrated by a mother, often with medical knowledge or training; the father may be a passive colluder and an uninvolved or absent parent (Schreier & Libow, 1993). Most such mothers present with a personality disorder (histrionic and borderline types), engage in self-harm, and have a history of factitious or somatoform disorder (Bools, Neale, & Meadow, 1994). Medically, the involvement with professionals is extensive and atypical, and may appear implausible. Less is known about this form of abuse than about others, and prevalence rates have not been determined. In a 1991 U.S. survey of 316 pediatric neurologists and gastroenterologists, 273 confirmed cases and 192 suspected cases were reported (Schreier & Libow, 1993). In a U.K. prospective survey of pediatricians, the incidence in children under 1 year old was 2.8 per 100,000 (McClure, Davis, Meadow, & Sibert, 1996).

THE NEGLECTED CHILD

As noted earlier, child neglect denotes deficiencies in caretaking obligations that harm a child's psychological and/or physical health (Dubowitz & Black, 1994; National Research Council, 1993; Pagelow, 1997; for reviews, see Erickson & Egeland, 2002; Hildyard & Wolfe, in press). Neglecting behaviors encompass educational, supervisory, medical, physical, and emotional domains. In severely neglecting families, there are typically no routines for eating, sleeping, bathing, and household cleaning. Living areas may be littered with decaying materials. Food may only be available on a random basis. There may be a failure to properly immunize and medically care for children. Children may be left unsupervised for hours or abandoned for days. Although most drowning and near-drowning cases (bathtubs, pools) occur when children are unsupervised, these tend to be classified as accidental deaths and injuries; some incidents may, however, constitute neglect (Kaufman & Henrich, 2000). In children under the age of 2 years, the most prominent form of neglect is failure to thrive (FTT; for a detailed discussion, see Lyons-Ruth, Zeanah, & Benoit, Chapter 13, this volume).

Physical Signs

Because child neglect is an act of omission rather than commission, there are usually fewer physical signs. With infants, these may include severe diaper rash, dehydration, diseases related to malnutrition, and delayed psychomotor skills. In older children, signs may include dental decay; fatigue and listlessness; recurrent ear infections; poor physical care indicators (e.g., accumulated ear wax, foul body odor, unclean clothes, frequent lice infestations); and inadequate physical development.

Cognitive and Behavioral Development

Similar to physically abused children, neglected children tend to differ from nonabused children on measures of language ability and intelligence (Hildyard & Wolfe, in press). Given the low level of educational input and parental feedback in the primary care environment of physically and/or emotionally neglected children, their cognitive and academic achievement has been found to be worse than that of other maltreated groups. Erickson and Egeland (2002) have recently reviewed findings from their longitudinal study of at-risk families, followed from infancy to late adolescence. Overall, children who were physically neglected had high rates of school failure and dropout, and the emotionally neglected group had high rates of psychopathology (i.e., 90% received a psychiatric diagnosis, with 73% displaying comorbidities). Cognitive and academic deficits were found across development, from infancy (e.g., Egeland & Sroufe, 1981b) and toddlerhood (e.g., Egeland, Sroufe, & Erickson, 1983) through to school age (e.g., Erickson et al., 1989) and adolescence (e.g., Egeland, 1997). Specifically, even when gender and welfare status were controlled for, maltreated children scored significantly lower in reading and math achievement, received more suspensions, received more disciplinary referrals, and repeated a grade more often than matched control children did. Also, maltreated children in general and physically neglected children in particular showed lower academic initiative (e.g., working independently, persistent, responsive to directions) than controls.

Rowe and Eckenrode (1999) found a pattern of academic difficulties across the years in a sample of maltreated children, the majority of whom were neglected. Compared to nonmaltreated children, these children were at greater risk for repeating kindergarten and first grade, which is consistent with lower school readiness. From second through sixth grade, maltreated and nonmaltreated children were similar in terms of first-time grade failure. Residential mobility mediated the relationship between reported child maltreatment and academic performance (Eckenrode, Rowe, Laird, & Brathwaite, 1995): maltreating families averaged twice as many moves during the children's school-age years.

Studies with matched controls indicate the presence of maltreatment-related cognitive deficits in the areas of delayed language, cognitive development, low IQ, and poor school performance (e.g., Perez & Widom, 1994; Shonk & Cicchetti, 2001; Widom, 1998; for a review of studies over the past three decades, see Veltman & Browne, 2001). In a study of 6-year-old children in low-income families who were recruited from inner-city pediatric clinics, a history of both FTT and maltreatment was related to greater impairment in school performance and cognitive functioning than among children with neither of these experiences (Kerr, Black, & Krishnakumar, 2000). In a prospective study of extremely low-birthweight infants, Strathearn, Gray, O'Callaghan, and Wood (2001) found that substantiated neglected infants showed a significantly progressive decline in their cognitive function over time (at 1, 2, 3, and 4 years), and had significantly smaller head circumference at 2 and 4 years (but not at birth), as compared to the nonmaltreated group. These authors found that disability (defined as cerebral palsy, blindness, or deafness) was not associated with a higher rate of CPS referral. Although Sullivan and Knutson (2000) did find that disability status was related to maltreatment, rates for children with physical disability status were lower than for children with cognitive-based or behavioral disabilities.

In observed interactions, neglected toddlers showed little persistence and enthusiasm, much negative affect and noncompliance, and little positive affect, yet were found to be highly reliant on their mothers. As preschoolers, these neglected children showed poor impulse control and were found to be highly dependent on teachers for support and nurturance (Erickson et al., 1989). Koenig, Cicchetti, and Rogosch (2000) found that neglected children displayed more negative affect during an observed clean-up session that followed a free-play period (physically abused children were not significantly different from controls). One interpretation of interactional differences may be that neglected children are in a stronger position than physically abused children to express negative affect directly in interactions with their caregivers. Similar interactional themes are found in observational studies of children with FTT and their families (Benoit, 2000). These mothers show fewer positive behaviors, less affect, more negative perceptions of their infants, and more adult insecure attachment patterns; have experienced more maltreatment themselves in childhood (physical and sexual abuse, neglect) and adulthood; and have more mental illness (e.g., anxiety, depression).

Socioemotional Development

Like physically abused children, most neglected children form insecure attachments with their caregivers (Crittenden, 1985, 1992; Egeland & Sroufe, 1981a). Consequently, some neglected children never learn strategies for engaging adults and for independently exploring their environments, tending to be passive interactants (Crittenden & Ainsworth, 1989). The passivity of neglected children often extends to their peer domain (Hoffman-Plotkin & Twentyman, 1984). Neglected children, however, have been rated by teachers and parents as having more internalizing behaviors (withdrawal, sadness) than comparison children (Hoffman-Plotkin & Twentyman, 1984; Manly et al., 2001). The extent to which such withdrawal from relationships indicates differences in psychological difficulties (e.g., depression, anxiety, repressed anger), acquired social skills (e.g., social reciprocity), motivation, or cognitive–affective abilities remains to be fully understood. In regard to the last-mentioned point, Pollak et al. (2000) demonstrated that physically neglected children accurately recognized emotions less frequently than did nonmaltreated or physically abused children, even after receptive language abilities were controlled for. Neglected children displayed deficits in discriminating among emotions (e.g., neglected children saw greater similarity between happy and sad expressions than did the other groups) that were not attributable to problems at the visual–

perceptual level, but rather at the level of understanding particular emotion displays. Neglected children, then, would seem to be exposed to fewer emotional learning opportunities and greater restriction of parental affect.

THE SEXUALLY ABUSED CHILD

Reviews of the child sexual abuse literature converge in identifying a range of common symptoms and adjustment problems (e.g., Beitchman et al., 1991; Berliner & Elliot, 2002; Finkelhor & Browne, 1988; Hartman & Burgess, 1989; Kendall-Tackett, Williams, & Finkelhor, 1993; Kendall-Tackett & Eckenrode, 1996, 1997). Sexual abuse is often related to specific symptoms of sexualized behavior, as well as clinical indications of aggression, depression, withdrawal, and anxiety. The range of symptoms can be meaningfully described in reference to (1) acute symptoms, representing a primary stress response to the abuse trauma; and (2) secondary symptoms, representing an accommodation and adaptation to the abuse experience.

Acute Symptoms of Sexual Abuse

Many of the acute symptoms of sexual abuse resemble children's common reactions to stressors. Rather than being directly related to the sexual offense per se, such stress-related problems may be connected to related (but nonsexual) aspects of the abuse, such as other forms of abuse by adults (physical, emotional); bullying by peers (teasing, physical assaults); stressful living conditions (domestic violence, criminal activity, substance misuse); and more subtle sexually abusive behaviors (exposure to sexual activity by adults, seductive parenting). Acute symptoms of the onset of child sexual abuse can be best detected by those individuals who are most familiar with the child's level of functioning, because these symptoms represent a *change* in behavior and disruption of previous competencies (Hartman & Burgess, 1989). Parents, relatives, teachers, coaches, and friends of the child may note symptoms of distress across physical, psychological, and behavioral dimensions signifying that "something is different."

Acute physical symptoms or signs include headaches, stomachaches, appetite changes, vomiting, sensitivity to touch in specific areas, genital complaints, and urinary tract infections. Gynecological problems in children, such as infections, perineal bruises and tears, or sexually transmitted diseases, are signs specific to sexual abuse (Asher, 1988). Frothingham et al. (2000) reported that at an 8-year follow-up, sexually abused youths were more likely to experience chronic health problems than controls. A community survey of women visiting a family practice clinic showed childhood sexual abuse history to be associated with a greater number of poor health indicators (overweight, heavier amount of smoking, earlier onset of smoking, more sexual partners, fewer Pap smears), gynecological problems (yeast infections, pelvic pain, pelvic inflammatory disease, pregnancy complications), breast disease, and higher scores on a somatization scale (Springs & Friedrich, 1992). Similarly, Newman et al. (2000) found that in their sample of patients presenting to a health maintenance organization (n = 602), sexually abused women reported significantly more physical symptoms, gastrointenstinal problems, pain, disability over the past month, and physician visits over the past year than did nonabused women. Medical chart review indicated more outpatient visits over a 2-year period for the sexually abused group. These authors controlled for childhood physical abuse, suggesting the lasting physical health effect of sexual abuse.

Disruptions to physical/sexual development can occur as a function of the emotional abuse within the sexual context. Finkelhor and Browne (1988) conceptualize this as "traumatic sexualization," referring to the process in which a child's sexuality is shaped in developmentally inappropriate and interpersonally dysfunctional ways. It may be more prominent in situations where force is used, a sexual response is evoked from the child, and the child is enticed to participate. Sexualized behaviors include persistent sexualized behavior (e.g., touching, exposing self or other, excessive masturbation), age-inappropriate knowledge of sexual activity, and/or pronounced seductive or promiscuous behavior. Friedrich (1993), using a parent report inventory tapping child sexual behavior, found a greater incidence of sexually related problems (e.g., "French-kisses," "uses sexual words") among sexually abused preschool children, as compared to the normative sample. In a retrospective chart review for child and adolescent psychiatric inpatients, sexually abused youths had elevated rates of hypersexual, exposing, and victimizing sexual behaviors (McClellan et al., 1996). These youths were more likely to have been chronically sexually abused, and more likely to have experienced physical abuse and neglect as well. Early age of onset of sexual abuse (before age 7) was the most significant predictor of inappropriate sexual behaviors. In a study of youths in foster care (mean age of 16 years), severity of sexual abuse was associated with recent HIV risk behaviors (e.g., consensual sexual intercourse; anal sex; traded sex for food, money, or a place to stay; etc.), even when the contributions of other childhood traumas and emotional and behavioral problems were taken into account (Elze, Auslander, McMillen, Edmond, & Thompson, 2001).

Psychological symptoms may further include emotional over- or underreactivity (e.g., panic, blunted affect); difficulty focusing and sustaining attention; and withdrawal in interest and participation from usual activities. These symptoms of distress may be associated with a decline in school performance, behavior, and peer relations. Sexual abuse has been related to poorer cognitive performance, as indicated by poorer teacher ratings of overall academic performance and of being a competent learner (high task orientation, low learning problems); parent ratings of dissociation/distractibility; and greater school avoidance (e.g., absences, teacher ratings of shy/anxious) (Trickett, McBride-Chang, & Putnam, 1994). Behavioral symptoms may include regression to behaviors of earlier levels of development (enuresis, encopresis, clinging, excessive crying, tantrums, fearfulness); sleeping problems and nightmares; self-destructive behaviors (self-injury, risk-taking behaviors); hyperactivity; and truancy, running away from home, or pseudomaturity (for a review, see Berliner & Elliot, 2002).

Secondary Symptoms of Sexual Abuse

Enduring symptoms of sexual abuse may be complicated by the disclosure and discovery process (Hartman & Burgess, 1989) and by the extended involvement of official agents (e.g., child protection, police, and court systems; Friedrich, 1990). In contrast with acute symptoms, a more identifiable clustering of secondary symptoms appears along trauma-specific dimensions. For example, abuse-specific fears (e.g., fear of being alone, fear of men), idiosyncratic fears related to the specific abuse events (e.g., fear of the bathroom), and trauma symptoms (e.g., McLeer, Deblinger, Atkins, Foa, & Ralphe, 1988; Wolfe, Gentile, & Wolfe, 1989; Wolfe, Sas, & Wekerle, 1994) may develop. Depressive symptoms have been noted in childhood and adulthood among survivors (e.g., Koverola, Pound, Heger, & Lytle, 1993; Zuravin & Fontanella, 1999). Studies have found that abuse-related feelings and perceptions predict higher levels of PTSD symptoms (e.g., Deblinger, Steer, & Lippmann, 1999; Fiering, Taska, & Lewis, 1998).

A main factor that mitigates the negative effects of sexual abuse is a child's experience of a positive relationship with the mother, as seen in maternal support and protective actions (Kendall-Tackett et al., 1993; Kendall-Tackett & Eckenrode, 1996, 1997). Maternal warmth was found to be a stronger predictor of adult adjustment than were several child sexual abuse variables (e.g., duration of abuse, number of incidents; Peters, 1988). In their 3-year follow-up of a sample of 61 sexually abused children following their testifying in court, Sas, Hurley, Hatch, Malla, and Dick (1993) similarly found that perceived support by mothers was one of the most important mediators of sexually abused children's adjustment over time.

Table 14.1 summarizes the range of child characteristics associated with physical abuse, neglect, and sexual abuse, based on the preceding discussions.

DEVELOPMENTAL ISSUES IN CHILD MALTREATMENT

Because child maltreatment is a private event as well as a personal invasion, it can have a wide range of impact on development. As Herman (1992) notes in regard to abuse,

> The child trapped in an abusive environment is faced with formidable tasks of adaptation. She must find a way to preserve a sense of trust in people who are untrustworthy, safety in a situation that is unsafe, control in a situation that is terrifyingly unpredictable, power in a situation of helplessness. Unable to care for or protect herself, she must compensate for the failures of adult care and protection with the only means at her disposal, an immature system of psychological defenses. (p. 98)

Maltreatment challenges all domains of development, given the task of processing a highly affective aversive experience that may be ongoing. There are common developmental issues to emerge for the traumatized child that are non-

TABLE 14.1. Range of Child Characteristics Associated with Physical Abuse, Neglect, and Sexual Abuse

Dimension of development	Physical abuse	Neglect	Sexual abuse
Physical	Minor: Bruises, lacerations, abrasions Major: Burns, brain damage, broken bones	Failure-to-thrive symptoms: Slowed growth, immature physical development	Physical symptoms: Headaches, stomachaches, appetite changes, vomiting; gynecological complaints
Cognitive	Mild delay in areas of cognitive and intellectual functioning; academic problems; difficulties in moral reasoning	Mild delay in areas of cognitive and intellectual functioning; academic problems; difficulties in moral reasoning	No evidence of cognitive impairment; self-blame; guilt
Behavioral	Aggression; peer problems; "compulsive compliance"	Passivity; "hyperactivity"	Fears, anxiety, PTSD-related symptoms; sleep problems
Socioemotional	Social incompetence; hostile intent attributions; difficulties in social sensitivity	Social incompetence; withdrawal, dependence; difficulties in social sensitivity	Symptoms of depression and low self-esteem; "sexualized" behavior; behaviors that accommodate to the abuse (e.g., passive compliance; no or delayed disclosuse)

specific to maltreatment type. These include cognitive adaptations (cognitive vigilance, dissociation, social-cognitive deficits); socioemotional adaptations (conceptualization of the self, conceptualization of the other, affect regulation); and family dynamics.

Cognitive Adaptations

The maltreated child must embark on creating some defensive structure, which may involve various cognitive adaptions. Cognitive distortions (deYoung & Lowry, 1992) and disruption to a success-based orientation (Cicchetti et al., 1988) have been noted. Other cognitive adaptations include cognitive vigilance, dissociation, and social-cognitive deficits, which are discussed here.

Cognitive Vigilance

As Herman (1992) discusses, hypervigilance includes not only constant scanning of the environment, but also development of the ability to detect subtle variations in it, to alert the child about possible abuse. Children can become adept at processing nonverbal communication, such that facial, intonational, and body language cues signifying danger states (e.g., adult anger, sexual arousal, intoxication, or dissociation) seem to be automatically processed without much conscious awareness. Indeed, a maltreated child can learn to respond to danger signals because they have evoked a feeling of alarm, without being able to verbally label or identify such cues. In other words, it appears that the "feeling state" is most accessible to the child. However, once alarmed, the maltreated child must make quiet efforts at escape, avoiding visible displays of agitation and, instead, effortfully attempting to be inconspicuous—avoiding the perpetrator if possible, or placating or complying if necessary.

Some evidence supports maltreated children's sensitivity to a particular class of affective cues—unresolved anger. Hennessy, Rabideau, Cicchetti, and Cummings (1994) found that children with a history of maltreatment and exposure to domestic violence reported greater fear following videotaped presentations of interadult anger than did matched low-socioeconomic-status (low-SES) children who were exposed to domestic violence. However, this heightened emotional reaction occurred in the context of unresolved (but not resolved) anger, suggesting that maltreated children are particularly sensitive to cues of conflict termination. These researchers suggest that the placating behaviors often observed in maltreated children may represent fear-based attempts to calm or soothe angry parents, so as to avoid becoming the recipient of parental aggression. In a psychophysiological experimental, Pollak, Cicchetti, Klorman, and Brumaghim (1997) found that maltreated children evidenced different brain event-related potentials (ERPs), specifically P300, as compared to nonmaltreated controls when exposed to angry or happy visual depictions. Maltreated children had larger ERP amplitude in response to the angry than to the happy stimulus, consistent with a more efficient or preferential cognitive processing of such negative affect. Thus maltreated children appear to be primed for detecting negative affect.

Dissociation

"Dissociation" denotes the situation of altering one's usual level of self-awareness, in an effort to escape an upsetting event or feeling (Trzepacz & Baker, 1993). It is a normal reaction to an emotionally overloaded situation, enacted in the service of self-preservation when neither resistance nor escape is possible (Herman, 1992). With dissociation, the child diverts attention away from the maltreatment (especially sexual or physical abuse), psychologically escaping from it. This process can include actively pretending to be somewhere or someone else, experiencing amnesia, and having the ability to "cut off" pain perception from parts of the body. The cognitive outcome of dissociation is a fragmentation of abuse-related information in memory, such that informational details may be separated from each other and from affective and physiological responses. This fragmentation can translate into patchy and disorganized event recall, seemingly illogical associations, and seemingly extreme affective reactions, such as extreme rage in reaction to relatively minor interpersonal "offenses." The trauma may lead to the experience of intense emotion without clear memory of an event, accompanied in some instances by flat affect.

Although children often emit dissociative experiences (e.g., daydreaming, forgetfulness, attentional shifts), essential features of atypical dissociation include amnestic periods, trance-like states, and marked changes in behavior and functioning (e.g., abruptly disrupted play) (Putnam, 1993). Friedrich, Jaworski, Huxsahl, and Bengtson (1997) compared nonabused controls, nonabused psychiatric clients, substantiated sexually abused clients, and suspected sexually abused clients on self-reported dissociation symptoms. All three clinical groups scored significantly higher than the normal controls, with no significant differences among clinical groups. In predicting dissociation symptoms, the duration and nature of the sexual abuse were significant contributors beyond age and gender. Young adolescents with a longer duration and greater severity of abuse were more likely to endorse dissociative symptomatology. Trickett, Noll, Reiffman, and Putnam (2001) found that dissociation at initial assessment (referral within 6 months of disclosure) described youths who had experienced abuse by multiple perpetrators (nonbiological father figures or other relatives) that was probably accompanied by physical violence, in contrast to those who had experienced chronic incest by a single perpetrator with low physical violence (all sexual abuse involved genital contact). When data were collapsed across subgroups, sexually abused girls had greater dissociation in adolescence at the follow-up assessment 7 years later.

Dissociation does not apply only to sexually abused children, however. Macfie, Cicchetti, and Toth (2001) examined dissociation among maltreated and nonmaltreated preschoolers, using a narrative story stem completion task. Developmentally, an integrated self would be evident in toddlerhood and the preschool period. Normative, nonmaltreating experiences facilitate this process to create a sense of self, separate but connected to others. In contrast, maltreatment experiences may promote the development of a dissociated self, with concomitant disruptions in the normal integration of memories, perceptions, and identity; this development supports denial, amnesia for the experiences, blurring of self and fantasy characters, and grandiose self-representations. Macfie et al. found that maltreated preschoolers did have higher dissociation scores than nonmaltreated controls. These differences described the sexually abused and physically abused groups, but were less striking for the neglected group. The nature of these differences indicates an increasing level of dissociation over the two time points (initial assessment and 1 year later). This finding does not indicate a "recovery" or greater subsequent coherence in the self, and raises the preschool period as a possible time of "sensitivity" for self-consolidation versus self-fragmentation.

Social-Cognitive Deficits

Social cognition is an important dimension of development to consider, because it may mediate the link between maltreatment experiences and the child's subsequent social behavior. Domains of social cognition can include inferences about the thoughts, feelings, and intentions of others, as in person perception and causal attributions (Smetana & Kelly, 1989). For example, in the domain of affective cognitions, maltreated preschoolers have been found to have greater difficulties with affect recognition than their peers (e.g., Camras, Ribordy, Spaccarelli, & Stefani, 1986). This may be a function of a lower mastery of verbal expressiveness about inner feelings. To illustrate, Cicchetti and Beeghly (1987) found that maltreated toddlers used fewer "internal state" words (e.g., talking about the feelings and emotions of self and other—"Ouch," "I be good," "You hurt my feelings") than their nonmaltreated counterparts in interactions with their mothers, and they spoke less often about their negative internal states. Furthermore, the maltreated children produced fewer utterances about negative affect and about physiological states (hunger, thirst). These researchers suggest that inhibition of emotional language may be adaptive in a maltreating environment, because its expression may function as a parental trigger for maltreatment. That is, certain classes of children's affect (e.g., distress) may not be tolerated in maltreating families, and this may be reflected in maltreated children's inappropriate responses to other-distress (e.g., Main & George, 1985).

Alternatively, maltreating parents may be poor models for children in their decoding abilities, perhaps overlabeling affects as negative. Cicchetti (1990) found similarities in the level of emotional language of maltreated and insecurely attached children, which again emphasizes the relational context as a main teaching environment for the child about emotional states, labeling of emotions, and affective perspective taking. Beeghly and Cicchetti (1994) clarify that toddlers at greatest risk for delayed internal-state language were maltreated children with insecure attachments, as compared to maltreated toddlers with secure attachment and comparison toddlers with insecure attachment. This suggests that maltreatment occurring within a generally problematic relational context is particularly toxic for young children's developing sociocommunicative abilities.

Thus cognitive development among maltreated children may be altered by their experiences to such an extent that various adaptational strategies, such as hypervigilance and dissociation, form to become a cognitive "style" that is highly responsive to signs of personal danger. Maltreated children, though, have difficulties verbally describing their experiences. *Ipso facto*, when the environment changes (as when a child starts school), such strategies are no longer adaptive, making cognitive flexibility more challenging.

Socioemotional Adaptation

Maltreatment requires a child to make social and emotional adjustments that may compromise development. This is especially true of much abuse, since part of the abuser's intent is to achieve acceptance, even willingness, on the child's part. This process can entail the use of coercive strategies to ensure psychological control over the child including fear-based tactics (e.g., threatening greater harm to the child or others) and tactics aimed at destroying the child's sense of self (e.g., verbally denigrating the child). For many abused children, these abuser behaviors occur within (and sometimes contribute to) the context of an insecure attachment to parental figures (Aber & Allen, 1987). This attachment context is important to understanding the impact of child abuse, because the child's conceptualization of self and of others in relationships represents both a belief system and a relationship prototype (Waters, Posada, Crowell, & Lay, 1993).

Conceptions of the Self

Maltreated children appear to struggle with a core deficit in the self—including poor self-integration, self-destructiveness, low self-esteem, low self-efficacy, self-blame, and negative affect toward the self, as seen in depression and suicidal ideation. Finkelhor and Browne (1988) identify the sense of "powerlessness" as being a salient component to the disruption of the self, as well as the process of "stigmatization," where negative connotations about the maltreatment experience become incorporated into the child's self-image. In neglect, a child's personal power or self-efficacy is diminished by his or her low value and status as a recipient of inadequate care. In child physical abuse, power is usurped from the child as a function of the invasion to his or her physical space and subjugation. The child's self-efficacy may be further diminished when his or her attempts to avoid or end the abuse meet with no or limited success. Thus the emotional undercurrent to the self as a function of childhood maltreatment is one of disrespect, being valued only as an "object," and lack of self-determination.

Limited work has been directed to self-conceptualization, especially as it evolves over time and with new salient experiences (e.g., romantic relationship formation). Awareness of a negative or "bad" sense of self was inferred from findings in which maltreated toddlers responded to their mirror reflections with neutral or negative affect more often than controls did (Schneider-Rosen & Cicchetti, 1991). Furthermore, chronic negative self-esteem and a low sense of self-efficacy are reported clinically among sexual abuse survivors, although self-esteem is not a strong discriminator between samples of abused and nonabused adults (Kendall-Tackett et al., 1993). Cicchetti, Rogosch, Lynch, and Holt (1993) found that school-age maltreated children (predominantly physically abused and/or neglected) showed lower ego resiliency (i.e., more fragile egos) than their nonmaltreated counterparts; no significant differences in self-esteem were found. Studies in the 1980s addressing the issue of self found that young maltreated children inhibited negative affect (Cicchetti & Beeghly, 1987; Crittenden, 1988), with Crittenden (1988) noting that some maltreated children displayed false positive affect. Toth, Cicchetti, Macfie, and Emde (1997), using a narrative story stem task to elicit material considered to reflect internalizations of their maltreating and other caregiving experiences, found that maltreated children expressed more negative maternal and self-representations than did nonmaltreated children in their completions of the stories. Physically abused children had higher levels of negative self-representations, and neglected children had lower levels of positive self-representation. Thus maltreated children are challenged to develop an integration of positive and negative aspects of the self and realistic self-appraisal (Cole & Putnam, 1992).

These issues may generalize to other domains. For instance, persistence in problem solving is less among maltreated children than among cognitively comparable controls (Egeland & Sroufe, 1981b; Gaensbauer, 1982). Also, a child's achievement may be met with acceptance and positive regard from others outside the maltreating environment, but the child's ability to take credit for and appreciate these sentiments is limited by his or her sense of self as "bad." In extreme cases, these alternate views of the self form the core of alternate personalities (Herman, 1992) and dissociative identity disorder (American Psychiatric Association, 2000).

Studies converge in identifying self-blame as an important construct for understanding symptomatology in children. Self-blame may serve a preventative function; that is, a child may know "better" what to do next time or how to prevent further maltreatment (Janoff-Bulman, 1979). However, the literature on sexually abused children in particular suggests that greater self-blame is associated with greater psychological distress (Wolfe et al., 1994; Fiering et al., 1998). In a recent report, McGee, Wolfe, and Olson (2001) found that in a CPS sample, most teens spontaneously attributed blame to the perpetrators. When the teens were probed about their own possible role, however, most physically/emotionally abused teens identified "misbehavior," and most sexually abused teens identified failure to prevent the abuse. Physically/emotionally abused youths showed a relationship between abuse severity and self-blame. Self-blame cognitions decreased with increased abuse severity, and self-blame negative affect also increased with severity among females. Also, self-blame was inversely related to perpetrator blame. Across all forms of maltreatment, self-blaming affect added unique variance to the prediction of internalizing problem scores. For physical/emotional abuse and sexual abuse, self-blaming affect also predicted externalizing problems. These authors suggest that *feeling* one is to blame for maltreatment may be more salient than *thinking* one is to blame, in terms of adjustment. In a similar vein, Dembo et al. (1990) found that the relationship between maltreatment and teen substance abuse was mediated by a self-derogation construct. Fiering, Taska, and Lewis (1998, 2002) found support for a model in which shame and a self-blaming attributional style mediated the relationship between number of abusive events and depressive symptoms, self-esteem, and eroticism among sexually abused children and adolescents

Herman (1992) argues that the functional value of self-blame in a child's interpretation of physical or sexual abuse is to absolve parents of blame and responsibility, thereby preserving the attachment relationship. Toward this end, the child may use other strategies in addition to self-blame, including minimalization, rationalization, suppression of thoughts, denial, and dissociative reactions. The meaning of the abuse may be changed from bad to "less bad," or even "good"—an interpretation that may be conveyed directly to the child by others in his or her environment (i.e., positive benefits or rewards, experience of pleasure, etc.). This process of adaptive misperception of adult behavior and self-blame is not unique to abused children, however. It also differentiates preschool children who are anxiously attached from those who are securely attached to their caregivers, and such reactions are considered to be a strategy that serves attachment (Waters et al., 1993).

Conceptions of Others

Research suggests that sexual abuse involving fathers and stepfathers is experienced as more traumatic than that involving non-relative males (Finkelhor & Browne, 1988). Finkelhor and Browne (1988) discuss this in terms of the betrayal dynamic of sexual abuse perpetrated by trusted persons, on whom the children were in some way dependent (see also Freyd's trauma betrayal theory, discussed subsequently). Betrayal involves the degree to which children feel their confidence was gained through manipulation and coercion, as well as the position of trust or authority held by the perpetrators. Since it is understood that caretakers take care of their children, any type of maltreatment may be experienced as a betrayal (including child abuse by persons involved with community institutions and organizations; Wolfe, Jaffe, Jette, & Poisson, 2002). As a consequence, a child's interpersonal needs may be compromised by intense and contradictory feelings of need for closeness and the fear of it (e.g., Dodge, Pettit, & Bates, 1994). For example, Wolfe et al. (1989) found that sexually abused children tended to report that in their belief systems, sexual abuse was a pervasive phenomenon and that adults were generally exploitative of children. On a projective storytelling task in another study, maltreated children's responses were characterized by difficulty resolving relationship problems and negative interpersonal expectations more often than comparison children, even when family SES and child IQ were controlled for (McCrone, Egeland, Kalkoske, & Carlson, 1994). Using a storytelling/completion task, Waldinger, Toth, and Gerber (2001) found that neglected preschoolers represented others as hurt, sad, and anxious more often than did physically abused, sexually abused, or nonabused controls. Abused/neglected children, as compared to controls, represented the self as angry and opposing others more often. Thus, over the course of development, this process may translate into interpersonal wariness, idealization, and conflict; affectively labile interpersonal interactions; and indiscriminate interpersonal relationships.

The disruption in relatedness caused by child maltreatment can also lead to general interpersonal patterns of withdrawal/isolation and anxious clinging (Hartman & Burgess, 1989). For example, some physically abused children (Friedrich & Einbender, 1983) and neglected and sexually abused children (Friedrich, 1990) indiscriminately seek affection, readily engaging strangers. Lynch and Cicchetti (1991) found that physically abused and neglected children showed a high degree of proximity seeking to mothers, teachers, and peers, suggesting their anxiety about closeness to others. In addition, maltreated children show a high preponderance of insecure attachment to their caregivers—particularly the disorganized/disoriented type—as compared to nonmaltreated children (e.g., Barnett et al., 1999; Carlson, Cicchetti, Barnett, & Braunwald, 1989; Schneider-Rosen, Braunwald, Carlson, & Cicchetti, 1985). We (Wekerle & Wolfe, 1998) found that adolescents' self-perceived insecure attachment style interacted with maltreatment history to predict violence perpetration and maltreatment in teen partnerships.

Another disruption in relatedness is heightened conflict. For example, McCloskey and Stuewig (2001) found that although children exposed to domestic violence did not differ on the number of friends they claimed or their frequency of peer contact, the child witnesses reported feeling more lonely and having more conflict with a close friend. The mothers of these children also reported their children to have more problems with friends than mothers from nonviolent families reported about their children. Likely contributors to such peer conflict are problems with aggression, as would be expected, given social learning influences and learned relational schemas. The increased aggressiveness of some maltreated children extends into delinquency during adolescence (Hotaling, Straus, & Lincoln, 1990; Widom, 1989b), including assaultive behavior toward others in general (Herrenkohl, Egolf, & Herrenkohl, 1997) and dating partners in particular (Wolfe et al., 1998; Wekerle et al., 2001). Interestingly, Toth et al. (2000) found that the link between maltreatment and externalizing problem behaviors was partially mediated by conflictual themes, as elicited by a storytelling task (the direct effect of maltreatment on externalizing problems remained significant). Differences in school achievement have not explained the association between chronic maltreatment and aggression (Bolger & Patterson, 2001).

Finally, maltreated children are at greater risk for peer rejection. A prospective, longitudinal design of three cohorts of public school children distinguished those who were identified as maltreated children in a statewide central registry of substantiated cases from a matched comparison group (Bolger & Patterson, 2001). Maltreated children were predominantly neglected (75%) and physically/emotionally abused (64%), with neglect only and overlapping neglect/abuse the most common patterns, and most maltreated children received one substantiated report. Based on annual sociometric testing, chronically maltreated children (5 years or more of maltreatment) experienced peer rejection more often on a single assessment occasion, as well as consistently across childhood to early adolescence. The longer maltreatment continued, the more likely a child was to be rejected repeatedly by peers over time. For example, 73% of the nonmaltreated children, 64% of the children maltreated up to 5 years, and 50% of the children maltreated for 5 years or more were classified as never being rejected by peers. Importantly, the relationship between maltreatment and peer rejection was accounted for in part by aggressive behavior for both boys and girls, whereas social withdrawal did not account for this relationship. These researchers concluded that chronicity rather than type of maltreatment best predicted aggression and rejection by peers. Chronic maltreatment by caregivers emerged as a significant predictor of both high levels of aggression and repeated peer rejection across the school years. One suggested mechanism for the maltreatment–aggression–peer rejection pathway is a coercive pattern of parent–child interactions; that is, the propensity to employ a coercive, aggressive interactional style with peers has probably been "trained up" in the family of origin.

Affect Regulation

A child's self-regulation of affect involves the ability to modulate, modify, redirect, and otherwise control emotions (especially intense ones) in a way that facilitates adaptive functioning (Cicchetti, Ganiban, & Barnett, 1990). Two categories of emotion regulation problems are (1) modulation difficulties (i.e., inability to alter emotion intensity with self-soothing strategies, etc.) and (2) experiential avoidance (i.e., inability to accept or tolerate affect, and hence efforts to avoid, control, or suppress the experiencing of emotion) (Cicchetti, Ackerman, & Izard, 1995). For maltreated children, affective issues seem in particular to involve difficulties with modulation, resulting in experiencing affective extremes, and the more fundamental difficulty of lack of awareness of body states or physiological responses (Herman, 1992).

Modulation difficulties can be seen in extreme depressive reactions and intense angry outburts. Considering depressive symptomatology and the timing of maltreatment, Thornberry, Ireland, and Smith (2001) found that any maltreatment during adolescence, as compared to childhood-only maltreatment, increased the risk for depressive symptoms in adolescence. Maltreatment experiences during either period were related to risk for internalizing disorder. Cicchetti and Rogosch (2001) found that maltreated children, as compared to sociodemographically matched, nonmaltreated children, were more likely to show clinical-level internalizing behavior problems (e.g., elevated self-reports of depression or teacher-rated internalizing problems). Furthermore, cortisol dysregulation was found in these internalizing maltreated children, in that higher cortisol levels were noted in the morning, afternoon, and on daily average. The typical cortisol pattern is that the highest level is evident at the time of awakening, with a decline to low levels by sleep onset. Because cortisol levels would be elevated in response to acute trauma, internalizing maltreated children's patterns would suggest chronic hyperactivity of the limbic–hypothalamic–pituitary–adrenocortical (LHPA) axis, which may indicate the presence of brain impairment (e.g., neuronal damage, neuronal loss in the hippocampus, retarded myelination, atypical synaptic pruning).[1] DeBellis, Baum, et al. (1999) found that maltreated prepubertal children with PTSD and comorbid depressive disorder evidenced dysregulation of the LHPA axis. Others have found a reduction in cortisol reactivity among maltreated preschool children, as well as lower social competence, as compared to nonmaltreated controls (e.g., Hart, Gunnar, & Cicchetti, 1995); these findings suggest cortisol dysregulation and an association with poorer socioemotional functioning. (For a review of studies on the psychobiology of the child maltreatment–depression connection, see Kaufman & Charney, 2001.)

Difficulties with affect regulation may lead to maladaptive and self-destructive behaviors in an attempt to manage the painful affect or avoid it. For example, Herman (1992) suspects from her clinical observations that child self-injurious behavior may be a pathological form of self-soothing, replacing intolerable psychological pain with physical pain. She postulates that a compulsion to self-mutilate is preceded by a strong dissociative state, tends to develop before puberty, and is often a source of shame and is practiced in secret. Other maladaptive attempts at negative affect regulation among survivors include purging and vomiting; compulsive sexual behavior; compulsive risk taking or exposure to danger; and alcohol and drug use (Beitchman et al., 1991). The functional value of such maladaptive behaviors may include positively reinforcing a negative self-construct, escaping from emotional numbing, and self-medicating aversive affective states by decreasing negative and increasing positive affect (Stewart & Israeli, 2002). Substance misuse may also bolster self-esteem, increase a sense of peer affiliation, and reduce feelings of isolation (Bensley, Van Eenwyk, & Simmons, 2000; Kendler et al., 2000). Two of the most prevalence self-destructive behaviors in adolescence are risky sexual practices and substance misuse.

"Sleeper" effects of maltreatment have been suggested as those that emerge subsequently when developmental maturity for their expression has been reached, as in the case of sexual dysfunction (e.g., Beitchman et al., 1992). The domain of risky sexual behaviors includes early entry into sexual activity, lack of protection during sex, a high number of sexual partners, and early pregnancy and prostitution. Childhood maltreatment has been found to be a risk factor for subsequent engagement in prostitution (e.g., Farley & Barkan, 1998; Widom & Kuhns, 1996) and teen pregnancy (e.g., Gershenson et al., 1989), as well as teenage parental status in both males and females (e.g., Herrenkohl, Herrenkohl, Egolf, & Russo, 1998). Other studies, though, have found that maltreatment is not a necessary and sufficient antecedent for teen promiscuity, pregnancy (e.g., Widom & Kuhns, 1996), or prostitution (e.g., Nadon, Koverola, & Schludermann, 1998). In a retrospective cohort study of boyhood exposure to maltreatment and risk of impregnating a teenage girl (n = 4,127 men), Anda et al. (2001) reported that 32% endorsed physical abuse, 15% endorsed sexual abuse, and 11% had witnessed domestic violence. Compared to no maltreatment, each of these maltreatment types significantly increased the risk of impregnation, by 70% to 140%. Although the mechanisms are yet unclear, such risk behaviors may reflect a means of regulating affect (induction of positive affect, distraction from negative affect). Because proper protection against pregnancy is not used, these behaviors may be functionally reinforcing a negative view of self and others (i.e., not worthy of protection), and poor skill development in terms of harm prevention.

For many maltreated youths, risky sexual practices overlap with other risk behaviors considered to assist with affect regulation (Stewart & Israeli, 2002), notably heavy substance use. In studies of collegiate females, experiencing date rape is associated with a history of childhood sexual abuse, a greater number of sexual partners, and heavier alcohol consumption (Abbey, 2000). It has been suggested that one long-term implication of early maltreatment is the increased likelihood of "drifting" into higher-risk situations and engaging in a greater array of risky behaviors (Wekerle & Wolfe, 1998). In a study of pregnant or parenting adolescent females, age at first pregnancy was predicted by family risk factors (drinking problem, physical abuse) and individual risk factors (early age of intoxication, early age of first wanted sexual experience). Furthermore, younger age at first unwanted sexual experience predicted earlier entry into wanted sexual experience (Kellogg, Hoffman, & Taylor, 1999). Similary, familial violence was predictive of rapid repeat pregnancy among low-income adolescent females (Jacoby, Gorenflo, Wunderlich, & Eyler, 1999).

Teens with histories of maltreatment have a much greater risk of substance misuse (Kilpatrick et al., 2000), and for females, child maltreatment and teen dating violence uniquely predict alcohol and drug use (Wekerle, Hawkins, & Wolfe, 2002). Consistently, the link between child maltreatment and youth substance use is reported in large surveys (Bensley, Spieker, Van Eenwyk, & Schoder, 1999; Chandy, Blum, & Resnick, 1996b). In a study comparing sexually abused males to females, males reported greater substance use before and during school, greater weekly alcohol and marijuana use, and more binge-drinking episodes (five or more drinks/occasion) than females (Chandy, Blum, & Resnick, 1996a). Furthermore, being physically abused, in addition to experiencing sexual abuse, increased the likelihood of binge drinking (Luster & Small, 1997) and the use of multiple substances (Harrison, Fulkerson, & Beebe, 1997). Finally, substantiated early abuse or neglect (before age 12) is related to subsequent arrest for an alcohol or drug violation as an adult, but not as a juvenile (Ireland & Widom, 1994).

Family Dynamics

The concept of family is challenging in the case of child maltreatment, as it is an often changing constellation—given such factors as mother-led households, varying parental figures and caretakers, child removal, perpetrator exit, transient involvement of extended families and friends, abrupt changes in interpersonal relationships, professional involvement, and so forth. In short, the family may not be a stable unit, and various family members may have maltreatment histories of various and overlapping types (Howes, Cicchetti, Toth, & Rogosch, 2000). A pattern of compromise and undervaluing of children within the family can be seen across maltreatment types. A common factor is the family climate of coercion and abuse of power, with concomitant low levels of prosocial behavior. Maltreated children often show role reversal with their mothers, taking on a caregiving role (e.g., Macfie et al., 1999), and are noted to have poor problem-solving strategies (e.g., Azar, Barnes, & Twentyman, 1988; Hansen, Pallotta, Tishelman, Conaway, & MacMillan, 1988). Thus a child's experience of helplessness may stem from the fact that the child is powerless in changing his or her home environment or the maltreatment itself. Similarly, the climate of domination seems to extend to the social isolation of the family; the social life of the child can be restricted as a result of the need to keep the home situation out of public view. Friedrich (1990) comments on the family context of abuse in particular (especially recurrent abuse) as one of insensitive, marginal parenting, although some parents and children may "perform" as superficially appropriate in interactions (Crittenden, 1988).

Interactional studies of maltreating families have generally supported this view, showing lower levels of verbal communication, especially positive verbalizations (Aragona & Eyberg, 1981; Burgess & Conger, 1978); deviant affective displays, such as a constricted range of affect and affective lability (Gaensbauer, Mrazek, & Harmon, 1980); and a lack of behavioral synchrony, such as maternal intrusiveness, punitiveness, or nonresponsiveness (Crittenden & Bonvillian, 1984; Crittenden, 1988; Mash, Johnson, & Kovitz, 1983). Dolz, Cerezo, and Milner (1997) observed that mothers at risk for child maltreatment (i.e., as indicated by scores on a child abuse potential inventory) made fewer neutral approaches and more indiscriminate responses to their children's prosocial behavior, even when educational differences were controlled for. This study highlights that in addition to greater aversiveness, maltreating parents miss opportunities to socialize their child through praise of appropriate behavior and fewer non-affect-laden interactional bids (for a review of interactional studies, see Cerezo, 1997).

Howes et al. (2000) observed the in-home interactional style of neglecting, physically abusive, sexually abusive, and low-income comparison families, each with a target preschool child. In the maltreating families ($n = 42$), the majority of children experienced emotional maltreatment and neglect, with over half experiencing physical abuse and 26% of children being sexually abused. The sexually abusive families had significantly greater frequency of anger than the neglecting, physically abusive, or control families. Also, these sexually abusive families were more chaotic, had lower role clarity, and showed less adaptive/flexible interpersonal strategy use than the other groups (most often different from controls). Neglecting and physically abusive families were not distinguishable on family-level variables (e.g., anger regulation, positive affect, chaos, organization, reaching common goals, adaptive relational style), based on a brief, structured interaction. The deception and betrayal particular to sexual abuse may signal a more extensive family breakdown, with role reversal being a dominating yet unstable family pattern.

DISORDERS IN ADULTHOOD

Although child maltreatment often poses major challenges to a child's cognitive, emotional, and behavioral coping strategies, many such children and adolescents still remain capable of becoming well-functioning adults (e.g., Finkelhor & Browne, 1988). However, evidence from community sample studies attest to the clinical reality that childhood maltreatment can result in significant negative sequelae that persist into adulthood (Cicchetti et al., 2000). Thus, although many maltreatment survivors can function adequately in later life, the lives of others can be replete with serious psychological distress and disturbance. This conclusion is supported by the awareness that many adult psychiatric patients have been maltreated as children (e.g., Carmen, Rieker, & Mills, 1984; Fossati, Madeddu, & Maffei, 1999; Scott, 1992).

Generally speaking, adolescents and adults with histories of physical abuse are at increased risk of developing interpersonal problems accompanied by aggression and violence (Malinosky-Rummell & Hansen, 1993). This relationship between being physically abused as a child and becoming abusive toward others as an adult supports the cycle-of-violence hypothesis, which infers that those subjected to violence become perpetrators of violence (Widom, 1989b). Those with histories of sexual abuse, in contrast, are more likely to develop chronic impairments in self-esteem, self-concept, and emotional and behavioral self-regulation, including severe outcomes such as PTSD, depression, and dissociative states (Putnam & Trickett, 1993). As adulthood approaches, the developmental impairments stemming from child maltreatment can lead to more pervasive and chronic psychiatric disorders, including panic and other anxiety disorders, depression, eating disorders, sexual problems, substance use disorders, and personality disturbances (Brown, Cohen, Johnson, & Smailes, 1999; Flisher, Kramer, Hoven, & Greenwald, 1997; Kendler et al., 2000; MacMillan et al., 2001). For instance, a prospective study of children with documented child abuse and neglect found that they had a fourfold increased risk for personality disorder, as compared to those without a maltreatment history. A wide range of personality disorders was noted (i.e., antisocial, borderline, dependent, depressive, narcissistic, paranoid, and passive–aggressive), even when parental education and psychiatric disorders were controlled for (Johnson, Cohen, Brown, Smailes, & Bernstein, 1999; Johnson, Smailes, Cohen, Brown, & Bernstein, 2000). Particular associations include the link between officially reported physical abuse cases and a pattern of antisocial behavior in adolescence and adulthood (Cohen, Brown, & Smailes, 2001). Community surveys have highlighted the salient risk to mothers; childhood abuse is associated with more mood, anxiety, and substance use disorders in both single and married mothers, increasing the odds for psychopathology two- to threefold (Lipman, MacMillan, & Boyle, 2001).

We now examine six prominent adult outcomes of maltreatment—substance misuse, mood and affect disturbances, posttraumatic-stress-related problems, sexual adjustment, criminal and antisocial behavior, and eating disorders—and note similarities and differences in these outcomes according to particular forms of maltreatment whenever appropriate.

Substance Abuse

While a causal relationship has not been demonstrated, studies have consistently found that women who misuse alcohol and other drugs are likely to have a history of sexual and/or physical abuse and/or neglect as children; the literature for men remains equivocal (for reviews, see Langeland & Hartgers, 1998; Wekerle & Wall, 2002c). About two out of three women entering substance abuse treatment have a maltreatment history (Dunn, Ryan, & Dunn, 1994; Miller, Downs, & Testa, 1993; Resnick, Kilpatrick, Dansky, Sanders, & Best, 1993). In a study of substance-using women who were admitted to a community-based family service agency (n = 171, with most being single, low-income mothers), it was found that half experienced sexual and/or physical abuse in childhood, with the majority (82%) abused by relatives. Maltreated women had higher drug use severity and psychological distress levels than nonmaltreated women (Kang, Magura, Laudet, & Whitney, 1999). In a similar study of teens and young adults presenting to an addiction treatment agency (n = 287), half of females reported a history of childhood sexual and/or physical abuse, with 64.7% using substances to cope with the maltreatment (Ballon, Coubasson, & Smith, 2001). For males, about a quarter reported a physical abuse history and about 10% reported being sexually abused, with 37.9% reporting using substances to cope with the maltreatment. Self-medication for maltreatment-related distress (e.g., Stewart & Israeli, 2002) would seem to characterize a substantial number of treatment-seeking addicted persons.

Longitudinal research considering substance use problems and childhood maltreatment have yielded inconsistent results, in part due to varying methodology. Prospective research by Widom and colleagues (e.g., Widom, Ireland, & Glynn, 1995) found that neither sexual or physical abuse history increased the risk of alcohol problems, although having a parent with an alcohol/drug problem did. For females, after controls for parental alcohol/drug problems, child sexual and physical abuse, childhood poverty, race, and age, a history of childhood neglect predicted number of lifetime alcohol-related symptoms, but not lifetime diagnosis. Another longitudinal study, but with a community sample and self-reported maltreatment, found that 43.5% of the sexually abused females met diagnostic criteria for alcohol abuse or dependence in young adulthood, as compared to 7.9% of the nonabused females. Similar associations were not found for child physical abuse (Silverman, Reinherz, & Giaconia, 1996). Kendler et al. (2000) found a nearly threefold increase for alcohol and drug dependence among women who retrospectively reported childhood sexual abuse, as compared to those who did not. Using both official and self-reports of maltreatment, Cohen et al. (2001) found elevated substance misuse in young adulthood for officially reported child physical abuse and retrospectively reported sexual abuse cases, but not for officially identified neglect cases. Another longitudinal community study of men and women found that self-reported childhood sexual abuse was associated with more alcohol use problems in adulthood (Galaif, Stein, Newcomb, & Bernstein, 2001). Finally, in a prospective study of African American women with a documented history of child sexual abuse, heavy drinking was more prevalent than it was in estimates from comparative population surveys (Jasinski, Williams, & Siegel, 2000). Although maltreatment and substance use disorders overlap, greater prospective work needs to be completed where both maltreatment and substance misuse is assessed comprehensively to capture acute and chronic forms, as well as taking into account the range of potential confounds (e.g., parental psychopathology beyond substance abuse) (Wekerle & Wall, 2002a).

Mood and Affect Disturbances

Emotional trauma resulting from the chronic rejection, loss of affection, betrayal, and feelings of helplessness that may accompany chronic maltreatment by trusted adults may be responsible for the emotional and behavioral disturbances shown among child, adolescent, and adult survivors. If symptoms of depression and mood disturbance go unrecognized among those who were sexually or physically abused and/or neglected in childhood, they are likely to increase during late adolescence and adulthood (Brown et al., 1999; Cohen et al., 2001; Kolko, 1992). In an important cotwin cohort study, a history of child sexual abuse increased the likelihood of obtaining a lifetime diagnosis of major depression, suicidal ideation, and past suicide attempt (as well as increasing the rates of conduct disorder, panic disorder, and alcoholism) for both genders (Dinwiddie et al., 2000). For women, the presence of childhood sexual abuse more than doubled the risk for major depression; for men, it nearly quadrupled the risk for depression. Concordance for childhood sexual abuse was not greater for identical than for fraternal twins, indicating that genetic effects did not play a significant role for either men or women. Rates of major depression and suicidal ideation (as well as conduct disorder) among adult survivors were higher when both cotwins were abused than if the study respondent alone reported childhood sexual abuse. This latter finding suggests that the link between child sexual abuse and adult depression is in part due to the influence of shared familial factors.

In another population-based twin study that controlled for parental psychopathology and family background factors, Kendler et al. (2000) found an approximately twofold increase in major depressive disorder (as well as generalized anxiety and panic disorders) among women who reported a childhood history of sexual abuse, compared to women who did not. In these cotwin studies there were few significant findings among twin pairs who were discordant for sexual abuse history, raising the possibility that shared familial factors influenced the risk of psychopathology; however, sexual abuse was assessed in a limited fashion (e.g., retrospectively, in a single question) and did not consider other types of maltreatment experiences.

Community surveys using retrospective recall have found an elevated lifetime risk for major depression in women, but not men, where there is a history of physical and/or sexual abuse; a trend for physically abused males has been found (MacMillan et al., 2001). MacMillan et al. note that females reporting physical abuse are more likely to have coexisting sexual abuse than males, raising the issue of whether females are exposed to more types of maltreatment. The sex difference in depressive symptoms has been advanced as a feature of greater child sexual abuse representation among women (Whiffen & Clark, 1997). In a study of community couples, Whiffen, Judd, and Aube (1999) found that intimate relationships moderated the relationship between child sexual abuse and depressive symptomatology; an intimate relationship that was perceived as high in quality appeared to act as a buffer.

Depressive symptoms are a serious concern, as they can lead to life-threatening suicide attempts and self-mutilating behavior (Kaplan, Pelcovitz, Salzinger, Mandel, & Weiner, 1997). Dinwiddie et al. (2000) found that a history of childhood sexual abuse increased the odds ratio for a serious suicide attempt greater than sevenfold for both genders. In a study of women presenting for nonemergency, routine gynecological medical care, prior suicide attempts were significantly higher in women who endorsed a childhood history of either sexual abuse, physical abuse, emotional abuse, or witnessing domestic violence than they were in women who did not endorse any type of maltreatment (Wiederman, Sansone, & Sansone, 1998). No significant relationship was found with experiencing physical neglect, although the endorsement rate was lowest for this type of maltreatment. In a logistic regression predicting suicide attempts, only sexual abuse and physical abuse remained significant predictors. In a study of college women measuring self-reported depression, suicide attempt, PTSD symptoms, and childhood maltreatment, women who witnessed domestic violence had significantly higher depression and trauma scores than did their nonmaltreated counterparts (Maker, Kemmelmeier, & Peterson, 1998). No significant differences were found for suicide attempts. Furthermore, it was noted that witnessing overlapped with physical abuse, sexual abuse, and paternal alcohol and other drug use. Thus it would seem that sexual and physical abuse, in particular, are related to suicide attempts.

Posttraumatic-Stress-Related Problems

A significant number of men and women who have been subjected to severe physical or sexual abuse during childhood suffer long-term stress-related disorders. About a third of individuals who were sexually abused, physically abused, or neglected as children meet criteria for lifetime PTSD (Widom, 1999). PTSD-related symptoms are also more likely in cases of abuse if the abuse was chronic and the perpetrator relied on some method of coercion or trickery to force compliance (Rodriguez, Ryan, Kemp, & Foy, 1998; Wolfe et al., 1994). In a study of college women, after controls for demographic variables (age, ethnicity, parental occupation, family mental health risks, presence of adult maltreatment), childhood abuse added 9% variance to the prediction of self-reported PTSD symptoms, and witnessing domestic violence added a further 2% of unique contribution (Feerick & Haugaard, 1999). Thus, although maltreatment in childhood is a distal variable, it remains a significant direct predictor of PTSD symptoms in adulthood. Another consideration would be how PTSD interacts with other problems. For example, Brady, Killeen, Saladin, Dansky, and Becker (1994) compared women with PTSD and substance use disorders to those with only substance use disorders, and found that those in the combined-disorder group were more likely to have experienced childhood sexual and physical abuse and to have greater addiction severity. It has been suggested that substance misuse exacerbates PTSD symptomatology (e.g., Stewart & Israeli, 2002).

Sexual Adjustment

A history of any type of maltreatment among males is a significant risk factor for inappropriate sexual behaviors, alienation, and social incompetence in adolescence (Haviland, Sonne, & Woods, 1995; Wolfe, Scott, Wekerle, & Pittman, 2001). Women with childhood histories of sexual abuse, in particular, are more likely to report difficulties in adulthood related to sexual adjustment—ranging from low sexual arousal to intrusive flashbacks, disturbing sensations, and feelings of guilt, anxiety, and low self-esteem concerning their sexuality (Davis & Petretic-Jackson, 2000; Meston & Heiman, 2000). In a survey study of undergraduates, frequency of childhood sexual abuse was related to a higher frequency of intercourse, a greater variety of sexual experiences, and greater frequency of masturbation, but lower subjective sexual drive (Meston, Heiman, & Trapnell, 1999). These findings are consistent with sexual traumatization (Finkelhor & Browne, 1988) and with a sexualization of relationships; that is, a sexually abused child was rewarded for sexual behavior, and this may promote the use of sexual behavior as an interpersonal strategy in adulthood.

Because their normal development of self-awareness and self-protection was compromised, adult survivors of child sexual abuse may become less capable of identifying risk situations or persons, or knowing how to respond to unwanted sexual or physical attention. Consequently, they are more likely to be subjected to further violence in adulthood, such as rape or domestic violence (Kendall-Tackett et al., 1993; Kendall-Tackett & Eckenrode, 1996, 1997; Humphrey & White, 2000; Tyler, Hoyt, & Whitbeck, 2000). Also, compromised self-protection ability may relate to the risk for unintended pregnancy. A community survey study found that the strongest association between childhood maltreatment and first unintended pregnancy was for psychological abuse, followed first by witnessing physical abuse of the mother, and then by physical abuse. Women who experienced four or more types of maltreatment were 1.5 times more likely to have an unintended first pregnancy during adulthood than nonmaltreated women, even after marital status and age at first pregnancy were controlled for (Dietz et al., 1999).

Criminal and Antisocial Behavior

Although many persons convicted of heinous crimes and child abuse report significant histories of child abuse and neglect, most maltreated children do not go on to commit crimes. As longitudinal studies demonstrate, there is a significant connection between early maltreatment (before age 12) and subsequent arrest as a juvenile or an adult (Widom, 1989a) or engaging in sexual and physical violence as a young adult, especially for males (Feldman, 1997). A history of maltreatment is associated with an earlier mean age at first offense; a higher frequency of offenses; a higher proportion of chronic offenders (Widom, 1989b, 2000); and a greater frequency of self-reported violence and delinquency (Kelley, Thornberry, & Smith, 1997; Smith & Thornberry, 1995). Beyond the contribution of socioeconomic factors, a history of maltreatment increases the likelihood of gang membership (Thompson & Braaten-Antrim, 1998). Heck and Walsh (2000), in a study of European American males processed by Idaho juvenile probation authorities (n = 388), found that child maltreatment history had a greater impact on violent delinquency (i.e., rape, assault) than did type of family structure, SES, Verbal IQ, family size, or birth order. Maltreatment was also predictive of property crime (e.g., burglary, theft) and misbehavior (e.g., truancy, running away), and emerged as the most powerful predictor of overall delinquency. In a longitudinal, inner-city community study, maltreatment was related to property and violence offenses, and the risk of court contact was about double for maltreated individuals as compared to nonmaltreated controls (Stouthamer-Loeber, Loeber, Homish & Wei, 2001). In this study, the maltreatment predominantly involved substantiated neglect, emotional maltreatment, or physical abuse, with most perpetrators family members. Given that antisocial and aggressive behavior precedes delinquency, Stouthamer-Loeber et al. examined the sequencing of officially detected maltreatment and delinquency, and found that CPS involvement tended to precede or co-occur with overt (e.g., physical fighting, rape) and covert (e.g., lying, property damage, theft) antisocial behavior problems. For instance, in the case of physical fighting, there was over a fourfold increase in likelihood when maltreatment was present than when it was not. Overall, these findings suggest a different process underlying the transition to delinquency for maltreated versus nonmaltreated children.

One consideration for a mediator of such delinquency outcomes (in addition to PTSD symptomatology noted earlier) may be relationship functioning—in particular, the success or failure of close romantic relationships during adolescence. Indeed, girls and boys who grew up in violent homes report more violence (especially verbal abuse and threats) toward their dating partners, as well as toward themselves (Wolfe, Wekerle, Reitzel-Jaffe, & Lefebvre, 1998; Wolfe et al., 2001). Dating violence during adolescence, and a past history of family violence, are strong prerelationship predictors of intimate violence in early adulthood and marriage (O'Leary, Malone, & Tyree, 1994). A history of childhood sexual or physical abuse is associated with more than 3.5 times greater risk of involvement in adult domestic violence (Coid et al., 2001). Thus adolescence may be an important prevention window for disrupting a trajectory toward continued relationship violence, as it may represent the initiation period in the formation of a violent dynamic in intimate partnerships.

In addition, a disturbingly high number of abused children—approximately 30%—carry the pattern of abusiveness from childhood into adulthood (Kaufman & Zigler, 1989). However, methodological problems exist in the case of physical abuse, with at least one study showing that low-SES women are a nearly 13 times more likely to abuse their children (for a review, see Ertem, Leventhal, & Dobbs, 2000). With families reported to CPS, history of substance misuse is a salient comorbid factor, identified as a leading problem in 85% of state CPS agencies (Wang & Harding, 1999). Drug and alcohol misuse by one or both caretakers was the strongest direct predictor of re-reports to CPS among cases closed after investigation (Wolock & Magura, 1996). What role, if any, substance misuse plays in the intergenerational transmission remains unclear. Growing up with power-based, authoritarian methods—even if they do not result in physical injuries or identified maltreatment—can be toxic to relationship and social patterns. Remarkably, the amount of routine violence (frequently being hit with objects or physically punished) one experiences as a child is significantly associated with violent delinquent behavior later on (Straus & Donnelly, 1994). This connection is especially noteworthy, given the previous description of how routine violence toward children is commonplace throughout North America.

Eating Disorders

Early clinical suspicions that child sexual abuse could be an underlying cause of eating disorders among some individuals have been supported by ongoing investigations of this important issue. Conceptually, bingeing or purging (a symptom of an eating disorder) and self-mutilation (a feature of borderline personality disorder) have been considered to be maladaptive tension-reducing activities (Briere & Runtz, 1991), reflecting maladaptive self-conceptualizations (Steiger, Leung, & Houle, 1992). Based on a general population sample, women with bulimia nervosa were about three times more likely to have been sexually abused as children than were women without the disorder (35% and 12.5%, respectively) (Garfinkel et al., 1995). Similar findings have been reported among population samples of school-age youths; that is, youths at risk for disordered eating reported more negative perceptions of their families and parents, and more sexual or physical abuse experiences (Neumark et al., 2000). In addition, sexually abused children report many of the early risk signs of eating disorders, such as higher levels of weight dissatisfaction and of purging and dieting behavior (Wonderlich et al., 2000). In a study of college women, Tripp and Petrie (2001) found support for their conceptual model of sexual abuse and eating disorders. Sexual abuse predicted higher levels of bodily shame, which in turn predicted increases in body disparagement (low body satisfaction, greater body degradation and loathing), which were predictive of eating disorder symptoms.

The above described connections between child maltreatment and mental disorders should be tempered by the awareness that maltreatment is a general risk factor for psychopathology, rather than a *specific* risk factor for eating disorders, antisocial behavior, or other disturbances. Such events are not uncommon in the background of individuals with eating disorders, as well as those with other psychiatric disorders. Presumably, childhood maltreatment is associated with many undesirable adolescent and adult outcomes, of which these the six types of disorders we have described here are prominent.

THEORETICAL FRAMEWORKS LINKING CHILD PSYCHOPATHOLOGY AND MALTREATMENT

The impact of maltreatment on a child's development was first assumed to be invariably negative and disruptive, until researchers began to recognize that maltreatment does not affect each child in a predictable or consistent fashion. Diverse outcomes are especially understandable when positive mediators of adjustment (such as supportive relatives or the child's coping abilities) and moderators (such as the developmental timing of the maltreatment) are taken into consideration (Cicchetti & Rizley, 1981; Sroufe & Rutter, 1984). Systemic influences—including parental marital/couple violence, separation of family members, and an aversive "everyday" environment (e.g., impoverished parent–child interactions, high levels of household "traffic,"multiple residential moves, low educational stimulation, etc.)—also vary in their consistency over time, and may synergistically and uniquely contribute to a maltreated child's maladaptation. Furthermore, the maltreatment and environmental problems are embedded in a relational context. The *unique* impact that maltreatment has on child development may be difficult to separate from other family and environmental forces (Wolfe, 1999). The following theories explaining the effects of maltreatment on children's development take into account developmental processes and how they might interact with maltreatment. Two major theoretical perspectives are presented: (1) the childhood trauma model, which focuses on learning theory; and (2) developmental psychopathology, which includes developmental traumatology.

Childhood Trauma Model

Theoretical concepts emerging from the study of the psychological processes underlying an individual's reaction to traumatic events provide further clarification of the nature of PTSD-related disorders or symptomatology. The contributions of Horowitz (1986), of Foa and colleagues (e.g., Foa & Kozak, 1986; Foa, Steketee, & Rothbaum, 1989), and of Briere (e.g., Briere, 1992, 1996, 2002) focus on conditioning principles and escape/avoidance mechanisms. The relational context as the prime learning environment is emphasized in betrayal trauma theory (Freyd, 1994, 1996). A common postulate of these models centers on the individual's efforts to integrate a traumatic event into an existing cognitive schema. During this process, PTSD symptoms arise; either intrusions (Horowitz, 1986) or phobic avoidance (Foa & Kozak, 1986) is viewed as a primary symptom. The functional value of such symptoms is to allow for slower assimilation of trauma information, given the overwhelming cognitive–affective nature of the trauma. These viewpoints have not gone without criticism, since differences in the features of the abuse, such as the presence of danger, violence, or coercion versus seduction, have not been adequately considered (Finkelhor, 1988).

Learning-based mechanisms may account for the manner in which a traumatic experience can result in an individual's long-term response that continues well beyond the original stressor (Baum, O'Keefe, & Davidson, 1990). The process of conditioning—that is, the manner by which traumatic episodes become associated with particular eliciting stimuli (e.g., odors, places, persons)—can lead to maladaptive or atypical reactions (e.g., flight-or-fight "overreactions"). Repetitive acute episodes occur on an irregular basis and, as such, are more resistant to extinction due to their unpredictability and intensity (Wolfe & Jaffe, 1991). In addition to conditioning, major and minor stressful life events (referred to as "secondary stressors") often occur as a result of the original traumatic event. For example, disclosure of sexual abuse gives rise to both immediate events (e.g., change in living arrangements, arrest of the perpetrator) and long-term events (e.g., loss of contact with the perpetrator) that also play a role in reducing an individual's coping resources. According to Baum et al. (1990), "new" stressful events may be sparked by intrusive imagery of the original trauma. The individual's recollections of the trauma in dreams or thoughts serve to renew the potency of the original stimuli and create generalization to other, previously unrelated events (e.g., dating in adolescence). These secondary stressors may support a chronic, stress-filled lifestyle that makes habituation to the original stressor(s) more difficult.

Briere's self-trauma model (e.g., Briere, 1992, 1996, 2002) accords self-dysfunction and the increased potential for retraumatization key roles. Because maltreatment impairs self-capacities, it leads to reliance on avoidance strategies, which in turn preclude the further development of self-capacities. This negative cycle is exacerbated by the self-healing need to process conditioned emotional responses via reexperiencing and reenactments. This process further overwhelms self-capacities and produces distress. At its core, maltreatment reduces the likelihood of encountering benign interactive experiences that would promote positive self-development. Instead, the maltreated child psychologically attenuates or avoids certain attachment interactions, developing broad negative self-schemas. This impairs functioning in terms of negative preverbal assumptions and relational schemas; conditioned emotional responses to maltreatment-related stimuli; implicit/sensory memories of maltreatment (e.g., sensory reexperiencing); narrative or autobiographical memories of maltreatment; suppressed or "deep" cognitive structures involving maltreatment-related material; and inadequately developed affect regulation skills. For example, conditioned emotional responses may elicit "out-of-the-blue" negative affect, in which the specific trigger may remain unclear to the maltreated individual, given the nonverbal nature of the conditioning. It is also postulated that verbally mediated memory material may be most aversive, since it activates associated nonverbal feelings, implicit/sensory memories, and maltreatment-related schemas. Through processes such as distraction and dissociative compartmentalization, thought suppression regarding the maltreatment may be achieved. The low capacity to control and tolerate strong negative affect may contribute to the use of affect avoidance strategies, such as dissociation, substance misuse, or external tension-reducing behavior (e.g., inappropriate or excessive sexual activity, eating, aggression, self-injury).

Freyd's (1994, 1996) betrayal trauma theory bridges the trauma and cognitive science literatures in addressing the motivations for, and mechanisms resulting in, impairment in memory for the maltreatment. Freyd asserts that knowledge is multistranded, with different kinds of knowing that can occur simultaneously. She points out that pain is a motivator for behavior change and that human beings have a system of natural analgesia. Dissociation during trauma and traumatic amnesia are considered psychological defenses against psychological pain. Behind the motivation to dampen felt pain is a goal more closely related to survival than to pain relief per se. A central factor is that the traumatization occurs while the child is in a situation of dependence. Because of the survival importance of attachment to caretakers to the developing child, attachment goals are important to maintain even when social betrayals are detected. Freyd (1997, p. 27) notes that "child abuse is especially likely to produce a social conflict or betrayal for the victim. If a child processes the betrayal in the normal way, he or she will be motivated to stop interacting with the betrayer. However, if the betrayer is a primary caregiver, it is essential that the child not stop inspiring attachment." The mediator in the maltreatment–dissociation link is the threat to the attachment system. Thus the knowledge gets isolated (memory repression, dissociation, unawareness), and the information gets blocked from ready retrieval (e.g., it may be partially blocked as seen in blunted affective responses). This process leads to a disruption in awareness and autobiographical memory. This continued information blockage contributes to later interpersonal distrust and difficulties in accurately assessing aspects of interpersonal and intrapersonal reality.

There is preliminary support for the belief that the closeness of the child and perpetrator is related to the probability of some degree of amnesia for childhood sexual abuse, with amnesia rates for parental abuse higher than those for nonparental abuse (see Freyd, 1996). Freyd and DePrince (2001) summarize their laboratory studies using a Stroop color-naming paradigm with college students; they have found that "high dissociators" (i.e., students with high levels of dissociation) have impaired attentional capacities in tasks of selective attention, but not divided attention. High dissociators also have impaired memory for affectively laden words (e.g., "incest"), but not neutral words, as compared to low dissociators (i.e., the time to name the color of the word is a function of the threat level of the word). High dissociators endorse three times as much trauma in their history as low dissociators do. These findings suggest that divided attention is a mechanism by which the flow of information is controlled.

The implication of betrayal theory is that there are two conceptually independent dimensions of trauma. The dimension of life threat may involve the symptoms of fear, anxiety, hyperarousal, and intrusive memories. The dimension of social betrayal may relate to the symptoms of dissociation, amnesia, numbing, and abusive relationships. Survivors of childhood maltreatment have learned to cope with an inescapable social conflict by being disconnected internally. Freyd and DePrince (2001) note that treatment goals for the social betrayal dimension include a focus on social relationships and related cognitive mechanisms promoting internal integration and more intimate external connections.

Developmental Psychopathology

General Description and Some Examples of Applications

Maltreatment as a special instance of major parent–child conflict was seldom studied until the field of developmental psychopathology turned its attention toward these phenomena (e.g., Aber & Cicchetti, 1984; Cicchetti, 1989; Cicchetti & Toth, 1995). Developmental psychopathology is an organizational framework for understanding that a child's poor resolution of one stage of development will lead to a greater *probability* of incompetence in subsequent tasks or milestones (Cicchetti et al., 1988; Cicchetti & Rogosch, 1996; Sroufe & Fleeson, 1986). Therefore, to understand the effects of maltreatment on children's progressive vulnerability and nonoptimal development over time, it is necessary to place their experiences in a broader context that includes their perceptions of their families' emotional climate; their previous experiences with conflict and abuse; their interpretations of violence and maltreatment; their available coping abilities and resources to countermand stress and inadequate caregiving; and the stability of toxic or growth-supportive environmental factors (Cicchetti & Tucker, 1994; Crittenden & Claussen, 2002; Wolfe & Jaffe, 1991). Developmental psychopathology also considers transactions among the biological, cognitive, affective, representational, and interpersonal domains of the individual. It recognizes that biological processes influence psychological functioning, and that psychological experience influences biological structure and function. Developmental traumatology (discussed below) is an excellent exemplar of developmental psychopathology moving in the direction of integrating neurobiological and psychosocial mechanisms.

Developmental psychopathology centers on the dynamic interplay of risk and protective factors in contributing to the organization of an individual and formation of the individual's particular developmental trajectory. Rather than a single prototype, different pathways are likely to exist in cases where there is marked vulnerability to psychopathology. In other words, diverse outcomes are likely to emerge from child maltreatment. Thornberry et al. (2001) provide support for a developmental psychopathology approach. In their longitudinal study, these investigators were able to classify the period of maltreatment and compare these as they relate to diverse outcomes. Children who experienced early-only maltreatment (birth to age 5) appeared to be a fairly resilient group with regard to adolescent outcomes. In contrast, those experiencing chronic maltreatment and adolescent-only maltreatment evidenced the widest range of maladaptation in late adolescence, including increased general delinquency, drug use, internalizing problems, and teen pregnancy. These authors suggest that substantiated maltreatment ending in the preschool years may be responsive to intervention, and that if the negative effects of maltreatment are not reinforced, then its effects may dissipate. Empirical support is consistent with this notion. A follow-up study of families that received a home-visiting intervention found no relation between number of maltreatment reports and early-onset problem behaviors (e.g., binge drinking, arrests, sexual intercourse, smoking marijuana, etc.) for maltreated youths receiving the intervention, whereas a significant relationship did exist in the no-intervention maltreated group (Eckenrode et al., 2001).

Cole and Putnam (1992) provide a specific example of the application of developmental psychopathology to the study of sexual abuse. They argue that incest has a unique negative impact on domains of the self and related social functioning; it is thus linked to adult disorders that have self-impairments and social impairments as core features (e.g., borderline personality disorder, multiple personality disorder [now known as dissociative identity disorder], and somatization, eating, and substance use disorders). These researchers also consider the developmental stage at which abuse begins as influential in symptom structure. For example, school-age children may be particularly vulnerable to guilt and shame, given their increased introspective abilities. Thus the timing of the maltreatment within a child's developmental context is an important consideration (Cicchetti & Manly, 2001).

Developmental Traumatology

Recently, the biological bases underlying the impairment associated with child maltreatment have been explored. In part, this reflects the accumulation of neurobiological studies showing that stress stimulates the formation of gene products, which then influence cellular processes responsible for gene expression, protein formation, and associated biological and behavioral change (for a review, see Yehuda, Spertus, & Golier, 2001). In addition, it is being driven by research demonstrating that early environmental events can lead to lasting effects on brain structure and function, and hence on biopsychosocial functioning throughout the life span (Bremner & Vermetten, 2001). Developmental traumatology is the study of the interactions among the complex factors of genetic constitution, psychosocial environment, and critical periods of vulnerability and resiliency in individuals experiencing child maltreatment, with the aim of disentangling the effect of trauma on neurobiological development (DeBellis & Putnam, 1994; DeBellis, 2001). Stress, known to influence gene expression, is responsible for initiating a predictable physiological response. In contrast to an acute event, chronic stress linked with the threat of or actual revictimization, is thought to impair the functioning of the body's stress-responsive systems. These systems include the immune system, the neurotransmitter systems (e.g., noradrenergic, serotonergic, and dopaminergic systems), the LHPA axis, and the sympathetic nervous system (e.g., activation of the fight-or-flight response). Also involved are such brain structures as the hippocampus (e.g., learning, memory, capacity for neuronal regeneration), amygdala (e.g., responding to fear-inducing stimuli in times of acute threat), and prefrontal cortex (e.g., planning, execution, inhibition of responses, extinction of fear response) (Bremner & Vermetten, 2001).

Child maltreatment encompasses a stressful acute event, as well as exposure to other stressful ongoing life circumstances (often including socioeconomically substandard and dangerous living situations, domestic violence, and parental psychiatric problems). High-level and long-term stress is detrimental to the optimal functioning of the body's stress response system and threatens sustained system dysfunction. Child maltreatment, whether acute or chronic, may generate changes in neurobiological systems that can result in augmented responses to subsequently experienced stressors. This can place survivors in vulnerable positions for the resurgence of PTSD and related problems.

Developmental traumatology advances the view that stress-induced changes in neurobiology underlie the development of psychopathology in maltreated children, and that the negative psychobiological sequelae of maltreatment may be more properly regarded as "an environmentally induced complex developmental disorder" (DeBellis, 2001, p. 540). There is evidence for its course over the life span. In a path-analytic design, a history of child sexual abuse was shown to be directly related to subsequent maltreatment in adulthood, as well as contributing substantially to adult PTSD symptoms (Nishith, Mechanic, & Resnick, 2000). In a prospective study of substantiated maltreatment in childhood, the prevalence of PTSD in the maltreated group (37.5% sexually abused, 32.7% physically abused, 30.6% neglected) exceeded that of the nonmaltreated, matched comparison group (20.4%) (Widom, 1999). Thus the best predictor of future maltreatment may be childhood maltreatment; that is, vulnerability to maltreatment may play a reciprocal role with PTSD symptom experience.

The extreme stress associated with maltreatment may cause changes in brain development and structure, which may explain some of the symptoms of psychological trauma (Glaser, 2000). Figure 14.1 depicts the developmental traumatology model (DeBellis, 2001) and the specific pathways hypothesized to be affected by experiencing traumatizing levels of child maltreatment. As can be seen from the model, maltreatment-related PTSD is hypothesized to lead to alterations of the catecholamines (norepinephrine, epinephrine, dopamine) and the LHPA axis. Much of the current research has focused on atypical cortisol levels in maltreated children, as compared to their nonmaltreated counterparts. As a result of hormones flooding the brain before and after a stressful period, the hippocampus—the part of the brain that deals with short-term memory and, possibly, the coding and retrieval of long-term memory—may be functionally impaired. The hippocampus is particularly sensitive to high levels of cortisols, which circulate for hours or days after stress. Low cortisol is linked with emotional numbing, and spasms of high cortisol coincide with disturbing memories (Heim et al., 2000). After prolonged stress, cortisol levels become depleted, and the feedback systems that control hormone levels in the brain may become dysfunctional. Stress floods the brain with cortisol; the brain in turn resets the threshold at which cortisol is produced, so that ultimately it circulates at a dramatically low level. The neuroendocrine system becomes highly sensitive to stress (DeBellis, Keshavan, Spencer, & Hall, 2000).

Research relevant to the subsequent pathways depicting ensuing changes in brain metabolism and adverse effects on brain development, with postulated compromised outcomes (see Figure 14.1), are accumulating—especially in the areas of cognitive functioning. For example, electroencephalographic examination of severely maltreated children found altered brain development, suggesting decreased cortical differentiation (Ito, Teicher, Glod, & Ackerman, 1998). Bremner et al. (1997) compared 17 patients with PTSD related to childhood maltreatment and 17 case-matched controls, and found that the maltreated group had a statistically significant 12% reduction in left hippocampal volume. In similar work with children with PTSD, no reduction in hippocampal volume was found, but a smaller intracranial and cerebral volume was noted (DeBellis, Keshavan, et al., 1999). A smaller intracranial volume may be tied to neuronal loss and consequent lower IQ. It is suggested that chronic PTSD may be a factor in determining hippocampal volume reduction, and that early stressors (e.g., maltreatment) may contribute to changes in the morphology of the hippocampus (Bremner & Vermetten, 2001). Bremner et al. (1995) found deficits in hippocampal-based declarative memory functioning (e.g., as assessed by the Wechsler Memory Scale) in adults with a history of childhood physical and sexual abuse as compared to nonmaltreated controls. Furthermore, a 1-year course of treatment with a selective serotonin reuptake inhibitor (paroxetine) resulted in an improvement in hippocampal-based verbal declarative memory in adults (Bremner & Vermetten, 2001). A methodological problem remains from the cross-sectional nature of most studies, in that premaltreatment assessment is required to assess change due to maltreatment (MacMillan & Munn, 2001). Thus this model requires further research that includes an assessment of maltreated children with and without PTSD, using a prospective, longitudinal design.

Developmental traumatology considers the key mediator linking childhood maltreatment and subsequent psychopathology in childhood, adolescence, and adulthood to be PTSD (see also Fletcher, Chapter 7, this volume). PTSD is regarded as a gateway illness and contributor to a wide range of problems of behavioral and affective dysregulation—often seen in other conditions, such as attention-deficit/hyperactivity disorder (ADHD), oppositional defiant disorder (ODD), conduct disorders, depression, and substance use disorders (DeBellis, 2001). A recent study of consecutive admissions to a child psychiatry outpatient unit found that a history of physical or sexual abuse was related to ODD and ADHD. The group with combined ODD and ADHD (n = 40) had the highest prevalence rate of maltreatment: 73% were physically maltreated, and up to 31% were sexually maltreated. When symptoms that overlap among the disorders were taken into account, ODD (but not ADHD) continued to be related to PTSD (Ford et al., 2000). These authors advance that maltreatment and subsequent PTSD may exacerbate ODD. Greater work is needed to assess whether PTSD is indeed a mediating or moderating factor in the link between child maltreatment and diagnosed psychiatric disorders.

Developmental traumatology is also concerned with trauma symptoms that are subclinical or below diagnostic threshold—not just PTSD per se—as a possible mediating factor (DeBellis, 2001). In contrast to most psychiatric diagnoses, PTSD requires an etiological agent, the traumatic event. However, many individuals exposed to trauma do not subsequently meet the criteria for a psychiatric disorder. Also, traumatic events (interpersonal and otherwise) are more prevalent than PTSD. Thus the presence of a trauma may be a necessary, but not sufficient, condition to account for PTSD (Breslau, Davis, Andreski, & Peterson, 1991;

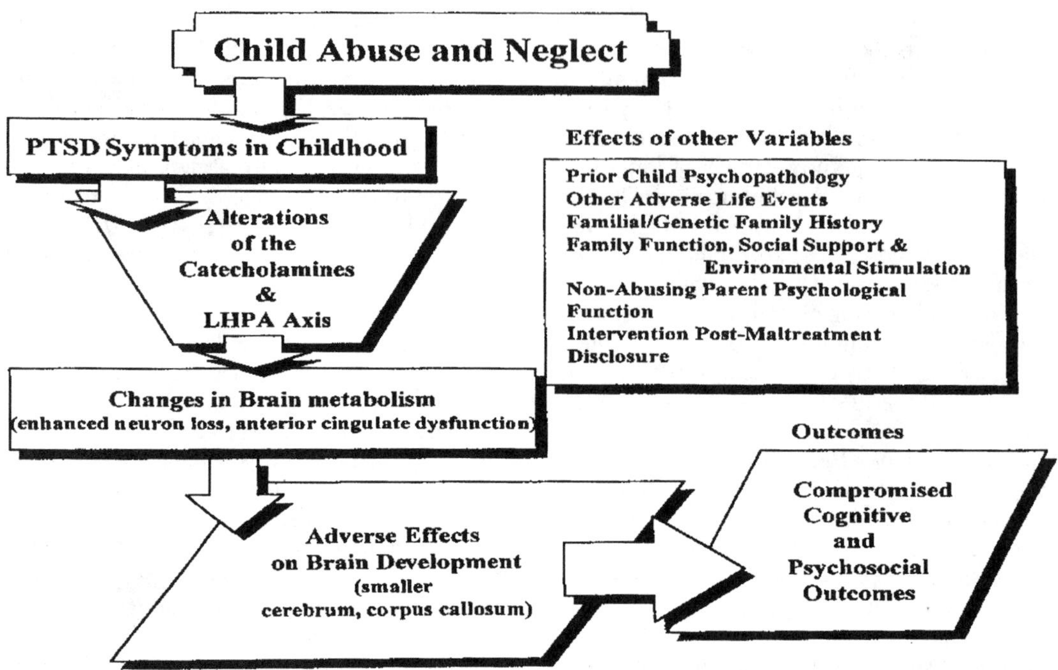

FIGURE 14.1. A developmental traumatology model of biological stress systems and brain maturation in maltreated children. In this model compromised neurocognitive and psychosocial outcomes are understood as results of adverse brain development. From DeBellis (2001, p. 552). Copyright 2001 by Cambridge University Press. Reprinted by permission.

Kessler, Sonnega, Bromet, Hughes, & Nelson, 1995). The DSM-IV defines exposure to an extreme traumatic stressor as involving personal experience of an event, witnessing an event, or learning about an event affecting a family member or close associate. Applied to child maltreatment, PTSD could therefore arise from direct maltreatment, witnessing maltreatment, and/or learning about familial maltreatment. The stress response can further be described as acute (i.e., symptoms lasting less than 3 months), chronic (i.e., symptoms lasting 3 months or longer), or delayed-onset (i.e., symptoms beginning 6 months or more after the traumatic event).

A traumatic event can be reexperienced in a variety of ways, commonly with recurrent and intrusive recollections of the event, distressing dreams of the event, or a sense of reliving the event (e.g., a dissociative flashback episode). Reexperiencing symptoms may involve bodily sensations as well as mental imagery. Intrusions occur spontaneously and involuntarily, and can be stimulated by seemingly minor connections. The DSM-IV identifies that intense psychological distress and physiological reactivity to internal or external trauma cues may occur as reexperiencing symptoms. Children may display more generalized reexperiencing, as in a frightening dream, without recognizable content. The compulsion to repeat the trauma can be regarded as a means of accomodating to, and ultimately integrating, the anxiety-provoking traumatic event, whereby a feeling and sense of efficacy and power can be restored (Herman, 1992). However, there is an emotional cost to reliving the trauma, given the intensity of distressing affect and consequent threat to and burden on coping. These intrusive DSM-IV Criterion B symptoms are thought to reflect a disorder of serotonin regulation, as the serotonin system is implicated in the regulation of mood and aggression (DeBellis, 2001).

The second symptom class pertains to persistent avoidance of stimuli linked to the trauma and the numbing of general responsiveness. These include efforts to avoid internal (thoughts, feelings) or external (persons, places) cues associated with the trauma; impaired recall of an important aspect of the trauma; diminished interest in significant activities; feelings of estrangement from others; constricted affect; and a sense of a foreshortened future. Events may continue to register in awareness, but with alterations in the perceptual processes, including affective detachment ("emotional anesthesia") (Herman, 1992). With such numbing, time sense may be changed as in slow motion, and there may be a sense of the unreal—either as if events were part of a bad dream (derealization), or as if events were occurring outside of oneself or one's body, as unreal or unfamiliar (depersonalization). The DSM-IV notes that the ability to feel emotions associated with intimacy, tenderness, and sexuality may be especially reduced. The mechanism postulated as underlying these Criterion C avoidant and dissociative symptoms is dysregulation of the endogenous opiate system and its links with dopamine systems (DeBellis, 2001). In a neuroimaging study of maltreated children, there were significant findings linking the corpus callosum (the major structural connector between the right and left hemispheres of the brain) and dissociative symptoms, suggesting possibly lessened communication ability in the corpus callosum (DeBellis, Keshavan, et al., 1999).

The third category of symptoms involves the occurrence of increased arousal and anxiety that were not present before the trauma. These may include hypervigilance, an exaggerated startle response, irritability or angry outbursts, difficulty concentrating or completing tasks, and sleep problems (which may be due to recurrent nightmares). It has been found that maltreated children (physically and/or sexually abused) are twice as active at night as normal and depressed children, having more difficulty falling and staying asleep (Glod, Teicher, Hartman, & Harakal, 1997). These Criterion D symptoms are considered to be mediated by dysregulation of the three catecholamine systems and the LHPA axis (DeBellis, 2001). A working hypothesis in these ongoing investigations relates to the priming of the LHPA axis. Consequent to the trauma, this system will hyperrespond during a subsequent acute stress (e.g., a recurrence of maltreatment). However, this primed system would also show chronic compensatory adaptation, which may be implicated in greater depressive as well as dissociative symptoms over the longer term. Clinically referred maltreated youths with chronic PTSD who were less than 1 year postdisclosure evidenced significant differences in catecholamine levels than nonmaltreated controls with overanxious disorder and normal controls. These catecholamine concentrations were positively correlated with trauma duration and PTSD symptom severity (DeBellis, Baum, et al., 1999).

In addition to the formal criteria, the DSM-IV lists associated features of PTSD, especially those following from an interpersonal stressor such as childhood sexual or physical abuse. These include physical symptoms (headaches), impaired affect modulation; self-destructive and impulsive behavior; dissociative symptoms; psychosomatic complaints; feelings of ineffectiveness, shame, despair, or hopelessness; feeling permanently damaged; a loss of previously sustained beliefs; hostility; social withdrawal; feeling constantly threatened; impaired relationships with others; or a change in personality characteristics. Such associated symptoms may be present in adulthood. For example, Arnow, Hart, Hayward, Dea, and Taylor (2000) reported that women who reported exposure to both sexual and physical abuse were more likely to present with chronic and acute pain complaints (most frequently headaches) than those who reported only sexual abuse. These persistent associated symptoms have been linked with structural changes in the brain, such as a stress-induced promotion of neuronal loss. DeBellis, Keshavan, et al. (1999) found that maltreatment duration (most subjects with longer-duration maltreatment also experienced multiple forms, particularly sexual abuse and witnessing domestic violence) correlated positively with lateral ventricular enlargement, which would be consistent with neuronal loss. Furthermore, as noted above, greater intracranial and cerebral volume reductions in maltreated children with PTSD than in nonmaltreated controls have been found; the fact that these brain measures correlated positively with age of onset, and negatively with maltreatment duration and PTSD symptoms, suggests that neurodevelopmental compromises may occur at critical junctures and may be cumulative.

DeBellis (2001) outlines seven postulations that underlie a developmental traumatology approach and that guide research in this area:

1. There are limited ways that the brain and biological stress systems can respond to overwhelming stressors.
2. In maltreatment, the nature of the stressor is a dysfunctional and traumatized interpersonal relationship. As such, subtle interpersonal cues (e.g., indices of interpersonal trust) may trigger the trauma response.
3. Maltreatment in childhood may be more detrimental than adulthood trauma, given its

potential to compromise development across multiple systems (e.g., behavioral, cognitive, emotional).

4. The biological stress system response will be based on individual differences (e.g., genetics); on the parameters of the stressor (e.g., severity, frequency); and on whether the system can maintain homeostasis in the context of severe and/or chronic stress, or whether it permanently changes in response to the stressor.

5. PTSD symptoms are normative responses to severe stressors.

6. Changes in biological stress systems cause psychiatric symptoms, particularly symptoms of PTSD. Lack of PTSD symptoms after experiencing a severe stressor will be associated with little psychopathology.

7. When trauma occurs during development, chronic PTSD symptoms represent a trajectory to more severe comorbidity and impaired cognitive and psychosocial functioning. The PTSD-mediated pathway underlies the intergenerational transmission of maltreatment via the presence of adverse brain development, consequent parental mental illness, and adverse parenting processes.

Thus, the chronic mobilization of the stress response in maltreating environments is considered a key cause of persistent negative neurological effects. Maltreated children who do not develop psychopathology following trauma exposure, then, may not have undergone such neurobiological changes. This may be consequent to an array of factors, including positive and "corrective" environmental experiences (such as attachment security or the child's perception and derived meaning of the maltreatment) that mitigate the stress response (e.g., by lowering the reactivity of the LHPA axis to stress) (Bremner & Vermetten, 2001; DeBellis, 2001; Glaser, 2000). For example, a study of maltreated youth in the community and in the child welfare system found that teens who failed to endorse their maltreatment experiences as "abuse" obtained lower levels of self-reported trauma symptoms than did those who classified themselves as having been "abused" (Wekerle, Wolfe, et al., 2001).

Whereas low rates of PTSD are observed in children who experience single and/or noninterpersonal traumatic events, high rates of symptomatology are associated with chronic and/or severe maltreatment (Yehuda, Halligan, & Grossman, 2001). Retrospective and prospective research finds increased rates of PTSD symptoms in those with a history of childhood maltreatment (Boney-McCoy & Finkelhor, 1996; Widom, 1999), including physical abuse (Silverman et al., 1996; Widom, 1999), sexual abuse (Wolfe et al., 1994; Widom, 1999), and neglect (Widom, 1999). PTSD incidence rates in nonclinical samples as assessed within 2 months following disclosure have been 36% (sexual abuse; McLeer et al., 1998) and 39% (physical abuse; Famularo, Fenton, & Kinscherff, 1994), with a third of those positive for PTSD continuing to meet criteria at a 2-year follow-up (Famularo, Fenton, Augustyn, & Zuckerman, 1996). Between 25% and 50% of children and adolescents with histories of maltreatment involving sexual abuse or combined sexual and physical abuse meet criteria for PTSD (McCloskey & Walker, 2000; Wolfe et al., 1994). In a prospective longitudinal study, Widom (1999) found that at the 20-year follow-up mark, maltreatment experiences continued to predict lifetime PTSD even after controls for family, individual child, and lifestyle confounds, with sexual abuse remaining highly significant. Considering gender differences, Kessler et al. (1995) report a greater lifetime PTSD rate for women than for men who have experienced molestation, witnessing violence, neglect, or physical abuse.

Although the diagnosis of PTSD appears to apply to a substantial minority of maltreated children, further research is needed to assess the extent of subclinical PTSD and how it affects neurobiological development. A dimensional study of PTSD may suggest contributory roles for individual clusters of symptoms (Criterion B, reexperiencing and intrusion; Criterion C, avoidance; Criterion D, hyperarousal) in multisystem developmental delays or deficits (DeBellis, 2001). To emphasize, although the existing research has focused on PTSD, the proposed keystone mediator consists of PTSD *symptoms* in childhood, rather than a diagnosis of PTSD per se.

Future work needs to consider the mediational role of trauma symptoms in the prediction of subsequent outcomes. One study (Wekerle, Wolfe, et al., 2001) found that the relationship between childhood maltreatment on the one hand, and violence both by and toward a dating partner on the other, was mediated by self-reported trauma symptoms in two samples of adolescent females: youths from a community sample, and youths on active CPS caseloads. For adolescent males, trauma symptoms added unique variance but did not achieve mediator status. These results support the value of considering PTSD symptoms as potential targets for reassessment when there is a history of child maltreatment, in an effort to reduce and prevent negative sequelae.

Understanding the psychobiology of maltreatment, in addition to the brain circuits and neuroendocrine systems that play a role in consequent psychopathology, remains a research priority for determining targets for treatment and early intervention. Brain maturation proceeds in an expectable sequential fashion. When expected experiences are absent (as in neglect), or when nonexpected experiences occur (as in abuse), maturation may proceed in atypical ways that may result in compromised functioning. There remains a need to decipher developmentally sensitive periods as they pertain to age of onset of maltreatment, as well as differences between acute and chronic maltreatment. From a clinical perspective, chronic (multiple-event) and acute (single-event) maltreatment would seem to result in two distinct PTSD patterns, with greater memory for details and less denial, numbing, and dissociation when an acute traumatic event is experienced (for a discussion, see Terr, 1991). Furthermore, earlier work has supported these two PTSD types (e.g., Famularo, Kinscherff, & Fenton, 1990; Kiser, Heston, Millsap & Pruitt, 1991). Additional studies on the relationship between PTSD (and other psychiatric disorders) and child maltreatment are presented in the following sections.

ETIOLOGY

The consensus is that child maltreatment does not result from any single risk factor or etiological process that provides a necessary or sufficient basis for such behavior (National Research Council, 1993). Most models seeking to explain physical abuse and neglect, in particular, have focused their attention on the nature of the parent–child relationship and the factors that influence the normal formation of a healthy, child-focused relationship. Models of child sexual abuse, in contrast, have looked for evidence of deviant sexual histories of the adult offender, as well as environmental and cultural risk factors that play a role in promoting the exploitation of children. Below are some of the major etiological factors that have been identified as part of this complex process.

Information-processing models have been applied to parenting, in recognition of the cognitive demands placed on the individual parent. These models focus on the internal processes in the parent, where child behavior *A* leads to parental behavior *B*. Typically, sequential stages of information processing are suggested, proceeding from parental attention to and perception of child behavior to the selection and implementation of a parental response. Four models focus on different abuse phenomena, with Crittenden's (1993) model centering on neglectful families, and Bugental's (1993), Milner's (e.g., 1993, 1998, 2000), and Dodge and colleagues' (e.g., Dodge, 1980; Dodge, Lochman, Laird, Zelli, & the Conduct Problems Prevention Research Group, 2002) models emphasizing physically abusive families.

Crittenden (1993) argues that neglectful parenting can occur as a function of a range of information-processing deficits: "Neglect occurs when there is a pattern in which mental processing is aborted before appropriate and necessary parental behavior is undertaken" (p. 32). Specifically, this pattern of deficits can include perceptual and interpretive "misses," in which the parent either does not perceive that the child is in need or, having accurately perceived a need, makes an inaccurate interpretation. This pattern can also include situations where child distress is misinterpreted (e,g., seeking attention) or is unrealistically interpreted, as in cases of overestimating the child's ability to care for him- or herself. Further deficits can occur at the response stage, where the neglectful parent "knows" a response is required but cannot develop a response strategy, or selects a response but fails to implement it. Thus the neglectful parent is considered to have a systematic bias toward not perceiving, not accurately interpreting, and/or not appropriately and effectively responding to direct child signals of need, as well as to contextual signals (e.g., time since last meal, mealtime).

Crittenden (1993) suggests a variety of parental factors that make these information-processing deficits more likely, such as parental depression, narcissism, mental retardation, a low sense of self-efficacy, and inappropriate belief systems (e.g., a belief in early child independence). For example, a depressed neglectful parent may have a perceptual bias for automatically processing negative affective information that is linked to depressive withdrawal and avoidance behaviors. The depression will make more effortful cognitive processes, such as reflecting on the range of possible causes for child misbehavior (e.g., physical illness, lack of attention or understanding, need for assistance, etc.), less likely. This perceptual deficit is further linked to "higher-order" cognitive variables, such as a parent's internal models of relationships, developed from his or her own experiences of being parented (Bowlby, 1980). Thus a neglectful parent who has learned as a child that he or she is powerless in eliciting loving and caring responses from adults may come to detach from distress signals in his or her own child as the parents had to as a child, in an effort to avoid being overwhelmed by distress yet maintain physical proximity.

Like Crittenden, Bugental and colleagues (e.g., Bugental, 1993; Bugental & Goodnow, 1998; Bugental, Blue, & Lewis, 1990; Bugental, Lyon, Krantz, & Cortez, 1997; Bugental, Lewis, Lin, Lyon, & Kopeikin, 1999; Bugental, Lyon, et al., 1999) link information-processing deficits (in particular, a negative interpretive bias of personal powerlessness) to "higher-order" cognitive variables, such as stable, cognitive constructions about relationships. Physically abusive parents are proposed to interact with a "threat-oriented" relationship prototype, such that they are sensitive to and expect possible challenges to their authority. Given their own low perceived power, they are hypervigilant for dominance challenges. As a consequence, there is an elevated risk for invoking aversive response strategies to defuse the perceived or feared power of others. Given the enduring and well-practiced (overlearned) nature of these schematic guides, aversive response strategies are rapidly and automatically accessed. Bugental centers on the power dynamics in abusive families, where parents attribute high levels of power to children, and children are placed in a reversed, parenting role. This role reversal leaves the children vulnerable to parental efforts to assume "counterpower" and make preemptive aggressive attacks, to counter perceived oncoming child hostile behavior. Women with low levels of perceived power attribute intentionality more often to ambiguous child behavior than to clearly responsive or unresponsive child behavior (Bugental, Lewis, et al., 1999). Thus abusive parents may see themselves as "victims" of aversive child behavior, which is perceived by the parents to be intentional and controllable by the children; therefore, they may minimize the severity of their actions as abusive. Parental aversiveness and abuse are seen as deriving from the parents' having a threat-oriented schema of interpersonal relationships, which may have originated from the parents' own early relationship experiences.

Several empirical studies support aspects of Bugental's proposed model. Compared to controls, abusive mothers were found to display higher levels of negative affect with their children, even during neutral or positive interactions (Bugental et al., 1990); moreover, the children of abusive parents showed speech patterns indicative of escalating levels of stress during interactions with their parents (Bugental & Lin, 1991, cited in Bugental, 1993). In an effort to control the stimulus of the child, Bugental and associates have observed adults "interacting" with a computer-simulated child on a computer-based teaching task. Women who were categorized as low in perceived control exhibited greater physiological arousal (heart rate, electrodermal activity) and negative affect to computer-simulated "unresponsive" child behaviors, and minimal levels of arousal and negative affect with responsive children, as compared to controls (Bugental, 1993). Thus women who perceive their power as low are more autonomically reactive to potential challenges to their authority.

Bugental, Lewis, et al. (1999) have clarified the importance of ambiguous control. Women with low perceived power, when placed in a situation of ambiguous (as compared to high or low) control, used higher levels of punitive force. This relationship was partially mediated by the elevated levels of autonomic arousal. The punitive response may temporarily reduce the perceived power threat. Children respond to low-power women with greater attentional disengagement, which is mediated by the ambiguous communication style of low-power women (Bugental, Lyon, et al., 1999). Experimentally induced adult ambiguity (in face and voice) was related to low levels of child attentional engagement, which may represent a means for children to regulate their distress. However, the reduced attention may impair the response formulation process. Furthermore, with experimentally manipulated stress (e.g., making judgments during engagement in a concurrent task), low-power women rated their children as in a position of greater power. This association did not hold in a nonstress context. These findings suggest the potential for a perpetuated defensive interactional style that lacks clarity in intent and purpose—one in which the adult views the interaction with the child as a "contest" to be won, and is especially vulnerable under stress and ambiguous cues.

In Dodge and colleague's social information-processing model (e.g., Dodge, 1980; Dodge et al., 2002; Zelli & Dodge, 1999), emphasis is placed on patterns of encoding (e.g., hypervigilance to self-threats, deficits in attention to relevant cues) that take on features of an acquired personality characteristic—stable over time, with high internal consistency. Patterns link processing with affective and behavioral responses, such that rapid encoding of threat cues may lead to activation of attributions of hostile intent (e.g., the assumption that the child is misbehaving "on purpose"), angry reactions, instrumental goal setting (e.g., revenge or "win" goals), ready accessing of aggressive responses, and selecting and enacting an aggressive response (e.g., hitting the child). As applied to a parent, this would reflect knowledge garnered from his or her history of interaction with the child, as well as personal knowledge from his or her own historical interactions (e.g., a childhood history of being harshly parented). Compared to nonmaltreating parents, abusive parents are expected to utilize "data bases" or latent knowledge structures stored in memory that contain more negative knowledge about the child—negative, aggression-prone perceptual, interpretive, and response biases—possibly within a context of poor understanding of emotions (Dodge et al., 2002).

Milner (e.g., 1993, 1998, 2000) describes a social information-processing model of physically abusive parenting in which parental cognition and motivation are given central roles. Abusive parents are thought to be less attentive to child behavior in general. As such, they are considered to be "faulty discriminators." For example, the finding that abusive mothers are equally highly reactive to a crying and a smiling infant (e.g., Frodi & Lamb, 1980) has been interpreted as suggesting that the abusive parent perceives *the child* as an aversive stimulus, failing to perceive accurately the distinct features of child behavior. Furthermore, Milner postulates that the personal "distress" of abusive mothers (resulting from both child-related and non-child-related events) decreases their perceptual abilities, such that greater inaccuracy in child-related perceptions results. In this model also, maternal depression in abusive mothers is cited as an important factor in accounting for a negative bias in abuse-relevant cognitive activities. For example, a lower threshold for perceived child misbehavior is suggested to be a function of depressive symptomatology.

The importance of parental perception of child behavior is indicated by Milner's proposing a direct path from perception to abusive parenting, via automatic processing. Automatic processing reflects rapid cognitive processing that is believed to occur outside of conscious awareness and to involve low demands on attention; because it is difficult to modify or suppress (especially under stress or threat), such processing generally proceeds to completion. Hence, automatic processing is likely to be invoked under the low-attention condition presumed to be present in abusive parents. Milner notes that such rapid processing may account for the nature of abusive behavior: immediate, rapid, and explosive parental reactions, and a lack of consideration of mitigating details about the child. In accounting for abusive rather than aversive parental behavior, Milner places emphasis on the parent's estimation of "wrongness." That is, an abusive parent not only may perceive child problem behavior and attribute responsibility and negative intent to the child, but may also evaluate the behavior as "very wrong" and thus as deserving severe parental disciplinary actions.

Maltreating mothers in one study did report higher levels of perceiving child behavior as negative; they also inferred greater child responsibility, reported more anger and stress, and endorsed more punitive punishments. In regression analyses, the strongest proximal predictor of endorsed punishment was how angry a mother felt toward a misbehaving child. Support has thus been found for the pathway in which perceived negativity of child behavior predicts inferences of child responsibility, inferred child responsibility influences maternal anger, and maternal anger predicts maternal punishment (Graham, Weiner, Cobb, & Henderson, 2001). In considering parents scoring as having high potential for committing child abuse, Nayak and Milner (1998) found that even when IQ was controlled for, such mothers showed neurocognitive deficits in the areas of conceptual ability, cognitive flexibility, and problem-solving skill. These differences dissipated when depression and anxiety were also controlled, suggesting that physically abusive behavior is not dominantly related to parental cognitive functioning. Indeed, Caselles and Milner (2000) found that such high-risk mothers perceived children's conventional and personal transgressions as more wrong, expected less compliance from their own children, and appraised their disciplinary responses as less appropriate. Also, when presented with a noncompliant child, high-risk mothers rated the child's behavior as more stressful (Dopke & Milner, 2000). This theoretical model, though, remains to be tested among sample of substantiated maltreating parents.

OVERVIEW OF ADULT AND CHILD CHARACTERISTICS

Child Risk Characteristics

Little research has been conducted into the possible role that a child may play in his or her own maltreatment (Ammerman, 1992). Rather than "victim blaming," however, these few studies seek to distinguish any characteristics a child might display that would place the child "at risk" of an adult's becoming neglectful or either physically or sexually abusive. Certain child factors may increase the potential for maltreatment only in the presence of other important causal factors, such as those noted above. Both longitudinal and comparative studies, however, have failed to discern any child characteristics—such as age or gender, temperament, low birthweight, hyperactivity, or conduct problems—that clearly increase the risk of maltreatment, once environmental and adult factors are controlled for (National Research Council, 1993). Factors that make it more difficult for a child to rebuff sexual abuse attempts in particular include an emotionally vulnerable child (e.g., an emotionally and/or physically deprived, compliant, or quiet child), the use of coercion and/or seduction, the child's having witnessed parental conflict, the child's lack of education about sexual abuse, and the general social powerlessness of children. If subtler coercion methods (e.g., purchasing candy) are not successful, violence may be used. This can also be deceptive to a child, as in the offender's framing abuse as "discipline." Often the actual sexual behavior takes place only after a period of "grooming" or gradual indoctrination into sexual activity (Conte, 1992), suggesting that many sexually abusive adults are "sophisticated, calculating, and patient" (Singer, Hussey, & Strom, 1992, p. 884). In the case of neglect, a child's early feeding problems or irritability may place an increased strain on the parent's limited child care ability, which sets in motion a pattern of caregiver withdrawal from the child and a concomitant escalation in the child's dependency needs and demandingness (Drotar, 1992). Similarly, a physically abused child may learn from an early age how to elicit attention from his or her parent through aversive means (crying, hitting, clinging, etc.), which escalates in intensity due to the parent's further decline in appropriate child management and stimulation (for a review, see Wolfe, 1999).

Adult Characteristics

Abuse and Neglect in General

Studies of abusive parents have supported the development of the cognitive-behavioral models presented above. In a review of studies comparing abusive and nonabusive parents on psychological variables, Wolfe (1999) concluded that although abusive parents may not manifest any distinguishable personality or psychiatric disorders, they do exhibit behavioral differences and lifestyle patterns indicative of incompetence in the role of child rearing (see also Black, Heyman, & Smith-Slep, 2001, and Milner, 1998, for reviews on physical abuse perpetration; see Flett & Hewitt, 2002, for a novel review on personality theory and empirical evidence). Abusive parents are not as effective or successful as nonabusive parents in the parenting role, in terms of either teaching their children new behaviors or controlling child problem behavior. Abusive parents are less flexible in their choices of disciplinary techniques, and often fail to match their choice of discipline to a child's misdeed and the situation. Their overreliance on physical punishment as a control strategy, in combination with limited child management skills, is intensified by their failure to develop social supports to alleviate stress and to assist in family problem solving.

Empirical findings also suggest that both overcontrolled (e.g., obsessive) and undercontrolled (e.g., aggressive) parental responses may be present along with, or precipitants of, child- and family-mediated stress. Individual adult characteristics—such as low tolerance for stress, inappropriate or inadequate models or learning opportunities, and a poor repertoire of life skills—may be important psychological processes that are involved in determining the expression of these stressful life events. Furthermore, it is highly probable that abusive parents' perceptions of adverse family and environmental conditions are exacerbated by their failure to use social supports and to develop social networks.

In a 17-year longitudinal study of 644 families, Brown, Cohen, Johnson, and Salzinger (1998) reported that three factors uniquely predicted physical abuse: low maternal involvement, early separation of the child from the mother, and perinatal problems. Two other factors—maternal young age and maternal sociopathology—predicted risk for physical abuse, sexual abuse, and neglect. Similarly, Bishop and Leadbeater (1999) found maternal depression, quality of social support from friends (low number of friends, contact with friends, and quality of friendship), and quality of current relationships (i.e., more negative) to be unique predictors of maltreatment status. These authors note that few maltreating mothers listed professionals as part of their formal social support system, despite higher-frequency and more varied service use. What remains unclear is how service use intersected with depression and relationship problems. It does, however, highlight the need to advocate for psychopharmacological and psychotherapeutic addressing of maternal depression.

Neglectful parents have received far less attention than physically and sexually abusive ones (Drotar, 1992), perhaps because omissions of proper caretaking behaviors are more difficult to describe and detect. Hillson and Kuiper (1994), in their description of a stress-and-coping model of physical abuse and neglect, convincingly argue that neglectful caregivers engage in varying degress of behavioral disengagement (i.e., reducing their efforts to remove, avoid, or cope with a stressor). Neglectful parents may also engage in activities aimed at distracting themselves from the current stressor, in an effort to cope. These depictions of neglectful parenting, framed within a stress-and-coping model, are generally consistent with the existing empirical evidence. Schumacher, Smith-Slep, and Heyman (2001) reviewed literature on the risk factors for neglect. Factors with moderate to strong effect sizes included fertility (e.g., more births, more unplanned conceptions), maternal self-esteem, impulsivity, lack of social support, daily stress, substance use disorder diagnosis, and poverty status.

In many other ways, however, the parental characteristics (e.g., depression) and lifestyle choices (e.g., substance abuse) overlap. For instance, a positive association between substance abuse (past or current) and scores on a child abuse potential inventory for both mothers and fathers have been noted (Ammerman, Kolko, Kirisci, Blackson, & Dawes, 1999). In a prospective study, Chaffin, Kelleher, and Hollenberg (1996) found that parental substance abuse predicted parents' self-report of child physical abuse and neglect, even after controls for several confounds (including antisocial personality). Depression was a risk factor for physical abuse but not neglect, once confounds such as substance use disorder diagnoses were controlled for. These authors conclude that there is a direct effect for substance misuse, and also that substance misuse may be a mediator of the depression–neglect connection.

From this overview, we can highlight three key elements that stand out as common etiological features concerning the parent's role in child abuse or neglect: (1) the manner in which the parent interacts with the child on an everyday basis; (2) the frustration–aggression relationship that is learned by the parent in relation to child rearing, which accounts for the rapid and often uncontrollable escalation from annoyance to rage; and (3) the cognitive, social-informational processes that explain the distorted beliefs and attributions underlying a parent's actions (Wolfe, 1999). Social-interactional, social information-processing, and arousal–aggression processes are useful in explaining the constant changes in the behavior of family members in response to events within or outside of the family unit. Child maltreatment can best be explained as the result of an interaction between the parent and child within a system that seldom provides alternative solutions (e.g., through exposure to appropriate parental models, education, and supports) or clear-cut restraints (e.g., maltreatment laws, sanctions, and consequences). Importantly, a focus on the more distal events that may shape the child-rearing environment (e.g., poverty, stress, etc.) and an integration with neurobiological findings (discussed earlier) have not been accomplished to date.

Sexual Abuse

Research has shown pedophiliac adults in general and incest offenders in particular to be heterogeneous groups, with an undercurrent being the association of violence and aggression with sexual abuse (Hartman & Burgess, 1989). Perpetrators of child sexual assaults are overwhelmingly male; data suggest that the majority of female offenders are usually in coercive relationships with male offenders (Friedrich, 1990). Mother involvement in cases of incest spans the continuum from active participation and encouragement (considered to be very rare), to denying the abuse and siding with the offender (a minority of instances), to supporting the child's disclosure and terminating the partner relationship, although sometimes in an ambivalent or defensive manner (Salter,

1988). The cycle-of-violence hypothesis is limited in sexual abuse. The rate of self-reported history of sexual abuse among offenders is between 20% and 30%, with lower rates emerging when polygraph verification is used (Chaffin, Letourneau, & Silovsky, 2002). Although various mechanisms have been advanced (e.g., identification with the abuser, dissociative states, trauma reenactments), it would seem that a salient characteristic for offenders with a history of sexual abuse may be increased levels of deviant sexual arousal. A maltreatment history may portend an earlier onset of offending and selection of younger children, and diverse pathways can exist—for example, embedded in a broad range of social rule violations, low social competency, opportunity taking, or experimentation (for a review, see Chaffin et al., 2002).

Critical features in classifying perpetrators identified from the literature include offense factors (such as degree of violence used, emphasis on coercion vs. seduction, relationship to the child, and age of the child), as well as offender factors (such as level of education, preoffense social and occupational adjustment, criminal history, personality traits, and substance misuse) (Hartman & Burgess, 1989). Personality features, on the other hand, are quite heterogeneous, and there is no single defining personality profile for either the juvenile or adult sex offender (Chaffin et al., 2002). Notably, a study of 246 male juvenile sex offenders (Becker, Kaplan, Tenke, & Tartaglini, 1991) reported that 42% of the subjects reported appreciable depressive symptomatology. Such symptoms, moreover, were higher in relation to the offender's own history of sexual or physical abuse. Prentsky, Harris, Frizell, and Righthand (2000) found that one salient difference between juvenile and adult offenders may be deviant sexual interest, which was not strongly predictive in juveniles. Instead, antisocial indicators seem more pertinent (e.g., psychopathy, delinquency) among youthful offenders. A treatment caution emerges from a study in which individuals who scored high on psychopathy and who were rated positively by treating clinicians were found to be more likely to reoffend sexually; this suggests the ability to engage convincingly in treatment, yet show no positive gain in outcome (Seto & Barbaree, 1999).

Finkelhor (1984) has identified the principal individual and situational conditions that foster child sexual abuse. Four offender preconditions are proposed as necessary before a sexual assault on a child can occur: (1) the motivation for sexual abuse (e.g., sexual arousal to children); (2) overcoming internal inhibitors (e.g., use of alcohol/drugs, impulsivity); (3) overcoming external inhibitors (e.g., lack of parental supervison of the child, opportunities to be alone with the child); and (4) overcoming the child's resistance (e.g., coercion through gifts, taking advantage of the child's curiosity). Finkelhor (1986) proposes that the first two conditions are necessary for abuse to occur; that is, the perpetrator must be inclined to abuse and uninhibited about it. This is consistent with the notion that the offender bears responsibility for the abuse. These perpetrator characteristics are considered to be fostered by societal practices, such as the erotic portrayal of children in mainstream advertising and in pornography, and the tolerance of male domination (Friedrich, 1990).

CURRENT ISSUES AND FUTURE DIRECTIONS

The developmental implications for children who have been abused or neglected have been emphasized throughout this chapter, in an effort to establish the significance and interconnectedness of these events vis-à-vis developmental psychopathology and the perpetuation of violence. These different forms of violence and maltreatment, although multiply determined, share common causes and outcomes; most importantly, the formation of healthy relationships is significantly impaired. This relational theme has emerged throughout the review and discussion of physical abuse, neglect, and sexual abuse, and one of the prominent issues in the field is establishing adequate services and supports for families and children that may serve to strengthen parent–child relationships and protect children from exploitation and harm. In closing, we discuss some ideas pertaining to this current direction of early identification and prevention.

How Can We Improve Our Definitions and Understanding of Different Forms of Maltreatment?

Defining child maltreatment in a manner that encompasses all of the social, methodological, and practical concerns poses a major challenge to research in this area. Typically, researchers have somewhat arbitrarily defined their groups of interest in a dichotomous manner, based on the most salient presenting characteristics of each child or family (e.g., evidence of physical abuse). However, this practice disguises other experiences these children may have had, resulting in a nonspecific categorization of maltreating families. Moreover, this common strategy treats each different type of maltreatment as singular independent variables, when in reality such events often co-occur and are highly related. The categorical approach, therefore, fails to identify other relevant factors (such as other forms of maltreatment or family experiences) that can have a synergistic or unique impact on a child's development.

Researchers have also expressed dissatisfaction with current methodology in defining child maltreatment (Cicchetti & Manly, 2001; Manly et al., 2001). A categorization approach to defining forms of maltreatment obscures differences in the severity of the different forms, and ignores the frequent co-occurrence of several forms in the lives of children (McGee & Wolfe, 1991). Furthermore, studies have reported considerable overlap among the types of maltreatment experienced. For example, Lewis, Lovely, Yeager, and Femina (1989) reported that among their follow-up sample of 95 young adults previously incarcerated for violent and nonviolent crimes, 60% (n = 57) both had been abused and had witnessed extraordinary family violence. These findings indicate that unique or nonoverlapping forms of maltreatment are atypical.

How Are We Currently Responding to Child Maltreatment?

The reduction or elimination of child maltreatment and related forms of family violence may be more readily achieved through a wide range of family support, education, and health promotion efforts (Wekerle & Wolfe, 1993; Thompson, 1995). In contrast to the view that offenders can be identified and controlled, an inclusionary (prevention) perspective strives to raise the level of understanding and skill among the broadest section of the population. Building healthy relationships is the central theme associated with violence prevention and enhanced family functioning. However, treatment needs will never be entirely supplanted by prevention, and continued investigation into efficacious treatment of maltreating parents will remain important (for treatment reviews, see Azar & Gehl, 1999; Chaffin et al., 2002).

Recently, our understanding of the causes and the developmental course of violence against women and children has grown significantly, allowing prevention efforts to be generated from a reasonable knowledge base. The developmental traumatology approach would argue for a national policy for general mental health screening (not just screening for PTSD) for all parents and children involved in CPS or law enforcement agencies, in cases where the perpetrator is not in a caregiving role (DeBellis, 2001). Given the cognitive and learning developmental risks to maltreated children, a developmental screening tool for children would be important to include. Medical examination and diagnoses need to be routine expectations for any child clinical presentation. This may be especially true for cases emerging in educational settings; for instance, school nurse examination should be available when abuse or neglect is suspected.

Global dimensions such as severity and chronicity, rather than type, of maltreatment are predictive of the severity of behavior problems (Manly, Cicchetti, & Barnett, 1994). Intervention for behavior problems, in particular, has been identified as a prime mental health need of maltreated children. In a study of children entering custody in Tennessee, the majority of whom were under the supervision of child welfare, a substantial number obtained scores in the clinical range (82%) on at least one of the three scales of the Child Behavior Checklist (parent and teacher report)—that is, Internalizing, Externalizing, and Total Behavior Problems (Glisson, 1994, 1996). In a review of studies of the foster care population, externalizing behaviors emerged as a prevalent clinical issue (Pilowsky, 1995). Similarly, a recent study (Shaffer, Fisher, Lewis, Dulcan, & Schwab-Stone, 2000) reported that among youths who had been declared dependents of the courts between ages 6 and 18, 41.8% qualified for one or more DSM-IV diagnoses, with the largest proportion meeting criteria for the disruptive behavior disorders (e.g., 16.1% for conduct disorder, 22.2% for ODD) as compared to internalizing problems (e.g., 8.6% for anxiety disorders, 5.2% for mood disorders). Since externalizing disorders constitute a predominant cause for referral for mental health services, child maltreatment assessment would seem prudent.

Few child-focused agencies, including CPS agencies, routinely evaluate the history of maltreatment in adult caregivers, in addition to parental mental health. For example, children with a history of family disruption and violence have been shown to be at an elevated risk of either experiencing or perpetrating violence toward others, especially during middle to late adolescence and adulthood (Dutton, 1988; Widom, 1989a, 1989b). Straus and Kantor (1994), using state records of offenses coupled with detailed histories of child rearing, contend that maltreatment experiences (including "milder" forms of corporal punishment) constitute the single most significant risk factor for subsequent relationship violence in adulthood. Thus it is believed that maltreatment experiences in one's family of origin create a vulnerability for further maltreatment by others (especially among young women), as well as a propensity to use power and control as a means of resolving conflict (especially among young men; Wolfe, Wekerle, Reitzel-Jaffe, & Gough, 1995).

Whenever dating violence or domestic violence is a consideration, maltreatment should be considered as well. For instance, whereas treatments for substance-abusing adults in couples consider partner violence, the adults' maltreatment histories and the presence of child maltreatment, either historically or currently, are not typically considered. In addition to prior maltreatment experiences, the risk of either experiencing or perpetrating violence increases as a result of negative influences from peers (i.e., condoning violence); the absence of compensatory factors (e.g., success at school, healthy relationships with siblings or friends, etc.); and the relative lack of alternative sources of information that serve to counteract existing biases, attitudes, and beliefs (Jessor, 1993). A thorough and comprehensive maltreatment evaluation is a necessity for all child and youth front-line health, education, mental health, justice, and CPS agencies. One is far more likely to discover what one looks for than what one prefers to overlook. Among the myriad of relevant factors, child maltreatment needs to be among those included for systematic consideration.

Although child maltreatment prevention has been attempted, it has met with only varying degrees of success. Tertiary prevention or treatment studies to prevent recidivism with identified abusive parents have reported some degree of success at improving child-rearing skills and knowledge of development, although limited follow-up data, evidence of recidivism, and high costs of delivery contribute to the inadequacy of this form of "prevention" (Wolfe & Wekerle, 1993). However, interventions with maltreating parents have not tended to operate with a multidisciplinary team perspective, and it may be prudent for CPS personnel to adopt a similar approach (e.g., ensuring psychiatric screening, including assessment of substance misuse and domestic violence, for all investigated parents). Selected or targeted prevention efforts, which range from interventions with high-risk to low-risk parents and expectant parents, favor assisting parents and children at an earlier point in time and have maintained gains over extensive follow-up periods (e.g., Olds et al., 1997, 1998; Olds, Hill, Robinson, Song, & Little, 2000). These wide-ranging strategies, and home-visiting approaches in particular, have demonstrated feasibility, cost-effectiveness, and effectiveness (Brust, Heins, & Rheinberger, 1998; Wekerle & Wolfe, 1993; Thompson, 1995). With multiproblem families, home visiting provides direction to families in terms of service linkage, child physical health care and monitoring, enhanced parent–child interactions, and the prevention of physical abuse and neglect.

Universal prevention of child abuse, the least studied approach, has largely focused on educational strategies aimed at teaching school-age children and youth about violence issues. Evaluations of such programs are typically limited to demonstrations of knowledge gain, attitude change, behavioral intentions, and self-reported outcomes. Behavioral gains supporting the preventative nature of such programs vis-à-vis child-rearing ability have not been evaluated, however. Sexual abuse prevention that focuses on educating parents and children would seem to have some effectiveness (for a review, see Finkelhor, Asidigian, & Dzuiba-Leatherman, 1995); however, the main concern for such programs is that they place the weight of responsibility on the individual child to resist, deter, or avoid assault (Reppucci & Haugaard, 1989). When the perpetrator of child sexual abuse is a determined adult, this is untenable as a dominant prevention strategy. If the child is not responsible for the abuse, the child can hardly be responsible for its prevention.

From these beginnings, child maltreatment prevention efforts have been reorganized around the principle of building upon strengths and developing protective factors in an effort to deter maltreatment (Helfer, 1982). This principle underscores the importance of the relational context to prevention. That is, learning to relate to others, especially intimates, in a respectful, nonviolent manner is a crucial foundation for building a child maltreatment prevention strategy

(Garbarino, Drew, Kostelny, & Pardo, 1992; Wekerle & Wolfe, 1993). "There can now be no dispute that maltreatment experiences are harmful for children" (Cicchetti & Rogosch, 1997, p. 798). What remains most dramatic is the fact that these maltreatment experiences are unnecessary. Two of our most salient windows of opportunity may be (1) adolescence and the formation of healthy intimacy and protection skills, and (2) the first pregnancy in a young family (Wekerle & Wolfe, 1998). Ideally, in taking a broader view of maltreatment beyond the individual child, we may shift our focus to intervening in mediating factors that are being established empirically (e.g., PTSD symptomatology is a promising consideration), and adopt a family services and support orientation to address the needs of all family members and enhance family dynamics. Efficient assessment, efficacious intervention, and effective prevention of child maltreatment are reasonable and achievable goals, and maltreating families and their children deserve nothing less.

ACKNOWLEDGMENTS

This work was supported in part by grants and fellowships from the Ontario Mental Health Foundation (Christine Wekerle, David A. Wolfe); the Canadian Institutes for Health Research (Christine Wekerle); U.S. National Institutes of Health Youth Violence Consortium (David A. Wolfe); and the Social Sciences and Humanities Research Committee (Christine Wekerle). We thank Dr. Harriet MacMillan, Ms. Valerie Hart, and Ms. Goldie Millar for their valuable support and assistance.

NOTE

1. The LHPA axis is the pathway connecting the hypothalamus (a structure in the brain) to the adrenal and pituitary glands. The hypothalamus secretes corticotropin-releasing hormone (CRH), which then stimulates the pituitary gland to secrete adrenocorticotropic hormone (ACTH). ACTH is released into the blood, leading to the stimulation of the adrenal cortex to produce and release the steroid cortisol into the circulation. Specific brain centers receive cortisol and send messages via the LHPA axis to regulate the level of cortisol. Cortisol level is elevated in response to stress; cortisol actions include suppressing the immune response, increasing the level of circulating glucose, dampening fear responses to the stressor, and adversely affecting the hippocampus (Glaser, 2000).

REFERENCES

Abbey, A. (2000). Adjusting to infertility. In J. Harvey & E. Miller (Eds.), *Loss and trauma: General and close relationship perspectives* (pp. 331–344). Philadelphia: Brunner–Routledge.

Aber, J. L., & Allen, J. P. (1987). Effects of maltreatment on young children's socioemotional development: An attachment theory perspective. *Developmental Psychology, 23*, 406–414.

Aber, J. L., & Cicchetti, D. (1984). The socio-emotional development of maltreated children: An empirical and theoretical analysis. In H. Fitzgerald, B. Lester, & M. Yogman (Eds.), *Theory and research in behavioral pediatrics* (Vol. 2, pp. 147–205). New York: Plenum Press.

Alexander, P. C. (1992). Application of attachment theory to the study of sexual abuse. *Journal of Consulting and Clinical Psychology, 60*, 185–195.

Alexander, P. C. (1993). The differential effects of abuse characteristics and attachment in the prediction of long-term effects of sexual abuse. *Journal of Interpersonal Violence, 8*, 346–362.

American Psychiatric Association. (2000). *Diagnostic and statistical manual of mental disorders* (4th edition, text rev.). Washington, DC: Author.

Ammerman, R. T. (1992). The role of the child in physical abuse: A reappraisal. *Violence and Victims, 6*, 87–101.

Ammerman, R. T., Kolko, D. J., Kirisci, L., Blackson, T. C., & Dawes, M. A. (1999). Child abuse potential in parents with histories of substance abuse disorder. *Child Abuse and Neglect, 23*, 1225–1238.

Anda, R. F., Felitti, V. J., Chapman, D., Croft, J., Williamson, D. F., Santelli, J., Dietz, P. M., & Marks, J. S. (2001). Abused boys, battered mothers, and male involvement in teen pregnancy. *Pediatrics, 107*(2), E19.

Appel, A. E., & Holden, G. W. (1998). The co-occurrence of spouse and physical child abuse: A review and appraisal. *Journal of Family Psychology, 12*, 578–599.

Appelbaum, A. S. (1977). Developmental retardation in infants as a concomitant of physical child abuse. *Journal of Abnormal Child Psychology, 5*, 417–423.

Aragona, J. A., & Eyberg, S. M. (1981). Neglected children: Mother's report of child behavior problems and observed verbal behaviors. *Child Development, 52*, 596–602.

Arnow, B. A., Hart, S., Hayward, C., Dea, R., & Taylor, C. B. (2000). Severity of child maltreatment, pain complaints and medical utilization among women. *Journal of Psychiatric Research, 34*, 413–421.

Asher, S. J. (1988). The effects of childhood sexual abuse: A review of the issues and evidence. In L. Walker (Ed.), *Handbook on sexual abuse of children* (pp. 3–18). New York: Springer.

Azar, S. T., Barnes, K. T., & Twentyman, C. T. (1988). Developmental outcomes in abused children: Consequences of parental abuse or a more general breakdown in caregiver behavior? *Behavior Therapist, 11*, 27–32.

Azar, S. T., & Gehl, K. S. (1999). Physical abuse and neglect. In R. T. Ammerman & M. Hersen (Eds.), *Handbook of prescriptive treatments for children and adolescents* (pp. 329–345). Boston: Allyn & Bacon.

Ballon, B. C., Coubasson, C. M. A., & Smith, P. D. (2001). Physical and sexual abuse issues among youths with substance use problems. *Canadian Journal of Psychiatry, 46*, 617–621.

Barahal, R., Waterman, J., & Martin, H. P. (1981). The social cognitive development of abused children. *Journal of Consulting and Clinical Psychology*, *49*, 508–516.

Barnett, D., Ganiban, J., & Cicchetti, D. (1999). Maltreatment, negative expressivity, and the development of type D attachments from 12 to 24 months of age. *Monographs of the Society for Research in Child Development*, *64*, 97–118.

Barstow, D. G. (1999). Female genital mutilation: The penultimate gender abuse. *Child Abuse and Neglect*, *23*, 501–510.

Baum, A., O'Keefe, M., & Davidson, L. (1990). The case of traumatic stress. *Journal of Applied Social Psychology*, *20*, 1643–1654.

Becker, J. V., Kaplan, M. S., Tenke, C. E., & Tartaglini, A. (1991). The incidence of depressive symptomatology in juvenile sex offenders with a history of abuse. *Child Abuse and Neglect*, *15*, 531–536.

Beeghly, M., & Cicchetti, D. (1994). Child maltreatment, attachment, and the self system: Emergence of an internal state lexicon in toddlers at high social risk. *Development and Psychopathology*, *6*, 5–30.

Beitchman, J. H., Zucker, K. J., Hood, J. E., DaCosta, G. A., Akman, D., & Cassavia, E. (1992). A review of the long-term effects of child sexual abuse. *Child Abuse and Neglect*, *16*, 101–118.

Benoit, D. (2000). Feeding disorders, failure to thrive, and obesity. In C. H. Zeanah, Jr. (Ed.), *Handbook of infant mental health* (2nd ed., pp. 339–352). New York: Guilford Press.

Bensley, L. S., Spieker, S. J., Van Eenwyk, J., & Schoder, J. (1999). Self-reported abuse history and adolescent problem behaviors: II. Alcohol and drug use. *Journal of Adolescent Health*, *24*, 173–180.

Bensley, L. S., Van Eenwyk, J., & Simmons, K. W. (2000). Self-reported childhood sexual and physical abuse and adult HIV-risk behaviors and heavy drinking. *American Journal of Preventive Medicine*, *18*, 151–158.

Berliner, L., & Elliot, D. (2002). Sexual abuse of children. In J. E. B. Myers, L. Berliner, J. Briere, C. T. Hendrix, C. Jenny, & T. A. Reid (Eds.), *The APSAC handbook on child maltreatment* (pp. 55–78). Thousand Oaks, CA: Sage.

Bishop, S. J., & Leadbeater, B. J. (1999). Maternal social support patterns and child maltreatment: Comparison of maltreating and nonmaltreating mothers. *American Journal of Orthopsychiatry*, *69*, 172–181.

Black, D. A., Heyman, R. E., & Smith-Slep, A. M. (2001). Risk factors for child physical abuse. *Aggression and Violent Behavior*, *6*, 121–188.

Bolger, K. E., & Patterson, C. J. (2001). Developmental pathways from child maltreatment to peer rejection. *Child Development*, *72*, 549–568.

Boney-McCoy, S., & Finkelhor, D. (1996). Is youth victimization related to trauma symptoms and depression after controlling for prior symptoms and family relationships?: A longitudinal, prospective study. *Journal of Consulting and Clinical Psychology*, *64*, 1406–1416.

Bools, C., Neale, B., & Meadow, R. (1994). Munchausen syndrome by proxy: A study of psychopathology. *Child Abuse and Neglect*, *18*, 773–788.

Bowlby, J. (1980). *Attachment and loss: Vol. 3. Loss: Sadness and depression*. New York: Basic Books.

Brady, K. T., Killeen, T., Saladin, M. E., Dansky, B., & Becker, S. (1994). Comorbid substance abuse and posttraumatic stress disorder: Characteristics of women in treatment. *American Journal on Addictions*, *3*, 160–164.

Bremner, J. D., Randall, P. R., Capelli, S., Scott, T., McCarthy, G., & Charney, D. S. (1995). Deficits in short-term memory in adult survivors of childhood abuse. *Psychiatry Research*, *59*, 97–107.

Bremner, J. D., Randall, P., Vermetten, E., Staib, L., Bronen, R. A., Capelli, S., Mazure, C. M., McCarthy, G., Innis, R. B., & Charney, D. S. (1997). MRI-based measurement of hippocampal volume in posttraumatic stress disorder related to childhood physical and sexual abuse: A preliminary report. *Biological Psychiatry*, *41*, 23–32.

Bremner, J. D., & Vermetten, E. (2001). Stress and development: Behavioral and biological consequences. *Development and Psychopathology*, *13*, 473–489.

Breslau, N., Davis, G. C., Andreski, P., & Peterson, E. (1991). Traumatic events and post-traumatic stress disorder in an urban population of young adults. *Archives of General Psychiatry*, *48*, 216–222.

Briere, J. (1992). *Child abuse trauma: Theory and treatment of the lasting effects*. Newbury Park, CA: Sage.

Briere, J. (1996). *Therapy for adults molested as children* (2nd ed.). New York: Springer.

Briere, J. (2002). Treating adult survivors of childhood abuse: Further development of an integrative model. In J. E. B. Myers, L. Berliner, J. Briere, C. T. Hendrix, C. Jenny, & T. A. Reid (Eds.), *The APSAC handbook on child maltreatment* (pp. 175–203). Thousand Oaks, CA: Sage.

Briere, J., & Runtz, M. (1991). The long-term effects of sexual abuse: A review and synthesis. *New Directions on Mental Health Services*, *51*, 3–13.

Bross, D. C., Miyoshi, T. J., Miyoshi, P. K., & Krugman, R. D. (2000). *World perspectives on child abuse: The fourth international resource book*. Denver, CO: Kempe Children's Center and the International Society for Prevention of Child Abuse and Neglect.

Brown, E., & Kolko, D. (1999). Child victims' attributions about being physically abused: An examination of factors associated with symptom severity. *Journal of Abnormal Child Psychology*, *27*, 311–322.

Brown, J., Cohen, P., Johnson, J. G., & Salzinger, S. (1998). A longitudinal analysis of risk factors for child maltreatment: Findings of a 17-year prospective study of officially recorded and self-reported child abuse and neglect. *Child Abuse and Neglect*, *22*, 1065–1078.

Brown, J., Cohen, P., Johnson, J. G., & Smailes, E. M. (1999). Childhood abuse and neglect: Specificity of effects on adolescent and young adult depression and suicidality. *Journal of the American Academy of Child and Adolescent Psychiatry*, *38*, 1490–1496.

Bruised and abused. (2001, January 29). *U.S. News and World Report*, p. 6.

Brust, J., Heins, J., & Rheinberger, M. (1998). *A review of the research on home visiting*. (Available from Health Care Coalition on Violence, 2829 Verndale Avenue, Anoka, MN 55303)

Bryk, M., & Siegel, P. T. (1997). My mother caused my illness: The story of a survivor of Munchausen by proxy syndrome. *Pediatrics*, *100*, 1–7.

Bugental, D. B. (1993). Communication in abusive relationships: Cognitive constructions of interpersonal power. *American Behavioral Scientist*, *36*, 288–308.

Bugental, D. B., Blue, J., & Lewis, J. (1990). Caregiver beliefs and dysphoric affect to difficult children. *Developmental Psychology*, *26*, 631–638.

Bugental, D. B., & Goodnow, J. G. (1998). Socialization processes. In W. Damon (Series Ed.) & N. Eisenberg

(Vol. Ed.), *Handbook of child psychology: Vol. 3. Social, emotional, and personality development* (5th ed., pp. 389–462). New York: Wiley.

Bugental, D. B., Lewis, J. C., Lin, E., Lyon, J., & Kopeikin, H. (1999). In charge but not in control: The management of teaching relationships by adults with low perceived power. *Developmental Psychology, 35*, 1367–1378.

Bugental, D. B., Lyon, J., Krantz, J., & Cortez, V. (1997). Who's the boss? Differential accessibility of dominance ideation in parent-child relationships. *Journal of Personality and Social Psychology*, 72(6), 1297–1309.

Bugental, D. B., Lyon, J. E., Lin, E., McGrath, E. P., & Bimbela, A. (1999). Children "tune out" in response to ambiguous communication style of powerless adults. *Child Development*, *70*(1), 241–230.

Burgess, R., & Conger, R. (1978). Family interaction in abusive, neglectful and normal families. *Child Development, 19*, 1163–1173.

Caldwell, R. A. (1992). *The costs of child abuse vs. child abuse prevention: Michigan's experience* [Online]. Available: http://www.msu.edu/user/bob/cost.html

Camras, L. A., Ribordy, S., Spaccarelli, S., & Stefani, R. (1986, August). *Emotion recognition and production by abused children and mothers*. Paper presented at the meeting of the American Psychological Association, Washington, DC.

Carlson, B. E. (2000). Children exposed to intimate partner violence: Research findings and implications for intervention. *Trauma, Violence, and Abuse, 1*, 321–342.

Carlson, V., Cicchetti, D., Barnett, D., & Braunwald, K. G. (1989). Finding order in disorganization: Lessons from research on maltreated infants' attachments to their parents. In D. Cicchetti & V. Carlson (Eds.), *Child maltreatment: Theory and research on the causes and consequences of child abuse and neglect* (pp. 494–528). New York: Cambridge University Press.

Carmen, E. H., Rieker, P. P., & Mills, T. (1984). Victims of violence and psychiatric illness. *American Journal of Psychiatry, 141*, 378–383.

Caselles, C. E., & Milner, J. S. (2000). Evaluation of child transgressions, disciplinary choices, and expected child compliance in a no-cry and crying infant condition in physically abusive and comparison mothers. *Child Abuse and Neglect, 24*, 477–491.

Cerezo, M. A. (1997). Abusive family interaction: A review. *Aggression and Violent Behavior, 2*, 215–240.

Chaffin, M., Kelleher, K., & Hollenberg, J. (1996). Onset of physical abuse and neglect: Psychiatric, substance abuse, and social risk factors from prospective community data. *Child Abuse and Neglect, 20*, 191–203.

Chaffin, M., Letourneau, E., & Silovsky, J. F. (2002). Adults, adolescents, and children who sexually abuse children: A developmental perspective. In J. E. B. Myers, L. Berliner, J. Briere, C. T. Hendrix, C. Jenny, & T.A. Reid (Eds.), *The APSAC handbook on child maltreatment* (pp. 205–232). Thousand Oaks, CA: Sage.

Chandy, J. M., Blum, R. W., & Resnick, M. D. (1996a). Female adolescents with a history of sexual abuse: Risk outcome and protective factors. *Journal of Interpersonal Violence, 11*, 503–518.

Chandy, J. M., Blum, R.W., & Resnick, M. D. (1996b). Gender-specific outcomes for sexually abused adolescents. *Child Abuse and Neglect, 20*, 1219–1231.

Cicchetti, D. (1989). How research on child maltreatment has informed the study of child development: Perspectives from developmental psychopathology. In D. Cicchetti & V. Carlson (Eds.), *Child maltreatment: Theory and research on the causes and consequences of child abuse and neglect* (pp. 377–431). New York: Cambridge University Press.

Cicchetti, D. (1990). The organization and coherence of socioemotional, cognitive, and representational development: Illustrations through a developmental psychopathology perspective on Down syndrome and child maltreatment. In R. Thompson (Ed.), *Nebraska Symposium on Motivation: Vol. 36. Socioemotional development* (pp. 266–375). Lincoln: University of Nebraska Press.

Cicchetti, D., Ackerman, B. P., & Izard, C. E. (1995). Emotions and emotion regulation in developmental psychopathology. *Development and Psychopathology, 7*, 1–10.

Cicchetti, D., & Beeghly, M. (1987). Symbolic development in maltreated youngsters: An organizational perspective. In *New directions for child development:Vol. 36*. (pp. 5–29). San Francisco: Jossey-Bass.

Cicchetti, D., Ganiban, J., & Barnett, D. (1990). Contributions from the study of high risk populations to understanding the development of emotion regulation. In K. Dodge & J. Garber (Eds.), *The development of emotion regulation* (pp. 1–54). New York: Cambridge University Press.

Cicchetti, D., & Manly, J. T. (2001). Operationalizing child maltreatment: developmental processes and outcomes. *Development and Psychopathology*, 13(4), 755–757.

Cicchetti, D., & Olsen, K. (1990). The developmental psychopathology of child maltreatment. In M. Lewis & S. M. Miller (Eds.), *Handbook of developmental psychopathology* (pp. 261–279). New York: Plenum Press.

Cicchetti, D., & Rizley, R. (1981). Developmental perspectives on the etiology, intergenerational transmission, and sequelae of child maltreatment. In D. Cicchetti & R. Rizley (Eds.), *New directions for child development: Vol. 11. Developmental perspectives on child maltreatment* (pp. 31–55). San Francisco: Jossey-Bass.

Cicchetti, D., & Rogosch, F. A. (1996). Equifinality and multifinality in developmental psychopathology. *Development and Psychopathology, 8*, 597–600.

Chiccetti, D., & Rogosch, F. A. (1997). The role of self-organization in the promotion of resilience in maltreated children. *Development and Psychopathology*, 9(4), 797–815.

Cicchetti, D., & Rogosch, F. A. (2001). The impact of child maltreatment and psychopathology on neuroendocrine functioning. *Development and Psychopathology, 13*, 783–804.

Cicchetti, D., Rogosch, F. A., Lynch, M., & Holt, K. D. (1993). Resilience in maltreated children: Processes leading to adaptive outcome. *Development and Psychopathology, 5*, 629–647.

Cicchetti, D., & Toth, S. (1995). A developmental psychopathology perspective on child abuse and neglect. *Journal of the American Academy of Child and Adolescent Psychiatry, 35*, 42–50.

Cicchetti, D., Toth, S., & Bush, M. (1988). Developmental psychopathology and incompetence in childhood: Suggestions for intervention. In B. B. Lahey & A. E. Kazdin (Eds.), *Advances in clinical child psychology* (Vol. 11, pp. 1–77). New York: Plenum Press.

Cicchetti, D., Toth, S. L., & Maughan, A. (2000). An ecological-transactional model of child maltreatment. In A. J. Sameroff, M. Lewis, & S. Miller (Eds.), *Handbook of developmental psychopathology* (2nd ed., pp. 689–722). New York: Plenum Press.

Cicchetti, D., & Tucker, D. (1994). Development and self-regulatory structures of the mind. *Development and Psychopathology, 6,* 533–549.

Claussen, A. H., & Crittenden, P. M. (1991). Physical and psychological maltreatment: Relations among types of maltreatment. *Child Abuse and Neglect, 15,* 5–18.

Cohen, P., Brown, J., & Smailes, E. (2001). Child abuse and neglect in the development of mental disorders in the general population. *Development and Psychopathology, 13,* 981–999.

Coid, J., Petruckevitch, A., Feder, G., Chung, W., Richardson, J., & Moorey, S. (2001). Relation between childhood sexual and physical abuse and risk of revictimisation in women: A cross-sectional survey. *Lancet, 358,* 450–454.

Cole, P. M., & Putnam, F. W. (1992). Effect of incest on self and social functioning: A developmental psychopathology perspective. *Journal of Consulting and Clinical Psychology, 60,* 174–184.

Conte, J. R. (1992). Has this child been sexually abused? Dilemmas for the mental health professional who seeks the answer. *Criminal Justice and Behavior, 19,* 54–73.

Crittenden, P. (1988). Relationships at risk. In J. Belsky & T. Nezworski (Eds.), *Clinical implications of attachment theory* (pp. 136–174). Hillsdale, NJ: Erlbaum.

Crittenden, P. M. (1985). Maltreated infants: Vulnerability and resilience. *Journal of Child Psychology and Psychiatry, 26,* 1299–1313.

Crittenden, P. M. (1992). Children's strategies for coping with adverse home environments: An interpretation using attachment theory. *Child Abuse and Neglect, 16,* 329–343.

Crittenden, P. M. (1993). An information-processing perspective on the behavior of neglectful parents. *Criminal Justice and Behavior, 20,* 27–48.

Crittenden, P. M., & Ainsworth, M. D. S. (1989). Child maltreatment and attachment theory. In D. Cicchetti & V. Carlson (Eds.), *Child maltreatment: Theory and research on the causes and consequences of child abuse and neglect* (pp. 432–463). New York: Cambridge University Press.

Crittenden, P. M., & Bonvillian, J. D. (1984). The relationship between maternal risk status and maternal sensitivity. *American Journal of Orthopsychiatry, 54,* 250–262.

Crittenden, P. M., & Claussen, A. (2002). Developmental psychopathology perspectives on substance abuse and relationship violence. In C. Wekerle & A.-M. Wall (Eds.), *The violence and addiction equation: Theoretical and clinical issues in substance abuse and relationship violence* (pp. 48–67). New York: Brunner–Routledge.

Crittenden, P. M., & DiLalla, D. L. (1988). Compulsive compliance: The development of an inhibitory coping strategy in infancy. *Journal of Abnormal Child Psychology, 16,* 585–599.

Davis, J. L., & Petretic-Jackson, P. A. (2000). The impact of child sexual abuse on adult interpersonal functioning: A review and synthesis of the empirical literature. *Aggression and Violent Behavior, 5*(3), 291–328.

DeBellis, M. D. (2001). Developmental traumatology: The psychobiological development of maltreated children and its implications for research, treatment, and policy. *Development and Psychopathology, 13,* 539–564.

DeBellis, M. D., Baum, A., Birmaher, B., Keshavan, M., Eccard, C. H., Boring, A. M., Jenkins, F. J., & Ryan, N. D. (1999). Developmental traumatology: Part I. Biological stress systems. *Biological Psychiatry, 45,* 1259–1270.

DeBellis, M. D., Keshavan, M. S., Clark, D. B., Casey, B. J., Giedd, J. N., Boring, A. M., Frustaci, K., & Ryan, N. D. (1999). Developmental traumatology: Part II. Brain development. *Biological Psychiatry, 45,* 1271–1284.

DeBillis, M. D., Keshavan, M. S., Spencer, S., & Hall, J. (2000). N-acetylaspartate concentration in the anterior cingulate in maltreated children and adolescents with PTSD. *American Journal of Psychiatry, 157,* 1175–1177.

DeBellis, M. D., & Putnam, F. (1994). The psychobiology of childhood maltreatment. *Child and Adolescent Psychiatry Clinics of North America, 3,* 663–678.

Deblinger, E., Steer, R. A., & Lippmann, J. (1999). Maternal factors associated with sexually abused children's psychosocial adjustment. *Child Maltreatment, 4,* 13–20.

Dembo, R., Getreu, A., Williams, L., Berry, E., LaVoie, L., Genung, L., Schmeidler, J., Wish, E. D., & Kern, J. (1990). A longitudinal study of the relationships among alcohol use, marijuana/hashish use, cocaine use, and emotional/psychological functioning problems in a cohort of high-risk youths. *International Journal of the Addictions, 25,* 1341–1382.

deYoung, M., & Lowry, J. A. (1992). Traumatic bonding: Clinical implications in incest. *Child Welfare, 71,* 165–175.

Dietz, P. M., Spitz, A. M., Anda, R. F., Williamson, D. F., McMahon, P. M., Santelli, J. S., Nordenberg, D. F., Felitti, V. J., & Kendrick, J. S. (1999). Unintended pregnancy among adult women exposed to abuse or household dysfunction during their childhood. *Journal of the American Medical Association, 282,* 1359–1364.

Dinwiddie, S., Heath, A. C., Dunne, M. P., Bucholz, K. K., Madden, P. A. F., Slutske, W. S., Bierut, L. J., Statham, D. B., & Martin, N. G. (2000). Early sexual abuse and lifetime psychopathology: A co-twin-cohort study. *Psychological Medicine, 30,* 41–52.

Dodge, K. A. (1980). Social cognition and children's aggressive behavior. *Child Development, 51,* 162–170.

Dodge, K. A., Lochman, J. E., Laird, R., Zelli, A., & the Conduct Problems Prevention Research Group. (2002). Multidimensional latent-construct analysis of children's social information processing patterns: Correlations with aggressive behavior problems. *Psychological Assessment, 14,* 60–73.

Dodge, K. A., Pettit, G. S., & Bates, J. E. (1994). Effects of physical maltreatment on the development of peer relations. *Development and Psychopathology, 6,* 43–55.

Dolz, L., Cerezo, M. A., & Milner, J. S. (1997). Mother–child interactional patterns in high- and low- risk mothers. *Child Abuse and Neglect, 21,* 1149–1158.

Dopke, C. A., & Milner, J. S. (2000). Impact of child compliance on stress appraisals, attributions, and disciplinary choices in mothers at high and low risk for child physical abuse. *Child Abuse and Neglect, 24,* 493–504.

Drotar, D. (1992). Prevention of neglect and nonorganic failure to thrive. In D. J. Willis, E. W. Holden, & M. Rosenberg (Eds.), *Prevention of child maltreatment: Developmental and ecological perspectives* (pp. 115–149). New York: Wiley.

Dubowitz, H., & Black, M. (1994). Child neglect. In R. M. Reece (Ed.), *Child abuse: Medical diagnosis and management* (pp. 279–297). Philadelphia: Lea & Febiger.

Dunn, G. E., Ryan, J. J., & Dunn, C. E. (1994). Trauma symptoms in substance abusers with and without histories of childhood abuse. *Journal of Psychoactive Drugs, 26,* 357–360.

Dutton, D. (1988). *The domestic assault of women: Psychological and criminal justice perspectives.* Vancouver: University of British Columbia Press.

Eckenrode, J., Rowe, E., Laird, M., & Brathwaite, J. (1995). Mobility as a mediator of the effects of child maltreatment on academic performance. *Child Development, 66,* 1130–1142.

Eckenrode, J., Zielinski, D., Smith, E., Marcynyszyn, L. A., Henderson, C. R., Jr., Kitzman, H., Cole, R., Powers, J., & Olds, D. (2001). Child maltreatment and the early onset of problem behaviors: Can a program of nurse home visitation break the link? *Development and Psychopathology, 13,* 873–890.

Egeland, B. (1997). Mediators of the effects of child maltreatment on developmental adaptation in adolescence. In D. Cicchetti & S. Toth (Eds.), *Rochester Symposium on Developmental Psychopathology: Vol. 8. Developmental perspectives on trauma: Theory, research, and intervention* (pp. 403–434). Rochester, NY: University of Rochester Press.

Egeland, B., & Sroufe, A. (1981a). Attachment and early maltreatment. *Child Development, 52,* 44–52.

Egeland, B., & Sroufe, A. (1981b). Developmental sequelae of maltreatment in infancy. In R. Rizley & D. Cicchetti (Eds.), *New directions for child development: Vol. 11. Developmental perspectives on child maltreatment* (pp. 77–92). San Francisco: Jossey-Bass.

Egeland, B., Sroufe, A., & Erickson, M. (1983). The developmental consequences of different patterns of maltreatment, *Child Abuse and Neglect, 7,* 459–469.

Elze, D. E., Auslander, W., McMillen, C., Edmond, T., & Thompson, R. (2001). Untangling the impact of sexual abuse on HIV risk behaviors among youths in foster care. *AIDS Education and Prevention, 13,* 377–389.

Emery, R. E., & Laumann-Billings, L. (1998). An overview of the nature, causes, and consequences of abusive family relationships. *American Psychologist, 53,* 121–135.

English, D. J., Marshall, D. B., Brummel, S., & Orme, M. (1999). Characteristics of repeated referrals to child protective services in Washington State. *Child Maltreatment, 4,* 297–307.

Erickson, M. F., Egeland, B., & Pianta, R. (1989). The effects of maltreatment on the development of young children. In D. Cicchetti & V. Carlson (Eds.), *Child maltreatment: Theory and research on the causes and consequences of child abuse and neglect* (pp. 647–684). New York: Cambridge University Press.

Erickson, M. F., Sroufe, L. A., & Egeland, B. (1985). The relationship between quality of attachment and relationship problems in preschool in a high-risk sample. In I. Bretherton & E. Waters (Eds.), Growing points of attachment theory and research. *Monographs of the Society for Research in Child Development, 50*(1–2, Serial No. 209), .

Erickson, M. F., & Egeland, B. (2002). Child neglect. In J. E. B. Myers, L. Berliner, J. Briere, C. T. Hendrix, C. Jenny, & T. A. Reid (Eds.), *The APSAC handbook on child maltreatment* (pp. 3–20). Thousand Oaks, CA: Sage.

Ertem, I. O., Leventhal, J. M., & Dobbs, S. (2000). Intergenerational continuity of child physical abuse: How good is the evidence? *Lancet, 356,* 814–819.

Famularo, R., Fenton, T., Augustyn, M., & Zuckerman, B. (1996). Persistence of pediatric post traumatic stress disorder after 2 years. *Child Abuse and Neglect, 20,* 1245–1248.

Famularo, R., Fenton, T., & Kinscherff, R. (1994). Maternal and child posttraumatic stress disorder in cases of maltreatment. *Child Abuse and Neglect, 18,* 27–36.

Famularo, R., Kinscherff, R., & Fenton, T. (1990). Symptom differences in acute and chronic presentation of childhood post-traumatic stress disorder. *Child Abuse and Neglect, 14,* 439–444.

Farley, M., & Barkan, H. (1998). Prostitution, violence, and posttraumatic stress disorder. *Women and Health, 27*(3), 37–49.

Feerick, M. M., & Haugaard, J. J. (1999). Long-term effects of witnessing marital violence for women: The contribution of childhood physical and sexual abuse. *Journal of Family Violence, 14,* 377–398.

Feldman, K. W. (1997). Evaluation of physical abuse. In M. Helfer, R. Kempe, & Krugman R. (Eds.), *The battered child* (5th ed., pp. 175–220). Chicago:University of Chicago Press.

Fiering, C., Taska, L., & Lewis, M. (1998). The role of shame and attributional style in children's and adolescents' adaptation to sexual abuse. *Child Maltreatment, 3,* 129–142.

Fiering, C., Taska, L., & Lewis, M. (2002). Adjustment following sexual abuse discovery: The role of shame and attributional style. *Developmental Psychology, 38,* 79–92.

Finkelhor, D. (1984). *Child sexual abuse: New theories and research.* New York: Free Press.

Finkelhor, D. (1986). Sexual abuse: Beyond the family system approach. In T. S. Trepper & M. J. Barrett (Eds.), *Treating incest: A multiple systems perspective* (pp. 53–65). New York: Haworth Press.

Finkelhor, D. (1988). The trauma of child sexual abuse: Two models. In G. E. Wyatt & G. J. Powell (Eds.), *Lasting effects of child sexual abuse* (pp. 61–82). Beverly Hills, CA: Sage.

Finkelhor, D., Asidigian, N., & Dzuiba-Leatherman, J. (1995). The effectiveness of victimization prevention instruction: An evaluation of children's responses to actual threats and assaults. *Child Abuse and Neglect, 19,* 141–153.

Finkelhor, D., & Browne, A. (1988). Assesesing the long-term inpact of child sexual abuse: A review and conceptualization. In L. Walker (Eds.), *Handbook on sexual abuse of children* (pp. 55–71). New York: Springer.

Finkelhor, D., & Dziuba-Leatherman, J. (1994). Victimization prevention programs: A national survey of children's exposure and reactions. *Child Abuse and Neglect, 19,* 129–139.

Flett, G. L., & Hewitt, P. L. (2002). Personality factors and substance abuse in relationship violence and child abuse: A review and theoretical analysis. In C. Wekerle & A.-M. Wall (Eds.), *The violence and addiction equation: Theoretical and clinical issues in substance abuse and relationship violence* (pp. 68–101). New York: Brunner-Routledge.

Flisher, A. J., Kramer, R. A., Hoven, C. W., & Greenwald, S. (1997). Psychosocial characteristics of physically abused children and adolescents. *Journal of the American Academy of Child and Adolescent Psychiatry, 36,* 123–131.

Fluke, J. D., Yuan, Y. T., & Edwards, M. (1999). Recurrence of maltreatment: An application of the National Child Abuse and Neglect Data System (NCANDS). *Child Abuse and Neglect, 7,* 633–650.

Foa, E. B., & Kozak, M. J. (1986). Emotional processing of fear: Exposure to corrective information. *Psychological Bulletin, 99,* 20–35.

Foa, E. B., Steketee, G., & Rothbaum, B. O. (1989). Behavioral/cognitive conceptualizations of post-traumatic stress disorder. *Behavior Therapy, 20,* 155–176.

Ford, J. D., Racusin, R., Ellis, C. G., Daviss, W. B., Reiser, J., Fleischer, A., & Thomas, J. (2000). Child maltreatment, other trauma exposure, and posttraumatic symptomatology among children with oppositional defiant and attention deficit hyperactivity disorders. *Child Maltreatment, 5,* 205–217.

Fossati, A., Madeddu, F., & Maffei, C. (1999). Borderline personality disorder and childhood sexual abuse: A meta-analytic study. *Journal of Personality Disorders, 13,* 268–280.

Francis, C. R., Hughes, H. M., & Hitz, L. (1992). Physically abusive parents and the 16–PF: A preliminary psychological typology. *Child Abuse and Neglect, 16,* 673–691.

Freyd, J. J. (1994). Betrayal-trauma: Traumatic amnesia as an adaptive response to childhood abuse. *Ethics and Behavior, 4,* 307–329.

Freyd, J. J. (1996). *Betrayal trauma: The logic of forgetting childhood abuse.* Cambridge, MA: Harvard University Press.

Freyd, J. J. (1997). Violations of power, adaptive blindness and betrayal trauma theory. *Feminism and Psychology, 7,* 22–32.

Freyd, J. J., & DePrince, A. P. (2001). Perspectives on memory for trauma and cognitive processes associated with dissociative tendencies. *Journal of Aggression, Maltreatment, and Trauma, 4,* 137–163.

Friedrich, W. N. (1990). *Psychotherapy of sexually abused children and their families.* New York: Norton.

Friedrich, W. N. (1993). Sexual behavior in sexually abused children. *Violence Update, 3,* 1, 5, 7.

Friedrich, W. N., & Einbender, A. J. (1983). The abused child: A psychological review. *Journal of Consulting and Clinical Psychology, 12,* 244–256.

Friedrich, W. N., Jaworski, T. M., Huxsahl, J. E., & Bengtson, B. S. (1997). Dissociative and sexual behaviors in children and adolescents with sexual abuse and psychiatric histories. *Journal of Interpersonal Violence, 12,* 155–171.

Frodi, A., & Lamb, M. (1980). Child abusers responses to infant smiles and cries. *Child Development, 51,* 238–241.

Frothingham, T. E., Hobbs, C. J., Wynne, T. M., Yee, L., Goyal, A., & Wadsworth, D. J. (2000). Follow up study eight years after diagnosis of sexual abuse. *Archives of Disease in Childhood, 83,* 132–134.

Gaensbauer, T. J. (1982). Regulation of emotional expression in infants from two contrasting caretaking environments. *Journal of the American Academy of Child Psychiatry, 21,* 163–171.

Gaensbauer, T. J., Mrazek, D. A., & Harmon, R. J. (1980). Emotional expression in abused and/or neglected infants. In N. Frude (Ed.), *Psychological approaches to child abuse* (pp. 120–135). London: Batsford.

Galaif, E. R., Stein, J. A., Newcomb, M. D., & Bernstein, D. P. (2001). Gender differences in the prediction of problem alcohol use in adulthood: Exploring the influence of family factors and childhood maltreatment. *Journal of Studies on Alcohol, 62,* 486–493.

Garbarino, J., Drew, N., Kostelny, K., & Pardo, C. (1992). *Children in danger.* San Francisco: Jossey-Bass.

Garfinkel, P. E., Lin, E., Goering, P., Spegg. C., Goldbloom, D. S., Kennedy, S., Kaplan, A. S., & Woodside, D. B. (1995). Bulimia nervosa in a Canadian community sample: prevalence and comparison of subgroups. *American Journal of Psychiatry, 152*(7), 1052–1058.

Garland, A. F., Hough, R. L., Landsverk, J. A., McCabe, K. M., Yeh, M., Granger, W. C., & Reynolds, B. J. (2000). Racial/ethnic variations in mental health care utilization among children in foster care. *Children's Services: Social Policy, Research, and Practice, 3,* 133–146.

Gershenson, H. P., Musick, J. S., Ruch-Ross, H. S., Magee, V., Rubino, K. K., & Rosenberg, D. (1989). The prevalence of coercive sexual experience among teenage mothers. *Journal of Interpersonal Violence, 4,* 204–219.

Glaser, D. (2000). Child abuse and neglect and the brain: A review. *Journal of Child Psychology and Psychiatry, 41,* 97–116.

Glisson, C. (1994). The effects of services coordination teams on outcomes for children in state custody. *Administration in Social Work, 18,* 1–23.

Glisson, C. (1996). Judicial and service decisions for children entering state custody: The limited role of mental health. *Social Service Review, 70*(2), 257–281.

Glod, C. A., Teicher, M. H., Hartman, C. R., & Harakal, T. (1997). Increased nocturnal activity and impaired sleep maintenance in abused children. *Journal of the American Academy of Child and Adolescent Psychiatry, 36,* 1236–1243.

Graham, S., Weiner, B., Cobb, M., & Henderson, T. (2001). An attributional analysis of child abuse among low-income African American mothers. *Journal of Social and Clinical Psychology, 20,* 233–257.

Graham-Bermann, S. A. (2000). Evaluating interventions for children exposed to family violence. *Journal of Aggression, Maltreatment and Trauma, 4,* 191–216.

Hansen, D. J., Pallotta, G. M., Tishelman, A. C., Conaway, L. P., & MacMillan, V. M. (1988). Parental problem-solving skills and child behavior problems: A comparison of physically abusive, neglectful, clinic, and community families. *Journal of Family Violence, 4,* 353–368.

Harrison, P. A., Fulkerson, J. A., & Beebe, T. J. (1997). Multiple substance use among adolescent physical and sexual abuse victim. *Child Abuse and Neglect, 21,* 529–539.

Hart, J., Gunnar, M., & Cicchetti, D. (1995). Salivary cortisol in maltreated children: Evidence of relations between neuroendocrine activity and social competence. *Development and Psychopathology, 7,* 11–26.

Hartman, C. R., & Burgess, A. W. (1989). Sexual abuse of children: Causes and consequences. In D. Cicchetti & V. Carlson (Eds.), *Child maltreatment: Theory and research on the causes and consequences of child abuse and neglect* (pp. 95–128). New York: Cambridge University Press.

Haviland, M. G., Sonne, J. L., & Woods, L. R. (1995). Beyond posttraumatic stress disorder: Object relations and reality testing disturbances in physically and sexually abused adolescents. *Journal of the American Academy of Child and Adolescent Psychiatry, 34*(8), 1054–1059.

Heche, A. (2001). *Call me crazy.* New York: Scribner.

Heck, C., & Walsh, A. (2000). The effects of maltreatment and family structure on minor and serious delinquency. *International Journal of Offender Therapy and Comparative Criminology, 44,* 178–193.

Heim, C., Newport, D. J., Heit, S., Graham, Y. P., Wilcox, M., Bonsall, R., Miller, A. H., & Charles, B. (2000). Pituitary–adrenal and autonomic responses to stress in women after sexual and physical abuse in childhood. *Journal of the American Medical Association, 284,* 592–597.

Helfer, R. E. (1982). A review of the literature on the prevention of child abuse and neglect. *Child Abuse and Neglect, 6,* 251–261.

Heller, S. S., Larrieu, J. A., D'Imperio, R., & Boris, N. W. (1999). Research on resilience to child maltreatment: Empirical considerations. *Child Abuse and Neglect, 23*, 321–338.

Hennessy, K. D., Rabideau, G. J., Cicchetti, D., & Cummings, E. M. (1994). Responses of physically abused and nonabused children to different forms of interadult anger. *Child Development, 65*, 815–828.

Herman, J. L. (1992). *Trauma and recovery: The aftermath of violence—from domestic abuse to political terror*. New York: Basic Books.

Herrenkohl, E. C., Herrenkohl, R. C., Egolf, B. P., & Russo, M. J. (1998). The relationship between early maltreatment and teenage parenthood. *Journal of Adolescence, 21*, 291–303.

Herrenkohl, R. C., Egolf, B. P., & Herrenkohl, E. C. (1997). Preschool antecedents of adolescent assaultive behavior: A longitudinal study. *American Journal of Orthopsychiatry, 67*, 422–432.

Hildyard, K., & Wolfe, D. A. (2002). Child neglect: Developmental issues and outcomes. *Child Abuse and Neglect, 26*, 679–695.

Hillson, J. M. C., & Kuiper, N. A. (1994). A stress and coping model of child maltreatment. *Clinical Psychology Review, 14*, 261–285.

Hoffman-Plotkin, D., & Twentyman, C. T. (1984). A multimodal assessment of behavioral and cognitive deficits in abused and neglected preschoolers. *Child Development, 55*, 794–802.

Horowitz, M. J. (1986). *Stress response syndromes* (2nd ed.). Northdale, NJ: Aronson.

Hotaling, G. T., Straus, M. A., & Lincoln, A. J. (1990). Intrafamily violence and crime and crime outside the family. In M. A. Straus & R. J. Gelles (Eds.), *Physical violence in American families: Risk factors and adaptations to violence in 8,145 families* (pp. 431–470). New Brunswick, NJ: Transaction.

Howes, P. W., Cicchetti, D., Toth, S. L., & Rogosch, F. A. (2000). Affective, organizational, and relational characteristics of maltreating families: A systems perspective. *Journal of Family Psychology, 14*, 95–110.

Humphrey, J. A., & White, J. W. (2000). Women's vulnerability to sexual assault from adolescence to young adulthood. *Journal of Adolescent Health, 27*, 419–424.

International Labor Organization. (2001). Reports on facts, pros and cons of child labor. Available online http://www.ilo.org/public/english/z30actra/child/index.htm

Ireland, T., & Widom, C. S. (1994). Childhood victimization and risk for alcohol and drug arrests. *International Journal of the Addictions, 29*, 235–274.

Ito, Y., Teicher, M. H., Glod, C. A., & Ackerman, E. (1998). Preliminary evidence for aberrant cortical development in abused children: A quantitative EEG study. *Journal of Neuropsychiatry and Clinical Neurosciences, 10*, 298–307.

Jacoby, M., Gorenflo, D., Wunderlich, C., & Eyler, E. (1999). Rapid repeat pregnancy and experiences of interpersonal violence among low-income adolescents. *American Journal of Preventive Medicine, 16*, 318–321.

Janoff-Bulman, R. (1979). Characterological versus behavioral self-blame: Inquiries into depression and rape. *Journal of Personality and Social Psychology, 37*, 1798–1809.

Jasinski, J. L., Williams, L. M., & Siegel, J. (2000). Childhood physical and sexual abuse as risk factors for heavy drinking among African-American women: A prospective study. *Child Abuse and Neglect, 24*, 1061–1071.

Jessor, R. (1993). Successful adolescent development among youth in high-risk settings. *American Psychologist, 48*, 117–126.

Johnson, J. G., Cohen, P., Brown, J., Smailes, E. M., & Bernstein, D. P. (1999). Childhood maltreatment increases risk for personality disorders during early adulthood. *Archives of General Psychiatry, 56*, 600–606.

Johnson, J. G., Smailes, E. M., Cohen, P., Brown, J., & Bernstein, D. P. (2000). Associations between four types of childhood neglect and personality disorder symptoms during adolescence and early adulthood: Findings of a community-based longitudinal study. *Journal of Personality Disorders, 14*, 171–187.

Kang, S., Magura, S. Laudet, A., & Whitney, S. (1999). Adverse effect of child abuse victimization among substance-using women in treatment. *Journal of Interpersonal Violence, 14*, 657–670.

Kaplan, S. J., Pelcovitz, D., Salzinger, S., Mandel, F., & Weiner, M. (1997). Adolescent physical abuse and suicide attempts. *Journal of the American Academy of Child and Adolescent Psychiatry, 36*(6), 799–808.

Kaufman, J., Birmaher, B., Perel, J., Dahl, R., Stull, S., Brent, D., Trubnick, L., & Ryan, N. (1998). Serotonergic functioning in depressed abused children: Clinical and familial correlates. *Biological Psychiatry, 44*, 973–981.

Kaufman, J., & Charney, D. (2001). Effects of early stress on brain structure and function: Implications for understanding the relationship between child maltreatment and depression. *Development and Psychopathology, 13*, 451–472.

Kaufman, J., Cooke, A., Arny, L., Jones, B., & Pittinsky, T. (1994). Problems defining resiliency: Illustrations from the study of maltreated children. *Development and Psychopathology, 6*, 215–229.

Kaufman, J., & Henrich, C. (2000). Exposure to violence and early childhood trauma. In C. H. Zeanah, Jr. (Ed.), *Handbook of infant mental health* (2nd ed., pp. 195–208). New York: Guilford Press.

Kaufman, J., & Zigler, E. (1989). The intergenerational transmission of child abuse and the prospect of predicting future abusers. In D. Cicchetti & V. Carlson (Eds.), *Child maltreatment: Research and theory on the causes and consequences of child abuse and neglect* (pp. 129–150). New York: Cambridge University Press.

Kelley, B. T., Thornberry, T. P., & Smith, C. A. (1997, August). In the wake of childhood maltreatment. *OJJDP Juvenile Justice Bulletin*, pp. 1–15.

Kellogg, N. D., Hoffman, T. J., & Taylor, E. R., (1999). Early sexual experiences among pregnant and parenting adolescents. *Adolescence, 34*, 293–303.

Kempe, C. H., Silverman, F. N., Steele, B. F., Droegenmueller, W., & Silver, H. K. (1962). The battered child syndrome. *Journal of the American Medical Association, 181*, 17–24.

Kendall-Tackett, K. A., & Eckenrode, J. (1996). The effects of neglect on academic achievement and disciplinary problems: A developmental perspective. *Child Abuse and Neglect, 20*, 161–169.

Kendall-Tackett, K. A., & Eckenrode, J. (1997). The effects of neglect on academic achievment and disciplinary problems: A developmental perspective. In G. Kaufman Kantor & J. L. Jasinski (Eds.), *Out of darkness: Contemporary perspectives on family violence* (pp. 105–112). Thousand Oaks, CA: Sage.

Kendall-Tackett, K. A., Williams, L. M., & Finkelhor, D. (1993). Impact of sexual abuse on children. *Psychological Bulletin, 113*, 164–180.

Kendler, K. S., Bulik, C. M., Silberg, J., Hettema, J. M., Myers, J., & Prescott, C. A. (2000). Childhood sexual abuse and adult psychiatric and substance use disorders in women: An epidemiological and cotwin control analysis. *Archives of General Psychiatry*, *57*, 953–959.

Kerr, M. A., Black, M. M., & Krishnakumar, A. (2000). Failure-to-thrive, maltreatment and the behavior and development of 6–year-old children from low-income, urban families: A cumulative risk model. *Child Abuse and Neglect*, *24*, 587–598.

Kessler, R. C., Sonnega, A., Bromet, E., Hughes, M., & Nelson, C. B. (1995). Posttraumatic stress disorder in the National Comorbidity Survey. *Archives of General Psychiatry*, *52*(12), 1048–1060.

Kilpatrick, D. G., Acierno, R., Saunders, B., Resnick, H. S., Best, C. L., & Schnurr, P. P. (2000). Risk factors for adolescent substance abuse and dependence: Data from a national sample. *Journal of Consulting and Clinical Psychology*, *68*(1), 19–30.

Kiser, L. J., Heston, J., Millsap, P. A., & Pruitt, D. B. (1991). Physical and sexual abuse in childhood: Relationship with post-traumatic stress disorder. *Journal of the American Academy of Child and Adolescent Psychiatry*, *30*, 776–783.

Kivlin, J. D., Simons, K. B., Lazoritz, S., & Ruttum, M. S. (2000). Shaken baby syndrome. *Ophthalmology*, *107*, 1246–1254.

Koenig, A. L., Cicchetti, D., & Rogosch, F. A. (2000). Child compliance/noncompliance and maternal contributors to internalization in maltreating and non-maltreating dyads. *Child Development*, *71*, 1018–1032.

Kolko, D. J. (1992). Characteristics of child victims of physical violence: Research findings and clinical implications. *Journal of Interpersonal Violence*, *7*, 244–276.

Kolko, D. J. (2002). Child physical abuse. In J. E. B. Myers, L. Berliner, J. Briere, C. T. Hendrix, C. Jenny, & T. A. Reid (Eds.), *The APSAC handbook on child maltreatment* (pp. 21–54). Thousand Oaks, CA: Sage.

Kolko, D., Moser, J., & Weldy, S. (1990). Medical/health histories and physical evaluation of physically and sexually abused child psychiatric patents: A controlled study. *Journal of Family Violence*, *5*, 249–266.

Koverola, C., Pound, J., Heger, A., & Lytle, C. (1993). Relationship of child sexual abuse to depression. *Child Abuse and Neglect*, *17*, 393–400.

Langeland, W., & Hartgers, C. (1998). Child sexual and physical abuse and alcoholism: A review. *Journal of Studies on Alcohol*, *59*, 336–348.

Leiter, J., & Johnsen, M. C. (1997). Child maltreatment and school performance declines: An event-history analysis. *American Educational Research Journal*, *34*, 563–589.

Levine, S. (2001, April 9). The price of child abuse. *U.S. News & World Report*, pp. 58–59.

Lewis, D. O., Lovely, R., Yeager, C., & Femina, D. B. (1989). Toward a theory of the genesis of violence: A follow-up study of delinquents. *Journal of the American Academy of Child and Adolescent Psychiatry*, *28*, 431–436.

Lipman, E. L., MacMillan, H. L., & Boyle, M. H. (2001). Childhood abuse and psychiatric disorders among single and married mothers. *American Journal of Psychiatry*, *158*, 73–77.

Luster, T., & Small, S. A. (1997). Sexual abuse history and problems in adolescence: Exploring the effects of moderating variables. *Journal of Marriage and the Family*, *59*, 131–142.

Luthar, S. S., Cicchetti, D., & Becker, B. (2000). The construct of resilience: A critical evaluation and guidelines for future work. *Child Development*, *71*, 543–562.

Lynch, M., & Cicchetti, D. (1991). Patterns of relatedness in maltreated and nonmaltreated children: Connections among multiple representational models. *Development and Psychopathology*, *3*, 207–226.

Macfie, J., Cicchetti, D., & Toth, S. L. (2001). The development of dissociation in maltreated preschool-aged children. *Development and Psychopathology*, *13*, 233–254.

Macfie, J., Toth, S. L., Rogosch, F. A., Robinson, J., Emde, R. N., & Cicchetti, D. (1999). Effect of maltreatment on preschoolers' narrative representations of responses to relieve distress and role reversal. *Developmental Psychology*, *35*, 460–465.

MacMillan, H. L., Fleming, J. E., Streiner, D. L., Lin, E., Boyle, M. H., Jamieson, E., Duku, E. K., Walsh, C. A., Wong, M. Y.-Y., Beardslee, W. R. (2001). Childhood abuse and lifetime psychopathology in a community sample. *American Journal of Psychiatry*, *158*, 1878–1883.

MacMillan, H. L., Fleming, J. E., Trocme, N., Boyle, M. H., Wong, R., Racine, Y. A., & Beardslee, W. R., & Offord, D. R. (1997). Prevalence of child physical and sexual abuse in the community: Results from the Ontario Health Supplement. *Journal of the American Medical Association*, *278*, 131–135.

MacMillan, H. L., & Munn, C. (2001). The sequelae of child maltreatment. *Current Opinion in Psychiatry*, *14*, 325–331.

Main, M., & George, C. (1985). Responses of abused and disadvantaged toddlers to distress in agemates: A study in the day care setting. *Developmental Psychology*, *21*, 407–412.

Maker, A. H., Kemmelmeier, M., & Peterson, C. (1998). Long-term psychological consequences in women of witnessing parental physical conflict and experiencing abuse in childhood. *Journal of Interpersonal Violence*, *13*, 574–589.

Malinosky-Rummell, R., & Hansen, D. (1993). Long-term consequences of childhood physical abuse. *Psychological Bulletin*, *114*, 68–79.

Manly, J. T., Cicchetti, D., & Barnett, D. (1994). The impact of subtype, frequency, chronicity, and severity of child maltreatment on social competence and behavior problems. *Development and Psychopathology*, *6*, 121–143.

Manly, J. T., Kim, J. E., Rogosch, F. A., & Cicchetti, D. (2001). Dimensions of child maltreatment and children's adjustment: Contributions of developmental timing and subtype. *Developmental Psychopathology*, *13*, 759–782.

Mash, E. J., Johnson, C., & Kovitz, K. (1983). A comparison of the mother–child interactions of physically abused and non-abused children during play and task situations. *Journal of Clinical Child Psychology*, *12*, 337–346.

McCabe, C. F., & Donahue, S. P. (2000). Prognostic indicators for vision and mortality in shaken baby syndrom. *Archives of Ophthalmology*, *118*, 373–377.

McClellan, J., McCurry, C., Ronnei, M., Adams, J., Eisner, A., & Storck, M. (1996). Age of onset of sexual abuse: Relationship to sexually inappropriate behaviors. *Journal of the American Academy of Child and Adolescent Psychiatry*, *35*, 1375–1383.

McCloskey, L. A., & Stuewig, J. (2001). The quality of peer relationships among children exposed to family violence. *Development and Psychopathology*, *13*, 83–96.

McCloskey, L. A., & Walker, M. (2000). Posttraumatic stress in children exposed to family violence and single-event trauma. *Journal of the American Academy of Child and Adolescent Psychiatry, 39*, 108–115.

McClure, R. J., Davis, P. M., Meadow, S. R., & Sibert, J. R. (1996). Epidemiology of Munchausen syndrome by proxy, non-accidental poisoning, and non-accidental suffocation. *Archives of Disease in Childhood, 75*, 57–61.

McCrone, E. R., Egeland, B., Kalkoske, M., & Carlson, E. A. (1994). Relations between early maltreatment and mental representations of relationships assessed wth projective storytelling in middle childhood. *Development and Psychopathology, 6*, 99–120.

McFadyen, R. G., & Kitson, W. J. H. (1996). Language comprehension and expression among adolescents who have experienced childhood physical abuse. *Journal of Child Psychology and Psychiatry, 37*, 551–562.

McGee, R., & Wolfe, D. A. (1991). Psychological maltreatment: Towards an operational definition. *Development and Psychopathology, 3*, 3–18.

McGee, R., Wolfe, D. A., & Olson, J. (2001). Multiple maltreatment, attribution of blame, and adjustment among adolescents. *Development and Psychopathology, 13*, 827–846.

McGloin, J. M., & Widom, C. S. (2001). Resilience among abused and neglected children grown up. *Development and Psychopathology, 13*, 1021–1038.

McLeer, S. V., Deblinger, E., Atkins, M. S., Foa, E. B., & Ralphe, D. L. (1988). Post-traumatic stress disorder in sexually abused children: A prospective study. *Journal of the American Academy of Child and Adolescent Psychiatry, 27*, 650–654.

Meston, C. M., & Heiman, J. R. (2000). Sexual abuse and sexual function: An examination of sexually relevant and cognitive processes. *Journal of Consulting and Clinical Psychology, 68*(3), 399–406.

Meston, C. M., Heiman, J. R., & Trapnell, P. D. (1999). The relation between early abuse and adult sexuality. *Journal of Sex Research, 36*, 385–395.

Miller, B. A., Downs, W. R., & Testa, M. (1993). Interrelationship between victimization experiences and women's alcohol use. *Journal of Studies on Alcohol, 11*, 109–117.

Milner, J. S. (1993). Social information processing and physical child abuse. *Clinical Psychology Review, 13*, 275–294.

Milner, J. S. (1998). Individual and family characteristics associated with intrafamilial child physical and sexual abuse. In P. K. Trickett & C. J. Schellenbach (Eds.), *Violence against children in the family and community* (pp. 141–170). Washington, DC: American Psychological Association.

Milner, J. S. (2000). Social information processing and child physical abuse: Theory and research. In D. J. Hansen (Ed.), *Nebraska Symposium on Motivation: Vol. 46. Motivation and child maltreatment* (pp. 39–84). Lincoln: University of Nebraska Press.

Mohr, W. K., Lutz, M .J .N., Fantuzzo, J. W., & Perry, M. A. (2000). Children exposed to family violence: A review of empirical research from a developmental–ecological perspective. *Trauma, Violence, and Abuse, 1*, 264–283.

Morton, T. D. (1999). The increasing colorization of America's child welfare system: The overrepresentation of African-American children. *Policy and Practice of Public Human Services, 57*, 23–30.

Nadon, S. M., Koverola, C., & Schludermann, E. H. (1998). Antecendents to prostitution: Childhood victimization. *Journal of Interpersonal Violence*, 13(2), 206–221.

National Research Council. (1993). *Understanding child abuse and neglect*. Washington, DC: National Academy Press.

Nayak, M. B., & Milner, J. S. (1998). Neuropsychological functioning: Comparison of mother at high and low-risk for child abuse. *Child Abuse and Neglect, 22*, 687–703.

Neumark-Sztainer, D., Story, M., Hannan, P. J., Beuhring, T., & Resnick, M. D. (2000). Disordered eating among adolescents: Associations with sexual/physical abuse and other familial/psychosocial factors. *International Journal of Eating Disorders, 28*(3), 249–258.

Newman, M. G., Clayton, L., Zuellig, A., Cashman, L., Arrow, D., Dea, R., & Taylor, C. B. (2000). The relationship of childhood sexual abuse and depression with somatic symptoms and medical utilization. *Psychological Medicine, 30*, 1063–1077.

Nishith, P., Mechanic, M. B., & Resnick, P. A. (2000). Prior interpersonal trauma: The contribution to current PTSD symptoms in female rape victims. *Journal of Abnormal Psychology, 109*, 20–25.

Okun, A., Parker, J., & Levendosky, A. (1994). Distinct and interactive contributions of physical abuse, socioeconomic disadvantage, and negative life events to children's social, cognitive, and affective adjustment. *Development and Psychopathology, 6*, 77–98.

Olds, D., Eckenrode, J., Henderson, C. R., Jr., Kitzman, H., Powers, J., Cole, R., Sidora, K., Morris, P., Pettitt, L. M., & Luckey, D. (1997). Long-term effects of home visitation on maternal life course and child abuse and neglect: Fifteen-year follow-up of a randomized trial. *Journal of the American Medical Association, 278*, 637–643.

Olds, D., Henderson, C. R., Jr., Cole, R., Eckenrode, J., Kitzman, H., Luckey, D., Pettitt, L., Sidora, K., Morris, P., & Powers, J. (1998). Long-term follow-up of nurse home visitation on children's criminal and antisocial behavior: 15-year follow-up of a randomized controlled trial. *Journal of the American Medical Association, 280*, 1238–1244.

Olds, D., Hill, P., Robinson, J., Song, N., & Little, C. (2000). Update on home visiting for pregnant women and parents of young children. *Current Problems in Pediatrics, 30*, 107–141.

O'Leary, K. D., Malone, J., & Tyree, A. (1994). Physical aggression in early marriage: Prerelationship and relationship effects. *Journal of Consulting and Clinical Psychology, 62*(3), 594–602.

Pagelow, M. D. (1997). Child neglect and psychological maltreatment. In K. Barnett, C. Miller-Perrin, & R. Perrin (Eds.), *Family violence across the lifespan* (pp. 107–132). Thousand Oaks, CA: Sage.

Parker, J. G., & Herrera, C. (1996). Interpersonal processes in friendship: A comparison of abused and nonabused children's experiences. *Developmental Psychology, 32*, 1025–1038.

Pelcovitz, D., Kaplan, S. J., DeRosa, R. R., Mandel, F. S., & Salzinger, S. (2000). Psychiatric disorders in adolescents exposed to domestic violence and physical abuse. *American Journal of Orthopsychiatry, 70*, 360–369.

Perez, C. M., & Widom, C. S. (1994). Childhood victimization and long-term intellectual and academic outcomes. *Child Abuse and Neglect, 18*, 617–633.

Peters, S. D. (1988). Child sexual abuse and later psychological problems. In G. E. Wyatt & G. J. Powell (Eds.), *Lasting effects of child sexual abuse* (pp. 101–117). Newbury Park, CA: Sage.

Pilowsky, D. (1995). Psychopathology among children placed in family foster care. *Psychiatric Services, 46*, 906–910.

Pollak, S. D., Cicchetti, D., Hornung, K., & Reed, A. (2000). Recognizing emotion in faces: Developmental effects of child abuse and neglect. *Developmental Psychology, 36,* 679–688.

Pollak, S., Cicchetti, D., Klorman, R., & Brumaghim, J. T. (1997). Cognitive brain event-related potentials and emotion processing in maltreated children. *Child Development, 68,* 773–787.

Prentsky, R. A., Harris, B., Frizell, K., & Righthand, S. (2000). An actuarial procedure for assessing risk with juvenile sex offenders. *Sexual Abuse: Journal of Research and Treatment, 12,* 71–93.

Putnam, F. W. (1993). Dissociative disorders in children: Behavioral profiles and problems. *Child Abuse and Neglect, 17,* 39–45.

Putnam, F. W., & Trickett, P. K. (1993). Child sexual abuse: A model of chronic trauma. *Psychiatry: Interpersonal and Biological Processes, 56,* 82–95.

Radbill, S. X. (1968). A history of child abuse and infanticide. In R. E. Helfer & C. H. Kempe (Eds.), *The battered child* (pp. 3–17). Chicago: University of Chicago Press.

Reppucci, N., & Haugaard, J. (1989). Prevention of child sexual abuse: Myth or reality? *American Psychologist, 44,* 1266–1275.

Resnick, H. S., Kilpatrick, D. G., Dansky, B. S., Sanders, B. E., & Best, C. L. (1993). Prevalence of civilian trauma and post-traumatic stress disorder in a representative national sample of women. *Journal of Consulting and Clinical Psychology, 61,* 984–991.

Rodriquez, N., Vande Kemp, H., & Foy, D. W. (1998). Posttraumatic stress disorder in survivors of childhood sexual and physical abuse: A critical review of the empirical research. *Journal of Child Sexual Abuse, 17*(2), 17–45.

Rogosch, F. A., Cicchetti, D., & Aber, J. L. (1995). The role of child maltreatment in early deviations in cognitive and affective processing abilities and later peer relationship problems. *Development and Psychopathology, 7,* 591–609.

Rowe, E., & Eckenrode, J. (1999). The timing of academic difficulties among maltreated and nonmaltreated chidren. *Child Abuse and Neglect, 8,* 813–832.

Salter, A. C. (1988). *Treating child sex offenders and victims: A practical guide.* Beverly Hills, CA: Sage.

Salzinger, S., Feldman, R. S., Hammer, M., & Rosario, M. (1993). The effects of physical abuse on children's social relationships. *Child Development, 64,* 169–187.

Salzinger, S., Feldman, R. S., Ng-Mak, D. S., Mojoca, E., & Stockhammer, T. F. (2001). The effect of physical abuse on children's social and affective status: A model of cognitive and behavioral processes explaining the association. *Development and Psychopathology, 13,* 805–825.

Salzinger, S., Kaplan, S., Pelcovitz, D., Samit, C., & Krieger, R. (1984). Parent and teacher assessment of children's behavior in child maltreating families. *Journal of the American Academy of Child Psychiatry, 23,* 458–464.

Sas, L., Hurley, P., Hatch, A., Malla, S., & Dick, T. (1993). *Three years after the verdict: A longitudinal study of the social and psychological adjustment of child witnesses referred to the Child Witness Project* (Final report prepared for the Family Violence Prevention Division, Health and Welfare Canada, No. FVDS #4887-06-91-026). Ottawa: Health and Welfare Canada.

Schneider-Rosen, K., Braunwald, K., Carlson, V., & Cicchetti, D. (1985). Current perspectives in attachment theory: Illustrations from the study of maltreated infants. In I. Bretherton & E. Waters (Eds.), Growing points in attachment theory and research. *Monographs of the Society for Research in Child Development, 50*(1–2, Serial No. 209), 194–210.

Schneider-Rosen, K., & Cicchetti, D. (1991). Early self-knowledge and emotional development: Visual self-recognition and affective reactions to mirror self-image in maltreated and nonmaltreated toddlers. *Developmental Psychology, 27,* 471–478.

Schreier, H. A., & Libow, J. A. (1993). *Hurting for love: Munchausen by Proxy syndrome.* New York: Guilford Press.

Schumacher, J. A., Smith-Slep, A. M., & Heyman, R. E. (2001). Risk factors for child neglect. *Aggression and Violent Behavior, 6,* 231–254.

Scott, K. D. (1992). Childhood sexual abuse: Impact on a community's mental health status. *Child Abuse and Neglect, 16,* 285–295.

Sedlak, A. J., & Broadhurst, D. D. (1996, September). *Third national incidence study of child abuse and neglect: Final report.* Washington, DC: U.S. Department of Health and Human Services.

Seto, M. C., & Barbaree, H. E. (1999). Psychopathy, treatment behavior, and sex offender recidivism. *Journal of Interpersonal Violence, 14,* 1235–1248.

Shaffer, D., Fisher, P., Lucas, C. P., Dulcan, M. K., & Schwab-Stone, M. E. (2000). NIMH Diagnostic Interview Schedule for Children, Version IV (NIMH DISC-IV): Description of differences from previous versions, and reliability of some common diagnoses. *Journal of the American Academy of Child and Adolescent Psychiatry, 39,* 28–38.

Shalhoub-Kevorkian, N. (1999). The politics of disclosing female sexual abuse: A case study of Palestinian society. *Child Abuse and Neglect, 23,* 1275–1293.

Shirk, S. R. (1988). The interpersonal legacy of physical abuse of children. In M. Straus (Ed.), *Abuse and victimization across the lifespan* (pp. 57–81). Baltimore: Johns Hopkins University Press.

Shonk, S. M., & Cicchetti, D. (2001). Maltreatment, competency deficits, and risk for academic and behavioral adjustment. *Developmental Psychology, 37,* 3–17.

Silverman, A., Reinherz, H., & Giaconia, R. (1996). The long-term sequelae of child and adolescent abuse: A longitudinal community study. *Child Abuse and Neglect, 20,* 709–723.

Singer, M. I., Hussey, D. L., & Strom, K. J. (1992). Grooming the victim: An analysis of a perpetrator's seduction letter. *Child Abuse and Neglect, 16,* 877–886.

Smetana, J. G., Daddis, C., Toth, S. L., Cicchetti, D., Bruce, J., & Kane, P. (1999). Effects of provocation on maltreated and nonmaltreated preschoolers' understanding of moral transgressions. *Child Development, 55,* 277–287.

Smetana, J. G., & Kelly, M. (1989). Social cognition in maltreated children. In D. Cicchetti & V. Carlson (Eds.), *Child maltreatment: Theory and research on the causes and consequences of child abuse and neglect* (pp. 620–646). New York: Cambridge University Press.

Smetana, J. G., Kelly, M., & Twentyman, C. (1984). Abused, neglected, and nonmaltreated children's judgments of moral and social transgressions. *Child Development, 55,* 277–287.

Smetana, J. G., Toth, S. L., Cicchetti, D., Bruce, J., Kane, P., & Daddis, C. (1999). Maltreated and nonmaltreated preschoolers' conceptions of hypothetical and actual moral transgressions. *Developmental Psychology, 35,* 269–281.

Smith, C., & Thornberry, T. P. (1995). The relationship between childhood maltreatment and adolescent involvement in delinquency. *Criminology, 33*, 451–477.

Springs, F. E., & Friedrich, W. N. (1992). Health risk behaviors and medical sequelae of childhood sexual abuse. *Mayo Clinic Proceedings, 67*, 1–6.

Sroufe, L. A., & Fleeson, J. (1986). Attachment and the construction of relationships. In W. W. Hartup & Z. Rubin (Eds.), *Relationships and development* (pp. 51–71). Hillsdale, NJ: Erlbaum.

Sroufe, L. A., & Rutter, M. (1984). The domain of developmental psychopathology. *Child Development, 55*, 17–29.

Steiger, H., Leung, F. Y. K., & Houle, L. (1992). Relationships among borderline features, body dissatisfaction, and bulimic symptoms in nonclinical females. *Addictive Behaviors, 17*, 397–406.

Stewart, S. H., & Israeli, A. L. (2002). Substance abuse and co-occurring psychiatric disorders in victims of intimate violence. In C. Wekerle & A.-M. Wall (Eds.), *The violence and addiction equation: Theoretical and clinical issues in substance abuse and relationship violence* (pp. 102–126). New York: Brunner-Routledge.

Stouthamer-Loeber, M., Loeber, R., Homish, D. L., & Wei, E. (2001). Maltreatment of boys and the development of disruptive and delinquent behavior. *Development and Psychopathology, 13*, 941–956.

Strathearn, L., Gray, P. H., O'Callaghan, M. J., & Wood, D. O. (2001). Childhood neglect and cognitive development in extremely low birth weight infants: A prospective study. *Pediatrics, 108*, 142.

Straus, M. A., & Donnelly, D. A. (1994). *Beating the devil out of them: Corporal punishment in American families*. New York: Lexington Books/Macmillan.

Straus, M. A., & Gelles, R. J. (1986). Societal change and change in family violence from 1975 to 1985 as revealed by two national surveys. *Journal of Marriage and the Family, 48*, 465–479.

Straus, M. A., & Kantor, G. K. (1994). Corporal punishment of adolescents by parents: A risk factor in the epidemiology of depression, suicide, alcohol abuse, child abuse, and wife beating. *Adolescence, 29*, 543–561.

Sullivan, P. M., & Knutson, J. F. (2000). Maltreatment and disabilities: A population-based epidemiological study. *Child Abuse and Neglect, 24*, 1257–1273.

Terr, L. C. (1991). Childhood traumas: An outline and overview. *American Journal of Psychiatry, 148*, 10–20.

Thompson, K. M., & Braaten-Antrim, R. (1998). Youth maltreatment and gang involvement. *Journal of Interpersonal Violence, 13*, 328–345.

Thompson, R. A. (1995). *Preventing child maltreatment through social support: A critical analysis*. Thousand Oaks, CA: Sage.

Thornberry, T. P., Ireland, T. O., & Smith, C. A. (2001). The importance of timing: The varying impact of childhood and adolescent maltreatment on multiple problem outcomes. *Development and Psychopathology, 13*, 957–980.

Toth, S. L., Cicchetti, D., Macfie, J., & Emde, R. N. (1997). Representations of self and other in the narratives of neglected, physically abused, and sexually abused preschoolers. *Development and Psychopathology, 9*, 781–796.

Toth, S. L., Cicchetti, D., Macfie, J., Rogosch, F. A., & Maughan, A. (2000). Narrative representations of moral-affiliative and conflictual themes and behavioral problems in maltreated preschoolers. *Journal of Clinical Child Psychology, 29*, 307–318.

Toth, S. L., Manly, J. T., & Cicchetti, D. (1992). Child maltreatment and vulnerability to depression. *Development and Psychopathology, 4*, 97–112.

Trickett, P. K., McBride-Chang, C., & Putnam, F. W. (1994). The classroom performance and behavior of sexually abused females. *Development and Psychopathology, 6*, 183–194.

Trickett, P. K., Noll, J. G., Reiffman, A., & Putnam, F. W. (2001). Variants of intrafamilial sexual abuse experience: Implications for short- and long-term development. *Development and Psychopathology, 13*, 1001–1019.

Tripp, M., & Petrie, T. A. (2001). Sexual abuse and eating disorders: A test of a conceptual model. *Sex Roles: A Journal of Research, 44*, 17–32.

Trocmé, N., & Wolfe, D. A. (2001). *Child maltreatment in Canada: Selected results from the Canadian Incidence Study of Reported Child Abuse and Neglect*. Ottawa: Minister of Public Works and Government Services Canada.

Trzepacz, P. T., & Baker, R. W. (1993). *The Psychiatric Mental Status Examination*. New York: Oxford University Press.

Tyler, K. A., Hoyt, D. R., & Whitbeck, L. B. (2000). The effects of early sexual abuse on later sexual victimization among female homeless and runaway adolescents. *Journal of Interpersonal Violence, 15*(3), 235–250.

U.S. Department of Health and Human Services (DHHS), National Center on Child Abuse and Neglect. (2001). *Child maltreatment 1999: Reports from the states to the National Center on Child Abuse and Neglect*. Washington, DC: U.S. Government Printing Office. (Available online: http://www.axf.dhhs.goc/programs/cb/publications/cm99/high.htm)

United Nations Children's Fund (UNICEF). (2000). [Online]. Available: http://www.unicef.org/lac/ingles/urgente/deten.htm

United Nations (UN) General Assembly. (1989, November 17). *Adoption of a convention on the rights of the Child*. New York: Author.

Veltman, M. W. M., & Browne, K. D. (2001). Three decades of child maltreatment research: Implications for the school years. *Trauma, Violence, and Abuse, 2*, 215–239.

Waldinger, R. J., Toth, S. L., & Gerber, A. (2001). Maltreatment and internal representations of relationships: Core relationship themes in narratives of abused and neglected preschoolers. *Social Development, 10*, 41–58.

Wang, C. T., & Harding, K. (1999). *Current trends in child abuse reporting and fatalities: The results of the 1998 annual fifty state survey*. Chicago: National Committee to Prevent Child Abuse.

Waters, E., Posada, G., Crowell, J., & Lay, K. (1993). Is attachment theory ready to contribute to our understanding of disruptive behavior problems? *Development and Psychopathology, 5*, 215–224.

Wekerle, C., Hawkins, D. L., & Wolfe, D. A. (2002). *Child maltreatment and dating violence: Risk factors for adolescent alcohol and street drug use*. Manuscript submitted for publication.

Wekerle, C., & Wall, A.-M. (2002a). The overlap between intimate violence and substance abuse. In C. Wekerle & A.-M. Wall (Eds.), *The violence and addiction equation: Theoretical and clinical issues in substance abuse and relationship violence* (pp. 1–21). New York: Brunner-Routledge.

Wekerle, C., & Wall, A.-M. (2002b). Clinical and research issues in relationship violence and substance abuse. In C. Wekerle & A.-M. Wall (Eds.), *The violence and addic-*

tion equation: Theoretical and clinical issues in substance abuse and relationship violence (pp. 324–348). New York: Brunner-Routledge.

Wekerle, C., & Wall, A.-M. (Eds.). (2002c). *The violence and addiction equation: Theoretical and clinical issues in substance abuse and relationship violence*. New York: Brunner-Routledge.

Wekerle, C., & Wolfe, D. A. (1993). Prevention of child physical abuse and neglect: Promising new directions. *Clinical Psychology Review*, *13*, 501–540.

Wekerle, C., & Wolfe, D. A. (1998). The role of child maltreatment and attachment style in adolescent relationship violence. *Development and Psychopathology*, *10*, 571–586.

Wekerle, C., Wolfe, D. A., Hawkins, D. L., Pittman, A.-L., Glickman, A., & Lovald, B. E. (2001). Childhood maltreatment, posttraumatic stress symptomatology, and adolescent dating violence: Considering the value of adolescent perceptions of abuse and a trauma mediational model. *Development and Psychopathology*, *13*, 847–871.

Whiffen, V. E., & Clark, S. E. (1997). Does victimization account for sex differences in depressive symptoms? *British Journal of Clinical Psychology*, *36*, 185–193.

Whiffen, V. E., Judd, M. E., & Aube, J. A. (1999). Intimate relationships moderate the association between childhood sexual abuse and depression. *Journal of Interpersonal Violence*, *14*, 940–954.

Widom, C. S. (1989a). Does violence beget violence?: A critical examination of the literature. *Psychological Bulletin*, *106*, 3–28.

Widom, C. S. (1989b). The cycle of violence. *Science*, *244*, 160–165.

Widom, C. S. (1998). Child victims: Searching for opportunities to break the cycle of violence. *Applied & Preventive Psychology*, *7*(4), 225–234.

Widom, C. S. (1999). Posttraumatic stress disorder in abused and neglected children grown up. *American Journal of Psychiatry*, *156*, 1223–1229.

Widom, C. S. (2000, January). Childhood victimization: Early adversity, later psychopathology. *National Institute of Justice Journal*, pp. 2–9.

Widom, C. S., Ireland, T., & Glynn, P. J. (1995). Alcohol abuse in abused and neglected children followed-up: Are they at increased risk? *Journal of Studies on Alcohol*, *56*, 207–217.

Widom, C. S., & Kuhns, J. B. (1996). Childhood victimization and subsequent risk for promiscuity, prostitution, and teenage pregnancy: A prospective study. *American Journal of Public Health*, *86*, 1607–1612.

Wiederman, M. W., Sansone, R. A., & Sansone. L. A. (1998). History of trauma and attempted suicide among women in a primary care setting. *Violence and Victims*, *13*, 3–9.

Wolfe, D. A. (1999). *Child abuse: Implications for child development and psychopathology* (2nd ed.). Thousand Oaks, CA: Sage.

Wolfe, D. A., & Jaffe, P. (1991). Child abuse and family violence as determinants of child psychopathology. *Canadian Journal of Behavioural Science*, *23*, 282–299.

Wolfe, D. A., Jaffe, P., Jette, J., & Poisson, S. (2002). *Child abuse in institutions and organizations: Advancing professional and scientific understanding*. Manuscript submitted for publication.

Wolfe, D. A., Sas, L., & Wekerle, C. (1994). Factors associated with the development of posttraumatic stress disorder among child victims of sexual abuse. *Child Abuse and Neglect*, *18*, 37–50.

Wolfe, D. A., Scott, K., Wekerle, C., & Pittman, A.-L. (2001). Child maltreatment: Risk of adjustment problems and dating violence in adolescence. *Journal of the American Academy of Child and Adolescent Psychiatry*, *40*, 282–289.

Wolfe, D. A., & Wekerle, C. (1993). Treatment strategies for child physical abuse and neglect: A critical progress report. *Clinical Psychology Review*, *13*, 473–500.

Wolfe, D. A., Wekerle, C., Reitzel-Jaffe, D., & Gough, R. (1995). Strategies to address violence in the lives of high-risk youth. In E. Peled, P. G. Jaffe, & J. L. Edelson (Eds.), *Ending the cycle of violence: Community responses to children of battered women* (pp. 255–274). Newbury Park, CA: Sage.

Wolfe, D. A., Wekerle, C., Reitzel-Jaffe, D., & Lefebvre, L. (1998). Factors associated with abusive relationships among maltreated and nonmaltreated youth. *Development and Psychopathology*, *10*, 61–86.

Wolfe, V. V., Gentile, C., & Wolfe, D. A. (1989). The impact of sexual abuse on children: A PTSD formulation. *Behavior Therapy*, *20*, 215–228.

Wolock, I., & Magura, S. (1996). Parental substance abuse as a predictor of child maltreatment re-reports. *Child Abuse and Neglect*, *20*, 1183–1193.

Wonderlich, S. A., Crosby, R. D., Mitchell, J. E., Roberts, J. A., Haseltine, B., DeMuth, G., & Thompson, K. M. (2000). Relationship of childhood sexual abuse and eating disturbance in children. *Journal of the American Academy of Child and Adolescent Psychiatry*, *39*, 1277–1283.

World Health Organization (WHO). (1999, March). *Report of the consultation on child abuse prevention*. Geneva: Author.

Yehuda, R., Halligan, S.L., & Grossman, R. (2001). Childhood trauma and risk for PTSD: Relationship to intergenerational effects of trauma, parental PTSD, and cortisol excretion. *Development and Psychopathology*, *13*, 733–753.

Yehuda, R., Spertus, I. L., & Golier, J. A. (2001). Relationship between childhood traumatic experiences and PTSD in adults. In S. Eth (Ed.), *PTSD in children and adolescents* (pp. 117–158). Washington, DC: American Psychiatric Association.

Zelli, A., & Dodge, K. A. (1999). Personality development from the bottom up. In D. Cervone & Y. Shoda (Eds.), *The coherence of personality: Social-cognitive bases of personality consistency, variability, and organization* (pp. 94–126). New York: Guilford Press.

Zuravin, S. J., & Fontanella, C. (1999). The relationship between child sexual abuse and major depression among low-income women: A function of growing up experiences? *Child Maltreatment*, *4*, 3–12.

VI

EATING AND HEALTH-RELATED DISORDERS

CHAPTER FIFTEEN

Eating Disorders

G. Terence Wilson
Carolyn Black Becker
Karen Heffernan

Eating disorders consist of severe disturbances in eating behavior, maladaptive and unhealthy efforts to control body weight, and abnormal attitudes about body weight and shape. The two most well-established eating disorders are anorexia nervosa (AN) and bulimia nervosa (BN). The former is characterized by a refusal to maintain a normal body weight. The latter is characterized by recurrent episodes of binge eating and inappropriate behaviors designed to control body weight and shape, such as self-induced vomiting or laxative misuse. Dysfunctional attitudes toward body weight and shape are a prominent feature of both disorders. Disorders that are closely related to AN and BN, but do not meet all of the formal diagnostic criteria, are classified as "eating disorder not otherwise specified" (EDNOS) (Fairburn & Walsh, 2002). A large number of the patients seen in clinical practice would receive the diagnosis of EDNOS. However, the different variations of eating disorders that are grouped within this category are not well specified, and as a whole they have been relatively ignored in the clinical and research literature. The single exception, and perhaps the most common example of this category, is what the *Diagnostic and Statistical Manual of Mental Disorders*, fourth edition (DSM-IV) labels "binge-eating disorder" (BED) and designates in an appendix as a diagnosis provided for further study (American Psychiatric Association, 1994). This disorder is characterized by recurrent binge eating, in the absence of inappropriate weight control behaviors as in BN. In this chapter, we focus on the three disorders of AN, BN, and BED.

AN has been identified as a psychiatric disorder for well over a century (Gull, 1873). What we now know as BN was originally described by Russell (1979) in England. Shortly thereafter, "bulimia" was included as a disorder in the American Psychiatric Association's DSM-III in 1980. It is now widely accepted that BN emerged as a clinical disorder during the 1970s. This development can be seen in an analysis of referrals to prominent centers for the treatment of eating disorders in different countries (Fairburn, Hay, & Welch, 1993). For example, in Toronto the referral rates for AN between 1975 and 1986 were relatively stable, but there was a noticeable increase in referral rates for BN. The alternative view is that BN had simply not previously come to the attention of mental health professionals. According to this line of reasoning, either the disorder had been overlooked or misdiagnosed by clinicians, or people only began seeking treatment in the 1970s. These possibilities seem implausible.

The inclusion of BED within the category of EDNOS in DSM-IV (American Psychiatric Association, 1994) was in response to reports of large numbers of patients who engaged in binge eating, but who did not meet the diagnostic criteria for BN (Spitzer et al., 1992). Most patients with this disorder are overweight. In fact, Stunkard (1959) had identified the problem of binge eating in obese patients in terms very similar to the current description of BED. But this problem was largely overlooked until the 1990s.

It is important to emphasize that obesity itself is neither a psychiatric disorder nor an eating disorder (Devlin, Yanovski, & Wilson, 2000). Nonetheless, many mental health professionals continue to view obesity as a form of eating disorder. This only further stigmatizes obese people, whose condition is better viewed as a complex metabolic disorder rather than simply a behavioral problem (Wadden & Stunkard, 2002). Obese individuals may develop eating disorders, and a small fraction of patients with BN are obese. A much larger minority of obese patients engage in binge eating and receive the diagnosis of BED, as we discuss below.

DEFINITIONAL AND DIAGNOSTIC ISSUES

Binge Eating

The terms "binge" and "binge eating" refer to a form of overeating that is a core feature of the eating disorders. Binge eating occurs across the weight spectrum and is one of the diagnostic criteria of AN (the binge-eating/purging subtype), BN, and BED. DSM-IV (American Psychiatric Association, 1994, pp. 549 and 731) defines binge eating as "characterized by both of the following: (1) eating, in a discrete period of time (e.g., within any 2-hour period), an amount of food that is definitely larger than most people would eat during a similar period of time and under similar circumstances[; and] (2) a sense of lack of control over eating during the episode (e.g., a feeling that one cannot stop eating or control what or how much one is eating)." The DSM-IV requirement that a binge consist of a large amount of food is now inconsistent with the findings of several studies indicating that the amount of food consumed is not the cardinal characteristic of a binge (Pratt, Niego, & Agras, 1998). For example, Rosen, Leitenberg, Fisher, and Khazam (1986) found that one-third of their patients, who otherwise satisfied diagnostic criteria for BN, reported consuming fewer than 600 kilocalories per binge, with no relationship between the size of the self-reported binge and the accompanying anxiety.

The DSM-IV definition was adapted from the Eating Disorder Examination (EDE; Fairburn & Cooper, 1993), a semistructured clinical interview that is the "gold standard" for assessing eating disorders. Research has shown that when members of the lay public use the word "binge" to describe their eating, they are referring to the sense of loss of control and not the amount of food consumed (Beglin & Fairburn, 1992). Similarly, a study of 60 women diagnosed with BED showed that the only criterion used by the majority (82%) to define a binge was the experience of loss of control (Telch, Pratt, & Niego, 1998). It is most important that in any assessment of disordered eating, both the assessor and the patient share the same, unambiguous meaning of the nature of a binge.

The most comprehensive and valid scheme for classifying binge eating and other forms of overeating is provided by the EDE. "Objective bulimic episodes" are what the DSM-IV criteria describe as binge eating. "Subjective bulimic episodes" are similar, except that the amount of food eaten is not objectively large. The EDE terms "objective overeating" and "subjective overeating" describe parallel episodes of perceived overeating, except that there is no loss of control. These different patterns of actual and perceived overeating are not mutually exclusive. Patients with BN and BED engage in both objective and subjective bulimic episodes.

Anorexia Nervosa

DSM-IV criteria for AN are listed in Table 15.1. In contrast to previous diagnostic schemes, DSM-IV (American Psychiatric Association, 1994) has subdivided AN on the basis of the presence or absence of binge eating and purging into a "binge-eating/purging type" (in which there are regular episodes of binge eating or purging) and a "restricting type" (in which binge eating and purging do not occur regularly). The basis for this distinction is the evidence that, compared with the restricting group, those who regularly binge or purge tend to have stronger personal and family histories of obesity and higher rates of so-called "impulsive" behaviors, including stealing, drug misuse, deliberate self-harm, and lability of mood (Garner, 1993).

Bulimia Nervosa

The DSM-IV criteria for BN are presented in Table 15.2. DSM-IV subdivides BN into a "purging type" (in which there is either regular self-induced vomiting or regular misuse of laxatives

TABLE 15.1. Diagnostic Criteria for Anorexia Nervosa (AN)

A. Refusal to maintain body weight at or above a minimally normal weight for age and height (e.g., weight loss leading to maintenance of body weight less than 85% of that expected; or failure to make expected weight gain during period of growth, leading to body weight less than 85% of that expected).

B. Intense fear of gaining weight or becoming fat, even though underweight.

C. Disturbance in the way in which one's body weight or shape is experienced, undue influence of body weight or shape on self-evaluation, or denial of the seriousness of the current low body weight.

D. In postmenarcheal females, amenorrhea, i.e., the absence of at least three consecutive menstrual cycles. (A woman is considered to have amenorrhea if her periods occur only following hormone, e.g., estrogen, administration.)

Specify type:
Restricting Type: during the current episode of Anorexia Nervosa, the person has not regularly engaged in binge-eating or purging behavior (i.e., self-induced vomiting or the misuse of laxatives, diuretics, or enemas)
Binge-Eating/Purging Type: during the current episode of Anorexia Nervosa, the person has regularly engaged in binge-eating or purging behavior (i.e., self-induced vomiting or the misuse of laxatives, diuretics, or enemas)

Note. From American Psychiatric Association (1994, pp. 544–545). Copyright 1994 by the American Psychiatric Association. Reprinted by permission.

or diuretics) and a "nonpurging type" (in which such behavior is not present).

Two major community-based studies have provided mixed support for this form of subtyping. In the first study, Hay, Fairburn, and Doll (1996) studied a representative community-based sample of women between the ages of 16 and 35 years who met carefully assessed criteria for recurrent binge eating. Cluster analysis was then used to identify clinically meaningful subgroups from this sample, based on current eating disorder characteristics. Four subgroups emerged from this analysis, yielding a solution that was reproducible and had satisfactory descriptive and construct

TABLE 15.2. Diagnostic Criteria for Bulimia Nervosa (BN)

A. Recurrent episodes of binge eating. An episode of binge eating is characterized by both of the following:
   (1) eating, in a discrete period of time (e.g., within any 2-hour period), an amount of food that is definitely larger than most people would eat during a similar period of time and under similar circumstances
   (2) a sense of lack of control over eating during the episode (e.g., a feeling that one cannot stop eating or control what or how much one is eating)

B. Recurrent inappropriate compensatory behavior in order to prevent weight gain, such as self-induced vomiting; misuse of laxatives, diuretics, enemas, or other medications; fasting; or excessive exercise.

C. The binge eating and inappropriate compensatory behaviors both occur, on average, at least twice a week for 3 months.

D. Self-evaluation is unduly influenced by body shape and weight.

E. The disturbance does not occur exclusively during episodes of Anorexia Nervosa.

Specify type:
Purging Type: during the current episode of Bulimia Nervosa, the person has regularly engaged in self-induced vomiting or the misuse of laxatives, diuretics, or enemas
Nonpurging Type: during the current episode of Bulimia Nervosa, the person has used other inappropriate compensatory behaviors, such as fasting or excessive exercise, but has not regularly engaged in self-induced vomiting or the misuse of laxatives, diuretics, or enemas

Note. From American Psychiatric Association (1994, pp. 549–550). Copyright 1994 by the American Psychiatric Association. Reprinted by permission.

validity. Women in the first cluster showed a high frequency of self-induced vomiting and laxative misuse, high levels of dietary restraint, and marked concerns about body weight and shape. The women in the second cluster resembled those in the first, reporting a high frequency of objective bulimic episodes (i.e., binge eating) but little purging. They did, however, show high levels of dietary restraint and concerns about body weight and shape. Those in the third cluster had frequent subjective bulimic episodes and lower levels of purging, and those in the fourth had heterogeneous symptoms.

The Hay et al. (1996) data are consistent with the DSM-IV practice of subtyping BN according to the presence or absence of purging, since the women in the first two clusters may be regarded as having subtypes of the same core disorder rather than two separate disorders. This is because they differed mainly in terms of the severity of eating disorder features rather than the presence or absence of the features themselves. The only significant qualitative difference between the two clusters was the presence or absence of purging. Support for keeping the distinction between the purging and nonpurging types of BN rests on the finding of predictive validity: The women in the two clusters differed in their outcomes at 1 year.

The second population-based study failed to find any significant differences between individuals with BN who purged (self-induced vomiting or laxative abuse) and those who did not (Walters et al., 1993). This study compared 54 individuals who purged with 69 who did not, identified from interviews with over 1,000 pairs of twins from the population-based Virginia Twin Registry. No differences between the two groups emerged on a variety of demographic, weight-related, or personality variables. Nor were there differences in associated psychiatric disorders. In both groups, BN showed significant association with major depression, alcoholism, and AN. A strength of this study is that it examined twins, thereby allowing an analysis of genetic and nongenetic influences. Consistent with other evidence, Walters et al. (1993) found support for a genetic predisposition in BN—a finding we elaborate on below. But these data indicate that the presence of purging is not intrinsically part of this genetic predisposition. Walters et al. (1993) summarized their findings as follows:

> There was no significant association between MZ twins concordant for bulimia and purging. Purging bulimics do not appear to have a greater threshold along a liability continuum than nonpurging bulimics, because the cotwin of a purger was not at increased risk for bulimia than the cotwin of a nonpurger. If purging bulimia required a higher threshold than nonpurging, then the relatives of purgers should be at increased risk for the disorder. (p. 271)

These findings are not necessarily inconsistent with those of Hay et al. (1996). Indeed, the latter argue for the existence of a core disorder of BN, regardless of the presence of purging. Their conclusion that the subtyping based on purging versus nonpurging is warranted is based on their 1-year follow-up findings. Walters et al. (1993) did not include a test of the predictive validity of the distinction between purging and nonpurging.

DSM-IV also specifies that an individual with BN does not currently meet diagnostic criteria for AN. This has the effect of restricting the diagnosis of BN to those of average or above-average weight. The main reason for allowing the diagnosis of AN to trump that of BN concerns therapeutic implications. In the former, but not the latter, there is the need for weight gain. Furthermore, the therapeutic outlook is quite different. BN can be effectively treated in the majority of cases, with good prospects for a full and lasting recovery (Wilson & Fairburn, 2002). AN, however, remains a disorder that is resistant to successful long-term treatment (Garner, Vitousek, & Pike, 1997).

Binge-Eating Disorder

DSM-IV has included BED as an example within the general category of EDNOS and provided provisional diagnostic criteria for BED in its Appendix B (see Table 15.3). Individuals with this disorder engage in recurrent binge eating, but do not regularly engage in purging (Marcus, 1993). BED criteria do not specify any weight range, but preliminary data clearly indicate that BED, unlike BN, occurs predominantly in obese patients (Spitzer et al., 1992). Obese patients who binge are often referred to as "compulsive overeaters" in the clinical and popular literature. The literature has been marked by diagnostic variability and inconsistency in the identification of obese individuals with BED. The common denominator across the different diagnostic schemes is the phenomenon of binge eating.

The wisdom of identifying BED as a provisional new diagnosis has been widely debated. Some critics charged that it was premature to single out this particular subgroup of patients with

TABLE 15.3. Research Criteria for Binge-Eating Disorder (BED)

A. Recurrent episodes of binge eating. An episode of binge eating is characterized by both of the following:
   (1) eating, in a discrete period of time (e.g., within any 2-hour period), an amount of food that is definitely larger than most people would eat in a similar period of time under similar circumstances
   (2) a sense of lack of control over eating during the episode (e.g., a feeling that one cannot stop eating or control what or how much one is eating)

B. The binge-eating episodes are associated with three (or more) of the following:
   (1) eating much more rapidly than normal
   (2) eating until feeling uncomfortably full
   (3) eating large amounts of food when not feeling physically hungry
   (4) eating alone because of being embarrassed by how much one is eating
   (5) feeling disgusted with oneself, depressed, or very guilty after overeating

C. Marked distress regarding binge eating is present

D. The binge eating occurs, on average, at least 2 days a week for 6 months.

   Note: The method of determining frequency differs from that used by Bulimia Nervosa; future research should address whether the preferred method of setting a frequency threshold is counting the number of days on which binges occur or counting the number of episodes of binge eating.

E. The binge eating is not associated with the regular use of inappropriate compensatory behaviors (e.g., purging, fasting, excessive exercise) and does not occur exclusively during the course of Anorexia Nervosa or Bulimia Nervosa.

Note. From American Psychiatric Association (1994, p. 731).

EDNOS, and that additional research might reveal more useful or valid ways of classifying different subgroups of individuals with recurrent binge eating (Fairburn, Hay, & Welch, 1993). Other critics have suggested that there is definitional overlap between nonpurging BN and BED. Persons in both groups engage in binge eating, and recent research has shown that patients with BED are indistinguishable from those with AN and BN in terms of dysfunctional concern and preoccupation with body shape and weight (Wilfley, Schwartz, Spurrell, & Fairburn, 2000). However, research has shown that there are important differences between BED and BN.

BED differs markedly from both subtypes of BN on several important dimensions. Studies using both clinical and community samples have shown that women with BN consistently report significantly higher levels of dietary restraint than do those with BED (Striegel-Moore et al., 2001; Wilfley, Schwartz, et al., 2000). Whereas dieting precedes the onset of binge eating in virtually all cases of BN (Wilson, 2002), dieting often develops following the emergence of binge eating (Howard & Porzelius, 1999). In contrast to BN, BED is also significantly associated with obesity (Marcus, 1993). The majority of patients with BED are overweight or obese.

CLINICAL CHARACTERISTICS

Anorexia Nervosa

Core Psychopathology

A defining feature of AN is an extreme concern about body weight and shape. This is often described as a set of overvalued ideas about the importance of shape and weight, or a "morbid fear of fatness." Patients fear weight gain and may even feel overweight despite being emaciated. These concerns drive the rigid dieting or fasting that leads to dangerously low body weight. The severe dietary restriction (semistarvation) that defines AN results in several other clinical features of the disorder, including depressed mood, preoccupation with food, and ritualistic and stereotyped eating. These latter obsessional features resemble elements of obsessive–compulsive disorder (OCD). In fact, there is significant comorbidity between AN and OCD (Barbarich, in press).

Overactivity is a common characteristic of patients with AN. Excessive exercise is aimed at weight control via energy expenditure. But many patients also display a general restlessness that may not be under voluntary control (Beumont, 1995). In addition to obsessiveness, perfectionism and ascetism are common premorbid traits in patients with AN, and even persist in patients who subsequently overcome their eating disorder (Lilenfeld et al., 2000).

A principal feature of AN is the need for control (Slade, 1982). Fairburn, Shafran, and Cooper (1999) hypothesize that this need for control over eating is the primary feature of AN. Successful dieting or fasting is a means of achieving personal control over life in general. It also has a profound impact on other people in the person's environment, especially family members. Accounts of dysfunctional relationships within the families of patients with AN are commonplace (Vandereycken, 1995).

Another central feature of the psychopathology of AN is its ego-syntonic nature. It is more common for patients to come to professional attention because of the concerns of family members over their extreme weight loss than to seek help themselves. Consequently, there is a marked resistance to change; weight loss signifies for these patients a triumph of self-discipline, upon which their self-esteem depends, and weight gain is felt to be intolerable. This resistance to change is linked closely to the need for control.

Patients with the two subtypes of AN exhibit significantly different clinical characteristics. Those with the restricting subtype are highly controlled, rigid, and often obsessive. Those with the binge-eating/purging subtype alternate between periods of rigid control and impulsive behavior. The latter display significantly more psychopathology and are more likely to attempt suicide than the former.

Associated Psychopathology

Associated psychopathology is commonplace. We discuss this comorbidity below.

Medical Complications

Serious complications can emerge as a result of starvation and malnutrition in AN, beginning with the striking emaciation of these patients. Amenorrhea is invariably present in postmenarcheal patients, and other common physical signs include dry, sometimes yellowish skin (due to hypercarotenemia); lanugo (fine, downy hair) on the trunk, face, and extremities; sensitivity to cold; and hypotension, bradycardia, and other cardiovascular problems (Hsu, 1990).

Purging behaviors may result in enlarged salivary glands, erosion of dental enamel, and calluses on the dominant hand from repeated skin abrasion by teeth when a patient is using the hand to induce vomiting. More dangerously, chronic dehydration and electrolyte imbalance, particularly serum potassium depletion, may lead to hypokalemia, increasing the risk of both renal failure and cardiac arrhythmia. Osteopenia may also result from malnutrition and decreased estrogen secretion, and in early-onset AN there may be some retardation of bone growth, although with recovery this may be reversed by normal "catch-up" growth (Hsu, 1990). These potentially serious conditions make thorough medical assessment an essential part of treatment for AN.

Bulimia Nervosa

Core Psychopathology

The specific psychopathology of BN is similar to that of AN. Thus both disorders are characterized by dysfunctional concerns about body shape and weight. Individuals with BN are typically secretive about their disorder. Often a therapist is the first person to whom a patient with BN might have disclosed the problem. The reason is the intense guilt and shame these patients experience. Like those with AN, patients with BN show a cognitive style marked by rigid rules and absolutistic (all-or-nothing) thinking (Butow, Beumont, & Touyz, 1993). Patients view themselves as either completely in control or out of control, virtuous or indulgent. Food is either "good" or "bad."

However, there are important differences between the two disorders. First, BN occurs predominantly in normal-weight women, as described earlier. Second, BN is not ego-syntonic, as AN is. Although many patients with BN are ambivalent or fearful about giving up their eating disorder, they do not resist change to the extent that patients with AN do.

The eating behavior of patients with BN has been studied directly under controlled laboratory conditions by Walsh and his colleagues. Patients were instructed either to overeat or to eat normally on different occasions. Their eating was compared with that of control subjects free of any eating disorder, who were tested under the same instructions. In these studies, the patients were also asked to rate how typical these different episodes of overeating were of an actual binge (Walsh, 1993). They found that patients with BN ate significantly larger amounts of food than normal control subjects when instructed to overeat. However, the patients with BN did not differ from the normal controls in terms of relative percentages of macronutrients consumed. On average, patients consumed 47% of carbohydrates in their binge episode, compared with 46% in the controls' episode of overeating. The comparable figures for fat were 40% and 39%, respectively. These findings are consistent with those from other laboratories (Kaye et al., 1992).

The finding that patients with BN do not consume an abnormally large amount of carbohydrates during binges discredits the widespread myth that binge eating is caused by "carbohydrate craving." There is no empirical evidence to support this view, despite its continued popularity (Wilson & Latner, 2001). Typical binge foods (desserts and snacks) tend to be sweet with high fat content.

Associated Psychopathology

BN is associated with high rates of comorbid psychopathology, especially depression, substance use disorders, and personality disorders. This comorbidity is described below. Patients with BN are often stereotyped as disinhibited, impulsive people who not only lose control over food intake but also act out in other ways (e.g., substance misuse, sexual promiscuity). Some clinical findings indicate that some patients do have problems with impulse control (Lacey & Evans, 1986), but it is likely that they are a minority. Other clinical reports dispute this profile, showing low rates of acting-out behavior.

Medical Complications

Although the physical sequelae of BN can be serious, they are not nearly as severe as those of AN, characterized as the latter is by dangerously low body weight. Common physical complaints in BN include fatigue, headaches, puffy cheeks due to enlargement of the salivary glands, dental problems due to permanent erosion of teeth enamel, and finger calluses from stimulating the gag reflex to induce vomiting (Mitchell, 1995).

Electrolyte abnormalities, such as hypokalemia and hypochloremia, probably pose the most serious medical complication. Excessive laxative abuse entails the risk of a patient's becoming dependent on laxatives and suffering severe constipation on withdrawal, or even sustaining permanent damage to the colon. For these reasons, it is important that any patient who purges (by whatever means) be medically screened and have blood tests to assess electrolyte status and any fluid imbalance.

Binge-Eating Disorder

Core Psychopathology

The eating disorder psychopathology seen in BED overlaps with both AN and BN. Across all three disorders, self-worth is unduly influenced by body weight and shape (Striegel-Moore et al., 2001; Wilfley, Schwartz, et al., 2000). However, several differences set BED apart from AN and BN as discussed above. Moreover, in contrast to AN and BN, a significant number of patients with BED are male.

Laboratory studies have shown that obese patients with BED consume significantly more food than nonbingeing obese patients do when instructed either to binge or to eat normally (Marcus, 1993; Yanovski et al., 1992; Yanovski & Sebring, 1994). Consistent with the data from normal-weight patients with BN, obese patients with BED do not consume more carbohydrates during binge meals. Yanovski et al. (1992) found that their obese patients with BED consumed a greater percentage of calories as fat and a lesser percentage as protein during binge meals than patients without BED. Obese individuals with BED have more chaotic eating habits, exhibit higher levels of eating disinhibition (i.e., eating in response to emotional states), and suffer from significantly higher levels of eating disorder psychopathology than do obese persons without BED (Brody, Walsh, & Devlin, 1994; Eldredge & Agras, 1996; Wilson, Nonas, & Rosenblum, 1993; Yanovski et al., 1992). Obese persons who binge are also more likely than those who do not binge to report a history of weight cycling (Foster, Wadden, Kendall, Stunkard, & Vogt, 1996; Spitzer et al., 1992).

Associated Psychopathology

Patients with BED often have significant levels of associated Axis I and Axis II disorders as described below. This is one of the most robust differences between obese individuals who do and do not binge (Telch & Stice, 1998). However, the degree of associated psychopathology in patients with BED is often less than in patients with BN (Marcus, 1993; Wilfley et al., 2000). Studies of both clinic and community samples have shown that BED is associated with obesity (Bruce & Agras, 1992; Striegel-Moore, Wilfley, Pike, Dohm, & Fairburn, 2000). This association is not surprising, given that obese individuals with BED eat more than their counterparts without BED, both during and between binges (Yanovski & Sebring, 1994). Obesity is a major health problem in the United States. There is evidence that the presence of binge eating or BED may further complicate the treatment of obesity (Sherwood, Jeffery, & Wing, 1999; Yanovski, Gormally, Lesser, Gwirtsman, & Yanovski, 1994).

DEVELOPMENTAL COURSE AND PROGNOSIS

Anorexia Nervosa

AN typically strikes in adolescence, with evidence indicating bimodal points of onset at ages 14 and 18 years (American Psychiatric Association, 1994). The course and outcome are highly variable. Some individuals recover after a single episode. Others continue to show fluctuating patterns of restoration of normal weight and relapse. This fluctuating course is often punctuated by periods of hospitalization when these individuals' weight sinks to dangerously low levels. Still others gain weight but continue to experience BN or EDNOS. Finally, a significant minority never recover, and it is estimated that as many as 10% of patients may die from suicide or the medical complications of the disorder (American Psychiatric Association, 1994). In contrast to the other eating disorders discussed in this chapter, there are no well-established treatments that have been shown to promote lasting weight gain and recovery in these patients.

Both clinical experience and research findings suggest that adolescent patients with AN or relatively short duration respond more positively to treatment than adults, in whom the disorder has probably become chronic (Lock, le Grange, Agras, & Dare, 2001; Russell, Szmukler, Dare, & Eisler, 1987).

Bulimia Nervosa

Whereas AN typically first occurs in adolescence, the onset of BN extends from adolescence into early adulthood (Lewinsohn, Striegel-Moore, & Seeley, 2000). In most patients, binge eating develops during or after a period of restrictive dieting (Hsu, 1990); this is a consistent finding in clinical samples, and one that has implicated dieting in the etiology of the disorder as discussed below. The onset of purging typically follows the onset of binge eating.

The rigid and unhealthy dieting that precedes the development of binge eating in BN is driven by dissatisfaction with body shape and weight—the relentless desire to be thin (Fairburn, 1997; Stice, 2001). Furthermore, the presence of intense dissatisfaction with body shape and weight, together with disordered eating in early adolescence, is a significant predictor of depression in adolescent girls (Stice & Bearman, 2001).

DSM-IV states that the course of the disorder is chronic or intermittent, with periods of remission alternating with binge eating or purging (American Psychiatric Association, 1994). Fairburn, Cooper, Doll, Norman, and O'Connor (2000) conducted a 5-year study of a community-based cohort of women diagnosed with BN. Their ages ranged from 16 to 35 years, and they were rigorously assessed each 15 months. The cohort showed marked initial improvement over the first 15 months, followed by gradual improvement thereafter. At the 5-year follow-up, 15% met DSM-IV criteria for BN, while an additional 2% met criteria for AN, and 34% for EDNOS. At 5 years, fully 41% of the participants met diagnostic criteria for major depressive disorder. There was considerable instability in the eating disorder symptoms among the cohort; each year, roughly one-third remitted and another one-third relapsed.

Reliable predictors of response to treatment remain to be identified (Wilson & Fairburn, 2002). A diverse array of pretreatment patient characteristics have been proposed as predictor variables, including past history of AN or previous low body weight, low self-esteem, comorbid personality disorders, and severity of core eating disorder symptoms. The results across studies have been inconsistent, however, and are of little practical clinical value (Agras et al., 2000; Wilson & Fairburn, 2002).

A prospective study of the long-term outcome of BN, using state-of-the-art assessment, has shown that outcome is significantly determined by the type of treatment (Fairburn et al., 1993). This study compared the 5-year outcome of patients from two controlled outcome studies comparing behavior therapy (BT), cognitive-behavioral therapy (CBT), and focal psychotherapy (FPT). The BT group did poorly; 86%

were diagnosed as having an eating disorder according to DSM-III-R (American Psychiatric Association, 1987). These patients improved significantly at the end of the 5-month treatment program, but they relapsed within a year. This pattern is similar to that described by Keller, Herzog, Lavori, Bradburn, and Mahoney (1992) in their naturalistic study of clinical outcome. In contrast, patients treated with CBT or FPT fared well. The majority maintained the impressive improvement they exhibited at a 1-year follow-up (Fairburn, Jones, Peveler, Hope, & O'Connor, 1993), showing little tendency to relapse. Two-thirds no longer could be diagnosed with an eating disorder. These findings strongly dispute the notion that BN is a particularly refractory disorder that is marked by inevitable relapse. Specific psychological therapies do enable patients to make lasting recovery from this otherwise chronic disorder.

Binge-Eating Disorder

Evidence on the natural course of BED is mixed. In a 5-year prospective study, in which binge eating was assessed every 15 months, Fairburn et al. (2000) found that BED largely remitted over time. By the 5-year follow-up, the rate of BED had declined to 18%. The level of general psychiatric symptoms decreased by an average of 42%. Significantly, the rate of obesity among these individuals with BED increased from 20% to 39%.

In contrast, the McKnight longitudinal study of the course of eating disorders has obtained different results (W. S. Agras, personal communication, May 2001). Participants in this study were recruited from the community and assessed at 6-month intervals. The percentages of individuals with a full DSM-IV diagnosis of BED at follow-up years 1, 2, and 3 were 33%, 19%, and 18%, respectively. However, other related eating disorders within the EDNOS category increased to 57% in year 1, 63% in year 2, and 60% in year 3. Thus 78% of the cohort suffered from a DSM-IV eating disorder in year 3, with only 22% fully recovered.

Participants in the Fairburn et al. (2000) study were younger and less obese than those in the McKnight study, and exclusively female. The participants in the McKnight study more closely resemble the typical patient who seeks treatment in the United States and might have represented a more chronic sample. BED has proven to be stable and persistent during wait-list control periods of up to 6 months in controlled treatment outcome studies (Wilfley & Cohen, 1997).

The prognosis for the treatment of BED is good. A variety of psychological interventions have proved effective. Specialty psychological treatments (CBT and interpersonal psychotherapy) appear especially effective, with abstinence rates of roughly 60% at 1-year follow-up (Wilfley, Welch, et al., in press; Wilson & Fairburn, 2002). Although the evidence is more mixed, antidepressant medication has also been shown to have significant short-term effects in reducing BED (Wilson & Fairburn, 2002). In addition, traditional behavioral weight loss treatment has been shown to be effective (National Task Force on the Prevention and Treatment of Obesity, 2000; Stunkard, 2002).

Relatively little research has focused on identifying robust predictors of treatment outcome.

EPIDEMIOLOGY

Prevalence

Current estimates of the prevalence of AN range from 0.2% to 0.5% among young females, whereas the figure for BN is roughly 1–2% among young females (American Psychiatric Association, 1994). The prevalence of BED in the general population is 1.5–2.0% (Gotestam & Agras, 1995; Smith, Marcus, Lewis, Fitzgibbon, & Schreiner, 1998)—a figure similar to that for BN. Some 3% of obese persons in the general population meet criteria for BED (Smith et al., 1998) The presence of BED among obese patients seeking treatment is much higher. In two large multisite studies based on a self-report questionnaire, Spitzer, Yanouski, Wadden, and Wing (1993) reported a rate of 30% of BED in obese patients.

Some data suggest that the prevalence of eating disorders has risen over recent decades (Fairburn, Hay, & Welch, 1993). However, there is also the possibility that the increased rates reflect improved identification and reporting of eating disorder cases, rather than an actual increase (Hoek, 1995). It is also widely believed that eating disorders occur disproportionately more often among the middle and upper socioeconomic classes. Once again, it is unclear whether this reflects a true difference or greater access to health care among higher socioeconomic groups (Hoek, 1995).

Two general points should be noted regarding the prevalence of eating disorders. First, there appears to be an overrepresentation of eating disorders among those who not do respond to or cooperate with prevalence studies. In the Johnson-Sabine, Wood, Patton, Mann, and Wakeling (1988) study of adolescents, for example, there were no cases of AN detected in the sample, but there were at least two among those who declined to participate. This has been detected in other studies and would suggest that our current figures may be underestimating the true prevalence of eating disorders. Second, since prevalence rates in most studies are given only for cases meeting full diagnostic criteria, these do not provide a full picture of the degree of subclinical or "partial" morbidity in the population. Using a large community sample, Lewinsohn et al. (2000) compared girls who met full diagnostic criteria for AN or BN with those who had partial syndromes. For example, partial BN was defined as the presence of recurrent binge eating plus one additional criterion. The findings indicated that the two groups obtained similar results on various measures of psychopathology. Both differed significantly from a normal control group of adolescent females.

Gender Differences

Precise data on gender differences are hard to come by (Andersen, 1995). In clinical samples, approximately 5–10% of patients with eating disorders are males (Hoek, 1995). Whereas AN and BN predominantly afflict women, the female-to-male ratio among individuals with BED is 3:2 (Spitzer et al.,1992, 1993). Men and women with BED present very similar clinical profiles, with no differences on measures of specific eating disorder psychopathology (Tanofsky, Wilfley, Spurrell, Welch, & Brownell, 1997). However, males with BED may suffer from greater psychiatric comorbidity.

Sexual Orientation

Research on the role of sexual orientation in the development of eating disorders is relatively sparse. However, it is generally believed that homosexuality in males is a risk factor (Carlat, Camargo, & Herzog, 1997). This association has been explained by what is regarded to be the greater emphasis gay men place on physical appearance, body shape, and weight than heterosexual males. There is even less information on lesbians. Although some have claimed that being a lesbian protects a woman against eating disorders, the available data are mixed (Heffernan, 1996).

Meyer, Blissett, and Oldfield (2001) have hypothesized that it is level of masculinity or femininity that is linked to the development of eating disorders, rather than sexual orientation per se. A study of heterosexual and homosexual (male and female) college students provided support for this hypothesis, with a measure of femininity emerging as the variable most closely linked to disordered eating.

Athletes and Eating Disorders

It is widely believed that eating disorders are disproportionately common among female athletes (Brownell, Rodin, & Wilmore, 1992). Physical condition and build are closely tied to performance in most athletic activities. Consequently, both male and female athletes are likely to engage in weight control behaviors and abnormal eating for the purpose of enhancing performance, especially in sports such as horse racing or wrestling (which require the meeting of specific weight thresholds) and those such as gymnastics (which require low body weight). Men are less likely than women to be among the minority of athletes who do go on to develop an eating disorder, since they are more likely to engage in weight control behavior solely for instrumental purposes, and less likely to experience weight and shape as important aspects of their self-evaluation (Wilson & Eldredge, 1992). Surprisingly, however, most of the evidence is based on small and often poorly controlled studies. Rigorous, large-scale investigations with methodologically adequate measures are lacking.

Recently, Smolak, Murnen, and Ruble (2000) completed a meta-analysis of 34 studies in order to examine the relationship between athletic participation and eating disorders. The results showed that athletes were significantly more likely than nonathletes to have an eating disorder. However, the difference was small and the data were marked by heterogeneity. The group at highest risk for eating disorders consisted of elite female athletes in those sports that place an emphasis on thinness for purposes of either performance or appearance (e.g., ballet dancers, aerobic instructors, and cheerleaders). Contrary to previous analyses of the literature (e.g., Brownell

& Rodin, 1992) and some highly publicized case studies, gymnasts were no more vulnerable than nonathletes. Nonelite (noncompetitive) high school girls were less likely to have an eating disorder than nonathletes, and also reported less body image dissatisfaction.

Ethnicity and Eating Disorders

Clinical reports to date have indicated that eating disorders occur most frequently among white females (Hsu, 1990). However, Smolak and Striegel-Moore (2001) have argued that this stereotype may be inaccurate, and that there has been insufficient research on ethnic minorities in the United States.

Numerous studies have reliably shown that blacks report less body dissatisfaction than whites. The ideal body image of blacks is heavier and more flexible than that of whites. Blacks also experience less social pressure about their weight (Smolak & Striegel-Moore, 2001). Similarly, Hispanic females report less body dissatisfaction than whites, even though they and black women have the highest rates of obesity in the United States (National Heart, Lung, and Blood Institute, 1998).

Despite these differences in body image, blacks' rate of binge eating may be similar (Striegel-Moore et al., 2000). Indeed, unlike AN and BN, BED is as much of a risk for ethnically diverse women (particularly blacks) as for white women (Smith et al., 1998). However, among women reliably diagnosed with BED, blacks differ from whites on some associated eating disorder features. Consistent with other data, blacks in one study reported less dietary restraint and less concern for body shape and weight. Blacks also had a higher average body mass index and an increased frequency of binge eating (Pike, Dohm, Striegel-Moore, Wilfley, & Fairburn, 2001).

Considerable evidence exists indicating that the more "Westernized" young women from other cultures become, the more vulnerable they are to developing eating disorders. Presumably this acculturation process has its effect because they adopt the thin ideal of beauty and engage in dysfunctional dieting. For example, in a study of 369 female high school students at English-medium schools in Pakistan, Mumford, Whitehouse, and Choudry (1992) looked at 1-year prevalence and only found 1 case of BN. In a study of 204 Indian and Pakistani high school students living in England, there were 7 cases, amounting to a prevalence rate of 3.4% (Mumford, Whitehouse, & Platts, 1991). Similarly, a study that compared Arab female students at Cairo University with those at London University found higher levels of disturbed eating attitudes among those in London (Nasser, 1986). However, there is also evidence that the rates of eating disorders are as high in countries like Japan and Taiwan as in the United States (Nakamura et al., 1999).

ETIOLOGY

Biological Mechanisms

The biological factors involved in eating disorders are numerous. Because of the complex nature of eating and the mechanisms behind it, research into the biological aspects of eating disorders has had to examine the effects of dieting on neurobiology and neuroendocrine systems, in addition to identifying biological abnormalities in patients with eating disorders. Since eating behavior can effect changes in neurobiology and vice versa, determining causality has been a problem for researchers examining the biological bases of eating disorders. In many cases, it has not yet been determined whether the biological abnormalities seen in patients with eating disorders are secondary to the dysregulated eating behavior or whether they play a causal role. It is clear, however, that a number of neurochemical disturbances are associated with both BN and AN, and that disturbances frequently persist after recovery from either disorder.

Anorexia Nervosa

In general, studies have consistently reported low levels of cerebrospinal fluid (CSF) norepinephrine and its metabolite, 3-methoxy-4-hydroxyphenyl glycol (MHPG), in patients with AN (Fava, Copeland, Schweiger, & Herzog, 1989; Pirke, 1996). In the early stages of weight gain, norepinephrine levels appear to return to normal. These results have generally been interpreted as indicating that low norepinephrine concentrations in AN are the result of low body weight. A few studies indicate that patients with AN may enter treatment with normal or even elevated levels of norepinephrine. These levels, however, appear to drop within the first few weeks of treatment and dietary stabilization (Lesem, George, Kaye, Goldstein, & Jimerson,

1989; Pirke, 1996). Although weight gain appears to return norepinephrine levels to normal in the short term (Fava et al., 1989), individuals who have long-term weight recovery still exhibit reduced norepinephrine levels (Kaye, Ebert, Raleigh, & Lake, 1984; Pirke, 1996). There are several possible explanations for these findings (Pirke, 1996). First, the effects of starvation may be long-lasting. Second, disturbances in the noradrenergic systems of patients with AN may represent a premorbid trait. Third, ongoing restraint in long-term recovered patients may be responsible for reduced norepinephrine levels. This hypothesis is supported by data showing that many recovered patients still score high on restraint scales, and by studies of normal subjects suggesting that dietary restraint results in down-regulation of norepinephrine activity (Pirke, 1996).

Studies examining serotonergic functioning in patients with AN have yielded inconsistent results. Although Garner, Olmstead, Polivy, and Garfinkel (1984) found normal CSF levels of the serotonin metabolite 5-hydroxyindoleacetic acid (5-HIAA) in underweight patients with AN, a number of other studies have found reduced levels (Gwirtsman, Guze, Yager, & Gainsley, 1990; Kaye, Ebert, Gwirtsman, & Weiss, 1984; Kaye, Gwirtsman, George, Jimerson, & Ebert, 1988). These studies suggest that AN is associated with decreased serotonergic activity. Kaye et al. (1988) hypothesized that discrepant findings may have resulted from the fact that the subjects in the Garner et al. study had begun gaining weight, because weight gain in patients with AN is associated with a normalization of CSF 5-HIAA levels (Kaye et al., 1988). Patients who have maintained weight at normal levels for at least 6 months appear to exhibit elevated CSF 5-HIAA levels (Kaye, Gwirtsman, George, & Ebert, 1991; Kaye et al., in press), indicating increased brain serotonin activity. Although the reasons for this finding remain unclear, Kaye et al. (in press) have speculated that individuals with AN have premorbid elevated serotonergic functioning that is associated with anxiety, perfectionism, and obsessionality. According to Kaye et al.'s model, individuals with AN discover that dieting reduces their dysphoric mood, and accordingly find starvation reinforcing. This model suggests that a reduction in elevated serotonergic function is responsible for the reinforcing properties of starvation in individuals with AN.

In an attempt to test the above-described model, Kaye et al. (in press) conducted an acute tryptophan depletion study. Tryptophan is a precursor to serotonin, and tryptophan directly influences brain serotonin levels, with a decrease in the amount of tryptophan transported into the brain producing a decrease in serotonergic functioning. Participants in the study included women with AN, women who had recovered from AN, and healthy control women. Results indicated that both symptomatic patients and individuals who had recovered from AN experienced a significant reduction in anxiety after consuming a tryptophan-free amino acid mixture as compared to placebo. It remains unclear, however, whether disturbed serotonergic functioning is casually related to the development of AN.

Bulimia Nervosa

Disturbances in both the noradrenergic and serotonergic systems have also been observed in BN. Both systems are involved in the regulation of eating behavior, with norepinephrine activating feeding in general and serotonin inhibiting it. The bingeing behavior observed in BN is consistent with dysregulation in either or both of these systems (Kaye & Weltzin, 1991).

Disturbances in the noradrenergic systems of patients with BN have been a consistent finding, with most studies reporting reduced central and peripheral norepinephrine activity (Ferguson & Pigott, 2000). Studies have found lower levels of the norepinephrine metabolite MHPG in patients with BN than in controls (Pirke, 1990), as well as reduced plasma and CSF norepinephrine concentrations (Kaye & Weltzin, 1991; Kaye, Ballenger, et al., 1990; Kaye, Gwirtsman, et al., 1990), and increased adrenoreceptor capacity (Kaye & Weltzin, 1991; Pirke, 1990). Despite the consistent findings of noradrenergic system disturbance, it is still not clear whether the norepinephrine alterations cause BN or are a result of pathological eating behavior (Kaye & Weltzin, 1991; Pirke, 1990). Limited data suggest that noradrenergic changes are sustained even after recovery (Ferguson & Pigott, 2000).

In addition to disturbances in the noradrenergic systems, patients with BN also exhibit considerable abnormalities in serotonin function (Ferguson & Pigott, 2000). As noted above, serotonin plays a major role in inhibition of feeding. Serotonin agonists tend to produce satiety and decrease food intake, whereas serotonin antagonists increase meal size. The role of serotonin in the regulation of hunger and satiety has led researchers to hypothesize that bingeing behavior in BN is influenced by hyposerotonergic function (Jimerson, Brandt, & Brewerton, 1988; Kaye & Weltzin, 1991). Although a few studies have failed to find differences between patients with BN and controls in serotonin metabolite CSF levels (e.g., Kaye, Ballenger, et al., 1990), patients with BN appear to exhibit decreased serotonergic activity (Jimerson, Lesem, Kaye, Hegg, & Brewerton, 1990; Kaye & Weltzin, 1991; Pirke, 1990). Research also indicates that as bingeing frequency increases, serotonin metabolite levels decrease (Jimerson, Lesem, Kaye, & Brewerton, 1992), and that long-term recovery from BN is associated with elevated serotonin metabolite levels (Kaye, Greeno, et al., 1998). Such findings may indicate that the failure to find serotonin differences in some studies may be related to a lack of severity of bulimic symptoms in subjects. The finding that active BN is associated with reduced serotonergic function and long-term recovery is associated with increased functioning has led some to speculate that serotonergic functioning in individuals with BN is inherently poorly modulated, and that individuals with BN may engage in dietary restraint, bingeing, and purging in order to modulate mood and serotonin activity (Ferguson & Pigott, 2000; Kaye et al., 1998).

Studies of the serotonin precursor tryptophan also provide support for the role of serotonin in BN. As noted above, tryptophan directly influences brain serotonin levels. Dietary intake affects brain serotonin levels via tryptophan, and moderate dieting appears to lead to a decrease in plasma tryptophan (Anderson, Parry-Billings, Newsholme, Fairburn, & Cowen, 1990). Research also indicates that decreasing serotonergic activity via tryptophan depletion can trigger some symptoms of BN in vulnerable individuals. In an attempt to assess the role of tryptophan depletion in BN, Smith, Fairburn, and Cowen (1999) studied the effects of acute tryptophan depletion on women who had recovered from BN and healthy controls. Findings indicated that, in comparison with healthy controls, the recovered women who consumed a tryptophan-free amino acid mixture experienced an increase in depressive symptoms, body image concern, and fear of losing control over eating.

Tryptophan and the other five large neutral amino acids (LNAAs) are actively transported across the blood–brain barrier by a common transport system. The larger the ratio of plasma tryptophan to the other LNAAs, the more tryptophan is transported to the brain. Meals that are protein-rich decrease the tryptophan-to-LNAA ratio, whereas carbohydrate-rich meals, mediated by the effects of insulin, increase the ratio. Thus low-carbohydrate diets will produce lower brain serotonin levels (Kaye & Weltzin, 1991; Pirke, 1990). This dietary effect has been supported empirically in healthy dieting individuals (Cowen, Anderson, & Fairburn, 1992) and patients with BN have been found to have an unusually large drop in the plasma tryptophan-to-LNAA ratio after eating a protein-rich meal (Broocks, Fichter, & Pirke, 1988). Research also indicates that women appear to be more sensitive to the tryptophan-depleting effects of dieting than men (Cowen et al., 1992; Walsh, Oldman, Franklin, Fairburn, & Cowen, 1995), which is of interest, since women are more prone to both dieting behaviors and eating disorders than men. Combined with the results from other studies, these findings may indicate that BN is triggered in part by dieting-based decreases in serotonergic activity vulnerable individuals (Smith et al., 1999). In addition, it appears that serotonergic dysfunction may represent a common etiological basis for AN and BN.

Genetic Influences

Although both family and twin studies point to a genetic component in the development of eating disorders, the exact role that genetics play in the development of BN and AN remains unclear. Recent studies, however, do support the view that AN and BN share some etiological determinants (Strober, Freeman, Lampert, Diamond, & Kaye, 2000).

Anorexia Nervosa

Family studies, which assess the degree to which eating disorders cluster within families, have demonstrated a strong tendency for rates of both AN and BN to be elevated in the families of probands with AN as compared to controls (Lilenfeld et al., 1998; Strober et al., 2000). For example, in what is probably the largest family study to date targeting eating disorders, rates of AN and BN were, respectively, 11.3 and 4.2 times higher in female relatives of probands diagnosed with AN than in the female relatives of control probands (Strober et al., 2000). Although two studies have failed to find elevated rates of eating disorders in the families of probands with eating disorders, both studies suffered from such methodological shortcomings as small sample size and indirect assessment of eating disorders in family members (Strober, 1995). Overall, family studies seem to implicate some familial role in the transmission of eating disorders, and they support the possibility of a genetic predisposition to AN.

Although family studies are useful in determining whether genetics can be considered as possible etiological factors in the development of a psychiatric disorder, they do not allow for a separation of environmental and genetic factors. In order to address this issue and to separate out the role of a common environment, researchers often turn to the study of twin pairs. Twin studies, which compare concordance rates of disorders between monozygotic (MZ) and dizygotic (DZ) twins, allow for a separation of environmental and genetic components. Twin studies, however, suffer from a number of methodological difficulties that have resulted in some debate regarding the results of such studies (Bulik, Sullivan, Wade, & Kendler, 2000; Fairburn, Cowen, & Harrison, 1999).

Twin studies of AN are inherently difficult because it is a rare disorder (Bulik et al., 2000). Studies of twin pairs have produced mixed results, and heritability estimates for AN range from 0% to 70% (Fairburn, Cowen, & Harrison, 1999). Although one study provided support for a genetic predisposition to AN and found greater concordance for MZ twins than for DZ twins (Treasure & Holland, 1989), a later study found that the concordance rate for DZ twins was higher than that for MZ twins (Walters & Kendall, 1995). Thus, although some data implicate a genetic diathesis for AN, at this time the heritability of AN is unknown (Bulik, Sullivan, Wade, & Kendler, 2000; Fairburn, Cowen, & Harrison, 1999).

Bulimia Nervosa

Family studies also find increased rates of eating disorders among of relatives of probands with BN as compared with control probands (Lilenfeld et al., 1998; Strober et al., 2000). In particular, Strober et al. (2000) found that rates of BN and AN were, respectively, 4.4 and 12.3 times higher in female relatives of probands diagnosed with BN than in the female relatives of control probands. Strober et al. point out that the risk for AN was virtually equal in relatives of eating-disordered probands, regardless of which eating disorder a proband was diagnosed as having. The risk for BN was also roughly the same for relatives of probands with AN as for the relatives of probands with BN (Strober et al., 2000).

A number of studies have examined the heritability of BN by examining concordance rates between MZ and DZ twins. Heritability estimates for BN range from 0% to 83% (Fairburn, Cowen, & Harrison, 1999), and there is some disagreement regarding the best way to interpret these findings. As noted above, methodological aspects of twin studies can be challenging. In particular, it is often difficult to prove that the equal-environment assumption has been met. In other words, twin studies rely upon the assumption that MZ twins and DZ twins are equally exposed to environmental factors that are relevant to the development of an eating disorder. Such methodological issues contribute to disagreement regarding the interpretation of twin data (Fairburn, Cowen, & Harrison, 1999).

Childhood Experiences

Various personal and familial factors have been put forward as causes of eating disorders. Speculation about etiological factors has been based largely on clinical samples. This is an important limitation, because patients seeking treatment may not be representative of a majority of people with a disorder. A series of studies by the Oxford University group has remedied this and other methodological deficiencies in the study of the etiology of eating disorders (Fairburn, Cooper, Doll, & Welch, 1999; Fairburn et al., 1998; Fairburn, Welch, Doll, Davies, & O'Connor, 1997; Welch & Fairburn, 1996).

In the earliest study (Welch & Fairburn, 1996), these investigators used a case–control design; they recruited a representative community-based sample of 102 cases of BN, together with 204 individually matched normal controls and 102 psychiatric controls. The latter comprised mainly cases of depression. This psychiatric control group was needed to identify specific risk factors. Underscoring the importance of basing etiological analyses on community-based rather than clinical samples, the Oxford study revealed that roughly 75% of this sample had never received treatment for BN. It seems clear that we know most about what seems to be only a small subset of individuals with eating disorders who seek treatment. Another distinguishing feature of this well-designed series of studies was the use of state-of-the-art clinical interviews for screening and assessing the prevalence of BN and its possible risk factors.

Several important findings have emerged from this research. It is popularly believed that childhood sexual abuse (CSA) is a cause of eating disorders, although empirical support for this belief has been lacking. The Oxford studies found that CSA occurred more frequently in both the participants with BN and the psychiatric controls than in the normal controls (Welch & Fairburn, 1996). In other words, CSA is a general risk for psychopathology, but not a specific risk factor for BN. A later study by the Oxford group revealed similar findings for AN (Fairburn, Cooper, et al., 1999). In this study, participants with AN had increased rates of CSA as compared with normal controls, and a similar rate as compared with psychiatric controls.

Two more recent studies have also attempted to examine the role of CSA, using more refined methodology. In the first, children between the ages of 10 and 15 who were in treatment following reported CSA were compared to age-matched controls (Wonderlich et al., 2001). The purpose of the study was to examine mediators in the development of an eating disorder, and to reduce limitations of earlier studies (such as long recall periods and variability associated with age of CSA). Behavioral impulsivity mediated the relationship between CSA and weight dissatisfaction, food restriction, and purging behaviors. Drug use was also found to be a secondary mediator for restricting and purging behaviors. Wonderlich et al. (2001) noted that other predicted mediating variables, such as depression and perfectionism, did not emerge in the analyses. They hypothesized that two pathways to eating disturbance may exist, and that individuals with a CSA history may follow a different path than those without such a history.

The second recent study utilized a community-based random sampling strategy to examine how eating disorders develop in women with a history of CSA (Romans, Gendall, Martin, & Mullen, 2001). In a comparison of women with CSA prior to age 16 and women without a history of CSA, Romans et al. found that eating disorders were significantly more common in the women with CSA. Subsequent comparisons, however, focused on variables that distinguished those women with a CSA history who developed an eating disorder from those who did not. Results indicated that belonging to a more recent birth cohort, early onset of menarche, and paternal overcontrol independently increased eating disorder risk in those who experienced CSA. It is important to note that this study also supports previous studies in finding that CSA appears to be a general and not a specific risk factor for eating disorders. No CSA variables (e.g., nature and duration) independently increased the risk for eating disorders in the regression analyses.

Other childhood experiences have also been examined as possible risk factors for the development of eating disorders. The Oxford epidemiological studies found that many childhood risk factors appear to be general, as opposed to specific, risk factors for eating disorders. Among other childhood experiences examined in these studies, negative self-evaluation and perfectionism were identified as specific risk factors for the development of AN (Fairburn, Cooper, et al., 1999). The primary specific childhood risk factors for BN included negative self-evaluation and parental problems (Fairburn et al., 1997). No specific childhood risk factors were found for BED (Fairburn et al., 1998).

Personal and Family Weight History

Clinical reports have indicated that patients with BN commonly have a history of being overweight prior to onset, and are also more likely to come from families in which parents are overweight (Garfinkel, Moldofsky, & Garner, 1980). The Oxford epidemiological research has confirmed this association; both participant and parental obesity proved to be specific risk factors (Fairburn et al., 1997). Moreover, there is evidence of a dose–response effect: the greater the severity of the obesity, the stronger the risk factor. The significance of this association is strengthened by an additional finding. The only two predictors of outcome from a 5-year follow-up of the psychological treatment of BN were patients' premorbid and parental obesity (Fairburn et al., 1995). A likely explanation of this finding is that a tendency toward being overweight makes it more difficult for these women to achieve or maintain the thinness that is culturally valued, and therefore drives them to engage in more extreme weight control measures (e.g., rigid dieting) that put them at greater risk for BN.

The role of a personal or familial history of being overweight is less clear for AN. Although there is evidence of a higher prevalence of overweight parents among patients with the binge-eating/purging subtype of AN (DaCosta & Halmi,

1992), Fairburn, Cooper, et al. (1999) did not find either parental or childhood obesity to be a risk factor for AN. Childhood obesity, however, did emerge as a specific risk factor for binge eating disorder (Fairburn et al., 1998).

Family History of Psychopathology

Evidence from clinical samples of patients has suggested that a family history of depression or substance use disorders is a risk factor for BN. The Oxford study confirmed this association for substance misuse: Parental alcohol abuse was a specific risk factor in this community-based sample (Fairburn et al., 1997). This conclusion is strengthened by Strober's (1995) data showing that relatives of patients with BN or the binge-eating/purging subtype of AN had a three- to fourfold increase in lifetime of substance use disorders, compared with both relatives of normal controls and relatives of patients with AN of the restricting subtype.

Gender and the Sociocultural Context

The eating disorders are dramatically gender-related. Our contemporary Western sociocultural context is thought to determine this differential risk in direct and indirect ways. Whereas the ideal female weight has decreased over recent decades, both the average weight of women and the prevalence of eating disorders in the population have increased (Striegel-Moore, Silberstein, & Rodin, 1986). This discrepancy between the cultural ideal of thinness and the average weight of women contributes to the normative body dissatisfaction found among females. As Striegel-Moore (1995) has noted, Western culture also sells the premise that human weight is malleable, and that with enough hard work, anyone's body can be shaped to meet or at least approach the ideal. As a result, failure to reach the ideal is often viewed as a matter of personal failure.

Studies have shown that weight concern and body dissatisfaction are endemic among adolescent girls. Estimates of the percentage who diet range from 10% to 70% (Hsu, 1990). Moreover, there is evidence that concerns about being fat and attitudes similar to those of older adolescents regarding physical attractiveness, are to be found in children as young as 7 or 8 years (Hsu, 1990; Striegel-Moore et al., 1986). It is argued that the socialization of girls to evaluate themselves in terms of their appearance lays the groundwork for the low self-esteem and negative body image that result when they cannot meet the unrealistically thin ideal that is the standard of female beauty. Thus body dissatisfaction, internalization of the thin ideal, and pursuit of the thin ideal via dieting and other efforts are hypothesized to play a role in the development of eating disorders (Stice & Agras, 1998). Empirical support for this model comes from a number of prospective studies in which body dissatisfaction has been found to be among the most consistent predictors of later eating-disordered behavior (Thompson, Heinberg, Altabe, & Tantleff-Dunn, 1999). For example, in a 9-month prospective study of female adolescents, Stice and Agras (1998) found that in addition to dieting and negative affect, body dissatisfaction, perceived pressure to be thin, and internalization of the thin ideal predicted the onset of binge eating and compensatory behaviors.

Sociocultural norms regarding attractiveness may also be said to influence girls and women through their sex-role identification. Women's social conduct is shaped by pervasive notions of what it is to be "feminine"—that is, to be perceived, and to perceive oneself, as possessing the characteristics associated with the female sex-role stereotype. Striegel-Moore (1993) has argued that two aspects of our contemporary female sex-role stereotype have particular relevance to women's risk for eating disorders. First, beauty is a central aspect of "femininity"; girls learn early on that being "pretty" is what draws attention and praise from others, and girls in books and on television focus on their appearance while boys are playing and "doing." Small wonder that as early as fourth grade, body build and self-esteem are correlated for girls but not for boys (Striegel-Moore et al., 1986). A second aspect is women's interpersonal orientation. It has been argued that a woman's identity is organized as a "self-in-relation," and that her self-worth is closely tied to the establishing and maintenance of close relationships (Jordan, Kaplan, Miller, Stiver, & Surrey, 1991; Miller, 1976). Thus women's self-concept is interpersonally constructed: Girls' self-descriptions at age 7 years have been found to be more based on the perceptions of others than are boys' self-descriptions (Striegel-Moore et al., 1986). Consequently, women are said to derive significant self-worth from other's opinions and approval of them; and in our culture, social approval is significantly related to physical attractiveness (Hatfield &

Sprecher, 1985). Research has consistently shown a significant correlation between self-esteem and feelings about one's body, especially in women, for whom it is significantly related to how they are evaluated by others (Hsu, 1990). One study found that even lesbians, who generally take a more critical stance toward sociocultural norms regarding women and female sex-role stereotypes, were not sgnificantly different from heterosexual women in their attitudes about weight. Self-esteem was strongly related to feelings about one's body, and the prevalence of BN among lesbians was similar to that of heterosexual women (Heffernan, 1996).

Female Adolescent Development: Changes and Challenges

No single variable explains the onset of eating disorders, but research indicates that certain developmental transitions may help to explain the increased risk during adolescence.

Physical Maturation

Whereas physical maturation for boys involves the development of muscle and lean tissue, girls experience weight gain in the form of increased fat tissue during this period, which moves them further away from the culture's lean physical ideal (Striegel-Moore et al., 1986). Onset of menarche and breast development also occur at this time and have been found to be associated with increased dieting among 7th- to 10th-graders, independently of age (Attie & Brooks-Gunn, 1989). Recent research has indicated that early menarche is a specific risk factor for BN (Fairburn et al., 1997).

The task of integrating these changes into one's changing self-image may be especially difficult for girls who are "early developers." In addition to earlier weight gain than peers, which may prompt dieting, adjustment problems may result from parents who react with concern to their daughters' early sexual maturation (Hsu, 1990)—or, alternatively, from increased freedom to engage in experiences for which these girls may not be sufficiently mature cognitively or emotionally to cope (Striegel-Moore, 1993).

Development of Intimate Relationships

Some adolescent women may also feel ill prepared for initiation of adult sexual behaviors, and their anxiety may be heightened by parental unreadiness for this transition into womanhood in their daughters. The view that eating disorders represent phobic avoidance of adult sexuality (Crisp, 1980) has not been established empirically, however.

Development of Sense of Self

One of the psychosocial tasks of adolescence is the formation of one's own, coherent identity. Consistent with the characterizations of women's self-concept as interpersonally oriented, female adolescents have been found to be more self-conscious and concerned with how others view them than males are (Striegel-Moore et al., 1986). Identity deficits have long been a focus of theories regarding the development of eating disorders. Bruch (1973), for example, believed AN to involve underlying deficits in sense of self and autonomy, feelings of paralyzing ineffectiveness, a sense of emptiness, and lack of emotional awareness. Some studies have found elevated levels of personal ineffectiveness, lack of interoceptive awareness, and interpersonal distrust (Garner et al., 1984). Striegel-Moore (1993) has persuasively suggested that girls whose identity is insecure, and who are concerned about how others view them, may focus on physical appearance as a concrete way to construct an identity.

Dieting

"Dieting" here refers to rigid and unhealthy restriction of overall caloric intake, skipping meals, and excessive avoidance of specific foods in order to influence body weight and shape. Dieting is clearly linked to the development of AN and BN in young women. Clinical descriptions consistently indicate that patients with BN typically report that their binge eating began following a diet. An overall correlation exists between cultural pressure to be thin and prevalence of eating disorders, both across and within different ethnic groups (Hsu, 1990). Prospective research has also linked dieting to the development of eating disorders. In a representative sample of 15-year-old schoolgirls in London, those who dieted were significantly more likely than those who did not to develop an eating disorder with 1 year (Patton, 1988). Similarly, a population-based study of adolescents in Australia showed that girls defined as "severe dieters" were 18 times more likely to develop an eating disorder within 6 months than "nondieters." Even "moderate dieters" were at risk compared with those who did not diet (Patton, Selzer, Coffey, Carlin, & Wolfe, 1999).

Dieting may not be a risk factor for obese patients with BED. Such patients reliably report less dietary restraint than patients with BN (Yanovski & Sebring, 1994). Moreover, a large percentage of obese patients with BED report that their binge eating preceded dieting, whereas dieting almost always antedates binge eating in patients with BN. These findings, taken in conjunction with the data indicating that even severe caloric restriction does not exacerbate existing binge eating in obese patients, suggest that dieting has quite different effects in obese and normal weight individuals (National Task Force, 2000).

Dieting alone cannot account for the development of AN or BN. A majority of adolescent and young adult women in the United States actively diet, but only a small minority develop AN or BN. Dieting must interact with some other psychological or biological risk factor (Wilson, 1993).

Dieting has various biological and psychological consequences that may predispose persons to binge eating. Among biological effects, short-term dieting in women produces an increase in the prolactin response to the administration of L-tryptophan, which indicates disturbance in brain serotonin levels (Cowen et al., 1992). At the cognitive level, unrealistically rigid standards of dietary restraint, coupled with a sense of deprivation, may leave an individual vulnerable to loss of control after perceived or actual transgression of the diet. A lapse leads to an "all-or-nothing" cognitive reaction. In this phenomenon, the person attributes the lapse to a complete inability to maintain control, abandons all attempts to regulate food intake, and temporarily overeats.

Are Eating Disorders Addictions?

Eating disorders are often likened to addictive disorders, and indeed there appear to be some comparable features. As noted above, there is some evidence that binge eating may be used to modulate negative emotions. In addition, binge eating is associated by definition with a loss of control. Individuals with eating disorders also report "craving" various foods and are often preoccupied by food (Wilson & Latner, 2001). The addictive model of eating disorders, however, has been challenged on a number of points. There is little scientific evidence that eating disorders share the key features of addictive disorders—namely, tolerance, physical dependence, and withdrawal reactions. Reports of so-called "carbohydrate craving" by individuals with eating disorders are commonly cited as evidence that eating disorders are a type of addiction. Yet studies of craving consistently fail to find support for carbohydrate craving (Wilson & Latner, 2001). The concept of physical dependence on food does not add to our understanding of eating disorders, because all species of animals require food to survive. The concept of physical dependence on food is as meaningless as stating that individuals with eating disorders are physically dependent on water. Moreover, as Wilson and Latner note, the addictive model of eating disorders focuses almost exclusively on binge eating and fails to conceptualize other core features of eating disorders (e.g., overconcern with weight and shape, excessive dietary restraint).

Individual Personality Characteristics

Theorists since Bruch (1973) have described patients with AN as perfect and compliant children, lacking in an autonomous sense of self, for whom affective overcontrol and obsessiveness are attempts to compensate for these core deficiencies (Crisp, 1980; Selvini Palazzoli, 1985). These reports are largely anecdotal and often retrospective, but they have consistently been a part of the clinical impressions of this population. Although objective studies are sparse, partly because of the difficulty of separating stable personality factors from those that result from the illness, Strober (1980) has found confirmation for greater conformity, obsessiveness, control of emotionality, lack of personal effectiveness and adaptation to the maturational challenges of adolescence, and need for social approval among young women with AN.

Recent research has identified perfectionism as a trait that is integral to AN and BN. Patients with these eating disorders score more highly on measures of perfectionism than either normal controls or patients with anxiety or mood disorders (Kaye, Gendall, & Strober, 1998). Even more significantly, perfectionism has been shown to be a specific risk factor for both AN and BN, but not BED (Fairburn et al., 1997, 1998). And in a series of family genetic studies (Kaye et al., 2000; Lilenfeld et al., 1998, 2000), perfectionism has been shown to be genetically influenced and linked to the development of AN and BN.

The Role of the Family

In an early observational study, Minuchin, Rosman, and Baker (1978) identified five characteristic patterns of interaction in families of adolescents with AN: (1) enmeshment (in which family members are overinvolved with one another, and personal boundaries are easily crossed); (2) overprotectiveness (which hinders children's development of autonomous functioning); (3) rigidity (which causes families to feel threatened by changes that come with puberty and adolescence in their daughters); (4) conflict avoidance; and (5) poor conflict resolution. Minuchin and colleagues portrayed the daughter with AN as a "regulator" in the family system, overinvolved in parental conflict—either as the object of diverted conflict, or as a party drawn into coalition with one parent against the other.

Despite the echoing of these characteristics in the family literature, reliable empirical data are fragmentary (Strober & Humphrey, 1987) and inconclusive (e.g., Calam, Waller, Slade, & Newton, 1990; Waller, Slade, & Calam, 1990). One study (Kog, Vandereycken, & Vertommen, 1985) that attempted to operationalize the patterns of Minuchin et al. (1978) found high levels of enmeshment in families of both patients with AN and patients with BN, but evidence for the other patterns was weak, and there was considerable variability in its small sample of families. More importantly, the lack of controlled prospective studies makes it difficult to distinguish whether these family characteristics are a cause or consequence of the eating disorders.

Finally, the family functions to some extent as a mediator of the sociocultural values described earlier. Striegel-Moore et al. (1986) hypothesize that risk may be increased if family members (particularly female ones) model weight preoccupation and dieting, if weight is a form of evaluation and thinness is valued, and also if weight is believed to be something one can and should control. There are fewer studies of this more "ordinary" influence from the family, but Pike and Rodin (1991) found elevated scores on measures of disordered eating among girls whose mothers were more critical of their daughters' weight, compared to those whose mothers were accepting of their daughters' appearance. Along with Attie and Brooks-Gunn (1989), Pike and Rodin (1991) reported that mothers who diet are significantly more likely to have daughters who diet. In fact, both mothers and fathers on diets have been found to be significantly more likely to encourage dieting in their children than parents who are not dieting.

Fairburn et al. (1997) have provided support for the influence of family dieting as a risk factor. Findings indicate that (1) critical comments about patients' weight, shape, or eating, and (2) absence of, or tension during, family meals, are specific factors accounting for a sizable portion of risk for later BN. The Oxford group also found that a number of more general aspects of parenting were specific risk factors. These were frequent parental absence, underinvolvement, high expectations, criticism, and discord between parents. Thus, even though the possibility of recall bias in patients is acknowledged, this methodologically sophisticated study provides welcome empirical substantiation of family variables that have been implicated in previous theory and research on the etiology of BN. The later binge-eating study also found that critical comments about weight, shape, and eating emerged as a specific risk factor for BED (Fairburn et al., 1998).

COMMON COMORBIDITIES

Eating disorders co-occur with a number of other disorders, and prevalence studies indicate that individuals with eating disorders are, throughout their lifetimes, likely to exhibit the symptoms of other psychological disorders. For example, in one community study of adolescent girls, full-syndrome eating disorders were associated with a comorbidity rate of 90% (Lewinsohn et al., 2000). In particular, many studies report finding high rates of comorbid substance use, anxiety, and mood disorders (Grilo, Levy, Becker, Edell, & McGlashan, 1996). Although a number of theories have been proposed to link eating disorders and such disorders as depression and substance use disorders via a common etiology, many such theories have been discredited (Strober & Katz, 1987; Wilson, 1991; Wilson & Latner, 2001). Thus, while eating disorders frequently co-occur and share specific features with other disorders, most findings indicate that they are a separate and distinct class of psychological disorders.

Anorexia Nervosa

AN and substance use disorders have been found to co-occur, with prevalence rates of the latter disorders in patients with AN ranging from 0%

(Halmi et al., 1991) to 36% (Braun, Sunday, & Halmi, 1994). Although these numbers suggest a lower rate of substance misuse in AN as compared with BN, differences emerge depending on the subtype of AN studied. Findings have consistently reported significantly higher levels of substance misuse for the binge-eating/purging subtype than for the restricting subtype of AN (Wilson, 1991). For example, Laessle, Kittl, Fichter, Wittchen, and Pirke (1987) reported a 20% rate of alcohol abuse or dependence in the binge-eating/purging subtype, compared with 0% in the restricting subtype. These findings are supported by Braun et al. (1994), who found a 36% prevalence rate of substance dependence in the binge-eating/purging subtype as compared to 12% in the restricting subtype. Similarly, in a 10-year prospective study, Strober, Freeman, Bower, and Rigali (1996) found that adolescent patients with AN who were binge-eating at the time of intake (referred to by these authors as "intake binge eaters") were at increased risk of developing a substance use disorder, compared to "intake restrictors" and "pure restrictors." Strober et al. noted that the relative risk of developing a substance use disorder was 9.20 in their comparison of "intake binge eaters" versus "pure restrictors." The overall rate of substance use disorders in this adolescent sample was 19% at the end of the study.

Of all the anxiety disorders, OCD and social phobia are most commonly linked with AN (Barbarich, in press; Wonderlich & Mitchell, 1997). Obsessional tendencies in AN have been noticed by numerous observers and have been reported to predate the development of AN and to exist after weight restoration (Kaye, Weltzin, & Hsu, 1993). In a long-term follow-up study of patients with AN, Toner, Garfinkel, and Garner (1988) reported finding that 27% of symptomatic patients, 39% of improved patients, and 37% of asymptomatic patients evidenced lifetime OCD; in addition, each group showed a prevalence rate of over 15% within the previous year. Similarly, in a 6-year study of Swedish adolescent patients with AN, Rastam, Gillberg, and Gillberg (1996) found that 31% also met criteria for OCD. Among a sample of patients with OCD, Rubenstein, Pigott, L'Heureux, Hill, and Murphy (1992) found that 10% met criteria for lifetime AN, and that an additional 13% qualified for subthreshold lifetime AN.

Although a specific relationship between OCD and AN has been explored, anxiety disorders in general co-occur with AN, and a few studies have found higher rates of comorbidity with social phobia. For example, in a sample of 29 French subjects with AN, Godart, Flament, Lecrubier, and Jeammet (2000) found lifetime comorbidity rates of 55% and 21% for social phobia and OCD, respectively. Similarly, Halmi et al. (1991) reported a lifetime prevalence rate of 34% for social phobia as compared to 26% for OCD. Looking at anxiety disorders in general, Toner et al. (1988) found lifetime rates in their long-term follow-up study to range from 47% in asymptomatic patients with AN to 73% in symptomatic patients. Similarly, Godart et al. (2000) found that 83% of their sample with AN met criteria for an anxiety disorder at some point in their lives. This same study also found that 41% of the sample met criteria for three or more lifetime anxiety disorders. Unfortunately, the vast majority of studies have been conducted using clinical samples, and few have utilized a psychiatric control group. As Bulik (1995) has noted, these studies may all overestimate the actual comorbidity between anxiety disorders and eating disorders, since treatment-seeking individuals with eating disorders may in general experience more comorbidity than non-treatment-seeking individuals.

The high rates of anxiety disorders in AN have been used to argue against a specific relationship between eating disorders and anxiety or depressive disorders (Fornari et al., 1992), although findings generally show higher rates of depression than of anxiety disorders in anorexics (Fornari et al., 1992; Halmi et al., 1991; Herzog, Keller, Sacks, Yeh, & Lavori, 1992). Probably the most commonly cited comorbidity, depression, has been reported to co-occur with acute AN frequently, with prevalence rates ranging from 21% to 91% (Kaye et al., 1993). Problems with interpretation of these findings have been pointed out, however, since many of the symptoms associated with starvation closely resemble those of depression (Kaye et al., 1993).

In an attempt to clarify the relationship between mood disorders and AN, some researchers have attempted to examine the rates of depression in patients with AN after treatment. Toner et al. (1988) found no significant difference in the rates of mood disorders among symptomatic, improved, and asymptomatic patients with AN for the year prior to assessment, indicating that the relationship between AN and mood disorders does extend beyond the secondary effects of starvation.

A number of studies have also examined rates of comorbidity between personality disorders and eating disorders. Although the effects of a co-occurring personality disorder in patients with eating disorders have not yet been firmly established, some evidence does suggest that Cluster B personality disorder comorbidity may be associated with a poorer prognosis (Wonderlich & Mitchell, 1997). In general, reported rates of personality disorders in samples with AN range from 23% to 80% (Wonderlich & Mitchell, 1997). AN appears to be most commonly associated with anxious/fearful personality disturbance (Skodol et al., 1993; Wonderlich & Mitchell, 1997). For example, Braun et al. (1994) found that 30% of restricting patients met criteria for a Cluster C personality disorder, with avoidant personality being the most commonly comorbid disorder. No patient with restricting AN met full criteria for a Cluster B (i.e., borderline, antisocial, histrionic, or narcissistic) personality disorder. Thirty-three percent of those with the binge-eating/purging subtype of AN, however, met criteria for a Cluster B personality disorder, indicating possible differences between the AN subtypes.

Bulimia Nervosa

Many analogies have been drawn between BN and addictive disorders. On the surface, the pattern of bingeing exhibited by individuals with BN seems to share many features with substance misuse. Studies have, in fact, found that eating disorders and substance use disorders co-occur to a degree greater than that predicted by chance. Studies of normal-weight individuals with eating disorders consistently reveal significantly higher rates of past and present substance use problems than in the general population (Wilson, 1991), and prevalence rates of alcohol use disorders in treatment-seeking individuals with BN range from 30% to 50% (Dansky, Brewerton, & Kilpatrick, 2000).

As noted above, this apparent relationship between BN and substance misuse might simply reflect an increased tendency for persons with more than one problem to find their way into treatment. However, Kendler et al. (1991), in their examination of over 1,000 female twin pairs obtained from a population-based register, found that of the 123 subjects with BN, 15.5% had a lifetime diagnosis of alcoholism. Similarly, in a Canadian community sample, Garfinkel et al. (1995) found that 31% of individuals with full-syndrome BN also met criteria for alcohol dependence. Finally, using data from the National Women's Study, Dansky et al. (2000) also found significantly higher rates of alcohol dependence in women diagnosed with BN than in those without. These results indicate that BN and alcohol use problems co-occur even in the general population.

Even if a relationship between eating disorders and substance misuse does exist, there is the question of whether this association is a specific one. If eating disorders and substance use problems do occur together, then there should be a higher frequency of eating problems in individuals with substance use problems. This association has been found. In the largest study, Higuchi, Suzuki, Yamada, Parrish, and Kono (1993) reported finding that 11% of female patients and 0.2% of male patients in a sample of 3,592 patients admitted for alcohol abuse or dependence also had an eating disorder. Moreover, among female patients under 30 years of age, the rate of eating disorders was 72%. As Higuchi et al. note, this is approximately 24 times the estimated prevalence of eating disorders in young Japanese women.

Several explanations have been proposed to explain the possible relationship between eating disorders and substance misuse. Perhaps the most popular view is that a common genetic or biological vulnerability exists in some people, although its nature has yet to be determined. As Wilson and Latner (2001) note, however, comorbidity studies fail to support this notion, because the relationship between eating disorders and substance use disorders is not specific. Many other psychiatric disorders are also associated with increased rates of substance misuse. Wilson and Latner also point out that studies of familial transmission, particularly studies of the relatives of substance-misusing probands, do not support a common underlying mechanism.

Anxiety disorders are also frequently found to co-occur with BN, although findings vary as to prevalence rates (Schwalberg, Barlow, Alger, & Howard, 1992). Lifetime prevalence rates of any anxiety disorder range from 13% to 70% in clinical samples with BN (Wonderlich & Mitchell, 1997). In the Canadian community study, Garfinkel et al. (1995) found that 58% of those with full-syndrome BN met criteria for a lifetime anxiety disorders. Rates of panic disorder among those with BN have been found to range from 2% to 41% (Schwalberg et al., 1992), and reported rates of OCD range from 3% to 80% (Mitchell, Specker, & de Zwaan, 1991). Social phobia rates range from 17% to 59% (Lepine & Pelissolo, 1996). Although fewer studies have examined the prevalence of posttraumatic stress disorder (PTSD) in samples with BN, Dansky, Brewerton, Kilpatrick, and O'Neil (1997) found that the rate for current PTSD in women with BN was 13 times greater than the rate for BED. In this sample from the National Women's Study, current and lifetime rates for PTSD in women with BN were 21% and 37%, respectively. A limited number of studies have also examined the rates of eating disorders in patients with anxiety disorders, and Rubenstein et al. (1992) found the lifetime prevalence of BN among a sample of patients with OCD to be 5%, with an additional 11% of subjects showing subthreshold lifetime BN. Surprisingly, in this sample, rates of BN did not significantly differ between male and female subjects.

In an attempt to address the inconsistencies in the literature, Schwalberg et al. (1992) examined 20 patients with BN, 20 patients with social phobia, and 20 individuals with panic disorder for comorbidity between eating and anxiety disorders. Seventy-five percent of those with BN met DSM-III-R criteria for an additional diagnosis of one or more anxiety disorders; the most commonly diagnosed anxiety disorders in this population were generalized anxiety disorder and social phobia (Schwalberg et al., 1992). Elevated levels of eating disorders among the subjects with anxiety disorders were not found, arguing against a simple relationship between eating disorders and anxiety disorders (Schwalberg et al., 1992). Given the range of findings regarding anxiety disorder comorbidity prevalence rates among individuals with eating disorders, Schwalberg et al. (1992) caution that problems with differential diagnosis between anxiety disorders and eating disorders may lead to unreliability in studies examining such comorbidity.

Mood disorders and eating disorders have been commonly linked. Studies have found lifetime mood disorder prevalence rates among individuals with eating disorders ranging from 25% to 80% (Wonderlich & Mitchell,1997). Herzog et al. (1992) found that 50% of a sample of 98 patients with BN met criteria at intake for at least one mood disorder, with 63% being accounted for by major depression, Brewerton et al. (1995) found that 63% of 59 patients with BN met criteria for lifetime major depression. Braun et al. (1994) also reported elevated rates of mood disorders in a sample with BN; 69% of patients met criteria for any mood disorder, and 53% met criteria for major depressive disorder. Schwalberg et al. (1992), however, found no significant difference in the lifetime prevalence rates of mood disorders among individuals with BN, social phobia, or panic disorder, thus raising the possibility that the connection between mood disorders and eating disorders is nonspecific.

In an analysis of the data generated by the twin study of 1,033 female twin pairs (described above), Walters et al. (1992) examined the role of unique environment and genetics in the development of BN and major depression. "Unique environment" refers to environmental factors that are unique for each individual in a twin pair. Whereas unique environmental factors accounted for roughly half of the variation in both disorders, these factors were unrelated between the disorders. Thus the unique environmental factors that contribute to BN are specific and do not appear to contribute to depression, and vice versa. Genetic factors (which also accounted for roughly half of the variation in both disorders in this analysis), however, did not appear to be as specific. The genetic liabilities of the two disorders were correlated at .46, suggesting that some genes may influence the development of both disorders. As a result, this study implies that there is some genetic overlap between the two disorders—although BN and depression are clearly not identical conditions, since a portion of the genetic factors and all of the unique environmental factors appear to be specific to each disorder.

A number of studies have examined the prevalence of personality disorders in BN. On the surface, it appears that BN may be indicative of general impulsivity, such as that associated with some personality disorders (Skodol et al., 1993; Wonderlich & Mitchell, 1997). Studies examining the relationship between BN and borderline personality disorder, however, have produced inconsistent results, with prevalence rates of borderline personality disorder ranging from as little as 2% to over 50% in patients with BN (Skodol et al., 1993). Overall, reported prevalence rates of personality disorders in individuals with bulimia range from 21% to 77% (Wonderlich & Mitchell, 1997).

Skodol et al. (1993) have reported findings regarding the relationship between BN and specific personality disorders. In their study, both current BN and lifetime BN were found to be significantly associated with both schizotypal and borderline personality disorders. Avoidant personality disorder was associated with lifetime, but not current, BN. The strongest association between BN and a specific personality disorder was found with borderline personality disorder. Overall, BN was significantly associated with the Cluster B personality disorders (antisocial, borderline, histrionic, and narcissistic) in general, and lifetime BN was also associated with Cluster C disorders. Similarly, Braun et al. (1994) reported finding a rate of 31% for any Cluster B personality disorder in their sample of patients with BN. Full-syndrome and subthreshold borderline personality disorder were diagnosed in 25% and 35% of patients, respectively.

Binge-Eating Disorder

Studies have generally shown significantly greater levels of psychopathology in obese persons with BED than in obese individuals without BED, and rates of lifetime Axis I comorbidity range from 59% (Telch & Stice, 1998) to 77% (Wilfley et al., 2000). For example, Marcus et al. (1990) found that 60% of obese individuals who binged had a history of at least one psychiatric disorder, as opposed to 28% of obese persons who did not binge. Similarly, Schwalberg et al. (1992) reported a 64% lifetime prevalence of mood disorders and a 70% lifetime rate of anxiety disorders in their sample of obese patients who binged. In one of the largest and most recent studies of treatment-seeking patients with BED, Wilfley et al. (2000) found that 58% of 162 patients with BED met criteria for lifetime major depressive disorder. Thirty-three percent of the sample met criteria for a lifetime substance use disorder, and 29% met criteria for a lifetime anxiety disorder. This study is particularly interesting because it examined the relation between comorbidity and both eating disorder severity and treatment outcome. Although Axis I psychopathology was not related to either baseline severity or treatment outcome, Axis II psychopathology (particularly Cluster B personality disorders) was associated with increased binge eating at 1-year follow-up. The overall Axis II comorbidity rate in the sample was 37%, with 12% of patients meeting criteria for a Cluster B personality disorder.

Findings from the one large community study largely support the results from clinical studies. Telch and Stice (1998) reported a 49% lifetime prevalence of major depression in female participants with BED recruited from the community, as compared with 28% in female participants without BED who were also recruited from the community. This study also found elevated rates of lifetime Axis I and Axis II disorders in participants with BED as compared to those without it. Results from this community study provide some of the best evidence that BED is associated with comorbid psychopathology. The prevalence rate of any lifetime Axis I disorder (59%) in the participants with BED is quite comparable to the findings of the Marcus et al. (1990) study, which was conducted with a clinical sample. It should be noted, however, that there were no differences between the patient groups with and without BED in any of the other mood disorders or in any of the anxiety disorders, either current or lifetime. Comorbidity rates were also somewhat lower than those in other studies, such as that by Wilfley et al. (2000). As Telch and Stice (1998) note, the findings from their study suggest that true comorbidity rates may be lower than suggested by studies using clinical samples.

FUTURE DIRECTIONS

It is likely that the diagnostic criteria for eating disorders will be refined on the basis of continuing research. In particular, we can anticipate elaboration and development of criteria for problems that are currently lumped together in the category of EDNOS.

Innovative and increasingly sophisticated research is underway on the biological bases of the different eating disorders. Improved specification of the brain mechanisms involved in the development and maintenance of eating disorders is likely to result not only in more efficient pharmacological treatment, but arguably also in more effective use of psychological methods. Large-scale studies of the genetics of these disorders also promise to provide greater understanding.

Researchers are currently making headway in the development of more effective treatments. Finally, systematic treatment outcome research is focusing on AN. CBT has been shown to reduce relapse rates following the discharge of weight-restored patients with AN from a hospital (Pike, Walsh, Vitousek, Wilson, & Bauer, 2001). And in a particularly promising innovation, a new form of manual-based family therapy has been developed that appears to be extremely effective for adolescent patients with AN (Lock et al., 2001). It is currently being evaluated in controlled research in the United States.

Manual-based CBT is well established as the current treatment of choice for BN (Wilson & Fairburn, 2002). However, its efficacy is limited, and it fails to help a significant minority of patients. Research is underway that is designed to improve on currently available CBT, and to extend this evidence-based approach to BN-like disorders within the EDNOS category.

The challenge ahead for the treatment of BED is the associated problem of obesity. Current treatments are effective in eliminating binge eating and associated eating disorder psychopathology, but the obesity that characterizes the majority of these patients remains difficult to treat. Future research will be focused on the improved management of obesity (Wadden & Stunkard, 2002).

There is considerable interest in developing programs that prevent eating disorders. Most proposals focus on intervening in elementary or middle school curricula (Shisslak, Crago, Neal, & Swain, 1987). The problem, however, is that we do not yet know enough about the causes of eating disorders, or even their risk factors, to design effective interventions. Dieting is often discussed as a possible target of preventive programs, but most young women in Western society diet. Thus a prevention program would have to be aimed somewhat indiscriminately at most girls. It is premature to rush into investing in costly prevention programs that have insufficient theoretical or empirical justification. The preferred approach is to pursue research on risk factors, so that we can identify those children or adolescents who are most vulnerable to the development of eating disorders.

REFERENCES

Agras, W. S., Crow, S. J., Halmi, K. A., Mitchell, J. E., Wilson, G. T., & Kraemer, H. (2000). Outcome predictors for the cognitive-behavioral treatment of bulimia nervosa: Data from a multisite study. *American Journal of Psychiatry, 157*, 1302–1308.

American Psychiatric Association. (1980). *Diagnostic and statistical manual of mental disorders* (3rd ed.). Washington, DC: Author.

American Psychiatric Association. (1987). *Diagnostic and statistical manual of mental disorders* (3rd ed., rev.). Washington, DC: Author.

American Psychiatric Association. (1994). *Diagnostic and statistical manual of mental disorders* (4th ed.). Washington, DC: Author.

Andersen, A. E. (1995). Eating disorders in males. In K. D. Brownell & C. G. Fairburn (Eds.), *Eating disorders and obesity: A comprehensive handbook* (pp. 151–158). New York: Guilford Press.

Anderson, I. M., Parry-Billings, M., Newsholme, E. A., Fairburn, G. G., & Cowen, P. J. (1990). Dieting reduces plasma tryptophan and alters brain 5-HT function in women. *Psychological Medicine, 20*, 785–791.

Attie, I., & Brooks-Gunn, J. (1989). Development of eating problems in adolescent girls: A longitudinal study. *Developmental Psychology, 25*, 70–79.

Barbarich, N. (in press). Is there a common mechanism of serotonin dysregulation in anorexia nervosa and obsessive compulsive disorder? *Eating and Weight Disorders*.

Beglin, S. J., & Fairburn, C. G. (1992). What is meant by the term "binge"? *American Journal of Psychiatry, 149*, 123–124.

Beumont, P. J. V. (1995). The clinical presentation of anorexia and bulimia nervosa. In K. D. Brownell & C. G. Fairburn (Eds.), *Eating disorders and obesity: A comprehensive handbook* (pp. 151–158). New York: Guilford Press.

Braun, D. L., Sunday, S. R., & Halmi, K. A. (1994). Psychiatric comorbidity in patients with eating disorders. *Psychological Medicine, 24*, 859–867.

Brewerton, T. D., Lydiard, R. B., Herzog, D. B., Brotman, A. W., O'Neil, P. M., & Ballenger, J. C. (1995) Comorbidity of Axis I psychiatric disorders in bulimia nervosa. *Journal of Clinical Psychiatry, 56*, 77–80.

Brody, M. J., Walsh, B. T., & Devlin, M. J. (1994). Binge eating disorder: Reliability and validity of a new diagnostic category. *Journal of Consulting and Clinical Psychology, 62*, 381–186.

Broocks, A., Fichter, M. M., & Pirke, K. M. (1988). Effects of test meals on insulin, glucose, plasma large neutral amino acids and norepinephrine in patients with bulimia nervosa. *Proceedings of 3rd International Conference on Eating Disorders*, p. 242.

Brownell, K. D., & Rodin, J. (1992). Prevalence of eating disorders in athletes. In K. D. Brownell, J. Rodin, & J. H. Wilmore (Eds.), *Eating, body weight and performance in athletes* (pp. 128–145). Philadelphia: Lea & Febiger.

Brownell, K. D., Rodin, J., & Wilmore, J. H. (Eds.). (1992). *Eating, body weight and performance in athletes*. Philadelphia: Lea & Febiger.

Bruce, B., & Agras, W. S. (1992). Binge eating in females: A population-based investigation. *International Journal of Eating Disorders, 12*, 365–373.

Bruch, H. (1973). *Eating disorders: Obesity, anorexia nervosa, and the person within*. New York: Basic Books.

Bulik, C. M. (1995). Anxiety disorders and eating disorders: A review of their relationship. *New Zealand Journal of Psychology, 24*, 51–62.

Bulik, C. M., Sullivan, P. F., Wade, T. D., & Kendler, K. S. (2000). Twin studies of eating disorders: A review. *International Journal of Eating Disorders, 27*, 1–20.

Butow, P., Beumont, P., & Touyz, S. (1993). Cognitive processes in dieting disorders. *International Journal of Eating Disorders, 14*, 319–329.

Calam, R., Waller, G., Slade, P., & Newton, T. (1990). Eating disorders and perceived relationships with parents. *International Journal of Eating Disorders, 9*, 479–485.

Carlat, D. J., Camargo, C. A., & Herzog, D. B. (1997). Eating disorders in males: A report on 135 patients. *American Journal of Psychiatry, 154*, 1127–1132.

Cowen, P. J., Anderson, I. M.,, & Fairburn, C. G. (1992). Neurochemical effects of dieting: Relevance to eating and affective disorders. In G. H. Anderson & S. H. Kennedy (Eds.), *The biology of feast and famine: Relevance to eating disorders* (pp. 269–284). New York: Academic Press.

Crisp, A. H. (1980). *Anorexia nervosa: Let me be*. London: Plenum Press.

DaCosta, M., & Halmi, K. A. (1992). Classification of anorexia nervosa: Question of subtypes. *International Journal of Eating Disorders, 11*, 305–314.

Dansky, B. S., Brewerton, T. D., & Kilpatrick, D. G. (2000). Comorbidity of bulimia nervosa and alcohol use disorders: Results from the National Women's Study. *International Journal of Eating Disorders*, 27, 180–190.

Dansky, B. S., Brewerton, T. D., Kilpatrick, D. G., & O'Neil, P. M. (1997). The National Women's Study: Relationship of victimization and posttraumatic stress disorder to bulimia nervosa. *International Journal of Eating Disorders, 21*, 214–228.

Devlin, M. J., Yanovski, S. Z., & Wilson, G. T. (2000). Obesity: What mental health professionals need to know. *American Journal of Psychiatry, 157*, 854–866.

Eldredge, K. L., & Agras, W. S. (1996). Weight and shape overconcern and emotional eating in binge eating disorder. *International Journal of Eating Disorders, 19*, 73–82.

Fairburn, C. G. (1997). Eating disorders. In D. M. Clark & C. G. Fairburn (Eds.), *Science and practice of cognitive behaviour therapy* (pp. 209–242). Oxford: Oxford University Press.

Fairburn, C. G., & Cooper, P. J. (1993). The Eating Disorder Examination. In C. G. Fairburn & G. T. Wilson (Eds.), *Binge eating: Nature, assessment, and treatment* (pp. 317–360). New York: Guilford Press.

Fairburn, C. G., Cooper, Z., Doll, H. A., Norman, P., & O'Connor, M. (2000). The natural course of bulimia nervosa and binge eating disorder in young women. *Archives of General Psychiatry*, 57, 659–665.

Fairburn, C. G., Cooper, Z., Welch, S. L., & Doll, H. A. (1999). Risk factors for anorexia nervosa: Three integrated case–control comparisons. *Archives of General Psychiatry, 56*, 468–476.

Fairburn, C. G., Cowen, P. J., & Harrison, P. J. (1999). Twin studies and the etiology of eating disorders. *International Journal of Eating Disorders, 26*, 349–358.

Fairburn, C. G., Doll, H. A., Welch, S. L., Hay, P. J., Davies, B. A., & O'Connor, M. E. (1998). Risk factors for binge eating disorder: A community-based case–control study. *Archives of General Psychiatry, 55*, 425–432.

Fairburn, C. G., Hay, P. J., & Welch, S. L. (1993). Binge eating and bulimia nervosa: Distribution and determinants. In C. G. Fairburn & G. T. Wilson (Eds.), *Binge eating: Nature, assessment, and treatment*. (pp. 123–143). New York: Guilford Press.

Fairburn, C. G., Jones, R., Peveler, R. C., Hope, R. A., & O'Connor, M. (1993). Psychotherapy and bulimia nervosa: The longer-term effects of interpersonal psychotherapy, behavior therapy and cognitive behavior therapy. *Archives of General Psychiatry, 50*, 419–428.

Fairburn, C. G., Norman, P. A., Welch, S. L., O'Connor, M. E., Doll, H. A., & Peveler, R. C. (1995). A prospective study of outcome in bulimia nervosa and the long-term effects of three psychological treatments. *Archives of General Psychiatry*, 52, 304–312.

Fairburn, C. G., Shafran, R., & Cooper, Z. (1999). A cognitive behavioural theory of anorexia nervosa. *Behaviour Research and Therapy, 37*, 1–13.

Fairburn, C. G., & Walsh, B. T. (2002). Atypical eating disorders (EDNOS). In C. G. Fairburn & K. D. Brownell (Eds.), *Eating disorders and obesity: A comprehensive handbook* (2nd ed., pp. 171–177). New York: Guilford Press.

Fairburn, C. G., Welch, S. L., Doll, H. A., Davies, B. A., & O'Connor, M. E. (1997). Risk factors for bulimia nervosa: A community-based case–control study. *Archives of General Psychiatry, 54*, 509–517.

Fava, M., Copeland, P. M., Schweiger, U., & Herzog, D. B. (1989). Neurochemical abnormalities of anorexia nervosa and bulimia nervosa. *American Journal of Psychiatry, 146*, 963–971.

Ferguson, C. P., & Pigott, T. A. (2000). Anorexia and bulimia nervosa: Neurobiology and pharmacotherapy. *Behavior Therapy, 31*, 237–264.

Fornari, V., Kaplan, M., Sandberg, D. E., Matthews, M., Skolnick, N., & Katz, J. L. (1992). Depressive and anxiety disorders in anorexia nervosa and bulimia nervosa. *International Journal of Eating Disorders, 12*, 21–29.

Foster, G. D., Wadden, T. A., Kendall, P. C., Stunkard, A. J., & Vogt, R. A. (1996). Psychological effects of weight loss and regain: A prospective evaluation. *Journal of Consulting and Clinical Psychology, 64*, 752–757.

Garfinkel, P. E., Moldofsky, H., & Garner, D. (1980). The heterogeneity of anorexia nervosa: Bulimia as a distinct subgroup. *Archives of General Psychiatry, 37*, 1036–1040.

Garfinkel, P. E., Lin, E., Goering, P., Spegg, C., Goldbloom, D. S., Kennedy, S., Kaplan, A., & Woodside, D. B. (1995). Bulimia nervosa in a Canadian community sample: Prevalence and comparison of subgroups. *American Journal of Psychiatry, 152*, 1052–1058.

Garner, D. M. (1993). Binge eating in anorexia nervosa. In C. G. Fairburn & G. T. Wilson (Eds.), *Binge eating: Nature, assessment, and treatment* (pp. 50–76). New York: Guilford Press.

Garner, D. M., Olmstead, M. P., Polivy, J., & Garfinkel, P. E. (1984). Comparison between weight-preoccupied women and anorexia nervosa. *Psychosomatic Medicine, 14*, 255–266.

Garner, D. M., Vitousek, K. M., & Pike, K. M. (1997). Cognitive-behavioral therapy for anorexia nervosa. In D. M. Garner & P. E. Garfinkel (Eds.), *Handbook of treatment for eating disorders* (2nd ed., pp. 94–144). New York: Guilford Press.

Godart, N. T., Flament, M. F., Lecrubier, Y., & Jeammet, P. (2000). Anxiety disorders in anorexia nervosa and bulimia nervosa: Co-morbidity and chronology of appearance. *European Psychiatry, 15*, 38–45.

Gotestam, K. G., & Agras, W. S. (1995). General population-based epidemiological study of eating disorders in Norway. *International Journal of Eating Disorders, 18*, 119–126.

Grilo, C. M., Levy, K. N., Becker, D. F., Edell, W. S., & McGlashan, T. H. (1996). Comorbidity of DSM-III-R Axis I and II disorders among female inpatients with eating disorders. *Psychiatric Services, 47*, 426–429.

Gull, W. W. (1873). Anorexia hysterica (apoepsia hysteria). *British Medical Journal, ii*, 527.

Gwirtsman, H. E., Guze, B. H., Yager, J., & Gainsley, B. (1990). Fluoxetine treatment of anorexia nervosa: An open trial. *Journal of Clinical Psychiatry, 51*, 378–382.

Halmi, K. A., Eckert, E., Marchi, P., Sampugnaro, V., Apple, R., & Cohen, J. (1991). Comorbidity of psychiatric diagnoses in anorexia nervosa. *Archives of General Psychiatry, 48*, 712–718.

Hatfield, E., & Sprecher, S. (1985). *Mirror, mirror: The importance of looks in everyday life*. Albany: State University of New York Press.

Hay, P. J., Fairburn, C. G., & Doll, H. A. (1996). The classification of bulimic eating disorders: A community-based cluster analysis study. *Psychological Medicine*, *26*, 801–812.

Heffernan, K. (1996). Eating disorders and weight concern among lesbians. *International Journal of Eating Disorders*, *19*, 127–138.

Herzog, D. B., Keller, M. B., Sacks, N. R., Yeh, C. J., & Lavori, P. W. (1992). Psychiatric comorbidity in treatment-seeking anorexics and bulimics. *Journal of the American Academy of Child and Adolescent Psychiatry*, *31*, 810–818.

Higuchi, S., Suzuki, K., Yamada, K., Parrish, K., & Kono, H. (1993). Alcoholics with eating disorders: Prevalence and clinical course. A study from Japan. *British Journal of Psychiatry*, *162*, 403–406.

Hoek, H. W. (1995). The distribution of eating disorders. In K. D. Brownell & C. G. Fairburn (Eds.), *Eating disorders and obesity: A comprehensive handbook* (pp. 207–211). New York: Guilford Press.

Howard, C. E., & Porzelius, L. K. (1999). The role of dieting in binge eating disorder: Etiology and treatment implications. *Clinical Psychology Review*, *19*, 25–44.

Hsu, L. K. G. (1990). *Eating disorders*. New York: Guilford Press.

Jimerson, D. C., Brandt, H. A., & Brewerton, T. D. (1988). Evidence for altered serotonin function in bulimia and anorexia nervosa: Behavioral implications. In K. M. Pirke, W. Vandereycken, & D. Ploog (Eds.), *Psychobiology of bulimia nervosa* (pp. 83–89). Berlin: Springer-Verlag.

Jimerson, D. C., Lesem, M. D., Kaye, W. H., & Brewerton, T. D. (1992). Low serotonin and dopamine metabolite concentrations in cerebrospinal fluid from bulimic patients with frequent binge episodes. *Archives of General Psychiatry*, *49*, 132–139.

Jimerson, D. C., Lesem, M. D., Kaye, W. H., Hegg, A. P., & Brewerton, T. D. (1990). Eating disorders and depression: Is there a serotonin connection? *Biological Psychiatry*, *28*, 443–454.

Johnson-Sabine, E., Wood, K., Patton, G., Mann, A., & Wakeling, A. (1988). Abnormal eating attitudes in London schoolgirls—a prospective epidemiological study: factors associated with abnormal response on screening questionnaires. *Psychological Medicine*, *18*, 615–622.

Jordan, J. V., Kaplan, A. G., Miller, J. B., Stiver, J. P., & Surrey, J. L. (1991). *Women's growth in connection: Writings from the Stone Center*. New York: Guilford Press.

Kaye, W. H., Ballenger, J. C., Lydiard, R. B., Stuart, G. W., Laraia, M. T., O'Neil, P., Fossey, M. D., Stevens, V., Lessers, S., & Hsu, G. (1990). CSF monoamine levels in normal-weight bulimia: Evidence for abnormal noradrenergic activity. *American Journal of Psychiatry*, *147*, 225–229.

Kaye, W. H., Barbarich, B. S., Putnam, B. S., Gendall, K. A., Fernstrom, J., Fernstrom, M., McConaha, C. W., & Kishore, A. (in press). Anxiolytic effects of acute tryptophan depletion (ATD) in anorexia nervosa. *International Journal of Eating Disorders*.

Kaye, W. H., Ebert, M. H., Gwirtsman, H. E., & Weiss, S. R. (1984). Differences in brain serotonergic metabolism between nonbulimic and bulimic patients with anorexia nervosa. *American Journal of Psychiatry*, *141*, 1598–1601.

Kaye, W. H., Ebert, M. H., Raleigh, M., & Lake, R. (1984). Abnormalities in CNS monoamine ketabolism in anorexia nervosa. *Archives of General Psychiatry*, *41*, 350–355.

Kaye, W. H., Gendall, K., & Strober, M. (1998). Serotonin neuronal function and selective serotonin reuptake inhibitor treatment in anorexia and bulimia nervosa. *Biological Psychiatry*, *44*, 825–838.

Kaye, W. H., Greeno, C. G., Moss, H., Fernstrom, J., Fernstrom, M., Lilenfeld, L., Weltzin, T. E., & Mann, J. (1998). Alterations in serotonin activity and psychiatric symptoms after recovery from bulimia nervosa. *Archives of General Psychiatry*, *55*, 927–935.

Kaye, W.. H., Gwirtsman, H. E., George, D. T.,, & Ebert, M. H. (1991). Altered serotonin activity in anorexia nervosa after long-term weight restoration. *Archives of General Psychiatry*, *48*, 556–562.

Kaye, W. H., Gwirtsman, H. E., George, D. T., Jimerson, D. C., & Ebert, M. H. (1988). CSF 5-HIAA concentrations in anorexia nervosa: Reduced values in underweight subjects normalize after weight gain. *Society of Biological Psychiatry*, *23*, 102–105.

Kaye, W. H., Gwirtsman, H. E., George, D. T., Jimerson, D. C., Ebert, M. H., & Lake, C. R. (1990). Disturbances of noradrenergic systems in normal-weight bulimia: Relationship to diet and menses. *Biological Psychiatry*, *27*, 4–21.

Kaye, W. H., Lilenfeld, L. R., Berettini, W. H., Strober, M., Devlin, B., Klump, K. L., Goldman, D., Bulik, C. M., Halmi, K. A., Fichter, M. M., Kaplan, A., Woodside, D. B., Treasure, J., Plotnicov, K. H., Pollice, C., Rao, R., & McConaha, C. W. (2000). A search for susceptibility loci for anorexia nervosa: Methods and sample description. *Biological Psychiatry*, *47*, 794–803.

Kaye, W. H., & Weltzin, T. E. (1991). Neurochemistry of bulimia nervosa. *Journal of Clinical Psychiatry*, *52*, 617–622.

Kaye, W. H., Weltzin, T., & Hsu, L. K. G. (1993). Relationship between anorexia nervosa and obsessive compulsive behaviors. *Psychiatric Annals*, *23*, 365–373.

Kaye, W. H., Weltzin, T. E., Hsu, L. K. G., Bulik, C., McConaha, C., & Sobkiewicz, T. (1992). Patients with anorexia nervosa have elevated scores on the Yale–Brown Obsessive-Compulsive Scale. *International Journal of Eating Disorders*, *12*, 57–62.

Keller, M. B., Herzog, D. B., Lavori, P. W., Bradburn, I. S., & Mahoney, E. M. (1992). The naturalistic history of bulimia nervosa: Extraordinarily high rates of chronicity, relapse, recurrence, and psychosocial morbidity. *International Journal of Eating Disorders*, *12*, 1–10.

Kendler, K. S., MacLean, C., Neale, M., Kessler, R., Heath, A., & Eaves, L. (1991). The genetic epidemiology of bulimia nervosa. *American Journal of Psychiatry*, *148*, 1627–1637.

Kog, E., Vandereycken, W., & Vertommen, H. (1985). Towards a verification of the psychosomatic family model: A pilot study of ten families with an anorexia/bulimia nervosa patient. *International Journal of Eating Disorders*, *4*, 525–538.

Lacey, J. H., & Evans, C. D. H. (1986). The impulsivist: A multi-impulsive personality disorder. *British Journal of Addiction*, *81*, 641–649.

Laessle, R. G., Kittl, S., Fichter, M., Wittchen, H. U., & Pirke, K. M. (1987). Major affective disorder in anorexia nervosa and bulimia: A descriptive diagnostic study. *British Journal of Psychiatry*, *151*, 785–789.

Lepine, J. P., & Pelissolo, A. (1996). Comorbidity and social phobia: Clinical and epidemiological issues. *International Clinical Psychopharmacology*, *11*, 35–41.

Lesem, M. D., George, D. T., Kaye, W. H., Goldstein, D. S., & Jimerson, D. C. (1989). State-related changes in norepinephrine regulation in anorexia nervosa. *Biological Psychiatry, 25*, 509–512.

Lewinsohn, P. M., Striegel-Moore, R. H., & Seeley, J. R. (2000). Epidemiology and natural course of eating disorders: Young women from adolescence to young adulthood. *Journal of the American Academy of Child and Adolescent Psychiatry, 39*, 1284–1292.

Lilenfeld, L. R., Kaye, W. H., Greeno, C. G., Merikangas, K. R., Plotnicov, K., Pollice, C., Rao, R., Strober, M., Bulik, C., & Nagy, L. (1998). A controlled family study of anorexia nervosa and bulimia nervosa: Psychiatric disorders in first-degree relatives and effects of proband comorbidity. *Archives of General Psychiatry, 55*, 603–610.

Lilenfeld, L. R., Stein, D., Bulik, C. M., Strober, M., Plotnicov, K. H., Pollice, C., Rao, R., Nagy, L., & Kaye, W. H. (2000). Personality traits among currently eating disordered, recovered, and never ill first-degree female relatives of bulimic and control women. *Psychological Medicine, 30*, 1399–1410.

Lock, J., le Grange, D., Agras, W. S., & Dare, C. (2001). *Treatment manual for anorexia nervosa*. New York: Guilford Press.

Marcus, M. D. (1993). Binge eating in obesity. In C. G. Fairburn & G. T. Wilson (Eds.), *Binge eating: Nature, assessment, and treatment* (pp. 77–96). New York: Guilford Press.

Marcus, M. D., Wing, R. R., Ewing, L., Kern, E., Gooding, W., & McDermott, M. (1990). Psychiatric disorders among obese binge eaters. *International Journal of Eating Disorders, 9*, 69–77.

Meyer, C., Blissett, J., & Oldfield, C. (2001). Sexual orientation and eating psychopathology: The role of masculinity and femininity. *International Journal of Eating Disorders, 29*, 314–318.

Miller, J. B. (1976). *Toward a new psychology of women*. Boston: Beacon Press.

Minuchin, S., Rosman, B. L., & Baker, I. (1978). *Psychosomatic families: Anorexia nervosa in context*. Cambridge, MA: Harvard University Press.

Mitchell, J. E. (1995). Medical complications of bulimia nervosa. In K. D. Brownell & C. G. Fairburn (Eds.), *Eating disorders and obesity: A comprehensive handbook* (pp. 271–277). New York: Guilford Press.

Mitchell, J. E., Specker, S. M., & de Zwaan, M. (1991). Comorbidity and medical complications of bulimia nervosa. *Journal of Clinical Psychiatry, 52*, 13–20.

Mumford, D. B., Whitehouse, A. M., & Choudry, I. Y. (1992). Survey of eating disorders in English-medium schools in Lahore, Pakistan. *International Journal of Eating Disorders, 11*, 173–184.

Mumford, D. B., Whitehouse, A. M., & Platts, M. (1991). Sociocultural correlates of eating disorders among Asian schoolgirls in Bradford. *British Journal of Psychiatry, 158*, 222–228.

Nakamura, K., Hoshino, Y., Waranabe, A., Honda, K., Niwa, S., Tominaga, K., Shimai, S., & Yamamoto, M. (1999). Eating problems in female Japanese high school students: A prevalence study. *International Journal of Eating Disorders, 26*, 91–96.

Nasser, M. (1986). Comparative study of the prevalence of abnormal eating attitudes among Arab females of both London and Cairo universities. *Psychological Medicine, 16*, 621–625.

National Heart, Lung, and Blood Institute. (1998). Clinical guidelines on the identification, evaluation, and treatment of overweight and obesity in adults: The evidence report. *Obesity Research, 6*, 51S–209S.

National Task Force on the Prevention and Treatment of Obesity. (2000). Dieting and the development of eating disorders in overweight and obese adults. *Archives of Internal Medicine, 160*, 2581–2589.

Patton, G. C. (1988). The spectrum of eating disorders in adolescence. *Journal of Psychosomatic Research, 32*, 579–584.

Patton, G. C., Selzer, R., Coffey, C., Carlin, B., & Wolfe, R. (1999). Onset of adolescent eating disorders: Population-based cohort study over 3 years. *British Medical Journal, 318*, 765–768.

Pike, K. M., Dohm, F. A., Striegel-Moore, R. H., Wilfley, D. E., & Fairburn, C. G. (2001). A comparison of black and white women with binge eating disorder. *American Journal of Psychiatry, 158*, 1455–1460.

Pike, K. M., & Rodin, J. (1991). Mothers, daughters, and disordered eating. *Journal of Abnormal Psychology, 100*, 198–204.

Pike, K. M., Walsh, B. T., Vitousek, K., Wilson, G. T., & Bauer, J. (2001). *Cognitive behavioral therapy in the relapse prevention of anorexia nervosa*. Unpublished manuscript, Columbia University.

Pirke, K. M. (1990). Central neurotransmitter disturbances in bulimia (nervosa). In M. M. Fichter (Ed.), *Bulimia nervosa: Basic research, diagnosis and therapy* (pp. 223–234). Chichester, UK: Wiley.

Pirke, K. M. (1996). Central and peripheral noradrenalin regulation in eating disorders. *Psychiatry Research, 62*, 43–49.

Pratt, E. M., Niego, S. H., & Agras, W. S. (1998). Does the size of a binge matter? *International Journal of Eating Disorders, 24*, 307–312.

Rastam, M., Gillberg, C., & Gillberg, I. C. (1996). A six-year follow-up study of anorexia nervosa subjects with teenage onset. *Journal of Youth and Adolescence, 25*, 439–453.

Romans, S. E., Gendall, K. A., Martine, J. L., & Mullen, P. E. (2001). Child sexual abuse and later disordered eating: A New Zealand epidemiological study. *International Journal of Eating Disorders, 29*, 380–392.

Rosen, J. C., Leitenberg, H., Fisher, C., & Khazam, C. (1986). Binge-eating episodes in bulimia nervosa: The amount and type of food consumed. *International Journal of Eating Disorders, 5*, 255–257.

Rubenstein, C. S., Pigott, T. A., L'Heureux, F., Hill, J. L., & Murphy, D. L. (1992). A preliminary investigation of the lifetime prevalence of anorexia and bulimia nervosa in patients with obsessive compulsive disorder. *Journal of Clinical Psychiatry, 53*, 309–314.

Russell, G. F. M. (1979). Bulimia nervosa: An ominous variant of anorexia nervosa. *Psychological Medicine, 9*, 429–448.

Russell, G. F. M., Szmukler, G. I., Dare, C., & Eisler, I. (1987). An evaluation of family therapy in anorexia nervosa and bulimia nervosa. *Archives of General Psychiatry, 44*, 1047–1056.

Schwalberg, M. D., Barlow, D. H., Alger, S. A., & Howard, L. J. (1992). Comparison of bulimics, obese binge eaters, social phobics, and individuals with panic disorder on comorbidity across DSM-III-R anxiety disorders. *Journal of Abnormal Psychology, 101*, 675–681.

Selvini Palazzoli, M. (1985). *Self-starvation: From individual to family therapy in the treatment of anorexia nervosa* (A. Pomerans, Trans.). New York: Aronson.

Sherwood, N. E., Jeffery, R. W., & Wing, R. R. (1999). Binge status as a predictor of weight loss treatment outcome. *International Journal of Obesity, 23,* 485–493.

Shisslak, C., Crago, M., Neal, M. E., & Swain, B. (1987). Primary prevention of eating disorders. *Journal of Consulting and Clinical Psychology, 55,* 660–667.

Skodol, A. E., Oldham, J. M., Hyler, S. E., Kellman, H. D., Dodge, N., & Davies, M. (1993). Comorbidity of DSM-III-R eating disorders and personality disorders. *International Journal of Eating Disorders, 14,* 403–416.

Slade, P. (1982). Towards a functional analysis of anorexia nervosa and bulimia nervosa. *British Journal of Clinical Psychology, 21,* 167–179.

Smith, K. A., Fairburn, C. G., & Cowen, P. J. (1999). Symptomatic relapse in bulimia nervosa following acute tryptophan depletion. *Archives of General Psychiatry, 56,* 171–176.

Smith, D. E., Marcus, M. D., Lewis, C., Fitzgibbon, M., & Schreiner, P. (1998). Prevalence of binge eating disorder, obesity, and depression in a biracial cohort of young adults. *Annals of Behavioral Medicine, 20,* 227–232.

Smolak, L., Murnen, S. K., & Ruble, A. E. (2000). Female athletes and eating problems: A meta-analysis. *International Journal of Eating Disorders, 27,* 371–380.

Smolak, L., & Striegel-Moore, R. H. (2001). Challenging the myth of the golden girl: Ethnicity and eating disorders. In R. H. Striegel-Moore & L. Smolak (Eds.), *Eating disorders* (pp. 111–132). Washington, DC: American Psychological Association.

Spitzer, R. L., Devlin, M. J., Walsh, B. T., Hasin, D., Wing, R., Marcus, M., et al. (1992). Binge eating disorder: A multisite field trial of the diagnostic criteria. *International Journal of Eating Disorders, 11,* 191–203.

Spitzer, R. L., Yanovski, S. Z., Wadden, T., & Wang, R. (1993). Binge eating disorder: Its further validation in a multisite study. *International Journal of Eating Disorders, 13,* 137–153.

Stice, E. (2001). A prospective test of the dual-pathway model of bulimic pathology: Mediating effects of dieting and negative affect. *Journal of Abnormal Psychology, 110,* 124–135.

Stice, E., & Agras, W. S. (1998). Predicting onset and cessation of bulimic behaviors during adolescence: A longitudinal grouping analysis. *Behavior Therapy, 29,* 257–276.

Stice, E., & Bearman, S. K. (2001). Body-image and eating disturbances prospectively predict increases in depressive symptoms in adolescent girls: A growth curve analysis. *Developmental Psychology, 37,* 1–11.

Striegel-Moore, R. H. (1993). Etiology of binge eating: A developmental perspective. In C. G. Fairburn & G. T. Wilson (Eds.), *Binge eating: Nature, assessment, and treatment* (pp. 144–172). New York: Guilford Press.

Striegel-Moore, R. H. (1995). A feminist perspective on the etiology of eating disorders. In K. D. Brownell & C. G. Fairburn (Eds.), *Eating disorders and obesity: A comprehensive handbook* (pp. 224–229). New York: Guilford Press.

Striegel-Moore, R. H., Cachelin, F. M., Dohm, F. A., Pike, K. M., Wilfley, D. E., & Fairburn, C. G. (2001). Comparison of binge eating disorder and bulimia nervosa in a community sample. *International Journal of Eating Disorders, 29,* 157–165.

Striegel-Moore, R. H., Silberstein, L. R., & Rodin, J. (1986). Toward an understanding of risk factors for bulimia. *American Psychologist, 41,* 246–263.

Striegel-Moore, R. H., Wilfley, D. E., Pike, K. M., Dohm, F. A., & Fairburn, C. G. (2000). Recurrent binge eating in black American women. *Archives of Family Medicine, 9,* 83–87.

Strober, M. (1980). Personality and symptomatlogical features in young, nonchronic anorexia nervosa patients. *Journal of Psychosomatic Research, 24,* 353–359.

Strober, M. (1995). Family-genetic perspectives on anorexia nervosa and bulimia nervosa. In K. Brownell & C. G. Fairburn (Eds.), *Eating disorders and obesity: A comprehensive handbook* (pp. 212–218). New York: Guilford Press.

Strober, M., Freeman, R., Bower, S., & Rigali, J. (1996). Binge eating in anorexia nervosa predicts later onset of substance use disorder: A ten-year prospective, longitudinal follow-up of 95 adolescents. *Journal of Youth and Adolescence, 25,* 519–531.

Strober, M., Freeman, R., Lampert, C., Diamond, J., & Kaye, W. (2000). Controlled family study of anorexia nervosa and bulimia nervosa: Evidence of shared liability and transmission of partial syndromes. *American Journal of Psychiatry, 157,* 393–401.

Strober, M., & Humphrey, L. L. (1987). Familial contributions to the etiology and course of anorexia nervosa and bulimia. *International Journal of Eating Disorders, 5,* 654–659.

Strober, M., & Katz, J. L. (1987). Do eating disorders and affective disorders share a common etiology? A dissenting opinion. *International Journal of Eating Disorders,* 6, 171–180.

Stunkard, A. J. (1959). Eating patterns and obesity. *Psychiatric Quarterly, 33,* 284–292.

Stunkard, A. J. (2002). Binge-eating disorder and the night-eating syndrome. In T. A. Wadden & A. J. Stunkard (Eds.). *Handbook of obesity treatment* (pp. 107–124). New York: Guilford Press.

Tanofsky, M. B., Wilfley, D. E., Spurrell, E. B., Welch, R., & Brownell, K. D. (1997). Comparison of men and women with binge eating disorder. *International Journal of Eating Disorders, 21,* 49–54.

Telch, C. F., Pratt, E. M., & Niego, S. H. (1998). Obese women with binge eating disorder define the term binge. *International Journal of Eating Disorders, 24,* 313–318.

Telch, C. F., & Stice, E. (1998). Psychiatric comorbidity in women with binge eating disorder: Prevalence rates from a non-treatment-seeking sample. *Journal of Consulting and Clinical Psychology, 66,* 768–776.

Thompson, J. K., Heinberg, L. J., Altabe, M., & Tantleff-Dunn, S. (1999). *Exacting beauty: Theory, assessment, and treatment of body image disturbance.* Washington, DC: American Psychological Association.

Toner, B. B., Garfinkel, P. E., & Garner, D. M. (1988). Affective and anxiety disorders in the long-term follow-up of anorexia nervosa. *International Journal of Psychiatry in Medicine, 18,* 357–364.

Treasure, J., & Holland. A. (1989). Genetic vulnerability to eating disorders: Evidence from twin and family studies. In H. Remschmidt & M. H. Schmidt (Eds.), *Child and youth psychiatry: European perspectives* (pp. 59–68). New York: Hogrefe & Huber.

Vandereycken, W. (1995). The families of patients with an eating disorder. In K. D. Brownell & C. G. Fairburn (Eds.), *Eating disorders and obesity: A comprehensive handbook* (pp. 219–223). New York: Guilford Press.

Wadden, T. A., & Stunkard, A. J. (Eds.). (2002). *Handbook of obesity treatment.* New York: Guilford Press.

Waller, G., Slade, P., & Calam, R. (1990). Family adaptability and cohesion: Relation to eating attitudes. *International Journal of Eating Disorders, 9,* 225–228.

Walsh, B. T. (1993). Binge eating in bulimia nervosa. In C. G. Fairburn & G. T. Wilson (Eds.), *Binge eating: Nature, assessment, and treatment* (pp. 37–49). New York: Guilford Press.

Walsh, A. E., Oldman, A. D., Franklin, M., Fairburn, C. G., & Cowen, P. J. (1995). Dieting decreases plasma tryptophan and increases the prolactin response to *d*-fenfluramine in women but not men. *Journal of Affective Disorders, 33,* 89–97.

Walters, E. E., & Kendler, K. S. (1995). Anorexia nervosa and anorexic-like syndromes in a population-based female twin sample. *American Journal of Psychiatry, 152,* 64–71.

Walters, E. E., Neale, M. C., Eaves, L. J., Heath, A. C., Kessler, R. C., & Kendler, K. S. (1992). Bulimia nervosa and major depression: A study of common genetic and environmental factors. *Psychological Medicine, 22,* 617–622.

Walters, E. E., Neale, M. C., Eaves, L. J., Heath, A. C., Kessler, R. C., & Kendler, K. S. (1993). Bulimia nervosa: A population-based study of purgers versus nonpurgers. *International Journal of Eating Disorders, 13,* 265–272.

Welch, S. L., & Fairburn, C. G. (1996). Childhood sexual and physical abuse as risk factors for the development of bulimia nervosa: A community-based case control study. *Child Abuse and Neglect, 20,* 633–642.

Wilfley, D. E., & Cohen, L. R. (1997). Psychological treatment of bulimia nervosa and binge eating disorder. *Psychopharmacology Bulletin, 33,* 437–454.

Wilfley, D. E., Dounchis, J. Z., Stein, R. I., Welch, R. R., Friedman, M. A., & Ball, S. A. (2000). Comorbid psychopathology in binge eating disorder: Relation to eating disorder severity at baseline and following treatment. *Journal of Consulting and Clinical Psychology, 68,* 641–649.

Wilfley, D. E., Schwartz, M. B., Spurrell, E. B., & Fairburn, C. G. (2000). Using the Eating Disorder Examination to identify the specific psychopathology of binge eating disorder. *International Journal of Eating Disorders, 27,* 259–269.

Wilfley, D. E., Welch, R. R., Stein, R. I., Spurrell, E. B., Cohen, L. R., Saelens, B. S., Dounchis, J. Z., Frank, M. A., Wiseman, C. V., & Matt, G. E. (in press). A randomized comparison of group cognitive-behavioral therapy and group interpersonal psychotherapy for the treatment of binge eating disorder. *Archives of General Psychiatry.*

Wilson, G. T. (1991). The addiction model of eating disorders: A critical analysis. *Advances in Behavior Research and Therapy, 13,* 27–72.

Wilson, G. T. (1993). Relation of dieting and voluntary weight loss to psychological functioning. *Annals of Internal Medicine, 119,* 727–730.

Wilson, G. T. (2002). The controversy over dieting. In C. G. Fairburn & K. D. Brownell (Eds.), *Eating disorders and obesity: A comprehensive handbook* (2nd ed., pp. 93–97). New York: Guilford Press.

Wilson, G. T., & Eldredge, K. L. (1992). Pathology and development of eating disorders: Implications for athletes. In K. D. Brownell, J. Rodin, & J. H. Wilmore (Eds.), *Eating, body weight and performance in athletes* (pp. 115–127). Philadelphia: Lea & Febiger.

Wilson, G. T., & Fairburn, C. G. (2002). Eating disorders. In P. E. Nathan & J. M. Gorman (Eds.), *Treatments that work* (2nd ed., pp. 559–592). New York: Oxford University Press.

Wilson, G. T., & Latner, J. (2001). Eating disorders and addiction. In M. Hetherington (Ed.), *Food cravings and addiction* (pp. 585–605). Surrey, England: Leatherhead.

Wilson, G. T., Nonas, K. A., & Rosenblum, G. D. (1993). Assessment of binge-eating in obese patients. *International Journal of Eating Disorders, 13,* 25–34.

Wonderlich, S., Crosby, R., Mitchell, J., Thompson, K., Redlin, J., Demuth, G., & Smyth, J. (2001). Pathways mediating sexual abuse and eating disturbance in children. *International Journal of Eating Disorders, 29,* 270–279.

Wonderlich, S. A., & Mitchell, J. E. (1997). Eating disorders and comorbidity: Empirical, conceptual, and clinical implications. *Psychopharmacology Bulletin, 33,* 381–390.

Yanovski, S. Z., Gormally, J. F., Leser, M. S., Gwirtsman, H. E., & Yanovski, J. A. (1994). Binge eating disorder affects outcome of comprehensive very-low-calorie diet treatment. *Obesity Research, 2,* 205–212.

Yanovski, S. Z., Leet, M., Yanovski, J. A., Flood, M., Gold, P. W., Kissileff, H. R., & Walsh, B. T. (1992). Food selection and intake of obese women with binge eating disorder. *American Journal of Clinical Nutrition, 56,* 975–980.

Yanovski, S. Z., & Sebring, N. G. (1994). Recorded food intake of obese women with binge eating disorders before and after weight loss. *International Journal of Eating Disorders, 15,* 135–150.

CHAPTER SIXTEEN

Health-Related Disorders

Lizette Peterson
Kelle Reach
Shelly Grabe

Over the last decade, psychologists have made extraordinary strides (Olson, Mullins, Gillman, & Chaney, 1994), similar to those made by physicians, nurses, and others, in the identification and treatment of childhood health-related disorders during the last century. It is astonishing to recall that at one time even the process of handwashing was new, and modern medicine—with the development of antibiotics, immunizations, organ transplants, and even an understanding of psychoneuroimmunology (Cohen & Herbert, 1996)—has completely altered concepts of health and illness. The field of pediatric psychology is extremely diverse by comparison with that of five decades ago; it varies from intervening with children who are primarily healthy (e.g., assisting a healthy child to cope with an immunization to prevent disease and maintain good health), to working with children who have serious health problems due to unintentional injuries, and on to helping children with lifelong chronic diseases.

The field has developed a positive, preventive focus, such as working to help children and their families follow a healthy diet, avoid substance use, and generally establish a healthy lifestyle to prevent later health problems (Seligman, 1996). Pediatric psychologists initially focused on acutely or chronically ill children, with goals of ultimately improving all aspects of children's behavioral treatment. They did this by increasing the optimal application of diet and utilization of drugs, improving medication adherence, reducing nonorganic pain (e.g., headaches) maintained with secondary rewards, and decreasing pseudoseizures maintained by adult and peer attention. The field also assisted chronically ill children in coping with the many side effects of chronic conditions, such as the need to limit diet in phenylketonuria (PKU) or to test blood sugar in diabetes. Then pediatric psychology sought to expand its focus by becoming involved in other areas of the field, such as reducing the psychosocial sequelae of children's health-related disorders. Children can now receive help in many different ways, ranging from social skills self-training when they are deprived of normal peer contact to classroom education about the nature of a disorder such as diabetes or what can be expected for a child with cancer who is going to lose his or her hair. Teaching caring and "normalizing" peer responding can be invaluable. As can be seen from these varied activities, the area of health-related disorders ranges along a continuum of different conditions, challenges, and levels of severity.

Some of the problems discussed in this chapter are not truly "medical disorders," but may be conceptualized as medical stressors with which children and their parents must cope. These stressors range along a continuum from mild difficulties that are experienced by a majority of children (e.g., injections, eating enough fiber), to rare health problems that are life-threatening and include complicated, daily medical treatment (e.g., cystic fibrosis, PKU, sickle cell disease, diabetes), to serious unintentional injuries (which are currently the leading cause of death for children in the United States; Baker, O'Neill, Ginsburg, & Li, 1992; National Institute for Health Care Management, 2000).

The field of child health-related disorders differs from child psychopathology in its emphasis on the interaction between physical well-being and psychological disorders. Indeed, each of the physical problems discussed in this chapter has medical, psychological, and psychosocial components. Because of the importance of each component in the biopsychosocial model, the field of health-related disorders is truly an interdisciplinary field; it requires teamwork among psychologists, physicians, nurses, occupational and physical therapists, dietitians, public health officials, educators, chaplains, and administrators.

In this chapter, an effort is made to help the reader appreciate the diversity of this field and understand the particular challenges of working with children who have health-related disorders. In contrast to most of the other chapters in this book, which focus on single, specific problems, this chapter provides an overview of many disorders rather than an in-depth examination of a particular disorder. Thus we can only offer some basic examples of critical issues. We begin our discussion with an examination of the history of this diverse field.

HISTORICAL CONTEXT

Scientists have been interested in health-related disorders throughout the course of history. Early cultures not only were interested in the treatment of existing diseases, but were curious about the relationship among behavior, health, and the prevention of disease. The earliest records of Oriental, Islamic, Buddhist, Judaic, and Christian religions suggest an understanding of the relationship between personal habits (e.g., avoiding certain foods, moderating intake of food and drink, adhering to good sleep habits) and good physical health (Matarazzo, 1984). Early treatments were primitive, and often based on physicians' belief systems rather than scientific data (e.g., the use of leeches to bleed the "bad blood" from patients; this practice may have assisted briefly in patients with high blood pressure, but more often had negative effects on a body already weakened by a disease having nothing to do with amount of blood). Some treatments focused on dealing with existing plague conditions, such as burning the bodies of those who had died of smallpox, and these may actually have limited the spread of such diseases. In other instances, however, medical practitioners were very slow to instigate change based on empirical data. For example, in the mid-19th century, the theories of physician Ignaz Semmelweis predated Pasteur's germ theory and Lister's surgical antisepsis. Semmelweis argued repeatedly that puerperal fever, which was killing many women delivering babies in busy hospitals, could be reduced simply by the attending physicians' washing their hands between deliveries. However, women continued to die following childbirth as physicians refused to accept Semmelweis's suggestions of antiseptic handwashing between patients, and the ridicule of his work continued until after his death (Raju, 1999).

During the early part of the 20th century, attention turned to psychodynamic theory, which was utilized to explain such diverse conditions as child abuse and neglect, enuresis and encopresis, and somatoform disorders. Only in the second half of the century was the field open to several new developments in the field of pediatric health disorders, including growth of the field of psychoneuroimmunology, the increased application of behavior therapy, and increased understanding of the biopsychosocial model of health and disease.

The field of psychoneuroimmunology has been influential in helping scientists understand the link between psychological factors (such as stress and coping style) and biological systems (such as the immune system). It is now widely accepted that a large variety of stressors, such as maternal separation, bereavement, restraint, and crowding, affect a child's immune system (Cohen & Herbert, 1996; Kemeny & Laudenslager, 1999; Maier, Watkins, & Fleshner, 1994). Although such psychological processes as mood state and coping style may affect the immune system, this relationship is bidirectional, as immune processes themselves may influence the central nervous system and behavior. For example, it has been hypothesized that the immune system may activate the central nervous system in such a way as to cue increased perceptions of pain, which therefore may result in active behaviors that serve to reduce the pain (Maier et al., 1994).

Similar to the impact of psychoneuroimmunology on new developments in the field of medicine, the advent of behavioral theory and behavior therapy has had a strong influence on the field of health-related disorders. Operant conditioning models have been utilized to teach children very specific skills (e.g., pill swallowing, glucose testing, and compliance with a medical regimen), as well as to assist children in dealing with pain disorders and elimination disorders (e.g., encopresis). Classical conditioning models have been utilized to understand and treat such specific conditions as anticipatory nausea and certain types of feeding disorders.

Although professionals have relied primarily on traditional behavioral models, writings in the pediatric field have also increasingly emphasized a systems perspective (e.g., Hanson, 1992; Kazak, 1992; Mullins, Gillman, & Harbeck, 1992). Currently, the behavioral–systems model has gained popularity. This model retains the behavioral emphasis on thorough assessment, but it focuses (as do all behavioral methods) on the use of empirically based treatment approaches, and concern for treatment maintenance, implementation, generalization, and demonstration of techniques with differing populations (Peterson, Homer, & Wonderlich, 1982). In addition, this approach includes systems concepts, such as multiple levels of inquiry and intervention (e.g., biological, cognitive, affective, and behavioral, at the individual, family, and community levels). Finally, the behavioral–systems model recognizes that extremely complex patterns of interaction exist within a given system. Few such studies, however, have focused on medicine; most family systems research has been in the area of delinquency. This chapter considers the studies that exist, but the small number of such studies needs to be acknowledged.

Currently, interest in child health-related disorders and child psychopathology remains high. Several organizations have been formed to promote scientific inquiry in this field. The Society of Behavioral Medicine, the Society for Pediatric Psychology (which recently became Division 54 of the American Psychological Association), the Society of Behavioral Pediatrics, and the Association for the Care of Children's Health are a few examples of professional organizations devoted to furthering additional study of specific care in the area. Of course, several other major associations—such as the Society for Research in Child Development and the American Psychological Association's Division 7 (Developmental Psychology) and Division 37 (Child, Youth, and Family Services)—have always had recognition in this area. Texts too numerous to mention have been written to further our understanding of the role of child health disorders, and illustrate the richness of this field.

Thus, even since the first edition of this book, many large strides have been made in the understanding of childhood health-related disorders. Researchers have improved the knowledge base through empirical research in articles, chapters, and textbooks that describe the biological and psychological components of many chronic childhood illnesses. Although much of the research in this area has been descriptive and has focused on increasing clinicians' understanding about health-related disorders, research on effective interventions and prevention programs is beginning as well. In addition, there has been an emphasis on theory-driven research over the last several years.

Perhaps the largest change in children's health care research in the last two decades has been the realization that unidimensional theories will no longer suffice. Children's health problems must be viewed in the context of the child, the family, the community, and larger influences from national sources. Ethnic and neighborhood cultural influences are profound and must also be taken into account in diagnosis and treatment of childhood health-related disorders. It is clear that all such disorders are products of both organic and psychosocial problems; the fourth edition of the *Diagnostic and Statistical Manual of Mental Disorders* (DSM-IV; American Psychiatric Association, 1994) considers the general etiology of health-related disorders and the effects of psychological factors on medical conditions (see Table 16.1). We try to do justice to these distinctions, and also discuss some more specific DSM-IV diagnoses.

We begin our consideration of children's health problems (see Table 16.2 for an outline) with the most basic of child processes: nutrition. We consider food intake situations where intake is too little (e.g., nonorganic failure to thrive [NOFTT]) or too much (e.g., obesity); situations in which certain foods must be eliminated from the diet (e.g., PKU); and diseases in which feeding itself presents distinct problems (e.g., cystic fibrosis). We then consider elimination disorders (e.g., enuresis and encopresis).

Medical problems then receive focus, beginning with those having a primarily psychosocial etiology (e.g., sleep disorders, unintentional injuries, neglect, somatoform disorders). We next focus on problems with disease-based pain (e.g.,

TABLE 16.1. DSM-IV Criteria for Psychological Factors Affecting Medical Condition

A. A general medical condition (coded on Axis III) is present.

B. Psychological factors adversely affect the general medical condition in one of the following ways:

(1) the factors have influenced the course of the general medical condition as shown by a close temporal association between the psychological factors and the development or exacerbation of, or delayed recovery from, the general medical condition
(2) the factors interfere with the treatment of the general medical condition
(3) the factors constitute additional health risks for the individual
(4) stress-related physiological responses precipitate or exacerbate symptoms of the general medical condition

Choose name based on the nature of the psychological factors (if more than one factor is present, indicate the most prominent):

Mental Disorder Affecting ... **[*Indicate the General Medical Condition*]** (e.g., an Axis I disorder such as Major Depressive Disorder delaying recovery from a myocardial infarction)
Psychological Symptoms Affecting ... **[*Indicate the General Medical Condition*]** (e.g., depressive symptoms delaying recovery from surgery; anxiety exacerbating asthma)
Personality Traits or Coping Style Affecting ... **[*Indicate the General Medical Condition*]** (e.g., pathological denial of the need for surgery in a patient with cancer; hostile, pressured behavior contributing to cardiovascular disease)
Maladaptive Health Behaviors Affecting ... **[*Indicate the General Medical Condition*]** (e.g., overeating; lack of exercise; unsafe sex)
Stress-Related Physiological Response Affecting ... **[*Indicate the General Medical Condition*]** (e.g., stress-related exacerbations of ulcer, hypertension, arrhythmia, or tension headache)
Other or Unspecified Psychological Factors Affecting ... **[*Indicate the General Medical Condition*]** (e.g., interpersonal, cultural, or religious factors)

Note. From American Psychiatric Association (1994, p. 678). Copyright 1994 by the American Psychiatric Association. Reprinted by permission.

sickle cell disease), problems involving minor disease-related pain but with life-threatening potential (e.g., diabetes, epilepsy, asthma), and childhood cancer. We conclude by describing an example of a successful psychological response to a child health challenge: the reduction of pain related to disease and to medical procedures.

There is, within all of these themes, the possibility of teaching healthy personal habits (e.g., an appropriate diet may ward off both anorexia nervosa and obesity; successful toilet training can often forestall many types of elimination disorders). This successful early treatment may, when there is no organic problem, act as prevention.

NUTRITION-RELATED PROBLEMS

Food Intake Problems

Nonorganic Failure to Thrive

The literature within the areas of abuse and neglect has often focused on NOFTT. NOFFT is categorized by DSM-IV as feeding disorder of infancy or early childhood, and is discussed by Lyons-Ruth, Zeanah, and Benoit in Chapter 13 of this volume as a disorder of infancy (see Table 13.3 of that chapter for the DSM-IV diagnostic criteria). It is one of the most classic cases of care-

TABLE 16.2. Types of Child Health-Related Disorders Covered in This Chapter

Nutrition-related problems
- Food intake problems (e.g., NOFTT, obesity, PKU, cystic fibrosis); elimination disorders (e.g., enuresis and encopresis)

Medical problems with a primarily psychosocial etiology
- Sleep disorders (e.g., primary insomnia, breathing-related sleep disorder, nightmare disorder, sleep terror disorder); unintentional injuries; neglect; somatoform disorders (general syndromes, such as somatization disorder, undifferentiated somatoform disorder, and conversion disorder; specific recurrent pain disorders, such as headaches and recurrent abdominal pain)

Disease-based pain (e.g., sickle cell disease)

Disorders with minor disease-related pain but life-threatening potential (e.g., diabetes, epilepsy, asthma)

Childhood cancer

giver neglect of an infant or small child; it is also one of the most serious. As will be discussed later in this chapter, failure to supervise a child or neglect of a child's basic needs is difficult to demonstrate. NOFTT, in contrast, is ultimately a clearly measurable and easily definable form of neglect. Unfortunately, there are many organic reasons for a child's failure to gain weight and grow as expected, including iron deficiency, chronic diseases, chronic renal failure, liver disease, and recurring urinary tract infections. Even if the cause is organic, however, neglectful parents may not be receptive to medical interventions that they are held responsible to carry out (Wright & Talbot, 1996).

Some scientists have attempted to break childhood feeding problems down according to specific causes, categorizing them as structural (related to the child's feeding behavior), neurological (related to child physiology), and maternal behavior problems. Burklow, Phelps, Schultz, McConnell, and Rudolph (1998) found that 30% of the infants with feeding problems they observed showed structural, neurological, and maternal behavioral problems, 27% showed neurological and maternal behavioral problems, 12% showed maternal behavioral problems alone, 9% showed structural and maternal behavioral problems, and 19% showed structural and neurological causes. In 3% of the cases, the causes of the children's feeding problems could not be diagnosed. The authors' conclusion was that although mothers played a decisive part in feeding problems, the children's behavioral difficulties could also be contributed to low birthweight. Similarly, many other researchers note the dangerous combination of difficult-to-feed children and mothers who are not securely attached to their infants (Chatoor, Ganiban, Colin, Plummer, & Harmon, 1998).

Part of the problem in some families of children showing NOFTT is that no one caregiver takes primary responsibility for appropriate feeding. Another typical pattern is that there are feeding problems caused by caregivers' insensitivity to infants' cues of hunger. It is the combination of less than sensitive mothers with infants who refuse to feed on a regular schedule that results in the most serious problems (Hagekull, Bohlin, & Rydell, 1997), and this situation does not resolve over time. Hagekull et al. (1997) found that when maternal sensitivity was not well suited to the child, resulting in difficulty in feeding at 10 months, this problem was still present at 2 years of age.

Kerwin (1999) has suggested that for women who do not have experience in reading their infants' signs of hunger, there needs to be some sort of contingency management that leads to appropriate feeding, which in turn is positively reinforcing. Such mothers need to be taught to ignore children's refusal responses (turning the head away from the nipple, etc.) and to wait and offer food again. Having mothers reward infants for food acceptance by vocal or tactile cues, and ignore food refusal, seems to be the most effective combination. These mothers often need more than the usual amount of help, as their children may have learned to get attention not only by refusing food, but by demanding pureed food rather than solid food, vomiting or physically throwing solid food, and so on. Steady rewarding of appropriate eating, and ignoring rather than harshly punishing inappropriate responses to food, are essential. Obviously, early preventive intervention is preferable to treating ingrained habits.

Thus the extent to which deprivation and neglect can be attributed solely to the parent may have been overstated in the literature. Most authors now agree that a clear absence of appropriate food-offering behavior from the mother, in combination with a child who has low appetite and underdemanding food behavior, results in the worst symptoms of NOFTT (Wright & Birks, 2000). Caregivers of such children typically do not have secure attachments with their children, which makes the necessary interventions (reward by touch or voice for appropriate eating) even more difficult. For example, Ward, Lee, and Lipper (2000) found that within their sample, only 13% of children with NOFTT had secure attachments, in contrast with 58% of well-nourished youngsters who had secure attachments. Again, it was concluded that disorganized mother–child pairs in which the mother lacked skill or motivation and the child had operantly conditioned refusal and low appetite were the cases most likely to lead to NOFTT.

Often children have had a medical "workup" to rule out organic causes of failure to grow and gain weight as expected. After an extensive hospital stay to undergo medical tests, children with no organic cause for their low weight are then sent home with caregivers who may have received no additional assistance or only a few home visits in order to investigate and address the possibility of potential neglect. The past typical conceptualization of a child's failure to grow (by weight, length, and head circumference) in the absence of organic causes has been the assumption that the caregiver is feeding the infant inadequate calories (Hobbs & Hanks, 1996). NOFTT can continue to be serious even if the caregiver later receives help. The absence of appropriate nutrition early in life results not only in simple absence of growth, but also in decreases in normal growth hormone, which influences future growth (Hobbs & Hanks, 1996). These problems often show up early in life (almost always by 6 months of age, when the child fails to be introduced to solid food). However, it is often difficult to know what difficulties to ascribe to NOFTT. For example, some children with NOFTT suffer from mental retardation at birth, and this is almost certainly confused with minor intellectual difficulties caused by inadequate pre- and postnatal nutrition.

Interventions for NOFTT have shown the utility of individualized treatments using food diaries and other forms of support to encourage women to offer children at least three meals a day and three high-energy snacks (Moores, 1996). When one considers how demanding it is for the caregiver to encourage and reward appropriate eating—and then often as a result of his or her efforts to have the child's face pucker and turn away, or actually to have food thrown against the wall or on the floor—the improvements that have been documented show impressive change. Assistance from multiple sources, such as a pediatrician, a psychologist, and a dietary specialist, can also help to maintain positive outcomes.

Wright and Talbot (1996) have described an inverted pyramid in which most families of children with NOFTT need some minimal training in feeding; 50–80% need the efforts of a medical team to assist them; 20–30% need a home visitor to assist in modeling and praising appropriate feeding; and 5% of the children may need to be removed from the home because their caregivers are unable to provide sufficient nutrition to guard against long-term physical and psychological growth problems. Kerwin (1999) has provided one of the best reviews of this literature (with multiple studies described in detail in appendices), in which effective interventions involve modeling of correct feeding and rewarding the child, as well as rewarding the mother for successful feeding; such interventions are facilitated by ignoring inappropriate child responses. Again, Kerwin has concluded that in-home care and continuing consultation are essential to guarantee the maintenance of treatment effects. In any case, knowledge in the field of NOFTT has grown exponentially in the last decade, and we hope that it will continue to expand.

Our discussion now moves from efforts to ensure that children are ingesting an appropriate number of calories, to attempts to address an even more frequent problem in children—that of obesity, where a combination of too many calories taken in and too few expended can result in child health, psychosocial, and self-esteem problems.

Obesity

There are various methods for determining obesity in children. In the past, weight for age quickly gave way to underwater weighing, where fat could be detected because its density and weight differ from those of lean body mass. Some evaluations have relied on triceps skinfold measurement, which is an inexpensive way of determining subcutaneous fat. Currently, most researchers use body mass index (BMI; weight in kilograms/height in meters squared) as a reasonable compromise between cost and accuracy; a BMI over the 85th percentile is regarded as an index of overweight, and a BMI over the 95th percentile is seen as indexing severe obesity (Dietz & Bellizzi, 1999).

One child out of every five in the United States is overweight (Anand, 1998). Genes obviously contribute to obesity, but the degree to which genes control obesity is as yet undetermined (Bar-Or et al., 1998)—partly because, from the moment of conception, the embryo shares the mother's nutritional habits. Interestingly, both undernutrition and obesity during pregnancy can influence later obesity, as well as whether the mother breast-feeds rather than bottle-feeds (Maffeis, 2000). The food provided for children who are not overweight differs from that provided to obese children, and later, a child's age influences the child's eating habits as the child gains more independence. Older children and adolescents often prefer high-fat, easy-to-ingest snacks and meals (e.g., frozen and microwaveable foods and take-out food). Such snacks and meals often contain not only higher fat, but also a greater quantity of food than would be included in a typical family meal.

Furthermore, many children with high BMIs prefer inactive habits (such as watching TV and playing video games) to physical activities (Dietz, 1998a). Promoting the sense of obesity as a potential "epidemic" is the steady increase in children's and adolescents' weight as reported by the National Health and Nutrition Examination Survey (NHANES; Centers for Disease Control and Prevention, 2001). There has been a steady increase in the proportion of children overweight since National Health Examination Survey (NHES) II (1963–1965) and NHES III (1966–1970). In addition, NHANES II Phase 1 continued to show a steady increase, and Phases II and III (to 1994) also showed this trend (Centers for Disease Control and Prevention, 2001). In 1994, approximately 14% of U. S. children were overweight. Obesity not only differs across race or ethnicity, with African Americans more at risk (Dietz, 1998a); it differs within cultures as well. Normal physical characteristics, such as structure of fat tissue, energy, balance, metabolic rate, and central nervous system balance (Wishon, Bower, & Eller, 1983), are affected by being overweight, as noted previously. Weight typically increases with age (Moran, 1999), and thus so do increased cardiac risk factors, such as elevated cholesterol level and high blood pressure (McMurray, Harrel, Levine, & Gansky, 1995). Similarly, any acceleration of weight gain can cause orthopedic problems, such as tibia torsion, bowed legs, and skin disorders (Moran, 1999).

Such symptoms sound to most laypersons as if being overweight is entirely a physical matter, but few experts would agree with this conclusion. Most agree that chromosomal difficulties contribute to the problem, but these scientists concentrate, sensibly, on those factors that can be the focus of intervention prior to genetic interventions. (Genetic interventions for obesity that have been predicted for the future include exciting new techniques such as gene splicing and other direct forms of intervention on genotype; see Oeffner et al., 2001.) Regardless of etiology, obesity is a more serious medical problem than many people think. Public Law 94-142 determines what kinds of problems are eligible for the rehabilitation of disabled children, and severe obesity has been regarded as a legally defined disability (Wishon & Childs, 1984).

Some treatments for obesity can be as simple as taking the stairs instead of riding the elevator and walking to school instead of riding the bus (Strauss & Knight, 1999). There have been some very successful treatments once experimenters use this approach and are able to convince families of its merit. Communities are typically eager to offer interventions to families, if only the families are motivated to remain in treatment. Haddock, Shadish, Klesges, and Stein (1994) published a meta-analysis that examined the entrance of cognitive-behavioral therapy into the treatment of obesity. This meta-analysis concluded that there could be effective treatment (and, ultimately, prevention) of obesity, if families were willing to continue to be involved.

Effective treatment can include the treatment of comorbid psychological problems as well. Parents confuse side effects from gastronomical processes, including such issues as low blood sugar (Wishon et al., 1983), with the dysthymia or depression that often accompanies obesity (Dietz, 1998b). Girls tend to experience more negative affect than boys and are less inclined to burn off calories that will be converted into fat (Maffeis, 2000). Girls are also more concerned about their weight than are boys from middle childhood on to adulthood (Thelen, Powell, Lawrence, & Kuhnert, 1992). Thus obese children, especially girls, are more likely to have low self-esteem and to misuse substances than children who are not overweight (Strauss, 2000). In other words, they are especially at risk for problems encountered in adolescence. To summarize these materials, Epstein, Myers, Raynor, and Saelens (1998) wrote a landmark article on the prevention and behavioral treatment of obesity, and Haddock et al. (1994) contributed a meta-analysis on the topic that is highly recommended as an introduction to treatment in this area. One preferred mode of treatment is to work simultaneously on making exercises reinforcing and enjoyable. It focuses on self-monitoring, stimulus control, and rewards (Epstein et al., 1998).

There is also clear evidence that diet can be controlled with a simple three-part system. First, children must avoid foods with high fat or sugar content (e.g., candy—referred to as "red light" foods), limit high-carbohydrate and high-protein foods (e.g., pasta, chicken—referred to as "yellow light" foods), and eat primarily foods with high nutritional value (e.g., vegetables—referred to as "green light" foods). These dietary changes, plus an exercise program that can realistically be expected of a child in terms of both motivation and physical ability, have not only been shown to be effective immediately in weight loss; the loss has continued for years after program completion (Brownell, Kelman, & Stunkard, 1983; Epstein, Wing, Steranchak, Dickson, & Michelson, 1980). Some of these studies continue to show long-term success at 10 years, with 15% of the children (now adolescents) continuing to maintain their weight loss (Epstein, McCurley, Wing, & Valoski, 1990). Jelalian and Saelens (1999) used the current system of describing the utility of this combined treatment and pronounced it to be a "promising intervention," which is next to being the treatment of choice.

Thus far, we have considered problems whose prevention and treatment are fairly straightforward, despite the real-world difficulty in implementing them. This is in contrast to the diseases to be described next, in which dietary changes are vital for a child's well-being. These are no longer just issues of too few or too many calories, but of certain kinds of foods ingested during certain periods of time. Our first example is PKU—a disorder sufficiently widespread and disastrous when untreated that every child born in the United States in a hospital is tested for PKU, and has been for the last 40 years (Hellekson, 2001).

Phenylketonuria

PKU is a metabolic disorder caused by an autosomal recessive gene necessary for producing the enzyme phenylalanine hydroxylase, which is used to convert dietary phenylalanine to tyrosine. It is located on chromosome 12, and in its recessive form results in various degrees of severity in outcome (Koch, 1999). When individuals inherit recessive genes from both parents, they have a complete or near-complete deficiency of the liver enzyme phenylalanine hydroxylase. If untreated, this deficiency results in mental retardation, microencephialy, and seizures, in addition to behavioral abnormalities (Hellekson, 2001). PKU occurs in only one of every 15,000 U.S. infants, but the test to identify PKU is sufficiently straightforward (a blood stick) and the potential outcome so far-reaching that the test is done routinely in the United States on newborns, as noted above. Specialists suggest screening within 12 hours of birth. For children who show any signs of the disorder, continued screening 12–24 hours after birth and then at 3 months, 6 months, 9 months, 12 months, and at least yearly after this time is strongly recommended (Koch, 1999). PKU is more common in European Americans and Native Americans, and is less common in Hispanic Americans, African Americans, and Asian Americans.

Successful treatment has involved a fairly restricted diet. Treatment for PKU is important, because lifelong dietary treatment is necessary and the disorder becomes more difficult to treat as individuals age. The diet does differ from child to child, as some individuals develop a tolerance to phenylalanine later in life. There has now been a great deal published about when and how the diet can be restricted (Poustie & Rutherford, 2000). The major change is for a person with PKU to remain on protein substitutes taken evenly throughout the day (Wappner, Cho, Kronmal, Schuett, & Seashore, 1999); this is dissimilar to the dietary habits of most Europeans and North Americans. Children whose food intake is maintained with exact precision within the demands of the diet, which avoids all phenylalanines, will grow up completely normally, with no sign of the disorder. Children who completely fail to be provided with a special diet will rarely reach adolescence without serious physiological problems—among them, severe mental retardation (Leuzzi, Trasimeni, Gualdi, & Antonozzi, 1995).

The devastating outcomes resulting from a failure to implement a dietary intervention seem exceptionally unfortunate. Breast feeding, for example, protects an infant for the first few months. Although PKU is a lifetime disorder, protection to age 5 seems particularly important (Koch & Wenz, 1987), as children under 3 years of age show a direct effect of phenylalanine levels on many forms of cognitive function in addition to mental retardation (Arnold et al., 1998). Moreover, reviews of the existing literature suggest that such children have poorer motor control and excretory functioning (Arnold et al., 1998). Internalizing problems (e.g., depression, anxiety, and low self-esteem) may be seen either alone or associated with externalizing problems (including attention difficulties and aggressive disorders), and even with psychotic and autistic-like problems (Friedman, 1969; Sullivan & Chang, 1999).

Although the demands of PKU are relatively mild in comparison with those of some disorders we will discuss—in which medication must be balanced with diet (e.g., diabetes), or in which a child is entirely dependent on a medication that may or may not work (e.g., childhood cancer)—it would be a mistake to underemphasize the difficulty of keeping an apparently normal and healthy child on a rigid diet. In one study, parents of children with PKU rated dealing with the diet as the most stressful aspect of the illness, and acknowledged deviating from the diet from time to time (Awiszus & Unger, 1990). Temporal stress (e.g., a parent suddenly has to make a decision about a diet, as when a child begs to go on a picnic with the neighbors, who are ready to leave) causes more difficulty in remaining on the diet, as does more general life stress (Fehrenbach & Peterson, 1989). Given that much is known about how to determine individuals' levels of phenylalanine, future research may well focus on methods of implementing this complex and often difficult-to-control diet. An especial challenge is the necessity of teaching teens to take over their own diet, when their peers prefer food not allowed in the PKU diet and adolescents have no immediate symptoms to warn them of the long-term costs of neglecting the narrowly prescribed foods on the PKU regimen. Many teens actually go off the diet at this time without significant complications, but this may not be appropriate for some.

We next consider an equally serious disorder—one almost always resulting in premature death, and again requiring a special diet. Rather than requiring that a child get a full, normal diet (as in NOFTT), or get fewer calories and more exercise (as in obesity), or even avoid certain foods (as in PKU), cystic fibrosis is a disorder that requires an unusually large number of calories to keep a child in reasonably good health.

Cystic Fibrosis

Cystic fibrosis is caused by an autosomal recessive gene. It results in retarded growth due to loss of fat via malabsorption in the intestine. An insufficiency of pancreatic enzymes leads to this malabsorption of fat, which necessitates more nutrition than is typically the case (Simmons, Goldberg, Washington, Fischer-Fay, & Maclusky, 1995) and results in respiratory tract difficulties and eating problems (Cannella, Bowser, Guyer, & Borum, 1993). The child also shows enhanced energy requirements and excess urinary glucose. These symptoms—combined with abnormal salt metabolism, liver disease, and short-bowel syndrome—render the child consistently nutritionally challenged. Children with cystic fibrosis typically require 120–150% of normal minimal daily requirement for nutrition, involving high protein, use of dietary supplements, and (as a last resort) internal feeding (MacDonald, 1996; MacDonald, Holden, & Harris, 1991). Utilizing ASA guidelines as the "gold standard," Australians Anthony, Catto-Smith, Phelan, and Paxton (1998) have recommended monitoring nutritional standards at least four times a year by measuring height, weight, skinfold, and arm circumference.

Frequent checkups and dietary "tracks" (such as tests of the need for supplementary fat or carbohydrates) are among those interventions required for prolonging life and health as long as possible. In infancy, this often means supplementing normal breast or bottle feeding with additional fat or carbohydrates (Cannella et al., 1993). As with NOFTT, this becomes problematic because a child's propensity to avoid feeding often results in insecure attachment, which makes feeding a very unpleasant situation for the mother (Simmons et al., 1995). The likelihood of a child's premature death (Stark, Powers, Jelalian, Rape, & Miller, 1994) may also contribute to this lack of attachment.

It is not surprising that there should be family problems surrounding dinnertime for children who are steadily being required to eat more than they want. Sanders, Turner, Wall, Waugh, and Tully (1997) noted that nearly three-quarters of parents whose children have cystic fibrosis report mealtime problems, and that over 90% report problems with the children's physiotherapy compliance. Nasogastic blockage, reflux, and other medical side effects make eating particularly unpleasant. Moreover, distinct clinical improvement (such as weight gain and ability to eat normally) typically takes up to 6 months of treatment. Treatment also often involves a prolonged time to be removed from one's normal social system, as such feeding requires medical supervision, which limits a child's attending school and being involved in other activities. Certainly eating at camp, at parties, or with friends is rarely possible.

Both parents and children contribute to the feeding problems. Stark et al. (2000) noted that parents using oral feeding methods seem instinctively to use both effective and ineffective techniques at the table. On the one hand, parents provide more effective directions and verbal rewards for eating, which are helpful. On the other, they also tend to use what is usually a socially positive technique ("coaxing"), but in this case it is ineffective; instead of switching to more effective contingencies, they simply increase the amount of coaxing. Furthermore, children with cystic fibrosis spend a significantly longer time engaging in behaviors incompatible with eating (e.g., talking, leaving the table, and food refusal). Families exposed to extensive nutritional education plus management strategies increased their children's caloric intake by 1,034 calories per day. Management of a 91.7-kg increase in weight is the goal to be achieved and held over 3 and 6 months posttreatment (Stark et al., 2000).

Sanders et al. (1997) have recently suggested that compliance problems in children with cystic fibrosis relate to several aspects of family functioning; only a third of such problems have to do with feeding difficulties (and less than a third with difficulties in reaching the recommended daily intake of calories). There are also problems with compliance in general: Lower levels of expected verbal interactions characterize such children, while their caregivers often respond with a lower sense of self-efficacy. Nonaversive methods are suggested by Sanders et al. (1997) to increase compliance and feelings of self-efficacy, and to decrease feelings of inadequacy, helplessness, and uncertainty. Stark et al. (1994) have suggested didactic training, based on a review of family-specific situations drawn from videotaped actual meals. Such training includes using differential attention and contingent privileges, setting realistic expectations, and (where possible) substituting preferred foods with the same amounts of nutrition as nonpreferred foods.

Plainly, many parents of primarily healthy children as well as parents of children with serious disorders must focus on getting their children to take appropriate amounts of foods at appropriate times. It is therefore intriguing that one of the other major problems of parenting is, once the food is properly digested, to get a child to expel the foods that parents may have worked so steadfastly to get the child to ingest. The two most common forms of such problems are enuresis and encopresis; these disorders are covered next.

Elimination Disorders

Enuresis

The lack of bladder control occurs in all infants, but is regarded by most diagnostic systems (e.g., DSM-IV [see Table 16.3]; *International Classification of Diseases*, 10th revision, [ICD-10; World Health Organization, 1993]) as problematic when it occurs in preschool-age or older children during the day (daytime enuresis) or night (nocturnal enuresis or bedwetting). Enuresis only becomes a problem when the society in which the child lives designates that the child is old enough to be able to control his or her bladder during the day and night. The later the child develops bladder and bowel control in Western culture, the more negative the consequences the child must endure from family or friends (Cendron, 1999). About 15% of children become dry overnight each year of development, with 11% persistence of bedwetting to adulthood (Skoog, 1998). Between 5 and 7 million U. S. children each year have what is regarded as problematic nocturnal enuresis (i.e., bedwetting that is worthy of regular attention from child specialists and pediatricians; Cendron, 1999). Many more children remain dry during the daytime, when they are sensitive both to social criticism and to physical sensation; establishing nighttime control is much more difficult. "Primary" nocturnal enuresis is said to exist when a child has never been dry overnight. "Secondary" nocturnal enuresis refers to a case in which a child has been dry overnight for 6 months and then experiences further episodes of wetness (Butler, 1998). Enuresis may be at least in part influenced by genetic sources, and thus getting a family history can be very helpful. It is also influenced by sleep disorders, urodynamics, psychological factors, and developmental delay (Skoog, 1998).

TABLE 16.3. DSM-IV Criteria for Enuresis

A. Repeated voiding of urine into bed or clothes (whether involuntary or intentional).

B. The behavior is clinically significant as manifested by either a frequency of twice a week for at least 3 consecutive months or the presence of clinically significant distress or impairment in social, academic (occupational), or other important areas of functioning.

C. Chronological age is at least 5 years (or equivalent developmental level).

D. The behavior is not due exclusively to the direct physiological effect of a substance (e.g., diuretic) or a general medical condition (e.g., diabetes, spina bifida, a seizure disorder).

Specify type:
Nocturnal Only
Diurnal Only
Nocturnal and Diurnal

Note. From American Psychiatric Association (1994, pp. 109–110). Copyright 1994 by the American Psychiatric Association. Reprinted by permission.

Despite being toilet-trained, approximately 15–20% of 5-year-old children in the United

States become symptomatic at one time or another (Cendron, 1999). It is more common in boys than in girls (Costello et al., 1996) and is seen more often in high-risk families (such as larger families, those experiencing separations, or those with lower incomes). Those youths with behavioral problems such as thumbsucking (Byrd, Weitzman, Lanphear, & Auinger, 1996), internalizing problems such as anxiety (Butler, 1998), and externalizing disorders such as increased aggression (Byrd et al., 1996) are also at further risk for enuresis.

There have been a variety of interventions, from the most simple interventions (e.g., "Just let the child grow out of it") to overcorrection, where high rates of fluids are given and the child is wakened periodically; if the bed is found to be wet, the failure to waken and use the toilet is followed by rehearsing the correct responses a dozen or more times (Azrin & Thienes, 1978). However, it seems upsetting to some children to be forced to repeat the task, and overcorrection is very effortful. Changes in diet have also been used successfully, as have diet therapy and pharmacological treatment (e.g., desmopressin acetate). Perhaps the most popular intervention has been placing a pad under the child with a bell in it, which is set off by fluid lost by the child; this is referred to as the "bell and pad" treatment (Vogel, Young, & Primack, 1996). Interestingly, some scientists have argued that the child need not fully wake up for this treatment to be successful (Harari & Moulden, 2000).

Encopresis

Encopresis is a complex problem, typically involving cycles of diarrhea and constipation, resulting in soiling of clothes or bedsheets (see Table 16.4). Effecting an even balance of feces softness (liquid and solid) is difficult, and the child is often left with the alternative of using laxatives, which is followed by cramping and watery, diffcult-to-control diarrhea. However, when laxative and other interventions have been withdrawn, the child experiences cessation of bowel movements, followed by painful stools and the retention of the fecal material (often because it hurts to have a bowel movement). Increased drying out of the feces (the intestines continue to extract liquid while the fecal material is present) results in impaction, and the stool may become so difficult to pass that a physician may need to assist in its removal. Stark et al. (1997) have suggested that 3%

TABLE 16.4. DSM-IV Criteria for Encopresis

A. Repeated passage of feces into inappropriate places (e.g., clothing or floor) whether involuntary or intentional.

B. At least one such event a month for at least 3 months.

C. Chronological age is at least 4 years (or equivalent developmental level).

D. The behavior is not due exclusively to the direct physiological effects of a substance (e.g., laxatives) or a general medical condition except through a mechanism involving constipation.

Code as follows:
787.6 With Constipation and Overflow Incontinence
307.7 Without Constipation and Overflow Incontinence

Note. From American Psychiatric Association (1994, p. 107).

of all pediatric visits and a quarter of all pediatric gastrointestinal visits are focused on encopresis. Stark et al. (1997) note that to meet other and more serious definitions of encopresis, a child needs to average 3.67 soiling episodes, 4 independent bowel movements, and 1.67 parental-prompted bowel movements per week. Like enuresis, encopresis is best viewed developmentally; Stark et al. (1997) suggest that it influences 2.8% of 4-year-olds, 1.7% of 6-year-olds, and 1.6% of 10- to 11-year-olds. Over time, many more boys than girls (the ratio varies from 2.5:1 to 6:1) show signs of encopresis.

Physiological and psychological interactions need to occur in a social context to allow appropriate fecal movement. Adequate fiber and water intake; awareness of fecal cues; recognition and response to other abdominal bodily cues; and social knowledge concerning such skills as undressing, self-cleaning, and handwashing are all necessary for appropriate child bowel function. As noted previously, the fear of passing painful stools usually exists because they have become dried and impacted earlier, and are thus more difficult to pass; the child avoids doing so, which makes for greater water absorption and increased pain (McGrath, Mellon, & Murphy, 2000). Assisting the child with this discomfort (via biofeedback, suppositories, etc.) is also helpful.

Because of the number of factors clearly involved in encopresis (diet, family issues, pain, self-control), it is unclear whether psychological problems cause the physiological ones or vice versa, whether there is reciprocal causation, or whether some third variable results in both outcomes. Abrahamian and Lloyd-Still (1984) reported that 20% of children with encopresis have significant psychological problems in learning and employing appropriate bowel habits. Borowitz, Cox, and Sutphen (1999) contrasted siblings with and without clinical encopresis; they found that both groups showed difficulties, but that the siblings with encopresis typically had the most serious bowel habits, as well as comorbid behavioral problems.

Effective treatment has involved a number of different possibilities. As noted, increased fiber consumption is a relatively new and important component of avoiding encopresis (Stark et al., 1997). Most Americans, however, are not well informed about the fiber content of many foods and habitually break down much useful fiber through overcooking. It is difficult to successfully increase fiber content when one is unclear about what foods contain fiber. Americans often rate foods with scarcely any fiber (e.g., iceberg lettuce) as "roughage," and regard foods that are actually high in fiber (e.g., beans) as "starch." In summary, a complete behavioral program typically involves change in diet to include more fiber, biofeedback to aid the child in relaxing the external anal sphincter and pelvic floor during defecation, followed by a complete flushing of the system with laxatives, and then by behavior therapy (e.g., regular toilet sitting, stool diary). It is important to begin the processes of sphincter biofeedback with the judicious use of laxatives, to ensure that painful defecation is cleared up as soon as possible (Cox, Sutphen, Ling, Quillian, & Borowitz, 1996); however, it is vital that the overuse of laxatives be avoided, so that the child does not become dependent on them. This balance can be maintained by regular dietary habits and by following each successful defecation with reinforcement.

In all the psychosocial problems discussed to this point, there is a clear interaction between a physiological susceptibility in the child and a behavioral failure on the part of both the parent and the child to react appropriately to food intake or output. This formulation summarizes most of clinical child psychologists' contributions to the understanding of these disorders. The next section requires attention to physiological as well as behavioral components, but in quite a different way. Medical problems that have a primarily psychosocial etiology begin with psychological variables (e.g., stress, helplessness, lack of social support) and end with a physiological outcome.

MEDICAL PROBLEMS WITH A PRIMARILY PSYCHOSOCIAL ETIOLOGY

Sleep Disorders

The proportion of infants and children with sleep disorders ranges from 10.8% (Stein, Mendelsohn, Obermeyer, Amromin, & Benca, 2001) to over 50% (Anders & Eiben, 1997), depending greatly on the children's ages, the reporters, and the definition of sleep disorders used. Parents are accurate in terms of evaluating their children's overt behavior as checked with an actigraph (activity monitor), but are far less accurate in assessing the children's sleep quality. They tend to underestimate night wakenings and restorative sleep (Tikotzky & Sadeh, 2001). In one study, over 95% of severe sleep problems were reported by the children but not by the parents (Paavonen et al., 2002). DSM-IV diagnoses may be useful with children, but few infants and toddlers have sufficiently severe sleep problems to make a DSM-IV diagnosis warranted. We consider DSM criteria later in this section, for consistency with the rest of this book, but it is important to note the utility of other systems.

The *International Classification of Sleep Disorders: Diagnostic and Coding Manual* (American Sleep Disorders Association, 1990) defines "extrinsic sleep disorders" as including inadequate sleep hygiene, adjustment sleep disorder, inadequate sleep syndrome, and sleep onset association disorder. The manual also offers a method to rate duration and acuity criteria; this method, by defining the nature of the problem, indicates a method of intervention. Yet it has less psychometric support than some other measures. The *Diagnostic Classification of Mental Health and Developmental Disorders of Infancy to Early Childhood* (Zero to Three/National Center for Clinical Infant Programs, 1994) has similar clinical strengths (by the authors' report), but weak psychometrics. Some authors (e.g., Stein et al., 2001) have successfully used the Child Behavior Checklist, which has excellent psychometrics but is not constructed to focus on sleep disorders per se, and the portion of the overall inventory that does is somewhat limited. Thus many individuals are still using DSM-IV or some variant. For example, Gaylor, Goodlin-Jones, and Anders (2001) described a developmental classification score for toddlers and young children that relates to the DSM-IV category of dyssomnias, and breaks these down into sleep onset problems and night wakening problems—both seen as aspects of normal development early in life and at low levels, but as becoming more problematic with duration and number of required parental contacts. Thus considering the DSM-IV system seems valuable, as it remains the most widely known system to health care professionals and thus may more easily evolve into a system by which assessment may result more easily into not only an understanding of the disorder but a set of suggestions for intervention.

Primary Insomnia

DSM-IV criteria for primary insomnia are discussed by Lyons-Ruth et al. in Chapter 13 of this volume, and presented in Table 13.6 there. This is the most common of sleep disorders, occurring in 5–50% of children under the age of 3 (Anders & Eiben, 1997). It is characterized as difficulty falling asleep or staying asleep, and, as can be seen in Table 13.6, is most often defined by exclusion (i.e., it is *not* one of the other sleep disorders). Unfortunately, this often results in increased family tension, maternal depression, and maternal ambivalence rather than love toward the child (Reid, Walter, & O'Leary, 1999).

It is intriguing to note that in some cultures it is considered abusive to leave small children alone in the dark to cry, while in North American culture it is considered abnormal to allow a child to remain with the parents (Lutzker, 1998). Some scientists have suggested progressively lengthening the time a child is allowed to cry as a behavioral treatment. At first light, this might seem illogical; progressively lengthening the time until reward usually strengthens a behavior, rather than weakening it. The process makes behavioral sense if it is viewed as progressively desensitizing the parent to the child's crying rather than operating on the child, who is merely ultimately undergoing extinction. In any case, a recent study (Reid et al., 1999) found that progressively lengthened crying time before parental contact with the child was no better in hastening the child's sleep onset than merely telling the parent not to attend to the child, both of which were superior to no directions whatsoever. Time to sleep onset seems to decrease in most children as they mature and to be a developmentally specific behavior, as noted earlier.

Breathing-Related Sleep Disorder

Another type of sleep disorder is caused by a child's airways' being blocked when he or she lies down, which results in repeated obstruction of the airways. This condition is called breathing-related sleep disorder by DSM-IV (see Table 16.5) and sleep apnea by the medical community, and can occur in individuals from infancy to middle age. It is exacerbated by overlarge adenoids and/or tonsils, and in adults by overweight, which tends to result in a caving in of the air passages. Once the condition is correctly diagnosed by observing or electronically monitoring a child's breathing, it can be readily corrected, typically by removal of the adenoids and tonsils. In older individuals, there may be other tissue that requires removal. As might be imagined, sleep apnea is impervious to most of the usual treatments, and thus it is very important to rule it out if a typically effective treatment is ineffective.

Nightmare Disorder

Nightmare disorder (Table 16.6) is characterized by being wakened from periods of sleep in association with rapid-eye-movement (REM) sleep. The child typically, if old enough to be verbal, can explain that a frightening set of visualizations

TABLE 16.5. DSM-IV Criteria for Breathing-Related Sleep Disorder

A. Sleeping disruption, leading to excessive sleepiness or insomnia, that is judged to be due to a sleep-related breathing condition (e.g., obstructive or central sleep apnea syndrome or central alveolar hypoventilation syndrome).

B. The disturbance is not better accounted for by another mental disorder and is not due to the direct physiological effects of a substance (e.g., a drug of abuse, a medication) or another general medical condition (other than a breathing-related disorder).

Coding note: Also code sleep-related breathing disorder on Axis III.

Note. From American Psychiatric Association (1994, p. 573). Copyright 1994 by the American Psychiatric Association. Reprinted by permission.

TABLE 16.6. DSM-IV Criteria for Nightmare Disorder

A. Repeated awakenings from the major sleep period or naps with detailed recall of extended and extremely frightening dreams, usually involving threats to survival, security, or self-esteem. The awakenings generally occur during the second half of the sleep period.

B. On awakening from the frightening dreams, the person rapidly becomes oriented and alert (in contrast to the confusion and disorientation seen in Sleep Terror Disorder and some forms of epilepsy).

C. The dream experience, or the sleep disturbance resulting from the awakening, causes clinically significant distress or impairment in social, occupational, or other important areas of functioning.

D. The nightmares do not occur exclusively during the course of another mental disorder (e.g., a delirium, Posttraumatic Stress Disorder) and are not due to the direct physiological effects of a substance (e.g., a drug of abuse, a medication) or a general medical condition.

Note. From American Psychiatric Association (1994, p. 583).

TABLE 16.7. DSM-IV Criteria for Sleep Terror Disorder

A. Recurrent episodes of abrupt awakening from sleep, usually occurring during the first third of the major sleep episode and beginning with a panicky scream.

B. Intense fear and signs of autonomic arousal, such as tachycardia, rapid breathing, and sweating, during each episode.

C. Relative unresponsiveness to efforts of others to comfort the person during the episode.

D. No detailed dream is recalled and there is amnesia for the episode.

E. The episodes cause clinically significant distress or impairment in social, occupational, or other important areas of functioning.

F. The disturbance is not due to the direct physiological effects of a substance (e.g., a drug of abuse, a medication) or a general medical condition.

Note. From American Psychiatric Association (1994, p. 587).

and cognitions occurred, wakening the child. The topics of nightmares vary greatly, but can often be traced to children's fears at a certain age (e.g., very young children may have fears of monsters in the closet, whereas older children may have fears of failing at school; Gelfand & Peterson, 1985). As noted in Table 16.6, the diagnosis of nightmare disorder is made only when other conditions (such as delirium, posttraumatic stress disorder, and medication-related disorders) can be ruled out. Apparently related to but quite different from nightmare disorder is sleep terror disorder.

Sleep Terror Disorder

In sleep terror disorder (Table 16.7), the child experiences non-REM sleep, but suddenly may sit straight upright and scream or cry and may be inconsolable for as long as 30 minutes before relaxing and falling back to sleep (Thiedke, 2001). At such times, the child may act as though he or she does not recognize the parent, and thus soothing is very difficult. Because sleep terror disorder often occurs at times of stress, decreasing stress has been especially effective with such disorders, and diazepam (Valium) has been used in some children with some success. Unlike nightmares (which can occur at any age), sleep terror disorder occurs almost exclusively from ages 3 to 8, and more males than females show this disorder (Thiedke, 2001).

Although most parents respond somewhat automatically to sleep-disordered children with nurturance and positive regard, sleep disorders constitute one example of how a parent can be stressed and disaffected by a child's problems, and thus can respond with anger to the child. Children make continual demands on parents—not only regarding sleep, but also (as has been discussed) in regard to nutrition, toilet training, and so forth. All of these situations have the propensity to put parents at odds with their children and to make parents feel less positively about themselves because of their inability to control the children. We next discuss, in some detail, how disaffection from a child may result in a situation that is hazardous to the child's health.

Unintentional Injuries

Because another chapter of this book (Wekerle & Wolfe, Chapter 14) discusses child physical abuse per se, we discuss the other side of the coin in this chapter—how parents can inadvertently rather than deliberately injure their children. In many such cases, this is a product of the parents' inability to correctly evaluate appropriate levels of child supervision for a given situation. We specifically consider "unintentional injuries," most of which could have been avoided had a child received a reasonable amount of environmental modification (e.g., moving poisons to a shelf a child cannot reach, using child gates on the stairs so that children do not have to be supervised to avoid stairways, locking away or not owning loaded guns, etc.). We also consider situations in which supervision rather than barriers is necessary to keep the child safe (e.g., parking lots, beaches, etc.).

The research area of unintentional injuries has typically discriminated such child outcomes from abusive incidents. However, the majority of unintentional injuries are in fact instances of punishment that result in far greater injury than a parent supposed (e.g., the literature is replete with cases when a swat across the bottom sends a child head first through a glass door or into the sharp corner of a coffee table, or a bath that feels merely hot to a parent punishing a child for failure to use the bathroom results in third-degree burns on a susceptible infants' skin). For this reason, the "advertent" versus "inadvertent" dichotomy makes less sense than it appears to on the surface. These are parents who did not intend to do the damage that was done, but it occurred through their actions. In addition, as will be considered below, appropriately child-friendly environments and supervision can go a long way toward keeping children safe. In any case, this section describes some of the medical outcomes that appear "accidental" to many laypersons, but in actuality are due to action or lack of action by caregivers and thus require national interventions. These interventions range from educating caregivers to passing laws protecting children from dangerous furniture (e.g., cribs), toys, and containers of poisonous substances, as well as laws mandating the use of safety equipment (e.g., life-jackets on boats and child safety seats in cars).

Unintentional injuries are by far the most common cause of death in the United States, from infants to individuals approaching their mid-40s (Baker et al., 1992; National Institute for Health Care Management, 2000). Approximately 600,000 children require hospitalization due to injuries every year, and 16 million children receive emergency room treatment (Centers for Disease Control, 1990). Government epidemiologists estimate that professional treatment in direct costs totals $4.7 billion every year (Rice & MacKenzie, 1989); when indirect costs are included, this number rises to $7 billion a year (Centers for Disease Control, 1990). None of these statistics can reflect the psychological trauma to the children and their caregivers, such as pain and loss of valued activities (e.g., watching with a cast from the sidelines when a child has practiced all springtime to play a sport may be rated by the child as the most costly aspect of the injury).

There have been many methods of describing injuries—some directed toward etiology and risk factors (as epidemiologists have traditionally played a major role in injury research); others directed at methods of prevention; and still others focused on type of injury, often using medical records as a primary source of information. The major problem with almost all of the data on these injuries is that they rely on human memory—and memory is often fallible, due to guilt, the potential for litigation, and simply the emotional upset at the time at which the injury occurred.

In one study in which trained maternal observers recorded sufficient information to assist them in biweekly interviews, child and parent data were compared to demonstrate relatively high reliability of the data, and laboratory tests were used to establish the validity of the data. However, when the participants were asked at the end of the study to recall the number of injuries the children had encountered, statements ranged from comments such as "I only recall one or two," to "Let's see . . . he gets some kind of mark on him nearly every day . . . over six months that roughly equals 90 injuries" (Peterson, Harbeck, & Moreno, 1993). Even subsequent studies offering environmental cues ("Where were you living?", "Where did Rachael typically play?", "Who did she play with?", and "Who looked after her?"); developmental cues ("Now, Michael would have been around 2 then—do you remember when he started to walk?", "When was he toilet-trained?"); and temperament measures (which examined risk taking, attention deficit problems, etc.) did not result in any reason to regard the resulting injury reports as more accurate (Peterson, Moreno, & Harbeck-Weber, 1993). Apparently parents do have a better memory for the occurrence of medically attended injuries than for the occurrence of injuries for which treatment was not sought. However, injuries in which parents involve medical personnel happen relatively infrequently, so it is not possible to train observers to collect descriptions of a sufficient number of such injuries to afford a detailed understanding of the behavioral mechanisms of the injury events (typical antecedents, events, and consequences).

Moreover, although memories seem to be driven by parents' decisions to take children in for treatment, we have found that 10 times as many injuries do not result in medical treatment but have the same degree of severity as those that are treated (Peterson, DiLillo, Lewis, & Sher, 2002). In fact, our current lab contains data on over 4,000 injuries, with nearly 100 aspects of information on each injury. It is intriguing to find, furthermore, that parents rarely take steps to prevent an injury from recurring (Peterson et al., 2002), even if they regarded it as relatively serious. These data are similar to other data that focus on burned children (Hartsough & Lambert, 1985): Not only is the "once burned, twice shy" aphorism incorrect, but data suggest that most children experiencing a serious burn have already been treated for at least one previous burn.

This conceptualization and its formation become logical if one employs a conditioning perspective and considers the large number of times that children encounter the possibility of being burned and escape without an injury or with only a minor injury. Each such encounter allows a child to become further desensitized to the threat of being burned. Similar laboratory work in strongly controlled conditions used paramedics to validate that the videotaped scenes experienced by the children involved a high likelihood of serious injury. These data show that second-grade children were more accurate in terms of evaluating the extent of their injuries than were fourth-, sixth-, or eighth-grade children, or undergraduates (Peterson, Brazeal, Oliver, & Bull, 1997; Peterson, Gillies, Cook, Schick, & Little, 1994; Peterson, Oliver, Brazeal, & Bull, 1995). The younger children had, at least in concept, experienced fewer situations in which they had narrowly missed injury, and thus still had an accurate appreciation for the possibility of physical damage.

There is an extensive literature on treating trauma in children, but we focus here instead on the data suggesting methods of preventing injury from occurring. Most of our past work has been organized by differing levels, methods, types, and targets for preventive intervention (Damashek & Peterson, in press). The most far-reaching and probably the most effective level of prevention occurs at the federal or state level. The law requiring refrigerators to have doors that can be opened from the inside has saved countless children from asphyxiation (Robertson, 1983). Likewise, the Poison Prevention Packaging Act, which requires the use of child-resistant packaging and limits the number of pills within a single container, resulted in an abrupt and sustained decrease in child poisoning (Walton, 1982). More recently, all U.S. states have passed laws requiring child restraints in automobiles. However, different states have adopted differing degrees of enforcement of these laws. Until a few years ago, for example, Missouri's child safety seat law was a secondary traffic offense—one in which a family could be cited for safety seat violation only if the car was stopped for another reason. We observed in one of our studies a family in which the parents never utilized the child safety seat except during the 3-week period in which their car had a broken tail light, during which time the car could be stopped. After the tail light was repaired, the parents went directly back to not using a child safety seat. Recently the Missouri state legislature voted to make safety seat use a primary offense, and enforcement is likely to determine the effectiveness of the law (initial laws in other states resulted in compliance rates from 27% to 68%, and we hope that these numbers will continue to rise; National Highway Traffic Safety Administration, 1988).

Community-level interventions range from being very effective (such as replacing playground materials that can cut, trap or choke a child) to somewhat effective (e.g., more pedestrian injuries take place in the after-school and evening hours than any other time, and crossing guards positioned directly around the schools may help, but may also create a false sense of security when children must cross several unguarded streets). Teaching children safe pedestrian skills (e.g., Rivara, Booth, Bergman, Rogers, & Weiss, 1991) may be a way of extending protection of children and can contribute to lowered rates of injury, especially if skills instruction is paired with strong contingencies.

Very few studies have attempted to intervene at the family systems level to prevent injury, and this is unfortunate, given that such interventions would seem to be powerful safety devices. For very young children, providing strong contingencies—such as time out for dangerous behavior (Mathews, Friman, Barone, Ross, & Christophersen, 1987) and stickers or more major rewards for positive behaviors (Roberts, Fanurik, & Layfield,

1987)—would be ideal. Interventions that focus on increased education of parents, such as safety-based television programs, have resulted in only a 9% improvement in safety behavior (Colver, Hutchinson, & Judson, 1982). In contrast, studies that have given away safety materials have shown large improvements in safety behavior (Bablouzian, Freedman, Wolski, & Fried, 1997) and in the use of such safety tools as smoke alarms (DiGuiseppi & Higgins, 2000). Again, strong contingencies, one-on-one teacher-to-parent or teacher-to-child interventions, and giveaway systems make these program more effective.

Finally, a small number of studies have used praise, stickers, and other small tangible rewards to teach older children safety behavior. Jones and colleagues (e.g., Jones, Kazdin, & Haney, 1981) have conducted a number of studies teaching children to escape from home fires; in other studies, children have learned to identify emergencies and make emergency safety calls (Rosenbaum, Creedon, & Drabman, 1981). Our lab has used trained undergraduates (Peterson, 1984), school teachers (Peterson & Thiele, 1988), parents (Peterson, Mori, Selby, & Rosen, 1988), and even siblings (Peterson, Farmer, & Selby, 1988) to teach a variety of skills—such as safe screening of visitors to the home, safe food preparation, and dealing with minor emergencies (e.g., cuts and burns). However, it is our belief that none of these programs take the place of strong parental supervision, and anything that may allow parents to feel they need not offer such supervision may do more harm than good.

Neglect: Failure to Offer Appropriate Supervision

As has been noted earlier, of the various forms of child maltreatment, psychological neglect in the form of failure to offer appropriate supervision may be among the most dangerous and yet least reported child problems. We emphasize this form of neglect here (see Wekerle & Wolfe, Chapter 14, this volume, for a more general discussion). The most difficult part of planning preventive programs to avoid injury is that there are no established parameters for appropriate supervision. Peterson, Ewigman, and Kivlahan (1993) surveyed groups of pediatricians, child protection workers whose clients included maltreating parents, and a randomly selected sample of community mothers. There was very little agreement within or between any of these groups regarding appropriate levels of supervision across different types of situations around the home and neighborhood (ranging from playing quietly in a child's bedroom to playing in the street) for children of different ages. When a normal curve was formed and the bottom (most cautious) quarter and the top (most careless) quarter were removed, there remained no commonalities among the respondents, with one exception: Children who were below school age were judged as requiring nearly continuous supervision.

Some individuals have specialized in specific types of supervision and have found some of the risk factors. There are so many obstacles to child pedestrian safety that it is truly an area calling for attention. As another issue of supervision, not only age but also number of children and age of the supervisor are factors. Wills et al. (1997), for example, found that children were at higher risk for pedestrian injury if paired with a young caregiver or with no caregiver than if they traveled in larger groups. In addition, Wills et al. (1997) note that small children should never have their hands held when crossing the street with an adult; a child can too easily let go of the hand and bolt ahead. A firm grip above the wrist is far safer.

Somatoform Disorders

It is not uncommon for children and adolescents to present to the medical system with recurrent or persistent physical complaints, such as abdominal pain, dizziness, or headaches, for which an appropriate medical evaluation identifies no organic cause (although the symptom reports may be supported by parents). Other children may have a known organic disease, but present with symptoms disproportionate to the symptoms expected from their particular illness. Treatment of these children and their families is extremely challenging for both medical and mental health professionals. Unlike most of the disorders described in this chapter, which have been viewed as outside the purview of traditional psychiatry and clinical psychology, the problems experienced by these children have been given psychiatric diagnostic labels.

In DSM-IV, these heterogeneous disorders are grouped under the heading of somatoform disorders. Types of somatoform disorders included are somatization disorder (SD), undifferentiated somatoform disorder, conversion disorder, pain disorder, hypochondriasis, body dysmorphic disorder, somatoform autonomic dysfunction, and somatoform disorder not otherwise specified. The essential feature in these disorders is the presence of physical symptoms in the absence of organic pathology or known physiological mechanisms. In addition, strong presumption of a psychological component to the symptom is required. Mullins, Olson, and Chaney (1992) recently reported that approximately 12% of children referred to a pediatric inpatient consultation service met the DSM-III-R (American Psychiatric Association, 1987) criteria for a somatoform disorder.

Somatization Disorder

SD, which is perhaps the most chronic of the somatoform disorders, is defined by a long history of multiple physical complaints that occur over a several-year period and result in treatment seeking or in significant social, occupational, or other impairments. DSM-IV requires a minimum of eight symptoms from four categories (see Table 16.8 for the DSM-IV diagnostic criteria). SD is a chronic, fluctuating condition that rarely totally remits and results in consumption of a disproportionate amount of health care resources. Because these patients view themselves as seriously ill, their use of health care resources may be as high as nine times that of the general population (Smith, Monson, & Ray, 1986).

Unfortunately, most research on SD has been conducted with adults, and little information is available on children and adolescents. Adult studies suggest that prevalence rates vary widely, depending on the definitions used. For example, when full DSM-III criteria have been used, the prevalence rates have been very low (Escobar, Golding, & Hough, 1987; Swartz, Blazer, George, Woodbury, & Manton, 1988).

SD is more common in female than in male cohorts. The onset is typically during adolescence (Margo & Margo, 1994), and must occur before age 30 in order to meet DSM-IV criteria. Cultural factors are important in this disorder, as the symptom presentation may reflect cultural ideology. It should be noted that the criteria developed in DSM-IV are based on U.S. data and may not fully reflect SD in other cultures.

Treatment of SD is often complicated by comorbid psychiatric diagnoses. Estimates suggest that individuals with SD are also at high risk for major depression, generalized anxiety disorder, and phobic disorders (Brown, Golding, & Smith, 1990). In individuals with both SD and a depressive disorder, the SD typically precedes the mood disorder (Rief, Schaefer, Hiller, & Fichter, 1992). In addition to Axis I diagnoses, individuals with SD are also frequently diagnosed with Axis II personality disorders; avoidant, paranoid, self-defeating, and obsessive–compulsive are the most commonly diagnosed personality disorders in this population (Rost, Akins, Brown, & Smith, 1992).

As with many of the somatoform disorders, the etiology of SD is unclear. Researchers have speculated that SD is caused by somatic amplification, labile physiological reactions, distortions in somatic perception, high levels of somatic attention, suppression of emotions, and developmental and social factors (Kirmayer, Robbins, & Paris, 1994). However, few of these factors have received consistent empirical support. Empirical work does suggest the importance of social and developmental factors, with the finding that emotional neglect followed by childhood illness may lead to SD (Craig, Boardman, Mills, Daly-Jones, & Drake, 1993). Correlational research suggests that high levels of unexplained somatic symptoms are related to high levels of somatic attention and emotional inhibition (Larson & Chastain, 1990; Pennebaker, 1982; Robbins & Kirmayer, 1991). In addition to these individuals' prior experience of illness and greater focus on illness symptoms, individuals with SD have difficulty accurately detecting their internal body cues (Gardner, Morrell, & Ostrowski, 1990). It is likely that a complex interaction of multiple factors accounts for SD. Clearly, more research is needed on this costly disorder.

Undifferentiated Somatoform Disorder

As in SD, the defining criterion of undifferentiated somatoform disorder is the presentation of multiple physical complaints for which no organic cause can be found. This diagnosis is a residual category and is used for individuals with persistent somatic complaints (lasting a minimum of 6 months), who do not meet the criteria for SD (see Table 16.9).

Some evidence suggests that multiple somatic complaints in childhood and adolescence may constitute a precursor of SD (Ernst, Routh, & Harper, 1984; Routh & Ernst, 1984). Because a diagnosis of SD is highly unusual in prepubertal children, due to the requirement that one of the individual's symptoms be a sexual symptom, a diagnosis of undifferentiated somatoform dis-

TABLE 16.8. DSM-IV Criteria for Somatization Disorder

A. A history of many physical complaints beginning before age 30 years that occur over a period of several years and result in treatment being sought or significant impairment in social, occupational, or other important areas of functioning.

B. Each of the following criteria must have been met, with individual symptoms occurring at any time during the course of the disturbance:

(1) *four pain symptoms:* a history of pain related to at least four different sites or functions (e.g., head, abdomen, back, joints, extremities, chest, rectum, during menstruation, during sexual intercourse, or during urination)
(2) *two gastrointestinal symptoms:* a history of at least two gastrointestinal symptoms other than pain (e.g., nausea, bloating, vomiting other than during pregnancy, diarrhea, or intolerance of several different foods)
(3) *one sexual symptom:* a history of at least one sexual or reproductive symptom other than pain (e.g., sexual indifference, erectile or ejaculatory dysfunction, irregular menses, excessive menstrual bleeding, vomiting throughout pregnancy)
(4) *one pseudoneurological symptom:* a history of at least one symptom or deficit suggesting a neurological condition not limited to pain (conversion symptoms such as impaired coordination or balance, paralysis or localized weakness, difficulty swallowing or lump in throat, aphonia, urinary retention, hallucinations, loss of touch or pain sensation, double vision, blindness, deafness, seizures; dissociative symptoms such as amnesia; or loss of consciousness other than fainting)

C. Either (1) or (2):

(1) after appropriate investigation, each of the symptoms in Criterion B cannot be fully explained by a known general medical condition or the direct effects of a substance (e.g., a drug of abuse, a medication)
(2) when there is a related general medical condition, the physical complaints or resulting social or ccupational impairment are in excess of what would be expected from the history, physical examination, or laboratory findings

D. The symptoms are not intentionally produced or feigned (as in Factitious Disorder or Malingering).

Note. From American Psychiatric Association (1994, pp. 449–450).

order is more likely to be made with a younger population. Unfortunately, little research exists in children with this diagnosis; however, it is hypothesized that the etiology is similar to that of SD. Undifferentiated somatoform disorder occurs most commonly in women of low socioeconomic status (SES) (American Psychiatric Association, 1994). In contrast to children who present with multiple physical complaints and are given a diagnosis of SD or undifferentiated somatoform disorder, the children and adolescents to be considered next present with more focal complaints.

Conversion Disorder

The most common somatoform disorder seen in children is conversion disorder (Maloney, 1980; Mullins & Olson, 1990; Siegel & Barthel, 1986). The defining feature of conversion disorder is the presence of unexplained symptoms or deficits affecting voluntary motor or sensory function that suggest the presence of a neurological or other general medical condition. These symptoms typically do not conform to known anatomical pathways or physiological mechanisms. A thorough medical evaluation with an absence of organic findings is required before a diagnosis of conversion disorder can be made (see Table 16.10 for full diagnostic criteria).

Reported rates of conversion disorder vary from 11 per 100,000 to 300 per 100,000 in general population samples, and the disorder occurs more frequently in women than in men (American Psychiatric Association, 1994). According to DSM-IV, the onset of a conversion disorder generally occurs between late childhood and early adulthood. The diagnosis is rarely made in children below age 10 years; conversion symptoms in children below 10 years of age do occur, but these are usually limited to gait problems or seizures. The onset of symptoms in conversion disorder is acute, and symptoms typically remit within 2 weeks, with recurrence of symptoms in 20–25% of individuals. Spierings, Pels, Sijben, Gabreels, and Renier (1990) reported that of

TABLE 16.9. DSM-IV Criteria for Undifferentiated Somatoform Disorder

A. One or more physical complaints (e.g., fatigue, loss of appetite, gastrointestinal or urinary complaints).

B. Either (1) or (2):

(1) after appropriate investigation, the symptoms cannot be fully explained by a known general medical condition or the direct effects of a substance (e.g., a drug of abuse, a medication)
(2) when there is a related general medical condition, the physical complaints or resulting social or occupational impairment is in excess of what would be expected from the history, physical examination, or laboratory findings

C. The symptoms cause clinically significant distress or impairment in social, occupational, or other important areas of functioning.

D. The duration of the disturbance is at least 6 months.

E. The disturbance is not better accounted for by another mental disorder (e.g., another Somatoform Disorder, Sexual Dysfunction, Mood Disorder, Anxiety Disorder, Sleep Disorder, or Psychotic Disorder).

F. The symptom is not intentionally produced or feigned (as in Factitious Disorder or Malingering).

Note. From American Psychiatric Association (1994, pp. 451–452).

69 children aged 6–17 years diagnosed with conversion disorder, 72% reported improvement over time (only a portion of these children had received treatment), but 33% still had the same complaints. Although conversion disorder is perhaps the most common somatoform disorder in children, more research is needed on its etiology, prognosis, and treatment.

For children who present with a primary symptom involving pain rather than neurological symptoms, a diagnosis of pain disorder is more appropriate. As is seen in the next section, several forms of chronic childhood illness can be correctly labeled as pain disorders.

Pain Disorders

When an individual presents with a primary symptom of pain with no motor, sensory, or seizure symptoms, a diagnosis of pain disorder should be considered (see Table 16.11 for diagnostic criteria). In contrast to past editions of the DSM, DSM-IV (American Psychiatric Association, 1994) instructs clinicians to code pain disorder into one of the following three categories: (1) pain disorder associated with psychological factors, (2) pain disorder associated with both psychological factors and a general medical condition, and (3) pain disorder associated with a general medical condition. It should be noted that the last category, pain disorder associated with a general medical condition, is not considered a mental disorder and is coded on Axis III.

Certain types of pains in DSM-IV's first category of pain disorder are referred to as "recurrent pain" in the pediatric literature. Recurrent pain syndromes typically involve frequently occurring pain episodes (e.g., headaches, abdomi-

TABLE 16.10. DSM-IV Diagnostic Criteria for Conversion Disorder

A. One or more symptoms or deficits affecting voluntary motor or sensory function that suggest a neurological or other general medical condition.

B. Psychological factors are judged to be associated with the symptom or deficit because the initiation or exacerbation of the symptom or deficit is preceded by conflicts or other stressors.

C. The symptom or deficit is not intentionally produced or feigned (as in Factitious Disorder or Malingering).

D. The symptom or deficit cannot, after appropriate investigation, be fully explained by a general medical condition, or by the direct effects of a substance, or a culturally sanctioned behavior or experience.

E. The symptom or deficit causes clinically significant distress or impairment in social, occupational, or other important areas of functioning or warrants medical evaluation.

F. The symptom or deficit is not limited to pain or sexual dysfunction, does not occur exclusively during the course of Somatization Disorder, and is not better accounted for by another mental disorder.

Specify type of symptom or deficit:
With Motor Symptom or Deficit
With Sensory Symptom or Deficit
With Seizures or Convulsions
With Mixed Presentation

Note. From American Psychiatric Association (1994, p. 457).

TABLE 16.11. DSM-IV Diagnostic Criteria for Pain Disorder

A. Pain in one or more anatomical sites is the predominant focus of the clinical presentation and is of sufficient severity to warrant clinical attention.

B. The pain causes clinically significant distress or impairment in social, occupational, or other important areas of functioning.

C. Psychological factors are judged to have an important role in the onset, severity, exacerbation, or maintenance of the pain.

D. The symptom or deficit is not intentionally produced or feigned (as in Factitious Disorder or Malingering).

E. The pain is not better accounted for by a Mood, Anxiety, or Psychotic Disorder and does not meet criteria for Dyspareunia.

Code as follows:

307.80 Pain Disorder Associated with Psychological Factors . . .
307.89 Pain Disorder Associated with Both Psychological Factors and a General Medical Condition . . .

Note. The following is not considered to be a mental disorder and is included here to facilitate differental diagnosis.

Pain Disorder Associated with a General Medical Condition . . .

Note. From American Psychiatric Association (1994, pp. 461–462).

nal pains, or limb pains) that persist beyond a 3-month period. These pains occur in otherwise healthy children and are not symptomatic of an underlying physical disease. Two specific and often-seen forms of recurrent pain are discussed in more detail below.

Headaches. Childhood headache typically starts during Piaget's concrete operational stage (about 7–8 years of age), and prevalence increases with age (McGrath, 1990). There is an unusual interaction with age, in which younger boys report more headaches and also more painful headaches than younger girls, whereas the reverse is true as girls approach adolescence. For some children, headaches in the absence of physical origin (e.g., tumor, injury) vary widely in terms of recovery rate, from 3% to 80%. In one 23-year follow-up of school-age children with migraine headaches, Billie (1981) noted that over half of the children were symptom-free in young adulthood, although a sizable portion continued to have migraine-like symptoms. However, by age 30, a majority of them (60%) were again reporting headache. There have been few other long-term studies, and thus the conclusions raised here should be regarded with caution.

Bandura (1977) offered one of the earliest rationales for nonphysiologically based headache, noting that young children often report another family member with pain. Bandura suggested that if a child observes positive consequences due to pain, similar findings can be anticipated to be imitated. Craig (1983) found that under conditions of induced pain, healthy adults utilized the model of pain tolerance or intervention used in a family, supporting Bandura's model.

Harbeck and Peterson (1992) found that even preschool children could reasonably discuss their pain-related experience if interviewed patiently and allowed to use their own language (e.g., a headache was discussed by one child as "elephants dancing in my head"). Similarly, Burbach and Peterson (1988) noted that a child's cognitive development of the concepts of illness and the quality of pain (e.g., aching, stinging) involved in an illness are often related, and that some relationships can be found between delayed cognitive growth and a delayed understanding of illness; that is, children who have an immature concept of pain and quality of pain have a delayed understanding of illness. Wallander and Varni (1992) have noted that pain experienced when a child is too young to understand explanations regarding pain may result in future oversensitivity to pain. Behavior therapists have suggested that children should receive the support they need to deal with pain, but that parents must be careful not to allow strong secondary gain for reporting pain (e.g., a child treated by resting in a dark room during headache pain, rather than sitting with his or her mother watching television, may be less likely to have headaches in the future).

Recurrent Abdominal Pain. Recurrent abdominal pain (RAP) is another very common childhood pain disorder (Burke, Elliott, & Fleissner, 1999). It is typically defined by paroxysmal pain, occurring for three or more episodes over a 6-month period, resulting in a change in normal habits (Janicke & Finney, 1999). These children are noteworthy for their repeated visits to the doctor with nausea and vomiting, as well as abdominal pain; they also often have other pain disorders, such as headache and limb pain (Barr & Feuerstein, 1983; Walker, Garber, & Greene, 1994). The etiology of RAP typically is such that most individuals are never identified with an organic basis for their pain (Stickler & Murphy, 1979), even though the pain is so severe that it intrudes on a child's daily life (Hyams, Burke, Davis, Rzepski, & Andrulonis, 1996). The severity and the number of RAP symptoms seem strongly related to family systems issues, such as family stress (Ernst et al., 1984). Symptoms include lactose intolerance (Barr, Levine, & Watkins, 1979), and constipation (Whitehead, Engel, & Schuster, 1980), which differs from simple encopresis because of the disabling pain. As in headache, modeling has been implicated in the etiology of RAP (Robinson, Alverez, & Dodge, 1990), in addition to ineffectual coping skills (Walker et al., 1994). Being anxious, shy, and perfectionistic (Robinson et al., 1990) can also combine with irregular bowel habits to produce the kinds of symptoms seen in RAP.

For some years, children's general and separation anxieties were the focus of therapy for RAP. More recent research has shifted toward behavioral medicine, involving both physical and psychological treatment. For example, a study involving the use of a fiber supplement to increase the chance of normal bowel movements, and the maintenance of a "stomachache diary," demonstrated that a substantial number of children experienced a 50% reduction in frequency of attacks (Feldman, McGrath, Hodgson, Ritter, & Shipman, 1985). A second study, by Edwards, Finney, and Bonner (1991), combined the use of fiber with relaxation treatment. This multilevel study involved two control groups receiving either fiber and relaxation or relaxation alone and demonstrated that children had a very positive response to fiber but only a minimal response to relaxation alone. Today, combinations of reward for appropriate toileting behavior, fiber, and therapy have been found to treat RAP most successfully.

DISEASE-BASED PAIN

Some forms of pain are specific to an active disease process and can be readily diagnosed. One of the most common examples is considered next.

Sickle Cell Disease

Sickle cell disease is an autosomal recessive disease that at one time threatened to cripple if not kill most of the children who experienced it. Now, however, sickle cell disease has become a relatively treatable disorder. Appropriate medical supervision to limit pain and internal bleeding offers relief to individuals suffering from the significant bone and joint pain that is caused by vaso-occlusion in the small blood vessels. One in every 400–500 African Americans is dizygotic for the recessive gene, demonstrating that a large proportion of this ethnic group probably carries the disorder (Brown, Doepke, & Kaslow, 1993). Pain is a central aspect of the disorder, and it requires intermittent pharmacotherapy (Armstrong, Pegelow, Gonzalez, & Martinez, 1992) and behavioral pain control methods (Gil et al., 1997). As in all kinds of pain (especially those experienced by children), there is substantial interaction between personal adjustment and sickle cell pain. At risk are performance-based school behaviors (Chua-Lim, Moore, McCleary, Shah, & Mankad, 1993) and peer interactions (Kumar, Powars, Allen, & Haywood, 1976). The central support of the child's family, and careful judgments about how much responsibility over activity and medication a child should have at any given developmental level, are critical. Self-concept (Kumar et al., 1976) and self-efficacy (Jensen, Turner, & Romano, 1991) are results of sufficient balance between support and freedom. Coping with the disease, especially its pain and crippling side effects, involves both cognitive and behavioral components.

Mechanic (1983) suggests four distinct stages of understanding sickle cell disease: (1) organization of personal perception of symptoms; (2) interpretation of what the symptoms mean (given that 80% of children with sickle cell disease have had a stroke before age 15, there are differing levels of risk to be faced); (3) symptom expression or style of behavior observed when symptoms are present; and (4) performance of specific and personally effective behavior patterns in order to cope with symptoms. Developmental stage, of course, influences how a child is able to cope with the pain. Young children may withdraw and cry, while other children may be expressive. Some pain signifies internal bleeding that must be medically treated at once, and other pains may be merely symptomatic of past damage of the disorder, requiring no intervention. Recognizing how to teach redirection of pain once it is understood to be only symptomatic is vital. In addition, there is an increasing understanding that (as is true with most childhood diseases) the adjustment of the caregivers to life in general, and to the child's illness in particular, will have a strong influence on the child's coping. Brown et al. (2000) have recently described a model of adaptation showing relationships among children's coping, their disease adjustment, and the adjustment of their parents.

Similarly, Gil and her colleagues have discussed for over a decade a comprehensive approach to pain assessment among individuals who can expect a lifetime of pain (Gil, 1994; Wilson Schaeffer, Gil, & Porter, 1999). Her work continues to describe aspects of sickle cell disease, from medical management to psychological adjustment. She reports successful use of observational methods of pain behavior assessment in the hospital, with a goal of living as well as possible once a child returns to home and school life.

DISORDERS WITH MINOR DISEASE-RELATED PAIN BUT LIFE-THREATENING POTENTIAL

Such disorders as diabetes mellitus, epilepsy, or asthma are often described within the same sources as other diseases of childhood involving major disease-based pain (e.g., sickle cell disease) (McQuaid & Nassau, 1999). These illnesses have many aspects in common. Such children are at constant increased risk for psychological disorders (Lavigne & Faier-Routman, 1992), and the adjustment to the chronic illness appears to be less influenced by the severity of the illness than by surrounding psychological and environmental factors (Chaney et al., 1999). However, because pain is not a major element of these diseases, they are considered together in this part of the chapter.

Diabetes

Type I (insulin-dependent) diabetes is the most common endocrine disorder of childhood (Bennett, 1981). It is usually diagnosed in childhood (between 5 and 11 years of age), and occurs when the body is unable to metabolize carbohydrates due to eventual failure to synthesize insulin. Treatment involves a complex regimen of balancing insulin injections and dietary carbohydrates. Although there is little actual pain involved, the disease requires consistent testing and adherence to a complex regimen.

In the absence of adherence to the treatment protocol, two things can happen. If inadequate insulin is taken, the body literally begins to starve, despite any amount of food taken. With no insulin to inhibit fat breakdown, fatty acids and ketones begin to accumulate. The kidneys cannot eliminate the ketones entering the bloodstream, and ultimately this hyperglycemia results in ketoacidosis, coma, and death. Unfortunately, underdosing with insulin (such that food cannot be broken down to use or store as fat) is an easy way to lose weight, and this can be a dangerous practice. On the other side of the equation, if too much insulin is taken, food is burned at a disproportionate level. Hypoglycemia (too little blood sugar) results in a jittery, uncomfortable feeling, and ultimately in loss of consciousness and convulsions. Yet the closer a person is to achieving perfect glycemic control, the more hypoglycemia is risked (Davis, Keating, Byrne, Russell, & Jones, 1997). When it occurs, giving a high dose of sugar (such as juice or a candy bar) can be very helpful. It is essential that the treatment agent know whether hypo- or hyperglycemia is occurring (Davidson, 1991).

Because there is no cure for diabetes, children and their families face a lifetime of balancing insulin injections, food eaten, and exercise. The absence of good glycemic control can result in blindness, kidney failure, peripheral vascular disease (requiring amputation of a limb), and heart disease. Sometimes even the best attempts fail to result in good glycemic control, as blood glucose is influenced by illness and other factors beyond the family's control (Johnson & Perwien, 2002). Home monitoring of blood glucose is now considered far superior to urine testing, which has been used for many years. This practice relies on a finger prick, sometimes just with a specialized needle and sometimes with specialized equipment (resulting in diminished pain). The blood then is placed into a computerized meter that reports blood glucose.

As can be imagined, diabetes is accompanied by a number of psychiatric disorders, primarily internalizing problems such as depression, anxiety, and worry. Interestingly, however, in most families where social support is good, children and adolescents tend to adjust well after the first year of diagnosis. Kovacs, Obrosky, Goldston, and Drash (1997) reported that over a 10-year period, most children diagnosed with diabetes returned to a normal level on most indices of psychopathology. Some, however, remained depressed, anxious, or angry (characterized by acting out in general, or by being aggressive with siblings, parents, and even medical staff).

Children with diabetes and their families thus face not only physical but also psychological problems, as well as the need to deal with the changing demands of this disorder across time. It is difficult for infants and toddlers to understand that their eating patterns must be different from those of other children, and to understand the need for repeated procedures involving needles (finger sticks and injections). Furthermore, consider holidays such as Halloween with trick or treating, Christmas with candy canes and cookies, Valentine's Day with candy hearts, or Easter with chocolate bunnies: All of these treats are forbidden to a diabetic preschooler, who probably does not understand the prohibitions.

In preschool or elementary school, exposure to peers and a sense of "being different" must be dealt with; sports, spending a night with a friend, or going to a school party all must be more strongly supervised for a diabetic child (Johnson & Perwien, 2002). The paraphernalia that must be carried and used can be problematic, given society's increased concerns about drug abuse, and can be very upsetting to other children. During the preteen and early teenage years, there is more responsibility for life tasks in general, but even more responsibility is necessary for diabetic management (Hanson, De Guire, Schinkel, & Kolterman, 1995). This is likely due both to a youth's different lifestyle, with fewer regular meals and more "junk food," and to differences in insulin production at puberty (Cutfield, Bergman, Menon, & Sperling, 1990).

In summary, diabetes is a physically, psychologically, and socially challenging disorder. Because of its high frequency and many potential serious consequences, it has been one of the most highly studied of all childhood diseases. However, there are many other childhood disorders where (as in diabetes) the main challenges have not been pain, but other serious symptoms and symptom outcomes. This chapter considers two such disorders, epilepsy and asthma.

Epilepsy

There is a great deal of similarity between epilepsy and diabetes. Both conditions involve the need for careful administration of daily medication, parental monitoring of younger children, and frequent interactions with physicians (Williams et al., 2000). However, unlike diabetes, epilepsy is really a term for a set of symptoms that may have many different causes. The symptoms include seizures, lapses of consciousness frequently accompanied by muscular spasms, loss of bladder and/or bowel control, and other behavioral changes (e.g., eyes rolling up, confusion, becoming stiff, etc.). Epilepsy is the most frequent chronic neurological disorder in the United States (McLin, 1992), and most epileptic children show over 50% of the symptoms described above (Seidenberg & Berent, 1992).

Poor psychological and social adjustment characterizes children with epilepsy. These children often have lower self-esteem, higher levels of depression, and more school problems than children without epilepsy (Austin, 1988, 1989). These symptoms appear to be more serious in children from low-SES families (Hermann, Whitman, & Dell, 1989). Black and other minority children may also be more susceptible, although ethnicity may be confounded with lower SES (Carlton-Ford, Miller, Brown, Nealeigh, & Jennings, 1995). Boys are more likely to have epilepsy than girls, and older children are more likely to have psychological problems than younger children (Achenbach, Howell, Quay, & Conners, 1991).

Few studies of epilepsy exist to assist parents and their children in adjusting to the disorder and the unusual demands of the disease. Based on their work examining risk factors, researchers such as Carlton-Ford et al. (1995) suggest that early identification of the specific problems experienced by a child (e.g., medication compliance, mood disorder, social adjustment, educational difficulties, and family problems) may be necessary to assist in planning an effective, individualized treatment plan for the epileptic child.

Asthma

The third of the disorders selected as examples here, not surprisingly, has many similarities to the other two. Asthma, like epilepsy, involves unpredictable episodes, the need for adhering to a prescribed medication regimen, and frightening attacks in which a child may appear to be dying. Asthma also tends to be a chronic disorder (Austin, 1989).

We have begun the section on diabetes by noting that it is the most common endocrine disorder in children, and we have noted in the section on epilepsy that it is the most common neurological disorder. Asthma, however, is the most common childhood chronic disease overall in the United States (Weitzman, Gortmaker, Sobol, & Perrin, 1992). Not surprisingly, given its prevalence, it also has the greatest financial influence in terms of academic and medical costs (Gergen & Weiss, 1990). Asthma involves sudden "obstruction" of the airways, with reduced lung function, a large amount of mucosal secretions, coughing, fatigue, and hypoxia (lack of oxygen) that can result in death (Rietveld & Colland, 1999). Indeed, asthma results in 60,000 deaths in Western countries each year, and a large proportion of these deaths are among young people (Sears, 1997). However, some scientists believe that appropriate medical treatment "can convert it from a major handicap to a minor inconvenience" (Buston & Wood, 2000, p. 134).

Why, then, does asthma continue to be a major threat to children's health? It is partially because the decisions regarding appropriate medication and adherence to these rules are very difficult (Slack & Brooks, 1995). One study of school-age children showed that complete adherence in the 24 consecutively recruited children occurred in only 4.9 days; on a median of 41.8% of days, no doses were taken. Nearly half of the children failed to use their steroid inhalers at all for over a year at a time. When asked about their compliance, the youths dramatically overreported the doses taken (Bender, Milgrom, Rand, & Ackerson, 1998). Examining the reasons behind such poor compliance, Buston and Wood (2000) noted that children and adolescents often used denial, as there was no indication of their having a physical disease unless an asthmatic attack occurred. (Paradoxically, with many forms of asthma, the only way to prevent an attack ultimately is to take the required medication; in other forms, patients need only take the medication on demand, but if it is unavailable the results can be fatal. The difficulty is that for many children there is no consequence for failing to take prescribed medication.) A lack of belief in the prescribed medication regimen was also cited as a cause, but the most frequently cited cause was simply forgetfulness. Different medications must be taken frequently and on time. Given the absence of symptoms, it is difficult to fit any of the regimens we have discussed into a life full of academic, social, physical, and other demands experienced by growing children and adolescents. Other scientists look at systemic functions beyond what is going on with a child, and note that a negative family climate and a poor family organization also contribute to the extent of adherence problems (Bender et al., 1998).

Like other children with chronic illness, children diagnosed with severe asthma often show signs of worry, fear, and depression (Badoux & Levy, 1994). Similarly, like children with diabetes who have a specific fear of hypoglycemia, these children often have a disease-specific fear of suffocation. Unfortunately, high levels of difficulties regarding breathing may actually trigger an asthma attack (Janson, Bjornsson, Hetta, & Boman, 1994).

CHILDHOOD CANCER

Childhood cancer differs from all the other diseases that have been discussed thus far, in that sometimes pain is involved and sometimes it is not; differing types of cancer can occur throughout the developmental period; some forms go into remission, while others rarely do so; and perhaps it is the most feared of childhood diseases. Cancer is not a single disorder, and there are differences among almost all types of cancer. Acute lymphoblastic leukemia (ALL) has the highest base rate and is currently one of the most treatable of cancers, with a survival rate of 73%; the survival rate is over 90% for Hodgkin's disease. By contrast, some brain and bone tumors involve much more pain, longer treatment periods, and lower survival rates (Eiser, 1998).

The three most common forms of cancer treatment are chemotherapy (the use of chemicals that poison many cells but especially fast-growing cells, such as hair cells and cancer cells), radiation therapy, and surgery. Some tumors can be removed directly by surgery and are followed by chemotherapy or radiation therapy to ensure that the disease will not spread to bone marrow. Almost all children with cancer experience pain regularly from diagnostic procedures, which can be relatively minor (such as pain caused by a finger prick) to relatively severe (such as pain emanating from bone marrow aspirations, in which a large needle is forced into the iliac crest on the hip and bone marrow is withdrawn by the needle). Pain is relative, however; 10–33% of the variance in distress in lumbar puncture has been shown to be rated to high parent- and child-reported pain (Chen, Craske, Katz, Schwartz, & Zeltzer, 2000).

For most forms of childhood cancer, however, side effects from the treatments are the most unpleasant part of the disease, ranging from alopecia (hair loss) to nausea, and effects on mood (e.g., depression, sleep disturbance, and nightmares) (Eiser, 1998). For families, the combination of these negative short-term outcomes with the potential for recurrence and a fatal outcome has caused some of the most knowledgeable psychologists in the area to refer to living with cancer in the long run as living "under the sword of Damocles" (Koocher & O'Malley, 1981).

Finally, one of the tragedies of this long-term disease is that even if a child goes into remission, the child can be left with abnormal growth and endocrine function, compromised fertility (Eiser, 1998), psychosocial problems, diminished hearing, skin and skeletal abnormality, and cognitive damage from treatment (Kissen, 1996).

CHALLENGES TO CHILD HEALTH

The Need for Different Types and Levels of Interventions

This chapter has attempted to show the many different kinds of challenges for successful treatment of pediatric problems. Each disorder has a different cause, a different course, different demands on the family, and shifting demands across the developmental course. Most of the factors placing youths at risk for purely psychological disorders also seem related to risk for psychological sequelae of medical disorders (low SES, minority status, family problems, lower-than-normal intellect, etc.). Psychology has responded by conducting not only research that studies global systems in hospitals, but also specific research that attempts to solve some of the most difficult challenges for health-related disorders and implements those solutions by teaching them to all of the different caregivers involved.

For example, for a diabetic child, one moment there may be nothing apparently overtly wrong, but too large a dose of insulin may begin to cause hyperglycemia, resulting in coma and subsequent death. Because of this possibility, and because the nonfatal long-term effects of diabetes can include loss of sight or loss of limbs, there has been an enormous press to offer better than our "best guess." As a result, a number of new therapeutic options have been developed for children and adolescents with diabetes (see Tamborlane, Bonfig, & Boland, 2001, for details). One of the most exciting of these treatment alternatives is the continuous subcutaneous insulin infusion system. This alternative to multiple daily injections involves an insulin pump that is placed within the body and releases insulin as needed. The use of this system is rapidly increasing with children and even, in some extreme cases, with infants (Arkansas Children's Hospital, 2000; Hanas, 2001); it seems to be a very safe and effective treatment method. In addition, scientists have made available new forms of insulin, such as glargine (a soluble and long-acting insulin alternative that seems to avoid the sharp peaks of glucose seen in forms of insulin used earlier) and the experimental use of inhaled insulin (which allows a child to take a large insulin dose via pulmonary delivery before a meal, without having to take an injection before eating). New continuous glucose-sensing systems can optimize doses of insulin, however these are administered. The future promises more such solutions. It is thus extraordinarily important that there is a growing literature on the efficacy and any potential side effects of these new treatment alternatives.

As noted earlier, all of the diseases discussed in this chapter have aspects in common. Bennett (1994) reviewed 60 studies involving children and adolescents with various chronic medical conditions. Although none of the youths met criteria for clinical depression, an elevated risk for depressive symptoms was noted. There was variability in the extent of depressive symptoms even among children with the same disorder. However, children with certain kinds of chronic diseases, such as asthma, were at greater risk for personality disorders than children with such disorders as diabetes. Time since diagnosis, gender, and age were generally unrelated to depression. Severity of depression was related to number of hospitalizations and restriction in daily routines. It is clear that regular treatment—or, better still, prevention of depression—should be routine practice for any child with a chronic disease who shows signs of even subclinical depression.

In all of the diseases we have examined in this chapter, there is a need for interventions to assist children with psychological symptoms (which might include training in coping methods or social skills training), as well as for methods of assisting children with medical adherence (many clever examples of such methods have been developed, such as a beeper's sounding as a prompt to take medication). We also see the need for intervention with parents to increase their sense of efficacy and their skills in managing their children's problems, including regimen adherence. Bender et al. (1998) have made an excellent point in arguing that teaching is not enough; some sort of improvement in parents' own motivation and belief in their ability to assist their children, frequent rewards for such interventions, and help with regard to their own emotional problems may be vital. Systems-level difficulties (e.g., do siblings feel that the ill child gets all of the attention? does the husband feel the loss of his wife as the child demands attention?) must also be considered. Finally, consideration of how a child fits into the school, social institutions (church, sports, etc.), and the community at large seems critical. Coordinating interventions at all these levels seems an almost impossible task at this time, but psychologists have skills relevant to each of these levels of intervention. Dividing the challenges into manageable segments, and receiving political and financial support for such interventions, seem the final and potentially the most difficult challenges in planning successful, holistic interventions for chronically ill children.

Example of a Psychological Response to a Child Health Challenge: Decreasing Pain Related to Diseases and Procedures

We do not have space in this chapter to cover in detail all of the successful interventions devised for health-related disorders by psychologists, although we have tried to name many of them. Nevertheless, it does seem logical to give one example in detail of psychological advances made in the child health area, common to many diseases. Analgesic drugs have been referred to as "the mainstay" for pain relief in children (Walco, Sterling, Conte, & Engel, 1999). Professionals in this area have described an analgesic ladder, which at the lowest level begins with aspirin or acetaminophen; at a midpoint, narcotics such as codeine are prescribed for moderate pain; and opioids such as morphine are used for severe pain. There has been an unfortunate tendency to undermedicate children for many years. Psychologists have assisted the medical community in becoming aware that children tend to respond to pain differently from adults (e.g., children may move restlessly around when in substantial pain, whereas adults tend to lie still), and that there may have been some conceptual errors in considering children's pain (e.g., male infants were traditionally circumcised without anesthesia because it was believed that their unmyelinated axons could not carry pain reception in the way they would later in life; more recent theorists have argued that the short length of these axons compensates for the absence of their myelin sheaths, and thus that many infants may have been subjected to more pain than is warranted).

Although there have been some inroads into behavioral technology for certain kinds of pain, both procedure-related pain (e.g., Jay, Elliot, Fitzgibbons, Woody, & Siegel, 1995) and disease-related pain (e.g., Gil, 1994), especially chronic and intense disease-related pain, have continued to be treated with medication. However, it seems only sensible to conclude that many aspects of an individual child will make behavioral techniques for pain more or less effective. For example, Harbeck and Peterson (1992) found that children's expressions of pain were influenced by their age and by their families' experiences with pain. Chen, Zeltzer, Craske, and Katz (2000) reported that children's memories of lumbar puncture procedures increased with age, and that regardless of age, children with more negative memories tended to exaggerate these memories and to experience higher distress at subsequent lumbar punctures.

Numerous behavioral techniques have been used to alleviate children's disease- and procedure-related pain, including simple explanations, hands-on experience with medical tools, many kinds of modeling appropriate behavior (usually with a videotape or puppet), and other forms of coping (using imagery distraction, deep breathing, deep muscle relaxation, etc.). O'Byrne, Peterson, and Saldana (1997) demonstrated that in the last decade, the use of such psychologically oriented tools has more than tripled.

A surprising number of tactics have proven effective: "Classic" techniques include the use of medical toys as coping aids (Burstein & Meichenbaum, 1979), parents as coping coaches (Zastowny, Kirschenbaum, & Meng, 1986), party blowers to slow breathing and distract children during venipuncture (Manne et al., 1990), and cartoons to distract children from burn hydrotherapy (Elliott & Olson, 1983). Powers (1999) has recently argued that according to the Chambless criteria for evaluating "best practices," the behavioral techniques outlined here—particularly those that have been described as coping techniques (relaxation, distraction, imagery, and filmed modeling as used in Peterson & Shigetomi, 1981)—could be considered "well-established treatments" for the prevention of distress in brief but stressful medical procedures.

The future will undoubtedly hold even further improvements, as psychological techniques for helping children deal with pain are combined with faster-acting and more effective anesthetics (e.g., the topical anesthetic EMLA; Lander et al., 1996), and as clearer methods are developed for assigning children to the optimal coping techniques for them. This is an area that has shown a steady upward trajectory in the last two decades, and it seems only logical to anticipate further improvements to the challenge of preventing disease- and procedure-related distress in the future.

SUMMARY

Psychologists have been involved in treating an enormous variety of childhood health problems for years, and their knowledge of potentially critical mechanisms underlying such problems and potential methods of assisting children and families expands every day. Many serious challenges remain, but there is a growing contingency of psychologists who will work alongside nurses, dietitians, physicians, epidemiologists, and others to improve the life situations of ill or injured children.

REFERENCES

Abrahamian, R. P., & Lloyd-Still, J. D. (1984). Chronic constipation in childhood: A longitudinal study of 186 patients. *Journal of Pediatric Gastroenterology and Nutrition, 3*, 460–467.

Achenbach, T. M., Howell, C. T., Quay, H. C., & Conners, C. K. (1991). National survey of problems and competencies among four- to sixteen-year-olds. *Monographs of the Society for Research in Child Development, 56*(3, Serial no. 225).

American Psychiatric Association. (1987). *Diagnostic and statistical manual of mental disorders* (3rd ed., rev.). Washington, DC: Author.

American Psychiatric Association. (1994). *Diagnostic and statistical manual of mental disorders* (4th ed.). Washington, DC: Author.

American Sleep Disorders Association. (1990). *The international classification of sleep disorders: Diagnostic and coding manual*. Rochester, MN: Author.

Anand, R. (1998, October). Foreword. In *Childhood obesity: Causes and prevention*. Symposium conducted at the meeting of the Center for Nutrition Policy and Promotion, Washington, DC.

Anders, T. F., & Eiben, L. A. (1997). Pediatric sleep disorders: A review of the past 10 years. *Journal of the American Academy of Child and Adolescent Psychiatry, 36*, 9–20.

Anthony, H., Catto-Smith, A., Phelan, P., & Paxton, S. (1998). Current approaches to the nutritional management of cystic fibrosis in Australia. *Journal of Paediatrics and Child Health, 34*, 170–174.

Arkansas Children's Hospital. (2000). ACH physicians pioneer use of insulin pump for diabetic newborn [Online] Available: http://www.ach.uams.edu/whatscurrent/ach_physicians_pioneer_use_of_in.htm [2002, January 25].

Armstrong, F. D., Pegelow, C. H., Gonzalez, J. C., & Martinez, A. (1992). Impact of children's sickle cell history on nurse and physician ratings of pain and medication decisions. *Journal of Pediatric Psychology, 17*, 651–664.

Arnold, G. L., Kramer, B. M., Kirby, R. S., Plumeau, P. B., Blakely, E. M., Sanger Cregan, L. S., & Davidson, P. W. (1998). Factors affecting cognitive, motor, behavioral and executive functioning in children with phenylketonuria. *Acta Paediatrica, 87*, 565–570.

Austin, J. K. (1988). Childhood epilepsy: Child adaptation and family resources. *Journal of Child and Adolescent Psychiatric and Mental Health Nursing, 1*, 18–24.

Austin, J. K. (1989). Comparison of child adaptation to epilepsy and asthma. *Journal of Child and Adolescent Psychiatric and Mental Health Nursing, 2*, 139–144.

Awiszus, D., & Unger, I. (1990). Coping with PKU: Results of narrative interviews with parents. *European Journal of Pediatrics, 149*(Suppl.), S45–S51.

Azrin, N. H., & Thienes, P. M. (1978). Rapid elimination of enuresis by intensive learning without a conditioning apparatus. *Behavior Therapy, 9*, 342–354.

Bablouzian, L., Freedman, E. S., Wolski, K. E., & Fried, L. E. (1997). Evaluation of a community based childhood injury prevention program. *Injury Prevention, 3*, 14–16.

Badoux, A., & Levy, D. A. (1994). Psychologic symptoms in asthma and chronic urticaria. *Annals of Allergy, 72*, 229–234.

Baker, S. P., O'Neill, B., Ginsburg, M. J., & Li, G. (1992). *The injury fact book*. Lexington, MA: Lexington Books.

Bandura, A. (1977). *Social learning theory*. Englewood Cliffs, NJ: Prentice-Hall.

Bar-Or, O., Foreyt, J., Bouchard, C., Brownell, K. D., Dietz, W. H., Ravussin, E., Salbe, A. D., Schwenger, S., St. Jeor, S., & Torun, B. (1998). Physical activity, genetic, and nutritional considerations in childhood weight management. *Medicine and Science in Sports and Exercise, 30*, 2–10.

Barr, R. G., & Feuerstein, M. (1983). Recurrent abdominal pain in children: How appropriate are our clinical assumptions? In P. Firestone & P. McGrath (Eds.), *Pediatric and adolescent behavioral medicine* (pp. 13–27). New York: Springer-Verlag.

Barr, R. G., Levine, M. D., & Watkins, J. B. (1979). Recurrent abdominal pain of childhood due to lactose intolerance. *New England Journal of Medicine, 300*, 1449–1452.

Bender, B., Milgrom, H., Rand, C., & Ackerson, L. (1998). Psychological factors associated with medication nonadherence in asthmatic children. *Journal of Asthma, 35*, 347–353.

Bennett, D. S. (1994). Depression among children with chronic medical problems: A meta-analysis. *Journal of Pediatric Psychology, 19*, 149–169.

Bennett, P. H. (1981). The epidemiology of diabetes mellitus. In H. Rifkin & P. Raskin (Eds.), *Diabetes mellitus* (Vol. 5, pp. 87–94). Bowie, MD: Prentice-Hall.

Billie, B. (1981). Migraine in childhood and its prognosis. *Cephalgia*, *1*, 71–75.

Borowitz, S. M., Cox, D. J., & Sutphen, J. L. (1999). Differences in toileting habits between children with chronic encopresis, asymptomatic siblings, and asymptomatic nonsiblings. *Journal of Developmental and Behavioral Pediatrics*, *20*, 145–149.

Brown, F., Golding, J. M., & Smith, R. (1990). Psychiatric comorbidity in primary care somatization disorder. *Psychosomatic Medicine*, *52*, 445–451.

Brown, R. T., Doepke, K. J., & Kaslow, N. J. (1993). Risk–resistance adaptation model for pediatric chronic illness: Sickle cell syndrome as an example. *Clinical Psychology Review*, *13*, 119–132.

Brown, R. T., Lambert, R., Devine, D., Baldwin, K., Casey, R., Depke, K., Ievers, C. E., Hsu, L., Buchanan, I., & Eckman, J. (2000). Risk–resistance adaptation model for caregivers and their children with sickle cell syndromes. *Annals of Behavioral Medicine*, *22*, 158–169.

Brownell, K. D., Kelman, J. H., & Stunkard, A. J. (1983) Treatment of obese children with and without their mothers: Changes in weight and blood pressure. *Pediatrics*, *71*, 515–523.

Burbach, D. J., & Peterson, L. (1988). Children's concepts of physical illness: A review and critique of the cognitive developmental literature. In B. G. Melamed & K. A. Matthews (Eds.) *Child health psychology* (pp. 153–171). Hillsdale, NJ: Erlbaum.

Burke, P., Elliott, M., & Fleissner, R. (1999). Irritable bowel syndrome and recurrent abdominal pain: A comparative review. *Psychosomatics*, *40*, 277–285.

Burklow, K. A., Phelps, A. N., Schultz, J. R., McConnell, K., & Rudolph, C. (1998). Classifying complex pediatric feeding disorders. *Journal of Pediatric Gastroenterology and Nutrition*, *27*, 143–147.

Burstein, S., & Meichenbaum, D. (1979). The work of worrying in children undergoing surgery. *Journal of Abnormal Child Psychology*, *7*, 121–132.

Buston, K. M., & Wood, S. F. (2000). Non-compliance amongst adolescents with asthma: Listening to what they tell us about self-management. *Family Practice*, *17*, 134–138.

Butler, R. J. (1998). Annotation: Night wetting in children: Psychological aspects. *Journal of Child Psychology and Psychiatry*, *39*, 453–463.

Byrd, R. S., Weitzman, M., Lanphear, N. E., & Auinger, P. (1996). Bed-wetting in U. S. children: Epidemiology and related behavior problems. *Pediatrics*, *98*, 414–419.

Cannella, P. C., Bowser, E. K., Guyer, L. K., & Borum, P. R. (1993). Feeding practices and nutrition recommendations for infants with cystic fibrosis. *Journal of the American Dietetic Association*, *93*, 297–300.

Carlton-Ford, S., Miller, R., Brown, M., Nealeigh, N., & Jennings, P. (1995). Epilepsy and children's social and psychological adjustment. *Journal of Health and Social Behavior*, *36*, 285–301.

Cendron, M. (1999). Primary nocturnal enuresis: Current. *American Family Physician*, *59*, 1205–1214.

Centers for Disease Control. (1990). Special contribution: Childhood injuries in the United States. *American Journal of Disease of Children*, *144*, 627–648.

Centers for Disease Control and Prevention. (2001). Update: Prevalence of overweight among children, adolescents, and adults—United States, 1988–1994. In *Morbidity and Mortality Weekly Report* [Onlne]. Available: http://www.cdc.gov/mmwr//preview/mmwrhtml/00046647.htm [2001, April 20].

Chaney, J. M., Mullins, L. L., Uretsky, D. L., Pace, T. M., Werden, D., & Hartman, V. L. (1999). An experimental examination of learned helplessness in older adolescents and young adults with long-standing asthma. *Journal of Pediatric Psychology*, *24*, 259–270.

Chatoor, I., Ganiban, J., Colin, V., Plummer, N., & Harmon, R. J. (1998). Attachment and feeding problems: A reexamination of nonorganic failure to thrive and attachment insecurity. *Journal of the American Academy of Child and Adolescent Psychiatry*, *37*, 1217–1224.

Chen, E., Craske, M. G., Katz, E. R., Schwartz, E., & Zeltzer, L. K. (2000). Pain-sensitive temperament: Does it predict procedural distress and response to psychological treatment among children with cancer? *Journal of Pediatric Psychology*, *25*, 269–278.

Chen, E., Zeltzer, L. K., Craske, M. G., & Katz, E. R. (2000). Children's memories for painful cancer treatment procedures: Implications for distress. *Child Development*, *71*, 933–947.

Chua-Lim, C., Moore, R. B., McCleary, G., Shah, A., & Mankad, V. N. (1993). Deficiencies in school readiness skills of children with sickle cell anemia: A preliminary report. *Southern Medical Journal*, *86*, 397–402.

Cohen, S., & Herbert, T. B. (1996). Health psychology: Psychological factors and physical disease from the perspective of human psychoneuroimmunology. *Annual Review of Psychology*, *47*, 113–142.

Colver, A. F., Hutchinson, P. J., & Judson, E. C. (1982). Promoting children's home safety. *British Medical Journal*, *285*, 1177–1180.

Costello, E. J., Angold, A., Burns, B. J., Stangl, D. K., Tweed, D. L., Erkanli, A., & Worthman, C. M. (1996). The Great Smoky Mountains Study of Youth: Goals, design, methods, and the prevalence of DSM-III-R disorders. *Archives of General Psychiatry*, *53*, 1129–1136.

Cox, D. J., Sutphen, J., Ling, W., Quillian, W., & Borowitz, S. (1996). Additive benefits of laxative, toilet training, and biofeedback therapies in the treatment of pediatric encopresis. *Journal of Pediatric Psychology*, *21*, 659–670.

Craig, K. (1983). Modeling and social learning factors in chronic pain. In J. J. Bonica, A. Iggo, & U. Lindblom (Eds.), *Proceedings of the Third World Congress on Pain* (pp. 813–827). New York: Raven Press.

Craig, T. K. J., Boardman, A. P., Mills, K., Daly-Jones, O., & Drake, H. (1993). The South London somatization study: I. Longitudinal course and the influence of early life experiences. *British Journal of Psychiatry*, *163*, 579–588.

Cutfield, W., Bergman, R., Menon, R., & Sperling, M. (1990). The modified minimal model: Applications to measurement of insulin sensitivity in children. *Journal of Clinical Endocrinology and Metabolism*, *70*, 1644–1650.

Damashek, A., & Peterson, L. (in press). Child unintentional injury prevention. *Journal of Developmental and Behavioral Pediatrics*.

Davidson, M. B. (Ed.). (1991). *Clinical diabetes mellitus: A problem-oriented approach*. New York: Thieme Medical.

Davis, E. A., Keating, B., Byrne, G. C., Russell, M., & Jones, T. W. (1997). Hypoglycemia: Incidence and clinical predictors in a large population-based sample of children and adolescents with IDDM. *Diabetes Care*, *20*, 22–25.

Dietz, W. H. (1998a). Childhood weight affects adult morbidity and mortality. *Journal of Nutrition*, *128*, 411S-414S.

Dietz, W. H. (1998b, October). Childhood obesity: The contribution of diet and inactivity. In *Childhood obesity: Causes and prevention*. Symposium conducted at the meeting of the Center for Nutrition Policy and Promotion, Washington, DC.

Dietz, W. H., & Bellizzi, M. C. (1999). Introduction: the use of body mass index to assess obesity in children. *American Journal of Clinical Nutrition, 70*, 123S–125S.

DiGuiseppi, C., & Higgins, J. P. (2000). Systematic review of controlled trials of interventions to promote smoke alarms. *Archives of Disease in Childhood, 82*, 341–348.

Edwards, M. C., Finney, J. W., & Bonner, M. (1991). Matching treatment with recurrent abdominal pain symptoms: An evaluation of dietary fiber and relaxation treatments. *Behavior Therapy, 22*, 257–267.

Eiser, C. (1998). Practitioner review: Long-term consequences of childhood cancer. *Journal of Child Psychology and Psychiatry, 39*, 621–633.

Elliott, C. H., & Olson, R. A. (1983). The management of children's distress in response to painful medical treatment for burn injuries. *Behaviour Research and Therapy, 21*, 675–683.

Epstein, L. H., McCurley, J., Wing, R. R., & Valoski, A. (1990). Five-year follow-up of family-based behavioral treatments for childhood obesity. *Journal of Consulting and Clinical Psychology, 58*, 661–664.

Epstein, L. H., Myers, M. D., Raynor, H. A., & Saelens, B. E. (1998). Treatment of pediatric obesity. *Pediatrics, 101*, 554–570.

Epstein, L. H., Wing, R. R., Steranchak, L., Dickson, B., & Michelson, J. (1980). Comparison of family-based behavior modification and nutrition education for childhood obesity. *Journal of Pediatric Psychology, 5*, 25–36.

Ernst, A. R., Routh, D. K., & Harper, D. C. (1984). Abdominal pain in children and symptoms of somatization disorder. *Journal of Pediatric Psychology, 9*, 77–86.

Escobar, J. L., Golding, J. M., & Hough, R. L. (1987). Somatization in the community: Relationship to disability and use of services. *American Journal of Public Health, 77*, 837–840.

Fehrenbach, A. M. B., & Peterson, L. (1989). Parental problem-solving skills, stress, and dietary compliance in phenylketonuria. *Journal of Consulting and Clinical Psychology, 57*, 237–241.

Feldman, W., McGrath, P., Hodgson, C., Ritter, H., & Shipman, R. T. (1985). The use of dietary fiber in the management of simple, childhood, idiopathic, recurrent, abdominal pain. Results in a prospective, double-blind, randomized, controlled trial. *American Journal of Diseases of Children, 139*, 1216–1218.

Friedman, E. (1969). The "autistic syndrome" and phenylketonuria. *Schizophrenia, 1*, 249–261.

Gardner, T. M., Morrell, J. A., Jr., & Ostrowski, T. A. (1990). Somatization tendencies and ability to detect internal body cues. *Perceptual and Motor Skills, 71*, 364–366.

Gaylor, E. E., Goodlin-Jones, B. L., & Anders, T. F. (2001). Classification of young children's sleep problems: A pilot study. *Journal of the American Academy of Child and Adolescent Psychiatry, 40*, 61–67.

Gelfand, D. M., & Peterson, L. (1985). *Child development and psychopathology*. Beverly Hills, CA: Sage.

Gergen, P., & Weiss, K. (1990). Changing patterns of asthma hospitalization among children: 1979 to 1987. *Journal of the American Medical Association, 264*, 1688–1692.

Gil, K. M. (1994). Psychosocial aspects of sickle cell disease. *Journal of Health and Social Policy, 5*, 19–38.

Gil, K. M., Wilson, J. J., Edens, J. L., Workman, E., Ready, J., Sedway, J., Reading-Lallinger, R., & Daeschner, C. (1997). Cognitive coping skills training with sickle cell disease. *International Journal of Behavioral Medicine, 4*, 365–378.

Haddock, C. K., Shadish, W. R., Klesges, R. C., & Stein, R. J. (1994). Treatments for childhood obesity. *Annals of Behavioral Medicine, 16*, 235–244.

Hagekull, B., Bohlin, G., & Rydell, A. (1997). Maternal sensitivity, infant temperament, and the development of early feeding problems. *Infant Mental Health Journal, 18*, 92–106.

Hanas, R. (2001). Insulin pumps in children and adolescents. *Practical Diabetes International, 18*, S5–S6.

Hanson, C. L. (1992). Developing systemic models of the adaptation of youths with diabetes. In A. M. La Greca, L. J. Siegel, J. L. Wallander, & C. E. Walker (Eds.), *Stress and coping in child health* (pp. 212–241). New York: Guilford Press.

Hanson, C. L., De Guire, M. J., Schinkel, A. M., & Kolterman, O. G. (1995). Empirical validation for a family-centered model of care. *Diabetes Care, 18*, 1347–1356.

Harari, M. D., & Moulden, A. (2000). Nocturnal enuresis: What is happening? *Journal of Paediatrics and Child Health, 36*, 78–81.

Harbeck, C., & Peterson, L. (1992). Elephants dancing in my head: A developmental approach to children's concepts of specific pains. *Child Development, 63*, 138–149.

Hartsough, C. S., & Lambert, N. M. (1985). Medical factors in hyperactive and normal children: Prenatal, developmental, and health history findings. *American Journal of Orthopsychiatry, 55*, 190–201.

Hellekson, K. L. (2001). NIH consensus statement on phenylketonuria. *American Family Physician, 63*, 1430–1432.

Hermann, B. P., Whitman, S., & Dell, J. (1989). Correlates of behavior problems and social competence in children with epilepsy, aged 6–11. In B. P. Hermann & M. Seidenberg (Eds.), *Childhood epilepsies: Neuropsychological, psychosocial, and intervention aspects* (pp. 143–157). New York: Wiley.

Hobbs, C., & Hanks, H. G. I. (1996). A multidisciplinary approach for the treatment of children with failure to thrive. *Child: Care, Health and Development, 22*, 273–284.

Hyams, J. S., Burke, G., Davis, P. M., Rzepski, B., & Andrulonis, P. A. (1996). Abdominal pain and irritable bowel syndrome in adolescents: A community-based study. *Journal of Pediatrics, 129*, 220–226.

Janicke, D. M., & Finney, J. W. (1999). Empirically supported treatments in pediatric psychology: Recurrent abdominal pain. *Journal of Pediatric Psychology, 24*, 115–127.

Janson, C., Bjornsson, E., Hetta, J., & Boman, G. (1994). Anxiety and depression in relation to respiratory symptoms and asthma. *American Journal of Respiratory and Critical Care Medicine, 149*, 930–934.

Jay, S., Elliott, C. H., Fitzgibbons, I., Woody, P., & Siegel, S. (1995). A comparative study of cognitive behavior therapy versus general anesthesia for painful medical procedures in children. *Pain, 62*, 3–9.

Jelalian, E., & Saelens, B. E. (1999). Empirically supported treatments in pediatric psychology: Pediatric obesity. *Journal of Pediatric Psychology, 24*, 223–248.

Jensen, M. P., Turner, J. A., & Romano, J. M. (1991). Self-efficacy and outcome expectancies: Relationship to chronic pain coping strategies and adjustment. *Pain, 44*, 263–269.

Johnson, S. B., & Perwien, A. R. (2002). Insulin-dependent diabetes mellitus. In H. Koot & J. Wallander (Eds.), *Quality of life in child and adolescent illness: Concepts, methods, and findings*. Brighton, England: Brunner–Routledge.

Jones, R. T., Kazdin, A. E., & Haney, J. I. (1981). Social validation and training of emergency fire safety skills for

potential injury prevention and life saving. *Journal of Applied Behavior Analysis, 14*, 249–260.
Kazak, A. E. (1992). The social context of coping with childhood chronic illness: Family systems and social support. In A. M. La Greca, L. J. Siegel, J. L. Wallander, & C. E. Walker (Eds.), *Stress and coping in child health* (pp. 262–278). New York: Guilford Press.
Kemeny, M. E., & Laudenslager, M. L. (1999). Beyond stress: The role of individual difference factors in psychoneuroimmunology. *Brain, Behavior, and Immunity, 13*, 73–75.
Kerwin, M. E. (1999). Empirically supported treatments in pediatric psychology: Severe feeding problems. *Journal of Pediatric Psychology, 24*, 193–214.
Kirmayer, L. J., Robbins, J. M., & Paris, J. (1994). Somatoform disorders: Personality and the social matrix of somatic distress. *Journal of Abnormal Psychology, 103*, 125–136.
Kissen, G. (1996). Late effects of treatment on paediatric oncology. In P. Selby & C. Bailey (Eds.), *Cancer and the adolescent* (pp. 226–241). London: BMJ.
Koch, R. K. (1999). Issues in newborn screening for phenylketonuria. *American Family Physician, 60*, 1462–1466.
Koch, R. K., & Wenz, E. (1987). Phenylketonuria. *Annual Review of Nutrition, 7*, 117–135.
Koocher, G. P., & O'Malley, J. E. (1981). *The Damocles syndrome*. New York: McGraw-Hill.
Kovacs, M., Obrosky, D. S., Goldston, D., & Drash, A. (1997). Major depressive disorder in youths with IDDM: A controlled prospective study of course and outcome. *Diabetes Care, 20*, 45–51.
Kumar, S., Powars, D., Allen, J., & Haywood, L. J. (1976). Anxiety, self-concept, and personal and social adjustments in children with sickle cell anemia. *Journal of Pediatrics, 88*, 859–863.
Lander, J., Hodgins, M., Nazarali, S., McTavish, J., Ouellette, J., & Friesen, E. (1996). Determinants of success and failure of EMLA. *Pain, 64*, 89–97.
Larson, D. G., & Chastain, R. L. (1990). Self-concealment: Conceptualization, measurement and health implications. *Journal of Social and Clinical Psychology, 9*, 439–455.
Lavigne, J. V., & Faier-Routman, J. (1992). Psychological adjustment to pediatric physical disorders: A meta-analytic review. *Journal of Pediatric Psychology, 17*, 133–158.
Leuzzi, V., Trasimeni, G., Gualdi, G. F., & Antonozzi, I. (1995). Biochemical, clinical and neuroradiological (MRI) correlations in late-detected PKU patients. *Journal of Inherited Metabolic Disease, 18*, 624–634.
Lutzker, J. R. (1998). *Handbook of child abuse research and treatment*. New York: Plenum Press.
MacDonald, A. (1996). Nutritional management of cystic fibrosis. *Archives of Disease in Childhood, 74*, 81–87.
MacDonald, A., Holden, C., & Harris, G. (1991). Nutritional strategies in cystic fibrosis: Current issues. *Journal of the Royal Society of Medicine, 84*(Suppl. 18), 28–35.
Maffeis, C. (2000). Aetiology of overweight and obesity in children and adolescents. *European Journal of Pediatrics, 159*, S35–S44.
Maier, S. F., Watkins, L. R., & Fleshner, M. (1994). Psychoneuroimmunology: The interface between behavior, brain, and immunity. *American Psychologist, 49*, 1004–1017.
Maloney, M. J. (1980). Diagnosing hysterical conversion reactions in children. *Journal of Pediatrics, 97*, 1016–1020.
Manne, S. L., Redd, W. H., Jacobsen, P. B., Gorfinkle, K., Schorr, O., & Rapkin, B. (1990). Behavioral intervention to reduce child and parent distress during venipuncture. *Journal of Consulting and Clinical Psychology, 58*, 565–572.
Margo, K. L., & Margo, G. M. (1994). The problem of somatization in family practice. *American Family Physician, 49*, 1873–1879.
Matarazzo, J. D. (1984). Behavioral immunogens and pathogens in health and illness. In B. L. Hannonds & C. J. Scheirer (Eds.), *Psychology and health* (pp. 5–44). Washington, DC: American Psychological Association.
Mathews, J. R., Friman, P. C., Barone, V. J., Ross, L. V., & Christophersen, E. R. (1987). Decreasing dangerous infant behaviors through parent instruction. *Journal of Applied Behavior Analysis, 20*, 165–169.
McGrath, P. A. (1990). *Pain in children: Nature, assessment, and treatment*. New York: Guilford Press.
McGrath, M. L., Mellon, M. W., & Murphy, L. (2000). Empirically supported treatments in pediatric psychology: Constipation and encopresis. *Journal of Pediatric Psychology, 25*, 225–254.
McLin, W. M. (1992). Introduction to issues in psychology and epilepsy. *American Psychologist, 47*, 1124–1125.
McMurray, R. G., Harrel, J. S., Levine, A. A., & Gansky, S. A. (1995). Childhood obesity elevates blood pressure and total cholesterol independent of physical activity. *International Journal of Obesity, 19*, 881–886.
McQuaid, E. L, & Nassau, J. H. (1999). Empirically supported treatments of disease-related symptoms in pediatric psychology: Asthma, diabetes, and cancer. *Journal of Pediatric Psychology, 24*, 305–328.
Mechanic, D. (1983). Adolescent health and illness behavior: Review of the literature and a new hypothesis for the study of stress. *Journal of Human Stress, 9*, 4–13.
Moores, J. (1996). Non-organic failure to thrive: Dietetic practice in a community setting. *Child: Care, Health and Development, 22*, 251–259.
Moran, R. (1999). Evaluation and treatment of childhood obesity. *American Family Physician, 59*, 861–877.
Mullins, L. L., Gillman, J., & Harbeck, C. (1992). Multiple-level interventions in pediatric psychology settings: A behavioral–systems perspective. In A. M. La Greca, L. J. Siegel, J. L. Wallander, & C. E. Walker (Eds.), *Stress and coping in child health* (pp. 377–400). New York: Guilford Press.
Mullins, L. L., & Olson, R. A. (1990). Familial factors in the etiology, maintenance, and treatment of somatoform disorders in children. *Family Systems Medicine, 8*, 159–175.
Mullins, L. L., Olson, R. A., & Chaney, J. M. (1992). A social learning–family systems approach to the treatment of somatoform disorders in children and adolescents. *Family Systems Medicine, 10*, 1–5.
National Highway Traffic Safety Administration. (1988). *Observed safety belt use statistics by state*. Washington, DC: U.S. Department of Transportation.
National Institute for Health Care Management. (2000, August). Preventing childhood injuries for a bright future. *Action Brief*, pp. 1–2.
O'Byrne, K., Peterson, L., & Saldana, L. (1997). Survey of pediatric hospitals' preparation programs. Evidence of the impact of health psychology research. *Health Psychology, 16*, 147–154.
Oeffner, F., Korn, T., Roth, H., Ziegler, A., Hinney, A., Goldschmidt, H., Siegfried, W., Hebebrand, J., & Grzeschik, K. (2001). Systematic screening for mutations in the human necdin gene (NDN): Identification of two naturally occurring polymorphisms and association analysis in

body weight regulation. *International Journal of Obesity, 25*, 767–769.

Olson, R. A., Mullins, L. L., Gillman, J. B., & Chaney, J. M. (1994). *The sourcebook of pediatric psychology*. Boston: Allyn & Bacon.

Paavonen, E. J., Almquist, F., Tamminen, T., Moilanen, I., Piha, J., Raesaenen, E., & Aronen, E. T. (2002). Poor sleep and psychiatric symptoms at school: An epidemiological study. *European Child and Adolescent Psychiatry, 11*, 10–17.

Pennebaker, J. W. (1982). *The psychology of physical symptoms*. New York: Springer.

Peterson, L. (1984). The "Safe at Home" game: Training comprehensive prevention skills in latchkey children. *Behavior Modification, 8*, 474–494.

Peterson, L., Brazeal, T. J., Oliver, K. K., & Bull, C. A. (1997). Gender and developmental patterns of affect, belief and behavior in simulated injury events. *Journal of Applied Developmental Psychology, 19*, 531–546.

Peterson, L., DiLillo, D., Lewis, T., & Sher, K. (2002). Improvement in quantity and quality of prevention measurement of toddler injuries and parental interventions. *Behavior Therapy, 33*, 271–297.

Peterson, L., Ewigman, B., & Kivlahan, C. (1993). Judgments regarding appropriate child supervision to prevent injury: The role of environmental risk and child age. *Child Development, 64*, 934–950.

Peterson, L., Farmer, J., & Selby, V. (1988). Unprompted between subject generalization of home safety skills training. *Child and Family Behavior Therapy Journal, 10*, 107–119.

Peterson, L., Gillies, R., Cook, S., Schick, B., & Little, T. (1994). Developmental patterns of expected consequences for simulated bicycle injury events. *Health Psychology, 13*, 218–223.

Peterson, L., Harbeck, C., & Moreno, A. (1993). Measures of children's injuries: Self-reported versus maternal-reported events with temporally proximal versus delayed reporting. *Journal of Pediatric Psychology, 18*, 133–147.

Peterson, L., Homer, A. L., & Wonderlich, S. A. (1982). The integrity of independent variables in behavior analysis. *Journal of Applied Behavior Analysis, 15*, 477–492.

Peterson, L., Moreno, A., & Harbeck-Weber, C. (1993). "And then it started bleeding": Children's and mothers' perceptions and recollections of daily injury events. *Journal of Clinical Child Psychology, 22*, 345–354.

Peterson, L., Mori, L., Selby, V., & Rosen, B. (1988). Community interventions in children's injury prevention: Differing costs and differing benefits. *Journal of Community Psychology, 16*, 62–73.

Peterson, L., Oliver, K. K., Brazeal, T. J., & Bull, C. A. (1995). A developmental exploration of expectations for and beliefs about preventing bicycle collision injuries. *Journal of Pediatric Psychology, 20*, 13–22.

Peterson, L., & Shigetomi, C. (1981). The use of coping techniques to minimize anxiety in hospitalized children. *Behavior Therapy, 12*, 1–14.

Peterson, L., & Thiele, C. (1988). Home safety at school. *Child and Family Behavior Therapy, 10*, 1–8.

Poustie, V. J., & Rutherford, P. (2000). Dietary interventions for phenylketonuria. In *Cochrane Database of Systematic Reviews* [computer file]. Available: (2):CD001304 [2001, June 3].

Powers, S. W. (1999). Empirically supported treatments in pediatric psychology: Procedure-related pain. *Journal of Pediatric Psychology, 24*, 131–145.

Raju, T. N. (1999). Ignac Semmelweis and the etiology of fetal and neonatal sepsis. *Journal of Perinatology, 19*, 307–310.

Reid, M. J., Walter, A. L., & O'Leary, S. G. (1999). Treatment of young children's bedtime refusal and nighttime wakings: A comparison of "standard" and graduated ignoring procedures. *Journal of Abnormal Child Psychology, 27*, 5–16.

Rice, D. B., & MacKenzie, E. J. (1989). *Cost of injury in the United States: A report to Congress 1989*. San Francisco, CA: University of California, Institute for Health and Aging, and Johns Hopkins University, Injury Prevention Center.

Rief, W., Schaefer, S., Hiller, W., & Fichter, M. M. (1992). Lifetime diagnoses in patients with somatoform disorders: Which came first? *European Archives of Psychiatry and Clinical Neuroscience, 241*, 236–240.

Rietveld, S., & Colland, V. T. (1999). The impact of severe asthma on school children. *Journal of Asthma, 36*, 409–417.

Rivara, F. P., Booth, C. L., Bergman, A. B., Rogers, A. B., & Weiss, J. (1991). Prevention of pedestrian injuries to children: Effectiveness of a school training program. *Pediatrics, 88*, 770–775.

Robbins, J. M., & Kirmayer, L. J. (1991). Cognitive and social factors in somatization. In L. J. Kirmayer & J. M. Robbins (Eds.), *Current concepts of somatization: Research and clinical perspectives* (pp. 107–141). Washington, DC: American Psychiatric Press.

Roberts, M. C., Fanurik, D., & Layfield, D. A. (1987). Behavioral approaches to prevention of childhood injuries. *Journal of Social Issues, 43*, 105–118.

Robertson, L. S. (1983). *Injuries: Causes, control strategies, and public policy*. Lexington, MA: Lexington Books.

Robinson, J. O., Alverez, J. H., & Dodge, J. A. (1990). Life events and family history in children with recurrent abdominal pain. *Journal of Psychosomatic Research, 34*, 171–181.

Rosenbaum, M. S., Creedon, D. L., & Drabman, R. S. (1981). Training preschool children to identify emergency situations and make emergency phone calls. *Behavior Therapy, 12*, 425–435.

Rosenberg, D. A. (1987). Web of deceit: A literature review of Munchausen syndrome by proxy. *Child Abuse and Neglect, 11*, 547–563.

Rost, K. M., Akins, R. N., Brown, F. W., & Smith, G. R. (1992). The comorbidity of DSM-III personality disorders in somatization disorder. *General Hospital Psychiatry, 14*, 322–326.

Routh, D. K., & Ernst, A. R. (1984). Somatization disorder in relatives of children and adolescents with functional abdominal pain. *Journal of Pediatric Psychology, 9*, 427–437.

Sanders, M. J. (1999). Hospital protocol for the evaluation of Munchausen by proxy. *Clinical Child Psychology and Psychiatry, 4*, 379–391.

Sanders, M. R., Turner, K. M., Wall, C. R., Waugh, L. M., & Tully, L. A. (1997). Mealtime behavior and parent–child interaction: A comparison of children with cystic fibrosis, children with feeding problems, and nonclinic controls. *Journal of Pediatric Psychology, 22*, 881–900.

Schreier, H. A., & Libow, J. A. (1993). *Hurting for love: Munchausen by proxy syndrome*. New York: Guilford Press.

Sears, M. R. (1997). Descriptive epidemiology of asthma. *Lancet, 350*(Suppl.), 1–4.

Seidenberg, M., & Berent, S. (1992). Childhood epilepsy and the role of psychology. *American Psychologist, 47*, 1130–1133.

Seligman, M. E. P. (1996). Science as an ally of practice. *American Psychologist, 51*, 1072–1079.

Siegel, M., & Barthel, R. P. (1986). Conversion disorders on a child psychiatry consultation service. *Psychosomatics, 27*, 201–204.

Simmons, R. J., Goldberg, S., Washington, J., Fischer-Fay, A., & Maclusky, I. (1995). Infant–mother attachment and nutrition in children with cystic fibrosis. *Journal of Developmental and Behavioral Pediatrics, 16*, 183–186.

Skoog, S. J. (1998). Primary nocturnal enuresis: an analysis of factors related to its etiology. *Journal of Urology, 159*, 1338–1339.

Slack, M. K., & Brooks, A. J. (1995). Medication management issues for adolescents with asthma. *American Journal of Health-System Pharmacy, 52*, 1417–1421.

Smith, G. R., Jr., Monson, R. A., & Ray, D. C. (1986). Patients with multiple unexplained symptoms: Their characteristics, functional health, and health care utilization. *Archives of Internal Medicine, 146*, 69–72.

Spierings, C., Pels, P. J. E., Sijben, N., Gabreels, F. J., & Renier, W. O. (1990). Conversion disorders in childhood: A retrospective follow-up study of 84 inpatients. *Developmental Medicine and Child Neurology, 32*, 865–871.

Stark, L., J., Jelalian, E., Powers, S. W., Mulvihill, M. M., Opipari, L. C., Bowen, A., Harwood, I., Passero, M. A., Lapey, A., Light, M., & Hovell, M. F. (2000). Parent and child mealtime behavior in families of children with cystic fibrosis. *Journal of Pediatrics, 136*, 195–200.

Stark, L. J., Opipari, L. C., Donaldson, D. L., Danovsky, M. B., Rasile, D. A., & DelSanto, A. F. (1997). Evaluation of a standard protocol for retentive encopresis: A replication. *Journal of Pediatric Psychology, 22*, 619–633.

Stark, L. J., Powers, S. W., Jelalian, E., Rape, R. N., & Miller, D. L. (1994). Modifying problematic mealtime interactions of children with cystic fibrosis and their parents via behavioral parent training. *Journal of Pediatric Psychology, 19*, 751–768.

Stein, M. A., Mendelsohn, J., Obermeyer, W. H., Amromin, J., & Benca, R. (2001). Sleep and behavior problems in school-aged children [Electronic version]. *Pediatrics, 107*, e60.

Stickler, G. B., & Murphy, D. B. (1979). Recurrent abdominal pain. *American Journal of Diseases of Children, 133*, 486–489.

Strauss, R. S. (2000). Childhood obesity and self-esteem [Electronic version]. *Pediatrics, 105*, e15.

Strauss, R. S., & Knight, J. (1999). Influence of the home environment on the development of obesity in children [Electronic version]. *Pediatrics, 103*, e85.

Sullivan, J. E., & Chang, P. (1999). Review: Emotional and behavioral functioning in phenylketonuria. *Journal of Pediatric Psychology, 24*, 281–299.

Swartz, M., Blazer, D., George, L., Woodbury, M. A., & Manton, K. G. (1988). Somatization disorder in a community population. *American Journal of Psychiatry, 143*, 1403–1408.

Tamborlane, W. V., Bonfig, W., & Boland, E. (2001). Recent advances in treatment of youth with Type 1 diabetes: Better care through technology. *Diabetic Medicine: A Journal of the British Diabetic Association, 18*, 864–870.

Thelen, M. H., Powell, A. L., Lawrence, C., & Kuhnert, M. E. (1992). Eating and body image concerns among children. *Journal of Clinical Child Psychology, 21*, 41–46.

Thiedke, C. C. (2001). Sleep disorders and sleep problems in childhood. *American Family Physician, 63*, 277–284.

Tikotzky, L., & Sadeh, A. (2001). Sleep patterns and sleep disruptions in kindergarten children. *Journal of Clinical Child Psychology, 30*, 581–591.

Vogel, W., Young, M., & Primack, W. (1996). A survey of physician use of treatment methods for functional enuresis. *Journal of Developmental and Behavioral Pediatrics, 17*, 90–93.

Walco, G. A., Sterling, C. M., Conte, P. M., & Engel, R. G. (1999). Empirically supported treatments in pediatric psychology: Disease related pain. *Journal of Pediatric Psychology, 24*, 155–167.

Walker, L. S., Garber, J., & Greene, J. W. (1994). Somatic complaints in pediatric patients: A prospective study of the role of negative life events, child social and academic competence, and parental somatic symptoms. *Journal of Consulting and Clinical Psychology, 62*, 1213–1221.

Wallander, J. L., & Varni, J. W. (1992). Adjustment in children with chronic physical disorders: Programmatic research on a disability–stress–coping model. In A. M. La Greca, L. J. Siegel, J. L. Wallander, & C. E. Walker (Eds.), *Stress and coping in child health* (pp. 279–300). New York: Guilford Press.

Walton, W. W. (1982). An evaluation of the Poison Prevention Packaging Act. *Pediatrics, 69*, 363–370.

Wappner, R., Cho, S., Kronmal, R. A., Schuett, V., & Seashore, M. R. (1999). Management of phenylketonuria for optimal outcome: A review of guidelines for phenylketonuria management and a report of surveys of parents, patients, and clinic directors [Electronic version]. *Pediatrics, 104*, e68.

Ward, M. J., Lee, S. S., & Lipper, E. G. (2000). Failure-to-thrive is associated with disorganized infant–mother attachment and unresolved maternal attachment. *Infant Mental Health Journal, 21*, 428–442.

Weitzman, M., Gortmaker, S. L, Sobol, A. M., & Perrin, J. M. (1992). Recent trends in the prevalence and severity of childhood asthma. *Journal of the American Medical Association, 268*, 2673–2677.

Whitehead, W. E., Engel, B. T., & Schuster, M. M. (1980). Irritable bowel syndrome: Physiological and psychological differences between diarrhea-predominant and constipation-predominant patients. *Digestive Diseases and Sciences, 25*, 404–413.

Williams, J., Lange, B., Sharp, G., Griebel, M., Edgar, T., Haley, T., Frindik, P., Casey, S., & Dykman, R. (2000). Altered sleeping arrangements in pediatric patients with epilepsy. *Clinical Pediatrics, 39*, 635–642.

Wills, K. E., Christoffel, K. K., Lavigne, J. V., Tanz, R. R., Donovan, M., Kalangis, K., McGuire, P., White, B., Barthel, M., LeBailly, S., Klinger, C., Buergo, F., Stewart, K., Shwver, N., & Jenq, J. (1997). Patterns and correlates of supervision in child pedestrian injury. *Journal of Pediatric Psychology, 22*, 89–104.

Wilson Schaeffer, J. J., Gil, K. M., & Porter, L. (1999). Sickle cell disease pain. In A. R. Block, E. F. Kremer, & E. Fernandez (Eds.), *Handbook of chronic pain syndromes* (pp. 569–587). Mahwah, NJ: Erlbaum.

Wishon, P. M., Bower, R., & Eller, B. (1983). Childhood obesity: Prevention and treatment. *Young Children, 39*, 21–27.

Wishon, P. M., & Childs, R. E. (1984). Perspectives on obesity: The unknown handicap. *Early Child Development and Care, 17*, 185–198.

World Health Organization. (1993). *The ICD-10 classification of mental and behavioral disorders: Diagnostic criteria for research*. Geneva: Author.

Wright, C. M., & Birks, E. (2000). Risk factors for failure to thrive: A population-based survey. *Child: Care, Health and Development*, *26*, 5–16.

Wright, C. M., & Talbot, E. (1996). Screening for failure to thrive: What are we looking for? *Child: Care, Health and Development*, *22*, 223–234.

Zastowny, T. R., Kirschenbaum, D. S., & Meng, A. L. (1986). Coping skills training for children: Effects on distress before, during, and after hospitalization for surgery. *Health Psychology*, *5*, 231–247.

Zero to Three/National Center for Clinical Infant Programs. (1994). *Diagnostic classification of mental health and developmental disorders of infancy and early childhood* (*Diagnostic Classification: 0–3*). Washington, DC: Author.

Author Index

Subject Index

f indicates figure; *t* indicates table; *n* indicates note